# OTOLOGIC MEDICINE AND SURGERY

## Volume 1

# OTOLOGIC MEDICINE AND SURGERY

## Volume 1

**Edited By**

## PETER W. ALBERTI, M.B., B.S., Ph.D., F.R.C.S., F.R.C.S.(C)

Professor and Chairman
Department of Otolaryngology
Professor, Occupational Medicine
Member, Institute of Biomedical Engineering
University of Toronto Faculty of Medicine
Otolaryngologist-in-Chief
Mount Sinai and Toronto General Hospitals
Toronto, Ontario, Canada

## ROBERT J. RUBEN, M.D., F.A.C.S., F.A.A.P.

Professor and Chairman
Department of Otolaryngology
Professor, Department of Pediatrics
Member, Department of History of Medicine
Albert Einstein College of Medicine of Yeshiva University
Chairman, Department of Otolaryngology
Montefiore Medical Center
Director, Department of Otolaryngology
North Central Bronx Hospital
New York, New York

## CHURCHILL LIVINGSTONE
New York, Edinburgh, London, Melbourne   1988

**Library of Congress Cataloging-in-Publication Data**

Otologic medicine and surgery.

Includes bibliographies and index.
1. Ear—Diseases.  2. Ear—Surgery.  I. Alberti,
Peter W.  II. Ruben, Robert J., 1933–
[DNLM: 1. Ear—surgery.  2. Ear—surgery.  WV 200 0875]
RF121.085   1988         617.8         88-1022
ISBN 0-443-08275-8

© **Churchill Livingstone Inc. 1988**

Distributed in the United Kingdom by Churchill Livingstone, Robert Stevenson
House, 1–3 Baxter's Place, Leith Walk, Edinburgh EH1 3AF, and by associated
companies, branches, and representatives throughout the world.

Accurate indications, adverse reactions, and dosage schedules for drugs are provided
in this book, but it is possible that they may change. The reader is urged to review
the package information data of the manufacturers of the medications mentioned.

The Publishers have made every effort to trace the copyright holders for borrowed
material. If they have inadvertently overlooked any, they will be pleased to make the
necessary arrangements at the first opportunity.

Assistant Editor: *Nancy Terry*
Copy Editor: *Margot Otway*
Production Supervisor: *Sharon Tuder*

Printed in the United States of America

First published in 1988

To our wives
Yvonne Korshak-Ruben and Elizabeth Smith-Alberti

# CONTRIBUTORS

**Sharon M. Abel, Ph.D.**
Professor, Department of Otolaryngology, and Professor, Graduate Department of Speech Pathology; Institute of Medical Sciences and Institute of Biomedical Engineering, University of Toronto Faculty of Medicine, Toronto, Ontario, Canada

**Maxwell Abramson, M.D.**
Professor and Chairman, Department of Otolaryngology, Columbia University College of Physicians and Surgeons; Director, Otolaryngology Service, Columbia-Presbyterian Medical Center, New York, New York

**Kedar K. Adour, M.D.**
Senior Consultant and Director of Research, Department of Otolaryngology, Cranial Nerve Research Clinic, Kaiser Permanente Medical Center, Oakland, California

**Peter W. Alberti, M.B., B.S., Ph.D., F.R.C.S., F.R.C.S.(C)**
Professor and Chairman, Department of Otolaryngology; Professor, Occupational Medicine; Member, Institute of Biomedical Engineering, University of Toronto Faculty of Medicine; Otolaryngologist-in-Chief, Mount Sinai and Toronto General Hospitals, Toronto, Ontario, Canada

**Bruce S. Bauer, M.D., F.A.C.S.**
Assistant Professor, Department of Surgery, Northwestern University Medical School; Chief, Division of Plastic Surgery, Children's Memorial Hospital, Chicago, Illinois

**James E. Benecke, Jr., M.D.**
Assistant Professor, Department of Otolaryngology, University of Southern California School of Medicine; Associate, Otologic Medical Group, Inc., House Ear Institute, Los Angeles, California

**LaVonne Bergstrom, M.D., F.A.C.S., F.A.A.P.**
Professor, Department of Surgery, Division of Head and Neck Surgery, University of California, Los Angeles, UCLA School of Medicine, Los Angeles, California

**Charles D. Bluestone, M.D.**
Professor, Department of Otolaryngology, University of Pittsburgh School of Medicine; Director, Department of Pediatric Otolaryngology, Children's Hospital of Pittsburgh, Pittsburgh, Pennsylvania

**Joann Bodurtha, M.D.**
Assistant Professor, Department of Human Genetics and Pediatrics, Virginia Commonwealth University Medical College of Virginia, Richmond, Virginia

**John B. Booth, M.B., B.S., F.R.C.S., A.K.C.**
Hunterian Professor, Royal College of Surgeons of England; Associate Lecturer, Institute of Laryngology and Otology, University of London; Consultant E.N.T. Surgeon, The London Hospital; Civil Consultant Otologist, Royal Air Force, London, England

**Derald E. Brackmann, Ph.D.**
Clinical Professor, Department of Otolaryngology, University of Southern California School of Medicine; Otologic Medical Group Inc., House Ear Institute, Los Angeles, California

**Barbara Canlon, M.S.**
Research Associate, Kresge Hearing Research Institute, University of Michigan, Ann Arbor, Michigan; Department of Physiology, Karolinska Institute, Stockholm, Sweden

**John Chong, M.D.**
Assistant Professor, Department of Clinical Epidemiology and Biostatistics, McMaster University Faculty of Health Sciences, Hamilton, Ontario, Canada

**Noel L. Cohen, M.D.**
Professor and Chairman, Department of Otolaryngology, New York University School of Medicine; Chief, Department of Otolaryngology, Bellevue Hospital Center, New York, New York

**Thomas F. DeMaria, Ph.D.**
Assistant Professor, Department of Otolaryngology, Otologic Research Laboratories, Ohio State University College of Medicine, Columbus, Ohio

**John V. Donlon, Jr., M.D.**
Assistant Clinical Professor, Department of Anesthesiology, Harvard Medical School, Boston, Massachusetts

**Jean-Jacques Dufour, M.D., F.R.C.S.(C)**
Associate Clinical Professor, Department of Surgery, Division of Otolaryngology, University of Montreal Faculty of Medicine; Director, Section of Neurotology, Notre-Dame and Ste. Justine Hospitals, Montreal, Quebec, Canada

**David A. F. Ellis, M.D., F.R.C.S.(C), F.A.C.S.**
Associate Professor, Department of Otolaryngology, University of Toronto Faculty of Medicine; Staff, Toronto Western Hospital, Toronto, Ontario, Canada

**Abraham Eviatar, M.D., F.A.C.S.**
Professor and Chief, Department of Otolaryngology, Jack D. Weiler Hospital of the Albert Einstein College of Medicine of Yeshiva University, New York, New York

**Lydia Eviatar, M.D.**
Associate Professor, Departments of Pediatrics and Neurology, State University of New York at Stony Brook Health Science Center School of Medicine, Stony Brook, New York; Chief of Pediatric Neurology, Schneider Children's Hospital of Long Island Jewish Medical Center, New Hyde Park, New York

**Bernt Falk, M.D., Ph.D.**
Consultant, Department of Otolaryngology, Vastervik Hospital, Vastervik, Sweden

**Joseph C. Farmer, M.D., F.A.C.S.**
Associate Professor, Department of Surgery, Division of Otolaryngology; Faculty, F.G. Hall Laboratory of Environmental Research, Duke University School of Medicine, Durham, North Carolina

**W. P. R. Gibson, M.B., B.S., M.D., F.R.C.S.**
Professor and Head, Department of Otolaryngology, University of Sydney, Sydney, New South Wales, Australia

**Cameron A. Gillespie, M.D., F.A.C.S.**
Fellow, Department of Surgery, Division of Otolaryngology, Duke University School of Medicine; Commander, Medical Corps, United States Navy, Durham, North Carolina

**Diane Giraudi-Perry, Ph.D.**
Assistant Professor, Department of Otolaryngology, Albert Einstein College of Medicine of Yeshiva University, New York, New York

**Michael E. Glasscock III, M.D., F.A.C.S.**
Clinical Professor, Department of Surgery (Otology and Neurotology), Vanderbilt University School of Medicine, Nashville, Tennessee; Clinical Professor, Department of Otolaryngology, University of Tennessee College of Medicine, Memphis, Tennessee

**Malcolm D. Graham, M.D.**
Staff Physician, Greater Detroit Otology Center, Detroit, Michigan

**Ronald E. Gristwood, Ch.M., F.R.C.S.(Edin), F.R.A.C.S.**
Consultant Otorhinolaryngologist, Royal Adelaide Hospital, Adelaide, South Australia

**Aina Julianna Gulya, M.D.**
Associate Professor of Surgery, Otology and Neurotologic Surgery, Department of Surgery, Division of Otolaryngology/Head and Neck Surgery, George Washington University School of Medicine and Health Sciences, Washington, D.C.

**Robert V. Harrison, Ph.D.**
Associate Professor, Department of Otolaryngology, University of Toronto Faculty of Medicine; The Hospital for Sick Children, Toronto, Ontario, Canada

**Andrew R. Harwood, M.B., Ch.B., F.R.C.P.(C)**
Radiation Oncologist, Romagosa Radiation Oncology Center, Lafayette, Louisiana

**Jonathan W. P. Hazell, M.A., M.B., B.Chir., F.R.C.S.**
Senior Lecturer, Department of Neuro-otology, University College, University of London; Honorary Consultant Neuro-otologist, University College Hospital; Consultant Neuro-otologist, Royal National Institute for the Deaf; Honorary Consultant, Department of Audiological Medicine, Royal National Throat, Nose and Ear Hospital, London, England

**Dikran Horoupian, M.D.**
Professor, Department of Pathology, Stanford University School of Medicine; Director of Neuropathology, Stanford University Medical Center, Stanford, California

**Cheng C. Huang, Ph.D.**
Associate Professor, Department of Otolaryngology, Columbia University College of Physicians and Surgeons, New York, New York

**Ivan M. Hunter-Duvar, Ph.D.**
Professor, Department of Otolaryngology, University of Toronto Faculty of Medicine; The Hospital for Sick Children, Toronto, Ontario, Canada

**Martyn L. Hyde, Ph.D.**
Associate Professor, Department of Otolaryngology, University of Toronto Faculty of Medicine; Director, Silverman Audiologic Research Laboratory, and Director of Audiological Development, Otologic Function Unit, Mount Sinai Hospital and Toronto General Hospital, Toronto, Ontario, Canada

**Brian Johnstone, Ph.D.**
Associate Professor, Department of Physiology, University of Western Australia, Nedlands, West Australia

**Jack M. Kartush, M.D.**
Staff Physician, Greater Detroit Otology Center, Detroit, Michigan

**Edward E. Kassel, D.D.S., M.D., F.R.C.P.(C)**
Assistant Professor, Department of Radiology, University of Toronto Faculty of Medicine; Neuroradiologist, Sunnybrook Medical Centre, Toronto, Ontario, Canada

**Thomas J. Keane, M.B., M.R.C.P.I., F.R.C.P.(C)**
Associate Professor, Departments of Radiology and Otolaryngology, University of Toronto Faculty of Medicine; Radiation Oncologist, The Princess Margaret Hospital, Toronto, Ontario, Canada

**Sam E. Kinney, M.D.**
Head, Section of Otology and Neurotology, Department of Otolaryngology and Communicative Disorders, The Cleveland Clinic Foundation, Cleveland, Ohio

**Yosef P. Krespi, M.D.**
Professor and Director, Department of Surgery, Division of Otolaryngology, State University of New York Health Science Center at Brooklyn College of Medicine; Chairman, Department of Otolaryngology, Long Island College Hospital, Brooklyn, New York

**Barbara Kruger, Ph.D.**
Director of Speech and Hearing, Department of Otolaryngology, Division of Audiology, Albert Einstein College of Medicine of Yeshiva University, New York, New York

**Toni M. Levine, M.D.**
Assistant Professor, Department of Otolaryngology, State University of New York Health Science Center at Brooklyn College of Medicine; Chief, Division of Otolaryngology, King's County Hospital, New York, New York

**Harry Levitt, Ph.D.**
Professor, Doctoral Program in Speech and Hearing Sciences, The Graduate School and University Center of the City University of New York, New York, New York

**David J. Lim, M.D.**
Professor, Department of Otolaryngology, and Director, Otologic Research Laboratories, Ohio State University College of Medicine, Columbus, Ohio

**Frank E. Lucente, M.D.**
Professor and Chairman, Department of Otolaryngology, New York Medical College, Valhalla, New York; Chairman, Department of Otolaryngology–Head and Neck Surgery, New York Eye and Ear Infirmary, New York, New York

**Paul F. A. Maderson, Ph.D., D.Sc.**
Professor, Department of Biology, Brooklyn College of the City University of New York, Brooklyn, New York

**Bengt Magnuson, M.D., Ph.D.**
Associate Professor, Department of Otolaryngology, Linkoping University Hospital, Linkoping, Sweden

**Gregory J. Matz, M.D.**
Professor and Chairman, Department of Otolaryngology, Division of Head and Neck Surgery, Loyola University of Chicago Stritch School of Medicine, Maywood, Illinois; Chief, Department of Otolaryngology, Veterans Administration Hospital, Hines, Illinois

**John T. McElveen, Jr., M.D.**
Assistant Professor, Department of Otolaryngology, Duke University School of Medicine, Durham, North Carolina

**Leslie Michaels, Ph.D., F.R.C.Path., F.R.C.P.(C)**
Professor, Department of Pathology, Institute of Laryngology and Otology, University of London; Professor, Department of Histopathology, University College and Middlesex School of Medicine; Director, Department of Pathology and Bacteriology, Royal National E.N.T. Hospital, London, England

**Robin P. Michelson, M.D.**
Clinical Professor, Department of Otolaryngology, University of California, San Francisco, School of Medicine, San Francisco, California

**Andrew W. Morrison, M.B., Ch.B., F.R.C.S., D.L.O.**
Lecturer in Otolaryngology, University of London; Honorary Consulting Otologist, Department of Otolaryngology, The London Hospital, London, England

**Walter E. Nance, M.D., Ph.D.**
Professor and Chairman, Department of Human Genetics, Virginia Commonwealth University Medical College of Virginia, Richmond, Virginia

**Arlene C. Neuman, Ph.D.**
Research Scientist, Center for Research in Speech and Hearing Sciences, The Graduate School and University Center of the City University of New York, New York, New York

**Drew M. Noden, Ph.D.**
Professor, Department of Anatomy, New York State College of Veterinary Medicine, Cornell University, Ithaca, New York

**Arnold M. Noyek, M.D., F.R.C.S.(C), F.A.C.S.**
Professor, Departments of Otolaryngology and Radiology, University of Toronto Faculty of Medicine, Toronto, Ontario, Canada; Senior Consultant in Otolaryngology, Faculty of Medicine, Technion University, Israel Institute of Technology, Haifa, Israel; Staff Otolaryngologist and Staff Radiologist (Otolaryngology), Mount Sinai Hospital; Staff Otolaryngologist, Sunnybrook Medical Centre, Toronto, Ontario, Canada

**Dennis P. O'Leary, Ph.D.**
Professor, Department of Otolaryngology–Head and Neck Surgery and Department of Physiology and Biophysics, University of California, Los Angeles, UCLA School of Medicine, Los Angeles, California

**Agnete Parving, M.D.**
Director, Department of Audiology, Copenhagen City Bispebjerg Hospital, Copenhagen, Denmark

**Myles L. Pensak, M.D.**
Assistant Professor, Department of Otolaryngology and Maxillofacial Surgery, Division of Otology and Neurotology, University of Cincinnati College of Medicine, Cincinnati, Ohio

**C. R. Pfaltz, M.D.**
Professor and Chairman, Department of Otorhinolaryngology, University of Basel Kantonsspital, Basel, Switzerland

**Jacques F. Poliquin, M.D., F.R.C.S.(C)\***
Professor and Chairman, Department of Otolaryngology, University of Ottawa School of Medicine, Ottawa, Ontario, Canada

---

\* Deceased.

**Michel Portmann**
Professor, Chief of Service, and Director of the University Clinic of Otorhinolaryngology, Université Bordeaux, Bordeaux, France

**Isabelle Rapin, M.D.**
Professor of Neurology and Pediatrics (Neurology), Department of Neurology, Albert Einstein College of Medicine of Yeshiva University, Bronx, New York

**Krista Riko, M.Sc.(App.)**
Assistant Professor, Department of Otolaryngology, University of Toronto Faculty of Medicine; Director, Otologic Function Unit, Mount Sinai Hospital and Toronto General Hospital, Toronto, Ontario, Canada

**Robert J. Ruben, M.D., F.A.C.S., F.A.A.P.**
Professor and Chairman, Department of Otolaryngology, Professor, Department of Pediatrics, and Member, Department of History of Medicine, Albert Einstein College of Medicine of Yeshiva University; Chairman, Department of Otolaryngology, Montefiore Medical Center; Director, Department of Otolaryngology, North Central Bronx Hospital, New York, New York

**Leonard Rybak, M.D., Ph.D.**
Associate Professor, Department of Surgery, Division of Otolaryngology, Southern Illinois University School of Medicine, Springfield, Illinois

**Gerhard Salomon, M.D.**
Director of the Audiological Clinic, Gentofte University Hospital, Hellerup, Denmark

**Jochen Schacht, Ph.D.**
Professor, Departments of Biological Chemistry and Otolaryngology, Kresge Hearing Research Institute, University of Michigan Medical School, Ann Arbor, Michigan

**Jerome D. Schein**
Adjunct Professor, Deafness Research and Training Center, New York University, New York, New York

**Mansfield F. W. Smith, M.D., M.S.**
Clinical Associate Professor, Department of Surgery, Division of Otolaryngology, Stanford University School of Medicine, Stanford, California

**Peter G. Smith, M.D., Ph.D., F.A.C.S.**
Assistant Professor, Department of Otolaryngology, Washington University School of Medicine; Assistant Otolaryngologist, Barnes Hospital; Attending Physician, Jewish Hospital of St. Louis; Consultant, Veterans Administration Hospital; Consultant, Missouri Crippled Children's Division, St. Louis, Missouri

**Gordon D. L. Smyth, D.Sc., M.D., M.Ch.(Hons), F.R.C.S., D.L.O.**
Consultant Surgeon, Eye and Ear Clinic, Royal Victoria Hospital, Belfast, Northern Ireland

**James B. Snow, Jr., M.D.**
Professor and Chairman, Department of Otorhinolaryngology and Human Communication, University of Pennsylvania School of Medicine, Philadelphia, Pennsylvania

**Heinrich Spoendlin, M.D.**
Professor and Head, Department of Otorhinolaryngology, University Hospital, Innsbruck, Austria

**Barbara A. Stahl, R.N.**
Chief Surgical Nurse, Otologic Medical Group, Inc., Los Angeles, California

**Takafumi Sugita, M.D.**
Visiting Associate Research Scientist, Department of Otolaryngology, Columbia University College of Physicians and Surgeons, New York, New York; Department of Otolaryngology, Jikei University School of Medicine, Tokyo, Japan

**Jun-Ichi Suzuki, M.D.**
Professor and Chairman, Department of Otolaryngology, Teikyo University School of Medicine, Tokyo, Japan

**J. Regan Thomas, M.D.**
Assistant Professor, Division of Facial Plastic Surgery, Department of Otolaryngology, Washington University School of Medicine, St. Louis, Missouri

**Jens Thomsen, M.D., Ph.D.**
Professor, Department of Otorhinolaryngology, Gentofte Hospital, Hellerup, Denmark

**Mirko Tos, M.D., Ph.D.**
Professor and Chairman, Department of Otorhinolaryngology, Copenhagen University, Copenhagen, Denmark; Department of Otorhinolaryngology, Gentofte Hospital, Hellerup, Denmark

**Thomas R. Van De Water, Ph.D.**
Professor, Department of Otolaryngology, and Associate Professor, Department of Neuroscience, Developmental Otobiology Laboratory, Albert Einstein College of Medicine of Yeshiva University, New York, New York

**Alfred D. Weiss, M.D.**
Assistant Clinical Professor, Department of Neurology, Harvard Medical School; Assistant Neurologist, Massachusetts General Hospital; Assistant in Otolaryngology (Otoneurology), Massachusetts Eye and Ear Infirmary, Boston, Massachusetts

**Laura Ann Wilber, Ph.D.**
Professor of Audiology and Hearing Impairment, Department of Communicative Sciences and Disorders, Northwestern University, Evanston, Illinois; Coordinator of Audiologic Research, Northwestern University Medical School, Chicago, Illinois

**Wesley R. Wilson, Ph.D.**
Professor, Department of Speech and Hearing Sciences, University of Washington, Seattle, Washington

# PREFACE

Otology is a science of many disciplines. Ranging over medical and nonmedical specialties, its diversity is at once its strength and weakness. The various specialties provide a wealth of information about ear disease and hearing science, but the fragmented nature of otologic sciences has made it difficult for practitioners to draw upon these resources.

Many works exist that emphasize surgery of the ear, audiology, rehabilitation, basic sciences, otoneurology, and otologic medicine. There are, in addition, books and monographs on subjects that pertain to otology, such as aerospace medicine, central nervous system disorders, and rehabilitation. However, there is no compilation that covers all otologic medicine and surgery.

This book is designed as a working text and reference for physicians and other health professionals in the fields of ear disease and hearing science. We hope it will close the gap between the disciplines of audiology, otology, and auditory rehabilitation and foster an integrated approach to the diagnosis and management of hearing disorders and diseases of the ear. *Otologic Medicine and Surgery* is intended as a systematic presentation of the underlying basic science, clinical diagnostic methods and techniques, biology of disease processes, and management of the disorders and diseases that affect the human ear, hearing, and balance.

To consolidate the current findings from the various otologic disciplines, we have assembled an international group of contributors from among the foremost specialists in each field. We have also tried to balance European medical audiology and North American interventionist otology to give a broad perspective of available modalities of treatment.

*Otologic Medicine and Surgery* begins with nine chapters on the basic sciences. The next section consists of 11 chapters dealing with various techniques and methodologies for obtaining diagnoses. The following 14 chapters present the biology of diseases, including anatomic pathology and disease processes. The remaining half of the book, 38 chapters, presents the therapy and management of diseases of the ear by medical, surgical, and public health interventions.

In editing this book we have taken as our goal to bring together all aspects of otology and the hearing sciences so that the discipline may be viewed as a whole. We hope the present work succeeds in uniting the disparate parts of otology and relating them to the discoveries of contemporary science and, in so doing, contributes to the current and future prevention, cure, and management of otologic disorders.

*Peter W. Alberti*
*Robert J. Ruben*

# ACKNOWLEDGMENTS

*Otologic Medicine and Surgery* could only have come about because of the genius and efforts of countless people who have served directly or indirectly as teachers and role models for the editors. We want to especially acknowledge several who have had a significant impact on our own intellectual and medical development. These are

Sir Charles A. Ballance

Georg von Békésy

John E. Bordley

Alfred J. Columbre

Stacy R. Guild

Jean M. G. Itard

Julius Lempert

Adam Politzer

Joseph Toynbee

Ernest G. Weaver

# CONTENTS

## Volume 1

# Volume 2

# Section 1

# BASIC SCIENCE

# Embryology of the Ear: Outer, Middle, and Inner

1

**Thomas R. Van De Water**
**Drew M. Noden**
**Paul F. A. Maderson**

This chapter discusses the mechanisms of embryogenesis that act during the formation of the components of the ear and their relationships during development.

## OUTER EAR

The outer ear consists of the auricle (pinna), the external acoustic canal and the cuticular (epidermal, epithelial) layer of the tympanic membrane. These structures derive from the ectoderm and cephalic mesenchyme tissues of the first branchial groove and the surrounding first (mandibular) and second (hyoid) branchial arches (Fig. 1-1).

The external acoustic canal is formed by invagination and medial growth of the first branchial groove to form a funnel-shaped pit, the primary external acoustic canal. This occurs in man at approximately the fourth gestational week. It is at this time that the ectoderm of the primary auditory pit comes in close contact with the endoderm of the

dorsal division of the first pharyngeal pouch (the tubotympanum). This close relationship between the invaginating branchial groove and outpocketing pharyngeal pouch is transient. The invagination of the branchial groove continues, but due to growth and elaboration of the craniofacial mesenchyme, the surfaces of the forming external auditory canal are forced together and appear as a strand of epithelial cells (the meatal plate) that terminates in a disc-like swelling near the lower wall of the developing tympanic (middle ear) cavity. Formation of this false core of epithelial cells occurs around the eighth week of fetal development and is the anlage of the secondary external acoustic meatus. At about the 28th week of development, a lumen forms in this secondary auditory meatal plate due to separation of the epithelial layers, and it becomes a medial extension of the lumen of the primary external acoustic canal. The disc-like swelling, which is found at the end of the secondary external acoustic canal, becomes the epidermal layer of the developing tympanic membrane (Fig. 1-2). The primary external acoustic canal is the anlage of the cartilaginous portion of the canal, and the secondary external acoustic

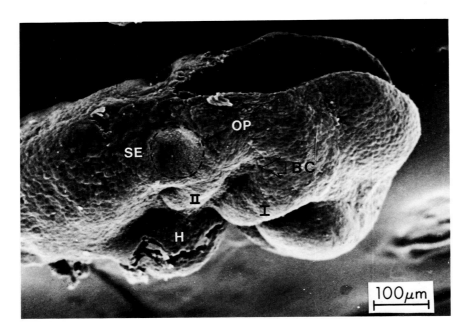

**Fig. 1-1.** Top view of the anlage of the external ear in an 8½-day-old embryo, showing first *(I)* and second *(II)* branchial arches separated by the first branchial cleft *(BC)*. The otic placode *(OP)* is seen as a depression in the surface ectoderm *(SE)*. The heart *(H)* at this stage is located externally.

canal corresponds to the bony portion of this structure. Information drawn from articles of Hammar,[1] Altmann,[2] Arey,[3] and Van De Water et al[4] was employed in formulating this description.

The development of the auricle from six hillocks arising equally from the hyoid and mandibular arches on either side of the first branchial cleft was described by His.[5] Hammar[1] called these hillocks of His "ridges" and reported his modified version of the genesis of the auricle. On the basis of data from congenital anomalies of the outer ear used in conjunction with normal embryologic material, Wood-Jones and Wen[6] asserted that the entire auricle, except the tragus, is of hyoid arch origin. In their description,[6] the hillocks of the hyoid arch fuse and form the posterior auricular fold, which extends beyond the dorsal limit of the first branchial cleft and then extends in a ventral direction, depressing the growth of the anterior fold formed by the fusion of the mandibular arch hillocks. The suppressed anterior fold was said to contribute only to the formation of the tragus.

Streeter[7] observed that the hillocks of His had been described for mammals with varying types of auricles and also reported that the hillocks are present during embryonic development in reptiles, amphibians, and birds, none of which develop distinct auricles. It was Streeter's opinion that too much significance had been placed on the hillocks, which are transitory and incidental in nature rather than fundamental to the formation of the auricle. Emphasizing the different topographic relationships between the hillocks, and the canal and tympanum, Presley[8] has concluded that the external otic tissues of reptiles and mammals are not homologous. Streeter stated that the auricle may be entirely of hyoid origin, but since his human material did not corroborate such a supposition, he[7] continued to describe the tragus as being of mandibular arch origin. Using a new method of flattening the auricular cartilage in a comprehensive comparative study, Boas[9] demonstrated that the tragus is a part of the posterior border of the ear cartilage, which is rolled so that the proximal portion lies over the anterior edge. Boas' technique was used in a study of the development of the auricle in the Dachs rabbit.[10] In the adult, the cartilage of the auricle is a single continuum. Crary[10] confirmed Streeter's[7] suggestion that it arose from a continuous, intact primordium. The tragus arises from the mandibular arch, and mesenchyme from the second and third hillocks on the mandibular arch migrate to the hyoid arch during organogenesis (Figs. 1-3 and 1-4).

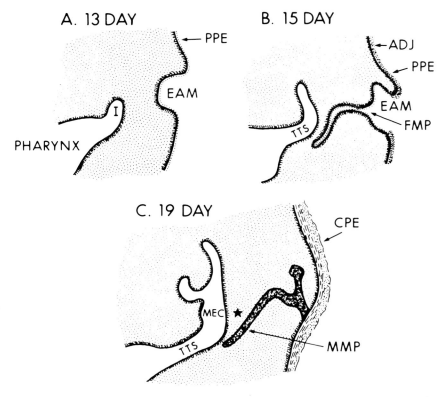

**Fig. 1-2.** Diagrammatic presentation of the development of the external auditory meatus and meatal plate in **(A)** 13-day-old, **(B)** 15-day-old, and **(C)** 19-day-old mouse embryos. Initially (13th day), the epidermal histology of the adjacent, nonotic skin *(ADJ)* is the same as that lining the external auditory meatus *(EAM)* and over the presumptive pinnal tissues *(PPE)*. By the 15th day the tubotympanic sulcus *(TTS)* has grown dorsal from the pharyngeal pouch *(I);* its endodermal lining approaches the presumptive meatal plate *(FMP)*. The lumen of the latter may still be patent distally, but its epidermis, like that of the meatus, bears only a single layer of superficial peridermal cells, while that of the pinna *(PPE)* and the adjacent skin now have several layers of peridermal cells. By 19 days, the lumen of the external meatus and the enlarged meatal plate *(MMP)* have become completely occluded. The epidermis of the pinna and the adjacent skin show the first signs of cornification beneath the multilayered periderm, while the meatal plate appears as a simple plate, but is in fact two younger epidermes lying en face. The star indicates the approximate location of the presumptive tympanic tissues, which lie between the meatal plate and the developing middle ear cavity *(MEC)*. *CPE* cornified peridermal epithelium.

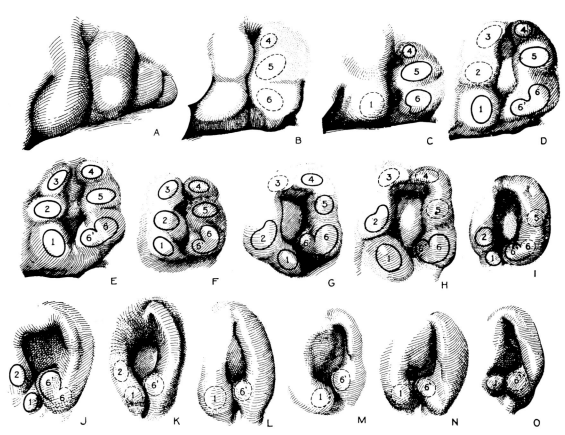

**Fig. 1-3.** A diagrammatic interpretation of the transitory occurrence of the branchial hillocks of His and the coincidental changes in the mandibular (first) and hyoid (second) arches. These stages cover the period of transition from simple branchial arches to the establishment of the primitive auricle. The hillocks are interpreted as transitory foci of the rapidly proliferating cells of the mesenchymal primordium of the auricle. They are considered to be incidental, rather than fundamental, to the development of the auricle. These observations are based on photographs of staged human embryo auricles (Streeter[7]) from the Carnegie Collection: (**A** to **C**) embryos 5 to 11 mm; (**D** to **G**) embryos 13 to 14 mm, (**H** to **K**) embryos 15 to 18 mm; (**L** to **O**) embryos 18 to 33 mm. Varying magnifications were used to represent the structures to about the same size. (Modified from Streeter GL: Development of the auricle in the human embryo. Contrib Embryol Carnegie Inst 14:111, 1922.)

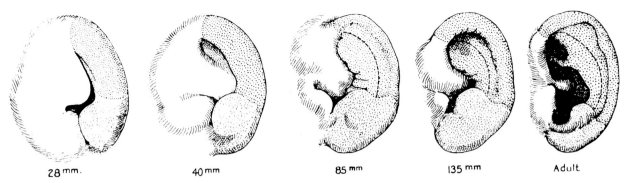

28 mm.   40 mm   85 mm   135 mm   Adult

**Fig. 1-4.** Drawings representing the development of the human auricle from its primitive form to the adult type. That portion of the auricle derived from the mandibular (first) arch is indicated in a lighter tone and is relatively greater in the earlier stages; the portion derived from the hyoid (second) arch is stippled and is shown to increase in the later stages; the broken line represents the approximate junction of the anthelix and scapha-helix. (Modified from Streeter, GL: Development of the auricle in the human embryo. Contrib Embryol Carnegie Inst 14:111, 1922.

## MIDDLE EAR

The middle ear comprises the middle fibrous layer and inner mucosal layer of the tympanic membrane, the ossicular chain (malleus, incus, and stapes), auditory (pharyngotympanic or eustachian) tube, and middle ear cleft. The middle fibrous layer of the tympanic membrane derives from the cephalic mesenchyme cells that lie between the outer epidermal component of the tympanic membrane and the inner endodermal (inner) layer of the developing tubotympanic cavity. The formation of the tympanic membrane of the frog depends on the presence of the annular tympanic cartilage.[11] Other visceral cartilages, especially the quadrate, can induce the formation of a membrane when in contact with the skin of the frog; cartilage of the appendicular skeleton is also effective but much less active. This induction is probably mediated by some chemical quality of the cartilage,[11] because cartilage that has been killed by various chemical and physical treatments still retains its inductive influence.

The ciliated, columnar cells forming the inner layer of the tympanic membrane are endodermal in origin and originate from the epithelial cells of the inpocketing dorsal division of the first pharyngeal pouch. Studies by Jaskoll and Maderson[12] and Jaskoll[13] have confirmed the endodermal nature of the ciliated, columnar cells that form the inner layer of the tympanic membrane.

The middle ear cleft and auditory (eustachian) tube were described by Hammar[1] to develop solely from the dorsal division of the first pharyngeal pouch. This was widely accepted until Frazer[14–16] contended that there were also contributions from the second arch endoderm and the dorsal division of the second pharyngeal pouch. Altmann, in his review article[2] on developmental mechanics of the ear gave credence to Hammar's theory.[1] From a study of the development of the human tubotympanic recess, Kanagasuntheram[17] concluded that migration of the first arch tissues into the area of the first pouch occurs during the 10- to 20-mm stages. This author also claimed that during this stage the contributions from the second arch and pouch diminish in importance so that the tubotympanic recess and tube are formed solely from first pouch tissues.[17] The following concept of middle ear cleft development emerges. The major endodermal contribution to the developing middle ear space is the dorsal division of the first pharyngeal pouch as was stated by Hammar,[1] and the second pharyngeal pouch is a transient contributor to the tubotympanic cavity and eustachian tube.

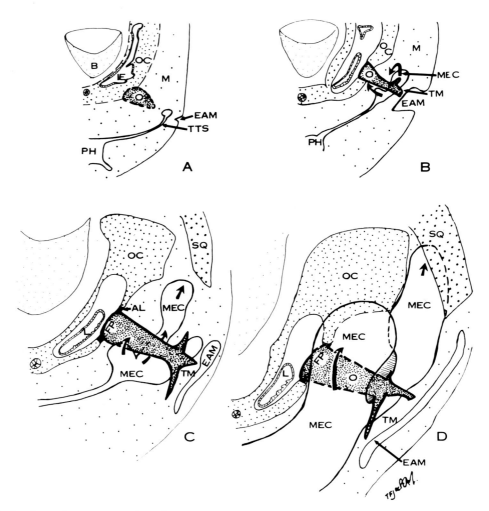

**Fig. 1-5.** A schematic representation of the development of the amniote middle and external ear. While based mainly on a study of chick embryonic development, it essentially resembles the major stages of development in all amniotes. **(A)** The tubotympanic sulcus *(TTS)*, an extension of the hyoid pouch, is growing dorsolaterally from the pharynx *(PH)* beneath the otic capsule *(OC)*, in the general direction of an ectodermal depression, the anlage of the external auditory meatus *(EAM)*. At this time, mesenchymal condensations representing the anlage(n) of the ossicle(s) *(O)* may be seen surrounded by mesenchyme *(M)*. **(B)** The single columella (reptiles and birds) — or the ossicular chain (mammals) *(O)* — now runs through the mesenchyma from a fenestra ovalis close to the lagena of the cochlea *(L)* to the presumptive tympanic region *(TM)*. The tubotympanic sulcus has grown dorsally directed pouches anterior and posterior to the ossicle(s), which represent the first indications of the developing middle ear cavity *(MEC)*. The external auditory canal may have reached its maximum relative depth at this time, or further depression may occur later in development, especially in mammals and birds. **(C)** As the middle ear cavities continue their dorsal growth and enlargement, the footplate *(FP)* of the columella (mammalian stapes) becomes suspended by a presumptive annular ligament *(AL)* within the fenestra ovalis. In birds and reptiles, the continued lateral expansion of the middle ear cavities is beginning to compress the mesenchyme against the ectoderm of the presumptive tympanum. In mammals, the development of the meatal plate may delay this event until much later in embryonic development, or even postnatally. **(D)** As the mesenchyme is removed, the endodermal epithelium of the middle ear cavity encroaches upon the ossicle(s). In mammals, joint differentiation between the ossicles would be well advanced at such a time, and ossification would have begun in any amniote embryo. *B,* hindbrain; *IE,* inner ear: *SQ* squamosal.

The fate of the mesenchyme, which originally occupies the region of the tympanic cavity, and the associated problem of the germ layer origin of the epithelium lining the mature tympanic cavity have been sources of contention for some years.[4,13,18] We may now be reasonably certain of two facts. First, the entire epithelial lining of the tympanic cavity is of endodermal origin. Second, since although it appears that the cavity expands by simple growth of the epithelium, the fate of the mesenchyme differs in different species. Jaskoll and Maderson[12] have shown that it is a minor site of hemopoiesis in birds; the mesenchyme differentiates either as blood cells or as vascular endothelia, which drain into the nearby jugular vein; cell death is either absent or of minor importance. A similar situation probably exists in lizard embryos (Maderson, preliminary observations). By contrast, no evidence of sinus vascularization or hemopoiesis is

apparent in mammals, and cell death predominates.[12,19]

A schematic representation of the development of an amniote middle ear cavity, based mainly on a study of chick embryos,[12] but essentially representing all amniotes, is presented in Figure 1-5. The problem of the evolutionary origin of the bones of the mammalian middle ear has aroused great interest in many biomedical disciplines.

Goodrich[20] reviews the original theories of Meckel[21] and Reichert[22] and analyzes the formation of the ossicular chain from the vantage points of a comparative morphologist. The modern version of Reichert's theory states that the mammalian stapes, incus, and malleus derive respectively from the reptilian columella auris, quadrate, and articular. The corollaries of this contention are that the malleus and incus develop from first arch mesenchyme and the stapes from second arch mesen-

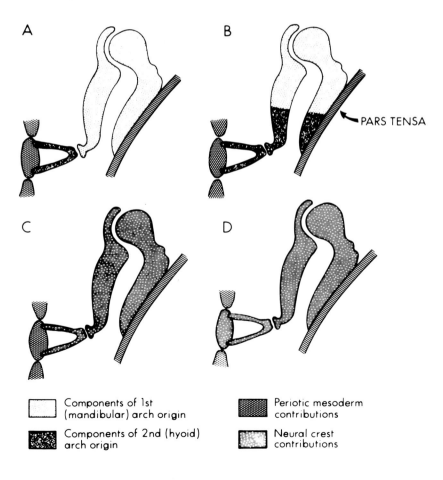

**Fig. 1-6.** Diagrammatic presentation of two major theories of embryonic origins of the auditory ossicles in mammals. **(A)** and **(B)** refer to conflicting theories regarding branchial arch origins of the ossicles; **(C)** and **(D)** deal with Mesoderm versus Neural Crest contributions to the footplate.

PARS TENSA

Components of 1st (mandibular) arch origin

Components of 2nd (hyoid) arch origin

Periotic mesoderm contributions

Neural crest contributions

chyme; the auditory capsule may or may not contribute to the formation of the stapedial footplate (Fig. 1-6A). An alternative view, presented by Strickland et al.,[23] suggests that the first branchial arch contributes to both the malleus and incus, whereas the second arch mesenchyme contributes to the formation of all three ossicles (Fig. 1-6B). The following facts concerning the origins of the auditory ossicles of man are evident in both of these presentations:

1. The major source of the ossicles and their associated structure is the neural crest mesenchyme of the first (mandibular) and second (hyoid) branchial arches.
2. The auditory capsule (mesodermal mesenchyme) plays a role in the formation of the stapedial base and oval window.

Controversy still exists as to the definitive origins of the tissues that form the ossicles and related structures. Anson and Bast,[24] using a wax reconstruction technique, stated that the head of the malleus and main body of the incus derive from first arch (Meckel's) mesenchyme, while the manubrium of the malleus, long process of the incus, and the stapes derive from second arch (Reichert's) mesenchyme (Fig. 1-6B). The lamina stapedius and the annular ligament were described as originating via degeneration of cartilaginous tissues of the otic capsule. Studies on other species have suggested further complications. In the mouse, the incus and malleus are said to derive from the upper part of the blastema of the mandibular arch, the stapes from the dorsal medial portion of the hyoid.[25] Jenkinson[25] claims that the only contribution from the auditory capsule is the lamina stapedius (Fig. 1-6D), but in the rabbit, Fuchs[26] claims that the stapedial footplate derives from the capsule (Fig. 1-6C). In the bird it has been claimed that the stapedial footplate derives from the capsule, the remainder of the ossicle from the second branchial arch[27,28] (Fig. 1-6C). Hanson and his colleagues[28] reiterated their previously published reports that the head of the malleus and body of the incus, including the short process, are derived from first arch mesenchyma. The manubrium of the malleus and long process of the incus, as well as the entire stapes, with the exception of the lamina stapedius portion of the base, are of second branchial arch origin (Fig. 1-6D). These anatomic observations were backed up by some congenital anomalies of the middle ear observed by these investigators (i.e., frequent partial insertion of the stapedial tendon into the long process of the incus). A more extensive study of congenital malformations of the

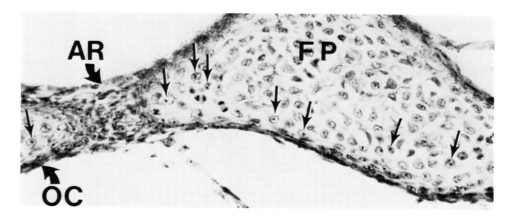

**Fig. 1-7.** Footplate *(FP)* of the columella auris of a chicken-quail chimera. The transplant was of quail somitomeres 6 and 7 (mesodermal tissue), which are located beneath and caudal to the otic placode. The arrows indicate cartilage cells in which the quail marker is obvious (heterochromatic body). The developing annular ring *(AR)* and otic capsule *(OC)* also contain quail cells. This illustrates that in the avian species the footplate receives a significant contribution from periotic mesoderm.

middle ear reported by Hough[29] supports the branchial arch origins of the ossicles and their related structures as put forth by Anson and Bast[24] and Hanson et al.[28] Alberti[30] described in detail the blood supply of the incudostapedial joint and the lenticular process. This work also supports the branchial arch derivations of the ossicular chain as put forth by Anson and Bast[24] and Hanson et al.[28]

The subtle complexities of the problem of interpreting descriptive and experimental data pertaining to the embryonic origin of the amniote stapedial footplate have been reviewed previously.[4] Although the avian footplate undoubtedly shows unique features by comparison with its assumed

mammalian homologue,[12] so that data derived from birds must be applied to mammals only with caution, interesting facts have been reported from studies on birds.[31] Analysis of chicken-quail embryonic chimeras have shown that the avian columella contains both neural crest and mesoderm cells[31,32] (Fig. 1-7), the latter being most numerous in the footplate. Such a contribution would not have been predicted from models assuming branchial arch origins of amniote ossicles, and the evidence might be taken as indicating "evolutionary opportunism" such as is seen in other posterior cranial elements in birds.[32] The avian footplate chondrifies simultaneously with the otic capsule,[12] whereas that in the

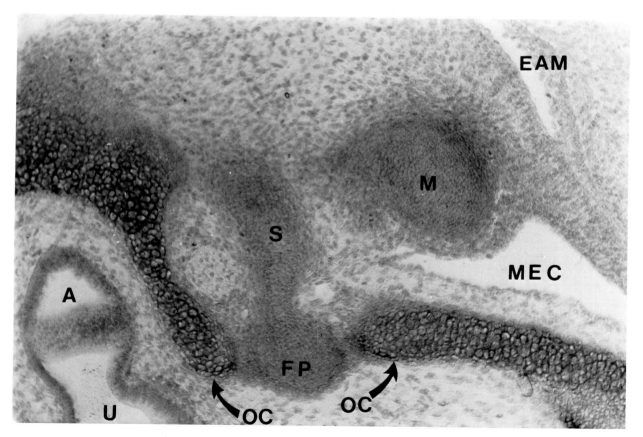

**Fig. 1-8.** An immunocytochemical localization of type 2 collagen in a 16-day-old embryonic mouse otic capsule *(OC)*. The presence of reaction product staining indicates the presence of type 2 collagen. The otic capsule has a denser concentration of reaction product than the footplate *(FP)* of the stapes *(S)*. The stapedial footplate has a staining pattern identical to the neural crest components of the ossicular chain. The malleus *(M)* and stapes are seen at this plane of section, which passes through the utricle *(U)* and the ampulla *(A)* of the anterior semicircular duct. The developing middle ear cavity *(MEC)* and external auditory meatus *(EAM)* are also present.

developing mouse (Van De Water TR, Galinovic-Schwartz V: Unpublished observations) follows the pattern of the assumed neural crest mesenchyma of the ossicular chain, which is delayed with respect to the capsule (Fig. 1-8). As concluded previously,[4] final answers to questions concerning evolutionary homologies and specific embryonic origins of putative neural crest derivatives in mammals must await technical advances permitting execution of appropriate manipulations. Summaries of current theories pertaining to these issues with respect to mammalian ear ossicles are shown in Figure 1-6.

## INNER EAR

The inner ear consists of the vestibular and auditory portions of the membranous labyrinth, the auditory (spiral) and vestibular (Scarpa's) portions of the eighth nerve ganglion, and the surrounding bony labyrinth.

Induction of the inner ear is a gradual process involving diverse inductor tissues, and continued induction after placode formation is essential for

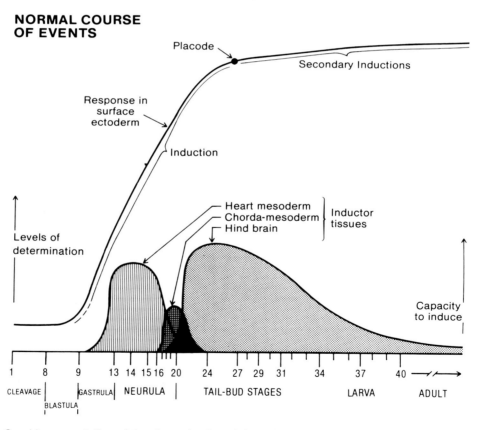

**Fig. 1-9.** Graphic presentation of the determination of the otic placode in amphibian embryos (Modified from Jacobson A: Inductive processes in embryonic development. Science 152 (No. 3718):25-34, 1966. Copyright 1966 by the American Association for the Advancement of Science.)

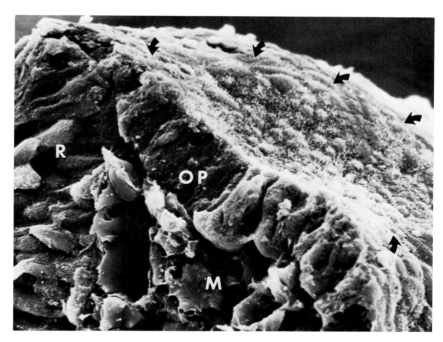

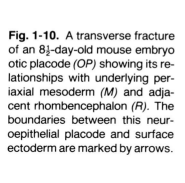

**Fig. 1-10.** A transverse fracture of an 8½-day-old mouse embryo otic placode *(OP)* showing its relationships with underlying periaxial mesoderm *(M)* and adjacent rhombencephalon *(R)*. The boundaries between this neuroepithelial placode and surface ectoderm are marked by arrows.

complete differentiation and growth. The process of otic placode determination has been best studied in amphibians.[33,34] There is a sequence of three overlapping inductive interactions of head surface ectoderm with heart mesoderm, chorda meso-

derm, and hind brain (rhombencephalon) tissues (Fig. 1-9). Because early inductive events of sensory receptors tend to be conserved, it may reasonably be assumed that a similar series of tissue interactions are responsible for the determination of the

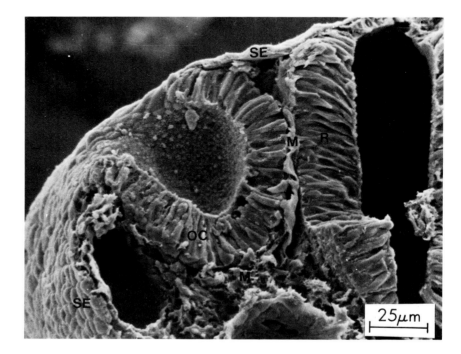

**Fig. 1-11.** An otic cup *(OC)* and its relationships to cephalic mesenchyma *(M)*, surface ectoderm *(SE)*, and the rhombencephalon are presented in this scanning electron micrograph of a transverse fracture of the head area of a 9-day-old mouse embryo. *R*, rhombencephalon.

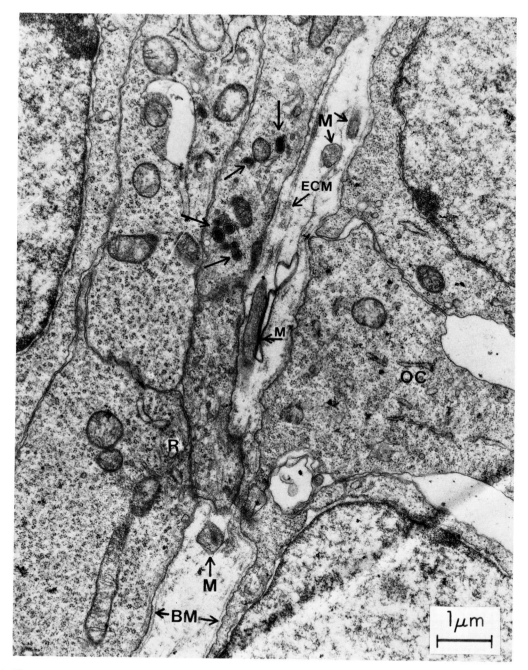

**Fig. 1-12.** An electron micrograph of the otic area of a 9-day-old mouse embryo. The area of closest apposition of the neuroepithelial components of the otic cup *(OC)* and adjacent rhombencephalon *(R)* show that direct cell-to-cell contact does not occur between these two tissues. The basement membranes *(BM)* are intact, and the clrft between these apposing tissues is rich in extracellullar matrix *(ECM)*. Intervening processes of cephalic mesenchyma cells *(M)* are present in this cleft, and dense core vesicles are seen *(arrows)* in the rhombencephalic tissue.

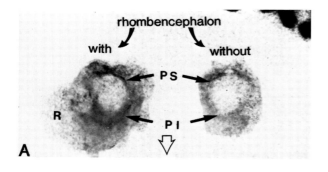

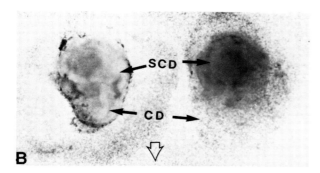

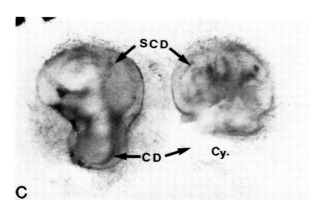

**Fig. 1-13.** Otocyst–rhombencephalon interaction. A sequence of micrographs of a pair of living 10½-day-old mouse otic explants: **(A)** Day of explantation: the morphology of both the with- and without-rhombencephalon explants is the same; pars superior *(PS)* and pars inferior *(PI)* areas are discernible. **(B)** 6 days in vitro: semicircular duct *(SCD)* development is equivalent in both explants, but cochlear duct *(CD)* formation is retarded in the without-rhombencephalon specimen. **(C)** 10 days in vitro: vestibular development is similar in both explants; dysmorphogenesis of the cochlear duct is evident with this structure expressing a cystic *(CY)* malformation. *R*, rhombencephalon.

mammalian otic placode (Fig. 1-10). As the otic placode invaginates to form an otocyst (Fig. 1-11), the neuroepithelial cells of this anlage come into close association with the neuroepithelial cells of adjacent rhombencephalic tissue. In amphibian embryos, direct contacts (focal gap junctions) occur between these two neuroepithelial cell populations,[35] but such have not been found in mammalian material (Fig. 1-12). A comparable period of development in humans is the fourth week of gestation.

The dependence of the development of the inner ear on the inductive influence of brain stem (rhombencephalon) tissue has been demonstrated by extirpation studies in both amphibian[36] and avian[37] embryos. In mammals, a temporal series of otocysts organ cultured with and without rhombencephalic tissue has demonstrated that this interaction is necessary for continued morphogenesis and cytodifferentiation of inner ear sensory structures.[38] The consequences of interrupting the inductive interactions that occur between otic anlage and brain stem tissue is evident in Figure 1-13. If these tissue interactions had been disrupted at an earlier stage, development of the entire membranous labyrinth would have been affected. A summarization of these results regarding temporal influence and the graded nature of the dysmorphogenesis that occurs when the tissue interactions are disrupted are presented in Figure 1-14. The temporal response of the developing inner ear (otocyst) to disruption of the inductive influence of brain stem tissue is graded, with the most severe malformations occurring in the earliest stage of otic development; older embryonic inner ears confine their expression of dysmorphogenesis and lack of cytodifferentiation to the area of the forming cochlea. These results clearly demonstrate the importance of otocyst–brain stem tissue interaction for the orderly development of the inner ear. A comparable period of development in humans is the fifth week of gestation.

As the otocyst separates from its close association with the developing brain, it becomes completely enveloped with cephalic mesenchyme, and at this stage (i.e., in humans 5½ to 6½ weeks of gestation) becomes dependent on the influences provided by the surrounding mesenchyme for continued development. During this period of otic development,

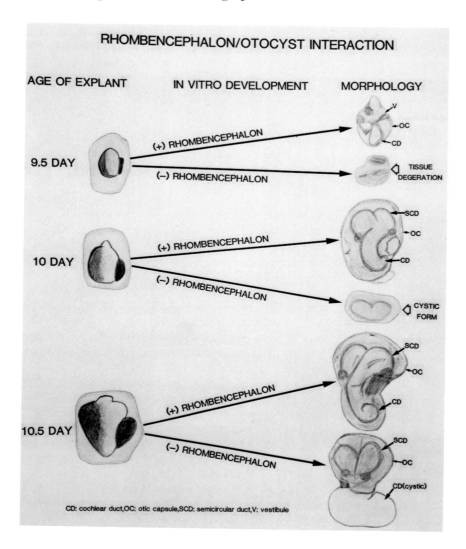

## RHOMBENCEPHALON/OTOCYST INTERACTION

AGE OF EXPLANT    IN VITRO DEVELOPMENT    MORPHOLOGY

9.5 DAY

(+) RHOMBENCEPHALON

(−) RHOMBENCEPHALON

V
OC
CD

TISSUE DEGERATION

10 DAY

(+) RHOMBENCEPHALON

(−) RHOMBENCEPHALON

SCD
OC
CD

CYSTIC FORM

10.5 DAY

(+) RHOMBENCEPHALON

(−) RHOMBENCEPHALON

SCD
OC
CD

SCD
OC
CD(cystic)

CD: cochlear duct,OC: otic capsule,SCD: semicircular duct,V: vestibule

**Fig. 1-14.** A pictorial summary of the results of a series of organ culture experiments of mouse otocyst–rhombencephalon explants versus otocyst explants that do not contain rhombencephalic tissue. The inner ear exhibits a graded response of dysmorphogenesis to the absence of the inductive influence that this brain stem tissue provides.

interactions between epithelial (otocyst) and periotic mesenchymal tissues predominate as the inductive influence on both the membranous and bony labyrinth. These epithelial–mesenchymal tissue interactions are reciprocal in nature and affect the morphogenesis and cytodifferentiation of both the tissue types that comprise the developing inner ear. Experiments[39] examining the effect of reduced mesenchymal mass on the morphogenesis and cytodifferentiation of both the tissue types that comprise the developing inner ear. Experiments[39] examining the effect of reduced mesenchymal mass on the morphogenesis and cytodifferentiation of inner ear explants have shown that a critical mass of

periotic mesenchyme must be present with the explanted otocyst for the support of normal development. A reduction in the periotic mesenchyme of otic explants results in varying degrees of labyrinthine malformations (Fig. 1-15), which correlate to the stage of development at which the mesenchymal mass was manipulated (Fig. 1-16). Other studies[40] using chick embryo otocysts confirm these results, which indicate the importance of periotic mesenchyme integrity on otic morphogenesis. Li and McPhee[41] showed that even a localized deficit of mesenchyme at the ventral tip of the otocyst could have a profound effect on morphogenesis of the cochlear duct (Fig. 1-17).

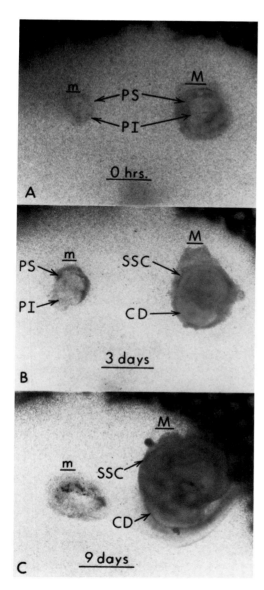

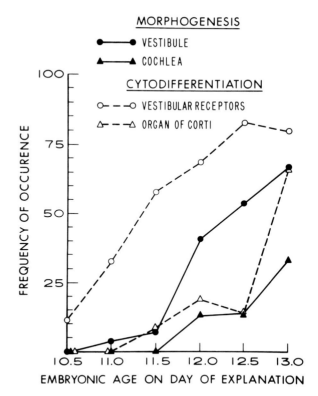

**Fig. 1-16.** A presentation of temporal aspects of the developmental consequences of periotic mesenchyma reduction on murine otic explant morphogenesis and cytodifferentiation into vestibular and auditory receptors.

**Fig. 1-15.** Otocyst–mesenchyma tissue interaction. A series of micrographs of a living pair of 11-day-old mouse otic explants with normal *(M)* and reduced *(m)* volume of periotic mesenchyma: **(A)** Day of explantation: the morphology of both explants is equivalent, each possessing both pars superior *(PS)* and pars inferior *(PI)* segments. **(B)** 3 days in vitro: the normal mesenchyma explant has developed both vestibular (semicircular ducts, *SCD*) and auditory (cochlear duct, *CD*) structures; the reduced mesenchyma explant has only expanded its cystic form *(CY)*. **(C)** 9 days in vitro: a membranous labyrinth complete with an otic capsule has developed from the *M* otic explant; in contrast, the *m* otic explant formed a flattened epithelial cyst.

The otocyst has been shown to be an essential factor in the formation of the cartilaginous otic capsule. Ablation of the otocyst results in the absence of an otic capsule in amphibian[42] and in avian embryos.[43] Organ culture studies[44,45] of mammalian otic capsule formation have demonstrated the importance of the otocyst in capsule formation and the role that it plays, both by inducing periotic mesenchyme to initiate chondrogenesis and in controlling its morphogenesis during capsule formation (Fig. 1-18).

In amphibian embryos there is strong experimental evidence[46,47] that the neurons of the vestibulocochlear ganglion are derived from the otic placode. Analysis of the vestibulocochlear ganglion complexes of mice with neural crest defects led Deol[47] to suggest that neural crest may make a strong contribution to formation of the vestibulocochlear ganglion in mammals. Recent evidence[48]

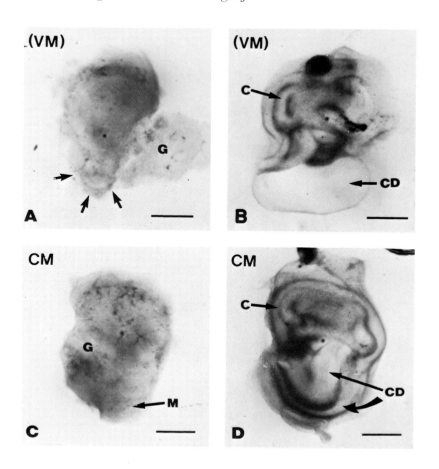

**Fig. 1-17.** The effect of a localized periotic mesenchyma deficiency in cochlear morphogenesis in 12-day-old mouse otic explants. **(A)** Day of explantation: an otic explant with ventral mesenchyma *(VM)* removed (arrows). **(B)** *VM* explant at 8 days in vitro: the vestibular labyrinth *(C)* has developed normally, but the cochlear duct *(CD)* is cystic and has not coiled. **(C)** Day of explantation. control otic explant *(CM)*: a normal amount of ventral mesenchyma *(M)* invests the tip of the cochlear duct anlage. **(D)** *CM* explant at 8 days in vitro: normal otic morphogenesis of both vestibular *(C)* and auditory *(CD)* portions of the inner ear. G, vestibulocochlear ganglion.

from quail-to-chick embryo transplants unequivocably demonstrates that in birds the vestibulocochlear ganglion complex is primarily of placodal origin and that the neural crest cells form all of the satellite and Schwann sheath cells of this ganglion (Fig. 1-19). Analysis of chimeric avian labyrinths that were not wholly derived from the placodal transplants[49] show that all of the neurons that form the vestibulocochlear ganglion have their origin in an area of the otic placode that will later form the medial wall of the utriculus (Fig. 1-20). The neurogenic foci that produces both vestibular and auditory neurons are either a common site or so close together that they appear to be either contiguous or overlapping. This means that most neurons of the vestibulocochlear ganglion have their origin in a portion of the membranous labyrinth different from that which forms most of their peripheral targets for innervation. This is an important concept

to consider when formulating a mechanism by which the vestibulocochlear ganglion sends dendrites back to their appropriate receptors within the developing inner ear. These data preclude from consideration the possibility that migrating presumptive neurons establish tracts that could later act as substrate guidance cues for the nerve growth cones of vestibulocochlear ganglion neurites as they grow to their appropriate target areas.

Interactions between nerves and other cells can either initiate or control molecular modifications in the other cells and/or the neurons. Nerves can have a trophic influence on organs that they innervate (i.e., taste buds).[50,51] Vestibulocochlear ganglion innervation of inner ear sensory structures was proposed to exert a trophic influence on their development, because the observed pattern of ingrowth to the cochlear duct preceded the pattern of cytodifferentiation of the organ of Corti.[52,53]

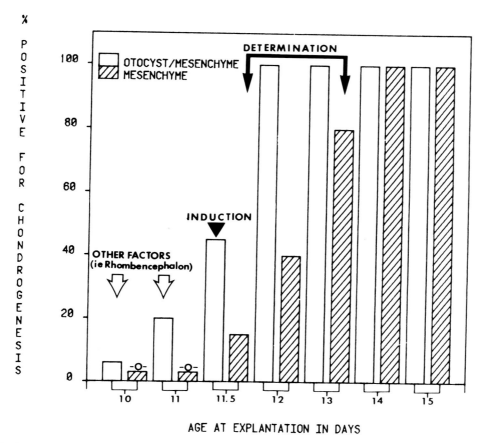

Fig. 1-18. A summary of murine otocyst-mesenchyma versus isolated periotic mesenchyma explant results showing the in vitro chondrogenic potential of periotic mesenchyme compared to periotic mesenchyma explants, that contain the otocyst (inductor tissue). The role of the otocyst in otic capsule formation is indicated on this histogram.

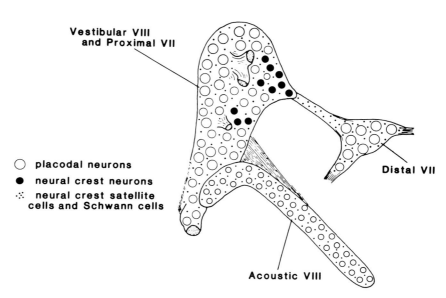

Fig. 1-19. Reconstruction of a right 7th and 8th (vestibulocochlear) cranial nerve ganglionic complex of a 12-day-old chick embryo indicating the origins of neurons, satellite cells, and Schwann sheath cells. These results are based on orthotopic transplantation of neural crest cells from quail embryos to chick embryo hosts.

19

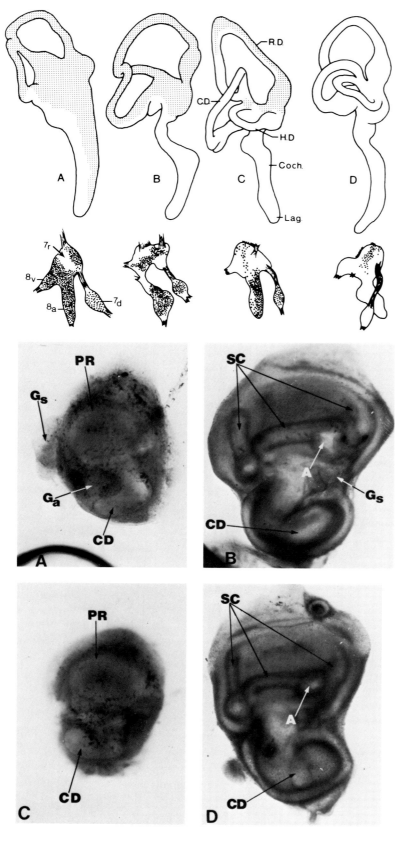

**Fig. 1-20. (A to D)** The patterns of labeling in reconstructed membranous labyrinths following grafting of small pieces of quail dorsolateral surface ectoderm **(A to C)** or neural crest tissue **(D)** at the midrhombencephalon level. Stippling indicates quail epithelium. Below are reconstructions of ganglia associated with the 7th and 8th cranial nerves in each of these four hosts. Dots indicate quail neurons. These reconstructions are used to map the origins both of each part of the membranous labyrinth and of the vestibular and acoustic neurons. *RD, HD,* and *CD* indicate rostral, horizontal, and caudal semicircular ducts; *Coch* and *Lag* are the cochlear duct and lagena, *7r* and *7d* are the proximal (root) and distal (geniculate) ganglia, respectively; *8a* and *8v* are the acoustic and vestibular ganglia, respectively.

**Fig. 1-21.** Vestibulocochlear ganglion, sensory receptor interaction: 13-day-old mouse inner ear explants. **(A, C)** Day of explantation; **(B, D)** after 8 days in vitro. The otic explant in **(A)** and **(B)** has an intact vestibulocochlear ganglion complex *(G_s,* vestibular part; *G_a,* cochlear part). The explant in **(C)** and **(D)** has had its vestibulocochlear ganglion excised prior to explantation. Removal of this ganglion has not adversely affected the morphogenesis of these inner ear explants. Areas that are fated to form vestibular structures *(PR)* and auditory structures *(CD)* are indicated in the otic explants at explantation in **(A)** and **(C)**. Developed semicircular canals *(SC),* their ampullae *(A),* and the coiled cochlea *(CD)* that formed during the 8 days of in vitro development are seen in **(B)** and **(D)**. *CD,* cochlear duct; *A,* Ampulla; *PR,* primary ridge; *SC,* semicircular canal.

This, coupled with the observation[54] that the oldest presumptive sensory cells of the organ of Corti were the last to undergo cytodifferentiation, gave credence to the proposal that a causal relationship existed between ingrowth of vestibulocochlear ganglion dendrites and cytodifferentiation of inner ear sensory receptors. This theory was a *fait accompli*, until it was tested experimentally using organotypic cultures of murine otocysts that had their vestibulocochlear ganglion complexes extirpated prior to explantation to organ culture.[55] The results of histologic quantification of sensory receptor development within these aganglionic otocysts were compared to otocysts cultured with intact vestibulocochlear ganglia (Fig. 1-21). These results (Figs. 1-22 and 1-23) clearly demonstrate that inner ear sensory receptors do not depend on nerve fiber ingrowth from the vestibulocochlear ganglion.

These findings have been confirmed in other systems,[56-60] most notably a recent study of aganglionic chick otocysts[60] transplanted to a chorioalantoic membrane site. These developing aganglionic chick otocysts have shown that even the pattern of stereocilia development of inner ear receptors remains unchanged in the absence of vestibulocochlear nerve fibers. The pattern of hair cell differentiation of otic sensory receptors is therefore considered to be intrinsic to the presumptive sensory cells and does not require the extrinsic stimulus of interaction with vestibulocochlear ganglion neuronal elements to cause its expression. In co-cultures of two otic explants that share a single vestibulocochlear ganglion (Fig. 1-24), Van De Water and Ruben[61] have shown that outgrowth of neurites from this single ganglion are received by areas of differentiating otic sensory structures in both otocysts (Fig. 1-25). This study,[61] combined with recent observation in elasmosbranch inner ears by Corwin,[62] support the theory proposed by Van De Water and Ruben[63] that differentiating otic sensory epithelium produce attractant fields, which guide the ingrowth of vestibulocochlear ganglion dendrites to their appropriate target sites within the developing inner ear.

Condensations of experimental results that define many of the embryologic mechanisms of vertebrate inner ear development have been presented in this chapter. These data are used to provide a comprehensive understanding of the interactions that occur between different components of the inner ear and how these tissue interactions result in orderly development of the vertebrate inner ear.

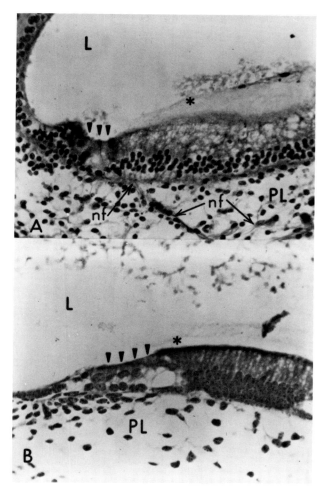

**Fig. 1-22.** Vestibulocochlear ganglion, sensory receptor interaction: Two 13-day-old mouse inner ear explants, after 8 days in vitro. **(A)** A with-vestibulocochlear ganglion explant showing Corti's organ with nerve fibers that have their origin from this ganglion complex. **(B)** A without-vestibulocochlear ganglion explant showing Corti's organ that has developed without any neural elements. The development of these sensory structures shows no major differences except for the lack of nerve fibers and ganglion cells in the aganglionic inner ears. *L,* lumen of the endolymphatic spaces; *nf,* nerve fiber; *PL,* perilymphatic spaces; arrowheads, organ of Corti; *,* tectorial membrane.

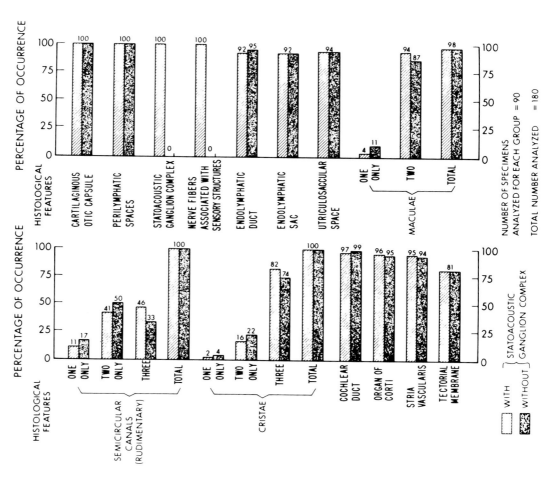

**Fig. 1-23.** The combined results of histologic quantification of mouse inner ear development within 11-, 12-, and 13-day-old with- and without-vestibulocochlear ganglion complex otic explants. These results show that vestibulocochlear ganglion removal has no major effect morphogenesis or cytodifferentiation of inner ear sensory receptors.

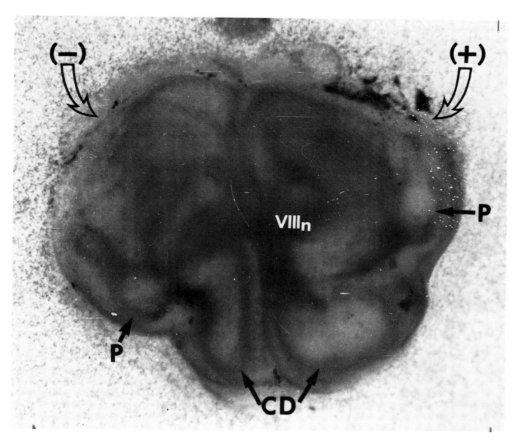

**Fig. 1-24.** Sensory receptor, vestibulocochlear ganglion interaction. Co-culture of two $12\frac{1}{2}$-day-old mouse otic explants that share a single vestibulocochlear ganglion complex *(VIIIn),* after 8 days in vitro. Right *(+)* otocyst was explanted with an intact ganglion complex; left *(−)* otocyst was explanted without its vestibulocochlear ganglion. Nerve fibers are present in the sensory structures of both otic explants. The cochlear ducts *(CD)* of the co-cultured otic explants and the location of a posterior semicircular canal ampulla *(P)* of the "with" ganglion otocyst are indicated. (Van De Water TR, Ruben RJ: Neurotrophic interactions during in vitro development of the inner ear. Ann Otol Rhinol Laryngol 93:558, 1984. With permission.)

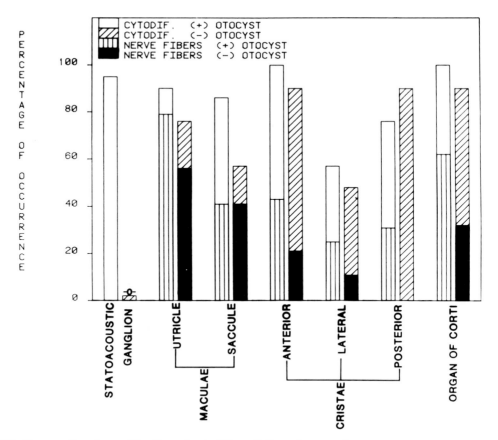

**Fig. 1-25.** The results of quantification of cytodifferentiation of mouse inner ear sensory receptors and the presence of nerve fibers in co-cultured 12½-day-old (+) and (−) vestibucochlear ganglion inner ear explants. The results clearly show that neurites are attracted to the areas of differentiating sensory receptors in the without-ganglion otic explants. (Van De Water TR, Ruben RJ: A possible embryonic mechanism for the establishment of innervation of inner ear sensory structures. Acta Otolaryngol (Stockh) 95:470, 1983. With permission.)

For clarity, a flow chart of these interactions is presented in Figure 1-26. Surface ectoderm of the cephalic area interacts in sequence with first chorda mesoderm and then rhombencephalic tissue to produce the first detectable form of the inner ear, the otic placode.[33,34] It is at this placodal stage of labyrinthine development that adjacent rhombencephalic tissue first comes into close apposition to the otic anlage.[35,38] The inductive interaction between the rhombencephalon and otic anlage has a major influence on otic morphogenesis until the late otocyst stage of development.[38] The rhombencephalon has also been suggested to play a role in the early events of periotic otic mesenchyme de-

termination.[39] The otocyst then plays a direct role in the determination of the chondrogenic phenotype of periotic mesenchyme and organization of its otic capsule,[44,45] which later acts as the template for the bony labyrinth. At this same period when the otocyst is influencing the mesenchyme, the mesenchyme in turn exerts a strong inductive influence on morphogenesis and cytodifferentiation of the membranous (otocyst) labyrinth.[39,41] This otocyst–mesenchyme reciprocal interaction is an excellent demonstration of the reciprocal nature of many of the inductive tissue interactions that control development of the inner ear. During formation of the vestibulocochlear ganglion, the otic epi-

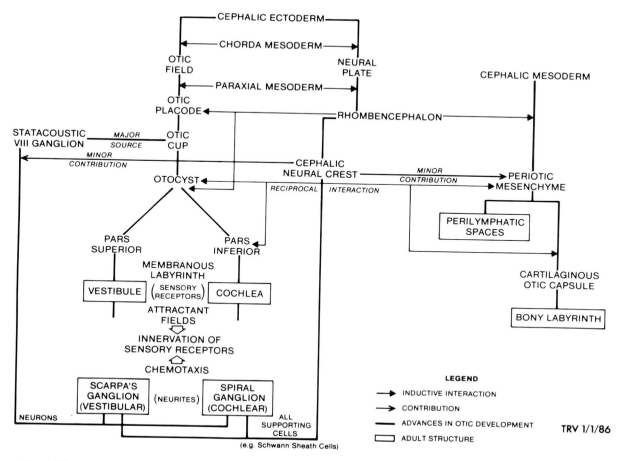

**Fig. 1-26.** A flow chart depicting the development interactions that influence and control organogenesis of a normal inner ear during its formation.

thelium at the otic cup stage produces most of its own neurons, which compose both the vestibular and cochlear portions of this ganglion,[48] while the neural crest contributes only a few neurons to Scarpa's (vestibular) ganglion and none to the spiral (cochlear) ganglion, but plays a major role in providing virtually all of the supporting cells for both of these ganglia that compose the vestibulocochlear ganglion complex.[48] The neurons of both the vestibular and cochlear portions of the vestibulocochlear ganglion appear to have a common site of origin within the otic epithelium,[49] even though the dendrites of these neurons will eventually in-

nervate quite different sites within the developing inner ear. Original postulations that ingrowth of vestibulocochlear ganglion dendrites to peripheral target epithelium might be a triggering event for the onset of cytodifferentiation of this otic sensory epithelium[52-54] has not stood up to experimental evaluation.[56-60] In contrast, further experimentation[61-63] has suggested that attractant fields produced by differentiating otic sensory epithelium and chemotaxis of vestibulocochlear ganglion neurons play important roles in the innervation of inner ear sensory receptors.

## REFERENCES

1. Hammar JA: Studien uber die Entwicklung des Vorderdarms und einiger angrenzenden Organe. I. Abtheilung: Allgemeine Morphologie der Schlundspalten beim Menschen. Entwicklung des Mittelohrraumes und des ausseren Gehorganges. Arch Mikr Anat 59:471, 1902
2. Altmann F: Normal development of the ear and its mechanisms. Arch Otolaryngol 52:725, 1950
3. Arey LB: Developmental Anatomy. 6th Ed. WB Saunders, Philadelphia, 1954
4. Van De Water TR, Maderson PFA, Jaskoll TJ: The morphogenesis of the middle and external ear. p. 147. In Gorlin RJ (ed): Morphogenesis and Malformation of the Ear. March of Dimes: Original Article Series. Vol. 16. Alan R Liss, New York, 1980
5. His W: Die Formentwickelung des ausseren Ohres. Anatomie menschlichern Embroyonen, 3:211, 1885
6. Wood-Jones F, Wen IC: The development of the external ear. J Anat 68:525, 1934
7. Streeter GL: Development of the auricle in the human embryo. Contrib Embryol Carnegie Inst 14:111, 1922
8. Presley R: Lizards, mammals and the primitive tetrapod tympanic membrane. Symp Zool Soc London 52:127, 1984
9. Boas JEV: Ohrknorpel und Ausseres Ohr der Saugetiere. Kopenhagen, 1912
10. Crary DD: Development of the external ear of the Dachs rabbit. Anat Rec 150:441, 1964
11. Helff OM: Studies on amphibian metamorphosis XVII influence of non-living annular tympanic cartilage on tympanic membrane formation. J Exp Biol 17:45, 1940
12. Jaskoll T, Maderson P: A histological study of the development of the middle ear and tympanum. Anat Rec 190:177, 1978
13. Jaskoll T: Morphogenesis and teratogenesis of the middle ear in animals. p. 9. In Levin LS, Knight CH (eds): Genetic and Enviromental Hearing Loss: Syndromic and Nonsyndromic. March of Dimes: Original Article Series. Vol. 16. Alan R Liss, New York, 1980
14. Frazer JE: The development of the human nasopharynx. Br Med J 1:1148, 1910
15. Frazer JE: The second visceral arch and groove in the tubotympanic region. J Anat 48:391, 1914
16. Frazer JE: The early formations of the middle ear and Eustachian tube: a criticism. J Anat 57:18, 1922
17. Kanagasuntheram R: A note on the development of the tubotympanic recess in the human embryo. J Anat 101:731, 1967
18. Van De Water TR, Ruben RJ: Organogenesis of the ear. p. 173. In Hinchcliffe R, Harrison D (eds): Scientific Foundation of Otolaryngology. Heinemann, London, 1976
19. Jaskoll T: The microscopic anatomy of dynamics of avian and mammalian middle ear development. Unpublished doctoral thesis, City University of New York, 1978
20. Goodrich ES: Studies on the Structure and Development of Vertebrates. Vol. 1. Dover Publishing, New York, 1958
21. Meckel JF: Handbuch der Menschlichen Anatomie. Vol. 4. Besondere Anatomie. Halle and Berlin, 1820
22. Reichert CB: Ueber die visceralbogen der Wirbelthiere im Allgemeinen und deren Metamorphosen bei den Vogeln und Saugethieren. Arch Anat Physiol Wiss Med 120, 1837
23. Strickland EM, Hanson JR, Anson BJ: Branchial sources of auditory ossicles in man. Arch Otolaryngol 76:100, 1962
24. Anson BJ, Bast TH: Development of the stapes of the human ear: illustrated in atlas series. Q Bull North Univ Med School 33:44, 1959
25. Jenkinson JW: Development of ear bones in the mouse. J Anat Physiol 45:22, 1911
26. Fuchs H: Bemerkungen uber die Herkunft und Entwickelung der Gehorknochelchen bei Kaninchen-Embryonen. Arch Anat Entwickelungsgesch, suppl., Anat, 1905
27. Reagan FP: The role of the auditory sensory epithelium in the formation of the stapedial plate. J Exp Zool 23:85, 1917
28. Hanson JR, Anson BJ, Stickland EM: Branchial sources of the auditory ossicles in man. Arch Otolaryngol 76:200, 1962
29. Hough JVD: Congenital malformations of the middle ear. Arch Otolaryngol 78:335, 1963
30. Alberti PWRM: Epithelial migration of the tympanic membrane. J Laryngolotol 78:808, 1964
31. Noden DW: The control of avian cephalic neural crest cytodifferentiation, I. Skeletal and connective tissues. Dev Biol 67:296, 1978
32. Maderson PFA, Noden D, Banks S: Developmental data in evolutionary problems: neural crest contributions to tetrapod ossicles. Anat Rec 202:117A, 1982
33. Yntema CL: An analysis of induction of the ear from foreign ectoderm in the salamander embryo. J Exp Zool 113:211, 1950
34. Jacobson AG: Inductive processes in embryonic development. Science 152:25, 1966

35. Model PG, Jarrett LS, Bonazzoli R: Cellular contacts between hindbrain and prospective ear during inductive interaction in the axolotl embryo. J Embryol Exp Morphol 66:27, 1981

36. Harrison RG: Relations of symmetry in the developing ear of *Amblystoma punctatum*. Proc Natl Acad Sci USA 22:238, 1936

37. Detwiler SR, Van Dyke RH: The role of the medulla in the differentiation of the otic vesicle. J Exp Zool 113:197, 1950

38. Van De Water TR, Conley E: Neural inductive message to the developing mammalian inner: contact mediated versus extracellular matrix interaction. Anat Rec 202:195A, 1982

39. Van De Water TR: Epithelial-mesenchymal tissue interactions effect upon development of the inner ear. Anat Rec 199:262, 1981

40. Orr MF, Hafft LP: The influence of mesenchyme on the development of the embryonic otocyst: an electron microscopic study. J Cell Biol 87:27a, 1980

41. Li CW, McPhee J: Influences on the coiling of the cochlea. Ann Otol Rhinol Laryngol 88:280, 1979

42. Lewis WH: On the origin and differentiation of the otic vesicle in amphibian embryos. Anat Rec 1:142, 1906

43. Kaan HW: The relationship of the developing auditory vesicle to the formation of the cartilage capsule in *Amblystoma punctatum*. J Exp Zool 55:263, 1950

44. McPhee J, Van De Water TR: A comparison of morphological stages and sulfated glycosaminoglycan production during otic capsule formation: in vivo and in vitro. Anat Rec 213:566, 1985

45. McPhee J, Van De Water TR: Epithelial-mesenchymal tissue interactions guiding otic capsule formation: the role of the otocyst. J Embryol Exp Morphol 97:1, 1986

46. Yntema CL: An experimental study of the origin of the cells which constitute the VIIth and VIIIth cranial ganglia and nerves in the embryo of *Amblystoma punctatum* J Exp Zool 75:75, 1937

47. Deol MS: The neural crest and the acoustic ganglion. J Embryol Exp Morphol 17:533, 1967

48. D'Amico-Martel A, Noden DW: Contributions of placodal and neural crest cells to avian cranial peripheral ganglia. Am J Anat 166:445, 1983

49. Noden DM: The use of chimeras in analyses of craniofacial development. p. 241. In LeDouarin N, McLaren R (eds): Chimeras in Development. Academic Press, Orlando, FL, 1984

50. Ranvier L: Traite Technique d'Histologie. F. Savy, Paris, 1875

51. Guth L: "Trophic" effects of vertebrate neurons. Neurosci Res Program Bull 7:1, 1969

52. Weibel ER: Zur Kenntnis der Differenzierungsvorgange in epithelia des Ductus Cochlearis. Acta Anat (Basel) 29:53, 1957

53. Sher A: The embryonic and postnatal development of the inner ear of the mouse. Acta Otolaryngol [Suppl] (Stockh) 285:1–77, 1971

54. Ruben RJ: Development of the inner ear of the mouse: a radiographic study of terminal mitoses. Acta Otolaryngol [Suppl] (Stockh) 220:1–44, 1967

55. Van De Water TR: Effects of removal of the statoacoustic ganglion complex upon the growing otocyst. Ann Otol Rhinol Laryngol [Suppl] 85: suppl. 33, 1–32, 1976

56. Jorgensen JM, Flock A: Non-innervated sense organs of the lateral line: development in the regenerating tail of the salamander *Ambystoma mexicanum*. J Neurocytol 5:33, 1976

57. Hirokawa N: Disappearance of afferent and efferent nerve terminals in the inner ear of the chick embryo after chronic treatment with β-Bungaratoxin. J Cell Biol 73:27, 1977

58. Van De Water TR et al: Development of the sensory receptor cells in the utricular macula. ORL J Otorhinolaryngol Relat Spec 86:297, 1978

59. Sans A, Chat M: Analysis of temporal and spatial patterns of rat vestibular hair cell differentiation by triated thymidine radioautography. J Comp Neurol 206:1, 1982

60. Corwin JT: Regeneration and self-repair in hair cell epithelia: experimental evaluation of capacities and limitations. p 291. In Ruben RJ, Van DeWater TR, Rafel EW (eds). Biology of Change in Otolaryngology. Elsevier Science Publishers B.V., Amsterdam, 1986.

61. Van De Water TR, Ruben RJ: Neurotrophic interactions during in vitro development of the inner ear. Ann Otol Rhinol Laryngol 93:558, 1984

62. Corwin JT: Auditory neurons expand their terminal arbors throughout life and orient toward the site of postembryonic hair cell production in the macula neglecta in elasmobranchs. J Comp Neurol 239:445, 1985

63. Van De Water TR, Ruben RJ: A possible embryonic mechanism for the establishment of innervation of inner ear sensory structures. Acta Otolaryngol (Stockh) 95:470, 1983

# Histology of the Ear and Temporal Bone

# 2

## Leslie Michaels

## TECHNICAL METHODS

### Removal at Autopsy

It is possible to use surgical specimens to examine the histology of some of the structures of the ear and temporal bone. The pinna and external auditory canal are removed mainly for the treatment of malignant neoplasms, the mastoid bone because of air cells, the malleus and incus are for drainage of chronic suppurative otitis media, and the stapes for otosclerosis. Parts of these specimens may be unaffected by the disease and may be suitable for histologic study of normal structures, but it is likely that most parts of the specimen will not be quite normal. Examination of normal cadaveric temporal bone specimens is, therefore, preferable for obtaining normal data. Autopsy and removal of the temporal bone should be carried as soon after death as possible. Useful information may, however, be obtained even after 20 hours and longer, particularly for studies of the bone or connective tissue structures. Autolysis is prevented to some degree if 20 percent formalin is injected into the middle ear through the tympanic membrane soon after death, although the injection will, of course, damage the tympanic membrane and some middle ear structures. The cadaver should be refrigerated as soon as possible after death.

### Standard Method

In order adequately to study the deeper part of the ear canal, the middle and the inner ear and the whole temporal bone should be removed as one block. The usual method of isolating the temporal bone at postmortem involves prior removal of the skull cap and brain.[1] During removal the dura should be treated carefully and left attached to the temporal bone in order not to damage the endolymphatic sac. The 7th and 8th cranial nerves should be cut at the orifice of the internal auditory canal, thus retaining portions of the nerve trunks within the temporal bone specimen. A vibrating electric saw is satisfactory for removing the petrous temporal bone. A triangular blade is preferable to the more commonly employed circular one. One horizontal and three vertical cuts are made with the saw (Figs 2-1 and 2-2), as follows;

1. The first cut is medial to the internal auditory meatus and extends vertically through the petrous temporal bone at right angles to the superior and posteromedial surfaces to a depth of approximately 2.5 cm.

2. The second cut is made parallel with the first and at least 2.5 to 3.0 cm posterolateral to it at the lateral end of the temporal bone. It also passes vertically to a depth of 2.5 cm. The removal of the whole of the endolymphatic sac requires a more lateral and deeper cut.
3. The third vertical cut is made connecting the forward ends of the two previous cuts, at the anterior extent of the middle cranial fossa
4. A horizontal cut is made underneath the petrous temporal bone at about 2.5 cm below the upper surface and parallel with it, to complete a block of bone measuring at least 2.5 × 2.5 × 2.5 cm. Again, in order to remove the complete endolymphatic sac, this cut has to be placed deeper. The block can be removed by gently "rocking" and cutting the ligamentous structures on its inferior surface. The block so removed will in-

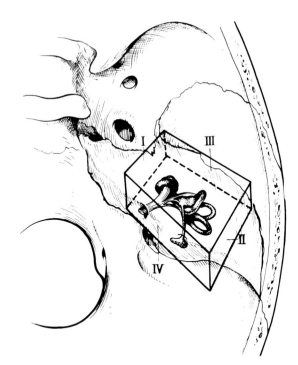

**Fig. 2-2.** Wedge of temporal bone removed for histologic examination. The outlines of the membranous labyrinth are drawn in. Roman numerals refer to the saw cuts required to remove the temporal bone. (Iurato S, Bredberg G, Bock G: Functional Histopathology of the Human Audio-vestibular Organ. Euro-data Hearing Project. Commission of the European Communities, 1982.)

clude a portion of the ear canal, the tympanic membrane, the middle ear, the labyrinthine structures, and the petrous portion of the 7th and 8th cranial nerves. By modifying the second cut, a wider excision may be made to include a portion of the squamous temporal bone and mastoid process as well as more of the external auditory canal. This is particularly advisable in children because of the smaller dimensions of the temporal bone. The further forward and medial the first cut is made, the larger is the portion of the eustachian tube obtained in the specimen.

## Schuknecht's Bone Plug Method

An alternative method is the bone plug method,[2] which necessitates the use of a hollow, cylindrical

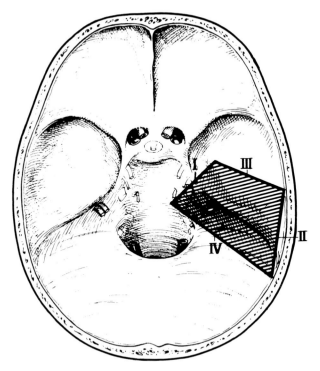

**Fig. 2-1.** Base of skull showing position of four saw cuts required in removal of temporal bone. (Iurato S, Bredberg G, Bock G: Functional Histopathology of the Human Audio-vestibular Organ. Euro-data Hearing Project. Commission of the European Communities, 1982.)

electrical vibrating saw 4.25 cm in diameter. The saw is centered on the arcuate eminence, and by drilling downward, a plug of bone is removed as far as the base of the skull. This contains the membranous labyrinth, but it is relatively easy to miss some of the middle ear and the endolymphatic sac.

After removing the specimen, plaster of paris may be inserted in the space previously occupied by the temporal bone. To assist the subsequent embalming process, it is recommended that the internal carotid arteries are ligated after removal has been completed.

When the specimen is removed, it is placed in fixative in a large screw-top plastic jar. For most purposes the fixative used may be buffered 4 percent formaldehyde solution. In some centers another fixative is preferred (e.g., Heidenhain Susa solution).[2]

## Preparation for Histologic Examination

Until recently the only satisfactory method available for histologic examination of the temporal bone was to decalcify and embed the bone in celloidin, and then subject it to serial sectioning. Removing parts of the temporal bone piecemeal and subjecting them to microscopic study is unsatisfactory because of the dense bony capsule surrounding most structures. An exception is the employment of surface preparations of basilar membrane for phase contrast microscopy. The only technique hitherto available for the exposure of inner ear structure required skilled drilling procedures.[3] A method has, however, recently been introduced whereby slices of the undecalcified bone are first examined. Representative parts are then subjected to light microscopy including histologic processing or (in suitably perfused material) examination of surface preparations.

### Method of Serial Sectioning after Celloidin Embedding

**Technique.** Fixation is required for approximately 4 weeks. The bone should be roughly sawn to size before fixation. The whole temporal bone is placed in 10 percent formic acid for a period of between 4 and 8 weeks, taking radiographs every week to check the progress of decalcification. After decalcification the final trimming of the specimen can be performed using a strong-bladed knife. This trimming process is very importat to allow sufficient diffusion of impregnating substances during the subsequent processing of the bone. The trimmed block should be not more than 4.0 cm long × 2.5 cm wide × 2.5 cm high. Dehydration of the whole specimen is then carried out, placing it for 1 day in ascending grades of alcohol and alcohol-ether as follows: 30, 50, 95, 100, 100 percent, equal parts alcohol and ether, equal parts of alcohol and ether, respectively.

Impregnation follows in celloidin dissolved in a mixture of equal parts of alcohol and ether. In my laboratory low viscosity nitrocellulose (LVN) is used.

For microtomy a long, heavy, stellite-tipped knife (Deloro Stellite, a subsidiary of British Oxygen Company Brentford, Middlesex, England), is preferable. This knife should be sharpened to a final cutting edge bevel of about 28 degrees. Sections are cut at 20 $\mu$m, and between 50 and 100 sections can be obtained from one bone. It is necessary to stain only every 10th section, keeping the intermediate sections interleaved in vellum tissue, which may be stored indefinitely with uncut blocks in 70 percent alcohol.

Sections may be stained with hematoxylin and eosin (preferably using Ehrlich's hematoxylin) and by a wide variety of other routine histologic methods.

### Disadvantages

Gross examination is an important requisite of the histologic analysis of all other organs. By sacrificing the whole temporal bone in serial sectioning of each specimen, histologic study of the ear has lacked an important dimension that may have impeded its development.

Before histologic examination, the temporal bone must be decalcified so that sectioning is not disturbed by the presence of bony masses. A weak solution of an acid such as formic, is used, as previously described, and the process takes at least 6 weeks. Marked alterations in the histologic appearances of some of the tissues occur as a result of this prolonged exposure. Many of the microscopic alterations ascribed to postmortem autolysis in serially sectioned temporal bones are in fact the result of damage by acid.

An adjunct of the gross preliminary examination of all other organs is the ability to carry out not only routine histologic sections but also special microscopic studies, including histochemistry and electron microscopy and also certain biochemical investigations on selected areas. These special studies are not possible when the whole temporal bone has been sacrificed to serial sections in celloidin.

Processing the whole temporal bone is extremely slow, since not only decalcification but also dehydration and embedding each require a long exposure. It takes at least 9 months from the autopsy for the stained serial sections to be made available. This discourages a sustained interest in research and teaching.

Serial sectioning of the embedded whole temporal bone is tedious and technically difficult. It demands a high degree of skill on the part of the histologic technician in cutting sections of constant high quality through the whole of this structure, which is both tough and at the same time contains fragile tissues.

Large numbers of serial sections are produced from a single temporal bone. Sometimes the serial examination of a specific portion of the temporal bone is useful, but more often most of the sections are not required. Storage of all of these is a serious problem; inexorable accumulation of containers filled with sections encroach on the available space of the laboratory.

### Transverse Slicing Method

A new method has been devised to obviate these disadvantages.[4] The temporal bone is removed at postmortem as previously described. Fixation occurs for a minimum of 4 days. The bone is then trimmed to about 2.5 × 2.5 × 2.5 cm. It is then mounted with molten dental wax on a glass plate measuring 6 × 2.5 cm with a thickness of approximately 0.5 cm. The surface to be presented for slicing is arranged perpendicular to the glass plate.

The glass plate, with the surface of the adherent temporal bone that is to be cut to the front, is now mounted on the metal plinth with dental wax, and this is fixed to the inner end of the lever of the slicing machine (Microslice 2 Precision Annular Saw, Cambridge Instruments, Ltd., Cambridge, England) (Fig. 2-3). This is a cutting machine with a circular steel blade, which is bolted to the machine at 16 points so that no lateral vibration takes place. Cutting proceeds around a circular inner opening where the blade is tipped with diamond dust. The cutting edge is lubricated by a continuous jet of cold water. The speed of the rotatory motor may be adjusted from low speeds up to 1,200 rpm by the left-hand knob on the front of the machine. The right-hand knob advances the lever with the specimen by the required length before each slice is made so that the thickness of the specimen can be regulated. Slices of 1, 2, or 3 mm thickness may be prepared. Slicing is carried out by gently lowering the weighted left-hand, counterpoised end of the lever so that the specimen rotates up and is applied against the cutting edge. With this system the specimen backs away from the blade when a particularly hard area is encountered, thereby avoiding excessive mechanical and thermal stresses. The slices adhere together and are removed from the machine after the whole temporal bone has been treated. A radiograph is made of each slice (4380 5N X-ray, Faxitron system, Hewlett Packard).

After careful examination of the slices with a hand lens and dissecting microscope, and after radiographic examination has been completed, selected areas of the whole or of a single slice may be subjected to celloidin or paraffin embedding for light microscopy, special histologic or histochemical study, or even electron microscopy (in the case of structures with a sufficient degree of preservation). In specimens that have been perfused through the perilymph, portions of basilar membrane or other parts of membranous labyrinth may be removed and examined by phase contrast or electron microscopy (see following discussion).

### Appearance of Microsliced Temporal Bone

Microslicing of the temporal bone results in a series of specimens in which all the main structures can be examined, and any gross pathologic changes may be detected and delineated (Figs. 2-4 to 2-6).

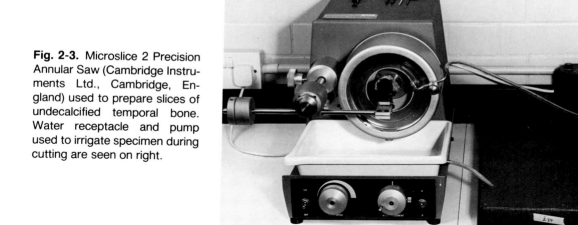

**Fig. 2-3.** Microslice 2 Precision Annular Saw (Cambridge Instruments Ltd., Cambridge, England) used to prepare slices of undecalcified temporal bone. Water receptacle and pump used to irrigate specimen during cutting are seen on right.

## Surface Preparation Method of Histologic Examination

Surface preparation method of histologic examination has been applied mainly to the analysis of the hair cells of the organ of Corti. Electron microscopy, particularly by the scanning method, is frequently used also to study specimens similarly obtained. The surface specimen technique is applicable only to temporal bones in which the perilymphatic space has been perfused by fixative within 10 hours after death, since the autolysis of the hair cells beyond that period of time renders them less suitable for this type of examination.

The technique of perilymphatic perfusion is described by Iurato et al.,[5] and the following details are summarized from that publication. The procedure is carried out directly on the cadaver as soon as possible after death. Using an ear speculum, the upper posterior part of the tympanic membrane is folded forward. With a curette any bony overhang is removed to expose the oval and round windows. The incudostapedial joint is divided, and the stapes is luxated from the oval window. It can be left in the middle ear, hanging from the stapedial muscle tendon, or removed for further study. The round window membrane is perforated with a small hook directed forward (in the direction of the eustachian tube).

A glass pipette of tip diameter 0.5 to 1.0 mm, or a syringe with an unsharpened needle of the same diameter is filled by aspiration with 1 to 2 ml of fixative solution at room temperature. The tip is directed toward the oval window, and the fixative is injected. This will produce a slight increase in pressure in the vestibule, and some fixative will enter the scala vestibuli and perfuse the cochlea. In this way the perilymphatic spaces are perfused for 15 minutes or at least 10 times. The fixative preferred for perilymphatic perfusion is "reduced Karnovsky" solution.[6]

## Technique of Sampling Membranous Labyrinth for the Surface Preparation Method

The method of drilling away the bony labyrinth to sample the membranous labyrinth is described by Johnsson and Hawkins.[3] The method is difficult, requiring special training and a detailed knowledge of temporal bone anatomy. Because of its difficulty, damage to membranous labyrinth is likely until the operator has acquired a high degree of skill in the procedure. Even then the drilling

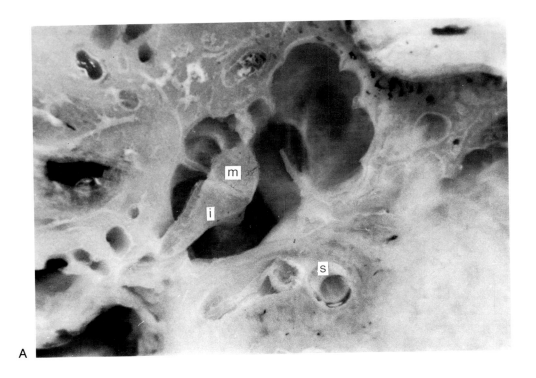

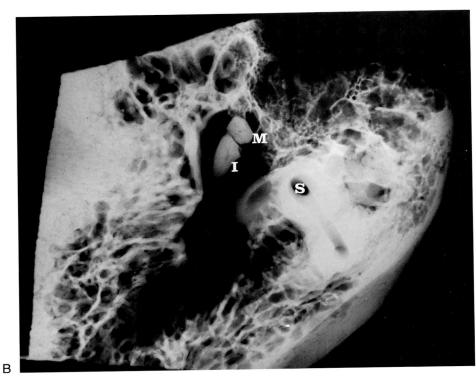

**Fig. 2-4. (A)** Horizontal microslice of temporal bone in attic region. *i*, short process of incus; *m*, malleus; *s*, superior semicircular canal. **(B)** Radiograph of same slice. *I*, incus; *M*, malleus; *S*, superior semicircular canal.

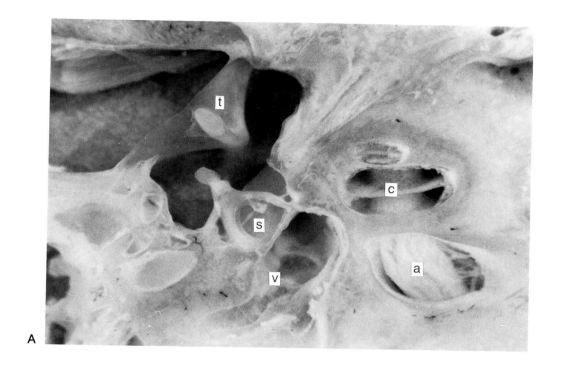

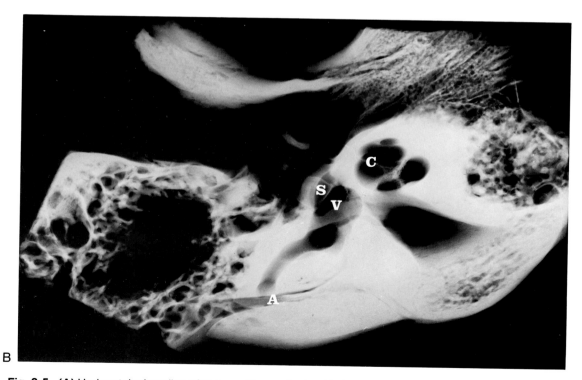

**Fig. 2-5. (A)** Horizontal microslice of temporal bone at a level below that of Fig. 2-4. *t*, tympanic membrane; *s*, stapes. Note attachment of stapedius tendon to posterior crus. *a*, acoustic nerve; *c*, basal coil of cochlea; *v*, vestibule. **(B)** Radiograph of same microslice. *A*, vestibular aqueduct; *C*, cochlea; *S*, stapes; *V*, vestibule.

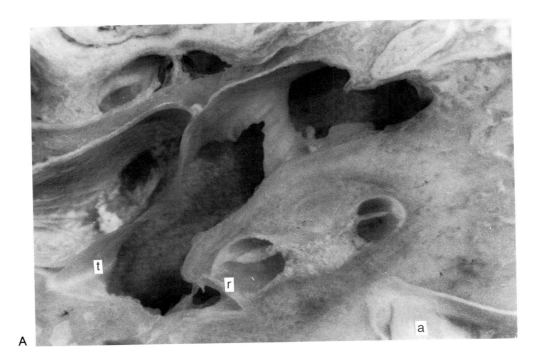

A

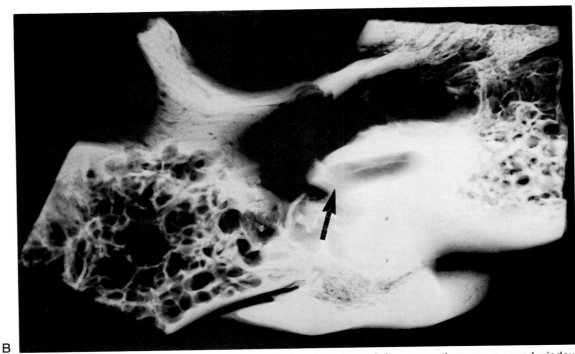

B

**Fig. 2-6. (A)** Microslice of temporal bone at a level below that of Fig. 2-6. *a*, acoustic nerve; *r*, round window membrane; *t*, tympanic membrane. **(B)** Radiograph of same slice. Arrow points to region of round window membrane.

method requires many hours of work. A further disadvantage is that in order to expose the membranous labyrinth by this method it is necessary to destroy other parts of the middle and inner ear. Thus, these parts are lost to routine microscopic study.

By contrast, the microsliced temporal bone prepared by the method previously described may be used to sample the membranous labyrinth without drilling and with only very slight damage to inner ear structures. Using this method the whole inner ear may be exposed within minutes. Moreover, there is no destruction of the rest of the ear. Thus, after portions of the inner ear have been selected and removed for the surface specimen technique, the rest of the temporal bone may undergo routine histologic study.

## PINNA: ELASTIC CARTILAGE AND PERICHONDRIUM

The pinna is composed of elastic cartilage with a covering of skin that follows all of the folds of the cartilage. The skin of the pinna contains three skin appendages: hair with sebaceous glands, eccrine sweat glands, and a few apocrine (ceruminous) glands. There is hardly any subcutaneous connective tissue in the pinna except in the ear lobe. Here the elastic cartilage is absent, and a pad of adipose tissue is present instead between the two layers of skin.

The elastic cartilage of the pinna, which is continuous with that of external auditory canal, is composed of chondrocytes and matrix that contains densely interwoven elastic fibers. The perichondrium, although important because it is the region from which the avascular cartilage is nourished by diffusion from a network of blood vessels, has a rather inconspicuous histologic appearance. In this area the basal layers of elastic cartilage cells merge with connective tissue. Small arteries and arterioles course in a plane parallel to the cartilage surface.

## EXTERNAL AUDITORY CANAL

The epidermis of the external auditory canal is continuous with that of the pinna, and, like the pinna epidermis, shows pronounced rete ridges in all areas except for the bony portion, where it is flat.

The skin over the cartilaginous portion shows two types of appendage: hair with sebaceous glands and apocrine (ceruminous) glands. Eccrine glands are absent. The skin of the bony portion shows only a few small hairs and sebaceous glands on the superior wall.

There are no special features of the epidermis, rete ridges, dermis, dermal papillae, hair follicles, and sebaceous glands of the external auditory canal, as compared with skin elsewhere in the body.

The ceruminous glands closely resemble apocrine glands found in the axilla and pubic skin. They are found in large numbers in the deeper portion of the dermis at a level below that of the sebaceous glands. It has been estimated that there are between 1,000 and 2,000 ceruminous glands in the average ear.[7] Each ceruminous gland is composed of a coiled tube situated just superficial to the perichondrium of the external auditory canal. The tube is continuous with a straight duct that passes into the dermis and opens into the luminal part of a hair follicle.

Two layers of cells are present in the ceruminous glands. The inner secretory layer is composed of cuboidal cells with abundant, eosinophilic cytoplasm. These cells display two special characteristics. First, they have buds of cytoplasm that bulge from the surface of the cell into the gland lumen. Variable degrees of pinching off of cytoplasm from these buds may be observed, and in some ceruminous gland lumina, eosinophilic secretion may be seen loose within the gland, representing fragments of cytoplasm sequestered from the cells (Fig. 2-7). This is a characteristic of apocrine secretion in which parts of the cell produce the secretion, as compared with the holocrine secretion of sebaceous glands in which whole sebaceous cells drop off to form the secretion, while eccrine (sweat)

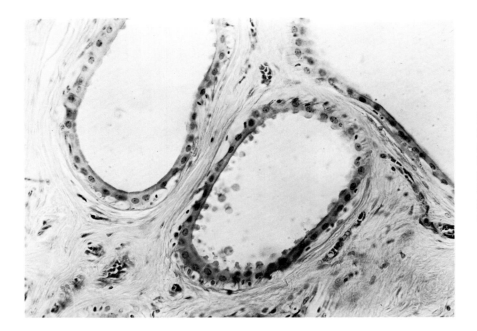

**Fig. 2-7.** Apocrine glands of external auditory canal. Note buds of cytoplasm projecting into the lumen. Some of these lie loose in the lumen. An outer myoepithelial layer may be identified in the glands. (H&E stain; original magnification ×500.)

gland secretion is a fluid product of the cells' metabolism. The second distinctive character is present in most secretory cells of ceruminous glands: yellowish-brown pigment granules, usually found near the luminal edge of the cell. These granules are acid fast, that is, they require strong staining methods, such as carbol fuchsin, and once stained, resist decolorization by acid. They also show reddish fluorescence when examined by ultraviolet light.

Peripheral to the secretory cells of the ceruminous gland is a second, flattened layer of cells forming a circle around the secretory cells. This is the myoepithelial layer. The nuclei of these cells are spindle shaped, and their cytoplasm eosinophilic. A layer of collagen is often present external to the myoepithelial cells separating the ceruminous gland tubules from the adjacent tissue. The duct of the ceruminous glands does not show apocrine or myoepithelial cells but is composed of two layers of cuboidal cells without an external fibrous layer. Toward its termination in a hair follicle (or sometimes on the skin surface), the duct develops multiple layers and may produce keratinizing epidermoid cells. Before puberty and in old age ceruminous glands are fewer in number.

## TYMPANIC MEMBRANE

The pars tensa is composed of an external layer of skin, a central collagenous zone formed by two layers of collagen and fibroblasts, and an internal mucosal layer.

The skin on the external surface is similar to that lining the bony portion of the external auditory canal. It shows a superficial stratum corneum, beneath which there is a zone of granular cells, the stratum granulosum, usually one layer thick; a stratum malpighii of "prickle" cells, which is usually four or five layers thick; and a single layer of basal cells, the stratum basale. There are no rete ridges or ceruminous glands; hair follicles and sebaceous glands are also absent. It is of interest that the histologic structure of the wall of a cholesteatoma sac is identical, even in the number of layers comprising the various components, to the normal epithelium of the tympanic membrane.[8] A thin lamina propria composed of connective tissue with capillaries lies beneath the epidermis.

The connective tissue layer of the normal pars tensa possesses a characteristic and unique architecture. It shows an external layer of radially arranged collagenous fibers and an internal layer in which these fibers are arranged circularly. In histologic sections of normal tympanic membrane, this two-layered structure can be easily recognized, and it is a mark of previous pathologic change that this layered microscopic structure is deformed or absent. Some elastic fibers are also present near the center and at the periphery of the membrane.[9]

The inner membranous surface, the mucosa of the middle ear, is composed of a single layer of cubical epithelium, which rests on a lamina propria of collagenous fibers and capillaries (Fig. 2-8).

The pars flaccida shows an epidermis in which the cell layers are rather more numerous than in the pars tensa, comprising up to 10 layers. The mucosa is similar in appearance to that lining the pars tensa. The intermediate, finely structured collagenous layers seen in the pars tensa are absent, however, and are replaced by a thicker zone of loose collagen and elastic fibers.

The periosteal connective tissue of the handle of the malleus is continuous with the central connective tissue layer of the tympanic membrane. The

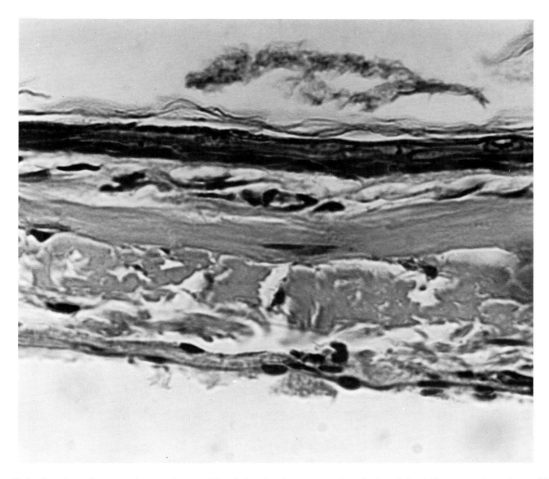

**Fig. 2-8.** Section of tympanic membrane. The following layers may be distinguished (from top down) stratified squamous epithelium, lamina propria, radially arranged collagenous fibers, circularly arranged collagen fibers (at right angles to former layer), lamina propria, middle ear epithelium. (H&E stain; original magnification ×800.)

mucosa of the tympanic membrane is reflected over the surface of the handle of the malleus (see following).

## EUSTACHIAN TUBE

The epithelial covering of the eustachian tube is one of pseudostratified columnar (respiratory) epithelium. Most of the cells are ciliated (Fig. 2-9). About one-fifth of the epithelial surface cells are goblet cells, that is, mucus secreting; the proportion is increased in association with middle ear infection.[10] The mucosa beneath the epithelium frequently contains lymphocytes. It has been suggested that lymphoid aggregates similar to pharyngeal tonsillar tissue are normal in the tube, and the term *Gerlach's tubal tonsil* has been applied to this feature, from the name of the author of one of its earliest descriptions. It is likely, however, that any accumulations of lymphoid tissue in the tubal mucosa are the result of inflammation. Nasopharyngeal lymphoid tissue never extends as far as the orifice of the eustachian tube.[11]

In the cartilaginous portion of the tube, there is a submucous layer containing abundant seromucinous gland acini. These are separated from the mucosa by a thin layer of elastic tissue. The seromucinous glands show acini lined by mucous cells with peripheral demilunes of serous cells, which contain darkly staining granules in their cytoplasm. Secretion from seromucinous glands passes along ducts that open through the mucosa on to the surface (Fig. 2-10).

The cartilaginous framework of the lateral portion of the eustachian tube is shaped like a shepherd's crook, the opening being below on vertical section. The cartilage is of hyaline type. The bone of the osseous portion is composed of thin lamellae. Medially, the mucosa of the osseous portion of the eustachian tube is separated from the carotid canal by a plate of bone, which I have observed in microscopic sections to be less than 1 mm in thickness. Squamous carcinoma growing from the epithelium of the middle ear and adjacent eustachian tube frequently penetrates the thin plate of bone to reach the carotid canal, where it tends to spread widely.[12]

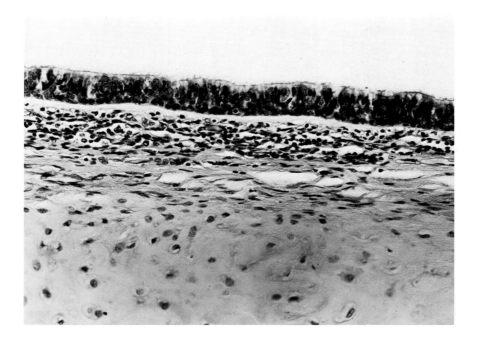

**Fig. 2-9.** Cartilaginous portion of eustachian tube near its middle-ear end. The epithelium is largely ciliated. The lamina propria shows a chronic inflammatory infiltrate; this is very common in the eustachian tube. Seromucinous glands are not present at this high level of the tube but are found nearer the pharynx (see Fig. 2-10). (H&E stain; original magnification × 500.)

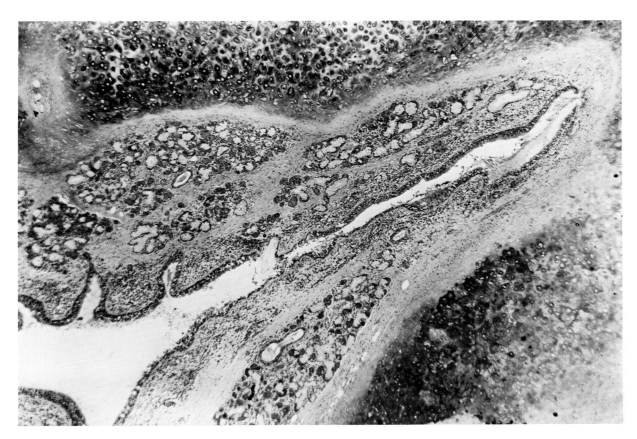

**Fig. 2-10.** Section of eustachian tube near the nasopharyngeal end. Note abundant seromucinous glands and outer cartilage layer. (H&E stain; original magnification ×50.)

An important sign in the radiologic assessment of squamous carcinoma of the middle ear is the presence of this intact bar of bone, which indicates that the neoplasm has not yet penetrated it.[13] There are air cells in the floor of the bony eustachian tube and frequently in the lateral wall, which also show thin bony plates.

## EPITHELIA OF THE MIDDLE EAR: VARIATION BY SITE

The epithelium of the respiratory tract is for the most part ciliated pseudostratified columnar. This epithelium is continued into the eustachian tube and the anterior part of the middle ear cavity immediately adjacent to it. More posteriorly, although zones of ciliated pseudostratified epithelium are present, much of the epithelial covering is of simple squamous or simple cuboidal type. Stratified squamous epithelium is not considered to be a feature of the "normal" ear, but it may be found in patches (squamous metaplasia) or as a cystic formation (cholesteatoma) in the abnormal middle ear. Gland formation is also not a feature of the normal middle ear mucosa but requires inflammatory change for its induction.[14]

Simple squamous epithelium or simple cuboidal epithelium lines the middle ear of the tympanic membrane, the posterior tympanic cavity, and the mastoid air cells. The cells form a single layer and in

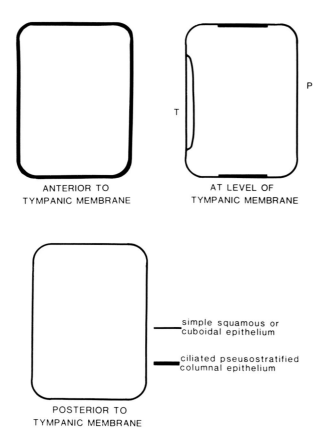

ANTERIOR TO
TYMPANIC MEMBRANE

AT LEVEL OF
TYMPANIC MEMBRANE

simple squamous or
cuboidal epithelium

ciliated pseusostratified
columnal epithelium

POSTERIOR TO
TYMPANIC MEMBRANE

**Fig. 2-11.** Ciliated pseudostratified epithelium in coronal sections at three different levels of normal tympanic cavity. *T*, tympanic membrane; *P*, promontory.

histologic section range from a flattened outline in the squamous type to a square outline in the cuboidal type.

Ciliated pseudostratified columnar epithelium shows nuclei at different levels and cells that are variable in shape. All cells extend down to the underlying basement membrane, but not all extend to the free surface (Fig. 2-11). Basal cells are present among columnar cells along the basement membrane; these are thought to possess regenerative ability on behalf of the epithelium. It is generally accepted that the cells reaching the surface may show cilia or mucous secretory granules or both. The capability of producing mucus and of moving it by ciliary activity exemplifies the main activity of this epithelium—the cleansing of the respiratory tract surface by the mechanism of a moving mucous stream.

The distribution of ciliated pseudostratified columnar epithelium was clearly worked out by Sadé[14] in a study of serial sections of temporal bones evenly distributed in ages ranging from 6 months to 95 years. Sadé considered the tympanic cavity in three zones: (1) anterior to the ear drum, (2) at the level of the ear drum, and (3) behind the ear drum. The eustachian tube is lined by ciliated epithelium, and this is continued over the medial wall, lateral wall, roof and floor of the tympanic cavity anterior to the drum. Two tracts of ciliated epithelium extend posteriorly from this region into the region at the level of the drum. One tract passes along the floor of the hypotympanum, and the other along the roof of the tympanic cavity. The anterior surface of the promontory is also frequently ciliated, and the middle part is sometimes so. A variable portion of the posterior part of the tympanic cavity shows extensions of these ciliated tracts. The posterosuperior part of the promontory, the posterior attic and aditus, the antrum and mastoid air cells are not ciliated in the normal ear. Sadé found the ciliary tracts to cover one third to two thirds of the middle ear lining. In children up to 4 years old, the ciliated pseudostratified epithelium is borne on papillary formations of the mucosa. These may also be frequently seen in the inner part of the eustachian tube.

As would be expected, the distribution of the mucous secretory cells closely parallels that of ciliated cells. Lim et al.[15] used the periodic acid Schiff and alcian blue stains to indicate "neutral mucopolysaccharides" with mucin and "acid mucopolysaccharides," respectively. Cells stained by either of these methods were found in the distribution shown in Table 2-1. The highest incidences of secretory cells were found in the eustachian tube and middle ear adjacent to it.

A study by Akaan-Penttila[16] in 20 newborn infants (live and stillborn) of gestational ages ranging from 25 to 40 weeks gave substantially similar results, except that goblet cells were very few. This would be expected, because goblet cells proliferate in any part of the respiratory epithelium when irritated by infective, gaseous, or vaporous agents or by hypersensitivity—factors that are more likely to occur over a period of years rather than in

Table 2-1. Incidence of Secretory Cells in Tympanic Cavity and Bony Eustachian Tube

| | |
|---|---|
| Bony Eustachian tube | 12% |
| Transitional area between eustachian tube and promontory | 10% |
| Hypotympanum | 10% |
| Promontory | 8% |
| Antrum (epitympanum) | 6% |
| Mastoid | <1% |

(Lim DJ et al: Distribution of mucus-secretory cells in the normal middle ear mucosa. Arch Otolaryngol 93:251, 1982.)

early infancy. In middle ears of earlier specimens, fetal loose connective tissue may be seen in some parts of the middle ear immediately beneath the epithelium. The connective tissue fills the middle ear earlier in fetal life but regresses toward the end of gestation and after birth. In the first year of life, subepithelial collections of myxoid tissue may still be found, particularly in the attic region of the middle ear.

that emanate from the tympanic cavity. The skeletal framework of each air cell is made up of a thin bony trabeculum composed of haversian systems of vascularized lamellar bone. This is covered by a thin periosteal layer of fibrous tissue on which the epithelium of the air cell rests. The epithelium is of cuboidal or a single layer of squamous epithelium (Fig. 2-12). Pseudostratified columnar epithelium rarely is found in the mastoid cells.

In the first year of life, when the air cell system is beginning to form by the pressure of the air-filled middle ear cleft from the attic region, round or irregular zones of connective tissue are seen in the bony wall of already-formed air cells. These "interstitial cell formations" are the first stage in the hollowing out of bone. Air-filled, epithelial-lined spaces push against these structures and eventually replace them.[17]

## MASTOID AIR CELLS

The mastoid air cells including the mastoid antrum are a network of intercommunicating spaces

## MIDDLE EAR CORPUSCLES

Pacinian corpuscles, often known as the corpuscles of Vater-Pacini, are found in many parts of the

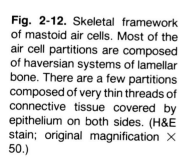

**Fig. 2-12.** Skeletal framework of mastoid air cells. Most of the air cell partitions are composed of haversian systems of lamellar bone. There are a few partitions composed of very thin threads of connective tissue covered by epithelium on both sides. (H&E stain; original magnification × 50.)

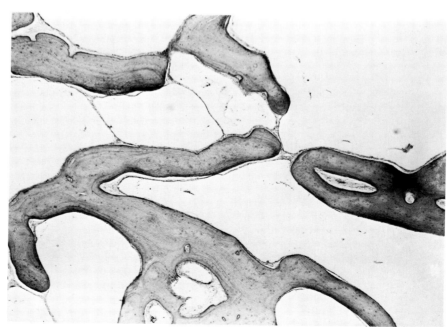

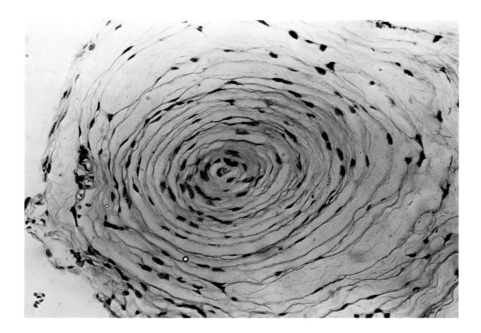

**Fig. 2-13.** Middle ear corpuscle from mucosa. The corpuscle is composed of many layers of concentric lamellae. (H&E stain; original magnification ×500.)

body under the deeper layers of the skin and under the mucous membranes of the conjunctiva, cornea, heart, mesentery, and pancreas and in loose connective tissue in general. Similar structures are often found in a subepithelial position in the tympanic cavity, where they are up to 1 mm in diameter. These corpuscles are not supplied by nerve fibers.[9] The corpuscle is composed of many layers of concentric lamellae (Fig. 2-13). The function of these structures in the middle ear is unknown.

## OSSEOUS TISSUES OF THE TEMPORAL BONE

The osseous tissues are among the most complex of the temporal bone in their development and histology. The bone surrounding the membranous labyrinth, which is the bony labyrinth or otic capsule, has a fine structure that is unique. Because the auditory ossicles and the mastoid air cells also show special features, it will be helpful to give the outlines of osteogenesis and of endochondral and membranous development of bones.

## Osteogenesis

Bone is composed of (1) an intercellular substance of collagen fibrils and amorphous protein with polysaccharides and crystalline mineral material, mainly calcium phosphate; (2) mesenchymal cells known as osteocytes. Osteocytes are derived from osteoblasts. Osteoclasts are multinucleate giant cells and represent fused histiocytic cells. These structures play an important part in the breakdown and molding of bone.

All bone formation occurs in the same way. It begins with the lining up of cells in loose connective tissue. These cells produce an eosinophilic substance which then becomes basophilic and is associated with the localization of randomly arranged collagen fibers. Calcium phosphate and other salts are then deposited in the ground substance. The osteoblasts are by now incorporated in the newly formed tissue and are known as osteocytes. The bone is at this stage "woven bone" and shows an irregular distribution of collagen fibrils. Remodeling and further development of this bone leads to a more regular distribution of the osteocytes and an ordered pattern of the collagen fibers into lamellae. The latter are arranged in a crisscross pattern. One lamella runs longitudinally in relation to the length of the bone, and the next runs circularly, and so on. This is adult or "lamellar" bone; the alternating directions of the fibers give rise to the regular, parallel striped effect when this type of bone is examined by polarized light.

Woven bone is always spongy, that is, it forms a network of thin trabeculae. Lamellar bone also forms a spongy network, as in the early arrangement of the medulla of a long bone. Compact bone, as in the cortex of a long bone, is formed by the apposition of layers of new bone on to the trabeculae of spongy lamellae until the supplying vessels are enclosed in a concentrically laminated tube of bone, known as a haversian system.

## Early Development of Bones

Bone, the tissue, is developed always in the same fashion by the mechanism previously described. Bones, the anatomic organs, are formed by this osteogenetic process following one of two different pathways. The first (endochondral ossification) commences with the development of a crude cartilaginous model of the bony organ. This is then followed by dissolution of the cartilage and its replacement by bone. In the second (membranous ossification) the precursor is connective tissue within which bone forms directly, without a cartilaginous model to be replaced.

In the initial ossification of the cartilage model of long bones, the perichondrium of the middle portion of the shaft forms a collar or "splint" of new woven bone. This eventually becomes lamellar bone, forming the circumferential lamellae under the periosteum, which is known as periosteal bone. The cartilage cells in this region of the shaft become pale and swollen, and the intercellular substance of the cartilage becomes basophilic and calcifies. Connective tissue from the ossifying collar of perichondrium grows into the degenerate cartilage lacunae. The swollen chondroctyes are removed by macrophages, and woven bone is laid down in the lacunae thus opened up. There is a stage in the development of all bones in which a mosaic of unabsorbed calcified ground substance of cartilage interweaves with newly formed bone. This is known as *intrachondrial* bone. In most bones the calcified cartilage matrix is completely resorbed

and replaced by immature bone. The subsequent bone formed in this way is known as *endochondral* bone. In the otic capsule the calcified cartilage matrix remains and is not absorbed (see following). The spaces in the newly formed spongy bone in the center of the diaphysis of a long bone are occupied by red bone marrow. Ossification in the metaphyseal end of the long bone and in the epiphysis occur along similar lines.

## Membranous Development

In the bones formed without a preceding cartilaginous model, a center of ossification develops within the connective tissue. When the major part of the particular bony structure has been completed, subsequent growth of the bone is in the region of the suture line. In the later stages of maturation of both this type of bone and endochondral bone, the woven bone is broken down by osteoblasts and replaced by lamellar bone. There is a continual process of breakdown and reconstruction of even the lamellar bone with growth and development.

## Otic Capsule

The bone of the otic capsule is extremely dense and has a unique histologic structure for an adult bone. The otic capsule surrounds and replicates the outline of the membranous labyrinth contained within it. Its dense structure is, perhaps, related to the necessity of protecting the extremely delicate acoustic and other vibrations of the fluids contained within it.

The otic capsule is formed from a preceding cartilaginous model like the long bones. Three layers may be recognized. The outer is the periosteal layer and corresponds to the circumferential lamella of long bones. The inner layer is similarly derived, although it is usually referred to as the endosteal layer of the otic capsule, suggesting correspondence to the layer next to the bone marrow of long bones. It does not strictly fall into that category but rather is an inner periosteal layer.

The middle layer has a unique structure, in that the calcified cartilage matrix is not removed when the lacunae of the degenerated cartilage cells are

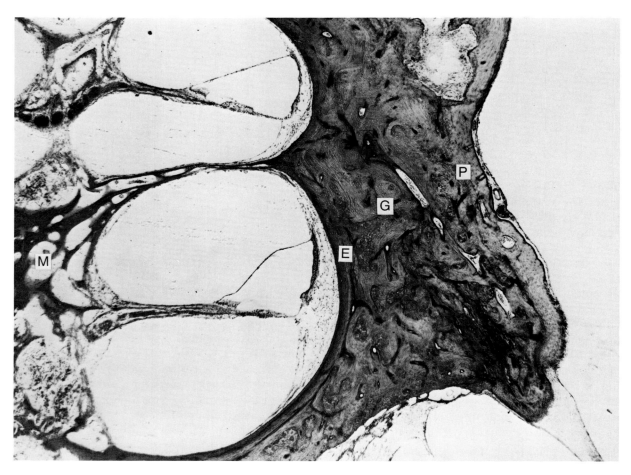

**Fig. 2-14.** Cochlea, bony cochlea, and modiolus. *E*, endosteal layer; *G*, intrachondrial layer containing globuli interossei; *M*, modiolus; *P*, periosteal layer. (H&E stain; original magnification ×50.)

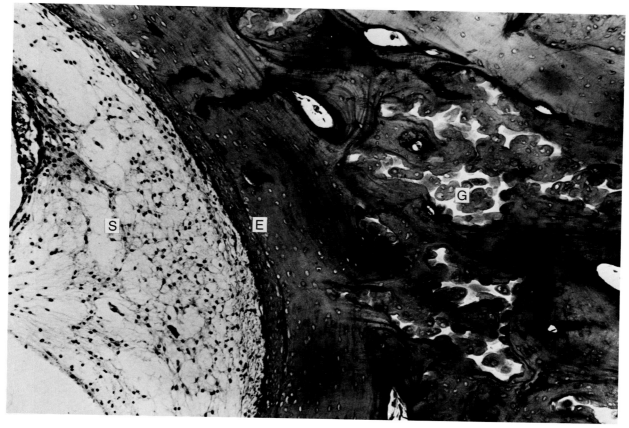

**Fig. 2-15.** Spiral ligament and adjacent bony cochlea. *E*, endosteal layer; *G*, intrachondrial bone showing globuli interossei; *S*, spiral ligament. (H&E stain; original magnification ×200.)

filled by primitive bone. This calcified matrix persists into adult life as the globuli interossei or globuli ossei characteristic of the otic capsule. The bony tissue in the first months of life is accompanied by red bone marrow, as in the development of long bones. This marrow is subsequently replaced by bone. The bone of the adult otic capsule, although not lamellated, is still somewhat more differentiated than woven bone. Thus, the middle layer otic capsule bone is characterized by (1) lack of removal and replacement of calcified cartilage matrix and (2) lack of removal and replacement of primitive bone. The two persisting tissues form a network of extremely hard consistency (Figs. 2-14 and 2-15).

## AUDITORY OSSICLES

The histologic appearance of the auditory ossicles results from the development of these structures along the general lines of a cartilage-derived long bone, with only a single center of ossification for each ossicle and no additional epiphyseal centers of ossification. The persistence of cartilage in certain situations in all three ossicles and the process of formation of the obturator foramen in the case of the stapes gives the ossicles a pro-

**Table 2-2.    Types of Bone and Persistence of Cartilage in the Parts of the Auditory Ossicles**

| | |
|---|---|
| **Stapes** | |
| Head | Endochondral bone |
| | Cartilaginous surface |
| Crura | Periosteal bone only |
| Footplate | Endochondral bone on tympanic surface |
| Stapediovestibular joints | Cartilage |
| **Incus** | |
| Body and long process | Outer covering of periosteal bone; inner core of endochondral bone; islands of intrachondrial bone occasionally retained |
| **Malleus** | |
| Head and upper handle | Outer covering of periosteal bone |
| | Inner core of endochondral bone |
| Articular process | Articular cartilage |
| Lower part of handle | Shell of cartilage (no periosteal bone); perichondrium merges with central fibrous tissue of tympanic membrane |
| | Inner core of endochondral bone |
| Anterior process | Membrane bone |

nounced histologic individuality.[18] Their special histologic features are listed in Table 2-2.

## Stapes

Cartilage is retained as a thin horizontal lamina on the vestibular aspect of the footplate and also covers the articular surfaces of the stapediovestibular joints. The vestibular surface of the stapes is lined by the single, flattened, thin, squamous layer of cells characteristic of the perilymph space. A thin layer of bone is applied exteriorly to the cartilage of the footplate, so that the latter is bilaminar in constitution (Fig. 2-16). This bony tissue is the residue of a considerable deposit of endochondral bone formed during early ossification of the stapes, most of which is eliminated during the development of the obturator foramen. The bilaminar footplate structure is sometimes interrupted by areas of cartilage that extend from the vestibular to the tympanic surface of the footplate.

The crura are formed of periosteal bone only (Fig. 2-17). Endochondral bone that covered the inner part of the crura is completely eliminated during fetal development of the obturator foramen.

The head of the stapes is composed of endochondral bone capped by a cartilage layer at the incudostapedial joint.

## Incus

The body and long process of the incus show a structure that is more like a typical long bone than is the stapes. There is an outer covering of periosteal bone and an inner core of endochondral bone, both showing well-formed haversian systems (Fig. 2-18). Both of these layers are subject to removal and production of new bone. These processes can occur at any age. Bone removal activity may give rise to pits on the surface of the incus, which should not be interpreted as the erosive effects of inflammation. The sites of fresh bony deposition are indicated by the presence of cement lines. Islands of intrachondrial bone similar to the globuli ossei of the otic capsule are sometimes found in the incus and malleus (Fig. 2-19).

The short process of the incus shows a tip of unossified cartilage that also covers the articular surfaces of the incus at its two joints.

## Malleus

The structure of the head and upper part of the handle of the malleus is similar to that of the body and long process of the incus, with an outer shell of periosteal bone and an inner core of endochondral bone. Most of the malleus handle does not have a shell of periosteal bone; instead there is a layer of retained cartilage. The handle merges with the middle collagenous layer of the tympanic membrane. Superiorly, the malleus handle is separated by a ligament, the inner core of which links the perichondrium of the handle to the middle layer of the tympanic membrane. This ligament is covered by middle ear epithelium. Lower down, the malleus handle is invested by the middle fibrous layer of the tympanic membrane, which divides equally medial and lateral to the handle (Fig. 2-20).[19] The inner core of the whole of the malleus handle is

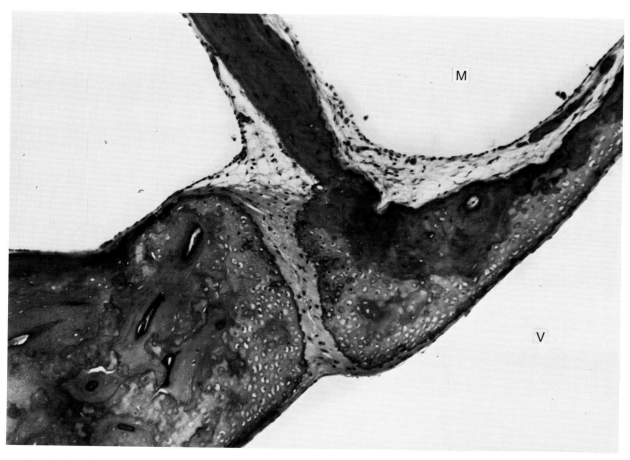

**Fig. 2-16.** Stapediovestibular joint, part of footplate of stapes, adjacent bony labyrinthine wall, and crus of stapes. The footplate shows a lamina of cartilage on its vestibular surface, which is continous with the cartilage of the articular surface of the stapediovestibular joint. *M*, middle ear cavity; *V*, cavity of vestibule. (H&E stain; original magnification ×200.)

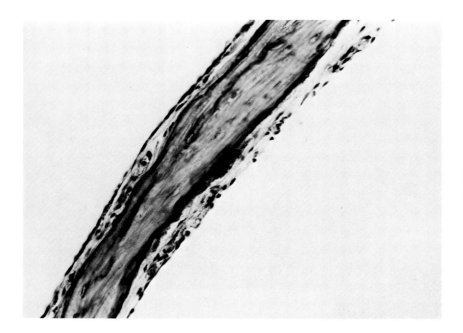

**Fig. 2-17.** Crus of stapes. It is composed of a thin layer of periosteal bone, covered by low epithelium. (H&E stain; original magnification ×250.)

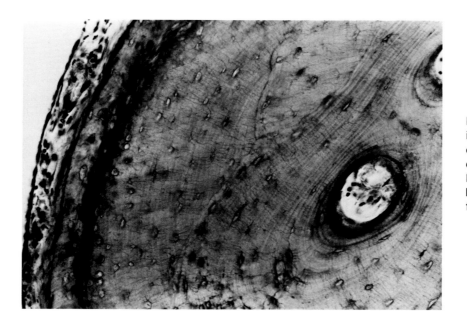

**Fig. 2-18.** Long process of incus. There is an outer covering of periosteal bone and an inner core of endochondral bone. Note surface flattened epithelium. (H&E stain; original magnification ×500.)

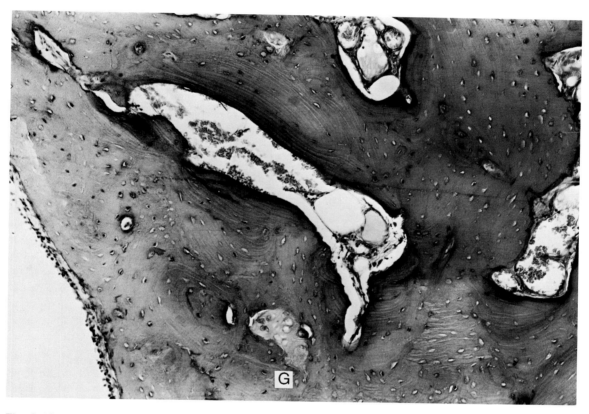

**Fig. 2-19.** Body of malleus, composed of haversian systems. *G,* an island of residual cartilage within bone (similar to globuli interossei). (H&E stain; original magnification ×200.)

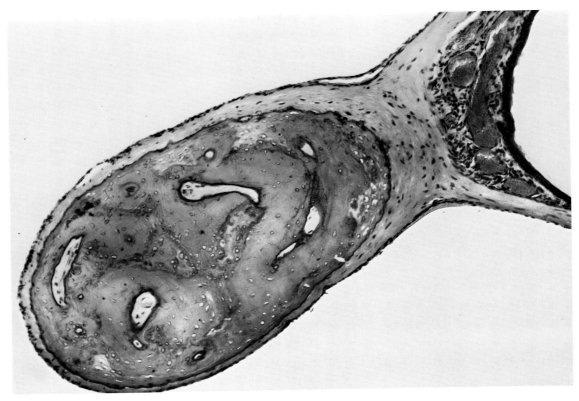

**Fig. 2-20.** Handle of malleus showing outer layer of cartilage in some areas. The handle is enveloped by fibrous tissue that is continuous with the middle layer of the tympanic membrane. (H&E stain; original magnification × 200.)

composed of endochondral bone like the rest of the malleus.

The articular process of the malleus is covered by cartilage.

The anterior process of the malleus is bone, which unlike the rest of the malleus, is formed in membrane early in fetal life and merges with the malleus soon after its formation. The malleus, like the incus, is subject to processes of breakdown and new formation during life, giving rise to excavations of the surface and irregular cement lines.

## MIDDLE EAR JOINTS

### Incudomalleal and Incudostapedial Joints

The incudomalleal and incudostapedial joints are diarthrodial, that is, they have a cavity that permits movement of the constituent bones at the articulation. The articular ends of the constituent

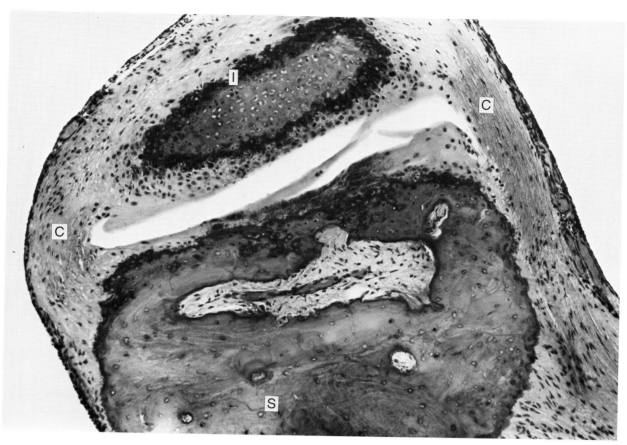

**Fig. 2-21.** Incudostapedial joint. The articular cartilage shows fraying and numerous particles of calcification. These are manifestations of advancing age. *C*, two sides of capsule; *I*, incus; *S*, stapes. (H&E stain; original magnification ×200.)

bone are covered by hyaline cartilage, the chondrocytes of which become progressively flattened toward the joint margin. The space between the articular ends is largely occupied by fibrocartilage, the articular disc. The joint capsule is lined on its outer surface by middle ear epithelium and on its inner surface by synovial membrane. The bulk of the capsule is composed of fibrous tissue with a very high content of elastic fibers.

Changes have been described in all the components of these two joints with advancing age. There is some audiologic evidence that these changes lead to an air bone gap for high tones.[20] The joint capsule shows hyalinization at first and later calcification, and similar changes are seen in the articular disc. The articular cartilage frequently shows fraying, vacuolation, and fibrillation even in some people less than 40 years of age. Later with more severe changes the articular cartilage becomes calcified. With further degeneration the joint becomes narrowed and eventually obliterated (Fig. 2-21).[21]

## Stapediovestibular Joint

The cartilaginous edge of the footplate of the stapes is bound to the cartilaginous rim of the vestibular window by a fibrous connection, the annular ligament. The stapediovestibular joint is classified as a synarthrosis; that is, a joint permitting little movement, and being lined by connective tissue is known as a *syndesmosis*. The annular ligament is composed of collagenous fibers radiating from footplate to vestibular window bone. Joint cavities, located mainly in the posterior pole of the annular ligament were found by Bolz and Lim in 70 percent of adult joints.[22] Prominent elastic fibers are present on the middle ear and vestibular surfaces of the joint.[23]

# MIDDLE EAR MUSCLES

## General Histology of Muscle

The stapedius and tensor tympani muscles are skeletal muscles composed of long fibers, each of which is a syncytium containing hundreds of nuclei — the sarcolemmal nuclei. These nuclei are situated immediately beneath the sarcolemmal sheath — the surface covering of the muscle fiber. In transverse section the fibers are polygonal. A

**Table 2-3. Bases of Four Systems of Classification of Skeletal Muscle**

Anatomic appearance
    Red versus white
    Dark versus light
    High or low granularity of the sarcoplasm on light microscopy
    Rich or poor in protoplasm
    Subcellular differences on electron microscopy
Physiological behavior
    Slow versus fast contraction on muscle fiber after stimulation
    High or low resistance to fatigue
Biochemical properties
    High or low respiratory activity
    High or low enzyme or chemical constituents
Histochemical features
    High or low enzyme content
    Enzyme profile

(Dubowitz V, Brooke MH: Muscle Biopsy: A Modern Approach. WB Saunders, Philadelphia, 1973.)

banded arrangement is easily seen on light microscopy, particularly in polarized light in which anisotropic and isotropic discs may be identified. The sarcolemmal sheath is composed of the cell membrane of the muscle fiber itself, together with a basement membrane of collagen reticulin fibers, which run into the delicate connective tissue framework of the muscle — the endomysium. This contains a network of capillary blood vessels and is continuous with the fibrous tissue that splits the muscle into bundles. Each muscle also contains muscle spindles, which are specialized structures consisting of striated fibers within a connective tissue capsule. The spindles are located in proximity to nerves or vessels and act as sensory organs to coordinate muscle activity and maintain tone.

Muscle fibers have been classified by a variety of morphologic and physiological methods, and the combination of the various methods in the assignment of a muscle into a particular category is a complex task.

Dubowitz and Brooke[24] have summarized the bases of four systems of classification of muscle (Table 2-3).

For histochemical typing, the adenosine triphosphatase reaction at pH 9.4 is recommended by Dubowitz and Brooke,[24] and on this basis, type 1 fibers have a high activity, and type 2 fibers low activity.

## Tensor Tympani

The tensor tympani muscle is composed of fibers in a penniform (i.e., feather-shaped) arrangement, with a central tendon composed of elastic tissue, from which muscle fibers radiate. The muscle often has a prominent content of adipose tissue, the function of which is not known, but which may serve to insulate the nearby cochlea from the electric effects of contraction. In some tensor tympani muscles, there is a striking sarcolemmal nuclear clustering and degeneration of muscle fibers. The significance of this change is not known (Figs. 2-22 and 2-23).

## Stapedius

Like the tensor tympani, the stapedius possesses a central elastic tendinous core into which the muscle fibers radiate (Fig. 2-24)

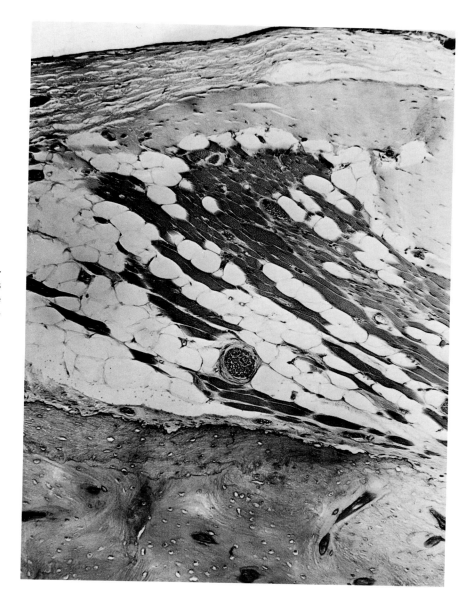

**Fig. 2-22.** Tensor tympani muscle with numerous adipose cells between the skeletal muscle fibers. (H&E stain; original magnification ×200.)

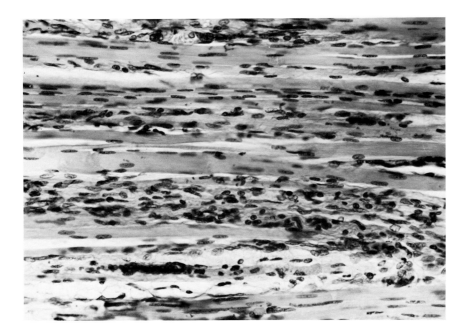

**Fig. 2-23.** Tensor tympani muscle showing clustering of sarcolemmal nuclei and degeneration of muscle fibers. (H&E stain; original magnification ×500.)

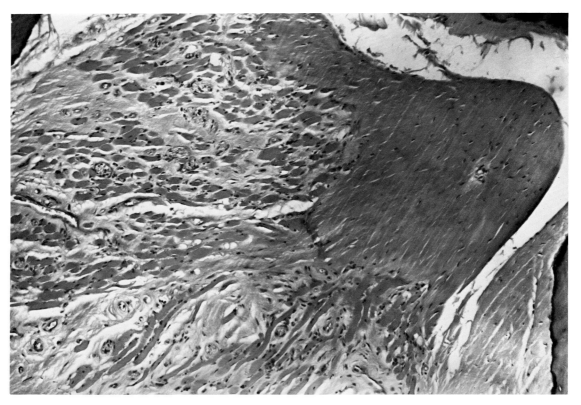

**Fig. 2-24.** Stapedius muscle and tendon. The skeletal muscle fibers and fibrous bands between the fibers radiate to a tendon on the right. (H&E stain; original magnification ×200.)

## Histochemical Typing of Middle Ear Muscles

Nothing is known about the histochemical status of the middle ear muscles in the human. Anderson[25] studied the stapedius and tensor tympani muscles of the guinea pig and cotton rat histochemically. He found that in both these animals the two muscles were heterogeneous in their fiber composition, containing both types 1 and 2 fibers. The arrangement differed also in the two species. Histochemical studies of the two muscles have been carried out in the two muscles of the horse, sheep, cow, pig, dog, cat, and rabbit.[26] Both types of fiber were found in the stapedius of all of these animals. In the tensor tympani, the situation was rather different. In the sheep, horse, rabbit, dog, and cat, both types of fiber were found in this muscle. In the cow and pig tensor tympani, however, it was very difficult to identify the different fiber types, because the number of fibers was small and most of the muscle was in the form of an intratympanic ligament. It would be expected that the human middle ear muscles, could they be studied by enzyme histochemical methods, would also show both types. Lyon and Malmgren[27] have carried out a more detailed histochemical enzyme profile on the stapedius muscle of the cat and found that fast fibers showing high respiratory activity were the major type. The authors suggest on this basis that the cat stapedius muscle is capable of intermittent contractions over long periods of time. The stapedial reflex, in the human, has been shown to decay following continuous noise exposure, and the ability for such repeated contractions would be of value during exposure to certain types of industrial noise.

## INNER EAR

The histologic structure of the membranous labyrinth, particularly that of the organ of Corti and the sensory structures of the vestibule and ampullae of the semicircular canals, are of prime importance in the description of microscopic appearances of temporal bone structures, because their morphology is closely related to the functions of hearing and balance. The relation of structure to function is, however, best appreciated for these locations by reference to the ultrastructural appearance. Since these are given in detail in Chapter 4, the present description of light microscopic appearances will be presented in summary form only.

## Cochlea

### Modiolus

The modiolus is composed of spongy bone. It is penetrated by blood vessels and nerve bundles of the cochlear branch of the 8th nerve.

### Spiral Ganglion

On the lateral side of the modiolus are located the cell bodies of the spiral ganglion (Fig. 2-14). These are bipolar neurons receiving impulses from the hair cells and relaying them to brain-stem nuclei. The ganglion cells are large structures with nuclei showing prominent nucleoli and cytoplasm filled with Nissl's granules (Fig. 2-25). Each nerve cell is surrounded by Schwann cells and myelin sheath. Ten percent of the nerve cells are said to be of particularly small diameter.[28]

Reduction of numbers of the spiral ganglion cells with advancing age has been well documented.[29] Guild et al.[29] devised an elaborate method for defining the numbers of spiral ganglion cells in relation to their position along the cochlear coils in serial sections. The authors found that with advancing age the ganglion cells in the basal coil region suffered the earliest and most severe change. This correlated with the audiometric findings of hearing loss for high tones in these patients. Subsequent studies of loss of spiral cells with advancing age have been on a semiquantitative basis,[30] but have all confirmed these findings.[31]

### Spiral Lamina

Emanating from the modiolus in a spiral manner is the spiral lamina, which separates the perilymph-containing space of the scala vestibuli from the similarly containing structure, the scala tympani. The inner zone of the spiral lamina is the

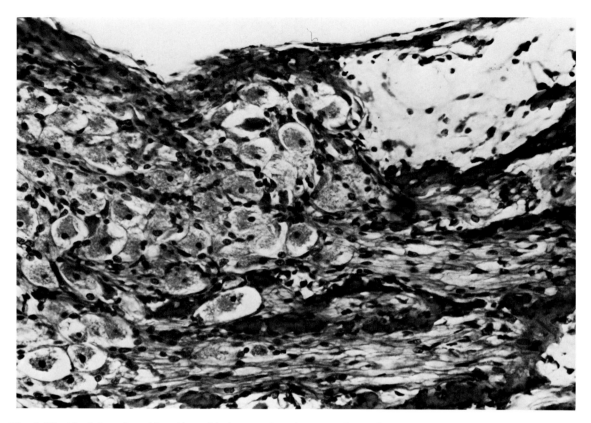

**Fig. 2-25.** Modiolus of cochlea. Note thin bony trabeculae, ganglion cells, and nerve fibers. (H&E stain; original magnification ×500.)

osseous spiral lamina, which contains thin trabeculae of bone and nerve fibers. The latter run from the organ of Corti and in the osseous spiral lamina unite to form prominent bundles that pass into the modiolus. These are especially prominent in the newborn (Fig. 2-26). Fine fibrils running spirally along the length of the osseous spiral lamina are also present, representing the efferent longitudinal nerve fibers. The outer zone of this lamina is known as the basilar membrane. At the attachment of the latter to the cochlear wall, the periosteal connective tissue is thickened to form the spiral ligament. This appears in histologic section as a crescentic structure with a protruding peak on the concave surface of the crescent to which the basilar membrane is anchored. It is composed of collagenous fibers with a few fibroblasts. The fibers blend with the endosteum of the cochlear bony wall and the

fibers of the basilar membrane. Pathologic changes such as the formation of spaces in this structure have been described, but these changes are common, and their significance doubtful.

### Reissner's Membrane

The cochlear canal is further subdivided by a thin membrane, Reissner's membrane, which extends from the spiral lamina to the outer wall of the bony cochlea (Fig. 2-27). This additional scala, the *scala media* or *cochlear duct*, is inserted between the other two. Reissner's membrane consists of two thin layers of cells. The inner layer on the scala media aspect is derived from the otocyst and is therefore ectodermal in origin; epithelial clusters are often observed by the surface preparation tech-

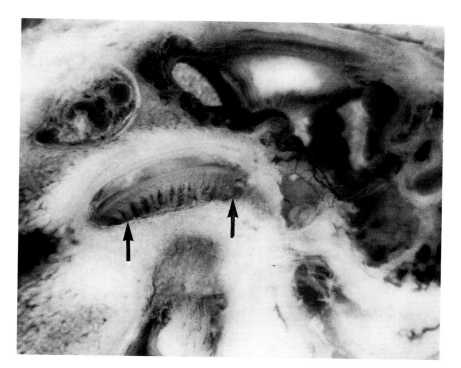

**Fig. 2-26.** Microslice of temporal bone from newborn infant in region of basal coil of cochlea (arrows). Note prominent bundles of nerve fibers running from the region of the organ of Corti toward the modiolus.

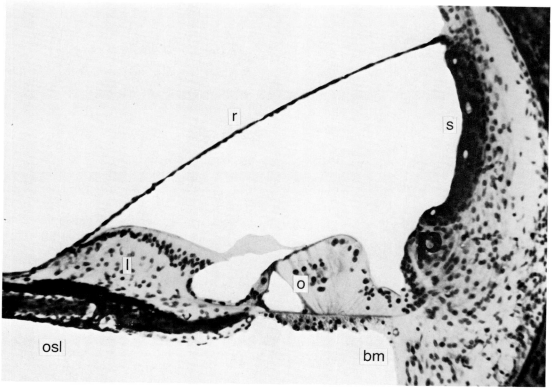

**Fig. 2-27.** Scala media of a monkey. *bm,* basilar membrane; *l,* spiral limbus; *o,* organ of Corti; *osl,* osseous spiral lamina; *p,* spiral prominence; *r,* Reissner's membrane; *s,* stria vascularis; *t,* tectorial membrane. (H&E stain; original magnification × 280.)

nique. The outer layer on the scala vestibuli side is mesodermal in origin; these cells are large, flat, and elongated. Blood vessels are occasionally found in the mesothelium of Reissner's membrane near the apex of the cochlea.[32]

### Stria Vascularis

The outer vertical wall of the triangle of the cochlear duct formed on the other two sides by Reissner's and basilar membranes is the stria vascularis. Under the light microscope, lightly staining basal cells and darkly staining epithelial-like marginal cells can be recognized in this structure (Fig. 2-27).

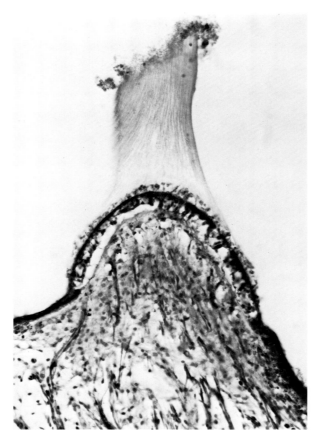

**Fig. 2-28.** Crista of lateral semicircular canal with cupula. (H&E stain; original magnification ×320.)

**Table 2-4.    Structures of Basilar Membrane**

| Name of Structure[a] | Remarks |
|---|---|
| Spiral prominence | Overlies spiral ligament |
| Cells of Claudius | — |
| Cells of Boettcher | Rest on basilar membrane beneath cells of Claudius |
| Cells of Hensen | Contain numerous globules of lipid in cytoplasm |
| Outer hair cells | Number of rows varies from three to five |
| Outer phalangeal cells (Deiters) | Interposed between outer hair cells. |
| Pillar cells enclosing tunnel of Corti | — |
| Inner hair cells | Single row |
| Spiral limbus | Bulge of periosteal connective tissue of the upper surface of the osseous spiral lamina; vertical arrangement of fibers to produce "auditory teeth of Huschke" |
| Interdental cells | On the upper margin of spiral limbus; secrete tectorial membrane |
| Tectorial membrane | Amorphous protein in which hairs of hair cells lie |

[a] See also Fig. 2-27.

### Basilar Membrane Structures

The main cells and structures of the basilar membrane are listed in Table 2-4, arranged from outer to inner aspects of the membrane.

### Sensory Areas of Ampullae

The epithelium of the floor of the three ampullae is formed into a transverse ridge, the crista, and represents the sensory epithelium. A viscous protein polysaccharide formation, known as the cupula, rests above each crista. The remainder of the ampullary and semicircular duct lining is composed of flattened cells (Fig. 2-28).

### Sensory Areas of Utricle and Saccule

The two main membranous structures of the vestibule, the utricle and saccule, show a large proportion of their lining to be composed of sensory epithelium, the maculae (Fig. 2-29). Overlying the hairs of the sensory cells of the maculae are large numbers of crystalline bodies, known as otoliths, which are composed of a mixture of calcium carbonate and a protein, suspended in jellylike polysaccharide.

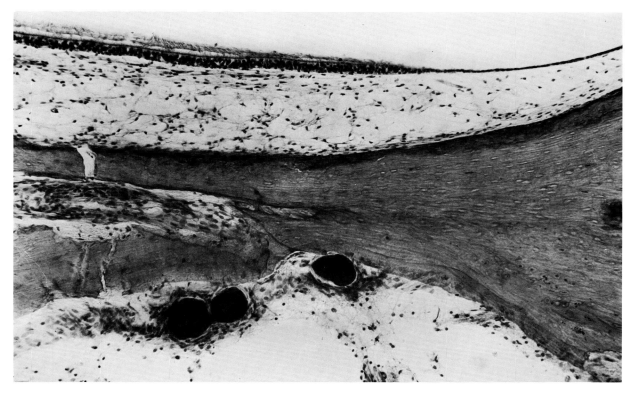

**Fig. 2-29.** Macula of the saccule. Note concentrically laminated structures (arachnoid villi) in internal auditory canal below. (H&E stain; original magnification ✕150.)

### Sensory Epithelium of Cristae and Maculae

Hair cells and supporting cells may be observed in both types of sensory epithelial areas. These structures and the means of their innervation are better seen electron microscopically and are described in detail elsewhere in this work.

### Vestibular Ganglion

The histologic structure of the vestibular ganglion is similar to that of the spiral ganglion with nerve cells (which are bipolar, although this is, of course, not seen in histologic section) and surrounding Schwann cells and myelin; Portmann et al.[28] find two types of nerve cell in this ganglion, one with basophilic cytoplasm and the other with paler cytoplasm.

### Surface Preparation of Organ of Corti

In surface preparations of specimens prepared from cases fixed by perilymphatic perfusion, the organ of Corti may be studied by placing pieces of basilar membrane flat on the slide and examining them by phase contrast microscopy. Fine microscopic details can be discerned by focusing at different levels.

### Round Window Membrane

The round window membrane is seen in histologic section in the depths of the round window fossa (Fig. 2-30). In horizontal sections the lowest part of the scala media is observed nearby across

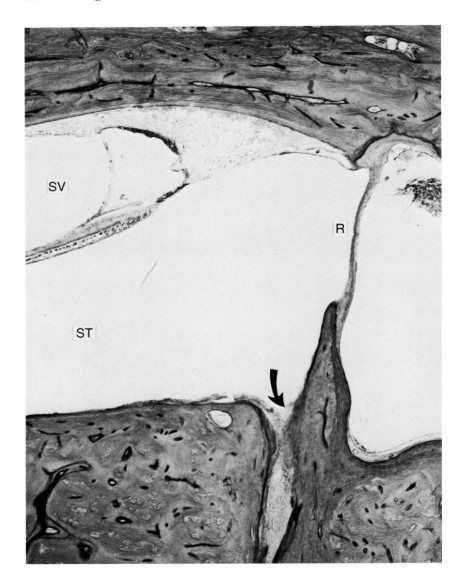

**Fig. 2-30.** Horizontal section of temporal bone in region of round window membrane (*R*). *SV*, scala vestibuli; *ST*, scala tympani. The orifice of the cochlear aqueduct is marked with an arrow. (H&E stain; original magnification × 50.)

the scala tympani, which terminates at the round window membrane. The cochlear aqueduct opens into the scala media also in this vicinity. The ampulla of the posterior semicircular canal is always present in the adjacent temporal bone. The round window membrane is composed almost entirely of elastic tissue. It is lined on its tympanic surface by cuboidal epithelium and on the scala tympani surface by the flattened cells covering the whole perilymph space.

## ENDOLYMPHATIC SAC

The endolymphatic duct arises from the saccule and utricle in the vestibule and passes through the vestibular aqueduct as a straight thin channel, which is lined by flattened cells. The endolymphatic sac is the terminal enlargement of the duct.

The sac is situated within the cranial meningeal tissue. It is described as having three portions: a proximal rugose portion; an enlarged flattened, intermediate portion; and a distal projection. The epithelium of the endolymphatic sac varies from low cuboidal in the proximal portion and distal projection to a high cuboidal or columnar type in the rugose portion. True villi with a vascular pedicle may be found in the rugose portion.[33]

## VESTIBULOCOCHLEAR NERVE

The vestibulocochlear nerve contains myelinated nerve fibers with a Schwann cell coating, the latter giving rise to the myelin. In the central nervous system the myelin coating of nerve fibers is produced by oligodendroglial cells. These cells persist into the vestibulocochlear nerve and are replaced by Schwann cells within the internal auditory canal. The transition takes place at the same level for the whole nerve at a variable distance from the porus. The Schwann cell nuclei are more abundant and larger than oligodendroglia, so that the transition appears as a line in section with more darkly staining nerve tissue on the peripheral side of the nerve replacing paler staining nerve on the central side (Fig. 2-31). The cochlear nerve in the internal auditory canal is reported to show fibers with a considerable variety of diameters between 1 and 9 $\mu$m. These may correspond to the large and small nerve cells of the spiral ganglion (see preceding discussions). Nerve fibers originating from the

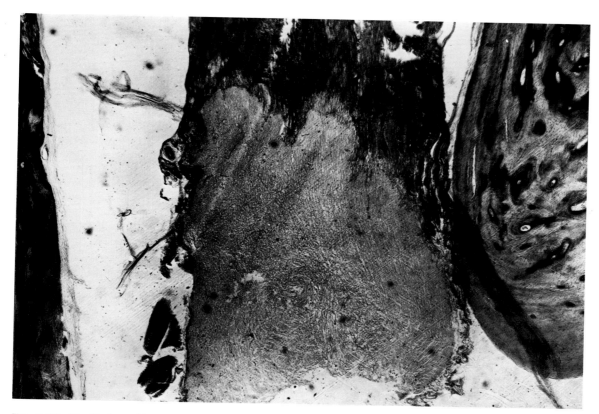

**Fig. 2-31.** Vestibulocochlear nerve in internal auditory canal showing transition from pale-staining glial area to darker neurilemmal area. (Periodic acid Schiff stain; original magnification $\times 50$.)

apex of the cochlea (low frequency) take up an axial position in the cochlear nerve, whereas those from the basal coil (high frequency) take up a peripheral position. The vestibular nerve contains fibers varying between 1 and 13 $\mu$m; the topography of the fibers is not known.[28]

bony portion it is surrounded by a sheath of connective tissue containing numerous blood vessels. The nervus intermedius shows fibers that are smaller than 8 $\mu$m. The geniculate ganglion contains two types of nerve cells that appear similar to the vestibular ganglion.[28]

## FACIAL NERVE, NERVUS INTERMEDIUS, AND GENICULATE GANGLION

Most of the fibers of the facial nerve are said to be large, between 8 and 10 $\mu$m in diameter. The facial nerve is myelinated throughout its extent. In its

## TEMPORAL BODIES

Temporal bodies are nodules of the same histologic structure as the carotid body, and they are found in the adventitia of the jugular bulb just below the floor of the middle ear, or in the canal of the tympanic nerve as far as the cochlear promon-

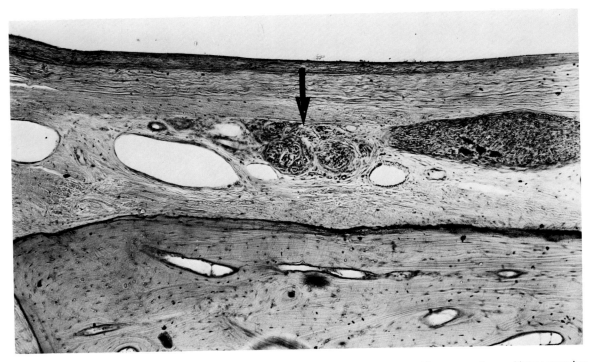

**Fig. 2-32.** Temporal body *(arrow)* in adventitia of jugular bulb. From temporal bone specimen. Note vascular character of this paraganglion and the thick nerve structure that is in contact with it. (H&E stain; original magnification ×126.)

tory. In a histologic study of 88 temporal bones, Guild[34] found 248 glomera with an average of 2.82 glomera per ear. The author also found that 135 glomera were associated with the tympanic branch of the glossopharyngeal nerve (Jacobson's nerve), and 113 with the auricular branch of the vagus nerve (Arnold's nerve).[34]

The histologic structure of the tympanic bodies is one of nests of polygonal darkly staining cells (chief cells) and a heavy vasculature (Fig. 2-32). There is a rich innervation of nonmyelinated nerve fibers of parasympathetic origin.[34] A variety of other cells have been described, mainly by electron microscopy.[35]

## ACKNOWLEDGMENTS

I am indebted to Mr. A. Frohlich for the technical work that is the necessary background for many of the descriptions and illustrations of this chapter.

## REFERENCES

1. Baker RD: Post Mortem Examination. Specific Methods and Procedures. WB Saunders, Philadelphia, 1967
2. Schuknecht HF: Pathology of the Ear. Harvard University Press, Cambridge, MA, 1974
3. Johnsson LG, Hawkins JE: A direct approach to cochlear anatomy and pathology in man. Arch Otolaryngol 85:599, 1967
4. Michaels L, Wells M, Frohlich A: A new technique for the study of temporal bone pathology. Clin Otolaryngol 8:77, 1983
5. Iurato S, Bredberg G, Bock G: Functional Histopathology of the Human Audio-vestibular Organ. Euro-data Hearing Project. Commission of the European Communities, 1982
6. Karnovsky MJ: A formaldehyde-glutaraldehyde fixative of high osmolality for use in electron microscopy. J Cell Biol 27:137A, 1965
7. Perry ET: The human ear canal. Charles C Thomas, Springfield, IL, 1957
8. Michaels L: Pathology of cholesteatoma: a review. J R Soc Med 72:366, 1971
9. Lim DJ, Shimada T, Yoder M: Distribution of mucus—secretory cells in the normal middle ear mucosa. Arch Otolaryrgol 98:2, 1973
10. Tos M, Bak-Pedersen K: Goblet cell population in the pathological middle ear and Eustachian tube of children and adults. Ann Otol Rhinol Laryngol 86:209, 1977
11. Aschan G: The Eustachian tube. Histologic findings under normal conditions and in otosalpingitis. Acta Otolaryngol (Stockh) 4:295, 1954
12. Michaels L, Wells M: Squamous carcinoma of the middle ear. Clin Otolaryngol 5:235, 1980
13. Phelps PD, Lloyd GAS: Radiology of the Ear. Blackwell Scientific Publications, Oxford, Boston, 1983
14. Sadé J: Middle ear mucosa. Arch Otolaryngol 84:137, 1966
15. Lim DJ, Shimada T, Yoder M: Distribution of mucus-secretory cells in the normal middle ear mucosa. Arch Otolaryngol 98:2, 1973
16. Akaan-Penttila E: Middle ear mucosa in newborn infants. A topographical and microanatomical study. Acta Otolaryngol (Stockh) 93:251, 1982
17. Eckert-Mobius A: Microscopische Untersuchungstechnic und Histologie des Gehörorgans. p. 211. In Denker A, Kahler O (eds): Die Krankheiten des Gehörorgans. Erste Teil. Handbuch der Hals-Nasen-Ohren Heilkunde. Julius Springer, Berlin, JF Bergmann, Munich, 1926
18. Anson BJ, Donaldson JA: Surgical Anatomy of the Temporal Bone. 3rd Ed. WB Saunders, Philadelphia, 1981
19. Graham MD, Reams C, Perkins R: Human tympanic membrane—malleus attachment. Preliminary study. Ann Otol Rhinol Laryngol 87:426, 1978
20. Glorig A, Davis H: Age, noise and hearing loss. Ann Otol Rhinol Laryngol 70:556, 1961
21. Etholm B, Belal A: Senile changes in the middle ear joints. Ann Otol Rhinol Laryngol 83:49, 1974
22. Bolz EA, Lim DL: Morphology of the stapediovestibular joint. Acta Otolaryngol (Stockh) 73:10, 1972
23. Davies DV: A note on the articulations of the auditory ossicles and related structures. J Laryngol Otol 62:533, 1948
24. Dubowitz V, Brooke MH: Muscle Biopsy: A Modern Approach. WB Saunders, Philadelphia, 1973
25. Anderson SD: Peripheral aspects of the physiology of middle ear muscles. Symp Zool Soc Lond No. 37:69, 1975
26. Veggetti A et al: A comparative histochemical study of fibre types in middle ear muscles. J Anat 135:333, 1982

27. Lyon MJ, Malmgren LT: A histochemical characterization of muscle fiber types in the middle ear muscles of the cat. 1. The stapedius muscle. Acta Otolaryngol (Stockh) 94:99, 1982

28. Portmann M, Sterkers JM, Charachon R, et al: The internal auditory meatus. Anatomy, pathology and surgery. Churchill Livingstone, New York, 1975

29. Guild SR, Crowe SJ, Bunch CC, Polvogt LM: Correlations of differences in the density of innervation of the organ of Corti with differences in the acuity of hearing, including evidence as to location in the human cochlea of the receptors for certain tones. Acta Otolaryngol (Stockh) 15:269, 1934

30. Schuknecht HV: Further observations on the pathology of presbycusis. Arch Otolaryngol 80:369, 1964

31. Jorgensen MB: Changes of aging in the inner ear. Histological studies. Arch Otolaryngol 74:56, 1961

32. Watanuki K, Sato M, Kaku Y, et al: Reissner's membrane in human ears. Acta Otolaryngol (Stockh) 91:65, 1981

33. Arenberg IK, Marowitz WF, Shambaugh GE: The role of the endolymphatic sac in the pathogenesis of endolymphatic hydrops in man. Acta Otolaryngol [Suppl] (Stockh) 275, 1970

34. Guild SR: The glomus jugulare, a non-chromaffin paraganglion in man. Ann Otol Rhinol Laryngol 62:1045, 1953

35. Zak FG, Lawson W: The paraganglionic Chemoreceptor System. Physiology, Pathology, and Clinical Medicine. Springer-Verlag, New York, 1982

# Surgical Anatomy of the Ear and Temporal Bone

# 3

Malcolm D. Graham
Jack M. Kartush

The safety that comes of boldness and skill in surgical work cannot be attained without accurate anatomical knowledge. The surgical treatment of most of the bones of the skeleton have long been scientifically and successfully carried out before the minds of surgeons were awakened to a clear perception of the fact that in disease of the temporal bone the same systematic surgical treatment was equally applicable and even more urgently called for. The earlier operations on the temporal bone lacked the real basis of anatomical and pathologic knowledge, and in consequences were halting in execution and failures in result. Now, however, the temporal bone has been brought within the field of ordinary surgical practice. Consequently, many details which a few years ago were of purely anatomical interest are now matters of cardinal importance to the surgeon. A clear appreciation of the anatomy of the living temporal bone not only frees the surgeon from anxiety during the operation, but enables him to forecast and to follow the paths along which infection may spread through the bone.

—Sir Charles A. Ballance (1919)[1]

## TEMPORAL BONE ANATOMY

The paired temporal bones each articulate with the respective sphenoid, parietal, zygomatic and occipital bones, and each contributes to the middle and posterior cranial fossae.

Each temporal bone comprises four parts: mastoid, squamous, petrous, and tympanic.

### Superior Surface of the Temporal Bone

The superior surface of the temporal bone, although irregular, is generally featureless (Fig. 3-1). Usually a prominence, termed the arcuate eminence is apparent, which has an intimate but somewhat varying relationship to the superior semicircular canal.[2] The petrous ridge forms the attachment for the tentorium. The hiatus for the greater superficial petrosal nerve allows passage of

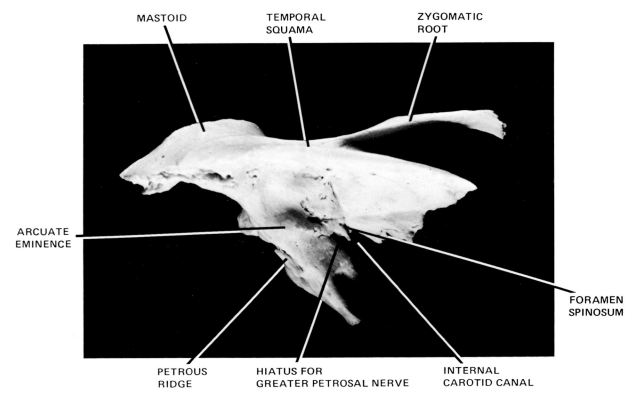

MASTOID   TEMPORAL SQUAMA   ZYGOMATIC ROOT

ARCUATE EMINENCE

FORAMEN SPINOSUM

PETROUS RIDGE   HIATUS FOR GREATER PETROSAL NERVE   INTERNAL CAROTID CANAL

**Fig. 3-1.** Surface anatomy of left temporal bone from above.

this nerve as it approaches the geniculate ganglion. Near the apex of the petrous portion of the temporal bone, the canal for the internal carotid artery is seen, and on the medial surface of the squamoustemporal bone, the impressions of branches of the middle meningeal artery are visible.

A full and accurate appreciation of the soft tissues and bony landmarks of the superior surface of the temporal bone are essential for the surgeon contemplating middle cranial fossa procedures.

## Lateral Surface

The lateral surface of the temporal bone is most familiar to the otologic surgeon (Fig. 3-2). Most operations on the tympanic membrane, middle ear, mastoid, vestibular labyrinth, and internal auditory canal are performed via this approach.

A postauricular incision readily reveals the mastoid cortex and, with slight anterior dissection, the spine of Henle, MacEwans' triangle, and the temporal line are readily observed. These landmarks allow identification of the underlying mastoid antrum. The temporal line marks the attachment of the temporal fascia and thus the inferior limits of the temporalis muscle.

The tympanic bone, although substantial inferiorly, is deficient superiorly, its anterior and posterior free edges forming the tympanosquamous and tympanomastoid sutures, respectively. Between these two suture lines, the skin of the external auditory canal is thick, vascular, and loosely attached to the underlying bone and is referred to surgically as the "vascular strip."

## Inferior Surface

The inferior surface reveals the carotid canal anteriorly and the impression for the jugular bulb posteriorly, separated by a bony ridge (Fig. 3-3).

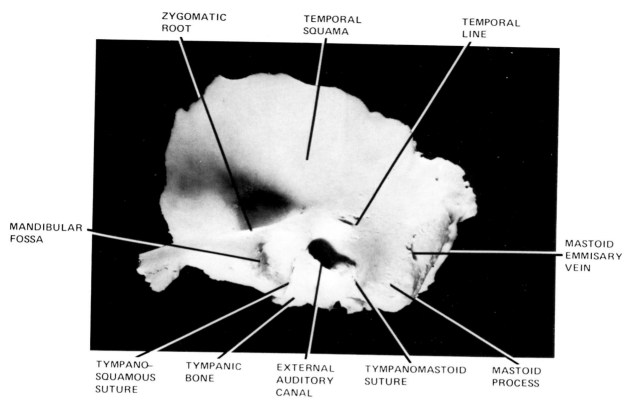

ZYGOMATIC ROOT

TEMPORAL SQUAMA

TEMPORAL LINE

MANDIBULAR FOSSA

MASTOID EMMISARY VEIN

TYMPANO-SQUAMOUS SUTURE

TYMPANIC BONE

EXTERNAL AUDITORY CANAL

TYMPANOMASTOID SUTURE

MASTOID PROCESS

**Fig. 3-2.** Surface anatomy of lateral aspect of temporal bone.

The mastoid tip is prominent, with the digastric muscle medially.

The styloid process is readily noted, with the stylomastoid foramen medially — the exit passage for the facial nerve.

### Anterior Surface

Knowledge of the anatomy of the petrous apex allows a clear understanding of the relationships between the internal carotid artery and the petrous apex air cell system medially and with the eustachian tube and semicanal for the tensor tympani muscle laterally (Fig. 3-4). Further laterally is the mandibular fossa, and superior to the carotid artery lies the hiatus for transit of the greater superficial petrosal nerve. The foramen spinosum, which lies

lateral to the eustachian tube and allows passage of the middle meningeal artery, is unclear because it lies within the line of disarticulation of the temporal bone from the remainder of the cranium.[3]

### Medial Surface

Retrolabyrinthine and suboccipital approaches to the cerebellopontine angle require an indepth knowledge of the anatomy of the medial temporal bone surface (Fig. 3-5). The internal auditory canal is divided laterally by vertical and horizontal crests. The jugular bulb lies below the internal auditory canal at a variable level occasionally separated by only 2 or 3 mm of bone. The endolymphatic sac lies just below and posterior to the operculum.

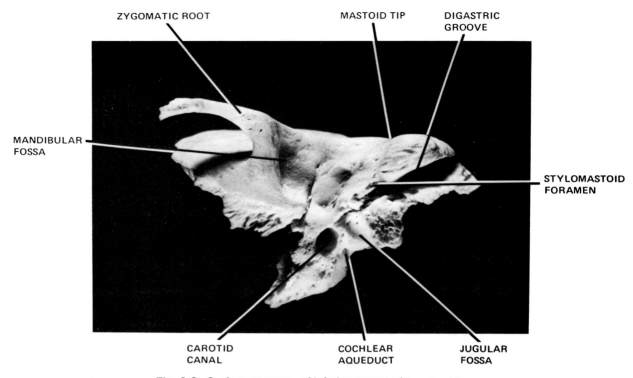

**Fig. 3-3.** Surface anatomy of inferior aspect of temporal bone.

ZYGOMATIC ROOT

MASTOID TIP

DIGASTRIC GROOVE

MANDIBULAR FOSSA

STYLOMASTOID FORAMEN

CAROTID CANAL

COCHLEAR AQUEDUCT

JUGULAR FOSSA

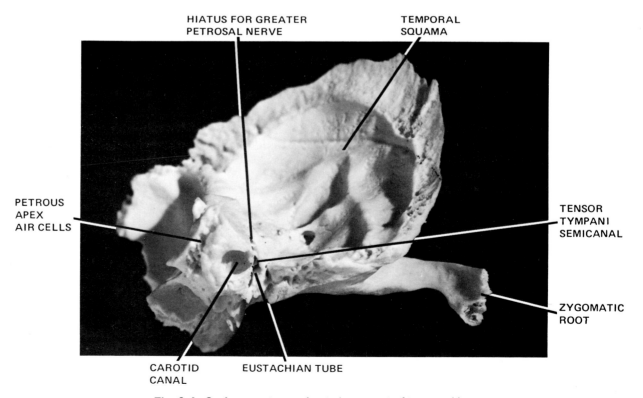

**Fig. 3-4.** Surface anatomy of anterior aspect of temporal bone.

HIATUS FOR GREATER PETROSAL NERVE

TEMPORAL SQUAMA

PETROUS APEX AIR CELLS

TENSOR TYMPANI SEMICANAL

ZYGOMATIC ROOT

CAROTID CANAL

EUSTACHIAN TUBE

70

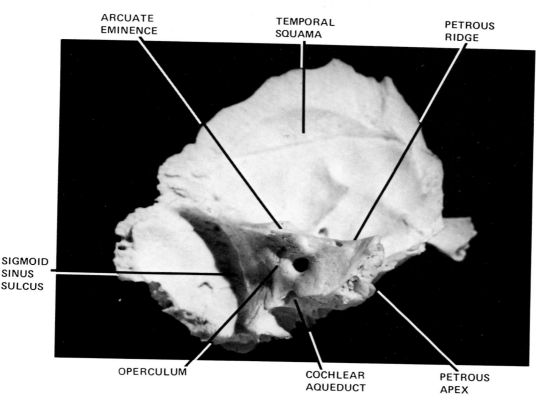

**Fig. 3-5.** Surface anatomy of medial aspect of temporal bone

## SURGICAL ANATOMY OF STRUCTURES WITHIN THE TEMPORAL BONE

### From Above

Surgical exposure of the temporal bone from the middle cranial fossa approach is considered by many otologic surgeons to be the most difficult technical procedure of all otologic operations.

The surgeon is seated at the patients' vertex and looks down on the floor of the middle cranial fossa (Fig. 3-6). Dura is elevated medially with the temporal lobe. Anteriorly, the middle meningeal artery arising from the foramen spinosum is visualized, and medially the greater superficial petrosal nerve. The dura is then elevated from behind forward, the dissector sweeping over the arcuate eminence and freeing the dura to its tentorial attachment along the petrous ridge. The internal auditory canal may be encountered by following the greater superficial petrosal nerve posteriorly toward the geniculate ganglion and subsequently following the labyrinthine portion of the facial nerve medially, posteriorly, and inferiorly until it enters the internal auditory canal. An alternative method is to skeletonize the superior semicircular canal, which lies at a 60 degree angle to the internal auditory canal after the method of Fisch. If the tegmen of the middle ear and antrum are removed, the ossicles, horizontal facial nerve, middle ear eustachian tube orifice, and the medial surface of the tympanic membrane can be readily visualized. The basal turn of the cochlea, the internal carotid artery, and the petrous apex marrow or air cell system is located anterior to the internal auditory canal.[5]

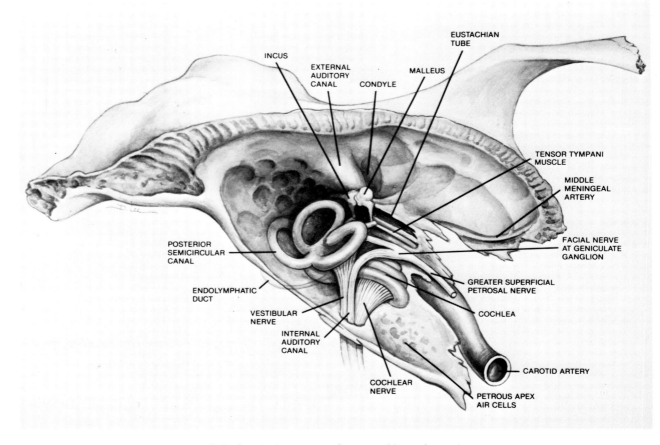

**Fig. 3-6.** Surgical anatomy of temporal bone from above.

## Lateral

The surface of the mastoid cortex should be removed of all soft tissue. With a large cutting burr, the cortex is removed, saucerizing the cavity and beveling over the middle fossa plate and the sigmoid sinus (Fig. 3-7). The sinodural angle is developed, and staying high and posterior, the mastoid antrum is exposed. Posterior bony canal wall is thinned, the zygomatic root of air cells developed, and the epitympanum exposed. The incus and head of the malleus are exposed, as is the facial recess, which gives good visualization of the stapes and the incudostapedial joint. The horizontal portion of the facial nerve passes superior to the stapes and inferior to the horizontal semicircular canal, mak-

ing a turn inferiorly at the genu. Then the posterior bony canal wall is removed as well as the posterior half of the tympanic membrane. The middle ear can be seen clearly, including the eustachian tube orifice, round and oval windows, promontory, and chorda tympani.

## SURGICAL ANATOMY OF THE FACIAL NERVE

For a complete visualization of the course of the intratemporal facial nerve, examination of the tem-

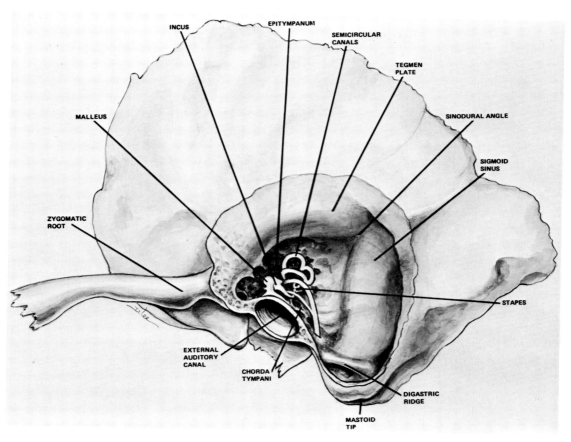

**Fig. 3-7.** Surgical anatomy of lateral temporal bone.

poral bone from the middle cranial fossa approach must complement examination via the lateral approach.

The facial nerve enters the internal auditory canal in the anterior superior compartment and immediately enters the labyrinthine facial nerve canal anterior to the vertical crest, or Bill's bar. The nerve passes anteriorly, laterally, and superiorly above the labyrinth, where it abruptly turns posteriorly and inferiorly into the middle ear. At this turn, or genu, the geniculate ganglion is found attached to the anterior surface of the facial nerve. As it passes into the middle ear, the nerve courses superiorly to the cochleariform process, stapes, and oval window and inferior to the horizontal semicircular canal (Fig. 3-8). Once it enters the mastoid segment, the nerve turns abruptly inferiorly

toward the stylomastoid foramen, where it exists to pass anteriorly and laterally into the parotid gland. The facial nerve sheath begins in the anterior middle ear, distal to the geniculate ganglion, and becomes progressively thicker to a maximum at the stylomastoid foramen.

## SURGICAL ANATOMY OF THE INTERNAL AUDITORY CANAL

The facial nerve enters the internal auditory canal in the anterior superior compartment to traverse the temporal bone and exit at the stylomas-

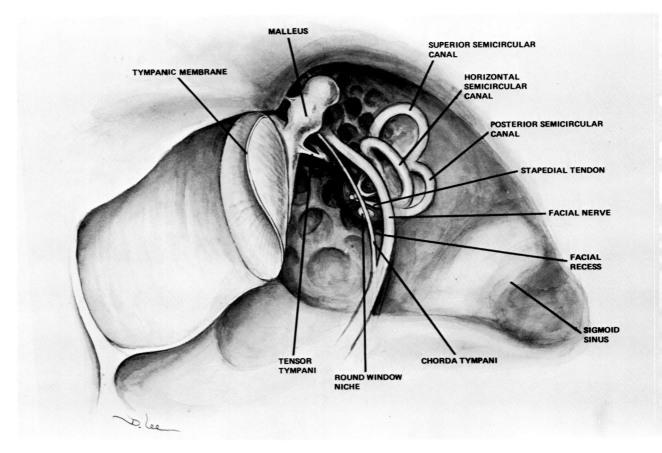

**Fig. 3-8.** Surgical anatomy of the tympanic and mastoid facial nerve.

toid foramen (Fig. 3-9). The vestibular and cochlear nerves also enter the internal auditory canal to supply the labyrinth. The superior vestibular nerve lies in the posterior superior compartment, and the inferior vestibular nerve lies in the posterior inferior compartment, sending a branch within the internal auditory canal, the singular nerve, to enter the singular foramen. The cochlear nerve lies in the anterior inferior compartment. Laterally, in the fundus of the internal auditory canal, the transverse crest separates the superior from inferior compartments, and set more laterally in the superior compartment is the vertical crest, or Bill's bar. The internal auditory canal has a posterior lip, roof, and floor but lacks an anterior lip.

## BLOOD SUPPLY OF THE LABYRINTH AND MIDDLE EAR

The arteries to the middle ear and ossicles are derived from branches of the external carotid system via the superior, inferior, anterior, and posterior tympanic arteries. The otic labyrinth is partly supplied by a single vessel of the internal auditory artery, a branch of the anteroinferior cerebellar artery from the basilar artery. This artery passes through the internal auditory canal and divides into three branches. The first of these is the vestibular

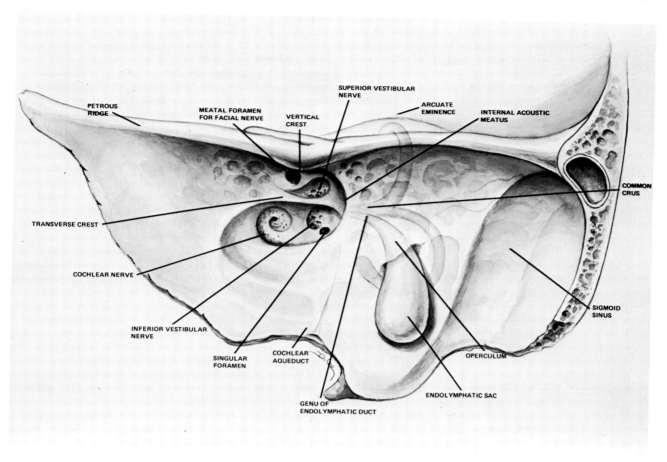

**Fig. 3-9.** Anatomy of internal auditory canal and medial right temporal bone.

artery, which supplies the vestibular nerve and parts of the saccule, utricle, and semicircular canals. The second branch is the vestibulocochlear artery, which supplies the basal turn of the cochlea, the greater part of the saccule, the body and lower part of the utricle, posterior semicircular canal, and parts of the lateral and superior semicircular canals. The third branch is the cochlear artery, which enters the modiolus, where it gives rise to the spiral arteries.

The venous drainage of the labyrinth is accomplished by three main veins and their branches, which ultimately drain into the lateral sinus.[6]

## MAJOR VESSELS RELATED TO THE TEMPORAL BONE

There are several venous sinuses adjacent to the temporal bone, the sinuses of the dura, the emissary veins to the mastoid, and sigmoid sinus.

The superior petrosal sinus runs from the cavernous to the sigmoid sinus and is enveloped by the attachment of the tentorium to the petrous ridge of the temporal bone. The inferior petrosal sinus also runs from the cavernous sinus and enters the anterior surface of the jugular bulb. The transverse (lateral) sinus runs anteriorly toward the mastoid process, where it turns inferiorly as the sigmoid sinus. The sigmoid sinus terminates at the internal jugular vein.[7]

The mastoid emmisary vein may be quite large and enters the mastoid emissary foramen posterior to the sigmoid sinus.

The carotid artery ascends in the neck and enters the inferior surface of the temporal bone, where it rapidly makes a sharp turn anteriorly toward the petrous apex and cavernous sinus. As it ascends in the middle ear, it forms the medial wall of the eustachian tube and passes medial to the tensor tympani muscle in its semicanal.

## CRANIAL NERVES RELATED TO TEMPORAL BONE

Cranial nerves 7 and 8 enter the internal auditory canal directly and have been discussed previously. Cranial nerves 3, 4, 5, 6, 9, 10, 11, and 12 enter the posterior cranial fossa, butting on or immediately adjacent to the temporal bone. The 3rd, 4th, and 6th cranial nerves enter the cavernous sinus adjacent to the petrous apex, whereas the 5th cranial nerve ganglion (Gasserian ganglion) lies on the apex of the petrous apex of the temporal bone before it branches into its three main divisions. The 9th, 10th and 11th cranial nerves exit the posterior fossa through the petro-occipital fissure and enter the pars nervosa of the jugular foramen prior to descending into the lateral neck. The 12th cranial nerve exits the cranium via the hypoglossal foramen, passes between the internal carotid artery and jugular bulb, descends in the neck, and passes to the carotid vasculature to innervate the tongue.[8]

## CONGENITAL ANOMALIES

The two parts of the hearing organ arise from different embryonic origins. The sensory labyrinth is derived from the ectodermal otocyst, whereas the sound-conducting system comes from the branchial or gill apparatus. Because of this very complex embryologic origin, it is not surprising that congenital anomalies may occur.

Auricular hypoplasia, external auditory canal atresia, and tympanic membrane absence or hypoplasia are relatively frequently encountered, whereas anomalies of the facial nerve and inner ear are far less common.

The mechanism by which these congenital malformations occur is largely unknown. Rubella toward the end of the first trimester of pregnancy has previously been implicated, and a significant number of anomalies were traced to the administration of thalidomide between 1959 and 1962.

Although these congenital anomalies may occur in successive generations within a single family, they generally occur as random, unilateral or bilateral events.[9]

## TEMPORAL BONE DEVELOPMENT WITH AGE

At birth the hearing mechanism is fully formed and of adult size, excluding the external auditory canal, which lacks a bony external auditory canal. The infants temporal bone consists of a relatively large squamous portion, which occupies the lateral inferior surface of the skull. The tympanic portion is an incomplete sulcus just large enough to support the annulus tympanicus, and there is no mastoid process. The antrum is well formed at birth; however, because the mastoid process is absent, the facial nerve emerges from the stylomastoid foramen onto the lateral surface of the skull, where it can be injured by the usual vertical postauricular incision. The mastoid process begins to develop during the second year of life by downward extension of the squamous portion to conceal the petrous portion and form the mastoid tip. The petrous portion of the temporal bone in the newborn varies from that of an adult. On the middle fossa surface of the newborn, the facial canal is not yet covered by bone in the region of the geniculate ganglion, and on the posterior surface there exists a large subarcuate fossa beneath the arch of the superior semi-circular canal. The lateral growth of the tympanic portion and mastoid process assume a vertical position in the adult. The stylomastoid foreamen and facial nerve are therefore deep and protected by the mastoid process.

## SUMMARY

The temporal bone harbors the organ of hearing and equilibrium. It is in intimate relation with the cerebrum and cerebellum. It is hallowed out for, or in close contact with, the lateral, sigmoid, petrosal, and cavernous sinuses, and the bulb of the internal jugular vein. It is tunneled for the internal carotid artery, and, like other bones, it is permeated with a network of minute vessels. It contains a complicated system of cavities lined with mucous membrane continuous with that of the pharynx. No wonder, then, that grave and even fatal illness should so often follow when the temporal bone is attacked by infective disease. (Ballance CA: Surgery of the Temporal Bone. Macmillan and Co. Ltd, 1919.)

## REFERENCES

1. Ballance CA: Surgery of the Temporal Bone. Macmillan and Company, Ltd., London 1919
2. Kartush, JM et al: The arcuate eminence: an anatomic review of its relationship to topographic orientation and middle fossa surgery. Ann Otol Rhinol Laryngol 94:25, 1985
3. Anson BJ, Donaldson JA: Surgical Anatomy of the Temporal Bone. WB Saunders, Philadelphia, 1981
4. Kartush JM, et al: Anatomic basis for labyrinthine preservation during posterior fossa acoustic tumor surgery. Laryngoscope 96:1024, 1986.
5. Pernkopf E: Atlas of Topographical and Applied Human Anatomy. WB Saunders, Philadelphia, 1963
6. Bast TH, Anson BJ: The Temporal Bone and the Ear. Charles C Thomas, Springfield, IL, 1949
7. Graham MD: The jugular bulb: its anatomic and clinical considerations in contemporary otology. Laryngoscope 87:105, 1977
8. Shaia FT, Graham MD: The hypoglossal nerve: its relationship to the temporal bone and jugular foramen. Laryngoscope 87:1137, 1977.
9. Shambaugh GE, Glasscock, ME: Surgery of the Ear. WB Saunders, Philadelphia, 1980

# Ultrastructure of the Middle and Inner Ear

# 4

Ivan M. Hunter-Duvar
Robert V. Harrison

Studies of the structure of the peripheral auditory system have progressed according to the technological development of microscopic techniques; our present knowledge, and therefore, this review, is largely based on transmission and scanning electron microscopic investigations. However, it is appropriate to recognize the pioneering contributions of early light microscopists. For example, early descriptions of tympanic membrane and middle ear structures were made by Shrapnell (1832),[1] Prussak (1867),[2] Rüdinger (1870),[3] Gerlach (1875),[4] and Politzer (1899).[5] The names of many early explorers of cochlear anatomy are familiar: Corti (1851),[6] Claudius (1856),[7] Hensen (1863),[8] Boettcher (1869),[9] and Retzius (1884).[10] Held (1926)[11] and Kolmer (1927)[12] completed detailed descriptions of the organ of Corti as seen by light microscopy. Early descriptions of the vestibular sense organs were made by Scarpa (1800),[13]

Schultze (1858),[14] and Odenius (1867),[15] followed by the systematic studies of Retzius (1884)[10] and Held (1909).[16]

With the introduction of transmission electron microscopy, more detailed studies were possible. Ultrastructural studies on the cochlea and vestibular system include those, for example, by Engström and Wersäll,[17] Engström et al.,[18] Wersäll,[19] Spoendlin,[20] Iurato,[21] Bredberg,[22] and Kimura.[23]

The development of the scanning electron microscope gave a new perspective to the study of the inner ear. The first of such investigations was made by Barber and Boyle (1968)[24] and have been followed by a number of detailed studies, for example, by Lim,[25,26] Bredberg et al.,[27] Hunter-Duvar,[28,29] Hunter-Duvar and Hinojosa,[30] Lindeman,[31] Smith and Tanaka,[32] and Harada.[33] This chapter draws on information obtained in many of these latter studies.

## THE MIDDLE EAR

### The Tympanic Membrane

From the pinna, the external auditory canal, about 2.5 cm long in adult man, leads to the tympanic membrane. The peripheral portion of the canal is formed with cartilaginous support and its dermal lining contains hair follicles and associated sebaceous glands. Sebaceous glands accumulate fatty material in their cytoplasm, and dead cells are cast off as sebum. Also present are modified apocrine glands (sudoriferous glands), secretions from which mix with sebum to form wax. Toward the tympanic membrane, the canal is bony with a thin dermal layer (Fig. 4-1).

In humans, the tympanic membrane is slightly conical in shape with an elliptic circumference. Along its major (vertical) axis it measures 9 to 10 mm, and its horizontal diameter is 8.5 to 9 mm.[34] Its total surface area is about 85 mm², but only an area of 55 mm² is normally displaced by sound waves.[35] In the central pars tensa area, the membrane is composed of radial and circular collagenous fibers, but these are interrupted in an area known as the pars flaccida, which is above its attachment to the manubrium of the malleus. The radial, fibrous layer radiates from the lower four-fifths of the manubrium of the malleus to the peripheral annulus of the tympanic membrane. The circular fiber layer arises partly from the short process of the malleus and partly from the manubrium of the malleus. This layer becomes more dense toward the annulus. The collagenous fiber layers are bounded by connective tissue layers and constitute the lamina propria of the tympanic membrane. The lamina propria is covered externally by an epidermal layer of stratified squamous epithelium, which is continuous with the skin of the external canal. This epidermis consists of a number of identifiable layers. the stratum cornium, stratum granulosum, stratum spinosum, and stratum basale. These components are shown in Figure 4-2, which is a cross-section of the

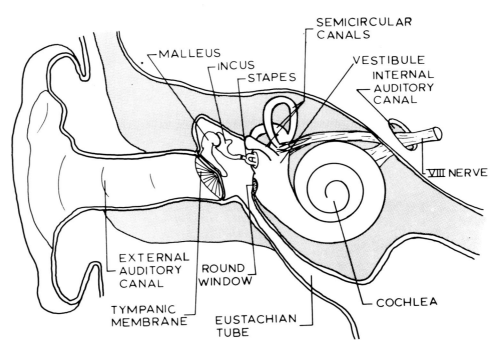

**Fig. 4-1.** Diagrammatic cross-section of the human outer, middle, and inner ear as viewed from the front. Bone is shown by the shaded area.

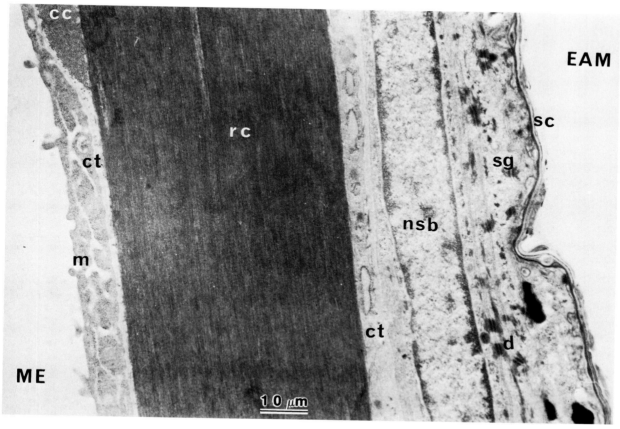

**Fig. 4-2.** Cross-section of pars tensa region of the tympanic membrane (guinea pig) as seen by transmission electron microscopy. The external auditory meatus *(EAM)* is to the right, the middle ear cavity *(ME)* to the left. Radial collagenous fibers *(rc)* and circular collagenous fibers *(cc)* are bounded by connective tissue *(ct)*. A mucosal epithelium *(m)* covers the internal surface. The epidermal layer is made up of stratum corneum *(sc)*, stratum granulosum *(sg)*, and stratum basale. The micrograph shows a large nucleus of this basal layer *(nsb)*. Also note desmosomes *(d)* between cells of the epidermal layer. (Courtesy of Dr. M. Hawke, Department of Otolaryngology, University of Toronto).

tympanic membrane of the guinea pig. The stratum granulosum contains keratin granules associated with fine cytoplasmic filaments attached to desmosomes. The latter are evident throughout the epidermal layer. The internal surface of the tympanic membrane is lined with a mucosal layer of ciliated squamous cells, some with an obvious centriole.

The pars flaccida is thicker than the pars tensa. Its lamina propria consists of irregularly arranged collagen and elastic fibers and many capillaries together with myelinated and unmyelinated nerve fibers. The epidermis is composed of 5 to 10 layers of desquamating epithelial cells. The mucous

membrane on the internal side is formed of simple squamous cells.

A number of detailed electron microscopic studies of tympanic membrane structure have been made in the guinea pig, [36,37] which has a structure similar to that of humans. [38]

## The Middle Ear Cavity

The middle ear (tympanic) cavity is approximately 2 cm³ in volume measuring about 15 mm anteroposteriorly and having a transverse diameter of 2 to 6 mm. The middle ear includes an upper cavity, the epitympanic recess, the roof of which is a thin plate of bone separating it from the middle cranial fossa. The epitympanum accommodates the head of the malleus and the short process of the incus. Much of its upper wall is an anchor point for ligaments that support the malleus.

Toward the lower (inferior) wall of the middle ear cavity is the eustachian tube orifice and the point of attachment for the tensor tympani muscle. The medial wall of the main cavity contains the oval and round window niches of the cochlea and the opening of the tympanic sinus. The latter lies between the bony labyrinth medially and the pyramidal eminence laterally. A hollow in the pyramidal eminence accommodates the stapedius muscle.

The middle ear cavity develops embryologically from the upper respiratory tract,[39] and its mucous membrane is somewhat similar to that of the respiratory tract. In electron microscopic studies,[40] five types of cells are found in the mucosa of the middle ear. These are (1) nonciliated cells without secretory granules, (2) nonciliated cells with secretory granules (including goblet cells), (3) the ciliated cells, (4) intermediate cells, and (5) basal cells. The distribution of cells is not uniform; ciliated cells are more abundant toward the lower (posterior) areas of the cavity.[41] The mastoid cavity has mainly simple cuboidal or squamous epithelium, although occasionally there are ciliated cells. The epitympanum has taller epithelial cells, which are often ciliated. The promontory has secretory and nonsecretory columnar cells, some ciliated cells and occasionally goblet cells.

A comprehensive description of the innervation and blood supply to the middle ear cavity is given by Schuknecht.[42]

## The Auditory Ossicles

Sound vibrations are transmitted from the tympanic membrane to the cochlear oval window by three auditory ossicles, namely the malleus, incus, and stapes (Fig. 4-3).

The malleus has a head, neck, lateral process, anterior process, and manubrium; the last attaches it to the tympanic membrane. It is the largest of the ossicles and weighs approximately 25 mg. The malleal head articulates with the body of the incus and is joined by incudomalleal ligaments. These articular surfaces are incompletely cartilaginous. The incus has a short process, which is attached to the fossa incudis; its long leg has a lenticular process at its end, which forms the incudostapedial joint. This joint has largely cartilaginous articular surfaces but becomes partly bony in adult life.

The stapes is the lightest of the ossicles, weighing about 3 mg. There are four main parts; the head, the posterior and anterior crura (bony struts), and the footplate. The footplate is flat, it covers the oval window to form the stapediovestibular articulation, which is held together by the annular ligament. The ossicles are held in position by ligaments to the malleus and incus as well as by the annular ligament.

## Middle Ear Muscles

The action of the ossicles is modified by two muscles: the tensor tympani and the stapedius. The tensor tympani is approximately 25 mm long. It lies mostly within a bony channel alongside the eustachian tube and arises from the superior wall of that channel as well as from the cartilage of the eustachian tube. Muscle fibers converge to form the tendon of tensor tympani, which turns laterally 90 degrees at the cochleariform process and attaches to the superior surfaces of the manubrium and the neck of the malleus. Muscle contraction draws the manubrium medially and puts tension on the tympanic membrane.

The tensor tympani is a typical striated muscle, with no smooth muscle fibers. The muscle fibers are relatively thick in humans with diameters between 5 and 32 $\mu$m. In the transition region between muscle and tendon, individual muscle fibers insert into tendonous fibers in a quill-like pattern. Fat globules are often present between muscle and tendon fibers in this region. The muscle fibers are richly supplied with mitochondria, which are often in bags formed by a bulging sarcolemma. The muscle receives its blood supply from the superior tympanic artery, a branch of the maxillary artery reaching the middle ear through the petrosquamous fissure. Rich innervation of tensor tympani is

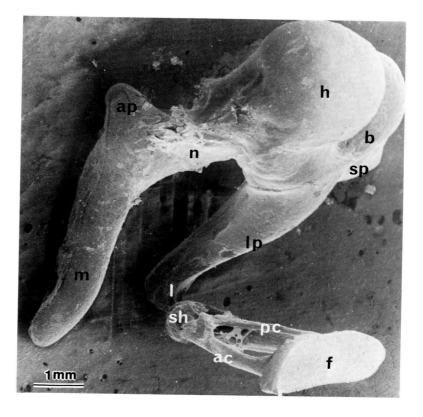

**Fig. 4-3.** Scanning electron micrograph of human middle ear ossicles. The malleus is made up of the head *(h)*, neck *(n)*, anterior process *(ap)*, and manubrium *(m)*. Parts of the incus are the body *(b)*, short process *(sp)*, long process *(lp)*, and lenticular process *(l)*. The main parts of the stapes are the footplate *(f)*, anterior crus *(ac)*, posterior crus *(pc)*, and the stapedial head *(sh)*.

from the mandibular branch of the trigeminal nerve.

The stapedius muscle lies in the hollow of the pyramidal eminence and arises from within this bony sulcus. The muscle has a length of only 6 mm. Muscle fibers converge into a round tendon, which attaches to the upper portion of the posterior crus of the stapes. Muscle contraction draws the anterior edge of the stapes footplate laterally.

The stapedius is the smallest striated muscle in mammals. Like the tensor tympani, the fibers contain an abundance of mitochondria, which accumulate in groups under the sarcolemma and in the motor endplate regions. It receives its blood supply from the posterior tympanic artery, a branch of the stylomastoid artery. The rich motor innervation of the stapedius muscle is by a branch of the facial nerve. The motor units are smaller than most muscles, indicating a fine regulation of muscle tension. There is some indication of sensory endings in the stapedius in the form of muscle spindles; however, the sensory innervation is not clearly understood.

There is a rich adrenergic plexus around the blood vessels of both tensor tympani and stapedius muscles. This adrenergic innervation originates at the superior cervical ganglion. A comprehensive review of middle ear muscle structure is provided by Densert and Wersäll.[43]

## The Round Window Membrane

The membrane of the round window is located at the base of the cochlea and separates the scala tympani from the middle ear cavity. The membrane has an epithelial layer on the middle ear side, then middle and inner layers. The epithelial layer is continuous with the mucous membrane over the promontory and consists of a single layer of regularly patterned flat cells. However, unlike the epithelium of the promontory, there are no cilia on the round window epithelium. The middle layer is formed by connective tissue, which includes fibrous cells, collagenous fibers, and elastic fibers.

The fibrous cells contain little cytoplasm and few intracellular organelles. Both collagenous and elastic fibers run across the minor axis of the round window. Between these large parallel strands are coarse and fine fibers which appear to connect the parallel ones together. Studies of the inner surface by scanning electron microscopy indicate a few layers of cells, the processes of which contact each other.

## The Eustachian Tube

The eustachian tube is about 35 mm long in adults. The osseous portion of the tube opens into the tympanic cavity at its anterior wall. The ostium measures 3 to 5 mm in diameter, gradually narrowing along its length. The epithelium of the tube is of ciliated columnar cells with an abundance of goblet cells. Below this layer the tunica propria consists of a basement membrane and loose connective tissue. The proximal portion of the tube is supported with crooked-shaped hyaline cartilages. Normally, the tube lumen is held passively closed by the cartilage and also by surrounding tissue pressure. During swallowing or yawning, three muscles, the tensor veli palati, levator veli palati, and the salpingopharyngeus, act to rotate and pull open the cartilages and, thus, the eustachian tube.[44] The most important muscle is the tensor veli palatini, which is innervated by the mandibular division of the trigeminal nerve. There have been several electron micrograph studies of the mucous membrane of the eustachian tube.[40,41,45,46] Lim and his colleagues[46] give a particularly good description. The lining consists of a mucous membrane of ciliated columnar epithelium interspersed with goblet cells and three layers of the tunica propria, namely a basement membrane, a lymphoid tissue layer, and a region containing compound tubuloalvealor glands. The surface of the ciliated columnar cell is lined with microvilli and cilia having classic 9 + 2 filamentous structure. At the base of each cilium is a basal foot; in each cell, basal feet are oriented in the same direction. Accumulations of glycogen granules are found in supra- and infranuclear areas, and a well-developed Golgi complex and scattered mitochondria are typical features. Adjacent epithelial cells are linked with desmosomes. Through-

out most of the tube, ciliated cells are dense, and their cilia are long and probably serve for clearance of debris. Mature goblet cells are of the classic goblet shape, with mucigen granules filling the extranuclear cytoplasm. The granules lose their limiting membranes as they migrate to the free cytoplasmic surface and are secreted into the eustachian tube lumen. Desmosomal structures bind the goblet cells to adjacent cells. Toward the pharyngeal portion, the epithelium has an increased number of nonciliated cells with short microvilli. These are simple squamous epithelial cells with few mitochondria, poorly developed Golgi apparatus, and no secretory granules. Toward the tympanic cavity there is a transition from columnar ciliated cells to simple cuboidal cells with fewer cilia. These cells have glycogen granules near the nucleus that are similar in distribution to those in the columnar cells. Together with these ciliated cells are cells containing numerous dark, large granules (1,500 to 2,700 Å; but smaller and denser than those of goblet cells). These cells have a Golgi apparatus and an abundant endoplasmic reticulum. At the eustachian tube orifice, these cell types give way to the simple squamous epithelium of the middle ear proper.

---

## THE INNER EAR

The mammalian inner ear consists of a series of membranous sacs and ducts (the membranous labyrinth) enclosed in a shell of bone (osseous labyrinth), which itself is largely embedded in the hard temporal bone. The membranous labyrinth is schematically illustrated in Figure 4-4. It contains the vestibular and auditory sensory epithelia and is largely filled with endolymph. Endolymph has an ionic composition similar to that found intracellularly (notably high potassium ion and low sodium ion concentrations). Between the membranous and osseous labyrinth is perilymph, which is high in sodium and low in potassium and is, therefore, similar to extracellular and cerebrospinal fluid.[47] To maintain the ionic differences between endolymph and perilymph, the membranous labyrinth is

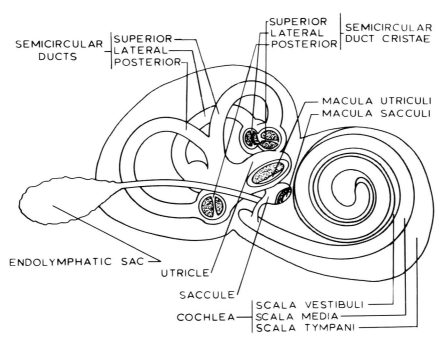

**Fig. 4-4.** Diagram of the inner ear showing the relative positions of the sensory epithelia. The endolymph-filled membranous labyrinth is shown unshaded.

bounded by epithelial layers having numerous occluding tight junctions.[48]

The vestibule of the labyrinth contains the macula sacculi, located in the spherical recess, and the macula utriculi in the elliptic recess. The sensory epithelia of these two otolithic organs are at right angles to each other. In humans, with head upright, the macula sacculi is in the vertical plane, and the utricle is in a horizontal plane. The size and shapes of the otolithic organs vary according to species.

Leading posteriorly from the vestibule are the semicircular canals. Each of the three canals makes two-thirds of a circle, and each has a plane approximately at right angles to the other two. The canals are 1 mm in diameter, and each opens up at one end into an ampulla containing the sensory epithelium. The nonampullated ends of the superior and posterior semicircular canals join at a common crus.

The spiral canal of the cochlea lies anteriorly to the vestibule. In humans, its axial length is about 5 mm, and the basal turn is about 10 mm across. Uncoiled, it measures approximately 35 mm and has just over $2\frac{1}{2}$ turns around the central modiolus.

The membranous labyrinth connects with the endolymphatic sac via a duct (the vestibular aqueduct) that lies in a bony niche on the posterior surface of the petrous bone and is in contact with the dura mater of the posterior fossa. The perilymphatic spaces of the bony labyrinth connect with the cerebrospinal fluid filled subarachnoid space via the fine cochlear aqueduct. This duct opens into the scala tympani at the base of the cochlea.

**The Cochlea**

Figure 4-5A is a scanning and Figure 4-5B is a cross-section view of the mammalian cochlea. The spiral cochlea is divided into three spaces: the scala vestibuli and scala tympani, which are filled with perilymph, and the scala media, which is part of the endolymphatic system. The scala media, its membranous boundary together with the sensory epithelium and supporting structures (organ of Corti) are sometimes collectively termed the membranous cochlear duct. The basal end of this duct

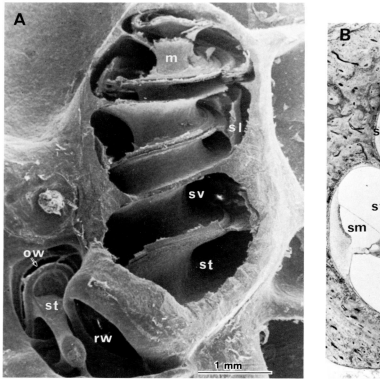
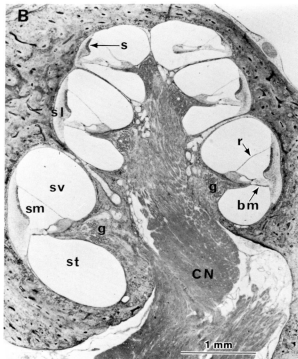

**Fig. 4-5. (A)** A scanning electron micrograph (chinchilla) and **(B)** a cross-sectional view (cat) of the cochlea. The round window *(rw)*, oval window *(ow)*, and stapes *(st)* are seen in **A**. The cochlear duct is separated into the scala tympani *(st)*, scala media *(sm)*, and scala vestibuli *(sv)* by Reissner's membrane *(r)* and the basilar membrane *(bm)*. Stria vascularis *(s)* is supported by the spiral ligament *(sl)*. Cochlear nerve fiber cell bodies are in the spiral ganglion *(g)*; their axons congregate within the modiolus *(m)* as the cochlear nerve *(CN)*.

(vestibular caecum) communicates with the saccule via the ductus reuniens. At the cochlear apex, the cochlear duct ends blindly; scala vestibuli and scala tympani join at the helicotrema.

Figure 4-6 is a scanning electron micrograph of the cochlear partition (chinchilla). In fixation, the tectorial membrane has shrunk back to reveal the reticular lamina of the organ of Corti and the outer and inner hair cell stereocilia.

### Reissner's Membrane

The cochlear duct is separated from scala vestibuli by Reissner's membrane, a thin (2 to 3 μm) membrane extending from the spiral limbus to the vestibular crest of the spiral ligament. The position of the membrane is most clearly seen in the cochlear cross-section of Figure 4-5B. Figure 4-7A shows a high magnification of part of Reissner's membrane. In the adult, it consists of two cellular layers: a single layer of polygonal epithelial cells on the scala media side and a flat mesothelial cell layer on the scala vestibuli side. Figure 4-7B is a scanning electron micrograph of this mesothelial surface. The cells have round nuclei, a little endoplasmic reticulum close to the nucleus, and a very thin, irregular layer of cytoplasm that appears to be discontinuous. Between the two cell layers is a basement membrane about 0.25 μm in thickness. On the endolymphatic surface there are numerous microvilli, particularly toward the osseus spiral lamina. The epithelial cells are bonded to each other

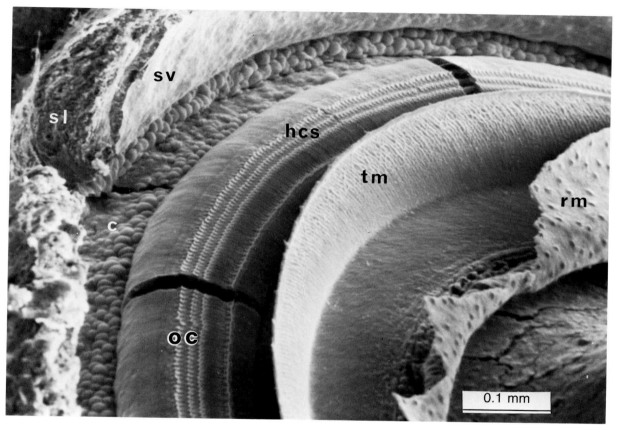

**Fig. 4-6.** Scanning electron micrograph of the surface of the (chinchilla) organ of Corti *(oc)*. The tectorial membrane *(tm)* has retracted due to fixation and reveals the hair cell stereocilia *(hcs)*. Part of Reissner's membrane *(rm)* remains. Outside the sensory epithelium are Claudius cells *(c)*. The stria vascularis *(sv)* is shown, supported by the spiral ligament *(sl)*.

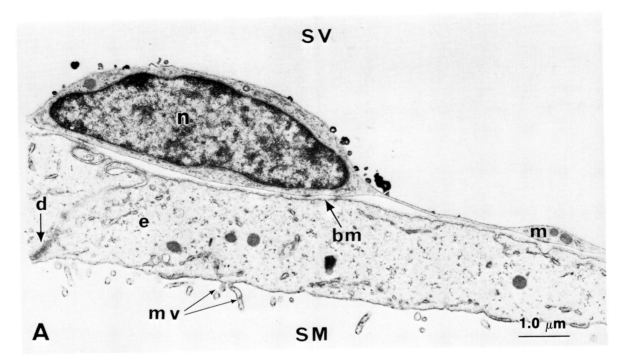

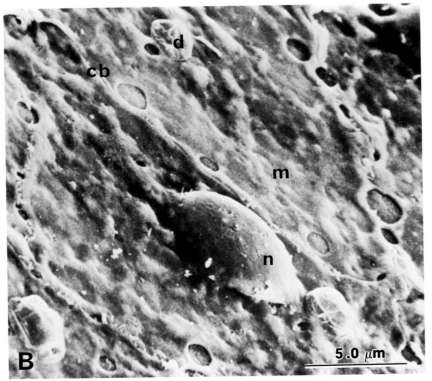

**Fig. 4-7. (A)** A transmission electron micrograph cross-section of Reissner's membrane. On the side of scala vestibuli *(SV)* is a thin mesothelial cell layer *(m)*. On the scala media *(SM)* side is an epithelial layer *(e)* with cells joined by tight junctions or desmosomes *(d)*. This epithelial surface is covered in microvilli *(mv)*. The two cell layers are separated by a basement membrane *(bm)*. *n*, cell nucleus. **(B)** A scanning electron micrograph of the mesothelial surface of Reissner's membrane showing the cell nucleus region *(n)* and the cell borders *(cb)*. There is often some debris *(d)* attached to the membrane. mesothelium *(m)*.

by numerous desmosomes (tight junctions, or zonula occludens). The cytoplasm of the epithelium is relatively thick with well-developed endoplasmic reticulum and Golgi complexes. There are numerous pinocytotic vesicles in the membrane, and in animals with cochlear damage there are large number of lysosomes in the epithelial layer, suggesting a possible role in endocytosis of cochlear debris.[49]

## The Tectorial Membrane

The tectorial membrane is an acellular matrix essentially composed of filaments, fibrils, and a homogeneous ground substance. It extends from the interdental cell region of the spiral limbus to the outer margin of the reticular lamina. In the unfixed state, the membrane appears to be a soft gel, the thickness of which increases from the base to apex of the cochlea. The fine structure of the membrane has been extensively studied by Iurato[50] and Lim.[51]

The outer zone of the tectorial membrane consists of a marginal band and a marginal net *(Randfasernetz)*, which is attached to the outermost row of Deiters cells or Hensen cells. Whether the outer margin forms a complete seal with the reticular lamina is not clear; there may be species differences in the extent of the attachment. The main body of the membrane is occupied by fibers that radiate from the inner zone inclined at about 30 degrees toward the apical turn of the cochlea. These fibers are 100 to 130 Å in diameter. Toward the outer margins of the tectorial membrane, the fibers run longitudinally. The fibers originate and terminate in a more dense homogeneous substance. Covering the surface of the fibrous layer is a covering net (Fig. 4-8A). On the underside a more homogeneous basal layer is present. Hensen's stripe is seen on the undersurface near the position of the inner hair cells (Fig. 4-8B). Small trabeculae may serve to anchor the tectorial membrane to the inner hair cell region of the organ of Corti. Hardesty's membrane occurs in the outer hair cell region (Fig. 4-8B). The fine structure of the tectorial membrane is much influenced by fixative and staining procedures used in its examination.

Recently, it has been suggested that the tectorial membrane consists only of (proto) fibrils without any homogeneous substance.[52] Two basic types of protofibrils have been described. Type A are straight, unbranched, about 100 Å thick, and constitute the middle zone of the tectorial membrane. Type B are branched, coiled 150 to 200 Å thick, and make up the marginal zone, covering net, and Hensen's stripe.

It is now clear that the tallest row of stereocilia of the outer hair cells may contact the tectorial membrane closely. The evidence for this is the observation by scanning electron micrography (Fig. 4-8B and C) of a W-shaped pattern of hollows on the underside (Hardesty's membrane) of the tectorial membrane.[51,53,54] It has been shown that such markings can persist (after hair cell degeneration), and this could represent an embryologic artifact.[54,55] It is less clear whether a similar attachment exists between the tectorial membrane and the inner hair cell stereocilia. If any contact exists, it is less firm than that with the outer hair cell stereocilia.

A useful review of tectorial membrane structure and function is given by Steel.[56]

### The Basilar Membrane

The cochlear duct is bounded on the scala tympani side by the basilar membrane, which is attached medially to the modiolus and laterally at the spiral ligament. The membrane is composed of fibrous material, ground substance, mesothelial cells, and some capillaries. The division between the basilar membrane and the organ of Corti is clear; the cells of the organ have a plasma membrane that appears to directly contact the inner surface of the basilar membrane. The membrane can be divided into two portions: the pars tecta (arcuate zone) extends from the region of the habenula perforata under the tunnel of Corti to the duct of the outer pillar cells. The pars pectinata stretches from outer pillar cells to the spiral ligament. Pars tecta consists of a band of radially directed fibrils 180 to 250 Å in diameter, which form a compact and uniform layer embedded in homogeneous ground substance. In the pars tecta, blood capillaries (vas spiralis) supported by coarse fibers may run longitudinally beneath the tunnel of Corti. In the pars pectinata, the membrane has two distinct fibrous layers (Fig. 4-9A). Of these two layers, the uppermost is situated immediately beneath the plasma membrane of the organ of Corti and has a

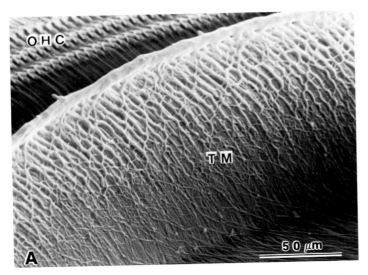

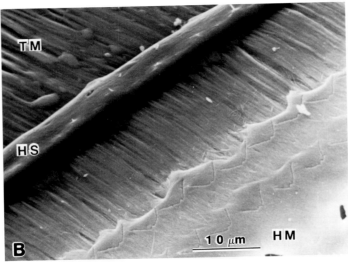

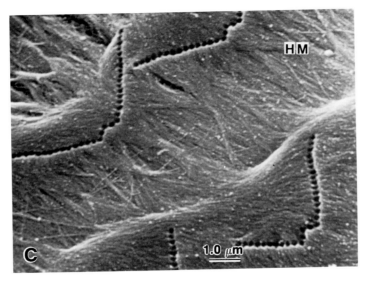

**Fig. 4-8. (A)** Scanning electron micrograph of the upper surface of the tectorial membrane *(TM)* showing the fibrous nature of the covering net. *OHC,* outer hair cells. **(B,C)** Scanning micrographs of the underside of the tectorial membrane *(TM)* showing Hensen's stripe *(HS)* and Hardesty's membrane *(HM)*. Hardesty's membrane bears clear W-shaped impressions corresponding to the tops of the tallest outer hair cell stereocilia.

**Fig. 4-9. (A)** Electron micrographic cross-section through the basilar membrane (pars pectinata) of the chinchilla. The section was made tangential to the cochlear spiral; thus, the upper radial fibers *(urf)* and lower radial fiber *(lrf)* lying in the homogeneous ground substance *(hgs)* are cut in cross-section. The large nuclei of the tympanic covering layer *(tcl)* are evident on the scala tympani *(ST)* side of the membrane, and on the upper side the Claudius cells *(c)* rest on a thin basement membrane *(m)*. **(B)** Scanning electron micrograph of the tympanic covering layer *(tcl)*. Just under and running perpendicular to this layer are the radial fibers *(rf)* of the basilar membrane.

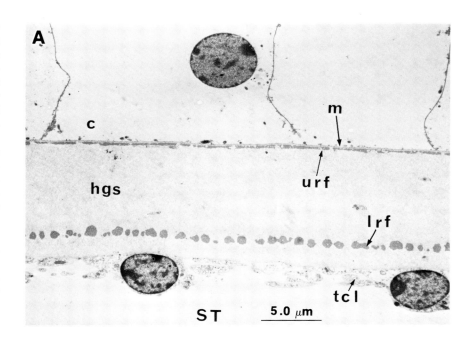

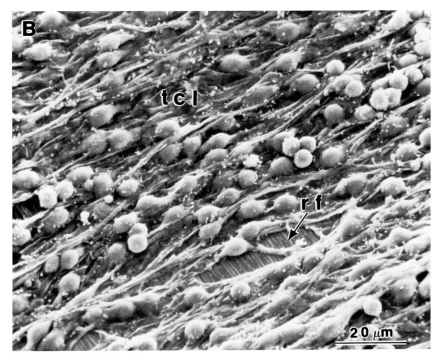

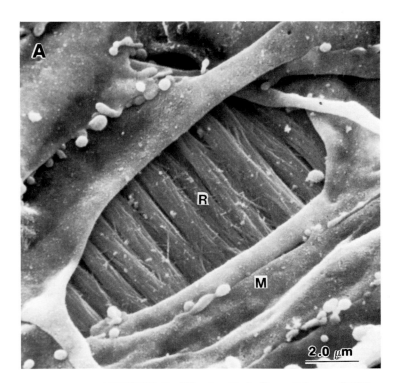

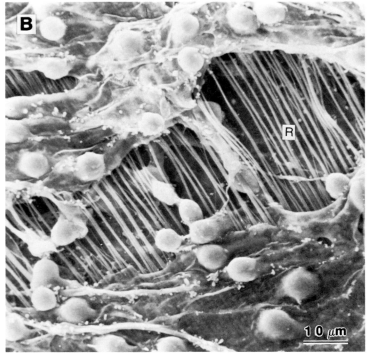

**Fig. 4-10.** Scanning electron micrographs of the tympanic surface of the basilar membrane at the base of the cochlea **(A),** compared with an apical turn **(B).** At the base, the mesothelial cells *(M)* of the tympanic covering layer and the radial fiber bundles *(R)* are more densely packed than at the apex.

depth of 600 to 800 Å. It is separated from the deeper and coarser layer by an (upper) homogeneous layer of unstructured matter. The lower fibrous layer is made up of numerous fibers, the larger of which tend to anastomize to some extent with each other. At the spiral ligament, the upper and lower fibrous layers join together. Both layers are made up of fibers ranging in size from 50 to 300 Å in diameter, which are often rectangular or diamond-shaped in cross-section. Under the lower fibrous layer, there is a second (lower) homogeneous layer of unstructured material. On the tympanic surface of the basilar membrane are the elongated

mesothelial cells of the tympanic covering layer (Fig. 4-9B). In the lower cochlear turns, these cells are longitudinally arranged, but in the apical turn they may also be orientated in a radial direction. The cytoplasm of the cells shows no unusual organization. It contains scattered mitochondria, free ribosomes, and small Golgi complexes. The structure of the basilar membrane shows graded differences along the cochlear length (Fig. 4-10A and B). Thus, at the base, fiber bundles are densely packed, as is the tympanic covering layer. Toward the apex, the fiber bundles and mesothelial cells are more loosely arranged.

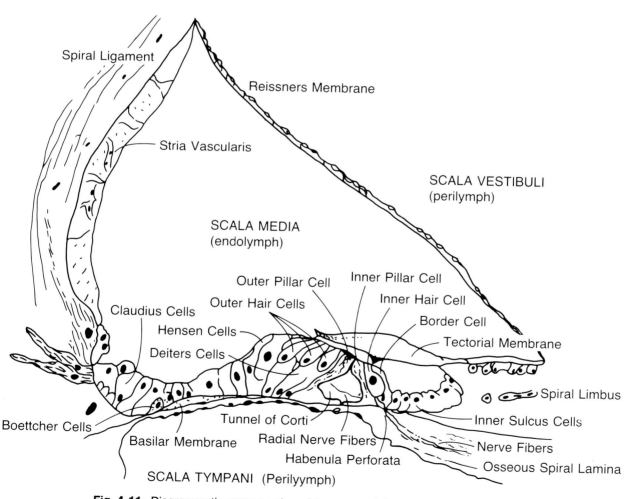

**Fig. 4-11.** Diagrammatic cross-section of the organ of Corti and related structures.

## The Organ of Corti

The organ of Corti[6] lies on the spiral basilar membrane and consists of sensory cells, supporting cells, and nerve fibers. A surface view of the (chinchilla) organ of Corti is given by the scanning electron micrograph in Figure 4-6. The tectorial membrane has lifted away from the reticular lamina to reveal the stereocilia of the hair cells. Along the length of the organ of Corti are two hair cell types, the inner hair cell forming one row and three to four rows of outer hair cells. In man, there are approximately 3,500 inner and 12,000 outer hair cells. Figure 4-11 shows a classic cross-sectional diagram of the organ of Corti and related structures. Each sensory and supporting cell type are described in detail in the following discussion.

**The Inner Hair Cells.**   The inner hair cell is flask shaped with a narrow apical region and a large cell body that is inclined toward the tunnel of Corti. The length of the inner hair cell is more or less constant throughout the cochlea. The cuticular surface is oval, with its long axis parallel to the cochlear length. A small area of the cell's apical surface is free of cuticle and in this area a basal body is usually found with a centriole just below it. During embryonic development, the inner hair cell has a kinocilium, which later disappears. The cuticular plate is 1 to 2 $\mu$m thick and supports the rootlets of approximately 60 sensory hairs or stereocilia. The scanning micrograph (Fig. 4-12A) shows the arrangement and size of stereocilia on the cuticular surface. These stereocilia extend to various lengths, depending on their position on each cell and on their cochlear location. The diameter of the stereocilia averages 0.1 $\mu$m and ranges up to 0.3 $\mu$m. The fibrous cores of the stereocilia penetrate the cuticular place as thin rootlets that sometimes reach the cytoplasm of the cell. The stereocilia (of all hair cell types) contain a number of structural proteins including actin and fimbrin, the latter cross linking the actin to form stiff filaments. In the cuticular plate, other proteins are present, including myosin. The presence of actin and myosin implies the possibility that a contractile mechanism may be important to the hair cell transduction process.[57]

A transmission electron microscopic cross-section through an inner hair cell is shown in Figure 4-12B. The cell is supported at its apex by the top of the inner pillar cells and the border cells of the inner sulcus. Below the cuticular plate, the intra-cuticular region is characterized by a well-developed endoplasmic reticulum and many mitochondria. Thin tubules extend from directly below the cuticle into the body of the hair cell, possibly down to the synaptic area.

In the region above the nucleus, there are many well-developed Golgi complexes and occasional lysosomes. Toward the outer wall of the cell is a single discontinuous membrane. This cell membrane is not as structured as that of the outer hair cell. The nucleus is spherical with one or two nucleoli. Near the nucleus, a few ribosomal cisterna are evident with associated groups of mitochondria. In general, mitochondria are round and scattered throughout the cytoplasm in contrast to the outer hair cells, where they are grouped in more specific regions.

The base of each inner hair cell contacts about 20 afferent nerve endings of inner radial fibers. These fibers come from the spiral ganglion via the habenula perforata, at which point they become unmyelinated. The afferent nerve endings contain some microtubule structures and large mitochondria. Their synapses with the hair cells are evident by thickenings of the postsynaptic membrane with less obvious thickening of the presynaptic membrane. The synaptic gap is typically about 145 Å. Associated with the presynaptic membrane (of the hair cell) are accessory synaptic vesicles up to 0.08 $\mu$m in diameter. Dense-cored vesicles are infrequent. There are few efferent endings contacting inner hair cells. Within the spiral plexus, below the sensory cells, radial afferent dendrites cross efferent inner spiral fibers. The latter are generally thin (0.1 $\mu$m) with swellings, filled with synaptic vesicles, which make contact with the afferent dendrites. These efferent synaptic regions contain small mitochondria and many densely cored vesicles. Details of the innervation pattern of the cochlea are given elsewhere (Chapter 5).

**The Outer Hair Cells.**   The outer hair cells are of cylindrical form and obliquely oriented (Fig. 4-13). Their length is position dependent; at the cochlear apex they are longer than toward the base of the cochlea. The sensory cells are supported at the apical cuticular region by the reticular membrane, and

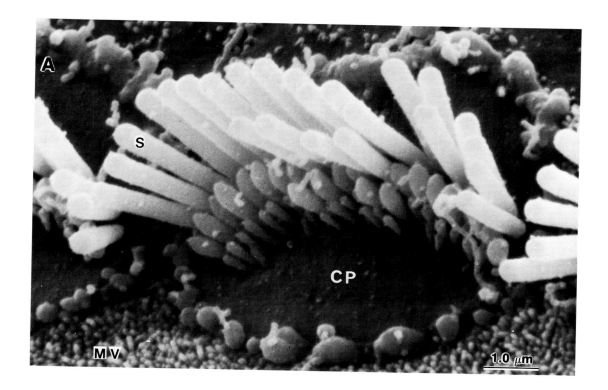

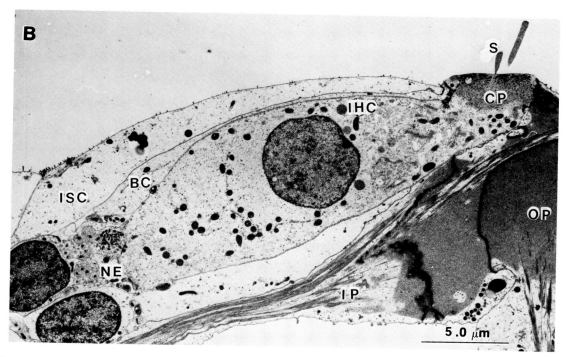

**Fig. 4-12.** **(A)** Scanning micrograph showing the arrangement of stereocilia *(s)* on the apical surface of an inner hair cell. *CP*, cuticular plate; *MV*, microvili of supporting cell. **(B)** Transmission micrograph through an inner hair cell *(IHC)* and supporting cells: *BC*, border cell; *IP*, inner pillar cell; *ISC*, inner sulcus cell; *OP*, outer pillar cell. The stereocilia *(S)* can be seen inserted into the cuticular plate *(CP)* at the cell apex. Mainly afferent nerve endings *(NE)* are seen in the synaptic area at the base of the cell.

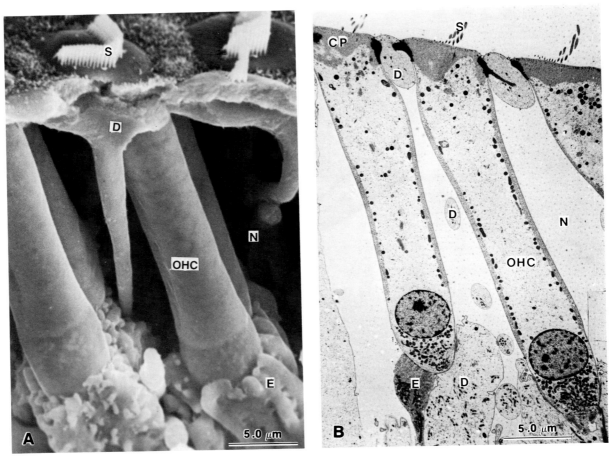

**Fig. 4-13. (A)** Scanning and **(B)** transmission micrographs of the outer hair cells *(OHC)*, their supporting Deiters cells *(D)*, and nerve endings *(E)*. The stereocilia *(S)* insert into the cuticular plate *(CP)* at the top of each cell. The sensory cells are almost totally surrounded by the extracellular space of Nuel *(N)*.

at their base they rest on supporting Deiters cells. The cuticular region is sealed into the reticular lamina with tight junctions (zonula occludens). The hair cells are, thus, almost entirely surrounded by extracellular (Nuel's) space. A dense cuticular plate holds 50 to 150 stereocilia arranged in W-shaped rows (Fig. 4-14). The stereocilia are largest in the outermost row (away from the modiolus); medially, their size tapers off. The average length of the stereocilia depends on cochlear position; thus, at the apex the largest are more than 6 $\mu$m long and at the base less than 2 $\mu$m. The number of stereocilia on outer hair cells decreases from coch-

lear base to apex. For example, in the squirrel monkey each cell has about 135 in basal turn, reducing to 80 in the third turn. Each stereocilium is club shaped, being narrow near to the cuticular plate (1,300 Å) and wider near the tip (3,200 Å). Between the stereocilia is an extensive array of cross-linkages. A large number of horizontal cross-links join stereocilia of the same and different rows together laterally, some distance below their tips. Also, the tip of each shorter stereocilium on the hair cell gives rise to a fine extension that joins the taller stereocilium of the next row. These features are best seen using glutaraldehyde fixation without

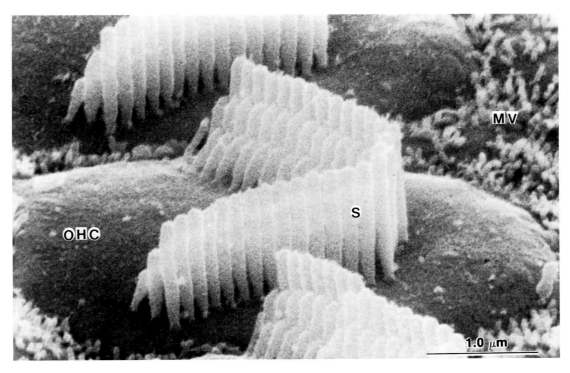

**Fig. 4-14.** The arrangement of stereocilia *(S)* at the surface of an outer hair cell *(OHC)*. The cell is surrounded by supporting cells having numerous microvilli *(MV)*.

osmium postfixation. A basal body and an underlying centriole is present in a gap in the cuticular plate. In some primate species, vestigial remains of a kinocilium can be found.

The stereocilia are covered by a thin plasma membrane. Each has a cylindrical core, and a dense, tubelike rootlet extends from the central core. The protoplasm contains long macromolecular fibers running the length of the hair, with a similar fibrillar structure in the core and rootlet. The cuticular plate is of a dense fibrillar material with a highly organized structure in the zone surrounding the stereocilia rootlets. As in the inner hair cells, actin and myosin proteins have been identified in these regions and these proteins have a structural and, possibly, a contractile role.[57]

The intracuticular region is rich in mitochondria and endoplasmic reticulum (Fig. 4-13B). The concentration of the latter is often termed the Hensen body. Lysosomes are found in increasing numbers relative to age or ototoxic damage. Glycogen-containing granules are found throughout the hair cell but particularly in the infracuticular region. The cell is bounded by a plasma membrane, and inside this run one or two discontinuous membranes making up subsurface cisternae. These are always 300 to 400 Å from the plasma membrane. Associated with these structures are large numbers of glycogen granules and mitochondria.

The outer hair cell nucleus is round or oval in cross-section with a nucleolus and a delicate chromatin network. The infranuclear region contains much glycogen, numerous mitochondria, and a complex endoplasmic reticulum with ribosomes (Fig. 4-13B). There are thin filamentous or tubular structures extending from the infracuticular region to the synaptic region, becoming especially evident near the latter. These filaments resemble neurotubules of nerve axons.

The outer hair cells are in contact with both ef-

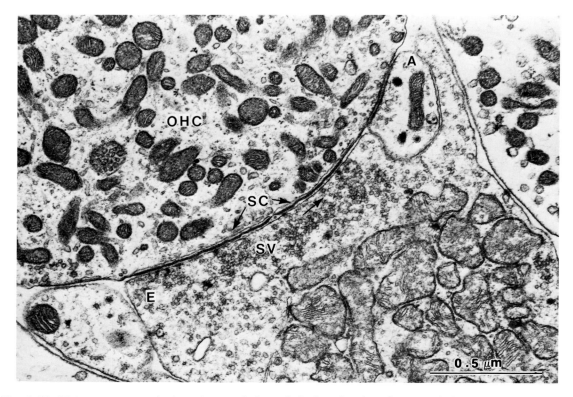

**Fig. 4-15.** High-power transmission micrograph through the basal region of an outer hair cell *(OHC)*. The figure shows a large efferent nerve ending *(E)* with presynaptic vesicles *(SV)* and subsynaptic cisternae *(SC)* on the hair cell side. A small bouton-like afferent synapse *(A)* is also shown with its characteristic thickening of both pre- and postsynaptic membranes and the lack of a subsynaptic cistern.

ferent and afferent nerve endings (Fig. 4-15). The efferent endings are those of the outer radial fibers. Their terminals are about 3 $\mu$m in diameter and, thus, larger than those of the afferents. In the basal turn of the cochlea, they are numerous in all rows of outer hair cells, but toward apical regions they progressively disappear from the peripheral rows of outer hair cells. Efferent endings may occur anywhere from the bottom of the hair cell to the level of the nucleus, as seen in the scanning micrograph of Figure 4-13A. The endings are rich in mitochondria, which tend to aggregate away from the synaptic gap. The endings also contain many vesicles, both of the small (300 to 400 Å) open-cored and larger (600 to 800 Å) dense-cored types (Fig. 4-15). The synaptic gap is typically about 190 Å wide. Associated with the efferent terminals are postsynaptic (hair cell) cisternae. These are evi-

dent in Figure 4-15. These subsynaptic cisternae are probably continuous with the subsurface system throughout the cell.

The afferent nerve endings are those of the outer spiral fibers and make up only about 10 percent of the afferent neurones in the spiral ganglion. Entering the cochlea at the habenula perforata, these fibers cross the tunnel close to the basilar membrane, turn at right angles at the Dieters cell region, and course some distance before contacting outer hair cells. The afferent synapse is small (1 $\mu$m) and boutonlike. At the site of the synapse, both plasma membrane and postsynaptic membrane are thickened, with a synaptic gap of about 150 Å (Fig. 4-15). There is no subsynaptic cisterna associated with the afferent synapse; however, there is often a synaptic bar or ring surrounded by small vesicles. Within the afferent nerve endings are vesicles of sizes similar to those found in the efferent endings; a few mitochondria are also evident.

**The Supporting Cells.** The sensory cells are supported by an elaborate system of cells. These were fully described by Retzius (1884)[10] and then Held (1926),[11] and more recently a detailed study has been made by Angelborg and Engström.[58] The cells clearly have a mechanical supporting function. To this end, pillar cells and Deiters cells contain a number of rigid structural proteins. The mechanical framework of the supporting cells seems well suited to transmit basilar membrane motion to the sensory region of the reticular lamina. The supporting cells may also serve a nutritive role.

**The Pillar Cells.** Transmission microscopy (Fig. 4-16) illustrates the supporting function of the pillar cells. The footplate of the inner pillar cell is anchored to the basilar membrane by an electron-

dense cementlike substance. From this base arises a slender (1 to 2 µm) but stiff cell body, which is filled with regularly arranged tubular tonofibrils and other microfilaments. At the surface of the organ of Corti is the head portion, which contacts with and supports the inner hair cells. The inner pillar cells also extend over the heads of the outer pillar cells and become the surface area of the pillar cells in the subtectorial space. The inner hair cells are surrounded and supported by the inner pillar cells and to a lesser extent the border cells of the inner spiral sulcus. On the modiolar side of the inner pillar cells are inner sulcus cells. These are relatively undifferentiated columnar cells with some microvilli at their free surface.

The outer pillar cells are similar in structure to the inner pillar cells in having a footplate giving rise to a supporting shaft. Near the surface of the organ of Corti, the head of the outer pillar attaches to the

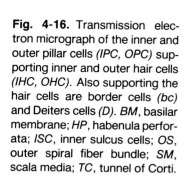

**Fig. 4-16.** Transmission electron micrograph of the inner and outer pillar cells *(IPC, OPC)* supporting inner and outer hair cells *(IHC, OHC)*. Also supporting the hair cells are border cells *(bc)* and Deiters cells *(D)*. *BM*, basilar membrane; *HP*, habenula perforata; *ISC*, inner sulcus cells; *OS*, outer spiral fiber bundle; *SM*, scala media; *TC*, tunnel of Corti.

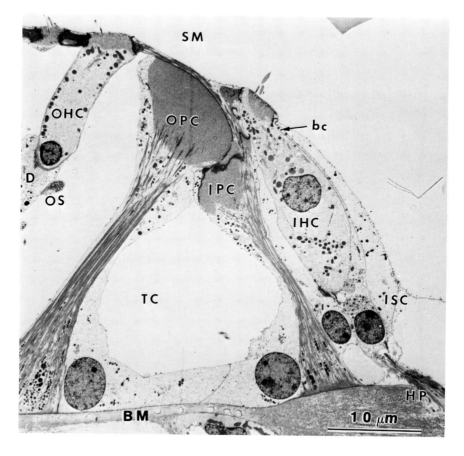

underside of the extensions of the inner pillar cell heads. They also extend between the tops of the first row of outer hair cells and form that portion of the reticular lamina.

For both inner and outer pillar cells and Deiters cells, the cell processes contain tubular tonofibrils with a diameter of about 275 Å as well as other microfilaments with a diameter of approximately 60 Å. The microtubules are bound to each other by thin bonds. One of the structural proteins of these microfibrils is actin.[57]

**Deiters Cells.** Deiters cells are attached to the basilar membrane below the outer hair cells and provide support for them. The main cell body and nucleus is below the hair cell level (Fig. 4-17). From this area arises a slender process containing tubular filaments and microfilaments similar to those found in the pillar cells. These filamentous structures appear to originate very near to the basilar membrane. At the surface of the organ of Corti, the cell forms a phalangeal process, which is part of the reticular lamina and supports the apical end of the second and third row of outer hair cells. The outer hair cell bodies are mainly surrounded by the fluid-filled spaces of Nuel. At the reticular surface, Deiters cells have abundant microvilli, especially at the cell borders. This contrasts with the pillar cells, which have relatively few microvilli.

**Hensen Cells.** Hensen cells are columnar cells lying next to the Deiters cells on the basilar membrane. They extend to the surface of the organ of Corti, where they have many microvilli (0.4 to 0.6 μm). The cells have generally few mitochondria and a poorly developed endoplasmic reticulum. In the guinea pig, toward the apical turn, Hensen cells are packed with large (5 to 10 μm in diameter) lipid granules. Adjacent Hensen cells have interdigitating plasma membranes and the cells contain pinocytotic vesicles. This, together with evidence that both Deiters and Hensen cells take up small particles, suggests that these cells may absorb cochlear debris.

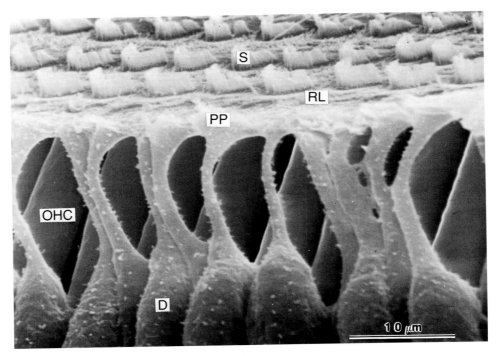

**Fig. 4-17.** Scanning micrograph showing the supporting function of the Deiters cells *(D)*. *OHC*, outer hair cells; *PP*, phalangeal process; *RL*, reticular lamina; *S*, stereocilia of OHC.

**Claudius Cells.** The organ of Corti is bounded on the strial side by the Claudius cells, which form a layer over the basilar membrane (Fig. 4-9A). These cells are not highly differentiated and have few mitochondria and microvilli. Toward the base of the cochlea, the Claudius cell area contains a group of so-called Boettcher cells forming a single cuboidal layer. These cells have invaginations and otherwise irregular contact with each other and with the basilar membrane, indicating a possible secretory or resorptive function. In addition, these cells contain numerous large granules and lysosomes.

### The Spiral Ligament

The spiral ligament forms the point of attachment of the basilar membrane with the cochlear wall and also supports the stria vascularis (Fig. 4-11). The major portion of the ligament is made up of loosely arranged connective tissue cells, fibrous bundles, and blood vessels. There are two main types of connective tissue cells (fibrocytes),

and these make many attachments with each other.[59] Areas near the stria vascularis and the spiral prominence are more cellular and contain large mitochondria. The spiral prominence is separated from the endolymphatic space by a surface epithelial cell layer.

### The Stria Vascularis

The stria is the major vascular area of the cochlea. It has three main layers: the marginal dark cell layer (chromophile), the intermediate light cell layer (chromophobe), and the basal cell layer. Within these layers runs a network of arterioles.

Figure 4-18 shows a cross-section of the stria vascularis from the chinchilla. The superficial stria is made up exclusively of the large marginal cells, which contain many mitochondria and have their nuclei close to the endolymphatic surface. There are numerous small microvilli on the endolymphatic surface. The cells have finger-like processes, which make intimate contact with the intermediate

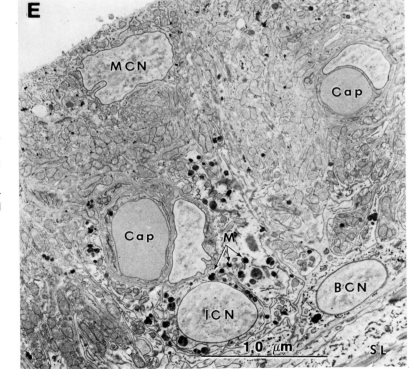

**Fig. 4-18.** Transmission micrograph of the stria vascularis of the chinchilla. *BCN*, basal cell nucleus; *Cap*, blood capillaries; *E*, endolymphatic space; *ICN*, intermediate cell nucleus; *M*, melanocytes; *MCN*, nucleus of marginal cell; *SL*, spiral ligament.

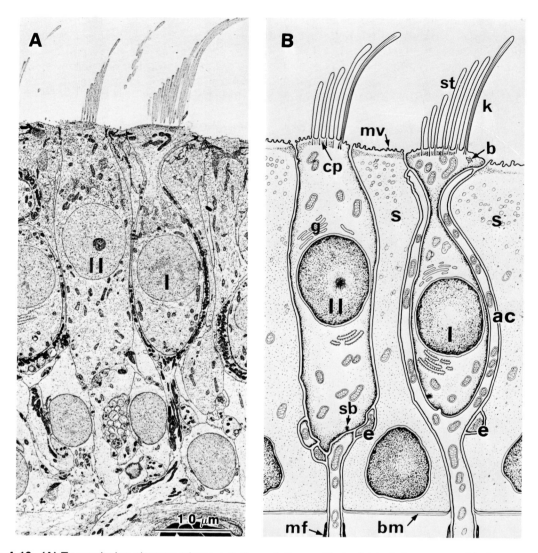

**Fig. 4-19. (A)** Transmission electron micrograph through the vestibular (utricular) sensory epithelium showing type I and type II hair cells. (Courtesy of Dr. R. Hinojosa, University of Chicago, Chicago, Illinois.) **(B)** Diagram of *A*. *ac*, afferent nerve chalice; *b*, basal body; *bm*, basement membrane; *cp*, cuticular plate; *e*, efferent nerve ending; *g*, Golgi complex; *k*, kinocilium; *mf*, myelinated nerve fiber; *mv*, microvilli; *S*, supporting cell; *sb*, synaptic body. *(Figure continues.)*

cells. These marginal cells constitute the major part of the stria. The cell bodies of the intermediate layer are smaller than those of the marginal cells. Cytoplasmic processes invade the marginal cells, and pinocytotic vesicles and melanin granules (within melanocytes) are common.

The basal cells opposite the spiral ligament are flat with long extensions into the intermediate and marginal cell layers. The cytoplasm of the basal cells is similar to the fibrocytes of the spiral ligament. The stria blood vessels have a continuous endothelial lining with an underlying basal lamina. The blood supply to the stria is from the spiral modiolar artery via vessels passing over scala vestibuli

## Vestibular Sense Organs

Vestibular sensory areas are found in the ampullae of each of the three semicircular canals, in the macula sacculi, and in the macula utriculi (Fig. 4-4). The three semicircular canals detect head rotation in space. The lateral canal lies close to the horizontal plane of the natural posture of the head, and the superior and posterior canals are in its vertical plane. These latter two vertical canals are joined in the crus commune. All three canals arise from the utricular sac, which provides fluid continuity for the canals as well as holding the utricular macula. The sensory epithelium of this organ lies in a horizontal plane and is used to detect the effects due to gravity and the static position of the head. Beneath and connected to the utricle is the saccule containing the vertically oriented saccular macula which has a role similar to that of the macula utriculi.

The vestibular system is innervated by the vestibular branch of the eighth cranial nerve. This is divided into superior and inferior branches. The superior branch supplies the superior and lateral canal cristae, the utricular macula, and part of the saccular macula. The inferior branch innervates the posterior canal crista and part of the saccular macula. The cell bodies of the afferent nerve fibers are contained in Scarpa's ganglion. Detailed descriptions of peripheral innervations have been made by Gacek.[64]

The sensory epithelia of all the vestibular organs contain two types of sensory cells[65] together with their blood supply, innervation, supporting cells, and accessory structures.[66,67] A detailed description of the type I and type II hair cells is given in the following sections; each vestibular organ is then considered separately.

### Type I Hair Cells

The type I sensory hair cell is flask shaped, having a rounded base, thin neck, and broader apical cuticular region. The shape and ultrastructure of the type I cell is illustrated in Figure 4-19. The cell body is almost totally surrounded by the afferent nerve chalice or calyx. One nerve ending sometimes encloses two or three adjacent or nonadjacent type I cells.

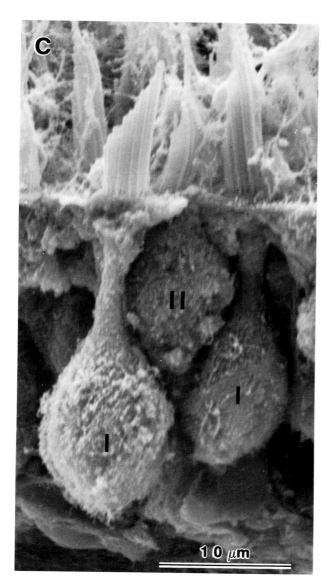

**Fig. 4-19** *(Continued).* **(C)** Scanning electron micrograph of the sensory epithelium showing type I and II hair cells.

to the lateral cochlear wall. Collecting venules in the wall of scala tympani return blood to the spiral modiolar vein. There are many detailed descriptions of the ultrastructure of stria vascularis[60–62] including studies of the vascular system.[63]

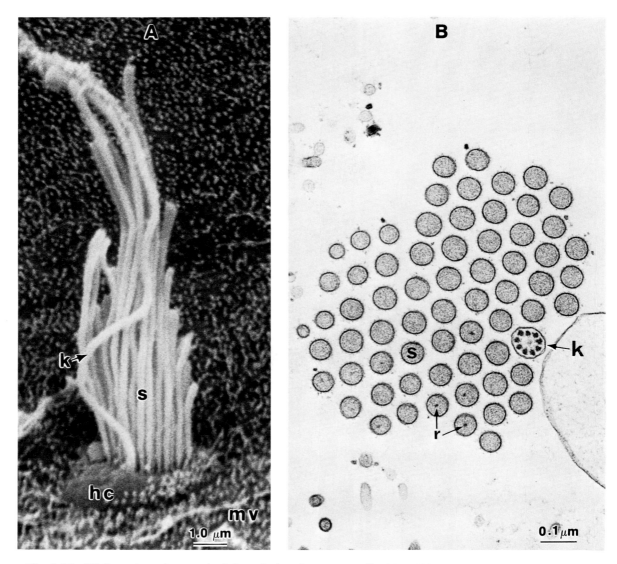

**Fig. 4-20. (A)** Scanning micrograph of the apical surface, stereocilia *(s)* and kinocilium *(k)* of a sensory hair cell *(hc)* from the macula utriculi. *mv*, microvilli of supporting cells. **(B)** A cross-section through the stereocilia *(s)* and kinocilium *(k)* of a vestibular hair cell made parallel to and near the cuticular plate. Rootlets *(r)* can be sen in some stereocilia.

The chalice is surrounded by supporting cells, which in turn, are anchored to a basement membrane. The upper surface of the cell holds between 20 and 100 stereocilia and one kinocilium (Fig. 4-20A and B). The stereocilia are arranged in regular rows at the cuticular surface and have varying length with the longest hairs close to the kinoci-lium. The stereocilium has a diameter of about 0.25 $\mu$m near its tip, but this is reduced to 0.1 to 0.15 $\mu$m at the level of the cuticular plate. The stereocilia are of different length according to sense organ; they are longest (up to 36 $\mu$m) in the cristae ampullaris, where they protrude into the cupula, and shortest in the maculae, where they are only a few microns in length. The stereocilia have a surface plasma membrane that is continuous with that of the hair cell. Along their length, blebs containing vesicles are often found, which appear to make contact with adjacent stereocilia. The stereocilia contain organized filaments of structural protein, such as actin, which penetrate the cuticular plate into which they are embedded. This cuticular plate is 1 to 1.5 $\mu$m in thickness and is made up of a fine granular or fibrillar material.

The kinocilium is of slightly larger diameter (0.25 to 0.3 $\mu$m) than the stereocilia and always much longer (Fig. 4-20). Its upper portion is embedded in the mesh of the otolithic membrane or the gelatinous cupula of the crista ampullaris. In cross-section (Fig. 4-20), the internal structure is the well-known nine double fibers surrounding a central two fibrils, although the latter are not always present throughout the kinocilium.

At the base of the kinocilium is a basal body, and a centriole is normally found in the vicinity. In this region, the cell has no cuticular plate.

The infracuticular region of the cell is rich in mitochondria and contains numerous vesicles and a poorly developed ribosomal endoplasmic reticulum. Very fine fibrillar structures arise close to the basal body of the kinocilium, and these have been traced through the cell as far as the synaptic region.

A large spherical nucleus without an obvious nucleolus is located in the center of the bulbous region of the cell. The nearby cytoplasm contains elongated mitochondria and a well-developed endoplasmic reticulum with Golgi complexes. The cytoplasm of the cell, in general, is rich in ribosomes and vesicles.

At the base of the cell, there are a number of ovoid mitochondria and few granulated membranes with ribosomes. Near the cell membrane, various synaptic bodies are found. The type I cell is innervated by the large afferent nerve chalice. The cytoplasm of the chalice contains many elongated mitochondria as well as nerve tubules and filaments that can end high up the chalice. At the lower end of the hair cell are synaptic structures, described as presynaptic vesicles surrounding synaptic bars, bodies, or balls. These are often found in a region of cell membrane invagination where the membranes of the nerve chalice and hair cell appear to join.

Efferent nerve endings synapse with the afferent chalice (Fig. 4-19). Within these efferent endings, mitochondria are smaller and more dense than those of the chalice.

## Type II Hair Cells

The type II hair cell is considered to be phylogenetically older than the type I cell. They are generally cylindrical or barrel shaped and vary considerably in length from about 10 $\mu$m to more than 45 $\mu$m (Fig. 4-19). The arrangement of cilia is almost identical to that found in type I cells (Fig. 4-20). The cuticular region is often a little thinner and less dense. The cytoplasm of type II cells contains the same organelles as described for type I cells, but the organelles of type II cells are more evenly distributed. The location of the nucleus varies from cell to cell but is usually within the middle third of the cell. A nucleolus is invariably evident.

Each type II cell contacts several afferent and efferent endings (Fig. 4-19). Several synaptic structures are associated with the afferent endings, including synaptic bars and balls and associated presynaptic vesicles. The afferent endings are sparsely granulated and contain large mitochondria. Efferent endings, on the other hand, are richly granulated, have smaller mitochondria, and are filled with synaptic vesicles of about 230 Å in diameter. Inside the plasma membrane of the hair cell, there is often a subsynaptic cisterna such as is found in cochlear hair cells (Fig. 4-15). Nerve endings tend to be unmyelinated inside the macula or crista, with myelination beginning below the basement membrane (Fig. 4-19).

## The Supporting Cells

The supporting cells reach from the basement membrane to the surface of the sensory epithelium, where they have a number of small (1 $\mu$m) microvilli. In some species a rudimentary kinocilium is evident. The surface area of the supporting cell contains some dense material that makes up the reticular lamina. There is some evidence of thin, supporting filaments within the cytoplasm, but these are not as highly organized as in cochlear supporting cells. The nuclei of the supporting cells are near the basement membrane, and the cytoplasm contains various organelles such as Golgi complexes, mitochondria, and lipid droplets. The

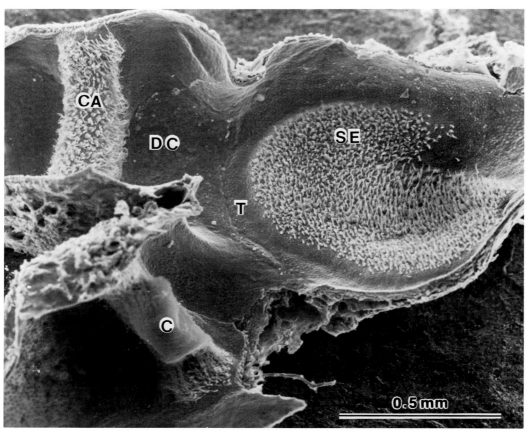

A

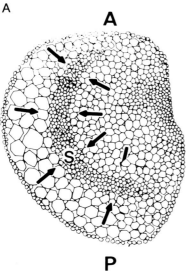

B

**Fig. 4-21. (A)** Scanning micrograph of the macula utriculi after removal of the otoconial layer. The sensory epithelium *(SE)* is bounded by a transitional cell region *(T)*. This figure shows the position of the utricle relative to the cristae ampullares *(CA)* of nearby semicircular canals. The cupula *(C)* remains intact on one crista. *DC*, dark cells. **(B)** Distribution and form of the overlying otoconia. The arrows indicate the orientation of the sensory hair cell cilia. In the macula utriculi, kinocilia are polarized toward the striola *(S)*. A, anterior; *P*, posterior. (B adapted from Lindeman HH: Studies on the Morphology of the Sensory Regions of the Vestibular Apparatus, Part 1. Advances in Anatomy, Embryology, and Cell Biology, Vol. 42. Springer-Verlag, Berlin, 1969.)

upper portion of the supporting cell often contains large numbers of spherical or ovoid granules, usually associated with ribosomes.

### The Utricle

In humans the utricle lies in the horizontal plane when the head is in an upright position. It lies superior to the saccule in the elliptic recess of the medial wall of the vestibule. The sensory epithelium (macula utriculi) is shell or kidney shaped as illustrated in Figure 4-21. In humans the area of the utricule is approximately 4 mm² and contains approximately 33,000 hair cells.[68] The cilia of the sensory cells (type I and II) are covered by a statoconial membrane that includes the otoconial layer.[66,67,69,70] The lower otoconia are embedded in the gelatinous layer, and above them surface otoconia are glued together with a gelatinous sub-

stance. Near the surface of the sensory epithelium is the subcupular meshwork, and above this is a so-called honeycomb layer. Collectively, these layers are termed the *intermediate mesh*. The mesh is organized to form many vesicle tubules into which the hair cell cilia project (Fig. 4-22). Scanning electron micrograph (Fig. 4-23B) shows the intermediate mesh after partial elevation of the otoconial layer. The shape and distribution of the otoconia of the utricle are shown by the inset of Figure 4-21. The otoconia are composed of calcium carbonate and have a specific gravity of approximately 2.7. Their general shape is cylindrical with pyramidal ends (Fig. 4-23A). The otoconia appear to be formed by macular supporting cells and accumulate on the intermediate mesh before fragmenting and migrating to areas of dark cells adjacent to the macula, where remnants are absorbed by pinocytotic activity.[71-73]

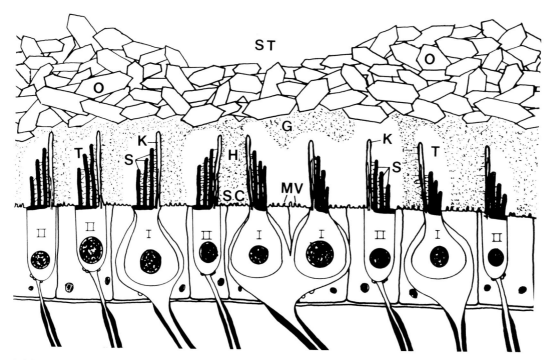

**Fig. 4-22.** Diagrammatic representation of the striola *(ST)* region of the macula utriculi. The otoconia *(O)* are part of the statoconial membrane. Below the otoconial layer is the intermediate mesh made up of three layers: the subcupular meshwork *(SC)*, the honeycomb layer *(H)*, and the gelatinous layer *(G)*. The mesh contains numerous tubules *(T)*, into which the kinocilia *(K)* and stereocilia *(S)* project. Type I and type II hair cells have their kinocilia oriented toward the striola region.

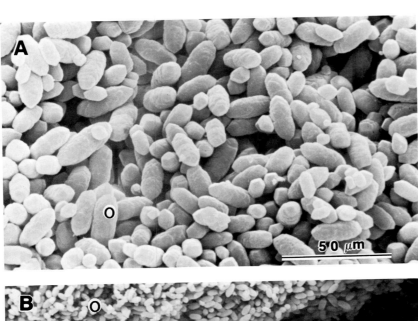

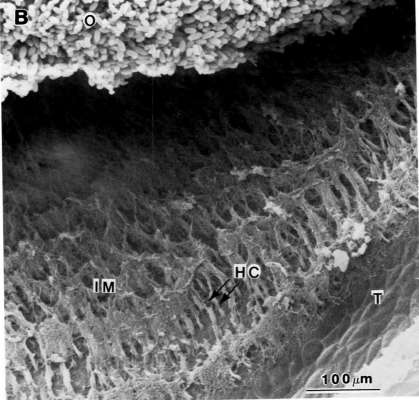

**Fig. 4-23.** Scanning electron micrograph of **(A)** utricular otoconia and **(B)** the intermediate mesh *(IM)* connecting the otoconia *(O)* to the sensory hair cell cilia *(HC)*. Bordering the macula utriculi is the transitional epithelium *(T)*.

The cilia of the sensory cells change their orientation along a narrow central area called the striola. In the macula utriculi the tallest stereocilia and the kinocilium face toward the striola (Figs. 4-21 and 4-22).

### The Saccule

With the head upright, the saccule is positioned vertically in the spherical recess of the vestibule.

The sensory epithelium has a hook-shaped form. In humans it has a surface area of about 2 mm² and contains approximately 18,000 hair cells.[68] In the scanning electron micrograph shown in Figure 4-24, the overlying otoconial layer has been removed to reveal the sensory epithelium. At the striola, the sensory hair cells change their orientation. In the macula sacculi, the kinocilium face toward the periphery; this is the opposite to that

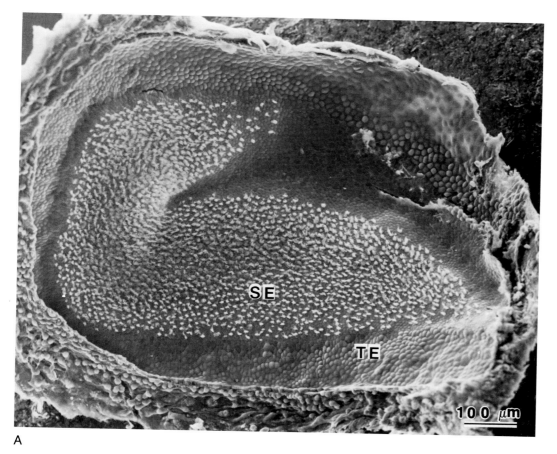

A

**Fig. 4-24. (A)** Scanning micrograph of the macula sacculi showing the sensory epithelium *(SE)* after removal of the statoconial layer. A transitional epithelium *(TE)* surrounds the sensory cell area. **(B)** In the sacculi, the sensory cells are oriented with their kinocilia away from the central striola *(s)*, as shown by the arrows. A, anterior; P, posterior. (B adapted from Lindeman HH: Studies on the Morphology of the Sensory Regions of the Vestibular Apparatus, Part 1. Advances in Anatomy, Embryology, and Cell Biology, Vol. 42. Springer-Verlag, Berlin, 1969.)

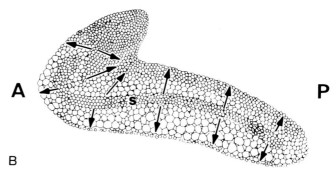

B

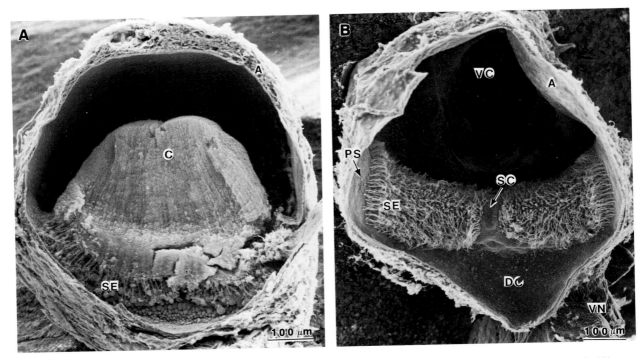

**Fig. 4-25.** Scanning electron micrographs of the crista ampullaris. **(A)** The opened semicircular canal ampulla (A) from the chinchilla; the cupula *(C)* covers the sensory epithelium. **(B)** The ampulla of a vertical canal (VC) from the rat; the cupula is removed to reveal the saddle-shaped sensory epithelium *(SE),* which is divided by the septum cruciatum *(SC)* in this species. *DC,* dark cell region; *PS,* planum semilunatum; *VN,* vestibular nerve.

found in the saccule. In the striola area, type I hair cells are more highly concentrated than in the periphery and, in general, the cilia are shorter.

## Crista Ampullaris

The ampulla of each semicircular canal contains a crista with a sensory epithelium that is best described as saddle shaped (Figs. 4-25 and 4-26). Both type I and type II hair cells are present, supported by cells resting on a basal lamina. Surrounded by connective tissue beneath the basal lamina are the blood capillaries and nerve fibers that supply the sensory epithelium (Fig. 4-26).

Over the surface of the crista, there are large variations in the density of hair cells. At the periphery the density is greatest; it reduces toward the center of the "saddle." Ciliary length also follows the same gradation, being considerably longer on peripheral sensory cells than on central sensory cells.

In each crista the orientation of sensory cells is in the same direction. In the ampulla for the lateral canal, crista polarization is toward the utricle, that is, the kinocilia are on the utricular side of the crista. For the anterior and posterior canals, polarization is away from the utricle. Some species (e.g., cat, dog, and rat) have a division across the cristae of the anterior and posterior canal ampullae called the septum cruciatum or eminentia cruciata in which there are no hair cells (Fig. 4-25B).

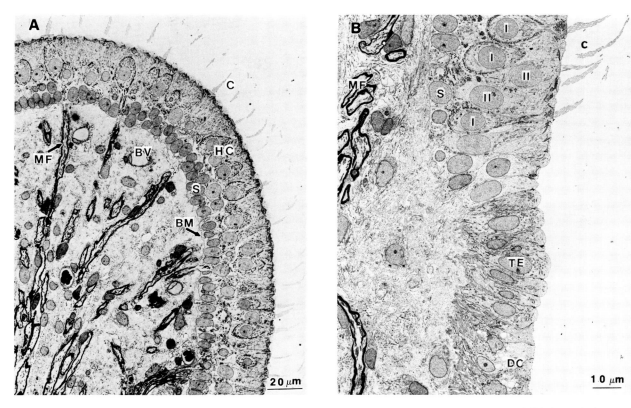

**Fig. 4-26.** Transmission micrograph of a vertical section **(A)** through the crista ampullaris and **(B)** through the transitional and dark cell epithelial areas. *BM*, basement membrane; *BV*, blood vessels; *C*, cilia of sensory hair cells; *DC*, dark cell region; *HC*, hair cells (type I and type II indicated in **B**); *MF*, myelinated nerve fiber; *S*, supporting cell nuclei; *TE*, transitional epithelium. (Courtesy of Dr. R. Hinojosa, University of Chicago, Chicago, Illinois.)

On the lateral wall of the crista ampullaris (Fig. 4-25B) is an area of flat, irregularly shaped, interdigitating epithelial cells. This area is half-moon shaped and is called the planum semilunatum. The bases of these cells have much infolding associated with a rich capillary network; thus, they have many of the characteristics of secretory cells.

**The Cupula.** Overlying the crista and extending to the inner epithelial wall of the ampulla is the cupula (Fig. 4-26A). This is a gelatinous mass containing mucopolysaccharide,[74,75] but whose precise structure is difficult to assess because of fixation and dehydration artifacts occurring in histologic preparation. The cupula appears to consist of fine (30 to 40 Å), unorganized filaments.[29,30] In addition, throughout the whole body of the cupula are fine canals that accommodate the long cilia of the hair cells. These canals are 3 to 5 $\mu$m in diameter at the basal part of the cupula and narrow to less than 1 $\mu$m toward its upper part. It is not clear whether or not the cupula adheres directly to the surface of the sensory epithelium. Some authors have described a subcupular space; however, this may be a fixation artifact. In species where the crista is separated by a septum cruciatum, the cupula is also divided into two sections.

**Transitional Epithelium.** The sensory epithelia of the saccule, utricle, and crista are surrounded by transitional cells. They appear to be similar to the supporting cells within the sensory areas but are a little smaller, have a more central nucleus, and have more evenly distributed organelles. The cells are cylindrical in shape and have a convex apical surface. These features can be seen in Figure 4-26.

**Dark Cells.**  In the utricle and crista, there are groups of cells lying peripheral to the transitional cell region called dark cells because of their microscopic appearance. The epithelial surface of these cells is relatively flat and polygonal in shape. Microvilli are present but not in great numbers and are concentrated toward the cell borders. Some of the cells contain a centriole. The cytoplasm of the cells stains darkly and contains numerous small mitochondria and large vacuoles. In the basal part of the cell, there is considerable interdigitation of the cytoplasm. It is common to find fragmented otoconia attached to the dark cells of the utricle and of the cristae; it is supposed that otoconia are absorbed in these areas.[71–73]

### Crista Neglecta

The crista neglecta is a small area of sensory epithelium similar to that of the crista ampullaris and found between the crista ampullaris of the posterior semicircular canal and the utricle. It is found occasionally in humans, and more often in other species.[42,76]

### Endolymphatic Duct and Sac

The endolymphatic duct extends from the junction of ducts from the utricle and the saccule (Fig. 4-27) on the medial side of the vestibule. It runs through the bony vestibular aqueduct and opens into the endolymphatic sac, which lies partly within the bony niche of the surface of the petrous bone and partly between the dura mater and the bone of the posterior fossa. The sac can be considered in three areas.[77] The distal portion, which is in intimate contact with the dura mater near to the transverse venous (sigmoid) sinus of the posterior fossa; the intermediate portion at the opening of the bony niche; and the proximal part within the bony niche.

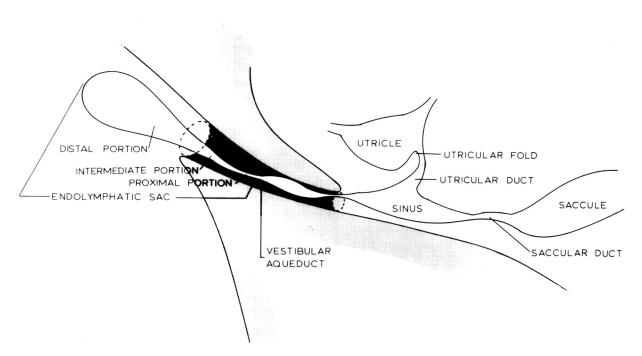

**Fig. 4-27.** Diagram of the endolymphatic sac and duct showing their major portions and connection to the membranous labyrinth.

The epithelium of the duct is of simple squamous or flattened cuboidal cells nesting on a basement membrane. The cytoplasm contains some ribosomes and lipid granules and a few evenly distributed mitochondria. The cell surface has a small number of microvilli projecting into the endolymph. The cells are not tightly contacted to each other, and the epithelium has been described as leaky.[78,79]

The proximal part of the sac is lined with more cuboidal epithelial cells with more inclusion bodies, notably lipid granules. The endolymphatic surface has more microvilli than in the duct, and some pinocytotic vesicles are present. The subepithelial tissue is more vascular than the duct.

The intermediate (rugose) portion has an epithelial lining of tall cylindrical cells. There are two basic cell types: (1) light cells, which contain numerous microvilli, many pinocytotic vesicles and abundant ribosomes, and are rich in mitochondria; and (2) dark cells, which have a dense cytoplasm and which are also rich in mitochondria but have a small number of microvilli, pinocytotic vesicles, and other cell inclusions. Adjacent cells have interdigitating membranes and tight junctions. The epithelial surface is highly infolded, and the lumen of the sac is sometimes difficult to determine. There is a rich capillary network near the epithelial layer.

The distal portion of the endolymphatic sac is thin and flat and has a largely cuboidal epithelial lining with cytoplasm resembling the light cells of the intermediate portion, perhaps with fewer microvilli and pinocytotic vesicles. Tight junctional connections between cells make it a relatively nonleaky epithelium.[78,79] The subepithelial tissue is richly vascularized.

The exact role of the endolymphatic sac remains unclear. However, it is evident from its ultrastructure that it is active in phagocytosis and fluid absorption.

## ACKNOWLEDGMENTS

The authors would like to thank Richard Mount and Brenda Rutledge for their assistance in preparing this manuscript.

## REFERENCES

1. Shrapnell H: On the form and structure of membrana tympani. London Med Gaz 10:120, 1832
2. Prussak A: Studien über die Anatomie des menschlichen Trommelfells. Arch Ohr Nas Kehlk Heilk 3:255, 1867
3. Rüdinger N: Beitrage zur Vergleichenden Anatomie und Histologie der Ohrtrompete. JJ Lentner, Munich, 1870
4. Gerlach J: Zur Morphologie der Tuba Eustachii. Mschr Ohrenheilk 9:48, 1875
5. Politzer A: Die Anatomische und Histologische Zergliederung des Menschlichen Gehororgans. Enke, Stuttgart, 1899
6. Corti A: Rercherches sur l'organe ee l'ouie des mammiferes. Z Wiss Zool 3:109, 1851
7. Claudius M: Bemerkungen über den Bauder hautigen Spiralleiste der Schnecke. Z Wiss Zool 7:154, 1856
8. Hensen V: Zur Morphologie der Schnecke des Menshen und der Säugethiere. Z Wiss Zool 13:481, 1863
9. Boettcher A: Uber Entwicklung und Bau des Gehörlabyrinths nach Untersuchungen an Säugetieran. Nova Acta Academiae Cesariae 35:1, 1869
10. Retzius G: Das Gehörorgan der Reptilien, der Vögel und der Säugethiere. Samson and Wallin, Stockholm, 1884
11. Held H: Die cochlea der Säuger und der Vögel, ihre entwicklung und ihr Bau. p. 467. In Bethe A (ed): Handbuch der Normalen und Pathologischen Physiologie. Vol. 11. :Springer-Verlag, Berlin, 1926
12. Kolmer W: Gehörorgan. p. 250. In von Mollendorf W (ed): Handbuch der Mikroskopischen Anatomie des Menschen. Vol. 3. Springer-Verlag, Berlin, 1927
13. Scarpa A: Anatomische Untersuchungen des Gehörs und Geruchs. Nürnberg, Germany, 1800
14. Schultze M: Uber die Endigungsweise des Hörnerver im Labyrinth. Arch Anat Physiol Wiss Med 1:343, 1858
15. Odenius MV: Uber das Epithel der Maculae acousticae beim Menschen. Arch Mikr Anat. 3:115, 1867
16. Held H: Untersuchungen über den feineren Bau des Ohrlabyrinthes der Wirbeltiere. Abh Sachs Ges Wiss (Liepzig) 31:193, 1909
17. Engström H, Wersäll J: The ultrastructural organization of the organ of Corti and of the vestibular sensory epithelia. Exp Cell Res 5:460, 1958

18. Engström H, Ades HW, Andersson A: Structural pattern of the organ of Corti. Almquist & Wiksell, Stockholm, 1966

19. Wersäll J: Studies on the structure and innervation of the sensory epithelium of the cristae ampullaris in the guinea pig. A light and electron microscopic investigation. Acta Otolaryngol [Suppl] (Stockh) 126:1, 1956

20. Spoendlin H: The organization of the cochlear receptor. Advances in Otolaryngology. Vol. 13. S. Karger AG, Basel, 1966

21. Iurato S: Submicroscopic Structure of the Inner Ear. Pergamon Press, New York, 1967

22. Bredberg G: Cellular pattern and nerve supply of the human organ of Corti. Acta Otolaryngol [Suppl] (Stockh) 236:1, 1968

23. Kimura R: The ultrastructure of the organ of Corti. p. 173. In Bourne GH, Danielli JF (eds): International Review of Cytology. Vol. 42. Academic Press, Orlando, FL, 1975

24. Barber VC, Boyle A: Scanning electron microscopic studies on cilia. Z Zelforsche 84:269, 1968

25. Lim D: Three dimensional observations of the inner ear with the scanning electron microscope. Acta Otolaryngol [Suppl] (Stockh) 255:1, 1969

26. Lim D. Vestibular sensory organs. A scanning electronmicroscopic investigation. Arch Otolaryngol 94:69, 1971

27. Bredberg G, Ades HW, Engström H: Scanning electron microscopy of the normal and pathologically altered organ of Corti. Acta Otolaryngol [Suppl] (Stockh) 301:1, 1972

28. Hunter-Duvar IM: An electron microscopic assessment of the cochlea. Acta Otolaryngol [Suppl] (Stockh) 351:1, 1978

29. Hunter-Duvar IM: An electron microscopic study of the vestibular sensory epithelium. Acta Otolaryngol (Stockh) 95:494, 1983

30. Hunter-Duvar IM, Hinojosa R: Vestibule: Sensory epithelia. p. 211. In Friedmann I, Ballantyne J (eds): Ultrastructure Atlas of the Inner Ear. Butterworth (Publishers), London, 1984

31. Lindeman HH: Anatomy of the otolith organs. Adv Otorhinolaryngol 20:405, 1973

32. Smith CA, Tanaka K: Some aspects of the structure of the vestibular apparatus. p. 3. In Nauton RF (ed): The Vestibular System. Academic Press, New York, 1975

33. Harada Y: Atlas of the ear by scanning electron microscopy. MTP Press, Lancaster, 1983

34. Wever E, Lawrence M: Physiological Acoustics. Princeton University Press, Princeton, NJ, 1954

35. Békésy G. von, Rosenblith W: The mechanical properties of the ear. In Stevens S (ed): Handbook of Experimental Psychology. John Wiley & Sons, New York, 1951

36. Harada Y: Scanning electron microscopic observation of the lamina propria of the tympanic membrane in guinea pig. Practica Otologica (Kyoto) 65:995, 1972

37. Kawabata I, Ishi H: Fiber arrangement in the tympanic membrane. Acta Otolaryngol (Stockh) 72:243, 1971

38. Lim DJ: Human tympanic membrane. Electron microscopic observation. Acta Otolaryngol (Stockh) 70:197, 1970

39. Procter B: The development of the middle ear spaces and their surgical significance. J Laryngol Otol 77:344, 1964

40. Hentzer E: Ultrastructure of the normal mucosa in the human middle ear, mastoid cavities and Eustachian tube. Ann Otol Rhinol Laryngol 79:1143, 1970

41. Shimada T, Lim DJ: Distribution of ciliated cells in the human middle ear. Ann Otol Rhinol Laryngol 81:203, 1972

42. Schuknecht HF: Pathology of the Ear. Harvard University Press, Cambridge, MA, 1974

43. Densert O, Wersäll J: The morphology of middle ear muscles in mammals. p. 111. In Keidel WD, Neff WD (eds): Handbook of Sensory Physiology. Vol 5/1. Springer-Verlag, Berlin, 1974

44. Procter B: Embryology and anatomy of the Eustachian tube. Arch Otolaryngol 86:503, 1967

45. Harada Y: Scanning electron microscopic study on the distribution of epithelial cells in the Eustachian tube. Acta Otolaryngol (Stockh) 83:284, 1977

46. Lim DJ, Paparella MM, Kimura RS: Ultrastructure of Eustachian tube and middle ear mucosa in the guinea pig. Acta Otolaryngol (Stockh) 63:425, 1967

47. Bosher SK, Warren RL: Observations on the electrochemistry of the cochlear endolymph of the rat: a quantitative study of its electrical potential and ionic composition as determined by means of flame spectrophotometry. Proc R Soc London [Biol] 171:227, 1968

48. Smith CA: Structure of the cochlear duct. p. 3. In Nauton RF, Fernandez C (eds): Evoked Electrical Activity in the Auditory Nervous System. Academic Press, New York, 1978

49. Hunter-Duvar IM: Reissner's membrane and endocytosis of cell debris. Acta Otolaryngol [Suppl] (Stockh) 231:24, 1978

50. Iurato S: Submicroscopic structure of the mem-

branous labyrinth. I The tectorial membrane. Z Zellforsch 51:105, 1960

51. Lim DJ: Fine morphology of the tectoral membrane: its relationship to the organ of Corti. Arch Otolaryngol 96:199, 1972

52. Kronester-Frei A: Ultrastructure of the different zones of the tectorial membrane. Cell Tissue Res 193:11, 1978

53. Hoshino T: Contact between the tectorial membrane and the cochlear sensory hairs in the human and the monkey. Arch Otorhinolaryngol 217:53, 1977

54. Hunter-Duvar IM: Morphology of the normal and the acoustically damaged cochlea. Scan Electron Microsc 2:421, 1977

55. Lim DJ: Fine morphology of the tectorial membrane. Fresh and developmental. p. 47. In Portmann M, Aran J-M (eds): Inner Ear Biology. INSERM Colloque, 68. INSERM, Paris, 1977

56. Steel KP: The tectorial membrane of mammals. Hear Res 9:327, 1983

57. Flock Å, Bretscher A. Weber K: Immunohistochemical localization of several cytoskeletal proteins in inner ear sensory and supporting cells. Hear Res 6:75, 1982

58. Angelborg C, Engström H: Supporting elements of the organ of Corti. Acta Otolaryngol [Suppl] (Stockh) 301:49, 1972

59. Takahashi T, Kimura RS: The ultrastructure of the spiral ligament in the Rhesus monkey. Acta Otolaryngol (Stockh) 69:46, 1970

60. Smith CA: Structure of the stria vascularis and spiral prominence. Ann Otol Rhinol Laryngol 66:521, 1957

61. Kimura R, Schuknecht H: The ultrastructure of the human stria vascularis. Part I. Acta Otolaryngol (Stockh) 69:415, 1970

62. Hinojosa R, Rodriguez-Echandia EL: The fine structure of the stria vascularis of the cat's inner ear. Am J Anat 118:631, 1966

63. Axelsson A: The vascular anatomy of the cochlea in the guinea pig and in man. Acta Otolaryngol [Suppl] (Stockh) 243:1, 1968

64. Gacek RR: The course and central termination of first order neurones supplying vestibular end organs in the cat. Acta Otolaryngol [Suppl] (Stockh) 254:1, 1969

65. Wersäll J: Studies on the structure and innervation of the sensory epithelium of the cristae ampullares

in the guinea pig. Acta Otolaryngol [Suppl] (Stockh) 126:1, 1956

66. Lindeman HH: Studies on the Morphology of the Sensory Regions of the Vestibular Apparatus, Part 1. Advances in Anatomy, Embryology and Cell Biology, Vol 42. Springer-Verlag, Berlin, 1969

67. Spoendlin H: Vestibular labyrinth. p. 264, In Bischoff A (ed); Ultrastructure of the Peripheral Nervous System and Sense Organs. Thieme, Stuttgart, 1970

68. Engström H, Bergstrom B, Ades HW: Macula utriculi and macula sacculi in the squirrel monkey. Acta Otolaryngol [Suppl] (Stockh) 301:75, 1972

69. Lindeman HH: Cellular pattern and nerve supply of the vestibular sensory epithelia. Acta Otolaryngol [Suppl] (Stockh) 244:86, 1967

70. Smith CA: Microscopic structure of the utricle. Ann Otol Rhinol Laryngol 65:450, 1956

71. Lim DJ: Formation and fate of otoconia. Ann Otol Rhinol Laryngol 82:23, 1973

72. Lim DJ: The development and structure of the otoconia. p. 245. In Friedmann I, Ballantyne J, (eds): Ultrastructural Atlas of the Inner Ear. Butterworth (Publishers), London, 1984

73. Anniko M: Development of Otoconia. Am J Otolaryngol 1:400, 1980

74. Igarasni M, Alford BR: Cupula, cupular zone of otolith membrane and tectorial membrane in the squirrel monkey. Acta Otolaryngol (Stockh) 68:420, 1969

75. Harada Y: The shape of the vertical canal crista in various animals. Equilibrium Res 32:82, 1974

76. Montandon P, Gacek R, Kimura R: Crista neglecta in the cat and human. Ann Otol Rhinol Laryngol 79:105, 1970

77. Lundquist P-G, Kimura RS, Wersäll J: Ultrastructure organization of the epithelial lining in the endolymphatic duct and sac in the guinea pig. Acta Otolaryngol (Stockh) 57:65, 1964

78. Bagger-Sjöbäck D, Lundquist P-G, Rask-Anderson H: Intracellular junctions in the epithelium of the endolymphatic sac. p. 127. In Vosteen K-H et al (eds): Meniere's Disease. Thieme, Stuttgart, 1982

79. Lundquist P-G, Rask-Anderson H, Galey FR, Bagger-Sjoback D: Ultrastructural morphology of the endolymphatic duct and sac. p. 309. In Friedmann I, Ballantyne J (eds): Ultrastructural Atlas of the Inner Ear. Butterworth (Publishers), London, 1984

# Biology of the Vestibulocochlear Nerve

# 5

## Heinrich Spoendlin

## STRUCTURAL ORGANIZATION

### Cochlear Nerve

Two systems of primary neurons connect the cochlea with the brain stem (Fig. 5-1): the afferent neurons with the bipolar ganglion cells, which form the spiral ganglion in Rosenthal's canal in the modiolus, and the efferent olivocochlear neurons, known as the olivocochlear bundle, originating in the homo- and contralateral superior olivary complex, as originally described by Rasmussen.[1] A third class of neurons consists of the adrenergic autonomic innervation, originating in the cervical sympathetic trunk.[2]

### Afferent Neurons

The number of afferent neurons varies considerably in different species; there are about 16,000 in bats, 36,000 in humans,[3] 50,000 to 60,000 in cats,[4,5] and about 250,000 in whales.[6] In the cochlear nerve the overwhelming majority of nerve fibers are myelinated, with diameters ranging from 4 to 6 $\mu$m in a unimodal distribution and a regular myelin sheath of about 50 lamellae, which is the structural basis of a uniform conduction velocity, probably a very important basic functional feature of the cochlear nerve. The nerve fibers are tonotopically arranged within the cochlear nerve according to their area of origin in the cochlea. From the spiral ganglion, they radiate in a radial direction through the osseous spiral lamina to the organ of Corti. The nerve fiber density as expressed in number of nerve fibers per unit of lengths of the organ of Corti shows the highest innervation density in the middle and lower basal turn with a gradual decrease in the apex and the hook area[7,8] (Fig. 5-2). All fibers lose their myelin sheath before entering the organ of Corti through the habenular openings.

In all mammalian species studied so far, namely the cat, the guinea pig, the rat, the rabbit, the chinchilla, the gerbil, the monkey, and the human, two distinct types of ganglion cells are found in the normal spiral ganglion; the great majority (90 to 95 percent) are large, bipolar type I cells and about 5 to 10 percent are smaller, type II cells with a number of distinctive features. The most common feature of the type II cells in all species is their smaller size and a lighter, more filamentous cytoplasm with fewer ribosomes or Nissl substance than the type I cells. (Fig. 5-3). A lack of myelin sheath around the

117

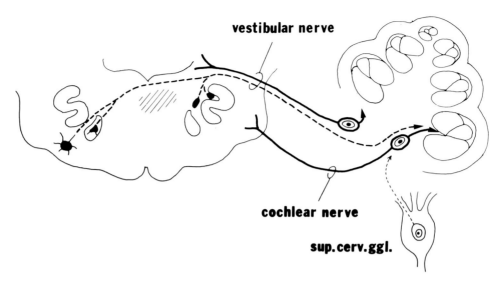

**Fig. 5-1.** Three innervation components of the inner ear. Solid lines indicate afferent neurons; thick dashed lines indicate efferent olivocochlear neurons; and thin dashed lines indicate adrenergic neurons from the superior cervical ganglion.

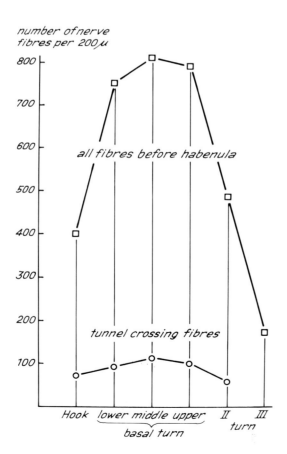

**Fig. 5-2.** Innervation densities of the organ of Corti in the cat. The maximum is in the middle and upper basal turn. The tunnel-crossing fibers represent about 15 percent of the entire nerve fiber population. In the human cochlea, the innervation density maximum is shifted toward the second turn.

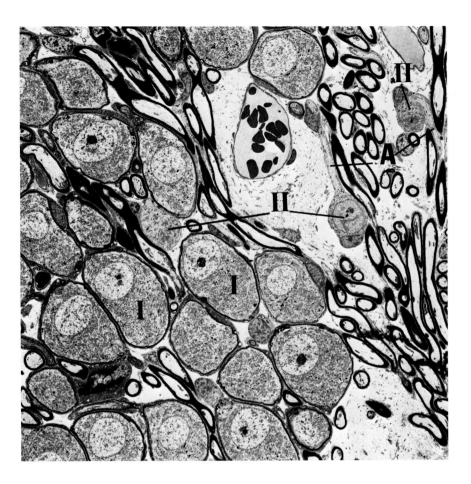

**Fig. 5-3.** Low magnification electron micrograph of a portion of the spiral ganglion of a cat with the myelinated type I *(I)* and unmyelinated type II *(II)* ganglion cells. The axons of the pseudo-monopolar type II ganglion cells are myelinated *(A).*

type II cells is a frequent but not constant finding. In the human there are just as many myelinated as unmyelinated small cells,[9] and in the cat some type II cells may have a thin myelin sheath. The eccentric position and the lobulation of the nucleus is typical in the cat, but lacking in rodents and humans. The suspicion that type II cells might just be spontaneously degenerating type I cells can be refuted by the fact that two types of ganglion cells are already present in the newborn kitten.[10] The type II neurons are predominantly pseudomonopolar, whereas the type I neurons are bipolar. The myelin sheath around the type I neurons of the cat is relatively thin, with an inner layer of loose and an outer layer of compact myelin. In the vicinity of the cell body the central process of the type I cells is much larger (with a diameter of about 2 $\mu$m) than

the peripheral process (with a diameter of about 1 $\mu$m). Up to the first node of Ranvier, the axon is surrounded by the same type of myelin as the perikaryon. Beyond the first node of Ranvier, the central as well as the peripheral axon is surrounded by the typical compact myelin of peripheral nerves with about 50 lamellae. The axons of the type II cells are unmyelinated and have a relatively large caliber close to the cell body, but they thin down considerably with increasing distance from the cell (Fig. 5-3).

The peripheral distribution of the afferent neurons is best studied after elimination of efferents by degeneration following transection of the olivocochlear efferent fibers within the vestibular nerve. The remaining afferent fibers are the inner radial fibers, the basilar fibers, and the outer spiral fibers. These fiber tracts obviously represent the afferent innervation of the organ of Corti (Fig. 5-4). The basilar fibers are the only afferent fibers reaching the area of the outer hair cells. They can be counted as they pass between the base of the outer pillars in tangential sections through this area. Evaluated over long distances of the cochlea, there is an average of one basilar fiber penetrating between two pillars, which amounts to a total of approximately 2,500 afferent fibers for the outer hair cells. This is an extremely small number, compared with the entire population of about 50,000 cochlear neurons in the cat cochlea. It means that only about 5 percent of all afferent cochlear

neurons are associated with the outer hair cell system, which represents more than three-quarters of the receptor cells of the cochlea. More evidence for the surprising 20 : 1 ratio of afferent innervation of inner and outer hair cells can be obtained by the reconstruction of the area of the inner hair cells after elimination of the efferent innervation. The great majority of all nerve fibers ending in the organ of Corti leads directly unbranched to the base of the nearest inner hair cell. Only about 1 fiber out of 20 turns outward to the outer hair cells.[5] After the demonstration of this surprising situation in the cat, similar ratios between neurons associated with the outer and inner hair cells have

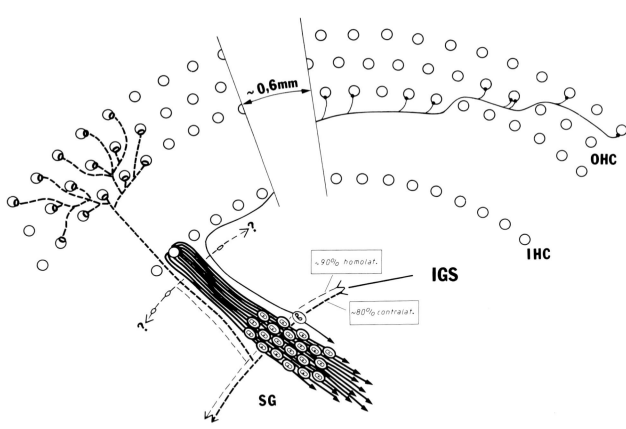

**Fig. 5-4.** Horizontal innervation schema of the organ of Corti. Thick solid lines indicate afferent neurons associated with the inner hair cells *(IHC)*; thin solid lines indicate afferent neurons associated with the outer hair cells *(OHC)*; thick dashed lines indicate efferent neurons from the intraganglionic spiral bundle *(IGS)* for the outer hair cells making direct synaptic contacts with the receptor cells; thin dashed lines indicate efferent neurons for the inner hair cell system making synaptic contacts with the afferent dendrites. *SG*, spiral ganglion.

been found in the guinea pig[5,11] and humans[12] (Fig. 5-4).

Within the habenula, fibers associated with the outer hair cells cannot be distinguished from the other fibers, but they are usually situated in the most distal portion of the habenular opening. Unlike the inner hair cell fibers, they take an independent spiral course immediately after the habenula for about five pillars, then they penetrate between the inner pillars to cross the bottom of the tunnel as basilar fibers and reach the area of the outer hair cells, where they form the outer spiral fibers, which gradually climb up toward the base of the outer hair cells. In its terminal portion, each fiber gives off collaterals, which end with afferent nerve endings at the base of outer hair cells. Each fiber sends collaterals to about 10 outer hair cells, and each outer hair cell receives collaterals from several outer spiral fibers, according to the principles of multiple innervation. The average spiral extension of the outer spiral fibers in the basalward direction amounts to about 0.6 mm. This peripheral innervation pattern is essentially confirmed in a recent Golgi study.[13]

The ultrastructure organization of the axoplasm varies to a certain extent between afferent fibers to outer and inner hair cells. The fibers for the outer hair cells contain mainly neurocanaliculi in their axoplasm, whereas the fibers for the inner hair cells contain predominantly neurofibrils. Each afferent ending at the inner hair cell usually forms one synaptic complex with a presynaptic bar of varying size. In the human several synapses can be observed in one nerve ending.[14] The afferent endings at the base of the outer hair cells, on the other hand, have no synaptic ribbons in the cat and only a few relatively small ones in the guinea pig and human. In more than 50 percent of the outer hair cells, Nadol[14] describes reciprocal synapses, where a single nerve ending of the nonvesiculated type poses two types of synaptic specialization of opposite polarity.

On the basis of location, caliber, and content of mitochondria, Liberman[15] distinguishes at the level of the inner hair cells different types of afferent dendrites, which he can correlate to the spontaneous discharge rate of the neurons by means of single neuron labeling. The larger fibers tend to have their endings at the distal circumference of the inner hair cells, whereas the smaller fibers end mostly on the modiolar side of the basal circumference of the inner hair cells. The average diameter of the radial fiber terminal is highly correlated with the spontaneous discharge of the unit. All 56 labeled neurons from 14 cats were neurons of type I associated with the inner hair cells. This strongly suggests that the activity of the outer hair cell innervation has never been sampled in any of the single-unit recordings from the auditory nerve, which is possibly due to the fact that the central axons of the type II neurons are probably not recordable, being unmyelinated and less than 0.5 $\mu$m in diameter.

The caliber of the fibers varies considerably along their course through the organ of Corti. Especially where the fibers pass mechanically important supporting structures such as the basilar membrane at the habenular region or the pillars, their diameter is considerably reduced and the axoplasm rather empty.

There is no morphologic evidence for direct functional interference between the afferent fibers from the inner and outer hair cells at any level. In no place are their direct contacts or even synapses between the axons of the two fiber systems. Within the habenular openings, all fibers are individually surrounded by processes of a special habenular satellite cell, which seems to take the role of the individual Schwann cells proximal to the habenula (Fig. 5-5).

In the spiral ganglion of the cat, no synaptic contacts between neurons could be found. However, in the spiral ganglion of the human and the monkey, synaptic contacts between small neurons and small unmyelinated fibers from the intraganglionic spiral bundle have been described.[16]

The neurons of the inner and outer hair cells differ not only in number, arrangement, and structure, but also in their metabolic behavior. The radial fibers to the inner hair cells are very susceptible to hypoxia in contrast with the outer spiral fibers, and aging changes are found predominantly within the type I neurons[17] (Fig. 5-6). All this suggests that the neurons of the inner and outer hair cells represent two different systems.

There is strong evidence that the type II neurons provide the afferent innervation of the outer hair cells, and the type I neurons provide the afferent

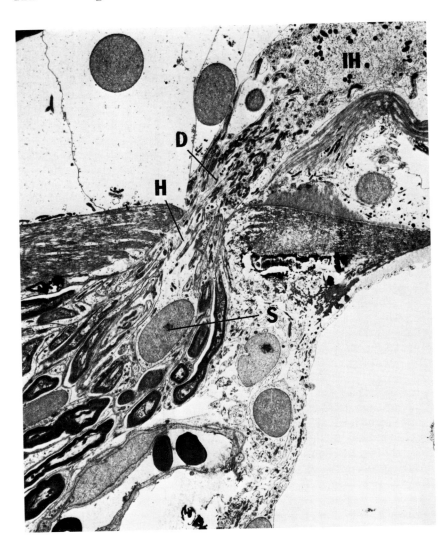

**Fig. 5-5.** Radial section through one habenular opening *(H)* showing the compressed nerve fiber bundle and the relatively large radial dendrites *(D)* to the inner hair cell *(IH)*. All nerve fibers lose their myelin sheath before the habenula. Within the habenula they are surrounded by a special satellite cell *(S)*.

innervation of the inner hair cells. The first suspicion of such a relationship came from the observation that the type II neurons and the afferent fibers to the outer hair cells both represent about 5 percent of the entire cochlear nerve population. Following transection of the 8th nerve in the inner acoustic canal, most type I neurons degenerate within several months, whereas the type II neurons remain morphologically unchanged in normal numbers. At the same time the afferent nerve supply of the outer hair cells also remains entirely unchanged. This led to the conclusion that the type II neurons provide the afferent innervation of the outer hair cells, whereas the type I neurons give rise to the radial fibers leading to the inner hair cells.[5,18] More recently these correlations could be directly demonstrated by horseradish peroxidase (HRP) labeling of cochlear neurons with iontophoretic injection of HRP into the cochlear nerve.[19] Additional support for the association of the type I neurons with the inner and the type II neurons with the outer hair cells is provided by the fact that retrograde degeneration of the type I cochlear neurons starts only after destruction of the inner hair cells but not after selective loss of the outer hair cells.

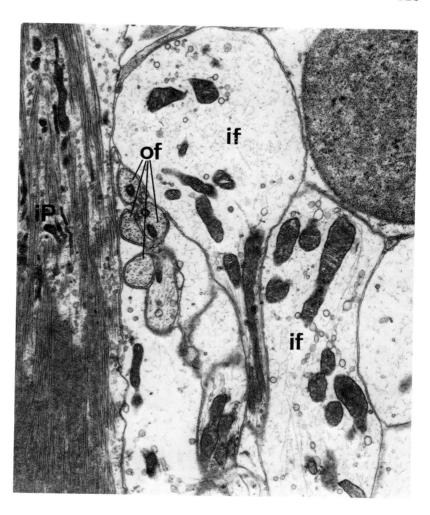

**Fig. 5-6.** Swelling of an afferent nerve fiber to the inner hair cell *(if)* under slight hypoxic conditions. The afferent fibers for the outer hair cells *(of)* are not affected. They run close to the inner pillars *(iP)*.

The observation that the type II axons are small in caliber and remain unmyelinated throughout their entire course is very important in respect to their function, but difficult to prove, since it is practically impossible to follow them over longer distances in normal animals.[18] To a limited extent this is possible with electron microscopy (**EM**) serial sections or with interference contrast microscopy of extra-thick sections following retrograde degeneration of the type I cells. In areas of the cochlea where, a long time after transection of the 8th nerve, only type II cells remain, we find almost exclusively unmyelinated nerve fibers in the osseous spiral lamina, which indicates that the peripheral axons of the type II neurons remain unmyelinated throughout their peripheral course.

To follow the central axon of type II neurons is more difficult. EM serial sections are only possible for limited distances. In light-microscopic preparations, the unmyelinated axons become extremely thin at a certain distance from the perikarya and are usually lost at the entrance of the modiolus. Because they are so small at this level, they will most probably remain very small and unmyelinated in their further centralward course within the cochlear nerve.

Unmyelinated fibers, on the other hand, are very rare within the normal cochlear nerve. There are two types of unmyelinated fibers. One type has a diameter of 0.2 to 0.5 $\mu$m, usually runs alone in its own Schwann sheath, and represents only 0.5 percent of the entire population. The other type is extremely small, with a diameter around 0.1 $\mu$m, usually runs in groups of several fibers in one Schwann sheath, and represents between 2 and 5 percent of the entire nerve fiber population. They closely resemble autonomic fibers (Fig. 5-7). It is more likely that the very small groups of somewhat larger fibers represent the central axons of the type II neurons. Their extremely small number and size are consistent with the impossibility of obtaining single-fiber recordings of them.[15] A complete and efficient connection of the type II neurons to the central nervous system seems therefore very questionable. The fact that the type II neurons undergo secondary retrograde degeneration after destruction of the organ of Corti but do not show any degeneration after transection of the cochlear nerve shows that the central axons are peculiar and unusual.

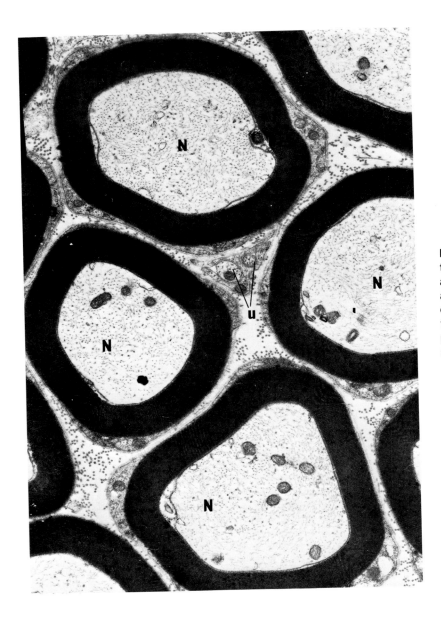

**Fig. 5-7.** Detail of some nerve fibers in the cochlear nerve trunk in the internal auditory canal showing the myelinated afferent neurons *(N)* of the inner hair cell system and some very small and few and unmyelinated fibers *(u)*, which possibly belong to the outer hair cell system, or are autonomic fibers.

A number of studies have been undertaken to inject HRP by various means into the cochlear nucleus or nerve, where the tracer is taken up by the axons and transported down to the nerve endings within the organ of Corti. There, it can be demonstrated by histochemical techniques. The results of such experiments have differed to some extent. In my experiments I found that the radial fibers to the inner hair cells were strongly labeled, but the outer spiral fibers or the afferent nerve terminals at the outer hair cells were not.[10,20] Leak-Jones and Snyder,[21] on the other hand, were able to demonstrate some nicely labeled outer spiral fibers and nerve endings at the base of the outer hair cells in cats. Similar results were obtained by Kiang et al.[19] Ruggero et al.,[22] in similar studies in chinchillas, found that the type II neurons were labeled but much less than the radial fibers of the type I neurons. Morest[23] could show by autoradiography that D-aspartate was transported from the cochlear nucleus to type II ganglion cells in cats.

These experiments suggest that the central axons of some type II neurons do indeed project into the cochlear nerve or even into the cochlear nucleus, but they do not say anything about the functional significance of these central connections. The extremely small number and size of the central axons of the afferent neurons of the outer hair cell system constitute a very poor information transmission system. In the small unmyelinated axons, saltatory action-potential conduction is not possible, so that the propagation of nerve potentials is presumably very slow with considerable decrement. There seems to be a direct correlation between fiber size, spontaneous activity, and sensitivity.[15] After section of the cochlear nerve in the cat, almost all type I neurons degenerate and disappear, and only the type II neurons, which represent the afferent innervation of the outer hair cell system, remain unchanged in normal numbers. In electrocochleographic recordings of such animals, no compound action potentials can be found in spite of the remaining normal type II neurons.[24] All this suggests that the main information transfer to the central nervous system relies on the inner hair cell system and that the outer hair cell system, which represents a great majority of all cochlear hair cells, has its main functional role at the level of the receptor cells, possibly by monitoring the receptor organ

electrically or mechanically, rather than in direct neural information transmission to the central nervous system. This is also illustrated by the extensive efferent innervation of the outer hair cells.

### Efferent Neurons

An efferent innervation of the cochlea has been known since Rasmussen[7] demonstrated a homo- and contralateral efferent olivocochlear bundle in the cat, rat, and opossum. An efferent innervation of the acoustic system originating in the brain stem is found in practically all species, from fish to mammals.[25]

With the application of HRP techniques, a clear and direct demonstration of the origin of the cochlear efferents was possible in the kitten,[26] the adult cat,[27] and the rat. With HRP labeling, between 1,400 and 1,600 efferent neurons were identified in the cat, more than double the number originally indicated by Rasmussen.[1] There are at least four different types of neurons located either in the lateral superior olivary nucleus (LSO), as very small fusiform cells deep in the hilus with a diameter of about $10 \mu m$ and somewhat larger cells medial to it, or in the medial nucleus of the trapezoid body (MNTB), as medium-sized, oval-shaped cells, and in the periolivary nucleus (PON), as very large, multipolar cells with a diameter up to $20 \mu m$. In the cat 85 to 90 percent of the neurons in the LSO are homolateral, whereas 70 to 80 percent of the larger neurons in the MNTB and PON are contralateral (Fig. 5-8).

The contralateral fibers cross the midline at the floor of the fourth ventricle. They join the homolateral bundle within the vestibular root and run with the vestibular nerve into the periphery before they cross over to the cochlear nerve deep in the inner acoustic canal through the anastomosis of Oort (vestibulocochlear anastomosis). The totality of efferent fibers can therefore best be selectively transected in the vestibular nerve without damage to the cochlear nerve. Within the modiolus they form the intraganglionic spiral bundle in the peripheral portion of the spiral ganglion, from where the fibers radiate to the organ of Corti. The efferent fibers are best identified in the anastomosis of Oort or in the intraganglionic spiral bundle,[27] where we

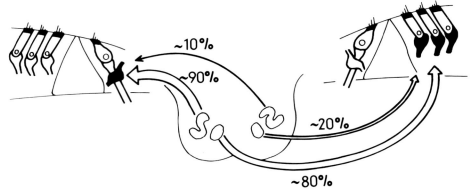

**Fig. 5-8.** Origin of the homolateral and contralateral olivocochlear efferent fibers for the outer and inner hair cell system.

found about two-thirds unmyelinated fibers of varying calibers.

By means of degeneration studies with selective transections of the olivocochlear fibers in the vestibular nerve or at the floor of the fourth ventricle, their peripheral distribution and terminations could clearly be demonstrated in the rat,[28] guinea pig,[29] the cat,[5] and chinchilla.[28] According to such studies, the large nerve endings at the outer hair cells, the upper tunnel radial fibers, and the inner spiral fibers belong to the efferent innervation.

The most striking finding is the enormous efferent innervation of the outer hair cells (Fig. 5-9), where on the basis of transmission electron microscopic serial sections[30] or with series of extra-thick sections observed at high-voltage electron microscopy, 6 to 10 large efferent endings at the base of each outer hair cell are found.[31] The efferent innervation of the outer hair cells decreases from base to apex and is less abundant in the second and third row of outer hair cells. The efferent nerve endings have enormous contact areas with the outer hair cell, about 10 times as large as the contact area of the afferent nerve endings with the hair cell. They have numerous synaptic contacts, in the cat almost exclusively with the hair cell and only exceptionally with an afferent dendrite. This certainly reflects the potential influence the efferents can have on the outer hair cells. The distribution of the efferents to the outer hair cells is essentially radial, and the tunnel-crossing fibers are relatively large, with an average diameter of 1 $\mu$m.

The efferents at the level of the inner hair cells are quite different. They form the inner spiral fibers and the tunnel spiral fibers. They are small, with diameters between 0.1 and 0.6 $\mu$m, the great majority about 0.2 $\mu$m. Their number increases from base to apex of the cochlea, in contrast to the efferents of the outer hair cells. The inner hair cell efferents generally number around 200 at any one place in the middle turn of the cat cochlea. The spiral extension and actual terminals are unknown. They form a plexus with the afferent dendrites, which penetrate through the spiral bundles on their way to the inner hair cells. Along their course these inner spiral fibers form varicose enlargements filled with synaptic vesicles partly surrounding the afferent dendrites. They have exclusively synaptic contacts, mostly "en passant," with afferent dendrites but not with the inner hair cells. In rodents one finds some exceptions to this rule.

In reconstructions of this area, Liberman[32] found that each afferent dendrite from the inner hair cell has up to 20 synaptic contacts with efferent inner spiral fibers. Even some afferents and efferents from the outer hair cells occasionally synapse with inner spiral efferents, and rarely, some synaptic contacts between efferents and afferents are found just above the habenula.

There is some evidence that the efferents for the inner and outer hair cells belong to two different systems. Morphologically, the efferents of the outer hair cells are large and radial and synapse predominantly with the receptor cells, whereas the

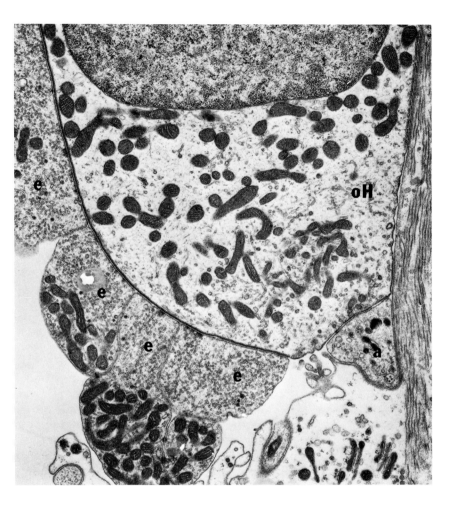

**Fig. 5-9.** Base of an outer hair cell *(oH)* with the numerous, very large efferent nerve endings *(e)* in a cat, showing a very large contact area with the inner hair cell and a much smaller afferent nerve terminal *(a)* with relatively poor synaptic differentiation.

efferents of the inner hair cell system have a spiral distribution and synapse exclusively with dendrites but not with the receptor cell. In addition, the inner hair cell efferents degenerate much slower than the efferents of the outer hair cell system. The most important evidence was provided in a study by Warr and Guinan.[33] Radioactive leucine or methionine was injected in the area of either the LSO or MNTB, using auditory-evoked potential recordings for orientation of the pipette. After 11 to 36 hours, the cochleae were evaluated by autoradiographic techniques, and the silver grains in the area below the inner hair cells and at the base of the outer hair cells were counted. After injection in the LSO, silver grains were found almost exclusively in the inner hair cell area, predominantly homolateral

but also some contralateral. After injection in the MNTB, most grains were found in the area of the contralateral outer hair cells, and only about 10 percent were found in the inner hair cell region, which might be due to passage of the outer hair cell efferents through this area.

These results are consistent with the degeneration studies according to which a midline lesion leads to degeneration of most efferents of the outer hair cells but has no effect or only partial effect on the efferents of the inner hair cell area. Whether or not the myelinated efferent fibers belong to the contralateral and the unmyelinated to the homolateral systems, as has been suggested, remains an open question. Considering that the olivocochlear efferent system consists of a number of different neural groups, the situation might be more complex. However, after midline lesions most of the remaining nerve fibers in the intraganglionic spiral bundle are unmyelinated.

Although there are definite electrophysiologically recordable and measurable efferent effects on the cochlear potentials,[34-36] there is very scarce and conflicting evidence concerning the physiological significance of the efferents in the hearing process.[27] Stimulation of the cross olivocochlear bundle was found to reduce the amplitude of the compound action potentials (CAP) to a maximum of an equivalent of 30 dB sound pressure. The same effect can be found in single-fiber recordings.[37] Stimulation of the crossed olivocochlear fibers also increases the cochlear microphonics to an equivalent of 2 to 3 dB.[34] Only a few experiments with uncrossed olivocochlear bundle stimulations have been done, and these show that the amplitude of the CAP is reduced correspondingly to a reduction in sound pressure of 6 to 7 dB,[38] but that the cochlear microphonics are not influenced.

The mode of action of the efferents might be by a change of the membrane resistance at the site of the synaptic contacts; this would explain the decrease of action potentials and the increase of the receptor potential. Although the crossed olivocochlear fibers are predominantly associated with the outer hair cells, and the great majority of all afferent neurons are associated with the inner hair cells, there is a clear effect of the stimulated crossed olivocochlear bundle on all afferent dendrites. This phenomenon can only be understood in connection with the general organization and functional significance of the outer hair cell system.[18,20]

The striking discrepancy between the extensive anatomic representation of the efferents in the organ of Corti and the physiologic effects has not yet been solved. A number of negative findings and the clinical observation that transection of the vestibular nerve in cases of Menière's syndrome did not induce any measurable changes of hearing led to the conclusion that under normal conditions the efferent system has no function.[39] Such a situation, however, seems very unlikely, because anatomically the efferent system is so well represented and highly developed that it is hardly conceivable that it would not have any functional significance. For a

feedback system, the latencies of more than 10 msec appear to be too long.

The evidence that the efferents are involved in a peripheral gating mechanism is uncertain, and the observation that the peripheral adaption of the cochlea is influenced by the efferents[40] has not been confirmed. Interaural influences seem to occur at the level of second-order neurons in the cochlear nucleus.[41] A number of behavioral experiments after transection of the crossed olivocochlear fibers have been reported. Dewson[42] found an impaired ability of stimulus discrimination, whereas Trahiotis and Elliot[43] found similar effects in the cat. Igarashi et al.,[44] on the other hand, found no effect on intensity and frequency discrimination, in contrast to earlier findings of Capps and Ades[45] in the squirrel monkey. Possible trophic functions are still hypothetical, and the same is the case for eventual feed-forward systems, which have been demonstrated in the vestibular system.

## Autonomic Innervation

The presence of an autonomic nerve supply to the inner ear has always been assumed. An unequivocal demonstration was so far only achieved for the sympathetic or adrenergic system, which can be best identified by means of the histochemical demonstration of its specific transmitter, noradrenaline. On the other hand, cholinergic parasymphathetic fibers can hardly be differentiated from somatic cholinergic fibers. In the ear they are, if present at all, possibly part of the olivochochlear efferent system.

The best way to show the adrenergic innervation is by histochemical demonstrations of noradrenaline after Falck et al.[46]

Using this technique, a dense continuous perivascular adrenergic plexus is found in the adventitia of the basilar artery, the inferior anterior cerebellar artery, the labyrinthine artery, and its greater modiolar branches. Further peripheral, the perivascular network disappears, and is not present in the osseous spiral lamina and the membraneous labyrinth.

On the other hand, a rich adrenergic nerve plexus is found independent of blood vessels. The most striking adrenergic nerve plexus is seen within the osseous spiral lamina in its peripheral zone, just before the habenula perforata. A great number of green fluorescent fibers with varicosities run between the other fibers of the cochlear nerve radially, independent of the blood vessels.[2] Whether those fibers sometimes penetrate the habenula cannot yet be decided, but they never appear to cross the tunnel of Corti to reach the outer hair cells. Most likely the great majority of them turn before entering the habenula to form the arcades of the terminal plexus. In combined preparations of ink perfusion of the blood vessels and histochemical demonstration of noradrenaline, such a plexus of adrenergic fibers is unquestionably shown in all turns. Only occasionally a fiber is seen to follow a blood vessel over a longer distance, which does not allow the conclusion that this is a perivascular innervation. The adrenergic fibers in the osseous spiral lamina are most conspicuous in the apical turn, where they can be followed through the entire length of the osseous spiral lamina. This corresponds possibly to the special autonomic innervation of the cochlear apex described by Palumbi.[47] There is, however, no adrenergic innervation in the other parts of the membranous labyrinth, especially not in the spiral ligament and the stria vascularis.

In the osseous spiral lamina, the adrenergic nerve fibers run predominantly between the myelinated fibers of the cochlear neurons without any closer relation to them. In the tympanic lip they usually run a certain distance from the blood vessels, the wall of which consists only of endothelium and some pericytes. These adrenergic fibers are of small size and have varicose enlargements filled with numerous dense-core vesicles that are between 600 and 1,200 Å in diameter. Such accumulations of dense-core vesicles are typical for the adrenergic system, and they can be enhanced by the administration of 6-hydroxydopamine, which accumulates very fast in adrenergic neurons.

The perivascular adrenergic innervation consists of several fascicles of very small nerve fibers in the adventitia and very few larger myelinated nerve fibers. All these fibers have no direct contacts to the smooth muscle cells of the vessel and no definite nerve endings, so that any sympathetic influence can only occur over distance by diffusion of the transmitter noradrenaline. The fact that there are some large, unmyelinated fibers indicates that

in this system also fast saltatory nerve conduction is possible.[2]

As shown by lesions in the cervical sympathetic chain, the adrenergic fibers of the cochlea, which are independent from blood vessels, originate in the superior cervical ganglion. The perivascular fibers, on the other hand, have their origin in the stellate ganglion, from which they reach the labyrinthine artery via the perivascular nerve plexus of the vertebral and basilar artery. There are, therefore, two different types of adrenergic innervation of the inner ear, one strictly perivascular, and the other independent of blood vessels originating in the superior cervical ganglion. The functional significance of both systems is not clarified, and thus far is only hypothetical.

## Vestibular Nerve

As in the cochlea, the vestibular apparatus also is provided with afferent, efferent, and autonomic innervation.

### Afferent Neurons

The vestibular afferent neurons, which connect the vestibular sensory epithelium with the vestibular nuclei in the brain stem, are bipolar neurons. The perikaryons are located in Scarpa's ganglion within the inner acoustic canal. The vestibular nerve is divided into two major portions, the superior division, innervating the lateral and superior crista and the macula utriculi, and the inferior division, innervating the macula sacculi and the posterior crista via the singular nerve.

The superior division is composed of about 12,000 neurons, and the inferior division of about 6,500 neurons. The diameter of the nerve fibers varies between 1 and 15 $\mu$m. The ampullary nerves contain more large fibers than the macular nerves. On the basis of the size of the ganglion cell as well as the size and position of the nucleus, two types of neurons can be distinguished: large neurons and small neurons, the latter making up only about 5 percent of the neural population in the superior division and 12 percent in the inferior division. Both types of neurons show varying degrees of myelination, from entirely missing to thick myelin sheaths.[48]

All fibers lose their myelin sheath when they enter the sensory epithelium through the basement membrane. Above the basement membrane, they form a horizontal plexus with considerable branching before they contact the sensory cells.

Two types of sensory cells are found in the vestibular sensory epithelia[49]:

1. The phylogenetically younger type I cells are found only in higher vertebrates, have a bottle shape, and are surrounded by a nerve chalice.
2. The phylogenetically older type II cells are found in all vertebrates and are connected with 10 to 20 individual small nerve endings.

Type II cells are usually associated with small nerve fibers and type I cells with large nerve fibers. The innervation ratio of sensory cells/nerve fiber is 2.6 for the superior crista, 3.1 for the posterior crista, 4.6 for the macula sacculi, and 5.6 for the macula utriculi.[50]

The sensory cells of the cristae obviously have a richer innervation than those in the maculae. In the cristae there are about 60 percent type I cells, whereas in the maculae type I and type II cells are equally represented. It is assumed that fibers innervating many hair cells will show a regular, spontaneous firing rate and fibers innervating only a few hair cells will show an irregular activity. Most fibers from the maculae have regular discharge patterns, whereas fibers from the cristae frequently show irregular firing. Since thin fibers innervating type II cells have more ramification and innervate a greater number of hair cells than thick fibers associated with the one type I cells, it is assumed that irregular firing units are the type I-associated fibers.

The receptor-neuron junction between nerve endings and type II cells is characterized by typical synaptic complexes with membrane thickenings and synaptic bars of variable forms. In the type I cells, there are two types of contacts between sensory cells and nerve chalice:

1. Areas with an irregular empty intercellular space with an average width of 200 Å and fusion of the unit membranes at certain spots. This type of receptor–neuron contact is mostly found in the supranuclear portion of the sensory cells. It is rather unspecific and closely resembles contacts between supporting cells.
2. Areas with a very regular intercellular space of 270 Å width filled with a dense amorphous material. The dense zones are very specific for the receptor–neuron contacts between type I cells and the nerve chalice and represent about 30 percent of the cell surface. Associated with these dense zones one frequently finds very large synaptic bars of various forms within the cytoplasm of the sensory cell. These specific dense zones probably serve a more efficient synaptic transmission and might be responsible for the degree of spontaneous activity, which is directly related to the sensitivity of the unit. The generally higher spontaneous activity of units in mammals compared to those of the more primitive vertebrates could be due to the presence of type I cells in mammals.

## Efferent Neurons

In type I units, the efferent endings sit exclusively at the nerve chalice with evidence of synaptic contacts. Usually, several efferent nerve endings are associated with one afferent nerve. They are never in direct contact with the sensory cell of type I. In the type II units, the efferent nerve endings may contact the sensory cell directly, but even their synaptic contacts are predominantly with the afferent nerve endings and nerve fibers, so that in the vestibular sensory epithelium the efferent contacts are almost exclusively axodendritic and not with the sensory cells, in contrast to the organ of Corti.

Functionally, the efferents of the vestibular system might be able to change the electrical polarization of the afferent neurons. As shown by Löwenstein[51] spontaneous activity of the afferent neurons can be changed by changing the electrical polarization. It would therefore be possible that the efferents, by changing the polarization of the afferent neurons, change the level of spontaneous activity and therefore the sensitivity of the units. Such an efferent control might be in part responsible for the phenomenon of adaptation, after effects, or preventive attenuation of the effect of vestibular stimuli during intentional movements.[52]

## Autonomic Innervation

Below the vestibular sensory epithelia, adrenergic nerve fibers can be demonstrated by the histochemical method of Falck et al.[46] These fibers do not seem to penetrate the basilar membrane, and they do not have direct contacts with the sensory cells. Also, in the vestibular ganglion, numerous adrenergic nerve fibers are found. As in the cochlea, there are perivascular adrenergic fiber systems and blood vessel-independent adrenergic nerve fibers. They seem to have the same origin as the autonomic fibers for the cochlea, whereas the blood vessel-independent nerve fibers originate in the superior cervical ganglion and the perivascular fibers originate in the stellate ganglion.[53] Nothing is known about their functional significance.

# DEGENERATION BEHAVIOR OF THE VESTIBULOCOCHLEAR NERVE

## Cochlear Nerve

Various conditions can lead to the degeneration of a neuron. If an intrinsic neuronal process causes its degeneration, the term *primary degeneration* may be used. If the degeneration is induced by an extrinsic factor such as a direct lesion of the neuron or severe damage of associated structures, the term *secondary degeneration* is used.

Injury to an axon is followed by two types of degeneration: (1) wallerian descending degeneration affecting the portion of the axon that has been separated from the perikaryon by the lesion, and (2) secondary retrograde degeneration, which affects the portion of the neuron containing the perikaryon (Fig. 5-10).

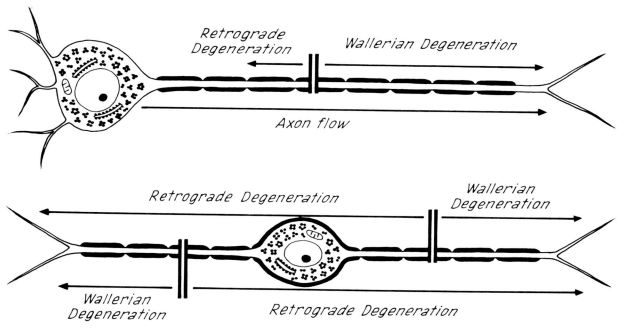

**Fig. 5-10.** Schema of types of degeneration after lesion of a neuron. *Top*, efferent motor neuron. *Bottom*, bipolar sensory neuron.

In motor or centrifugal neurons, which have their ganglion cell within the central nervous system, wallerian degeneration is very marked and within few hours leads to degeneration of the peripheral axon and the nerve endings, whereas retrograde degeneration affects only a very short segment of the central axon adjacent to the lesion where regeneration starts very early. This phenomenon is well-known to occur in the facial nerve and is probably also present in the olivocochlear efferent neurons.

Retrograde secondary degeneration, on the other hand, is a very slow phenomenon and affects the entire neuron including the ganglion cell body. It occurs typically in the pseudomonopolar and bipolar sensory neurons, including the cochlear neurons when their central or peripheral axon or dendrites are damaged. The percentage of affected neurons varies considerably among different nerves.

Secondary or retrograde degeneration affects about 50 percent of the neurons in the spinal nerves, about 90 percent of the neurons in the cochlear nerve, and only about 30 percent of the neurons in the vestibular nerve. In the cochlear neurons it is obviously sufficient to damage only the very peripheral terminal portions (i.e., the nerve endings of the peripheral dendrites) to induce such retrograde degeneration. One year after an acoustic overstimulation with 140 dB white noise for about 20 minutes or acute intoxication with amikacin with complete destruction of the organ of Corti, we find a very pronounced retrograde degeneration of the cochlear neurons with subtotal loss of spiral ganglion cells (Fig. 5-11).

Immediately after acute destruction of the organ of Corti by acoustic overstimulation, the remnants of the peripheral dendrites within the habenula appear to be swollen, and the axoplasm of the adjacent portions of the axons show considerable vacu-

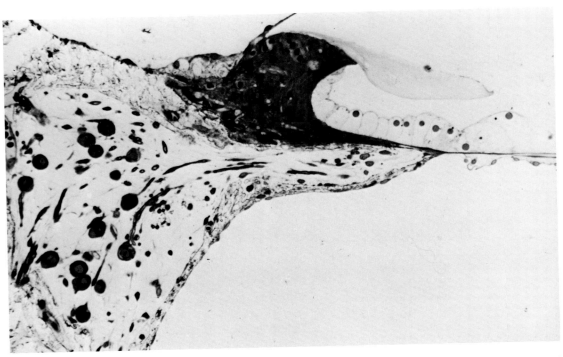

**Fig. 5-11.** Spiral ganglion of the basal turn of a rat cochlea 12 months after destruction of the organ of Corti by amikacin. About 90 percent of the ganglion cells have disappeared as a consequence of retrograde degeneration.

olization as the first sign of retrograde degeneration. The myelin sheath remains intact at this early stage. Four days later, however, the myelin becomes fragmented with the formation of individual myelin figures, secondary lysosomes, and complete disappearance of the axons. The ganglion cells within the spiral ganglion begin only a few weeks later to show signs of degeneration. There are great time differences in the progression of degeneration among the individual ganglion cells. For several weeks all stages and degrees of degeneration are found within the same spiral ganglion (Fig. 5-12). During the first few months, however, the great majority of ganglion cells will gradually

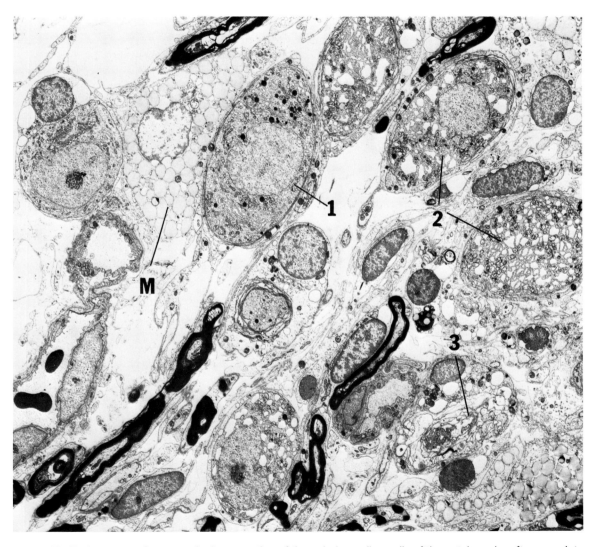

**Fig. 5-12.** Early stages of retrograde degeneration of the spiral ganglion cells of the cat 4 weeks after complete destruction of the organ of Corti by acoustic traumatization. Ganglion cells are found in different stages of degeneration. Some *(1)* have only lost their myelin sheath, others *(2)* show heavy vacuolization of the cytoplasm, and others *(3)* are in complete degeneration. There are many macrophages *(M)* between the degenerating ganglion cells.

and completely disappear. The products of this degradation are taken up by phagocytes.

The quantification of the cochlear neurons is best achieved on the basis of the block-surface technique.[54] In these surface preparations the organ of Corti can be evaluated exactly. In serial tangential sections through the corresponding areas of the osseous spiral lamina, the peripheral axons of the cochlear neurons can be counted,[7] and in extra-thick serial sections through the spiral ganglion, the spiral ganglion cells can be quantitatively evaluated and identified using the interference-contrast technique of Nomarski.[18] The type I ganglion cells and their derivatives, the type III cells, are characterized by a large size and a large, round central nucleus with a pronounced nucleolus. They are always bipolar with a thicker central and a thinner peripheral axon. The type II ganglion cells, on the other hand, appear to be pseudomonopolar, smaller, with an eccentric irregular nucleus and a less pronounced nucleolus, features that have been described and discussed in electron microscopic

studies (Fig. 5-3).[10] In general there is a good correlation between the figures obtained by counting the peripheral axons in the osseous spiral lamina and by counting the ganglion cells in extra-thick serial sections through the ganglion.

The typical time course of retrograde degeneration of the cochlear neurons is clearly demonstrated in rats where the organ of Corti has been completely destroyed by amikacin intoxication. The number of neurons has been evaluated at various time intervals after the destruction of the organ of Corti. The regression curve is asymptotic, reaching a final apparently stable value of about 10 percent surviving neurons after about 12 months (Fig. 5-13).[55] A similar time course of retrograde degeneration is found after section of the 8th nerve, where, however, only about 5 percent of the neurons survive.[56] The time course of retrograde degeneration seems to be related to the normal life span of the species. Retrograde degeneration proceeds much faster in animals with short normal life span than in species with longer life span such as

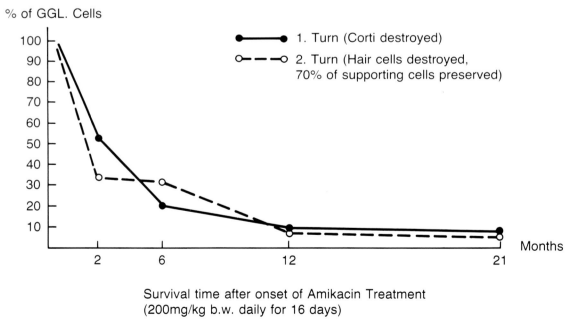

Survival time after onset of Amikacin Treatment
(200mg/kg b.w. daily for 16 days)

**Fig. 5-13.** Time course of retrograde degeneration after destruction of the organ of Corti by amikacin. There is no significant difference between the first turn, where the organ of Corti is completely destroyed, and the second turn, where the supporting cells of the organ of Corti are essentially preserved. *GGL*, ganglion cells.

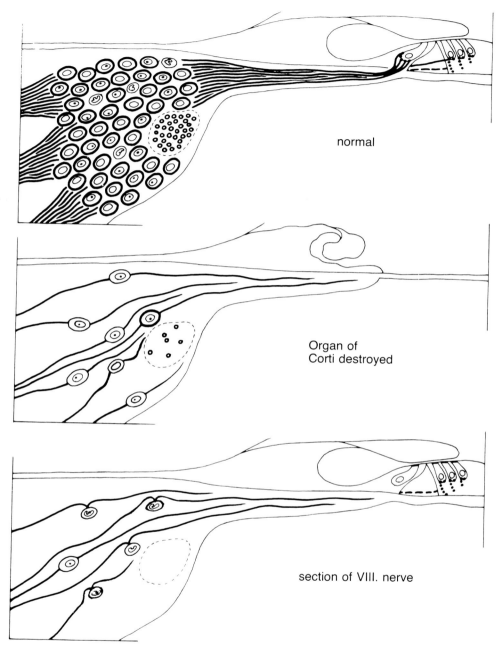

normal

Organ of
Corti destroyed

section of VIII. nerve

**Fig. 5-14.** Two different types of secondary retrograde degeneration after destruction of the organ of Corti and after section of the 8th nerve. After destruction of the organ of Corti, about 90 percent of the ganglion cells of types I and II degenerate. After section of the 8th nerve, only the great majority of the type I neurons associated with the inner hair cells degenerate, whereas the type II neurons associated with the outer hair cells, as well as the entire afferent nerve supply of the outer hair cells, remain in normal numbers and structure. A few neurons of the inner hair cell system always remain as unmyelinated type III neurons.

the human, where the degeneration seems to progress very slowly over years.

The transection of the 8th nerve in the inner acoustic canal also reveals other aspects of secondary retrograde degeneration (Fig. 5-14). The organ of Corti remains intact if the lesion did not interfere with the cochlear blood supply, as already described by earlier investigators.[57] Therefore, the reaction of the peripheral dendrites within the organ of Corti to section of the central axons of the

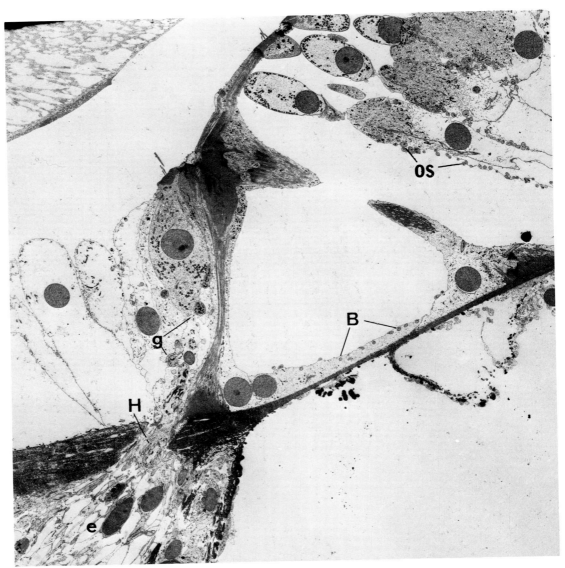

**Fig. 5-15.** Low magnification electron micrograph of the organ of Corti 8 months after transection of the 8th nerve in the internal auditory canal. The great majority of the nerve fibers in the osseous spiral lamina *(e)* have disappeared, and within the habenula *(H)* there are only very few remaining fibers. Some of them form the very few giant nerve fibers *(g)* below the inner hair cells as well as the basilar *(B)* and the outer spiral *(OS)* fibers of the afferent nerve supply of the outer hair cells.

neurons can be studied. Two weeks after transection of the 8th nerve, we find signs of degeneration in some fibers but considerable proliferation in others. Degeneration processes manifest themselves in vacuoles in the axoplasm and myelin figures, whereas proliferating processes usually are associated with an increased number of very small mitochondria and a considerable augmentation of the endoplasmic reticulum within the axoplasm. Secondary retrograde degeneration therefore appears to be a very complex necrobiotic process that extends over a long period of time. Four months after transection, degenerative processes clearly prevail. Most nerve fibers have disappeared in the osseous spiral lamina, and in the spiral ganglion only about 5 percent of the ganglion cells remain. All type I cells have disappeared. The remaining cells are of type II and type III, the latter of which are type I cells that have lost their myelin sheath. Below the base of the inner hair cells, all normal inner radial fibers are gone, and a few giant nerve fibers have appeared instead.[58] The giant fibers represent the peripheral portion of the few remaining myelinated nerve fibers within the osseous spiral lamina, which obviously belong to the few surviving type III ganglion cells. The afferent neurons of the outer hair cells, on the other hand, remain entirely normal with normal numbers. They belong to the type II neurons, which are unmyelinated and also remain in normal numbers (Fig. 5-15).[18]

Between 4 months and 1 year survival, little change occurs in the organ of Corti, but with longer survival times an increasing number of nerve fibers are found in the inner hair cell region, although in the osseous spiral lamina there are relatively very few predominantly unmyelinated nerve fibers remaining.[59,60] During this time, the remaining type III ganglion cells in the spiral ganglion are gradually reduced in number, along with the myelinated axons in the osseous spiral lamina.

In most animals with survival times of more than 1 year, this fiber proliferation in the area of inner hair cells is very pronounced, frequently exceeding by far the amount of nerve fibers in normal animals and giving sometimes the impression of neuroma formation, with several thousand nerve fibers densely packed together and filling the entire space below and around the inner hair cells (Fig.

5-16). The inner hair cells are frequently pushed aside by the overgrowing nerve fibers. The fibers are unmyelinated and are of various sizes, usually larger than the normal inner spiral fibers. In cases with relatively few proliferating fibers, they are all large in size, similar to the giant fibers observed earlier. The more numerous the proliferating fibers are, the more small-sized fibers are found among the larger ones.

These small-sized fibers appear to be ramifications of giant fibers. They run over large distances in spiral courses, making synaptic contacts with the inner hair cells. The actual spiral extension could not be determined. Between the larger fibers, a special type of satellite cell, normally not present, can be observed. It partially surrounds some fibers with small tentacle-like protrusions that have a very dark and dense cytoplasm. These satellite cells probably are extensions of the habenular satellite cells, which normally do not protrude above the level of the habenular openings.

In some animals with survival times of 2 years after section of the 8th nerve or after selective section of the cochlear nerve, abundant proliferation is not only observed at the level of the inner hair cells, but also at the base of the outer hair cells at some locations in the cochlea.[61] There, bundles of very small fibers are found close to the base of the outer hair cells. Occasionally it can be seen that they are ramifications of outer spiral fibers. Among these fibers large structures are also found, filled with secondary lysosomes, myelin figures, and degenerating membranes. Such degenerating elements may be very predominant even after survival times of 2 years. In such animals the afferent outer spiral fibers and the afferent nerve endings at the outer hair cells are numerically and structurally intact. The efferent fibers are completely missing in the animals in which the 8th nerve was sectioned, and entirely intact in the animals in which only the cochlear nerve was sectioned. The only neurons from which these proliferating fibers possibly can originate are afferent neurons associated with the outer hair cells. Some fibers form nerve endings at the base of outer hair cells with evidence of synaptic contacts, which surprisingly, frequently have the morphologic characteristics of efferent terminals.

In studying the spiral ganglion in animals with

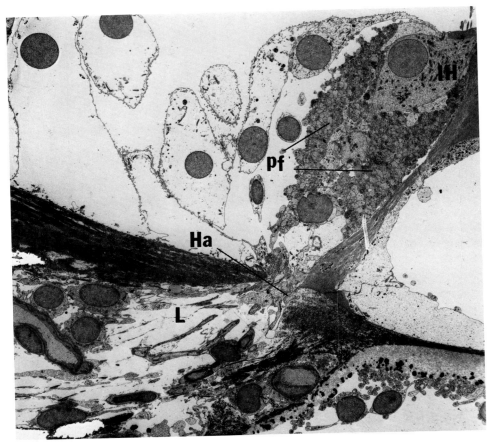

**Fig. 5-16.** Habenula *(Ha)* and inner hair cell *(IH)* 2 years after transection of the 8th nerve in the internal auditory canal. Most fibers in the osseous spiral lamina *(L)* are missing. Only very few predomonantly unmyelinated and some myelinated fibers remain. There is an enormous number of proliferating nerve fibers *(pf)* below the inner hair cells.

survival times of more than 4 months, the following observations can be made: after 4 months there is about an equal number of surviving type II and type III ganglion cells. Whereas the type II ganglion cells remain constant in number for survival times in excess of 4 months, there is a progressive reduction of type III ganglion cells, which seem to reach a very small asymptotic value after about 2 years. However, although they are very much reduced in number, we always found some surviving type III cells in animals with survival times of 2 years or greater (Fig. 5-14).[61]

Parallel to the reduction of the type III ganglion cells, the myelinated fibers in the osseous spiral lamina are gradually reduced with increasing survival times. In the case of transection of the cochlear nerve, they reach minimal values after 2 or more years. However, in the case of the combined transection of the cochlear and inferior vestibular nerves, the number of myelinated fibers surprisingly tends to increase again in animals with survival times of more than 1 year. In the spiral ganglion of such animals one finds a considerable number of predominantly very large, myelinated nerve fibers passing the ganglion without a ganglion cell body (Fig. 5-17). Most of them continue as large fibers through the osseous spiral lamina toward the organ of Corti, but some of them turn

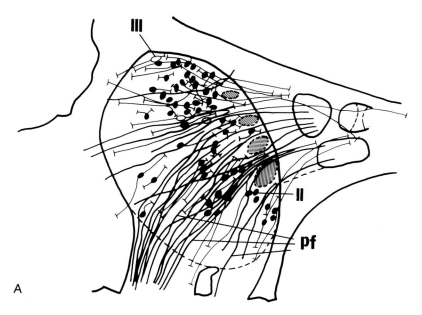

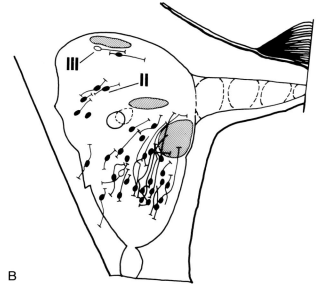

**Fig. 5-17.** Numerical evaluation of the nerve elements in the spiral ganglion of cats two years after nerve lesions in the inner acoustic canal 150-$\mu$m extra-thick serial sections observed with interference contrast microscopy are evaluated. The ganglion cells of type II *(II)* and type III *(III)* are represented with the peripheral and central axons as far as these fibers could be followed in these serial sections. The passing fibers *(pf)* through the spiral ganglion are represented by thick black lines. **(A)** Situation after transection of the cochlear and vestibular nerve. The great majority of surviving ganglion cells are of type II, (solid ovals) and only a few are type III, (open ovals). There is a great number of passing fibers, which run through the spiral ganglion without having a ganglion cell body and correspond most probably to regenerating fibers. **(B)** Situation after selective transection of the cochlear nerve. Again the great majority of surviving ganglion cells are of type II and only very few are of type III. There are practically no regenerating fibers passing through the spiral ganglion.

around to go backward toward the modiolus. In the osseous spiral lamina of such animals, there is an increasing number of myelinated and unmyelinated fibers as compared with animals with shorter survival times or selective section of the cochlear nerve. At the habenula not many fibers are found penetrating into the organ of Corti. Many fibers do not reach the habenular openings, and they return backward toward the lamina.

The increasing number of nerve fibers in the osseous spiral lamina more than 1 year after the transection of the 8th nerve and the new fibers crossing the spiral ganglion without a ganglion cell body obviously are the result of some sort of regeneration. The regenerating myelinated fibers in the spiral ganglion and within the osseous spiral lamina could theoretically originate in the remaining afferent neurons, in vestibular neurons whose axons have been transected, or in the olivocochlear efferent neurons. It is important to note that substantial regeneration of myelinated fibers is found only after combined lesions of the cochlear and vestibular nerve but not after selective lesions of the cochlear nerve (Fig. 5-17A and B). Regenerating afferent neurons are, therefore, practically excluded. Most of them have completely disappeared, including the perikarya, and the few remaining type III neurons provide only a small number of myelinated fibers in the osseous spiral lamina, as seen in animals with selective lesions of the cochlear nerve. The possibility, however, that some of these regenerating fibers originate from vestibular neurons, cannot be excluded. The vestibular neurons degenerate only to about 30 percent after transection of their axons; therefore, remaining neurons theoretically could regenerate and follow an abnormal course into the cochlea. However, not much is known about their regeneration power. Facial neurons, on the other hand, could regenerate. It is very unlikely that the regenerating fibers are of facial origin, however, because the facial nerve was carefully left intact during surgery and the animals showed no deficit of facial function after the intervention. Since motor or efferent neurons are known to have a very strong regeneration power, these regenerating, large myelinated fibers are most likely crossed olivocochlear efferent fibers, which in the combined lesions have been totally transected within the inferior branch of the vestibular nerve.

The most pronounced regeneration is found among the unmyelinated fibers. These fibers most probably are homolateral olivocochlear and autonomic fibers but also partly belong to the type II afferent fibers.

The available material shows that there is considerable regeneration and proliferation among the few surviving cochlear neurons after transection of the central axons and that there is strong evidence for fiber regeneration from the efferent or vestibular neurons.

Retrograde degeneration is found independent of the mechanism of damage to the organ of Corti, whether it is acoustic overstimulation, intoxication, or other types of damage.

The question about what induces the retrograde degeneration in the damaged organ of Corti can best be studied in long-surviving animals after various degrees of acoustic damage to the organ of Corti. In areas where only the outer hair cells are missing, there is practically no retrograde degeneration to be seen (Fig. 5-18). On the other hand, in the rare case where the outer hair cells are present but the inner hair cells are gone, there is a full-blown retrograde degeneration affecting most type I neurons with the disappearance of about 90 percent of the afferent neurons. The collapse or absence of the supporting structures in the organ of Corti, which was thought to be an important factor, does not seem to be essential for the initiation of retrograde degeneration. Retrograde degeneration is frequently found in the presence of perfectly normal supporting structures. The presence or absence of the supporting structures does not influence the degree of retrograde degeneration of amikacin-intoxicated rats with complete loss of hair cells (Fig. 5-12).[55] The loss of the inner hair cells seems to be the crucial event for the initiation of retrograde degeneration. Even though this might be correct in most cases, there are exceptions where we find retrograde degeneration in the presence of inner hair cells, or only very little retrograde degeneration where the inner hair cells are gone. Thus, the critical factor that initiates retrograde degeneration appears to be damage to the peripheral afferent dendrites associated with the inner hair cells. The afferent dendrites to the inner hair cells are very susceptible to many kinds of damaging influences, such as acoustic overstimulation, hypoxia, or others. They react in general with an enormous swelling, which leads eventually to the rupture of the axon membrane.[63]

## Vestibular Nerve

Much less is known about the behavior of the vestibular nerve than about the cochlear nerve. However, Ranson[62] has already noticed a much less pronounced degeneration of the vestibular nerve after transection of the vestibulocochlear nerve. More recently Spoendlin[63] and Richter[64] found that only about 30 percent of the vestibular neurons degenerate and disappear completely within 1 year after destruction of the vestibular sensory epithelia by labyrinthectomy. There is no

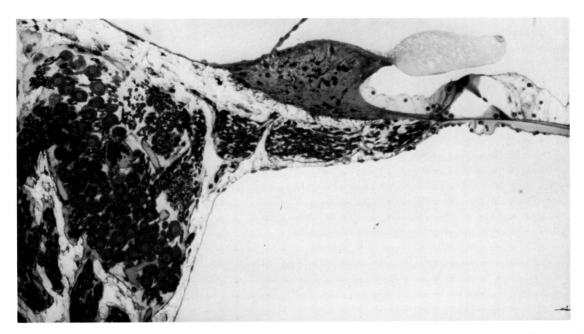

**Fig. 5-18.** Organ of Corti and spiral ganglion of a cat, in which the outer hair cells have been destroyed selectively. In this situation, practically no retrograde degeneration of the cochlear neurons occurs.

predominance of large or small neurons in degeneration. Their proportions remain unchanged, as they do in normal animals. The surviving 70 percent of neurons show some vacuolization in the cytoplasm and loss of myelin sheath, so that a higher percentage of the surviving neurons appear to be unmyelinated.

# PATHOLOGY OF THE VESTIBULOCOCHLEAR NERVE

The pathology of the 8th nerve is subdivided in the discussion here into conditions whose primary effect is on the neurons and those in which the alterations of the neurons occur secondary to pathologic changes in associated structures. However, these pathogenetic groups cannot always be clearly distinguished and are frequently combined.

## Primary Pathology of Neurons

### Genetic Disorders

Today, over 100 different types of genetic disorders associated with sensorineural deafness are known. About 50 percent of all cases with congenital deafness are genetically determined, about 10 percent with dominant and 40 percent with recessive inheritance.[65-67] In human cases only relatively little is known about the temporal bone pathology. The only cases where a clear primary degeneration of the cochlear neurons are shown in temporal bone histopathology are the cases of two profoundly deaf sisters suffering from Friedrich's ataxia.[68] There is a severe loss of cochlear neurons in the presence of a perfectly normal organ of Corti (Fig. 5-19).

In all other cases where the temporal bones have been examined, the neural degeneration is associated with severe pathologic changes of the organ of Corti or the cochlear duct. In a few congenital conditions known to be associated with sensorineu-

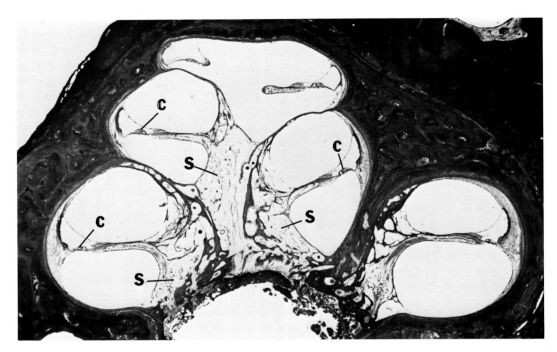

**Fig. 5-19.** Midmodiolar section of a cochlea of a case of Friedreich's disease, showing a normal organ of Corti *(C)* and a very pronounced degeneration of the ganglion cells in the spiral ganglion *(S)*, especially in the upper cochlear turns.

ral deafness, primary alteration of the cochlear neurons can be assumed, as for instance in Tay-Sachs disease with pathologic lipidosis, which seems to affect predominantly the neurons as shown in animal experiments with experimental lipidosis (see Metabolic Disturbances, below). Another congenital condition leading to primary disturbance of the cochlear neurons is von Recklinghausen's disease, a neurofibromatosis that frequently affects the cochlear nerve on both sides.

Recently, it has been shown that chronic pressure of the loop of the inferior-anterior cerebellar artery in the inner acoustic canal on the cochlear nerve at the site of transition from central glia cells to peripheral Schwann cells is the cause of certain cases of tinnitus by irritation of the cochlear neurons.

**Traumatic Alterations**

Direct traumatic damage of the cochlear neurons can happen in medial transverse fractures of the temporal bone or in the course of surgery in the inner acoustic canal. The consequence of selective transection of the cochlear neurons in the inner acoustic canal with preservation of the blood supply has been thoroughly studied in animal experiments. However, this type of selective damage to the neurons without involvement of blood supply would certainly be very rare in nature.

Direct injuries to neurons can also occur during the introduction of cochlear implants into the scala tympani, where, depending on the technique used, the osseous spiral lamina and the neurons in it can easily be damaged. This leads to further degeneration of the surviving cochlear neurons in already deaf ears. As I have seen after complete destruction of the organ of Corti, about 10 percent of cochlear neurons survive; they are reduced to about 3 percent when additional damage to the neurons in the osseous spiral lamina occurs, (Fig. 5-20) thus rendering an effective electrical stimulation of a totally deaf ear more difficult and more problematic.[69]

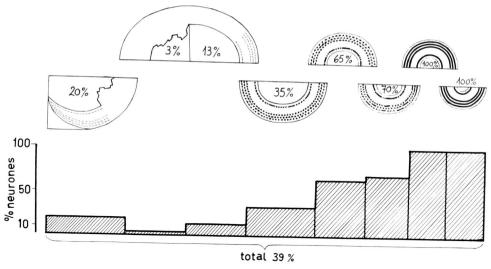

**Fig. 5-20.** Cochleogram of a cat cochlea 7 months after mechanical destruction of a portion of the lower basal turn, including the osseous spiral lamina. The number indicates the percentage of surviving ganglion cells, which is very low, with about 3 percent surviving in the area where the osseous spiral lamina has been destroyed. In the organ of Corti, a normal structure is represented by thick solid lines, selective loss of hair cells by dotted lines, and complete destruction of the organ of Corti by blank areas.

The effect of various types of mechanical damage to the cochlea is of considerable interest today because many surgical procedures increasingly involve inner ear structures. Three types of mechanical lesions have been made in cats: selective mechanical destruction of the organ of Corti in the lower basal turn, selective lesion of the nerve fibers in the osseous spiral lamina (in most cases in connection with a perforation of the lamina), and more extensive mechanical lesion of the basal turn including multiple fractures of the spiral lamina and destruction of the organ of Corti. After localized selective destruction of the organ of Corti we find, of course, a full-blown retrograde degeneration of the cochlear neurons in the area of the lesions. In addition, there is a selective loss of outer hair cells, a normal inner hair cell population, and practically no retrograde degeneration of the cochlear neurons in the greater portion of remaining cochlear turns. This result is in agreement with the original work of Schuknecht and Sutton,[70] who found a widespread loss of outer hair cells but only a restricted area of neuron degeneration after experimental lesions in the basal coil of the cochlea. If the

osseous spiral lamina is perforated with local destruction of the cochlear neurons but without touching the organ of Corti, we find the damage restricted to the immediate neighborhood of the lesion, whereas the rest of the cochlea remains entirely normal, including the outer hair cells. After extensive lesions involving the osseous spiral lamina and organ of Corti, there is also widespread damage to the organ of Corti, including inner and outer hair cells, and consequently considerable retrograde degeneration of the afferent neurons over large portions of the cochlea. In each group of lesions in four animals, we consistently found the respective patterns of pathology. This data might explain the astonishing observation that after most cases of cochleosacculotomy where only the osseous spiral lamina is penetrated by a small needle, there is very little hearing impairment.[71]

### Metabolic Disturbances

A number of metabolic disorders involving the peripheral nerves can also affect the cochlear neurons. Such disorders are mainly diabetes mellitus, uremia, and other disorders of lipid metabolism. However, not much is known about the histopathologic changes of the cochlear nerve in these conditions. One well-studied example is the experimental lipidosis induced by the administration of chlorphentermine, in which we find an enormous accumulation of secondary lysosomes in the cochlear neurons accompanied by a deterioration of cochlear function.[72]

Most ototoxic agents, such as aminoglycoside antibiotics, chinin, arsen, salicylate and others, seem to affect primarily the organ of Corti or the stria. Only very few may lead to a primary damage of the cochlear neurons.

### Infections

In severe meningitis, frequently the vestibulocochlear nerve is involved and damaged. In most cases, however, there is a combined lesion of neurons and blood supply or even diffuse labyrinthitis, leading usually to a complete destruction and obliteration of the cochlea.[69,73]

In herpes zoster oticus (Ramsay-Hunt syndrome), the viral infection is essentially and primarily localized in the geniculate ganglion. Collateral inflammatory processes, such as cell infiltrations and edema, however, frequently lead to changes in the cochlear, vestibular, and facial nerve — changes that are reversible only when the neurons do not degenerate.

### Tumors

All tumors compressing or invading the cochlear nerve can induce primary degeneration of the cochlear neurons. The best known and most frequent of these tumors are the schwannomas of the vestibulocochlear nerve, originating most frequently in the inferior division of the vestibular nerve and progressively involving the cochlear nerve by compression and invasion. In many cases the cochlear blood supply remains undisturbed, so that the organ of Corti and the stria remain intact and the cochlear neurons degenerate selectively.

## Secondary Pathology of Neurons in Inner Ear Disease

### Acoustic Trauma

The typical and pure case of secondary pathology of cochlear neurons is the secondary degeneration after acoustic-traumatic destruction of the organ of Corti.[63] The crucial factor to induce retrograde degeneration is the destruction of the inner hair cells. The degree of degeneration depends on the degree of cochlear damage. Complete loss of the organ of Corti leads to a more severe degeneration of cochlear neurons than selective loss of hair cells, and further damage such as rupture of Reissner's membrane, basilar membrane or damage to the stria has an even greater effect on the degeneration of the neurons.[74] The degenerating neurons correspond, of course, to the damaged area in the cochlea, which in most cases initially is located in the upper basal and lower second turn, corresponding to the 4,000 Hz dip in the audiogram (Fig. 5-21). Complete destruction of the cochlea by acoustic overstimulation is probably not possible. Some sensory elements with associated neurons always remain in the cochlear apex.

### Intoxication

Among the ototoxic substances that lead to inner ear damage, the aminoglycoside antibiotics differ considerably in their ototoxicity for the cochlear and the vestibular apparatus. Some are predominantly ototoxic and others vestibulotoxic. The most common aminoglycoside antibiotics are streptomycin, dihydrostreptomycin, kanamycin, gentamicin, tobramycin, sysomycin, amikacin, netilmicin, and dibekacin. The primary targets are the sensory cells, and, most probably, any neural degeneration is only secondary to the receptor organ damage, comparable to the situation in the acoustic trauma. According to some animal studies, the outer hair cells are predominantly affected in the basal turn with a gradually reduced toxic effect toward the cochlear apex, whereas the opposite is the case for the inner hair cells.[75]

The second important group of ototoxic substances are the diuretics such as ethacrynic acid,

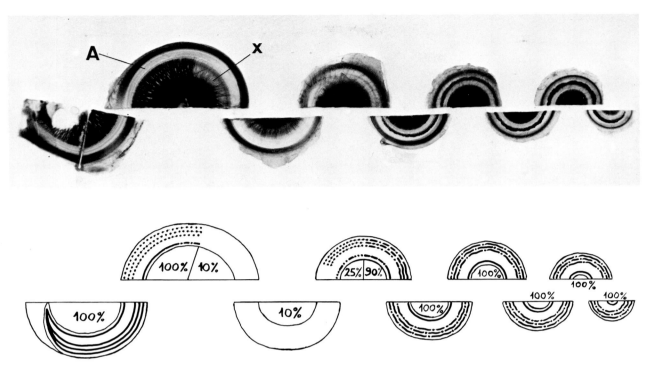

**Fig. 5-21.** Progenerary neurons in the upper basal and lower second term of the cochlea duct. Upper diagram microphotographed, lower diagram graphic reconstruction. *A*, cochlea duct; *X*, degenerating neurons.

furosemide, and carboanhydrase inhibitors (such as acetazolamide). Their primary morphologic effect is a very pronounced extracellular edema in the stria; it is usually reversible, but can eventually lead to irreversible membrane ruptures.[76] The functional consequence is depression of the cochlear potentials and the action potentials of the cochlear nerve.

Other less frequent ototoxic substances are chinin and its relatives as well as arsenic compounds.[77] Salicylates in higher dosage produce a pancochlear hearing loss that has no histopathologically detectable morphologic basis and is always reversible. Some antitumor drugs are also ototoxic to a certain extent. Cisplatin is known to produce mild sensorineural deafness if given in high doses. In animal experiments it could be shown that the drug's main targets are the hair cells, primarily the outer hair cells. Any neural degeneration seems to be secondary to the hair cell damage.[78]

**Inflammatory Processes**

Among the infectious processes, the viral labyrinthitis affects primarily the epithelial elements in the inner ear, namely the organ of Corti and the stria. The viruses known to produce labyrinthitis are essentially measels, mumps, influenza, and chicken pox, and other herpes viruses. Rubella infection of the mother also invades the embryo and causes severe malformation, including damage of the inner ear resulting in congenital deafness.

It is interesting to note that the various viruses affecting the inner ear have a different effect on the neurons. In cases of measels labyrinthitis, one finds pronounced secondary degeneration of cochlear neurons, whereas in many cases of mumps labyrinthitis, the neuronal population of the cochlea is well preserved.[3] The exact reason for this difference is not known but most probably has something to do with the tissue affinity of the viruses.

## Endolymphatic Hydrops

Spontaneous endolymphatic hydrops is a well-known entity of inner ear pathology in the human. It is the typical pathology of Menière's syndrome. In animals it can be produced by obliteration of the endolymphatic sac or duct. However, the pathogenesis or etiology of Menière's syndrome is not known. In the long run it leads primarily to a degeneration of sensory cells. Whether it is associated with primary pathologic alterations of the neurons remains an open question. A number of pathologic alterations in the spiral and vestibular ganglion in Menière patients have been reported, especially accumulation of pathologic lysosomes in the ganglion cells and atypical long-spaced collagen in the Schwann cells.[79] These alterations are, however, not specific and are also observed during the course of secondary degeneration.

## Genetic Disorders

Two types of genetic disorders can be distinguished. The first type comprises congenital malformations (dysplasias or aplasias) showing, mostly at birth, gross alterations of bony and membranous labyrinth, called Mondini-type pathology. This type of pathology is usually stable, nonprogressive, and might be associated with a considerably reduced number of cochlear neurons. The second type of genetic disorders consists of heredodegenerative processes (abiotrophy). The inner ear is fully developed but at any time postnatally begins to degenerate progressively.

These cases exhibit mostly a cochleosaccular degeneration called Scheibe type, which is restricted to the inferior portion of the labyrinth. In the Scheibe type of pathology, there is also a progressive neural degeneration. This type of pathology is especially well studied in the deaf white cat,[80,81] the Dalmatian dog,[82] and other animals with congenital pigment anomalies.[83] In these animals, progressive degeneration starts in the first days or weeks after birth. In the human, a typical example of this type of pigment anomaly associated with heredodegenerative deafness is the syndrome of Waardenburg. In the human, however, the onset and progression of inner ear degeneration can only be clinically assessed. In the rarely available temporal bones, only the final state of degeneration can be seen. Most authors have believed that the degeneration starts in the organ of Corti. Recently, however, evidence has been provided that primary neural degeneration also occurs parallel to the degeneration of the organ of Corti.[83]

## Combined Primary and Secondary Pathology

Frequently, primary and secondary pathology seem to be combined, in which case the mechanisms cannot be distinguished.

## Presbycusis

On the basis of the cochlear pathology, four types of presbycusis have been described[84]:

1. Sensory type of presbycusis with primary degeneration of the organ of Corti with secondary neural degeneration. This type of presbycusis shows a typical abrupt high-tone loss in the pure-tone audiogram that is associated with relatively good speech discrimination.
2. Neural type of presbycusis with primary degeneration of the cochlear neurons and relatively well-preserved organ of Corti. Here one finds a mildly descending audiometric pattern in the pure-tone audiogram that is associated with a relatively poor speech discrimination.
3. Strial type of presbycusis with predominant pathology in the stria and a pancochlear hearing loss.
4. Mechanical type of presbycusis. This type is merely postulated on the basis of missing pathologic changes in the cochlea in the presence of considerable sensorineural hearing loss.

Although a predominantly neural presbycusis with primary degeneration of neurons and intact organ of Corti as well as a primary sensory presbycusis with only secondary degeneration of neurons do exist, in most cases there is a combined neural pathology characterized by a scattered degeneration of neurons with neural rarefraction throughout the cochlear and, in addition, a degeneration of the organ of Corti at the basal end with pronounced secondary neural degeneration in this area. This type of pathology expresses itself in a pure-tone audiogram with regularly slightly descending pure-tone threshold curve from low to high frequencies combined with an abrupt high-tone loss.

In animal studies it has been found that the type I spiral ganglion cells degenerate predominantly with a relatively good preservation of type II ganglion cells.

## Vascular Disturbance

Impairment of the cochlear blood supply, acute or chronic, leads in general to damage of neurons as well as sensory cells. After sudden interruption of the cochlear blood supply, the complete disappearance of the action potentials occurs first, whereas the cochlear microphonics, the expression of hair cell function, remain to a certain degree over a longer time. This illustrates the extreme susceptibility of the cochlear neurons to hypoxia. The first morphologic alterations found in acute ischemia of the inner ear are enormous swellings of the terminal unmyelinated portions of the afferent neurons associated with the inner hair cells (Fig. 5-22). However, no early alterations are found in the afferent neurons associated with the outer hair cells. Irreversible damage and progressive degeneration of the neurons probably starts when the swollen terminal portions of the neurons burst. In animal experiments this occurs about 20 minutes after a complete interruption of the cochlear blood supply.

## Injuries

Severe injuries of the temporal bone, such as transverse fractures, lead in general to severe impairment of the blood supply and to direct damage to the membranous labyrinth as well as to the neurons. It results usually in complete or profound deafness with complete or partial obliteration of the cochlea and virtually total loss of neurons.

## Infections

Bacterial labyrinthitis, otogenic or meningogenic, usually causes a complete destruction of all

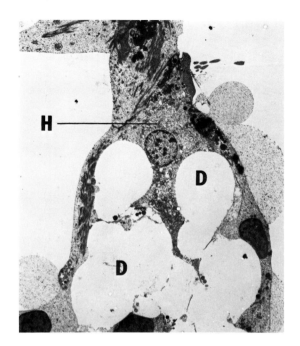

**Fig. 5-22.** Area of a human inner hair cell *(H)* with hypoxic postmortem changes, showing an extreme swelling of the afferent dendrites *(D)* associated with the inner hair cells.

components of the inner ear. If not fatal, it heals in most cases with a complete fibrous or bony obliteration of the cochlea and almost no surviving neurons.

## FUNCTIONAL IMPLICATIONS OF NERVE PATHOLOGY

As already stated, the type I cochlear afferent neurons are extremely sensitive to hypoxia. The interruption of oxygen or blood supply results in an almost immediate disappearance of the action potentials. Other metabolic disturbances of the neurons, such as those found in experimental lipidosis, lead to a reduction of the amplitude of the compound action potentials of the cochlear nerve.

The influence of neuron loss on pure-tone hearing and speech perception has been investigated in animal experiments and human temporal bones. Partial sections of the cochlear nerve in cats results in various degrees of neuronal loss.[57] The behavioral pure-tone threshold was still normal when the neuronal population was reduced by 50 percent and only slightly elevated when 90 percent of the neurons were lost, provided the cochlear blood supply was undisturbed and the endorgan remained intact. Some cases in human pathology may correspond to these experimental findings, for instance cases of Friedreich's ataxia. There might still be a relatively good pure-tone threshold in spite of the loss of most of the cochlear neurons in the presence of a normal organ of Corti. A similar situation can be found in certain cases of acoustic neuromas.

In contrast to pure-tone hearing, speech perception seems much more related to the number of available functional neurons, as found in studies with correlation between speech discrimination capacity and histopathologic findings in the corresponding temporal bones.[3]

Up to 10 years of age, the human cochlea contains an average of 36,000 spiral ganglion cells. After this age there is a gradual reduction of neurons; in the ninth decade of life, only 50 percent of the original neuron population remain.

The correlation of the ganglion cell population and the pure-tone threshold shows enormous individual variations. In cases with slight threshold elevations of 30 dB, one might find neuron populations from 17,000 to 36,000, probably due to various degrees of endorgan damage. However, in cases with normal pure tone thresholds, there were always at least 20,000 neurons.

In most cases with 20,000 neurons, there was a good speech discrimination of at least 90 percent. There are, however, exceptions with a speech discrimination of only 50 percent in spite of a neuron population of more than 30,000 or an almost normal speech discrimination with a neuron population of only 15,000. The great majority of cases with good discrimination have at least 3,000 ganglion cells in the apical turn of the cochlea.[85] Such studies lead to the conclusion, that for a useful speech discrimination a neuron population of minimal 10,000 is needed, 3,000 of which must be located in the apical turn.

# REFERENCES

1. Rasmussen GL: The olivary peduncle and other projections of the superior olivary complex. J Comp Neurol 84:141, 1946
2. Spoendlin H: Autonomic innervation of the inner ear. Adv Otorhinolaryngol 27:1, 1981
3. Otte J et al: Ganglion cell populations in normal and pathological human cochleae: implication for cochlear implantation. Laryngoscope 88:1231, 1978
4. Schuknecht HF: Neuroanatomical correlates of auditory sensitivity and pitch discrimination in the cat. p. 10. In Rasmussen GL, Windle WF (eds): Neural Mechanisms of the Auditory and Vestibular System. Charles C Thomas, Springfield, IL 1960
5. Spoendlin H: Innervation patterns in the organ of Corti of the cat. Acta Otolaryngol (Stockh) 67:239, 1969
6. Hall JG: Hearing and primary auditory centers of the whales. Acta Otolaryngol [Suppl] (Stockh) 224:1, 1966
7. Spoendlin H: Innervation densities of the cochlea. Acta Otolaryngol (Stockh) 73:235, 1972
8. Bohne BA, Kenworthy A, Carr CD: Density of myelinated nerve fibers in the chinchilla cochlea. p. 39. In Lim D (ed): Abstracts for the Association for Research in Otolaryngology, 1982
9. Ota CY, Kimura RS: Ultrastructural study of the human spiral ganglion. Acta Otolaryngol (Stockh) 89:53, 1980
10. Spoendlin H: Differentiation of cochlear afferent neurons. Acta Otolaryngol (Stockh) 91:451, 1981
11. Morrison D, Schindler RA, Wersäll J: Quantitative analysis of the afferent innervation of the organ of Corti in guinea pig. Acta Otolaryngol (Stockh) 79:11, 1975
12. Nomura Y: Nerve fibers in the human organ of Corti. Acta Otolaryngol (Stockh) 82:317, 1976
13. Dunn-Ginzberg R, Morest DK: A study of cochlear innervation in the young cat with the Golgi method. Hear Res 10:227, 1983
14. Nadol JB: Reciprocal synapses at the base of outer hair cells in the organ of Corti. Ann Otol Rhinol Laryngol 90:12, 1981
15. Liberman MC: Single neuron labeling in the cat auditory nerve. Science 216:1239, 1982
16. Kimura RS, Ota CY: Nerve fibers synapses on primate spiral ganglion. p. 82. In Lim D (ed): Abstracts for the Association for Research in Otolaryngology, 1981

17. Feldman M: Morphological observations on the cochleas of very old rats. p. 14. In Lim D (ed): Abstracts for the Association for Research in Otolaryngology, 1984

18. Spoendlin H: Neural connections of the outer hair cell system. Acta Otolaryngol (Stockh) 87:130, 1979

19. Kiang NYS, Rho JM, Northrop CC, et al: Hair cell innervation by spiral ganglion cells in adult cats. Science 217:9, 1982

20. Spoendlin H: The innervation of the outer hair cell system. Am J Otol 3:274, 1982

21. Leak-Jones PA, Snyder RL: Uptake transport of horseradish peroxidase by cochlear spiral ganglion neurons. Hear Res 8:199, 1982

22. Ruggero MA, Santi PA, Rich NC: Type II cochlear ganglion cells in the chinchilla. Hear Res 8:339, 1982

23. Morest DK: Retrograde axonal transport of D-aspartate from cochlear nucleus to type II spiral ganglion cells in the cat. p. 90. In Lim D (ed): Abstracts for the Association for Research in Otolaryngology, 1982

24. Spoendlin H, Baumgartner H: Electrocochleographic and cochlear pathology. Acta Otolaryngol (Stockh) 83:130, 1977

25. Strutz J: Der Ursprung der akustischen und vestibulären Efferenz bei Vertebraten. Habilitationsschrift 1983

26. Warr WB: The olivocochlear bundle: its origins and terminations in the cat. p. 43. In Naunton NF, Fernandez C (eds): Evoked Electrical Activity in the Auditory Nervous System. Academic Press, Orlando, FL, 1978

27. Spoendlin H: Efferent innervation of the cochlea. p. 163. In Bolis L et al (eds): Comparative Physiology of Sensory Systems. Cambridge University Press, Cambridge, England, 1984

28. Iurato S: Efferent fibers to the sensory cells of Corti's organ. Exp Cell Res 27:162, 1962

29. Smith CA, Rasmussen GL: Degeneration in the afferent nerve endings in the cochlea after axonal section. J Cell Biol 26:63, 1965

30. Spoendlin H: The organization of the cochlea receptor. Adv Otorhinolaryngol 13:1, 1966

31. Takasaka T, Shinkawa H, Watanuki K, et al: High-voltage electron microscopic study of the inner ear. Ann Otol Rhinol Laryngol [Suppl] 101:1, 1983

32. Liberman MC: Efferent synapses in the inner hair cell area of the cat cochlea: an electron microscopic study of serial sections. Hear Res 3:289, 1980

33. Warr WB, Guinan JJ, Jr.: Efferent innervation of the organ of Corti: two separate systems. Brain Res 173:152, 1979

34. Fex J: Augmentation of cochlear microphonics by stimulation of efferent fibers to the cochlea. Acta Otolaryngol (Stockh) 50:540, 1959

35. Desmedt JE, Monaco P: Mode of action of the efferent olivocochlear bundle on the inner ear. Nature 192:1263, 1961

36. Galambos RG: Suppression of auditory nerve activity by stimulation of efferent fibers to cochlea. J Neurophysiol 19:424, 1956

37. Wiederhold ML, Kiang NYS: Effects of electric stimulation of the crossed olivocochlear bundle on single auditory-nerve fibers in the cat. J Acoust. Soc. Am. 40:1427, 1970

38. Sohmer H: A comparison of the efferent effects of the homolateral and contralateral olivocochlear bundles. Acta Otolaryngol (Stockh) 62:74, 1966

39. Pfalz RKJ: Absence of a function for the crossed olivocochlear bundle under physiological conditions. Arch Klin Exp Ohr Nas Kehlk Heilk 193:89, 1969

40. Leibrandt CC: The significance of the olivocochlear bundle for the adaption mechanism of the inner ear. Acta Otolaryngol (Stockh) 59:134, 1965

41. Klinike R, Boerger G, Gruber J: The alteration of afferent, tone-evoked activity of neurons of the cochlear nucleus, following acoustic stimulation of the contralateral ear. J Acoust Soc Am 45:788, 1969

42. Dewson JH: Efferent olivocochlear bundle: some relationships to stimulus discrimination in noise. J Neurophysiol 31:122, 1968

43. Trahiotis C, Elliot DN: Behavioral investigation of some possible effects of sectioning the crossed olivocochlear bundle. J Acoust Soc Am 47:592, 1970

44. Igarashi M, Alford BR, Gordon WP, et al: Behavioral auditory function after transection of crossed olivo-cochlear bundle in the cat. II. Conditioned visual performance with intense white noise. Acta Otolaryngol (Stockh) 77:311, 1974

45. Capps MJ, Ades HW: Auditory frequency discrimination after transection of the olivocochlear bundle in squirrel monkeys. Exp Neurol 21:147, 1968

46. Falck B, Hillarp NA, Thieme G, et al: Fluorescence of catecholamines and related compounds condensed with formaldehyde. J Histochem Cytochem 10:348, 1962

47. Palumbi G: Particolare apparato nervoso recettore nella regione apicale della chiocciola dell'orecchio humano. Boll Soc Ital Biol Sper 26:136, 1950

48. Richter E, Spoendlin H: Scarpa's Ganglion in the cat. Acta Otolaryngol (Stockh) 92:423, 1981

49. Spoendlin H: Relation entre structure et fonction du récepteur vestibulaire. Acta Otorhinolaryngal Belg 29:75, 1975

50. Bergström B: The primary vestibular neurons. p.

270. In Friedmann I, Ballantyne J (eds): Ultrastructural Atlas in the Inner Ear. Butterworth (Publishers), London 1984

51. Löwenstein O: Peripheral mechanisms of equilibrium. Br Med Bull 12:114, 1956

52. Flock A: Efferent nerve fibres: postsynaptic action on hair cells. Nature 243:89, 1973

53. Spoendlin H, Lichtensteiger W: The adrenergic innervation of the labyrinth. Acta Otolaryngol (Stockh) 61:423, 1966

54. Spoendlin H, Brun JP: The block-surface technique for evaluation of cochlear pathology. Arch Otorhinolaryngol 208:137, 1974

55. Bichler E, Spoendlin H, Rauchegger H: Degeneration of cochlear neurons after amikacin intoxication in the rat. Arch Otorhinolaryngol 237:201, 1983

56. Spoendlin H, Suter R: Regeneration in the VIIIth nerve. Acta Otolaryngol (Stockh) 81:228, 1976

57. Schuknecht HF, Woellner R: Hearing losses following partial section of the cochlear nerve. Laryngoscope 63:441, 1953

58. Spoendlin H: Neuro-anatomy of the cochlea. Audiol Foniatr 1:1, 1978

59. Lindsay JR: Profound childhood deafness inner ear pathology. Ann Otol Rhinol Laryngol 31:257, 1969

60. Kerr A, Schuknecht HF: The spiral ganglion in profound deafness. Acta Otolaryngol (Stockh) 65:586, 1968

61. Spoendlin H: Nerve proliferation in the cochlea. p. 68. In Yasua Nomura (ed): Hearing loss and dizziness. Igaku-Shoin, New York, 1985

62. Ranson SW: Retrograde degeneration in the spiral nerves. J Comp Neurol Psychiatr 16:1 1950

63. Spoendlin H: Factors inducing retrograde degeneration of the cochlear nerve. Ann Otol Rhinol Laryngol [Suppl.] 112:76, 1984

64. Richter E: Scarpa's ganglion in the cat one year after labyrinthectomy. Arch Otorhinolaryngol 230:251, 1981

65. Danish J, Tillson J, Levitan M: Multiple anomalies in congenitally deaf children. Eugen Q 10:12, 1963

66. Fraser G: A study of causes of deafness amongst 2,355 children in special schools. p. 10. In Fisch L (ed): Research into Deafness in Children. Blackwell Scientific Publications, Oxford, 1964

67. Brown K: The genetics of childhood deafness. p. 177. In McConnell F, Ward P (eds): Deafness in Childhood. Vanderbilt University Press, Nashville, TN, 1967

68. Spoendlin H: Optic and cochleovestibular degenerations in hereditary ataxias. II. temporal bone pathology in two cases of Friedreich's ataxia with vestibulo-cochlear disorders. Brain 97:41, 1974

69. Spoendlin H: Anatomisch-pathologische Aspekte der Elektrostimulation des ertaubten Innenohres. Arch Otorhinolaryngol 223:1, 1979

70. Schuknecht HF, Sutton S: Hearing losses after experimental lesions in basal coil of cochlea. Arch Otolaryngol 57:129, 1953

71. Schuknecht HF: Cochleosacculotomy for Menière's disease: theory, technique and results. Laryngoscope 92:853, 1982

72. Bichler E, Spoendlin H: Experimental lipidosis of the inner ear. Arch Otorhinolaryngol 229:201, 1980

73. Paparella MM, Shigeru S: The pathology of suppurative labyrinthitis. Ann Otol Rhinol Laryngol 76:554, 1967

74. Spoendlin H: Retrograde degeneration of the cochlear nerve. Acta Otolaryngol (Stockh) 79:266, 1975

75. Kohonen A: Effect of some ototoxic drugs upon the pattern and innervation of cochlear sensory cells in the guinea pig. Acta Otolaryngol [Suppl] (Stockh) 208:1, 1965

76. Klinke R, Lahn W, Auerfurth H, Scholtholt J (eds): Ototoxic side effects of diuretics. Scand Aud [Suppl] 14:1, 1981

77. Rüedi L, Furrer W, Lüthy F, et al: Further observations concerning the toxic effects of streptomycin and quinine on the auditory organ of guinea pigs. Laryngoscope 62:333, 1952

78. Böheim K, Bichler E: Cisplatin induced ototoxicity: audiometric findings and experimental cochlear pathology. Arch Otorhinolaryngol 242:1, 1985

79. Ylikoski J, Collan Y, Palva T: Vestibular nerve in Menière's disease. Arch Otolaryngol 106:477, 1980

80. Bosher SK, Hallpike, CS: Observations on the histological features, development and pathogenesis of the inner ear degeneration of the white cat. Proc R Soc Edinb B (Nat Environ) 162:147, 1965

81. Mair IWS: Hereditary deafness in the white cat. Acta Otolaryngol [Suppl] (Stockh) 314:1, 1973

82. Lurie MH: The membranous labyrinth in the congenitally deaf collie and dalmatian dog. Laryngoscope 58:279, 1948

83. Schrott A, Spoendlin H: Pigment anomaly-associated inner ear deafness. Acta Otolaryngol (Stockh) 1987 (in press)

84. Schuknecht HF: Pathology of the Ear. Harvard University Press, Cambridge, MA, 1976

85. Pauler M, Schuknecht HF, Thornton AR: Correlative studies of cochlear neuronal loss with speech discrimination and pure-tone thresholds. Arch Otorhinolaryngol 243:200, 1986

# Biochemistry of the Inner Ear 6

Jochen Schacht
Barbara Canlon

## THE EARLY YEARS

Traditionally, research on audition has been kept in the disciplines of anatomy and electrophysiology, which laid the foundation for the knowledge of the basic mechanisms of hearing. Biochemical investigations were slow in developing but not because of a lack of awareness of their importance. Von Békésy,[1] for example, discussed the concept of several transformers in the ear where the terminal one was "a molecular transformer between the wall of the receptor and the sensitive molecular structures." Advances were hampered by technical difficulties of fluid and tissue sampling and lack of sensitive analytic techniques. Despite these limitations, Vinnikov and Titova[2] attempted to formulate a biochemical hypothesis of transduction as early as 1961. Although the details of their hypothesis proved incorrect, credit has to be given to these and other early pioneering studies for establishing an inner ear biochemistry. For a review of these early approaches, the reader is referred to Vosteen's monograph[3] as well as to the first book published on this topic, Rauch's "Biochemie des Hörorgans,"[4] and Schätzle's book on the histochemistry of the inner ear.[5]

Over the next two decades, a variety of new and sophisticated analytic techniques found their way into inner ear research. A major advance was the application of quantitative microanalytic techniques such as enzymatic cycling, developed by Lowry and his collaborators,[6] to cochlear structures by Matschinsky and Thalmann in 1967.[7] Today, with the availability of radiolabeled compounds, radioimmunoassays, high-performance liquid chromatography, and laser- and radiography-based microprobe analysis, to name a few, we have adequate means to study the molecular mechanisms of auditory and vestibular information processing and pathology.

At present, biochemical information about the inner ear is available primarily for the cochlea, and less for the vestibular system. Even "cochlear biochemistry" is a rather heterogeneous topic. It encompasses the study of sensory and supporting cells of the organ of Corti, and also of the cells of stria vascularis, spiral prominence, and spiral ligament—tissues whose physiological roles are distinctly different. Such investigations frequently obtain results from whole tissues rather than specialized cells, for example, through analysis of an organ of Corti preparation rather than of hair cells proper. In this chapter, we combine the information from various auditory and vestibular systems (mammalian cochlea, amphibian or fish lateral line canal organ, and insect ear) in order to synthesize a current biochemistry of the inner ear. It should be mentioned, however, that a number of studies have demonstrated that hair cell systems from different species may have different biochemical properties. Cross-species extrapolations sometimes necessitated by the lack of sufficient data from a single species are therefore to be undertaken with caution. This caveat applies to many aspects of auditory biochemistry and physiology and complicates the formulation of theoretic concepts.

Any treatment of the biochemistry of the inner ear will show overlap with areas that may be considered physiology or pharmacology. This is inevitable, because the boundaries of these disciplines are fluid and research into the problems of the inner ear has moved more and more toward interdisciplinary approaches. Conversely, some topics, although apparently related, have been excluded because they deserve more extensive coverage than could be afforded here — in particular, the pharmacology of inner ear fluids and potentials and the neurotransmitters.

## MEMBRANES AND MACROMOLECULES

The cell plasma membrane acts both as a barrier protecting the cell's microhomeostasis and as a site of communication with the environment. Transport of metabolites and ions, hormonal regulation, and cell recognition are some typical processes associated with the external membrane. Intracellular membranes enclose specific organelles such as mitochondria, or compose networks such as the Golgi apparatus. They provide metabolic compartmentalization and the site of complex biochemical reactions such as molecular syntheses, biologic oxidations, or respiration. Despite such a high degree of diversification and specialization, some generalizations can be made about membranes. Lipids and proteins are their primary components. These macromolecules are arranged in a "fluid mosaic"

where lipids form a bilayer into which proteins are inserted.[8] Lipids, predominantly phospholipids and cholesterol in varying ratios, confer electrical and chemical insulating properties to the membranes, whereas proteins may serve structural or specialized physiological functions as enzymes, carrier molecules, or hormone receptors. These concepts should apply also to the membranes of the inner ear. Specific and detailed biochemical analyses of cochlear cell membranes have only been performed in a few instances, and inferences as to possible events at the cell membrane frequently have to be made from whole cell analyses.

## Lipids

Early histochemical, as well as qualitative biochemical, analyses demonstrated that cochlear cells possess the normal complement of lipids: neutral lipids, phospholipids (phosphatidylethanolamine, phosphatidylserine, phosphatidylcholine, sphingomyelin, and lysophosphatidylcholine), fatty acids, and cholesterol without significant differentiation between various cochlear structures or cell types.[9] Studies by Schacht and his collaborators attempted to elucidate the functional aspects of the lipids of the inner ear. With radioactive orthophosphate $^{32}P_i$ as the precursor, they labeled phospholipids in the mature guinea pig cochlea,[10] the developing inner ear of the mouse,[11] the fish lateral line,[12] and the ear of the noctuid moth.[13] All structures showed a similar pattern of rapid $^{32}P$ incorporation, namely highest into phosphatidylinositol bisphosphate and phosphatidylinositol phosphate ("polyphosphoinositides"), and less into other phospholipids, primarily phosphatidate and phosphatidylinositol. Polyphosphoinositides in general constitute only a minor fraction of the total cell lipids, and the rapid $^{32}P$ labeling reflects their highly active metabolism. Considerably longer incubation times with $^{32}P$ are required to label the more abundant phosphoglycerides such as phosphatidylcholine and phosphatidylethanolamine because of their slower turnover. These can be more efficiently labeled with [$^3H$]glycerol,[14] which traces their de novo synthesis and thus reflects the large amount of these lipids in most cells.

Polyphosphoinositides are lipids enriched in the plasma membrane of neural and secretory tissues, and their turnover is responsive to neuromodulators and hormones that elevate intracellular calcium levels.[15,16] These physiological agents act at the cell membrane, where they initiate a reaction sequence that leads to the generation of a specific intracellular signal or "second messenger." The initial step in the action of, among others, acetylcholine (muscarinic), noradrenaline ($\alpha_1$), vasopressin ($v_1$), 5-hydroxytryptamine, and thrombin is thought to be a stimulation of phosphodiesteratic hydrolysis of membrane-bound phosphatidylinositol bisphosphate liberating diacylglycerol and inositol trisphosphate as second messengers and initiating a signal cascade, analogous to the adenylate cyclase/cyclic adenosine monophosphate (AMP) system. Diacylglycerol activates a specific protein kinase C and inositol trisphosphate mobilizes intracellular calcium stores. These two signals may then synergistically induce the cellular response (Fig. 6-1). Recent evidence suggests that visual excitation may be mediated by inositol trisphosphate as an intracellular messenger.[17] Whether cochlear phosphoinositide metabolism is responsive in such a fashion, and to which stimulus, remains to be established. There is evidence, however, that it may be involved in aminoglycoside toxicity (see the section Aminoglycosides, below) and possibly some aspect of auditory processing.

A stimulus-induced increase in $^{32}P$ labeling of phosphatidylinositol phosphate and phosphatidylinositol bisphosphate was measured in the ear of the noctuid moth.[13] This structure contains primary sensory cells and no efferent or afferent synapses. Only two bioelectric events, receptor and action potential, are triggered by the stimulus. Comparing the effect of pulsed tones to continuous tones, the latter leading to adaptation of the action potential, it was suggested that the increased label-

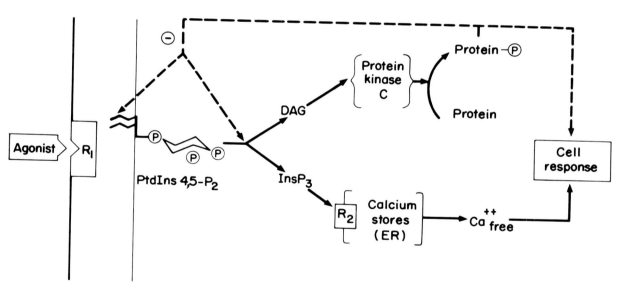

**Fig. 6-1.** Phosphoinositides as second messengers. Binding of the agonist to the receptor ($R_1$) at the outer plasma membrane of the cell stimulates the hydrolysis of phosphatidylinositol bisphosphate (PtdIns 4,5-$P_2$) to its products diacylglycerol (DAG) and inositol trisphosphate (InsP$_3$). InsP$_3$ acts on intracellular calcium stores ($R_2$) associated with the endoplasmic reticulum (ER) to release free $Ca^{2+}$, which triggers the intracellular response. DAG activates protein phosphorylation via protein kinase C. The resultant phosphorylated protein may modulate the cellular response or act as a negative feedback signal. (Modified by permission from Berridge MJ: Inositol triphosphate and diacylglycerol as second messengers. Biochem J 220:345, copyright © 1984 The Biochemical Society, London; and Nishizuka Y: Turnover of inositol phospholipids and signal transduction. Science 225:1365, 1984. Copyright 1984 by the American Association for the Advancement of Science.)

ing was associated with action potentials. An investigation of the guinea pig organ of Corti for sound-induced changes of lipid metabolism remained inconclusive because of the heterogeneity of the preparation analyzed.[12] Investigations at the hair cell level will be necessary to provide further answers.

Speculation of a specific role for phosphatidylinositol bisphosphate in transduction seem to have received support from recent immunohistochemical studies.[18] Antiserum against this lipid reacted preferentially with the cuticular plates and stereocilia of inner and outer hair cells, while cell bodies of sensory and supporting cells remained unreactive. However, some cross-reactivity of the antiserum with other lipids leaves these studies open to criticism. Phosphatidylinositol bisphosphate represents usually only 1 to 2 percent of total phospholipids, and even weak cross-reactivity with lipids of 20 to 40 times higher concentration may produce a strongly positive reaction at the cell membrane.

In addition to membrane-associated lipids, cells of the inner ear of some animal species, in particular Hensen's cells, contain "lipid droplets." Their lipidic nature was already suspected by Hensen[19] and later confirmed by histologic procedures. Their composition—triglycerides, cholesterol esters, and two phospholipids, sphingomyelin and phosphatidylethanolamine[20]—resembles that of transport or storage lipids, but the physiological role of these inclusion bodies is not known.

## Calcium-Binding Sites

An important feature of the plasma membrane of sensory cells is the mediation of electrical excitability through specific permeability changes. Davis' battery theory introduced the concept that deflection of the stereocilia changes the resistance of the hair cell membrane by modulating its ion pores.[21] This general concept is still valid, yet neither the molecular transducer nor the cellular site of transduction has been precisely delineated. Experiments with the lateral line organ[22] and the bullfrog vestibular system established that deflection of the hair cell bundle, specifically of the stereocilia (as opposed to the kinocilium)[23] indeed results in the receptor potential in the hair cells. Recently, Hudspeth and Jacobs[24] suggested that transduction begins near the distal ends of the stereocilia rather than at the apical surface of the hair cell proper, as previously assumed. Stimulus-induced extracellular potentials around the hair bundles of saccular hair cells of the bullfrog were larger near the top than the base. The presence of a high current density at the tips, however, may not necessarily correlate with a site of transduction; the current might be "funneled" to the base through the stereocilia.

In a biochemical approach to the problem of transduction, it seems important to consider calcium binding to hair cells as this ion modulates the permeability of excitable membranes. Based on the strong dependence of the cochlear microphonic on the $K^+$ concentration of endolymph, it is believed that this potential is based on the flow of $K^+$ through the outer hair cells.[25] Calcium is known to regulate specific $K^+$ permeability in a number of cells, including neurons, ganglia, smooth muscle, glands, and erythrocytes. Because the microphonic potential is dependent on extracellular calcium and because aminoglycoside antibiotics, which can act as calcium antagonists, suppress the microphonics in various hair cell systems,[26,27] it is reasonable to assume that calcium may be involved in the acoustic transduction mechanism. Studies of calcium localization in hair cells have not excluded either the stereocilia or the hair cell membranes as the site of transduction. Cytochemical and radiographic microanalysis[28] have found the highest concentration of calcium along the base of the kinocilium of the goldfish lateral line, but not of the bullfrog vestibular system. In the latter, and in the vestibular system of the guinea pig, staining for calcium was associated with the outer surface of stereocilia. Another study[29] attempted to identify binding sites by immunocytochemical reactions with an antibody against human cerebellar calcium-binding protein. The cuticular plates of both inner and outer cochlear hair cells of the rat reacted most heavily and more so than those of vestibular hair cells. With this specific assay, the presence of other types of calcium-binding proteins in hair cells was not precluded. Furthermore, phospholipids are known sites of calcium binding and contribute to the membrane-bound pool of this cation.

## Proteins

### Ear-Specific Proteins

The demonstration of proteins and protein synthesis in the cells of the cochlea was among the earliest histologic and autoradiographic findings. The impression gained from the qualitative and semiquantitative results was that of a more active metabolism in stria vascularis than in either the sensory or supporting cells of the organ of Corti. Detailed analyses were not undertaken until much later, when disc gel electrophoresis was used to separate individual proteins. Some 30 to 40 protein bands from the whole cochlea were resolved,[30] and different protein-synthesis patterns were demonstrated in cochlear tissues through the incorporation of radioactive methionine supplied by perilymphatic perfusion.[10] Greater resolution of more than 200 radiolabeled polypeptides from the stria vascularis of the guinea pig[31] was achieved with two-dimensional acrylamide gel electrophoresis. Two unique proteins were found in the organ of Corti[32] of the guinea pig and rat. These two organ-of-Corti-specific polypeptides (termed OCP-I and OCP-II) were soluble acidic proteins of molecular weight 37,000 daltons and 22,500 daltons, respectively. They were absent not only from other body tissues, but also from all other inner ear structures, including the macula sacculi. This led the authors to suggest that these proteins are not just characteristic of mechanoreceptors of the inner ear in general, but are specific of the more highly specialized auditory system. To date, localization of these intriguing peptides to sensory or supporting cells and their functional significance have not been reported.

### Contractile and Structural Proteins

Since the first description of organized filamentous actin in stereocilia of the crista ampullaris of frog and guinea pig by Flock and Cheung,[33] a variety of contractile and structural proteins have been found in cochlear and vestibular structures. Evidence from analytic, electron microscopic, and immunohistochemical studies indicate the presence of actin, myosin, tropomyosin, $\alpha$-actinin, fimbrin, prekeratin, and tubulin. Actin, myosin, tropomyosin, and $\alpha$-actinin are known as part of the contractile units of skeletal muscle. They also occur in nonmuscle cells, where they may serve structural or motile functions. Fimbrin is a cross-linking protein associated with actin in the filament bundles of microvilli; tubulin is the protein subunit of microtubules, those ubiquitous fibrillar organelles of the nervous system; prekeratin is a structural fibrous protein of ectodermal origin. These macromolecules in auditory systems have recently been reviewed in detail.[34-36]

The structural and functional role of these proteins in cochlear hair cells and stereocilia is currently receiving the most attention, but their occurrence is not limited to the sensory cells. In the stria vascularis, immunoreactivity in the basal epithelial layer shows actin, myosin (of the smooth muscle and nonmuscle type), and the actin cross-linking protein $\alpha$-actinin. These are also seen in specific regions of the superficial cell layer.[36] In the supporting cells of the mammalian organ of Corti, the structural organization seems to be based on four cytoskeletal proteins: actin, tubulin, prekeratin, and a protein with an $\alpha$-actininlike immunoreactivity.[37,38]

A different and unique composition of proteins has been reported for hair cells: actin is present in both stereocilia and cuticular plate, and fimbrin seems to be specific to the stereocilia whereas tubulin may be absent from them. Reports on this localization, however, are conflicting. Strong immunoreactivity to fimbrin antibodies was reported[37] in both stereocilia and cuticular plates of inner and outer hair cells of guinea pigs, but another study,[36] while confirming its presence in stereocilia, did not detect it in cuticular plates of auditory or vestibular hair cells (except for traces in outer hair cells). Tubulin was demonstrated in the cytoskeleton of hair cells of mice and guinea pigs[38] with antibodies purified by affinity chromatography. The antibody used by Flock et al.,[39] however, located it in supporting cells only, although microtubules can be seen electron optically in the cuticular plates of hair cells.[40] The cuticular plates of all species investigated also contained F-actin, nonmuscle type myosin, $\alpha$-actinin, and tropomyosin. In contrast, fimbrin and F-actin appear to be the only structural components in mammalian cochlear stereocilia. Myosin, reported to be present in stereocilia of inner and outer hair cells of the guinea pig cochlea,[41] was not confirmed by other investigators.[42] Such discrepancies can be attributed to different techniques and to different specificities, and sensitivities of the antibody reactions, and remain currently unresolved.

In the face of such uncertainties inherent in the demonstration of these proteins, it is difficult to judge whether other results represent genuine differences between species, between vestibule and cochlea, or between inner and outer hair cells. For example, nonmammalian stereocilia may additionally contain $\alpha$-actinin[36]; actin in the cuticular plate of vestibular and cochlear hair cells may differ in its cross-linkages, as suggested by differences in the intensity of its reactivity with myosin S1-fragment; and stereocilia of outer hair cells showed a much weaker immunoreaction for fimbrin than those of inner hair cells.[36]

The discussion on the function of actin in the cochlea centers around its role in the crucial locations of stereocilia and cuticular plate, where it may provide structural support or motility. The stereocilia are stiff structures, and it is their actin core that confers this stiffness.[33] Tilney et al.[43] analyzed in detail the physical parameters of actin in stereocilia of the cochlea of the alligator lizard, and the authors deduced from its geometry of packing and cross-linking, and from the insensitivity of the filament packing to calcium and adenosine triphosphate (ATP) (which control movement in intestinal microvilli), that stereocilia are rigid and not equipped to contract. Orman and Flock[44] found that the deflection of vestibular stereocilia by a fluid jet was decreased under conditions that are known to cause contraction in muscle, suggesting the possibility of an active control of the mechanical properties of stereocilia. Because stereocilia are interconnected at their tips and pivot around their base as stiff rods,[45] control mechanisms may well lie in the cuticular plate. Here, the presence of myosin would provide the second component to actin for a contractile system. Since tropomyosin, which in an interplay with calcium regulates actin–myosin interactions, was also demonstrated in the cuticular plate (at least of cochlear hair cells), the existence of a motile system has received considerable support. Troponin, however, which is also an essential component of the contractile system in striated muscle, has not been demonstrated. The existence of a motile system would be in accord with electrophysiological studies postulating a modulator of the physical characteristics of the basilar mem-

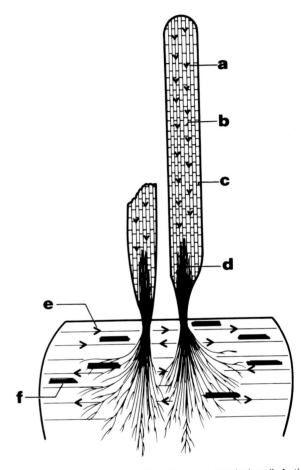

**Fig. 6-2.** Polarization of actin in the cochlear hair cell. Actin filaments in the stereocilia run in parallel strands (a) linked by perpendicular crossbridges (b). Lateral arms attach the actin filaments to the limiting membrane of the stereocilium (c). As the stereocilium tapers at the base, an electron-dense material becomes apparent (d). Polarization of actin in the cuticular plate runs perpendicular to that in the stereocilium (e) and myosin (f) is present in this region.[33–36] (Reproduced from Flock Å, Cheung AC: Actin filaments in sensory hairs of inner ear receptor cells. J Cell Biol 75:339, 1977, by copyright permission of The Rockefeller University Press and from Drescher DG (ed): Auditory Biochemistry. Courtesy of Charles C Thomas, Publisher, Springfield, IL, 1985.)

brane associated with outer hair cells.[46] Actin may then play a dual role in cochlear mechanics: structural rigidity for the ciliary core and motility for the cuticular plate-stereocilia system (Fig. 6-2).

## Enzymes

Three enzymes — carbonic anhydrase, $Na^+/K^+$-ATPase, and adenylate cyclase — have been extensively studied in the cochlea. They are discussed later in this chapter connection with their purported physiological functions (see the sections Regulation of Endolymph and Otoconia, below.)

## Proteins of the Tectoria

The tectorial membrane is a proteinaceous structure of the cochlea, an extracellular matrix consisting primarily of two types of fibrils.[47] Amino acid and x-ray diffraction analysis[48,49] suggested that the proteins are not of the collagen but more of the keratin type. Whether or not they are conjugated proteins has been a matter of controversy, since histochemical staining indicated a high glycoprotein content of the tectoria (see Schätzle[5]). Biochemical analyses found carbohydrates as minor components only.[48,50] Mucopolysaccharides constituted 0.1 percent of its dry weight.[51] More recent studies resolved tectorial proteins by sodium dodecyl sulfate (SDS) polyacrylamide gel electrophoresis into three major and a number of several minor protein compounds, and none of these showed reactions indicative of glycoproteins. This failure may, however, be attributed to a lack of sensitivity of the staining procedure, since more sensitive analyses by the same laboratory measured a carbohydrate content of 2.5 percent of dry weight.[52]

## Proteoglycans (Acid Mucopolysaccharides)

Proteoglycans are a group of structural macromolecules mostly found in "ground substance" or "intercellular cement" of connective tissue. These molecules are formed by a core protein to which polysaccharide chains (glycosaminoglycans, acid mucopolysaccharides) are covalently bound. About 95 percent of the molecule is polysaccharide, which determines the hydrophilic and viscoelastic properties of these compounds. Acid mucopolysaccharides were present in all cochlear tissues

investigated, and the lateral wall of the cochlea showed the highest content (0.5 percent of dry weight[53]) with chondroitin sulfate B (75 percent) and chondroitin sulfate A (12 percent) as the polysaccharide components.

Whether the diverse group of proteoglycans has biologic functions other than structural is speculative. Some suggestions have been made for an association of these compounds with hearing disorders, primarily because Hurler's syndrome, which can be accompanied by deafness, is a hereditary disorder of mucopolysaccharide metabolism. Also suggested was an involvement of the compounds in aminoglycoside ototoxicity because, like other polyanions, mucopolysaccharides can bind cationic drugs such as aminoglycosides. There is no evidence, however, that would assign a specific role to these compounds in inner ear physiology or pathology.

## INTERMEDIARY METABOLISM IN THE ORGAN OF CORTI AND STRIA VASCULARIS

### Cochlear Gradients

There are no known metabolic pathways unique to the cochlea, as is the case, for example, with the rhodopsin cascade in the retina. In the vestibular system, on the other hand, the formation and maintenance of the otoconia may be considered such a unique feature.

An intriguing property of cochlear tissues is the existence of longitudinal and transverse gradients of metabolites, which however, do not follow a consistent pattern. Glycogen concentrations increase about fourfold from the base to the apex of the cochlea, whereas phosphocreatine shows the opposite trend. There are no gradients in enzymes of carbohydrate metabolism that could account for the observed phenomenon.[54] No gradient appears to exist for ATP levels,[55] but $N^+/K^+$-ATPase has a differential distribution of decreasing concentration toward the apex.[56] Of the cyclic nucleotides, cyclic AMP occurs at similar levels in all turns of the cochlea, while cyclic guanosine monophosphate (GMP) gradually increases toward the base.[55] The latter corresponds to a gradient of enzymatic activity of acetylcholine metabolism, and supports for the cochlea the idea of cyclic GMP involvement in cholinergic mechanisms. Transverse gradients (between inner and outer structures of the organ of Corti) also exist for some compounds, for example, glycogen and cyclic GMP. These gradients may be a biochemical indicator of physiological differences between these structures or the base and apex of the cochlea, but at the moment their significance remains obscure.

## Energy Metabolism

Energy metabolism is the ability of a cell to synthesize high-energy compounds, primarily ATP, and use them for the maintenance and control of physiologic and biochemical activities. These include biosynthetic processes, maintenance of cellular resting potentials, mechanical work, neurotransmitter synthesis and release, and generation of bioelectric responses to stimuli. In all tissues, metabolism of ATP is highly regulated, and increased use is met by increased ATP production in order to maintain steady-state levels of this compound. Depending on the tissue and the physiologic state of the cell, carbohydrates, fatty acids, or amino acids can serve as exogenous energy sources, while glycogen represents an intracellular store of potential energy (Fig. 6-3).

Most investigations into cochlear energy-releasing and -consuming processes have been carried out in vitro. In vitro studies have the advantages of simplifying complex physiologic systems and easy manipulation of experimental conditions. Their disadvantage is that potentially important cellular control mechanisms or interactions between tissues, as well as between tissues and the surrounding biologic fluids, are lost, so that extrapolations to an in vivo situation have to be made with great care. For example, enzyme activities measured in vitro

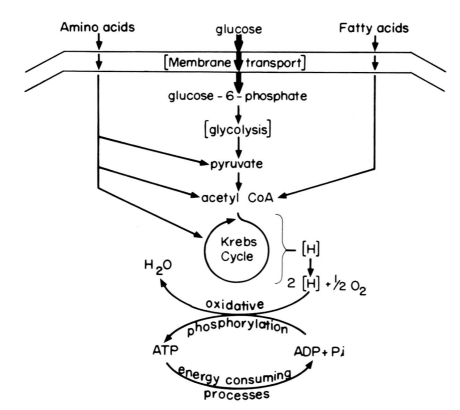

**Fig. 6-3.** Schematic representation of energy metabolism. Amino acids, glucose, and fatty acids may serve as energy sources, depending on the tissue and its physiologic or pathologic state. Their metabolism converges at several points and is ultimately linked to the generation of ATP via oxidative phosphorylation. Bold arrows indicate the pathways represented in the deoxyglucose technique of measuring "glucose utilization." Note that this measure can only reflect energy metabolism if (1) glucose is the main energy source of the cell, and (2) the deoxyglucose analog of glucose-6-phosphate is not metabolized to other intermediates.

are generally maximal activities determined under optimal substrate conditions. In vivo, enzymes almost never operate under such optimal conditions, but are restricted by substrate availability and complex cellular regulatory mechanisms.

In a description of cochlear energy metabolism, we are faced with fundamental differences in the function and the anatomy of the inner ear tissues. The organ of Corti, the site of transduction, is largely avascular, whereas the stria vascularis, considered responsible for the maintenance of the endolymphatic potential, is highly vascularized. This differentiation led to early speculations that the organ of Corti has a relatively low metabolic rate compared to a metabolically highly active stria vascularis. In vitro studies of $O_2$ consumption[57] seemed to bear out this hypothesis, but convincing evidence came from comparisons of the rate of energy consumption in vivo under ischemia.[58] The initial consumption of high-energy phosphates is about four times lower in the organ of Corti than in stria vascularis. On the other hand, the often propagated idea of anaerobic versus aerobic metabolism of these structures has little if any experimental background. Anaerobic metabolism is far less efficient in energy production than aerobic oxidative metabolism, puts a great demand on supply of energy sources, and leads to the formation of excess lactate. There is neither evidence for a high substrate/ATP ratio in the organ of Corti, nor is there evidence for unusually high concentrations of lactate dehydrogenase[58] or lactate. In perilymph, the lactate/pyruvate ratio is about equal to that in serum of guinea pigs.[59] Since there is also no apparent limitation of metabolism by oxygen supply (vascular and through the cochlear fluids), an aerobic, albeit low, metabolism of the organ of Corti would best fit available evidence.

Nervous and sensory tissue is metabolically highly active for the maintenance of transmembrane potentials and their restoration after stimulus-induced depolarization and for the synthesis and release of neurotransmitters. The reason for the exceptionally low metabolism of the organ of Corti has therefore long been a matter of speculation. It seems to be at least in part explained by the contribution of the stria vascularis to the physiology of the cochlea. Present biochemical and physiological evidence supports the idea that the ionic composition of endolymph and the endolymphatic potential are maintained by this tissue (see section on Regulation of Endolymph). Thus, a large proportion of the energy for the transduction process (essentially as postulated by Davis' "battery theory") seems provided by stria vascularis. What may amount to the first direct evidence for a stimulus-responsive strial metabolism is the finding that energy utilization in this tissue increases with sound stimulation in parallel with energy utilization in the organ of Corti.[60] The regulation of this "metabolic coupling" remains presently unknown, but feedback mechanisms sensitive to changes of the endocochlear potential or the $K^+$ concentration might be suggested. Processing of acoustic stimuli by the hair cells is accompanied by a decrease of the electrical impedance of the organ of Corti, probably resulting in $K^+$ fluxes across the hair cells. It is then the metabolic activity of stria vascularis that restores the ionic and electrical microhomeostasis of endolymph. The finding of a metabolic response of the nonsensory, nonneural stria vascularis to acoustic stimulation once again reveals the tissues of the cochlea as a closed and interdependent physiological and biochemical system and reminds us of the limitations of in vitro approaches to elucidate its complexities.

Under normal conditions, most nervous tissue relies primarily on glucose as the energy-providing substrate, and this seems generally to be true for the inner ear. The respiratory quotient for stria vascularis reflected preferential utilization of carbohydrates,[61] which are usually supplied via the vasculature. Under exceptional circumstances (such as substrate-free vascular perfusion) glucose provided from perilymph will adequately support strial metabolism. Normal levels of ATP in the organ of Corti are also maintained by perilymphatic glucose.[62]

On the other hand, the organ of Corti is a heterogenous tissue, and its cells are not biochemically uniform. Differences in enzyme concentrations (e.g., of lactate dehydrogenase and malate dehydrogenase) between different cell populations of the organ of Corti were among the early quantitative results of biochemical studies of the inner ear.[63] More strikingly, immunoreactivity to a neuron-specific enolase was found in inner but not in outer hair cells of the guinea pig cochlea,[64] indicating significant differences between the cell types. Thus, cellular variations may also exist in the preferential substrate of energy metabolism. Autoradiographic studies with deoxyglucose (a synthetic marker of glucose utilization) indeed demonstrated a high uptake into inner hair cells, but only little if any uptake into outer hair cells.[65]

The role of glycogen stores in the cochlear tissues does not seem to be clear. In the hair cells, they are postulated to give resistance to ischemic conditions.[58] Such an interpretation is complicated by the fact that in some species (e.g., mouse), hair cell glycogen is very low.[66] Furthermore, in the stria vascularis, glycogen cannot provide metabolic energy sufficient to maintain the endolymphatic potential.

### Acoustic Stimulation

Because of the intimate involvement of cellular metabolism with information processing, it is not surprising that cochlear energy metabolism is modulated by acoustic stimulation. Experimental evidence, however, was not provided until very recently, when cochlear glucose utilization was measured by the technique of "deoxyglucose trapping." Radiolabeled 2-deoxy-D-glucose is taken up in vivo by tissues and phosphorylated like the natural substrate, glucose. The phosphorylated glucose analog, however, is not further metabolized and effectively "trapped" in the cell. The rate of its accumulation reflects the rate of glucose utilization, which in turn is a measure of energy flux in the cell.[67] In contrast to this dynamic measurement, determinations of high-energy metabolites such as ATP provide information about their steady-state levels and not their turnover.

Steady-state levels of ATP are indeed maintained in the sensory cells of the organ of Corti under conditions of acoustic stimulation, including those leading to temporary threshold shifts.[68] Glucose utilization, on the other hand, was increased two- to threefold at moderate stimulation in the organ of Corti of the mouse[60] and about twofold in the gerbil.[69] Auditory nerve and inferior colliculus followed this response, in agreement with the well-established fact that stimulus processing increases the metabolic demand in neural tissues. Autoradio-

graphic analyses of the gerbil cochlea confirmed and extended these findings[65,70]: inner hair cells responded strongly to sound, whereas outer hair cells did not. This could be considered in support of the currently prevailing idea that inner hair cells are the primary sites of stimulus transduction while outer hair cells modulate the properties of the basilar membrane.[46,71] However, because a control of basilar membrane movement by contractile proteins in outer hair cells would also require energy for mechanical work, a better explanation could be a difference in the preferred energy substrate for outer hair cells. (For a detailed account of noise-induced changes of cochlear energy metabolism and an assessment of the deoxyglucose technique in the auditory periphery, the reader is referred to Schacht and Canlon.[72])

## OTHER COCHLEAR STRUCTURES

The spiral ligament has received little attention in biochemical studies, because its role in cochlear function is not clear. Nevertheless, this tissue may show some interesting biochemical features. For instance, carbonic anhydrase has its highest concentration in this tissue,[73] as has succinate dehydrogenase.[74] Aside from these and some other isolated observations, however, a "biochemistry" of the spiral ligament cannot be discussed.

Similarly, although histochemical and biochemical studies have dealt with Reissner's membrane[54,75] this tissue is not sufficiently characterized that we could describe its biochemistry.

## INNER EAR FLUIDS

### Analytic Studies

The inner ear contains several distinct fluids (or "lymphs") within anatomically well-defined boundaries: perilymph in the scala vestibuli and scala tympani of the cochlea and in the vestibular canals; endolymph in the scala media of the cochlea and in the endolymphatic duct and sac of the vestibular system. These are the classic and well-studied fluids. In addition, there exist a subtectorial lymph bounded by the tectorial membrane and the reticular lamina, inner sulcus lymph, and a Corti lymph in the tunnel of Corti whose physiology and chemistry are much more speculative. The existence of a subtectorial lymph as an independent fluid had frequently been challenged, but evidence has been presented[76] that the tectorial membrane establishes a separate compartment under this structure without free communication with endolymph.

The analysis of their composition shows a clear distinction between perilymphatic and endolymphatic fluids. Perilymph values resemble those of other extracellular fluids[77]: 140 mM Na$^+$, 4 mM K$^+$, and 0.6 mM Ca$^{2+}$. The characteristically low [Na$^+$] (Na$^+$ concentration) and high [K$^+$] in endolymph were first recognized by Smith et al.[78] However, due to technical difficulties in sampling, in particular of cochlear endolymph, precise values for the ionic concentrations were not established until much later. Bosher and Warren[79] reported 0.9 mM Na$^+$ and 154 mM K$^+$ for rat endolymph, and about 10 $\mu$M free Ca$^{2+}$.[80] Endolymph has the same pH value (approximately 7.3) as perilymph and blood but is hyposmotic to these two fluids.[77,81] While perilymph and cochlear as well as vestibular endolymph have been thoroughly analyzed, subtectorial and Corti lymph pose further experimental difficulties. They cannot be sampled by conventional approaches and require analysis in situ. Radiographic microanalysis and Laser Microprobe Mass Analysis (LAMMA) have provided the most reliable data. It appears that the lymphs in the inner sulcus and the subtectoral space have an endolymphlike composition, whereas those in the organ of Corti resemble extracellular fluid.[82] The methodology of specimen preparations of these fluids is a critical point. Small delays in freezing or temperature shifts during the subsequent preparation can cause diffusion of ions or movement of fluids. An additional limitation is that these techniques primarily yield ionic ratios and not absolute concentrations, so that it is not possible to present quantitative data at this time.

## Regulation of Perilymph

The regulation of the microhomeostasis of inner ear fluids has received extensive physiological and pharmacologic investigation, and some biochemical investigation. While the mechanisms of fluid origin have yet to be established, it is clear that both perilymph and endolymph have their own specific regulatory controls. The composition of perilymph was early taken to suggest its origin partially as an ultrafiltrate of plasma.[83,84] The kinetics of entry of radioactive K$^+$ and Cl$^-$ from plasma into cerebrospinal fluid (CSF) and perilymph was indeed consistent with a plasma origin of perilymph and the existence of a blood–perilymph barrier.[85] Other studies indicated that a significant portion of this lymph is also derived from CSF.[86] However, when large volumes of perilymph are sampled it is difficult to avoid contamination by CSF through the cochlear aqueduct. Dyes, when applied into the CSF in low volume and under controlled pressure, did not diffuse through the cochlear aqueduct,[87] negating a bulk flow between these compartments. Blocking the cochlear aqueduct was found to have no significant effect on the composition of perilymph,[88] yet it led to increased susceptibility of the organ of Corti of the basal turn of aminoglycosides, interpreted to be the result of a decreased turnover of perilymph.[89] A contribution by CSF, therefore, may exist but may be limited in the amounts or specificity of components transported. Perilymph is also not a mixture of plasma ultrafiltrate and CSF but has its own unique composition. Low-molecular-weight components such as amino acids may be present in higher concentration in perilymph than in either serum or CSF,[90] and proteins are not only quantitatively but also qualitatively different.[91] Thus, selective transport or resorption processes have to be postulated that remain to be elucidated.

## Regulation of Endolymph

Its ionic composition and high positive potential make the cochlear endolymph a unique extracellular fluid. Largely through the work of Konishi and his collaborators, the physiology and electrochemistry of ion and water movements have been well described.[92] The fluid compartments surrounding the endolymph are the perilymph of scala vestibuli and tympani and the vascular bed of the stria vascularis. The latter tissue has long been considered the primary site of maintenance of endolymphatic composition and potential.[93,94] Metabolic processes as a control of the ionic gradients in the cochlea were suggested by the fact that endolymphatic [K$^+$] declines and [Na$^+$] increases postmortem toward an equilibrium with the surrounding fluids, and the endocochlear potential (EP) assumes a negative value. Because the cochlear epithelium appears essentially freely permeable to water,[95] and because CL$^-$ movement is electrochemically coupled to the K$^+$ gradient, the processes that are driven by metabolic reactions are those of K$^+$ and Na$^+$ transport. The existence of two "pumps," an Na$^+$, K$^+$ pump in the basolateral membrane and a K$^+$ pump in the epithelial membrane of strial marginal cells, would best fit physiological and biochemical data.[96] In addition, other transport systems must exist for compounds that exhibit a concentration gradient between the various labyrinthine components, for example, calcium[81] or amino acids.[97] No attempts, however, have yet been made to characterize these processes, and we have to limit our discussions to the location and the molecular nature of Na$^+$ and K$^+$ transport.

Radiotracer experiments of water, K$^+$, and Cl$^-$ movement in the cochlea[85,95] have suggested that exchange of electrolytes between serum and endolymph does not take place directly but via perilymph. The intimate relationship between perilymph and endolymph is also demonstrated in experiments of perilymphatic perfusions with K-free media. The endolymphatic potential under this condition declines rapidly,[98] while it is maintained at normal values during K-free vascular perfusions.[99] This hypothesis then places active transport processes at endolymph/perilymph borders in the cochlear membranous labyrinth. However, judging from movement of radioactive K$^+$ and Na$^+$ from perilymph to endolymph, Konishi[92] concluded that the lateral wall is responsible for K$^+$ uptake and Na$^+$ excretion and that Reissner's membrane cannot be considered to play a major role in this process.

Three enzymes potentially regulating ion and fluid balance have been investigated in the cochlea, although any of a number of active transport systems, such as those known from transporting epithelia, may be operating. Cochlear Na$^+$/K$^+$-ATPase[100] and adenylate cyclase[101] have recently been reviewed, as has the distribution of carbonic anhydrase in the inner ear.[102] In the following discussion we briefly evaluate the involvement in cochlear physiology of each one.

Na$^+$/K$^+$-ATPase, an enzyme present in all epithelial membranes, transports Na$^+$ and K$^+$ against their electrochemical gradients across the membrane at the expense of ATP. It is an asymmetric electrogenic system generally operating at a ratio of three Na$^+$ transported for each two K$^+$. In the cochlea the enzyme has been demonstrated in the organ of Corti, Reissner's membrane, and stria vascularis, with the highest concentration in the last. The concentrations of the enzyme in stria vascularis, as well as in the tegmentum vasculosum of the chick (which has an analogous role), were comparable to those in other ion-transporting epithelia. By histochemical reactions and by binding of the specific inhibitor ouabain, the area of highest activity was localized to the basolateral infoldings of the strial marginal cells of the guinea pig.[103] A basolateral rather than luminal localization is typical for this enzyme in transporting epithelia. Strial ATPase also shows a concentration gradient decreasing in the apical direction.[104] It is intriguing that endolymphatic electrolyte composition, osmolality, and resting potential similarly show graded differences between the different turns,[77,81] but a connection between these observations must remain speculative.

The implication of Na$^+$/K$^+$-ATPase in cochlear ion balance was strengthened by studies linking the enzymatic activity to the maintenance of the endolymphatic potential. During postnatal development in the rat, Na$^+$/K$^+$-ATPase activity in stria rises about fourfold during the period when this potential develops.[105,106] Furthermore, in perfusions of the guinea pig cochlea, ouabain depressed the endocochlear potential in a dose-dependent manner similar to its inhibition of Na$^+$/K$^+$-ATPase in vitro.

The postulate of a "second pump"[96] was

prompted by experimental data that apparently could not be explained by the action of ATPase alone in maintaining electrochemical homeostasis. The ionic composition of the developing rat endolymph reaches adult values before the maturation of the endocochlear potential, only the latter coinciding with the development of ATPase. After acute ethacrynic acid intoxication,[107] recovery of EP was similar to that of $K^+$ flux but not of $Na^+$ flux. Although these data were compatible with the production of EP by an electrogenic $K^+$ transport, they could also be interpreted to indicate that endolymphatic ionic homeostasis is under the control of more than one mechanism.

The search for an additional regulating system focused on adenylate cyclase. A ubiquitous membrane-bound enzyme, adenylate cyclase is known to mediate the physiological effects of a variety of hormones and neuromodulators such as catecholamines, parathyroid hormone, vasopressin, and prostaglandins. Binding of the effector to specific receptors on the cell plasma membrane stimulates production of cyclic AMP inside the cell, which in turn alters enzymatic activities or membrane properties by a complex reaction cascade. Cyclic AMP may in a given tissue regulate metabolic pathways such as glycogen synthesis and utilization or lipolysis, or modulate ionic channels of the plasma membrane. Adenylate cyclase was present in all labyrinthine structures investigated, with high activity found in stria vascularis.[108–111] Because of the wide variety of physiological functions of this enzyme, its presence alone does not suggest participation in any specific processes. Speculations of its involvement in cochlear fluid balance in analogy to its role in the amphibian urinary bladder and the mammalian renal collecting tubules and duct[112] first came from studies of the ototoxicity of ethacrynic acid. Parallel effects of this loop diuretic on the endocochlear potential and on adenylate cyclase were consistent with such a proposition.[110] Later studies, however, disproved this hypothesis[113,114] (see also the section Ototoxicity in this chapter).

A connection between adenylate cyclase activity and control of endolymph volume was drawn from experiments in which cholera toxin, stimulant of the enzyme, was introduced into the scala media.[115] The conclusion that this led to an increase in endolymph production was reached indirectly through measurements of the dilution of the extracellular marker inulin injected into scala media. Subsequent studies of the endolymphatic pressure in guinea pigs seemed to corroborate the findings of increased endolymph volume after injection of cholera toxin into the scala media.[116] A difficulty in interpretation comes from the absence of direct histologic demonstration of hydrops and the fact that cochlear cyclic AMP levels were not measured in either study. They were determined by Thalmann and collaborators[117] after perilymphatic and endolymphatic application of cholera toxin. Perilymphatic application caused small changes in cyclic AMP in Reisser's membrane, while endolymphatic application did not significantly alter levels in any of the cochlear tissues. This finding apparently contradicted the assumption of a link between adenylate cyclase and cholera-toxin-induced alterations of endolymphatic volume. Cyclic AMP levels did rise in cochlear tissues when cholera toxin was combined with the phosphodiesterase blocker, theophylline. Stimulation in stria still was only two- to fourfold, whereas that in Reisser's membrane was 20- to 40-fold. This was an apparent paradox because Reisser's membrane is not considered to be so actively engaged in ion transport. The results, then, could indicate that either the cholera toxin – adenylate cyclase interaction is not correlated with cochlear ion and fluid transport activities, or that Reisser's membrane plays a hitherto unrecognized major role in cochlear physiology.

Developmental and histochemical evidence is consistent with a role of adenylate cyclase in cochlear fluid and electrolyte control. The enzyme in stria vascularis of the mouse increased its specific activity severalfold during the postnatal period in which the $Na^+$ and $K^+$ composition of endolymph reached mature values.[118] Histochemically, highest activity of the enzyme was shown in the contraluminal infoldings of the strial marginal cells.[119] This distribution is typical for epithelia in which adenylate cyclase is involved in ion transport: The enzyme is found at the basal membrane of the cell, accessible to hormones from the circulation, while the effect on ion and fluid permeability is exerted at the luminal membrane.[112] A previously reported localization of adenylate cyclase on the endolymphatic surface of stria[120] and thus inaccessible to control by circulatory hormones can be considered an artifact of the particular cytochemical technique employed.[101]

Because adenylate cyclase activity is under strict hormonal control, it is important to know the effectors of the strial enzyme. A "cochlear" adenylate cyclase was stimulated by the synthetic $\beta$-adrenergic agonist, isoproterenol, and by vasopressin (antidiuretic hormone).[121] Because the latter is a well-established stimulator of adenylate cyclase in epithelia engaged in the regulation of water resorption, this finding could be taken to support a similar cochlear role for the enzyme. The experiments, however, did not provide information about the tissue localization of the hormonal action, because a preparation of the total cochlear membraneous labyrinth was investigated.

Carbonic anhydrase catalyzes the equilibrium between $CO_2$ and carbonic acid, which dissociates into bicarbonate ($HCO_3^-$) and hydrogen ion. In several epithelia a $Cl^-/HCO_3^-$ exchange is mediated by this enzyme, and its activity can be linked to ion and water secretion and the production of aqueous humor. Extremely high concentrations of carbonic enhydrase in the cochlea[122] prompted speculations for a specific role in cochlear physiology. However, cochlear concentrations may be considerably lower than initially measured,[73] and enzymatic activity is also higher in spiral ligament than in stria vascularis, the latter being the expected site of high activity if the enzyme plays a specific role in endolymph regulation. Acetazolamide, intravenously administered to rats in quantities sufficient to inhibit carbonic anhydrase, did not alter $Na^+$ or $K^+$ concentrations in endolymph, but decreased EP and $Cl^-$ concentration, suggesting a decrement of active $H^+$ transport into endolymph. This active $H^+$ transport could, at least in part, be dependent on strial carbonic anhydrase.[77]

In summary, then, precise mechanisms of the control of endolymphatic microhomeostasis cannot be formulated yet. The involvement of $Na^+/K^+$-ATPase in regulating the electrochemical gradient seems firmly established. This activity alone is not sufficient to account for the complexities of cochlear physiology, but the participation of adenylate cyclase as another regulatory systems remains tentative. Carbonic anhydrase may participate in the control of acid–base balance, and more systems need to be explored.

---

# VESTIBULAR BIOCHEMISTRY

The vestibular apparatus is less frequently included in biochemical studies of the inner ear than the cochlea. There are no compelling reasons for this neglect. The differences in structure and function imply different metabolic features and a vestibular biochemistry in its own right. For example, the magnitude of the positive potential as well as the chemical composition of vestibular endolymph differs significantly from that of cochlear endolymph.[97,123] We should note that studies of ion transport and of enzymes and metabolites have been reported for both the mammalian[111,124,125] and the amphibian[126] vestibular system and that selected features of energy metabolism have been compared to the auditory system.[127] Overall, however, we lack comprehensive and specific approaches to a "vestibular biochemistry." The exception is to be found in one unique feature of the vestibular system, the otoconia.

## Otoconia

Otoconia are crystals of calcium carbonate in the form of calcite that are present in the gravity receptors of most vertebrates. Otoliths are calcium carbonate in the form of aragonite, often found as a large single crystal in fishes.[128,129] Otoconia have an active turnover of their calcium content. This was first deduced from the reduction in size and number of otoconia in aged humans and the in vitro exchange of $^{45}Ca$ between isolated otoconia and a bathing solution.[130] Although some incorporation of radioactive calcium was found into otoconia of young rats, this was initially not confirmed for adult mice.[131] More sensitive techniques later clearly demonstrated[132,133] calcium incorporation in vivo into otolithic membranes of adult gerbils and guinea pigs as well as calcium uptake and exchange in otoconia of young adult rats.[134] A dynamic behavior of otoconia was also suggested by studies of aminoglycoside-induced otoconial pathology. Streptomycin caused loss and morphologic alterations of saccular and utricular otoconia,[135] and incorporation of radioactive calcium was decreased significantly in saccular and utricular otolithic membranes after treatment of guinea pigs with streptomycin or neomycin,[134] an effect that may be accounted for by the calcium antagonism of aminoglycosides.

The calcium carbonate crystals also incorporate an organic matrix in their structure, which may be crucial for their mineralization. In all mineralized vertebrate tissues investigated so far, specific matrix proteins have been found containing the amino acid $\gamma$-carboxyglutamic acid. This includes the fish otolith[136] and probably rat otoconia.[129] Evidence from normal and pathologic calcifications in a variety of tissues in vivo, as well as in vitro studies with the isolated proteins[137,138] suggests that carboxyglutamate-containing calcium-binding bone proteins control nucleation and calcification processes. By extrapolation, a regulation of vestibular calcification deposits by such proteins seems likely, but other hypotheses, for example, glycoproteins as potential modulators of otoconial seeding and growth,[134] are also being discussed.

An enzyme involved in the deposition of calcium carbonate in some tissues is carbonic anhydrase, which is widely distributed in all parts of the labyrinth. In the cochlea it is found in the organ of Corti, intermediate and basal cells of stria vascularis, outer sulcus, and spiral ligament; in the vestibule, it was seen in supporting cells of all sensory epithelia, in the dark cells and transitional cells of the utricle, and saccule and epithelial cells of the endolymphatic sac.[102] Such a diverse localization of the enzyme does not provide clues to a specific role in calcium deposition in the inner ear. There is, however, indirect evidence pointing to a participation of carbonic anhydrase in the formation of otoconia.[139,140] The administration of inhibitors of this enzyme, such as acetazolamide, resulted in malformation of otoconia in developing chicks and mice. Zinc deficiency affects otoconial formation, and carbonic anhydrase is known to be zinc dependent (for a recent review see Lim[141]).

## PATHOLOGY

The elucidation of the causes of human inner ear pathology is a challenging task for the biochemist. While such pathologies are amply documented morphologically and audiologically, the biochemical discussion is presently restricted to animal models of a limited number of hearing disorders, primarily noise- and drug-induced hearing loss.

### Noise

The biochemistry of noise trauma is rather problematic. Levels of sound frequently used to induce pathology are likely to cause gross damage through mechanical disruption of tissues. Once destruction of a cell has set in, eventually all cellular reactions will become abnormal. This may explain why such a multitude of biochemical changes have been observed after noise exposure including effects on DNA, RNA, protein synthesis, enzymatic activities, concentration of metabolites, and membrane functions. In order to understand the molecular basis of noise-induced hearing loss, the primary mechanisms that cause the chain of events leading to cell death must be discovered. Here, however, we have few or no clues. The condition of "asymptotic temporary threshold shift" investigated by Thalmann and his collaborators,[68] nicely satisfies the requirement for an animal model of functional deficit without gross pathology. Here, however, ATP levels, one of the sensitive indicators of cellular viability, remain unchanged. The production of noxious metabolites such as lactate, as once suggested,[142] also does not seem to be a mechanism of action, because carefully controlled determinations of that compound did not detect changes of its level in inner ear fluids after noise trauma.[143] On the other hand, impairments of energy metabolism that may stress cellular physiology may not be totally ruled out. Localized capillary vasoconstriction has been postulated as a result of overstimulation leading to restricted oxygen and nutrient supply to cochlear tissues.[144] However, this concept is not clearly supported in other studies of the cochlear vasculature using different techniques.

While intense noise may reduce local blood supply in the cochlea of the guinea pig, the changes in the vasculature are small in number, and there is no regular pattern to the decreased blood flow.[145]

Changes in the cochlear electrolyte balance have been reported in noise-exposed animals. Konishi and his collaborators demonstrated that exposure of guinea pigs to noise led to changes of EP and endolymphatic $K^+$, possibly due to an altered K-conductance of the endolymph–perilymph barrier. Although these changes could be part of the traumatic mechanism, they were, however, dissociated from the suppression of the cochlear microphonics (CM). There was also no change in the $K^+$ concentration in the extracellular fluid of the organ of Corti, and the decrease of CM was speculated to be due to change in the properties of the hair cell membrane.[146,147]

Stereocilia may be a site of early damage by noise. Audiometric data appear to correlate well with damage to stereocilia from impulse noise[148] and narrow-band noise.[149] The structures can become flaccid and clumped, indicative of changes in their stiffness,[150] which apparently leads to decreased auditory sensitivity. Since stiffness, as mentioned earlier, is conferred by the actin core, noise-induced alterations of actin packing should be expected. Recently, work in the alligator lizard showed a decrease in the number of cross-linkages between adjacent actin filaments in the stereocilium corresponding to the degree of threshold shift.[151] Such damaged stereocilia may recover with time,[152] and this process may be important for an understanding of temporary noise-induced hearing loss. The underlying biochemical trigger for breaking and reforming the covalent actin cross-linkages remains to be established.

## Drugs

The number of drugs that are liable to cause temporary or permanent threshold shifts is large and ever increasing. These drugs belong to such various therapeutic classes as analgesics and antipyretics (salicylates, quinine), aminoglycoside antibiotics (neomycin, gentamicin), polypeptide antibiotics (viomycin, vancomycin), antineoplastic drugs (*cis*-dichlorodiamminoplatinum), metallo

compounds (arsenicals, mercurials), and diuretics (ethacrynic acid, furosemide). Their molecular structures are quite dissimilar, as are their effects on the cochlea (permanent or temporary hearing loss), their primary target tissue, and the type of pathology they induce.[153,154]

A few of these drugs have been investigated for the molecular mechanism of their toxicity. The same caution that applies to biochemical studies of noise pathology also applies to drug pathology. Once a cell is damaged by a drug, a wide variety of secondary metabolic pathologies can be observed. Although these may contribute to the eventual manifestation of toxicity, it is the primary reaction that needs to be determined. In the first place, those secondary reactions may be common to cell injury of a variety of origins and thus may not provide information as to a specific drug action; in the second place, prevention of the primary reaction is necessary to counteract the entire sequence of events and consequently the ototoxic action. Further complicating the elucidation of toxic mechanisms is the fact that drugs, when given at high doses, will frequently cause nonspecific effects (not related to the primary action) that may mask the specific pathologic mechanisms. It is not surprising then that a large number of biochemical effects have been reported in response to ototoxic drugs. For aminoglycosides, for instance, interactions with DNA, RNA, protein, lipid, and carbohydrate metabolism have been claimed. We examine here some hypotheses that have been advanced recently on the toxic actions of aminoglycosides, diuretics, and salicylates.

### Aminoglycosides

Despite the development of new and powerful drugs, the aminoglycosides are still and probably will continue to be widely used because of their efficacy against gram-negative bacteria. Binding to the bacterial membrane leading to permeability changes and ion fluxes has been established as an early event, but its relation to cell death remains unclear. The antibacterial efficacy of aminoglycosides has mostly been linked to a number of potential intracellular mechanisms including an interference with protein synthesis.[155,156] Such actions are apparently not exerted in the same fashion in mammalian cells because of the differences in molecular structure between prokaryotic and eukaryotic cells.

Nephrotoxicity and ototoxicity are major complications of aminoglycoside therapy. Although renal damage is reversible, insults to the inner ear are generally irreversible and permanent hearing loss will result. Since the early analytic studies of Voldrich[157] and Stupp,[158] the toxicity of aminoglycosides had been assumed to reside in their accumulation in inner ear fluids. Extensive pharmacokinetic analyses by Tran Ba Huy et al.[159,160] of gentamicin uptake into and clearance from endolymph and perilymph did not provide evidence for such a phenomenon. Perilymph and endolymph drug levels remained at a rather low and constant ratio to serum levels over a wide range of time and drug concentration. In guinea pig inner ear tissues, the levels of neomycin after 3 weeks of chronic systemic administration[161] were similar to levels in nonaffected organs such as liver or lung. Such results are incompatible with the idea that an overall accumulation of drug in the inner ear is the cause of the specific toxicity. Autoradiographic studies of acutely administered dihydrostreptomycin[162–164] or gentamicin[165] have shown a distribution of the drug among the various cochlear tissues but have failed to establish specific sites of accumulation. This does not preclude, however, that during chronic administration a preferential uptake (e.g., into hair cells) may occur.

Schacht and collaborators have postulated a multistep sequence of aminoglycoside toxicity that includes the binding to phosphatidylinositol bisphosphate, an acidic phospholipid, as a key reaction.[166,167] In animals receiving chronic injections or acute perilymphatic perfusions, metabolism of phosphatidylinositol bisphosphate in cochlear tissues was depressed,[10,168] and an inhibition of the turnover of this lipid was also demonstrated in vitro by ototoxic drugs but not by nonototoxic compounds.[169] Using techniques of affinity chromatography,[170] phosphatidylinositol bisphosphate was isolated on immobilized neomycin, supporting its receptorlike interaction with the drug.

The hypothesis (Fig. 6-4) suggests that the first event in the sequence of aminoglycoside toxicity is an electrostatic binding to negatively charged sites on the plasma membrane, such as acidic phospholipids, leading to a competitive and reversible displacement of calcium.[168] This inhibits calcium-dependent membrane functions, such as calcium-controlled membrane channels, and may account for acute effects. The next step is an energy-dependent uptake process into the cell[171] followed by the specific complex formation with phosphatidylinositol bisphosphate on the cytoplasmic site of the plasma membrane. This may disrupt membrane structure and permeability and result in abnormal ion fluxes lethal to the cell. The altered cellular permeability may also enable the drug itself to penetrate the cell, where it may exert further toxic actions such as interference with calcium or polyamine-regulated processes. It is, however, interesting to speculate that the binding to phosphatidylinositol bisphosphate interferes with the physiological role of this lipid since it leads to inhibition of its hydrolysis.[169] As mentioned previously, the hydrolysis of this lipid is implicated as the first step in the signal cascade triggered by a variety of hormonal stimuli. The selective damage to the kidney and specific cells of the ear may then be the consequence of two combined factors, the presence of an active transport system and of phosphatidylinositol bisphosphate.

Prevention or amelioration of aminoglycoside-induced hearing loss would be of considerable importance. Reversibility is not a common clinical experience but has been reported in some patients receiving gentamicin or streptomycin and kanamycin, particularly when drug administration was stopped shortly after onset of symptoms.[172–174] Combination of aminoglycosides with various pharmacologic agents has frequently been suggested for detoxification, but the results of these treatments have been largely unconvincing. Recently it was postulated[175] that kanamycin ototoxicity involves the formation of free radicals and that a free-radical scavenger, S-2(3-aminopropylamino)ethylphosphorothioate, lowered its toxicity. This report is difficult to evaluate because no measurements of drug levels in serum or in tissues were presented. For example, an effect of the first drug on the kidney causing increased excretion of the aminoglycoside might lower toxicity but it would also lower its antibacterial efficacy. Furthermore, another free radical scavenger, N-acetylcysteine, was ineffective as a protectant.[176] On the other

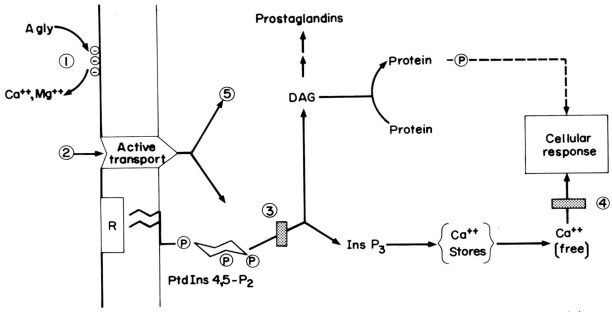

**Fig. 6-4.** Hypothesis of aminoglycoside toxicity. **(1)** The aminoglycoside (Agly) binds to negatively charged sites at the outer plasma membrane and displaces $Ca^{2+}$ and $Mg^{2+}$. This represents acute and reversible aminoglycoside effects. **(2)** The drug is taken up into the cell by an active transport system. **(3)** The drug binds to phosphatidylinositol bisphosphate (PtdIns $4,5-P_2$) and blocks its hydrolysis to inositol trisphosphate (InsP$_3$) and diacylglycerol (DAG), thereby interfering with the function of the phosphoinositide cascade (see Fig. 6-1) and the integrity of the membrane. R, receptor. **(4)** Calcium-dependent intracellular reactions are inhibited by the aminoglycosides. **(5)** Based on their high positive charge, aminoglycosides may also interfere with various other intracellular reactions (e.g., polyamine-regulated mechanisms, block of metabolism and function of negatively charged compounds such as RNA).

hand, elevated calcium concentrations in cochlear perfusions were able to prevent or reverse the loss of microphonic potential caused by gentamicin.[27] This was in good agreement with the suggestion that the first step in aminoglycoside toxicity is a reversible binding to the plasma membrane competitive with calcium. The experiments also showed that reversibility was limited to a narrow set of conditions determined by both concentrations of drug and duration of treatment. This result may explain the difficulty in reversing the ototoxic effect after chronic administration of aminoglycosides. Recently calcium has also been reported to be an effective antidote to gentamicin nephrotoxicity.[177] Such findings may not yet have immediate

clinical significance, but they provide an interesting basis for future research.

## Diuretics

Diuretics, like the aminoglycosides, exert actions on the kidney and on the inner ear. In the kidney, the loop diuretics ethacrynic acid and furosemide inhibit electrolyte absorption in the ascending loop of Henle. Morphologic investigations in the cochlea suggest the stria vascularis as the target issue, where edema is an early manifestation.[178,179] Cation permeability and transport are decreased, and the endocochlear potential turns negative.[107] These findings prompted investigations into the effect of ototoxic diuretics on presumed systems of ion and fluid regulation in the cochlea.

Cochlear $Na^+/K^+$-ATPase was first ruled out as target of ethacrynic acid or furosemide, and adenylate cyclase was suggested.[110] However, inhibition of the enzyme by several diuretics did not correlate with the ototoxicity of the compounds,[113] and measurements of cyclic AMP levels in stria vascularis during the early stages of ethacrynate intoxication conclusively dissociated the effect on the endocochlear potential from effects on the adenylate cyclase system.[114] Because neither $Na^+/K^+$-ATPase nor adenylate cyclase is the renal site of action of loop diuretics, these results were consistent with the pharmacologic similarity of inner ear and kidney. In fact, the cochlear uptake mechanism for diuretics may be similar to that in kidney. In the renal tubule, furosemide is transported by an active organic acid transport system from the blood to its site of action in the lumen. Recent electrophysiologic studies have shown that furosemide ototoxicity can be ameliorated or prevented by probenecid, an inhibitor of organic acid transport that reduces furosemide concentrations in the inner ear fluids.[180] Further extending the analogy to renal pharmacology, it may be suggested that these drugs act on the stria vascularis by inhibiting an active chloride transport, which may be their mechanism of renal action.[181]

### Salicylates

The ability of salicylates, commonly known in the form of acetylsalicylate as the drug aspirin, to suppress various forms of pain and inflammatory responses, has long been recognized. Reversible hearing loss or potentiation of a temporary hearing loss induced by loud sound are well-established side effects.[182] The pharmacologic action of aspirin is based on the inhibition of cyclooxygenase, an enzyme catalyzing the first step in the synthesis of prostaglandins from arachidonic acid. Tissues of the inner ear are capable of synthesizing prostaglandins, and injections of aspirin lowered the rate of synthesis and the levels of prostaglandins in the perilymph of guinea pigs.[183] It is, however, too early to tell whether there is indeed a causal relationship between prostaglandins and tinnitus and other aspects of aspirin ototoxicity.

## CLINICAL IMPLICATIONS

Our current knowledge of human hearing disorders is primarily based on otologic assessments that describe and classify disorders as well as on information extrapolated from postmortem histologic observations. These tests and studies cannot afford a direct insight into the biochemical disorders that may be associated with the particular hearing pathology. Animal experimentation is providing a wealth of information, but a major problem exists in the validity of extrapolations to the human ear. A most striking example of species differences is the susceptibility to the ototoxic drug dihydrostreptomycin that is shared by humans and the patas monkey but not by the macaque or by other laboratory animals.[184] The majority of biochemical reactions, however, in both the normal and pathologic state can be expected to be similar across species and the preceding example is presumably an exception.

Theoretic models derived from animal experimentation may well have implications for clinical treatments that go beyond direct toxicity assessment.[185] For example, from in vivo and in vitro studies it was predicted[186] that aminoglycosides alter membrane permeabilities. An autoradiographic study of the distribution of ethacrynic acid in the cochlea[187] supported this concept: when preceded by an injection of neomycin, ethacrynic acid reached three to five times higher concentrations in the inner ear of the mouse than when no aminoglycoside was given. This may indicate that aminoglycosides are generally capable of facilitating drug entry into susceptible tissues, which may become a potential clinical hazard if the second drug is an ototoxic agent.

Unfortunately, the benefit of animal models does not exist for some of the most common hearing disorders such as tinnitus, sudden hearing loss, or Menière's disease. However, surgically induced hydrops[188] is a promising approach to a cochlear pathology that has yet to be explored in biochemical investigations. The extent of the information that the studies of biochemical control of cochlear fluids will provide on Menière's disease and its management remains to be seen. There is no evidence yet linking enzymatic defects to this pathology, particularly since endolymph appears to be of normal composition in patients with Menière's disease.[189] Likewise, inner ear fluids in animals with experimental endolymphatic hydrops may contain normal levels of electrolytes,[190,191] although some studies show deviations.[192,193]

Presently, there exist no systematic biochemical studies of the human inner ear either in vitro or in vivo. The first seems primarily a problem of supply of normal and pathologic tissues because appropriate analytic techniques exist. The latter seems improbable at first sight, but recent advances in technology may have placed it within reach.

The deoxyglucose technique, which had been introduced to measure energy metabolism in the central nervous system of animals,[67] is now being used to study the metabolic activity of the central nervous system in humans.[194] A positron-emitting radiotracer (e.g., [18F]fluorodeoxyglucose) is injected into the patient, and its distribution in the central nervous system is monitored by using positron emission transaxial tomography (PETT). The results from the early human measurements confirm increased metabolic activities in those central nervous system structures that are expected to respond to a given physiologic stimulus.[195,196] Aberrant metabolic patterns have been reported in pathologies such as epilepsy or brain tumors.[197] Although this technique seems of great promise for clinical diagnosis and research, it has also been challenged for a number of reasons whose consideration would go beyond the scope of this review.[198]

With respect to applying the deoxyglucose technique to the auditory periphery, complications may arise mainly from the resolution limits of the PETT detectors. Currently, a resolution of the order of 7 mm can be achieved, which is the approximate dimension of the whole labyrinth. The petrous bone, however, may afford an advantage because it provides an area of low metabolic activity surrounding the inner ear. Some obvious applications of this method would be studies to determine whether or not certain human auditory pathologies such as Menière's disease, sudden hearing loss, or presbycusis are accompanied by a disorder of energy metabolism or blood flow. Animal experiments have already demonstrated altered metabolic responses to acoustic stimuli for various types of inner ear disorders.[69]

The 20 years since the publication of the first compendium of cochlear biochemistry by Rauch[4] and the last decade in particular have brought great advances in this discipline. From the broad base of information that has been built, we may now advance to the most challenging of research areas, that of the human auditory physiology and pathology.

## ACKNOWLEDGMENT

The writing of this chapter was concluded in the spring of 1985 and literature published through 1984 was considered in this review.

We wish to thank our colleagues who were so kind (or who felt coerced) to read and comment on this manuscript: Sandy Bledsoe, Ben Clopton, Joseph Hawkins, Alfred Nuttall, Fred Scheibe, Olivier Sterkers, and Hans-Peter Zenner. Their comments were most helpful and are incorporated in this chapter; we do not assume, however, that these colleagues necessarily agree with our interpretation of this biochemistry of hearing. It was also a pleasure to work with Susan Pierson-DiTomasso and Francine Hume, who patiently and expertly typed the many drafts of this manuscript.

Jochen Schacht's research—some of which is cited here—is currently supported by grants from the National Institutes of Health, RO1 NS13972 and PO1 NS05785.

## REFERENCES

1. Békésy G von: The gap between the hearing of external and internal sounds. Symp Soc Exp Biol 16:267, 1962

2. Vinnikov YA, Titova LK: Kortiev Organ. Isdatelstvo akademii Nauk SSR, Moskva-Leningrad, 1961

3. Vosteen KH: Neue Aspekte zur Biologie und Pathologie des Innenohres. Arch Ohren Nasen Kehlkopfheilk 178:1, 1961

4. Rauch S: Biochemie des Hörorgans: Einführung in Methoden und Ergebnisse. Thieme, Stuttgart, 1964

5. Schätzle W: Histochemie des Innenohres. Urban and Schwarzenberg, Munich, 1972

6. Lowry OH, Passonneau JV, Schulz DW, Rock MK: The measurement of pyridine nucleotides by enzymatic cycling. J Biol Chem 236:2746, 1961

7. Matschinsky FM, Thalmann R: Quantitative histochemistry of the organ of Corti, stria vascularis, and macula sacculi of the guinea pig. I. Sampling procedure and analysis of pyridine nucleotides. Laryngoscope 77:292, 1967

8. Singer SJ, Nicolson GL: The fluid mosaic model of the structure of cell membranes. Science 175:720, 1972

9. Scheibe F, Gerhardt HJ, Hache U, et al: Thin-layer chromatographic investigation of the lipids of inner ear and perilymph of the guinea pig. ORL J Otorhinolaryngol Relat Spec 35:96, 1973

10. Stockhorst E, Schacht J: Radioactive labeling of phospholipids and proteins by cochlear perfusion in the guinea pig and the effect of neomycin. Acta Otolaryngol (Stockh) 83:401, 1977

11. Anniko M, Schacht J: Phosphoinositides in the developing inner ear with reference to brain, kidney, and liver of the mouse. Int J Biochem 13:951, 1981

12. Schacht J: Phosphoinositides in the auditory system. p. 89. In Oosawa F (ed): Transmembrane Signaling and Sensation. Japan Societies Press, Tokyo 1984

13. Kilian P, Schacht J: Sound stimulates labeling of polyphosphoinositides in the auditory organ of the Noctuid moth. J Neurochem 34:709, 1980

14. Tachibana M et al: Effects of perilymphatically perfused gentamicin on microphonic potential, lipid labeling and morphology of cochlear tissues. Acta Otolaryngol (Stockh) 96:31, 1983

15. Berridge MJ: Inositol trisphosphate and diacylglycerol as second messengers. Biochem J 220:345, 1984

16. Nishizuka Y: Turnover of inositol phospholipids and signal transduction. Science 225:1365, 1984

17. Brown JE, Rubin LJ, Ghalayini AJ, et al: Myo-inositol polyphosphate may be a messenger for visual excitation in Limulus photoreceptors. Nature 311:160, 1984

18. Horikoshi T, Yanagisawa K, Yoshioka T: A highly specific staining of cochlear hair cells by TPI (triphosphoinositide) antibody. Proc Jpn Acad 60: series B, 157, 1984

19. Hensen V: Zur Morphologie der Schnecke des Menschen and der Säugetiere. Z Zool 13:481, 1863

20. Schiff M, Christiensen-Lou H: The nature of lipid globules in Hensen's cells. Ann Otol Rhinol Laryngol 76:624, 1967

21. Davis H: A model for transducer action in the cochlea. Cold Spring Harbor Symp Quant Biol 30:181, 1965

22. Flock A: Sensory transduction in hair cells. p. 395. In Loewenstein WR (ed): Handbook of Sensory Physiology. Springer-Verlag, New York, 1971

23. Hudspeth AJ, Jacobs R: Stereocilia mediate transduction in vertebrate hair cells. Proc Natl Acad Sci USA 76:1506, 1979

24. Hudspeth AJ: Extracellular current flow and the site of transduction by vertebrate hair cells. J Neurosci 2:1, 1982

25. Konishi T, Salt AN: Permeability to potassium of the endolymph – perilymph barrier and its possible relation to hair cell function. Exp Brain Res 40:457, 1980

26. Wersäll J, Flock A: Suppression and restoration of the microphonic output from the lateral line organ after local application of streptomycin. Life Sci 3:1151, 1964

27. Takada A, Schacht J: Calcium antagonism and reversitility of gentamicin-induced loss of cochlear microphonics in the guinea pig. Hear Res 8:179, 1982

28. Moran DT, Rowley JC, Asher DL: Calcium-binding sites on sensory processes in vertebrate hair cells. Proc Natl Acad Sci USA 78:3954, 1981

29. Rabie A, Thomasset M, Legrand C: Immunocytochemical detection of calcium-binding protein in the cochlear and vestibular hair cells of the rat. Cell Tiss Res 232:691, 1983

30. Drescher, DG: A review of general cochlear biochemistry in normal and noise-exposed ears. p. 111. In Henderson D et al (eds): Effects of Noise on Hearing. Raven Press, New York, 1976

31. Wenthold RJ, McGarvey ML: Analysis of proteins of the stria vascularis of the normal and the waltzing guinea pig. Acta Otolaryngol (Stockh) 90:66, 1980

32. Thalmann I et al: Organ of Corti-specific polypeptides. OCP-1 and OCP-11. Arch Otorhinolaryngol 226:123, 1980

33. Flock A, Cheung HC: Actin filaments in sensory

hairs of inner ear receptor cells. J Cell Biol 75:339, 1977

34. Flock A: Contractile and structural proteins in the auditory organ. p. 310. In Drescher DG (ed): Auditory Biochemistry. Charles C Thomas, Springfield, IL, 1985

35. Tilney LG, DeRosier DJ: The organization of actin filaments in the stereocilia of the hair cells of the cochlea. p. 261. In Drescher DG (ed): Auditory Biochemistry. Charles C Thomas, Springfield, IL, 1985

36. Drenckhahn D, Schäfer T, Prinz M: Actin, myosin and associated proteins in the vertebrate auditory and vestibular organs: Immunocytochemical and biochemical studies. p. 317. In Drescher DG (ed): Auditory Biochemistry. Charles C Thomas, Springfield, IL, 1985

37. Flock A, Bretscher A, Weber K: Immunohistochemical localization of several cytoskeletal proteins in inner ear sensory and supporting cells. Hear Res 7:75, 1982

38. Zenner HP: Cytoskeletal and muscle-like elements in cochlear hair cells. Arch Otorhinolaryngol 230:81, 1981

39. Flock A, Hoppe Y, Wei X: Immunofluorescence localization of proteins in semithin 0.2-1 $\mu$m frozen sections of the ear. Arch Otorhinolaryngol 233:55, 1981

40. Flock A, Cheung HC, Flock B, Utter G: Three sets of actin filaments in sensory cells of the inner ear. Identification and functional orientation determined by gel electrophoresis, immunofluorescence and electronmicroscopy. J Neurocytol 10:133, 1981

41. Marcartney JC, Comis SD, Pickles JO: Is myosin in the cochlea a basis for active motility? Nature 288:491, 1980

42. Drenckhahn D, Kellner J, Mannherz HG, et al: Absence of myosin-like immunoreactivity in stereocilia of cochlea hair cells. Nature 300:531, 1982

43. Tilney LG, DeRosier DJ, Mulroy MJ: The organization of actin-filaments in the stereocilia of the cochlear hair cells. J Cell Biol 86:244, 1980

44. Orman S, Flock A: Active control of sensory hair mechanics implied by susceptibility to media that induce contraction in muscle. Hear Res 11:261, 1983

45. Flock A, Strelioff D: Studies on hair cells in isolated coils from the guinea pig cochlea. Hear Res 15:11, 1984

46. Siegel JH, Kim DO: Efferent neural control of cochlear mechanics? Olivocochlear bundle stimulation affects cochlear biomechanical nonlinearity. Hear Res 6:171, 1982

47. Kronester-Frei A: Ultrastructure of the different zones of the tectorial membrane. Cell Tissue Res 193:11, 1978

48. Bairati A, Iurato S, Pernis B: Biophysical properties of the tectorial membrane (of Corti). Exp Cell Res 13:207, 1957

49. Iurato, S: Submicroscopic structure of the membranous labyrinth. I. The tectorial membrane. Z Zellforsch 52:105, 1960

50. Naftalin L, Spencer Harrison M, Stephens A: The character of the tectorial membrane. J Laryngol Otol 78:1061, 1964

51. Saito H, Daly JF: Quantitative analysis of acid mucopolysaccarides in the normal guinea pig cochlea. Acta Otolaryngol (Stockh) 69:333, 1970

52. Steel KP: Composition and properties of the mammalian tectorial membrane. p. 351. In Drescher DG (ed): Auditory Biochemistry. Charles C Thomas, Springfield, IL, 1985

53. Saito H, Nakamura A, Iida T: A comparison of acidic glycosaminoglycans in the inner ear and other organs: Electrophoretic microanalysis. Arch Otorhinolaryngol 214:149, 1976

54. Thalmann I, Matschinsky FM, Thalmann R: Quantitative study of selected enzymes involved in energy metabolism of the cochlear duct. Ann Otol Rhinol Laryngol, 79:12, 1970

55. Thalmann R, Paloheimo S, Thalmann I: Distribution of cyclic nucleotides in the organ of Corti. Acta Otolaryngol (Stockh) 87:375, 1979

56. Kuijpers W, Bonting SL: Studies on (Na$^+$-K$^+$)-activated ATPase. Localization and properties of ATPase in the inner ear of the guinea pig. Biochim Biophys Acta 173:477, 1969

57. Chou JT-Y, Rodgers K: Respiration of tissues lining the mammalian membraneous labyrinth. J Laryngol Otol 76:341, 1962

58. Thalmann R, Miyoshi T, Thalmann I: The influence of ischemia upon the energy reserves of inner ear tissues. Laryngoscope 82:2249, 1972

59. Scheibe F, Haupt H, Rothe E, et al: Laktat-und Pyruvat-Konzentrationen von Perilymphe, Blut und liquor cerebrospinalis des Meerschweinchens. Arch Otorhinolaryngol 232:81, 1981

60. Canlon B, Schacht J: Acoustic stimulation alters deoxyglucose uptake in the mouse cochlea and inferior colliculus. Hear Res 10:217, 1983

61. Marcus DC, Thalmann R, Marcus NY: Respiratory rate and ATP content of stria vascularis of the guinea pig in vitro. Laryngoscope 88:1825, 1978

62. Marcus DC, Kobayashi T, Rokugo M, et al: Support of cochlear metabolic and ion transport processes solely by perilymphatic perfusion. Hear Res 15:287, 1984

63. Thalmann R, Thalmann I, Comegys TH: Dissection and chemical analysis of substructures of the organ of Corti. Laryngoscope 30:1619, 1970

64. Altschuler RA, Reeks KA, Marangos PJ, Fex J: Neuron-specific enolase-like immunoreactivity in inner but not outer hair cells in the guinea pig cochlea. Neurosci Abs 10:191, 1984

65. Ryan AF: Anatomical measures of physiological parameters in the cochlea. p. 181. In Berlin C (ed): Hearing Science. College Hill, San Diego, CA, 1984

66. Thalmann R, Marcus DC, Thalmann I: Biochemistry of the inner ear. p. 83. In Gorlin RJ (ed): Morphogenesis and Malformation of the Ear. Alan R Liss, New York, 1980

67. Sokoloff L, Reivich RM, Kennedy C, et al: The $^{14}$C-deoxyglucose method for measurement of local cerebral glucose utilization. J Neurochem 28:897, 1977

68. Thalmann R: Quantitative biochemical techniques for studying normal and noise-damaged ears. p. 129. In Henderson D, Hamernik RP, Darshan S, et al (eds): Effects of Noise on Hearing. Raven Press, New York, 1976

69. Canlon B, Takada A, Schacht, J: Glucose utilization in the auditory system: cochlear dysfunctions and species differences. Comp Biochem Physiol [A] 78:43, 1984

70. Ryan AF, Woolf NK, Catanzaro A, et al: Deoxyglucose uptake patterns in the auditory system: metabolic response to sound stimulation in the adult and neonate. p. 401. In Drescher DG (ed): Auditory Biochemistry. Charles C Thomas, Springfield, IL, 1985

71. Dallos P: Cochlear physiology. Ann Rev Psychol 32:153, 1981

72. Schacht J, Canlon B: Noise-induced changes in cochlear energy metabolism. p. 389. In Drescher DG (ed): Auditory Biochemistry. Charles C Thomas, Springfield, IL, 1985

73. Drescher DG: Purification of a carbonic anhydrase from the inner ear of the guinea pig. Proc Natl Acad Sci USA 74:892, 1977

74. Spoendlin HH, Balogh K: Histochemical localization of dehydrogenases in the cochlea of living animals. Laryngoscope 73:1061, 1963

75. Ross MD: Glycogen accumulation in Reissner's membrane following chemical sympathectomy with 6-hydroxydopamine. Acta Otolaryngol (Stockh) 86:314, 1978

76. Konester-Frei A: Localization of the marginal zone of the tectorial membrane in situ, unfixed, and with in vivo-like milieu. Arch Otorhinolaryngol 224:3, 1979

77. Sterkers O, Saumon G, Tran Ba Huy P, et al: Electrochemical heterogeneity of the cochlear endolymph: effect of acetazolamide. Am J Physiol 246:F47, 1984

78. Smith CA, Lowry OH, Wu ML: The electrolytes of the labyrinthine fluids. Laryngoscope 64:141, 1954

79. Bosher SK, Warren RL: Observations on the electrochemistry of the cochlear endolymph of the rat: a quantitative study of its electrical potential and ionic composition as determined by means of flame spectrophotometry. Proc R Soc London 171B:227, 1968

80. Bosher SK, Warren RL: Very low calcium content of cochlear endolymph, an extracellular fluid. Nature 273:377, 1978

81. Sterkers O, Ferrary E, Amiel C: Inter- and intracompartmental osmotic gradients within the rat cochlea. Am J Physiol 247:F602, 1984

82. Anniko M, Lim D, Wroblewski R: Elemental composition of individual cells and tissues of the cochlea. Acta Otolaryngol (Stockh) 98:439, 1984

83. Schuknecht HF, Seifi el A: Experimental observations on the fluid physiology of the inner ear. Ann Otol Rhinol Laryngol 72:687, 1963

84. Schindler K: Perilymphe als Ultrafiltrat des Serums. Arch Ohren Nasen Kehlkopfheilkd 185:586, 1965

85. Sterkers O, Saumon G, Tran Ba Huy P, Amiel C: K, Cl and H$_2$O entry in endolymph, perilymph, and cerebrospinal fluid of rat. Am J Physiol 243:F173, 1982

86. Medina JE, Drescher DG: The amino acid content of perilymph and cerebrospinal fluid from guinea pigs and the effect of noise on the amino-acid composition of perilymph. Neuroscience 6:505, 1981

87. Kommoss J, Giebel W: Die Ausbreitung loslicher Substanzen nach Applikation in die cisterna cerebellomedularis. Arch Otorhinolaryngol 221:67, 1978

88. Kimura RS, Schuknecht HF, Ita CY: Blockage of the cochlear aqueduct, Acta Otolaryngol (Stockh) 77:1, 1974

89. Kimura RS, Maynard LB: Histopathological study of the cochlea with altered perilymph metabolism. Acta Otolaryngol (Stockh) 97:535, 1984

90. Thalmann R, Comegys TH, Thalmann I: Amino acid profiles in inner ear fluids and cerebrospinal fluid. Laryngoscope 92:321, 1982

91. Scheibe F, Diezel W, Haupt H, Hache U: Elekrophoretische Untersuchungen zur Proteinverteilung in der Meerschweinchen-Perilymphe. Acta Otolaryngol (Stockh) 81:68, 1976

92. Konishi T: Ion and water control in cochlear endolymph. Am J Otolaryngol 3:434, 1982
93. Bekesy G von: DC potentials and energy balance of the cochlear partition. J Acoust Soc Am 22:576, 1950
94. Tasaki I, Spiropoulos CS: Stria vascularis as source of endocochlear potential. J Neurophysiol 22:149, 1959
95. Konishi T, Hamrick PE, Mori H: Water permeability of the endolymph–perilymph barrier in the guinea pig cochlea. Hear Res 15:51, 1984
96. Sellick PM, Johnstone BM: Production and role of inner ear fluid. Prog Neurobiol 5:337, 1975
97. Thalmann R, Comegys TH, DeMott JE, Thalmann I: Steep gradients of amino acids between cochlear endolymph and perilymph. Laryngoscope 91: 1785, 1791, 1981
98. Konishi T, Kelsey E: Effect of potassium deficiency on cochlear potentials and cation contents of the endolymph. Acta Otolaryngol (Stockh) 76:410, 1973
99. Wada J, Kambayashi J, Marcus DC, Thalmann R: Vascular perfusion of the cochlea: effect of potassium-free and rubidium-substituted media. Arch Otorhinolaryngol 225:79, 1979
100. Ross MD, Ernst SA, Kerr TP: Possible functional roles of Na$^+$-ATPase and their relevance to Meniere's disease. Am J Otolaryngol 3:353, 1982
101. Schacht J: Adenylate cyclase and cochlear fluid balance. Am J Otolaryngol 5:328, 1982
102. Lim D, Karabinas C, Trune DR: Histochemical localization of carbonic anhydrase in the inner ear. Am J Otolaryngol 4:33, 1983
103. Kerr TP, Ross MD, Ernst SA: Cellular localization of Na$^+$/K$^+$-ATPase in the mammalian cochlear duct. Am J Otolaryngol 3:332, 1982
104. Kuijpers W, Bonting SL: Studies on (Na$^+$-K$^+$)-activated ATPase XXIV. Localization and properties of ATPase in the inner ear of the guinea pig. Biochim Biophys Acta 173:477, 1969
105. Kuijpers W: Na/K-ATPase activity in the cochlea of the rat during development. Acta Otolaryngol (Stockh) 78:341, 1974
106. Bosher SK, Warren RL: A study of the electrochemistry and osmotic relationships of the cochlear fluids in the neonatal rat to the time of development of the endocochlear potential. J Physiol (Lond.) 212:739, 1971
107. Bosher SK: The nature of the ototoxic actions of ethacrynic-acid upon the mammalian endolymph system. 1. Functional aspects. Acta Otolaryngol (Stockh) 89:407, 1980
108. Ahlström P, Thalmann I, Thalmann R, et al: Cyclic AMP and adenylate cyclase in the inner ear. Laryngoscope 85:1241, 1975
109. Kerr TP, Schacht J: Adenylate cyclase in the guinea pig cochlea. J Acoust Soc Am 57:S61, 1975
110. Paloheimo S, Thalmann R: Influence of "loop" diuretics upon Na$^+$/K$^+$-ATPase and adenylate cyclase of the stria vascularis. Arch Otorhinolaryngol 217:347, 1977
111. Bagger-Sjöbäck D, Filipek CS, Schacht J: Characteristics and drug responses of cochlear and vestibular adenylate cyclase. Arch Otorhinolaryngol 228:217, 1980
112. Strewler GJ, Orloff J: Role of cyclic nucleotides in the transport of water and electrolytes. Adv Cycl Nucl Res 8:311, 1977
113. Marks SC, Schacht J: Effects of ototoxic diuretics on cochlear Na$^+$/K$^+$-ATPase and adenylate cyclase. Scand Audiol S14:131, 1981
114. Thalmann I, Kobayashi T, Thalmann R: Arguments against a mediating role of the adenylate cyclase — cyclic AMP system in the ototoxic action of loop diuretics. Laryngoscope 92:589, 1982
115. Feldman AM, Brusilow SW: Effects of cholera toxin on cochlear endolymph production: model for endolymphatic hydrops. Proc Natl Acad Sci USA 73:1761, 1976
116. Feldman AM, Bittner HR, Brusilow SW: Measurement of the hydrostatic pressure of the cochlear compartments. Neurol Res 1:11, 1979
117. Thalmann I, DeMott JE, Ge XX: Effect of cholera toxin upon cyclic AMP (cAMP) levels in tissues lining cochlear duct. J Acoust Soc Am 71:S99, 1982
118. Anniko M, Spangberg ML, Schacht J: Adenylate cyclase activity in the fetal and early postnatal inner ear of the mouse. Hear Res 4:11, 1981
119. Zajic G, Anniko M, Schacht J: Cellular localization of adenylate cyclase in the developing and mature inner ear of the mouse. Hear Res 10:249, 1983
120. Duvall AJ, Santi PA, Hukee MJ: Cochlear fluid balance — a clinical/research overview. Ann Otol Rhinol Laryngol 89:335, 1980
121. Zenner HP, Zenner B: Vasopressin and isoproterenol activate adenylate cyclase in the guinea pig inner ear. Arch Otolaryngol 222:275, 1979
122. Erulkar SD, Maren TH: Carbonic anhydrase and the inner ear. Nature 189:459, 1961
123. Sellick PM, Johnstone BM: Differential effects of ouabain and ethacrynic acid on the labyrinthine potentials. Pflugers Arch 352:339, 1974
124. Thalmann R, Stroud MH, Anshutz LE: Energy metabolism of vestibular sensory structures. Adv Otorhinolaryngol 19:179, 1973
125. Morgenstern C, Amamo H, Orsulakova A: Ion

transport in the endolymphatic space. Am J Otolaryngol 3:323, 1982

126. Burnham JA, Stirling CE: Quantitative localization of Na-K pump sites in frog inner ear dark cells. Hear Res 13:261, 1984

127. Thalmann R: Metabolic features of auditory and vestibular systems. Laryngoscope 81:1245, 1971

128. Carlström D: A crystallographic study of vertebrate otoliths. Biol Bull 125:441, 1963

129. Ross MD, Pote KG: Some properties of otoconia. Philos Trans R Soc Lond [Biol] 304:445, 1983

130. Belanger LF: Autoradiographic visualization of in vitro exchange in teeth, bones, and other tissues, under various conditions. J Dent Res 32:168, 1953

131. Veenhof VB: The Development of Statoconia in Mice. Academie van Wetenschappen, Amsterdam, 1969

132. Preston RE, Johnsson L-G, Hill JH, et al: Incorporation of radioactive calcium into otolithic membranes and middle ear ossicles of the gerbil. Acta Otolaryngol (Stockh) 80:269, 1975

133. Mechigian I, Preston RE, Johnsson L-G, et al: Incorporation of radioactive calcium into otolithic membranes of the guinea pig after aminoglycoside treatment. Acta Otolaryngol (Stockh) 88:56, 1979

134. Ross MD: Calcium ion uptake and exchange in otoconia. Adv Oto Rhino laryngol 25:26, 1979

135. Harada Y, Sugimoto Y: Metabolic disorder of otoconia after streptomycin intoxication. Acta Otolaryngol (Stockh) 84:65, 1977

136. King K: Distribution of gamma-carboxyglutamic acid in calcified tissues. Biochim Biophys Acta 542:542, 1978

137. Lian JB, Hauschka PV, Gallop PM: Properties and biosynthesis of a vitamin K-dependent calcium binding protein in bone. Fed Proc 37:2615, 1978

138. Burnier JP, Borowski M, Furie BC, et al: Gamma-carboxyglutamic acid. Mol Cell Biochem 39:191, 1981

139. Purichia N, Erway LC: Effects of dichlorophenamide, zinc and manganese on otolith development in mice. Dev Biol 27:395, 1972

140. deVincentiis M, Marmo F: Inhibition of the morphogenesis of the otoliths in the chick embryo in the presence of carbonic anhydrase inhibitors. Experientia 24:818, 1968

141. Lim DC: Morphogenesis and malformation of otoconia: a review. p. 111. In Gorlin RJ (ed): Morphogenesis and Malformation of the Ear. Alan R Liss, New York, 1980

142. Schnieder, EA: A contribution to the physiology of the perilymph. III: on the origin of noise-induced

hearing loss. Ann Otol Rhinol Laryngol 83:406, 1974

143. Scheibe F, Haupt H, Hache U: Vergleichende Untersuchungen der Laktatkonzentration von Perilymphe, Blut and liquor cerebrospinalis normaler und schallbelasteter Meerschweinchen. Arch Otorhinolaryngol 214:19, 1976

144. Hawkins JE, Jr.: The role of vasoconstriction in noise-induced hearing loss. Ann Otol 80:903, 1971

145. Dengerink HA, Axelsson A, Miller JM, Wright JW: The effect of noise and carbogen on cochlear vasculature. Acta Otolaryngol (Stockh) 98:81, 1984

146. Salt AN, Konishi T: Effects of noise on cochlear potentials and endolymph potassium concentration recorded with potassium-selective electrodes. Hear Res 1:343, 1979

147. Konishi T, Salt AN: Electrochemical profile for potassium ions across the cochlear hair cell membranes of normal and noise-exposed guinea pigs. Hear Res 11:219, 1983

148. Slepecky N, Hamernik R, Henderson D, Coling D: Correlation of audiometric data with changes in cochlear hair cell stereocilia resulting from impulse noise trauma. Acta Otolaryngol (Stockh) 93:329, 1984

149. Liberman MC, Mulroy MJ: Acute and chronic effects of acoustic trauma: cochlear pathology and auditory nerve pathophysiology. p. 105. In Hamernik RP, Henderson D, Salvi R (eds): New Perspectives on Noise-Induced Hearing Loss. Raven Press, New York, 1982

150. Hunter-Duvar IM: Electron microscopic assessment of the cochlea. Acta Otolaryngol [Suppl] (Stockh) 351:1, 1978

151. Tilney LG, Saunders JC, Egelman E, et al: Changes in organization of actin filaments in the stereocilia of noise-damaged lizard cochlea. Hear Res 7:181, 1982

152. Mulroy MM, Whaley E: Structural changes in auditory hairs during temporary deafness. Scan Electron Microsc 1984:831

153. Hawkins JE, Jr.: Drug ototoxicity. p. 707. In Keidel WD, Neff WD (eds): Handbook of Sensory Physiology. Vol. 5. Topics. Springer-Verlag, Berlin, 1976

154. Hawkins JE, Jr., Preston RE: Vestibular ototoxicity. p. 321. In Naunton RF (ed): The Vestibular System. Academic Press, Orlando, FL, 1975

155. Hancock REW: Aminoglycoside uptake and mode of action — with special reference to streptomycin and gentamicin. I. Antagonists and mutants. J Antimicrob Chemother 8:429, 1981

156. Hancock REW: Aminoglycoside uptake and mode

of action—with special reference to streptomycin and gentamicin. II. Effects of aminoglycosides on cells. J Antimicrob Chemother 8:429, 1981

157. Voldrich L: The kinetics of streptomycin, kanamycin and neomycin in the inner ear. Acta Otolaryngol (Stockh) 60:243, 1965

158. Stupp HF: Untersuchung der Antibiotikaspiegel in den Innenohrflussigkeiten und ihre Bedeutung für die spezifische Ototoxizitat der Aminoglykosidantibiotika. Acta Otolaryngol [Suppl] (Stockh) 262:1, 1970

159. Tran Ba Huy P, Manuel C, et al: Pharmacokinetics of gentamicin in perilymph and endolymph of the rat as determined by radioimmunoassay. J Infect Dis 143:476, 1981

160. Tran Ba Huy P, Menlemans A, Wassef M, et al: Gentamicin persistence in rat endolymph and perilymph after a two-day constant infusion. Antimicrob Agents Chemother 23:344, 1983

161. Desrochers CS, Schacht J: Neomycin concentrations in inner ear tissues and other organs of the guinea pig after chronic drug administration. Acta Otolaryngol (Stockh) 93:233, 1982

162. Balogh K, Hiraide F, Ishii D: Distribution of radioactive dihydrostreptomycin in the cochlea. Ann Otol Rhinol Laryngol 79:641, 1970

163. von Ilberg C, Spoendlin H, Arnold W: Autoradiographical distribution of locally applied dihydrostreptomycin in the inner ear. Acta Otolaryngol (Stockh) 71:159, 1971

164. Portmann M, Darrouzet J, Coste Ch: Distribution within the cochlea of dihydrostreptomycin injected into the circulation. Arch Otolaryngol 100:473, 1974

165. Larsson B, Nilsson M, Tjälve H: The tissue disposition of gentamicin in rats. Acta Pharmacol Toxicol (Copenh) 48:269, 1981

166. Weiner ND, Schacht J: Biochemical model of aminoglycoside-induced hearing loss. p. 113. In Lerner SA, Matz GJ, Hawkins JE (eds): Aminoglycoside Ototoxicity. Little, Brown, Boston, 1981

167. Humes HD, Weiner ND, Schacht J: The biochemical pathology of aminoglycoside-induced nephro- and ototoxicity. p. 333. In Fillastre JP (ed): Nephrotoxicity and Ototoxicity of Drugs. Colloq. INSERM, Paris, 1982

168. Orsulakova A, Stockhorst E, Schacht J: Effect of neomycin on phosphoinositide labeling and calcium binding in guinea pig inner ear tissues in vivo and in vitro. J Neurochem 26:285, 1976

169. Schacht J: Inhibition of neomycin of polyphosphoinositide turnover in subcellular fractions of guinea pig cerebral cortex in vitro. J Neurochem 27:1119, 1976

170. Schacht J: Isolation of an aminoglycoside receptor from guinea pig inner ear tissues and kidney. Arch Otorhinolaryngol 224:129, 1979

171. Takada A, Bledsoe S, Schacht J: An energy-dependent step in aminoglycoside toxicity: prevention of gentamicin ototoxicity during reduced endolymphatic potential. Hear Res 19:245, 1985

172. Jackson GG, Arcieri G: The ototoxicity of gentamicin in man: a survey and controlled analysis of clinical experience in the United States. J Infect Dis 124:S130, 1971

173. Federspil P: Ubersicht über die in Deutschland beobachteten Fälle von Gentamicin-Ototoxizität. HNO 18:328, 1970

174. Tjernström O, Banck G, Belfrage S, et al: The ototoxicity of gentamicin. Acta Pathol Microbiol Scand [B], suppl., 241: 73, 1973

175. Pierson MG, Moller AR: Prophylaxis of kanamycin-induced ototoxicity by a radioprotectant. Hear Res 4:79, 1981

176. Bock GR, Yates GK, Miller J, et al: Effects of N-acetylcystein on kanamycin ototoxicity in the guinea pig. Hear Res 9:255, 1983

177. Humes HD, Sastrasinh M, Weinberg JM: Calcium is a competitive inhibitor of gentamicin-renal membrane binding interactions and dietary calcium supplementation protects against gentamicin nephrotoxicity. J Clin Invest 73:134, 1984

178. Quick CA, Duvall AJ: Early changes in the cochlear duct from ethacrynic acid: an electromicroscopic evaluation. Laryngoscope 80:954, 1970

179. Bosher SK: The nature of the ototoxic actions of ethacrynic acid upon the mammalian endolymph system. II. Structural-functional correlates in the stria vascularis. Acta Otolaryngol (Stockh) 90:40, 1980

180. Rybak LP, Green TP, Juhn SK, Morizono T: Probenecid reduces cochlear effects and perilymph penetration of furosemide in chinchilla. J Pharm Exp Ther 230:706, 1984

181. Burg MB: Tubular chloride transport and the mode of action of some diuretics. Kidney Int 9:189, 1976

182. McFadden D, Plattsmier HS: Aspirin can potentiate the temporary hearing loss induced by intense sounds. Hear Res 9:295, 1983

183. Escoubet B, Amsallem P, Ferrary E, Tran Ba Huy P: Prostaglandin synthesis by the cochlea of the guinea pig. Influence of aspirin, gentamicin, and acoustic stimulation. Prostaglandins 29:589, 1985

184. Hawkins JE, Jr., Johnsson L-G, Stebbins WC, et al: The patas monkey as a model for dihydrostreptomycin ototoxicity. Acta Otolaryngol (Stockh) 83:123, 1977

185. Wang BM, Weiner ND, Takada A, et al: Characterization of aminoglycoside-lipid interactions and development of a refined model for ototoxicity testing. Biochem Pharmacol 33:3257, 1984

186. Lodhi S, Weiner ND, Mechigian I, et al: Ototoxicity of aminoglycosides correlated with their action on monomolecular films of polyphosphoinositides. Biochem Pharmacol 29:597, 1980

187. Orsulakova A, Schacht J: A biochemical mechanism of the ototoxic interaction between neomycin and ethacrynic acid. Acta Otolaryngol (Stockh) 93:43, 1981

188. Kimura RS: Recent observations on experimental endolymphatic hydrops. p. 15. In Vorsteen K-H, Schuknecht H, Pfaltz CR et al (eds): Menière's Disease, Pathogenesis, Diagnosis and Treatment. Thieme, New York, 1981

189. Tran Ba Huy P: Electrophysiological and biochemical findings in four cases of Meniere's disease. Acta Otolaryngol (Stockh) 97:571, 1984

190. Konishi T, Kelsey E: Cochlear potentials and electrolyte contents in endolymphs in experimentally induced endolymphatic hydrops. J Acoust Soc Am 54:294, 1973

191. Giebel W, Bäck P, Glöggler FW, et al: Vorläufige Ergebnisse der Analyse von Innenohrflüssigkeiten bei Meerschweinchen mit experimentellem Hydrops. p. 51. In Jakobi H, Kuhl K-D, Lotz P (eds): Cochlea-Forschung. Martin-Luther-University, Halle, 1982

192. Nakamura T: Experimental obliteration of the endolymphatic sac and the perilymphatic duct. Nippon-Jibiinkoka-Gakkai-Kaiho 70:932, 1967

193. Silverstein H, Takeda T: Endolymphatic sac obstruction. Biochemical studies. Ann Otol Rhinol Laryngol 86:493, 1977

194. Reivich M, Kuhl D, Wolf A, et al: Measurement of local cerebral glucose metabolism in man with $^{18}$F-2-Fluor-2-Deoxy-D-Glucose. p. 190. In Ingrar DH, Lassen NA (eds): Cerebral Function, Metabolism and Circulation. Munksgaard, Copenhagen, 1977

195. Alavi A, Reivich M, Greenberg J, et al: Mapping of functional activity in brain with $^{18}$F-Fluoro-deoxyglucose. Semin Nucl Med 11:24, 1981

196. Mackay RS, Liaw HM: Metabolic mapping of functional activity in human subjects with the ($^{18}$F) fluorodeoxyglucose technique. Science 212:678, 1981

197. Rottenberg DA, Cooper AJL: Positron emission tomography of the central nervous system. Trends Biochem Sci 6:120, 1981

198. Fox JL: PET scan controversy aired. Science 224:143, 1984

# Physiology of Hearing

**7**

Brian Johnstone

The physiology of the ear may be conveniently divided into two functional systems. The primary, or direct, pathway in effect follows sound through the external and the middle ear into the cochlea, then on to the basilar membrane and hair cells, finally ending with the response of the 8th nerve. The secondary, or indirect, system involves the support functions that enable the primary pathway to fulfill its function. These support systems are the blood supply, the endolymph and perilymph production and reabsorbtion systems, and the autonomic and efferent nervous systems.

## THE OUTER EAR

The outer ear consists of the pinna, or external ear, and the external auditory canal. The main functional property of the outer ear is the role it plays in sound localization. The most important cues for sound localization are intensity and timing differences between the sound waves at the two ears. For instance, the sound wave from a source on the right will strike the right ear before the left, leading to a time delay. In addition, the sound could be more intense in the right ear due to the shadowing effect of the head. However, our ability to distinguish sounds above from those below, or those in front from those behind, is due to the operation of the pinna and concha. When the wave length of sound is short compared with the dimensions of the pinna, there will be a directional selectivity in the reception of sound, that is, the pinna is most useful in our detection of sound direction at the higher frequencies. Physical measurement shows that the pinna alters the sound pressure entering the ear in the 5-7 kHz region, depending on whether the sound is in front or behind, above or below. This contribution to localization is due to variations in the stimulus spectrum caused by the various folds and depressions. In summary then, our ability to localize sounds in space may be divided into three bands. At low frequencies, up to about 1 kHz, the phase delay of the wave front striking the ears, caused by the separation of the ears in space, is of primary importance. In the intermediate frequencies ranging from about 1 to 3 kHz, a significant head-shadowing effect takes place, so that the sound intensity striking the two ears will be different, depending on the position of the sound source in space. At high frequencies, from 5 kHz on up, it appears that the pinna plays a primary role and is particularly important in resolving sounds directly in front from those directly behind.

Since the tympanic membrane is located at the end of the external auditory canal, the sounds reaching it are affected by the acoustic characteristics of the canal as well as those of the pinna and the head. The external canal is similar to an organ pipe: open at one end and closed at the other. Such a tube resonates at a frequency with a wave length four times the length of the tube. Because the average length of the external canal is 2.5 cm, the fundamental mode of this pipe is calculated as $f$ = velocity of sound/4 L (in meters) = 343/4 × 0.025 = 3,430 Hz. At this resonant frequency, a pressure node occurs at the entrance of the canal and an antinode at the tympanic membrane. As a conse-

quence, there is a sound-pressure amplification at the closed end of the pipe. However, the external canal is not a perfect organ pipe, and its resonance is rather broad. Direct measurements of the sound pressure at the tympanic membrane, relative to free field sound a short distance away from the head, show that it is capable of a gain of up to 20 dB in the 2- to 5-kHz band. This correlates well with the fact that human hearing is most sensitive in this band. Another consequence of this resonance would be that audiograms performed under free field condition (minimum audible field), with earphones (minimum audible pressure), or with insert earphones in the canal would be expected to give somewhat different results, particularly in the 2- to 4-kHz region (Fig. 7-1). Care must be taken when

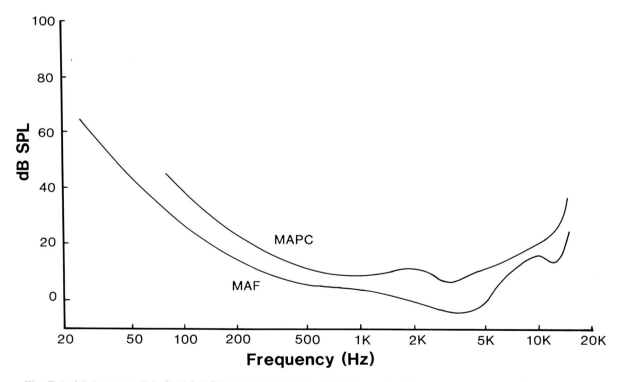

**Fig. 7-1.** Minimum audible field (MAF) is the threshold sound pressure level in free field measured in an anechoic chamber. Minimum audible pressure (MAPC) is the threshold measured with earphones calibrated in a standard 6 cc coupler or artificial ear. The thresholds are in decibels sound pressure level (SPL), which is a measure of the sound pressure with reference to the international standard of 0 db = 20 $\mu$Pa (= 0.0002 dyn/cm$^2$). The difference between the curves above 1 kHz is accounted for by the head and pinna diffraction plus ear canal resonance. At lower frequencies there is some masking by physiological noises picked up by the ear when it is covered by an earphone. In addition, binaural hearing (MAF) is somewhat better than monaural hearing (MAPC).

comparing audiograms under these different conditions that the equipment is calibrated and appropriately compensated for the effect of the disturbance of this resonance.

## THE MIDDLE EAR

Anatomically, the middle ear consists of the tympanic membrane and the three small bones, the ossicles, that conduct sound to the oval window. The malleus attaches to the tympanic membrane and to the incus, which is in turn attached to the stapes, the footplate of the stapes resting in the oval window. The motion of the tympanic membrane is transmitted through the ossicles and delivers a force to the fluids of the cochlea. The primary functional significance of the middle ear may be understood when we consider the physical properties of its two boundaries. Sound reaches the ear by way of the air, a gas. On the other hand, the organ of Corti is contained within the cochlear fluids, which may be considered as water (but see below). The difference between these two media is of considerable importance to the theory of hearing. Air offers less opposition to flow of sound energy than does water; that is, the air is of lesser impedance than water. The concept of impedance is extremely important to the understanding not only of the middle ear but to the whole of cochlear mechanics.

Impedance $(z)$ is the ratio of sound pressure $(p)$ to particle velocity $(v)$: $z = p/v$. The impedance of water is 4,000 times that of air, so for a sound going from air to water, 99.9 percent is reflected (see Appendix 7-1). This corresponds to an energy loss of $10 \log 4{,}000 = 30$ dB. (Note energy ratios in dB $= 10 \log(\text{ratio})$; pressure ratios in dB $= 20 \log(\text{ratio})$.) An important consequence of this is that a fish cannot hear a fisherman talking, unless the fisherman shouts very loudly.

The primary function of the middle ear is to reduce the impedance mismatch. The main principle used is that of the hydraulic transformer. When an amount of force is applied over a large area and the resultant motion is applied to a smaller area, this smaller area can in turn impart a large force, that is,

one obtains a pressure amplification in proportion to the area ratios. For the human, the areas of tympanic membrane and stapes are about 64 and 3.2 mm² respectively — a ratio of approximately 20 : 1. In addition, the malleus and incus make a lever ratio of about 1 : 2. Furthermore, the tympanic membrane is not a simple flat plate but is a curved membrane, and this increases the force applied to the manubrium by a factor of 2. Taking into account all these factors, a pressure transformer ratio of close to 50 : 1 results. This will give an impedance ratio of about 2,500, compared to the ideal ratio of 4,000, thereby reducing energy losses to only 3 dB. The implication of these calculations is that the middle ear does its job very well. However, the calculations assume that the impedance of the cochlea is the same as that of water. In fact, this is only correct at about 1 kHz, and at other frequencies other factors come into play.

It is obvious that the cochlea does not have a large fluid volume. Its dimensions are small compared with the wavelength of sound in water; therefore, its impedance will be complex, with the helicotrema, the impedance of the basilar membrane, and the impedance of the round window being the major determinants. The latest measurements in the cat suggest that the cochlear input impedance could be a fifth of that of the previously supposed large volume of water. The impedance match therefore is much better, and most of the energy is transmitted. While this seems very satisfactory, it is subject to the caveat that the impedance of the cochlea is a function of frequency. At low frequencies the stapes ligament also adds a strong stiffness component, and the impedance rises. Similarly, at high frequencies the basilar membrane impedance also rises and the inertial mass of the ossicles becomes important. It is therefore at the midfrequencies of about 1 to 4 kHz that the middle ear is most efficient.

The importance of considering the energy transfer comes when we look at the effect of middle ear pathology. Otosclerosis reduces the possibility of vibration and effectively makes the middle ear stiffer. This raises the low-frequency impedance and so causes a reduction in energy transfer and the familiar low-tone hearing loss. Disarticulation of the stapes naturally affects all frequencies, but the effect of fluid in the middle ear cavity can be complex. A small amount of viscous fluid around the stapes could affect the low frequencies (increased stiffness), but the middle ear full of fluid backing onto the eardrum will cause an air–water mismatch, which will affect a wide frequency band.

The fact that there is a significant reflection of sound at low frequencies underlies the concept of impedance audiometry. If a low tone of less than 1 kHz (220 Hz is often used) is fed into the ear, a significant amount of the energy is reflected. Anything that alters the stiffness of the middle ear will alter its impedance at low frequencies and therefore the amount of sound energy reflected back. A microphone placed near the eardrum will detect the reflected energy, and thus the change of impedance can be deduced. Such changes are brought about by pathology, the action of the middle ear muscles, and increases or decreases in static pressures in the middle ear. (The pressures alter the stiffness of the stapes ligament by forcing it in or out of the oval window.) It is theoretically possible that changes in basilar membrane impedance could be detected by measuring at high frequencies, but the technical difficulties seem enormous. Work in this area is for the future.

In summary then, the middle ear is a reasonable impedance transformer at middle frequencies, but below about 500 Hz the efficiency falls off at 6 to 12 dB per octave, and this substantially contributes to the poor absolute hearing thresholds at low frequencies. The efficiency at middle frequencies is further enhanced by the ear canal resonance and the effect of the pinna and head. At high frequencies the efficiency falls again due to the mass inertial effects of the middle ear and the rise in input impedance of the cochlea, which probably reflects the effect of the basilar membrane.

## COCHLEAR MECHANICS

The vibration of the stapes causes movement of the fluid in the scala vestibuli, which in turn moves the basilar membrane, then the fluid in scala tympani, and finally the round window. The movement of the fluid along the length of scala vestibuli is partially hindered by its inertia. As a result a pressure gradient is induced across the basilar membrane which is only released by its transverse movement, and finally movement of the round window.

At low stimulus frequencies, the pressure gradient across the membrane in the basal regions of the cochlea is resisted by the stiffness of the membrane. At more apical sites along the cochlea, however, the stiffness force decreases due to changes in the structure and dimensions of the organ of Corti. At a particular location along the cochlear the membrane stiffness and inertial forces cancel and the membrane moves freely. That is, the membrane resonates. This free transverse movement of the membrane effectively "short-circuits" the pressure gradient across it, precluding a pressure gradient at more apical regions, at that stimulus frequency. Without a pressure gradient no vibration exists beyond the place of the membrane resonance. Since the cancellation of the stiffness and inertial forces occurs at different places at different stimulus frequencies the free movement of the membrane is tonotopically arranged.

A classical view of hearing, advanced by Helmholtz, considered the basilar membrane to be a graded series of resonators like a piano or harp, with the radial fibers (of the basilar membrane) acting like strings. The appropriate strings, or places, would vibrate with the largest amplitude at their tuned, or resonant, frequency. The main problem with this model is that the high degree of tuning required necessitates a considerable inertia. That is, the strings would have to continue to vibrate for some time after the sound ceased. Also, with continual sinusoidal sound input, the theory predicts that standing waves should form on the basilar membrane.

Von Békésy directly observed the basilar membrane motion in response to sound input using a microscope and stroboscopic illumination (see von Békésy 1960[1] for all of his papers). He saw that waves travel down the cochlear partition only in one direction, and no standing waves were seen. Starting at the base, they travel toward the apex, building up an amplitude to a peak (Fig. 7-2), then are quickly damped with minimal afteroscillations. This seems to eliminate completely Helmholtz' ideas. The position of peak amplitude depends on

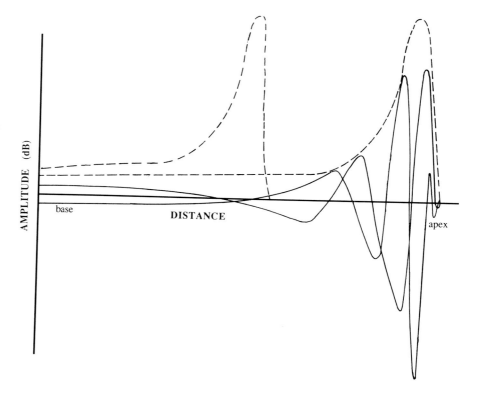

**Fig. 7-2.** A schematic diagram of the traveling wave at two instances in time. These waves can be regarded as side views of the basilar membrane frozen at two phases of a particular frequency of the sine wave. The envelopes (dotted) show the peak displacement as a function of distance for two frequencies.

frequency in a very regular manner, the logarithm of the frequency being approximately proportional to distance from the apex, so the maximum for higher frequencies is near the base, and for the lower frequencies it is near the apex. In the guinea pig basal turn, one octave corresponds to a distance of 2.5 mm.

More recent experiments using Mössbauer techniques, capacitance probes, and lasers have confirmed von Békésy's observations in essence. That is, a wave indeed does appear to travel along the cochlea from base to apex. A popular misconception regards the traveling wave as a bundle of energy moving down the basilar membrane, rather like a wave down a rope or whip when it is given a flick; this is inaccurate. The basilar membrane absorbs some energy from the pressure difference along its entire length up to the resonant point where most is absorbed. In addition, energy is propagated longitudinally through the fluid, due to the inertia of the fluid and its coupling with the membrane, especially near resonance. The relative amount of energy in each of these pathways is still in dispute, and some researchers would not agree with the following ideas:

1. The fluid coupling is probably significant only over a small distance in the vicinity of resonance.
2. Energy is not propagated from base to apex by the basilar membrane itself.

The name "traveling wave" has given the wrong impression to many people and can be considered somewhat of a visual illusion. Actually, any series of locally coupled resonators, with high frequencies at one end and low at the other, will appear to have a wave travel from high to low frequencies. This is principally a consequence of the fact that high-frequency resonators respond before low-frequency resonators, and the fluid coupling alters the shape and properties of the resonators so the system appears to be a traveling wave, similar to ocean waves approaching a shore.

The vibration of the basilar membrane has also been investigated by means of models, both mechanical and mathematical, and several clear statements can be made:

1. The vibration is a function of the stiffness of the membrane, viscosity of fluids, and effective mass of the membrane (the effective mass is not only that of the organ of Corti and structures on the basilar membrane but includes the fluid coupled to the basilar membrane), so that it has all the elements of a resonator.
2. The "wave" travels from base to apex because of the variation in stiffness (about 100 to 1) but the speed of propagation and the wave shape largely depend on the interactions with the fluid. This is because one part of the basilar membrane is coupled to neighboring parts by the adjacent fluid flows. They do not depend on the longitudinal coupling of the basilar membrane itself, which is small.
3. Most recent measurements[2] have shown that the basilar membrane is very sharply tuned and sensitive — much more so than can be accounted for by its mechanical and hydrodynamic properties. Some active process is needed in addition, and it is now thought that the outer hair cells assist as micromotors or muscles that react on the basilar membrane, pushing and pulling it in synchrony, so assisting its resonance and helping to largely overcome the viscous damping of the fluid (See Fig. 7-3A).

The longitudinal fluid coupling is only over short, adjacent segments and has the major effect of altering the resonance shape and characteristics, so that the response at a particular point of the basilar membrane increases gradually as frequency rises, peaking sharply at its characteristic frequency (CF) and then falling abruptly at higher frequencies. There are many practical consequences of the preceding ideas. For instance, if the basilar membrane is damaged at one point, it matters little for the rest. Aside from places very close to the damaged point, traveling waves on each side will be normal, hence a defect of mechanics will only have a local effect. Since the basilar membrane has all the properties of a resonator (i.e., mass, stiffness, and damping), then how does the traveling wave differ from Helmholtz' idea? Basically, only by the fluid coupling, which not only alters the response but causes increased damping after the sound has ceased and so prevents a long afterringing or oscillation. We might somewhat lightly consider the basilar membrane as a Helmholtz harp immersed in a bath.

The basilar membrane is not only very sharply tuned and sensitive but also nonlinear; that is, the basilar membrane vibration is not an exact copy of the sound input, and indeed many properties of 8th nerve responses and psychoacoustics can now be shown to be due to the mechanics of the basilar membrane. The nonlinearity manifests itself in several ways:

1. The amplitude of vibration grows less in proportion to an increase in sound pressure (compressive nonlinearity).
2. At high sound pressures the tuning is broader.
3. At very high sound pressures, the place of best vibration changes, moving more basally.
4. Two tones presented together interact so that a low-frequency tone inhibits, suppresses, or masks a higher tone. To a lesser extent, a high tone can suppress a lower tone if they are close in frequency.
5. Distortion products are produced. For instance, if two tones ($f1 + f2$, $f2$ being higher in frequency) are presented together, combination tones at various frequencies can be generated.

Combination tones include simple difference tones ($f2 - f1$) and a major complex difference tone ($2f1 - f2$). This latter is a consequence of a particular type of nonlinearity known as "essential" cubic nonlinearity. It is called an essential nonlinearity because the strength of the distortion tone rises directly in proportion to the strength of the primaries. In a simple cubic nonlinearity, they would rise three times as fast. The nonlinearity almost certainly resides in the transducer mechanism at the top of the outer hair cells (or in their stereocilia)[7]. This mechanism transduces cilia motion into electric current through the hair cells and it is probably this current which in turn stimulates or causes the active process.

A note on noise deafness. When a loud sound is presented, the peak of maximum basilar membrane

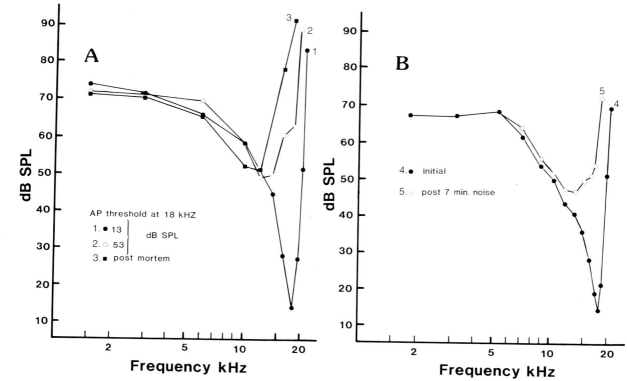

**Fig. 7-3.** A mechanical "threshold tuning curve" in the first turn of the guinea pig cochlea, measured with the Mössbauer technique. The ordinate is the sound pressure required to give a basilar membrane velocity of 0.06 mm/sec. *Curve 1:* This velocity (=3 nm at 18 kHz) elicits a neural response very close to threshold values for high-frequency nerve fibers. *Curve 2:* After experimental damage causing a 40-dB sensorineural loss at 18 kHz, an extra 40 dB of sound pressure is now needed to reach 0.06 mm/sec at this frequency. *Curve 3:* Postmortem response. This illustrates that when the threshold has shifted by 50 dB, the resultant motion is almost entirely passive and close to that of a dead cochlea. Until recently all measurements of basilar membrane motion were on dead or damaged cochleae. The low-frequency portion that is unaltered in curves 1, 2, and 3 is called the *tail* and the sharp, vulnerable portion is called the *tip* of the tuning curve. The difference between curves 1 and 3 is thought to be due to active processes in the outer hair cells. **(B)** Single nerve fiber tuning curves from a guinea pig. This nerve fiber innervates a similar place, as mechanically measured, to that for curve 3 *(curve 4).* A loud sound for 7 minutes was used to give a threshold shift of 30 dB, and the tuning curve was remeasured *(curve 5).* Note the correspondence to curves 1 and 2.

vibration moves basalward. Thus, loud noises induce pathology at a higher frequency than the presented sound. The resonance of the external canal is around 3 kHz, so a broad-band noise will show a spectral peak at this frequency at the tympanic membrane. When loud, broad-spectrum noises are presented, the upward shift on the basilar membrane combined with the resonance would produce pathology at higher frequencies, between 4 and 6 khz. This seems to be the best explanation of

the noise-induced hearing "notch," which usually occurs at 4 to 5 kHz.

The sharp tuning and high sensitivity and nonlinearity are physiologically vulnerable. Almost any insult to the cochlea (drugs, anoxia, loud sounds) will affect and reduce these properties. The sharp tuning and nonlinearity are almost certainly both due to the active process in the outer hair cells; anything that affects this action appears to have similar coordinate effects of reducing tuning, sensitivity, and nonlinearity. Hence, most cochlea damage that reduces threshold also reduces its frequency selectivity (sensorineural hearing loss). This explains much of the inadequacy of hearing aids when the hearing loss is more than 30 dB. The aid just boosts the sensitivity not the selectivity.

The new basilar membrane measurements indicate a threshold of hearing corresponding to the vibration of the basilar membrane of about 1 nm, considerably greater than previously thought. (von Békésy's calculation was 0.001 nm). The difference is due to the active process and nonlinearity, older measurements being made either at loud sounds or on damaged cochleas, both of which cause reduced sensitivity. For example, for a dam-

aged cochlea, 86 dB SPL may cause a vibration of 20 nm. Extrapolating to 9 dB, SPL (neural threshold) gives 0.001 nm for threshold. However, for an undamaged cochlea, 26 dB SPL causes a vibration of 20 nm, and thus the threshold equals 1 nm (Fig. 7-3, curve 2).

When a very low frequency is presented and basilar membrane vibration to an added high-frequency best place (CF) tone is measured, the high-frequency response is modulated by the low tone.

Displacements toward scala tympani are strongly inhibitory and toward scala vestibuli are mildly inhibitory (Fig. 7-4). Some studies of this phenomenon on the mechanical level have been made, and it appears that displacement of the basilar membrane

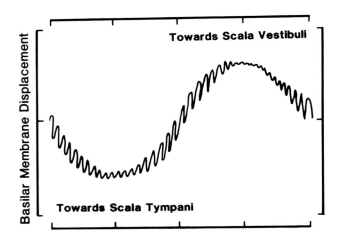

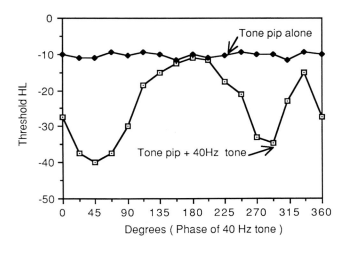

**Fig. 7-4.** A high tone and a low tone when presented together, interact on the basilar membrane at the high tone's best place or characteristic frequency. The high-tone response is reduced (modulated) twice per low-tone cycle. This modulation can be measured psychoacoustically and is often experienced musically, for example, when the longest pipe and a short pipe are sounded together on a pipe organ. Above 200 Hz the modulation sensation becomes smaller and a smooth inhibition or masking of the high tone is observed. The top diagram represents the response of a point on the basilar membrane when a high tone (the fine sinusoid) and a low tone (one cycle is represented) are presented together. The response of the high tone is suppressed at the peak of scala tympani and scala vestibuli motion. Displacement towards scala tympani is more effective. The lower diagram is from a psychophysical experiment. Short tone pips of 3 kHz were presented at a number of fixed positions in the phase of a 40 Hz tone and the threshold determined at each point. The top curve is when the 40 Hz tone is attenuated. The lower is when the 40 Hz tone is presented at 90 dB SPL. The ordinate is in hearing loss from an arbitrary zero. The abscissa represents fixed points on the phase of the 40 Hz tone. One cycle is represented. 45 degrees corresponds to maximum deflection of the basilar membrane towards scala tympani.

away from its rest position inhibits the active process and so reduces basilar membrane sensitivity. This effect has been measured with sounds up to several kHz and as low as 10 Hz and is the essence of two-tone suppression or masking. It probably exists down to static deflections and could be the cause of fluctuant hearing loss in endolymphatic hydrops (high and variable scala media pressure). When tones higher than the CF are presented, two-tone suppression is also evident, but the mechanism is possibly different in this range and not as well understood.

## TRANSDUCTION, NONLINEARITY, AND THE ACTIVE PROCESS

The detector elements for the basilar membrane motion are the hair cells residing on the organ of Corti, which is very firmly attached to the membrane by the arches of Corti and the reticular lamina. There are two types of hair cells, outer and inner. The inner hair cells form a single row, and their stereocilia are lined up in a gentle curve, whereas the outer hair cells lie in three rows, and their stereocilia are in a characteristic W-formation. These cells are motion detectors. A deflection of the hairs away from the center of the cell is excitatory, toward the center, inhibitory, and motion side to side has little effect. The inner hair cells receive 95 percent of the innervation of the 8th nerve, while the outer hair cells receive only 5 percent. This 5 percent is of a different type; the axons are very fine (less than 1 $\mu$m) and probably slow conducting. The main functions of the outer hair cells appear to be to actively assist the basilar membrane vibration, although some other function, such as moving the tectorial membrane, cannot be ruled out. How the hair cells are stimulated can be seen by simple geometry (Fig. 7-5A). Note that displacement across the width of the basilar membrane rather than along its length must now be considered. The basilar membrane, outer hair cell stereocilia, tectorial membrane and attachment of the tectorial membrane to the limbic lip form a parallelogram. As the basilar membrane vibrates

up and down, this parallelogram changes shape, and the hairs are deflected. The inner hair cells do not contact the tectorial membrane and are stimulated by the fluid flow in the subtectorial space, caused by the change of shape and volume of the parallelogram. Thus, the outer hair cells are stimulated by (and contribute to) basilar membrane displacement, and the inner hair cells by fluid flow, which is proportional to basilar membrane velocity (see Fig. 7-3A).

In 1965 Davis[3] proposed a model to account for the transduction by hair cells of stereocilia movement into a voltage change inside the cell. The top of the hair cell and its cilia reside in the endolymph in the scala media, whereas the base is in the perilymph. Endolymph is almost isotonic for KCl and has a positive potential, the endocochlear potential (EP), of about 80 mV with respect to perilymph. The inside of the hair cell, like any other cell, has a negative potential of 60 to 80 mV. Therefore, across the top of the cell and the stereocilia membrane is a potential difference of up to 60 mV. This large potential difference will drive a steady current (mainly of potassium ions) through the apical membrane resistance. It is hypothesized that movement of the stereocilia alters their membrane resistance and so alters the flow of current (Fig. 7-5B). This change of current must flow out across the base and lateral walls of the cell and causes a change of voltage across the membrane. These currents also flow along scala tympani and vestibuli and can be detected by an electrode on the round window. Such extracellular recordings are discussed later in this chapter.

A very fine microelectrode placed in an inner hair cell shows intracellular evoked potentials up to 30 mV for loud sounds. Recordings from outer hair cells have been less successful. However, they probably behave like the inner hair cells but develop less potential. As discussed previously, the basilar membrane is actively assisted in vibrating by some action of the outer hair cells. This activity is critically dependent on outer hair cell integrity and is very vulnerable. Drugs (furosemide, ouabain, aspirin, aminoglycosides), loud sounds, mechanical trauma, anoxia, and efferent stimulation (see later), all appear to affect outer hair cell function. The effect of outer hair cell malfunction is rather similar, irrespective of the cause. There is a

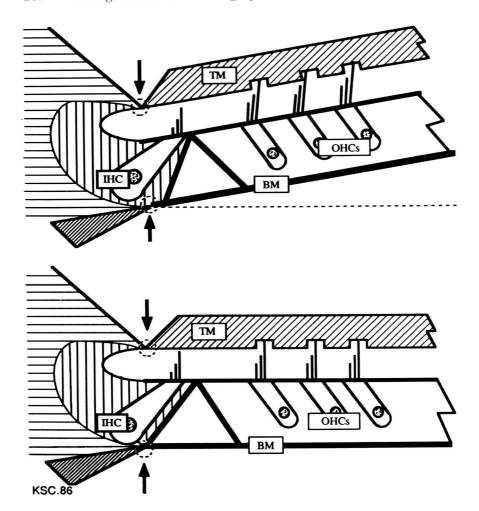

**Fig. 7-5. (A)** When the basilar membrane is displaced, the organ of Corti and the tectorial membrane move together and cause a shearing force on the stereocilia of the outer hair cells. BM, basal membrane; IHC, inner hair cell; OHC, outer hair cell; TM, tectorial membrane.

KSC.86

loss of basilar membrane sensitivity of up to 50 dB; the tuning at a particular point becomes broad and shifts to lower frequencies (i.e., the traveling wave for a particular frequency shifts basalward), and the basilar membrane vibration becomes linear.

The details of how the active process works is unknown. Somehow it must sense the movement of the stereocilia or the current flow and then make some movement of the outer hair cells or stereocilia in the right direction at the precise moment. Furthermore, it must do this at speeds of the order of 25 $\mu$sec to account for active processes at 40 kHz, the high-frequency limit for most mammals. No mechanism known at present can fulfill these requirements. Some first steps have been made in investigating this problem. Recently, Flock et al.[4] showed contraction of isolated outer hair cells to a variety of chemical stimuli and that the stereocilia and the lateral walls contain actin. Brownell et al.[5] showed that the cells move in response to slow, alternating electric fields. These motions of the hair cells are rather slow and only demonstrated under artificial conditions, but it is now known at least that the outer hair cells are capable of some sort of contraction. Since all similar experiments on inner hair cells have failed to show they are capable of any movement, the contractile behavior seems quite specific to outer hair cells.

Another consequence of the active process is the existence of "cochlear echoes." Using a sensitive

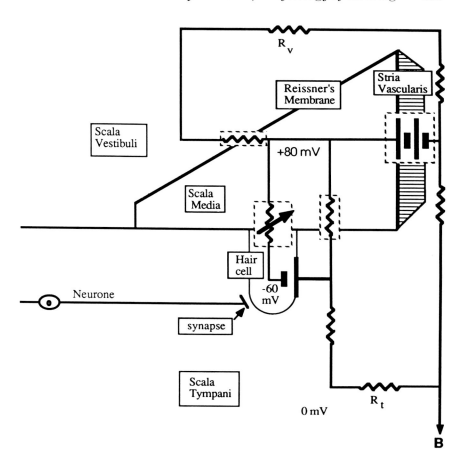

**Fig. 7-5** *(continued).* **(B)** The endocochlear potential together with the intracellular potential drive current through the hair cell. The movement of the hairs changes the resistance of the apical end and causes more or less current to flow. The changing current flows through fluids of the scala tympani ($R_t$) and scala vestibuli ($R_v$) and back through the stria vascularis to complete the circuit. The arrow labeled *B* indicates a pathway to the animal body, probably via the internal auditory canal. An electrode in the scala tympani (or on the round window) and a reference on the animal body will record the current flowing through $R_t$.

microphone in the external canal and computer-processing techniques, Kemp[6] demonstrated an emission from the tympanic membrane some 5 to 30 msec after presentation of a sharp click. Further work showed that this emission (echo) originated in the cochlea. Spontaneous emissions have also been found in many people. They are usually pure tones between 200 Hz and 2 kHz at levels of −10 to +10 dB SPL. Both the spontaneous emissions and the evoked emissions are reduced by procedures that reduce cochlear sensitivity. They can be masked, and their masking functions are similar to those of ordinary tones. It appears that the outer hair cells can become hyperactive and cause oscillations of the basilar membrane by themselves. Distortion tone emissions also can be evoked by presenting two simultaneous tones. The most readily evoked is the $2f1 − f2$ combination tone (or cubic difference

tone, e.g., 1 kHz + 1.2 kHz yields an 800-Hz combination tone). This combination tone is also easily heard psychoacoustically and can be measured in 8th-nerve responses. Procedures that eliminate its psychophysical perception (masking and deafness) also eliminate its emission. Thus, the cochlear echoes, distortion tones, and spontaneous emissions seem to be properties of the active (or over-active) process of the outer hair cells of the cochlea. It is of interest in this connection that frog saccular hair cells and turtle auditory papilla hair cells have been shown to have electrical oscillating properties, albeit at frequencies below 1 kHz.[7,8] Since some people have spontaneous cochlear emissions, the following questions arise: do people hear them? and what is the relationship to tinnitus? The evidence is rather scarce at the moment. However, only a few people have tinnitus that seems to match the emissions in frequency and behavior. Early hopes of finding large numbers of tinnitus sufferers with matching emission have not been fulfilled.

While the outer hair cell is of utmost importance to normal hearing, the inner hair cell, as the final step in the mechanicoelectrical transduction function of the cochlea, is crucial to all hearing. Russell and Sellick[9] provided the first intracellular recordings from inner hair cells. They found the receptor potential follows the sound input at low levels and low frequencies, but at loud sounds and high frequencies, several important changes take place. With a loud sinusoidal sound input, the depolarizing direction was much larger than the reverse; that is, the inner hair cell showed rectification (Fig. 7-6). At high frequencies, the alternating compo

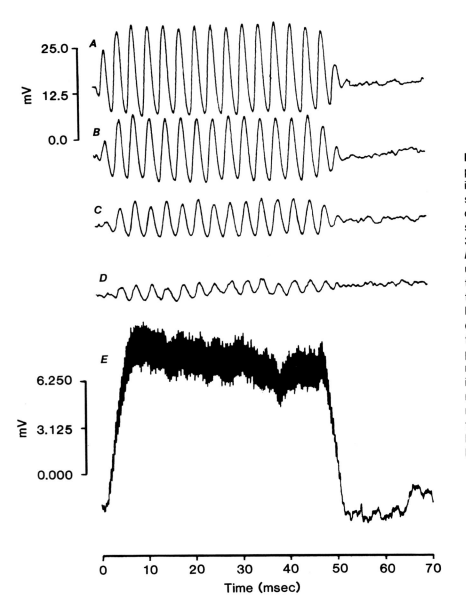

**Fig. 7-6.** Intracellular receptor potentials recorded from an inner hair cell. *A* to *D* are responses to a 300-Hz tone decreasing in intensity in 10-dB steps. *E* is the response to a 3-kHz tone at the same SPL as *B*. In response to symmetric sinusoidal sound pressure input, the depolarizing phase is two times greater than the hyperpolarizing phase. Each cycle is clear for the low tone, but at high frequencies the membrane capacitance filters the alternating response, markedly reducing it in amplitude compared to the rectified (DC) response. Such rectification of the receptor potentials is a common property of hair cells, even those from the lateral line of frogs.

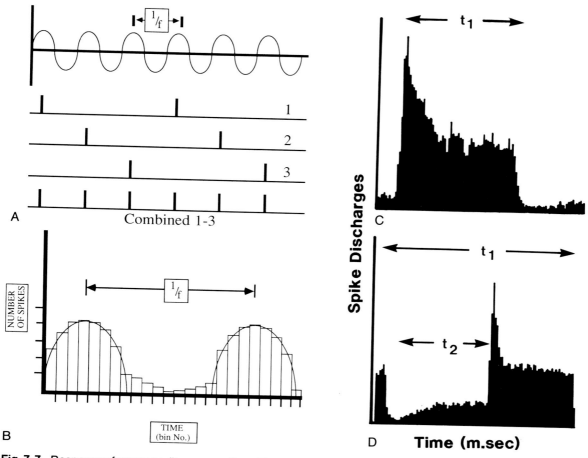

**Fig. 7-7.** Responses from an auditory nerve fiber. **(A)** For low-frequency tones, the nerve firing is phase locked to the sound. With repeated presentations, therefore, a cycle histogram can be built up that bears a recognizable relationship to the half-rectified version of the sound input. **(B)** High-frequency tone pips show a strong on-and-off effect, illustrating the adaptation of the hair cell–neuron synapse. **(C)** The addition of a second low-frequency tone pip to that of Fig. B shows the influence of two-tone inhibition. The nerve fiber does not respond to the second tone alone, but when the tones are presented together, the response to the first is severely depressed. **(D)** Rate intensity function for a single nerve fiber. Note the saturation firing rate and the limited dynamic range.

nent disappeared, and all that was left was the DC rectified component. It is a function of the membrane potential difference to cause the inner hair cell to release a chemical transmitter from its base onto the synaptic terminals of the 8th nerve. A depolarization releases transmitter, a hyperpolarization inhibits release. At low frequencies, nerve firing increases and decreases in sympathy with the alternating voltage in the inner hair cells. For loud

sounds, a nerve can generate an action potential on a 1-to-1 basis in synchrony with sound up to a frequency of about 300 Hz. As the frequency rises, the nerve fiber misses some cycles, but when it does fire it is in approximate register with the maximum depolarization of an inner hair cell (Fig. 7-7A). At higher frequencies the misses become more common, until by 4 kHz no synchrony is apparent. It is at frequencies above 500 Hz that the rectification in the inner hair cell becomes important. At these higher frequencies the rectified DC component is as great as the alternating voltage component. Thus during a tone the nerve fires continuously with a superimposed rhythm. Above 4 kHz, only the DC component is present, so transmitter is released continuously, and the nerve fires with no hint of rhythm or synchrony.

Recording from a single auditory nerve can reveal much complex activity. The time course of a response can be demonstrated by means of a post-stimulus histogram to a tone burst. These are generated by presenting a tone burst and then recording the occurrence of action potentials (APs) as a function of time after the tone onset. With many presentations, a histogram can be built up, showing the average activity of the nerve as a function of time. High-frequency tone bursts produce a sharp onset response (number of APs), which quickly decays to a steady state (Fig. 7-7B). This adaptation is a function of the synapse as no such decay is seen in the inner hair cell receptor potential. It is probable that the transmitter is glutamate or a small polypeptide incorporating glutamate and that in response to a steady depolarization of hair cells, transmitter release is large at first, then decays to a steady state. A sudden additional step increase in sound will cause another sharp additional initial response. The synapse therefore enhances changes in sound, thus increasing contrast, a common phenomenon in most sensory systems.

The threshold tuning curve of a single nerve fiber is defined by the intensity frequency points that just cause the nerve to respond. This curve can be modified if a second tone is presented simultaneously, the presence of the second tone causing suppression of the response to the first tone (suppression or masking) (Fig. 7-7C). It is possible to suppress a tone presented at the CF by a tone that does not excite the nerve by itself. Such suppression exists in inner hair cell responses and is a consequence of basilar membrane nonlinearity. It is important to notice that two-tone interactions occur in any nonlinear system. Even when the basilar membrane is linear (due to pathology), the inner hair cell is nonlinear at loud sounds, and the synapse itself shows rectification and nonlinearity. Both of these will cause two-tone inhibition or masking at higher sound levels.

## FREQUENCY ANALYSIS AND TWO THEORIES OF PITCH PERCEPTION

For many years there have been two basic theories as to how to code the frequency of a sound:

1. Volley or synchrony theory
2. Place theory

The volley theory states that the synchrony of a group of nerve fibers carries information about the frequency of the sound input and that higher centers can detect and recognize the average spike interval and so assign a frequency. The place theory relies on the fact that a nerve fiber only innervates one inner hair cell and so responds best to one place along the basilar membrane. When this place is stimulated, the cochleartopic organization of the nervous system, which exists all the way to the cortex, enables the assigning of a frequency according to which nerve fiber or cortical cell is stimulated. Recent results from patients implanted with electrical cochlear prostheses suggest that the volley theory is valid up to 300 Hz and the place theory principally above 4 kHz, and in between this range is a very grey area where both contributions seem important. The exquisite frequency discrimination of the auditory system is illustrated by the psychoacoustic experiments that show a frequency difference detection limit of 3 Hz at 1 kHz. Any theory has problems with such high performance. The above difference limen corresponds to a shift in excitation place of 20 $\mu$m, or about the width of two hair cells. It also corresponds to a time discrimination of 3 $\mu$sec, even though a single action potential lasts 1,000 $\mu$sec. It would seem that the central nervous system must average responses over a number of neurons and over a considerable number of cycles of the stimulus. At frequencies above 4 kHz, the ability to discriminate small changes in pitch is rather poor.

## INTENSITY ANALYSIS

Understanding the coding of intensity in the auditory system is a formidable problem. Normal hearing can achieve an effective range of 100 to 120 dB. The just noticeable increment of intensity ($\delta I$) is a linear function of base intensity ($I$) over this range, that is Weber's law ($\delta I/I = $ a constant) is valid over a 100-dB range. A single nerve fiber responds to an increase of sound above threshold by increasing its rate of firing, but after an increase of 30 to 40 dB in intensity, the fiber reaches maximum firing rate (Fig. 7-7D). Put another way, the effective dynamic range of a single fiber is only about 40 dB. Not all nerve fibers have the same threshold, however. Fibers with very low spontaneous rates make smaller synapses with the inner hair cells and have higher thresholds, but there seem to be too few with thresholds high enough to span the necessary range to account for the extraordinary dynamic range and accuracy of Weber's law. It has been hypothesized that the 5 percent of the 8th nerve fibers going to the outer hair cells may somehow aid in this coding, but as mentioned previously, these fibers are very small and slow

conducting, and it is doubtful that they can pass on information fast enough to contribute to Weber's law, which also holds for very brief stimuli.

Another effect of loud sounds is to enlarge the excitation pattern along the basilar membrane. As the intensity of a tone is increased, the pattern spreads basalward from the point of best frequency, and so more and more fibers are recruited. It is probable that loudness is a summation of firing rate and the number of active fibers. Loudness recruitment (an abnormally fast growth in the loudness function) is a characteristic of sensorineural hearing loss (Fig. 7-8A). For normal ears with sharp tuning, as the stimulus intensity is raised, the number of active fibers rises, at first slowly, then much faster as the tails of the more basalward fibers are activated (Fig. 7-8B). In sensorineural hearing loss, the sharp tips are lost (the active processes), but the tails (passive parts) are unchanged. Once threshold is reached, the basal fibers are readily activated by small further increases in intensity, and the number

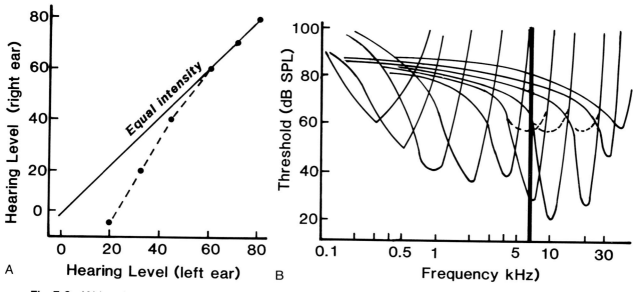

**Fig. 7-8. (A)** Loudness recruitment in a patient with sensorineural hearing loss in one ear. The loudness function (dashed line) is steep at first until it intersects the normal function (solid line); then it behaves normally also. **(B)** Sample neural tuning curves from a normal cochlea for a variety of frequencies. A tone of increasing intensity at 6 kHz (the solid vertical line) will activate a few fibers at first while only the tip segments of the curves are intersected and then very many more as the tails of the tuning curves are encountered. In the case of a sensorineural loss of 40 dB in the 4- to 20-kHz band, the tips of the tuning curves are lost (dotted lines). Now as the stimulus intensity is raised, no fibers are activated until 60 dB SPL is reached, then the number of fibers increases rapidly, soon approaching normal levels.

of active fibers soon approaches that of normal levels.

# THE ENDOLYMPHATIC SYSTEM

The endolymphatic system of the ear is a separate, membrane-enclosed system inside the bony walls of the cochlea and the labyrinth. It consists of the fluid-filled semicircular canals, utricle, saccule, endolymphatic sac and the cochlear duct or scala media. The endolymphatic system is surrounded by perilymphatic fluid, which has an ionic composition similar to cerebrospinal fluid (Table 7-1). The formation of the perilymph is still in some dispute and possibly varies from species to species. In the guinea pig, most of the perilymph appears to be formed from the cerebrospinal fluid (CSF), as the cochlear aqueduct is quite large and so a considerable fluid exchange can occur between the CSF and perilymph. The perilymph also is in contact with the blood supply to the inner ear and perilymph and plasma exchange takes place. Thus, perilymph may be considered to be a mixture of an ultrafiltrated plasma and CSF. In humans, the cochlear aqueduct appears to be somewhat restricted, or filled with some material, and it is possible that the perilymph-to-plasma exchange is the most dominant. The endolymph, in contrast, has a unique ion composition, something like that of intracellular fluid; that is, it has a high potassium and a low sodium concentration. A comparison of the various fluid properties of endolymph and perilymph is contained in Table 7-1. The most outstanding point of the endolymph is its very high potassium chloride composition and the extremely low sodium. Even more startling is the fact that the endolymph in the scala media is at a high positive potential of 80 mV with respect to perilymph. The endolymph composition of the saccule and the utricle is somewhat different, being a little less in potassium and quite substantially higher in sodium and also having only a small positive +5 to +10 mV potential with respect to perilymph. The ionic composition of the fluid in the endolymphatic sac is still controversial. It appears to be of a composition rather intermediate between endolymph and perilymph, with sodium and potassium being somewhat similar at about 70 mM each.

Any ion concentration different (C1, C2) can be recalculated into an equivalent electrical potential difference given by (for a singly charged ion) 58 log C1/C2 (in mV). Both voltage gradients and concentration gradients act in summation on an ion. When they are equal and opposite (E1 − E2 = 58 log C1/C2) the ion is said to be in equilibrium and it does not move. If it is not in equilibrium, then it will move and a flux of the ion will occur (see Appendix 7-2 for more details).

In the scala media, the concentration force (endolymph to perilymph) may be represented by Ce and Cp, and the potential difference by EP (perilymph is taken as reference). The equivalent concentration = 58 log Cp/Ce, and for the potassium ion (K$^+$) is 58 log 6/150 = −90 mV. This force drives K$^+$ out of endolymph. The EP is equal to 80 mV, an electric force also driving K$^+$ out of endolymph. Therefore, the total flux of K$^+$ is proportional to 80 − (−90) = +170 mV, driving potassium out of endolymph, a very high force, indeed (see Table 7-1).

Similarly for sodium, the Na$^+$ concentration equivalent = 58 log 138/1 = +140 mV. The total

**Table 7-1. Fluid Composition of the Inner Ear**

| Substance | Perilymph | Cochlear Endolymph | EP | Passive Flux | Utricular Endolymph | EP | Passive Flux |
|---|---|---|---|---|---|---|---|
| K$^+$ | 4 mM | 170 mM | | E to P | 150 mM | | E to P |
| Na$^+$ | 138 mM | 1 mM | +80 mV | P to E | 20 mM | +5 mV | P to E = 0? |
| Cl$^-$ | 135 mM | 150 mM | | P to E | 145 mM | | |
| H$_2$O | 300 mOsm | 320 mOsm | | P to E | ? | | ? |

Note that water flows from low osmolar solutions to high. The passive flux columns show the direction of movement. EP, endocochlear potential; E, endolymph; P, perilymph.

force is equal to $+80 - (+140)$, which is equal to $-60$ mV, that is, $Na^+$ has a net force driving it into endolymph.

For chloride ($Cl^-$), the concentration equivalent $= 58 \log 150/150 = 0$, but the EP $= +80$, so $Cl^-$ has a net force driving it into endolymph. A stable system for these three ions can only result if there is an active transport of the following:

1. $K^+$ into endolymph and
2. $Na^+$ out of endolymph and
3. $Cl^-$ out of endolymph

If the EP changes, then all of the ionic species are affected and variations in concentration or transport rates will occur.

In scala media, across the apical surface of the hair cells, there is a potential difference of about 160 mV composed of the $^+$EP and the negative intracellular potential of the hair cells. The concentration difference across the apical part of the hair cells for $K^+$ is approximately zero. Therefore, a $K^+$ current can be driven into the cells from scala media with this force of approximately 160 mV. In the utricle where the EP is low, the force is about 60 mV, less than half that of scala media. The ion pump, which controls the composition of the endolymph, appears to be situated in the marginal cells of the stria vascularis in the cochlea and in dark cells scattered throughout the boundaries of the utricle. All evidence points to an unusual potassium transport system in the cochlea, an "electrogenic pump." Most transport systems are close to electrically neutral. That is, the usual sodium potassium exchange pump in all cells where potassium is transported into and sodium out of the cells is close to a one-to-one exchange, so the net result is neutral. In the cochlea, potassium appears to be transported by itself and so generates a large potential difference. Indeed, the value of the EP in the cochlea is directly proportional to the rate of potassium transport and is very heavily dependent on metabolism. In the guinea pig, the potassium pump accounts for most of the inner ear oxygen consumption of $0.03 \, \mu l$ of $O_2$/min. Sudden anoxia causes the EP to decay to zero and reverse polarity to $-40$ mV within 2 minutes. The negative potential decays back to zero over some hours and is mainly due to the diffusion potential of the high endolymph $K^+$.

The long-term decay follows the equilibration of the $K^+$ between endolymph and perilymph. The diffusion potential, of course, is always present, so the true value of the electrogenic potential is $80 + 40 = 120$ mV.

Both ouabain and furosemide reduce EP. Ouabain, a specific $Na^+/K^+$ transport inhibitor, acting via the $Na^+/K^+$-ATPase enzyme, reduces EP at $10^{-6}$ M when perfused into perilymph but $10^{-4}$ M when perfused into scala media. Furosemide, a loop diuretic and K and Cl transport inhibitor, reduces EP when injected intravenously at $10^{-6}$ M but requires $10^{-4}$ M when perfused into perilymph and $10^{-3}$ M when perfused into scala media. Histochemically, $Na^+/K^+$-ATPase is localized at the base of the marginal cells. All these results suggest that the major active transport systems are located on the basal surface. In this case the marginal cells should have an intracellular potential more positive than endolymph (due to the $K^+$ electrogenic pump). Thus, endolymph would be considered as a part extension of the intracellular component of the marginal cells after diffusing through the luminal surface of these cells. Although measurements of the intracellular potential have been attempted, the results have been equivocal, and no definite statement can be made at present about its value.

So far only the radial flow (i.e., local formation of endolymph) has been discussed. Recent measurements of longitudinal flow in the guinea pig[10,11] indicate a value of up to 1 mm/min in the basal turn, corresponding to $1 \, \mu l/10$ min or a cochlear volume turnover of scala media in 15 to 30 minutes. This is a very high value, and details of how this occurs are still not understood. It is important to note that the bulk longitudinal flow must be due to a hydrostatic pressure gradient along the scala media, and this must be developed by osmotic pressure differences, causing water to flow into scala media. The hydrostatic pressure can be quite small. A gradient of about 0.1 mm of water per millimeter of duct is quite sufficient. However, a water flux into scala media of about $0.1 \, \mu l$/min is required. This water must flow across the scala media boundaries, probably across Reisner's membrane and be driven by an osmotic pressure difference. Values for osmotic pressure in perilymph and endolymph are 300 mOsm and 320 mOsm, respectively. This is a fairly strong force and certainly seems adequate to account for the measured flow.

A major question is what happens to the endolymph? It is usually assumed that it is absorbed in the endolymphatic sac, and disease or disabling the sac would cause malabsorbtion, a consequent increase in endolymphatic pressures, and endolymphatic hydrops. Experiments suggest that this is an oversimplification. Elimination of just the sac in guinea pigs only occasionally leads to hydrops, and then only after a long time. Blockage of the duct distal to the sac causes hydrops much more quickly, and a theory has been proposed[12] that most of the absorbtion takes place in the initial portion of the duct and only a small percentage is absorbed in the rugose portion or in the sac. Such an idea makes sense. A high volume flow in the cochlea (and the rest of the endolymphatic system), enables foreign bodies (bacteria, damaged cells, etc.) to be eliminated from the sensory areas quite quickly. These must be swept up into the endolymphatic duct, so the entrance to the duct should also have a high flow. However, once the foreign bodies are in the duct, only a very small flow is necessary to take them up to the rugose portion for phagocytosis. The sac itself may be only of vestigial use. In the amphibia, the sac is very large and full of otoconia. Reptiles have somewhat smaller sacs, which also contain otoconia, and it is smallest in mammals. A similar progression is also seen in the saccule, and it is very possible that both organs have changed in tandem to play a somewhat minor role in the physiology of the cochlea.

## BLOOD SUPPLY

In the guinea pig cochlea, blood flow has been measured at between 1 and 2 $\mu$l/min with a total blood volume of 10 $\mu$l. The blood vessels are very similar to those in the central nervous system, having a small autonomic innervation, a very large reactivity to $Pco_2$, and a small reactivity to other vasodilators. They only pass small molecules, being impermeable to curare and its derivatives, slightly permeable to sucrose, a little more permeable to mannitol, and highly permeable to glycerol and urea. This explains why glycerol and urea are more effective in testing for Menière's syndrome than mannitol, although mannitol should have more osmotic effect on scala media, as it is almost impermeable through Reissner's membrane. It is so slowly diffusable into perilymph, compared with urea and glycerol, that a high perilymph level in a reasonable time is not attained. Autonomic innervation of blood vessels has been identified in the spiral lamina but not as yet in the stria vascularis. Its role has not been firmly identified, and early work suggesting major blood vessel changes during loud sound has not been confirmed by later experiments. Speculations that autonomic fibers innervate the afferent nerve dendrites have also not been confirmed.

## EFFERENT SYSTEM

In the cat there are about 2,000 efferent fibers originating bilaterally in the superior olivary nuclei, one-third of which give rise to synaptic terminals on the base of the outer hair cells. These fibers are mainly crossed, and their transmitter is acetylcholine. The remainder innervate the dendrites under the inner hair cells. These are mainly uncrossed, and their transmitter is unknown but could be one of the met-enkephelins. Most of our knowledge about the efferent system applies to fibers going to the outer hair cells, because no unequivocal effect of those going to the inner hair cells has been reported. When the crossed olivocochlear bundle is electrically stimulated, effects on the neural threshold and cochlear microphonics can be measured. The effect is to reduce the active process of the outer hair cells, leading to an elevation of threshold only around the tip of the neural tuning curve. The small increase of cochlear microphonics is a consequence of the method of action on the outer hair cells. It increases the outer hair cell membrane permeability to chloride, decreasing membrane resistance, and thus the current flow through the hair cells is increased. This is recorded as an increase in round window cochlear microphonics. The outer hair cell efferents are sharply tuned, just like an auditory nerve fiber, and innervate at or close to an appropriate place on the basilar membrane (i.e., an efferent tuned to 10 kHz terminates at or near the 10 kHz region of the basilar membrane). In the anesthetized animal, they have a long latency of 10 msec or more and a low maximum firing rate of 50 spikes/sec. This seems rather odd, since an efferent action can only be seen at stimulus rates in excess of 100 shocks/sec. It is probable that there is a strong effect of anesthesia on the cell bodies of origin, either directly or by inhibitory activity coming down from higher centers. It is also odd that they are so few in number, and a single efferent, although sharply tuned, innervates a number of hair cells along many microns of the basilar membrane. The natural function of the efferent system on auditory performance is unknown. It has been hypothesized that it is activated during vocalization or is part of a feedback loop involving the outer hair cell afferents and controls the outer hair cell active process. However, evidence for these suggestions is completely lacking.

## SOUND-EVOKED POTENTIALS

When an electrode is placed on the round window and another reference electrode is somewhere outside the cochlea, three different electrical responses to sound can be recorded. They are the cochlear microphonics (CM), summating potential (SP), and neural responses (N1, N2) (Fig. 7-9). Of these, the CM is most easily observed and has been the subject of much investigation. It is recorded as an alternating voltage that matches the presented sound wave form with good fidelity. Despite nearly 50 years of research, many details of the round window-recorded CM are obscure. It is probably generated mainly by the outer hair cells, because if they are absent due to pathology, the CM is attenuated by 90 percent. However, noise-induced threshold shifts of less then 20 dB do not alter CM appreciably, and even anoxia quickly reduces CM by only one-half to one-third, from which value it slowly further decays to zero over an hour or more. It appears to be predominantly derived from the basal coil and does not give much information about any other region. Thus, it is of not much use as an index of cochlea function except for large losses in the more basal regions. However, it is directly proportional to the potential difference between the EP and the hair cell intracellular potential, so changes in EP are accurately reflected in CM amplitude. The CM grow linearly with intensity over a range of 70 dB (from about 0.5 $\mu$V to about 1,000 $\mu$V), and then flatten out, a further unexplained finding considering the essential basilar membrane nonlinearity at low sound levels. Some pathology lowers the sound pressures at which the flattening occurs, but no real correlation has been established. The converse always holds, namely an abnormally small CM always means damage to hair cells or a low EP.

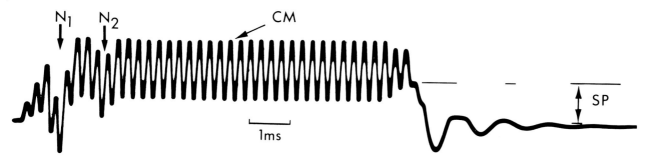

**Fig. 7-9.** Round window recorded potentials evoked by a 70-dB SPL, 4-kHz tone pip. Shown are the cochlear microphonics (CM), the N1 and N2 gross action potentials, and the DC shift of the CM from the base line, which is the summating potential (SP). Note the small neural response to the termination of the tone pip.

Unlike the alternating potential of the CM, the SP is a shift in the DC baseline and is best seen in a response to a 10 to 20 msec tone pip. Generally, the SP appears to be a rectified and smoothed derivation of the CM, and as such, it is part of the nonlinear response of the cochlea, with the polarity recorded at the round window usually being positive. However, there is much confusion over the labeling, because the SP commonly is given the sign that is recorded in the scala media, which is opposite to that in the scala tympani. It is essential that the convention used by clearly stated and understood. Under certain circumstances, usually at low sound pressures and low frequencies, the SP can be opposite in sign (negative at round window). With increasing sound pressure, the negative SP decreases and goes through zero, then reverses, becoming the positive SP and growing as large as 3 mV. The origin of the SP is still highly controversial, and it is probably a multicomponent response. One component is certainly the rectified current through the inner hair cell. This becomes prominent over 500 Hz and shows as a depolarization in the intracellular inner hair cell potential. It is a result of the decreased apical resistance with stimulation and so gives an increased current. An increase of current (scala media to scala tympani) shows up at the round window as a positive potential in scala tympani (and negative in scala media). No reverse potential has been recorded from the inner hair cells, and the negative round window SP may come from the outer hair cells, but this is uncertain. When the basilar membrane is displaced from its rest position, the inherent nonlinearity is increased. When the displacement is toward scala tympani, the negative round window SP is increased. This concept has been used in investigations of Menière's syndrome, and indeed, many Menière's patients seem to show an enhanced SP. However, there is a defect in the way most clinical recordings are made. Usually, a click is used as a stimulus, the click causing a ringing of the loudspeaker and so giving a damped oscillation lasting for a few milliseconds. Such a waveform would give an N1, N2, and an SP. The SP will decay quickly with time as the ringing decays, and presumably an enhanced SP would decay somewhat more slowly (i.e., last longer); therefore, measurements are made of the length (time) of the SP complex. The

problem is that often the neural N1 and N2s are altered and lengthened by pathology of various sorts, and because these potentials are of the same time span as the SP to this click, interpretation is not straightforward. This may be one reason why published correlations between SP and Menière's syndrome have been somewhat disappointing. A 10- to 20-msec tone pip would overcome this problem, measurements being made in the last 5 msec, well after the N1–N2 complex.

The two dominant waves of the neural response to a tone pip or click are known as N1 and N2. The first comes 1 msec after the start of the CM, the second about 1 msec later. With increasing intensity, N1 is first to appear followed by N2. At high intensities more responses appear and waveforms become complex. The N1 response is the sum of synchronous firings from a number of auditory nerves. With good equipment the N1 is just visible on an oscilloscope (visual detection threshold [VDT]) at sound levels close to thresholds. The response probably comes from activity as the nerves enter the internal auditory canal, because its amplitude is almost independent of frequency (or site of origin along the basilar membrane). This means that the N1 VDT to a tone pip can be used as an excellent approximation to hearing thresholds from the highest frequencies down to 2 kHz, where the lack of onset synchrony smears the response. Such a threshold is known as the cochlear action potential (CAP) threshold and is typically 5 dB above single nerve fiber thresholds and 10 dB above psychoacoustic thresholds. It is an extremely valuable response for investigative purposes, because small hair cell lesions of a few hundred microns in extent are detectable and changes in threshold with a precision of 6 dB are easily measured. A small amount of averaging, even 20 times, can increase this accuracy by 3 dB. A click response is often used to elicit N1, and this can be very useful; but it should be realized that most clicks have little energy above 12 kHz, and the click (CAP) threshold is derived from the most sensitive region of the hearing curve (central portion of the cochlea). This means that considerable pathology of the basal and apical coil can occur before click CAP threshold is altered, a fact that has caused much confusion. In man, probably due to the thickness of the cochlear bone, responses, usually recorded from the promontory, are of much smaller amplitude than in other animals, and in consequence, greater care and more averaging are often needed. Nonetheless the utility of electrocochleography is being increasingly recognized, particularly if tone pips are utilized.

## REFERENCES

1. Békésy, G. von: Experiments in Hearing. Wever EG, trans. and ed. McGraw-Hill, New York, 1960
2. Sellick PM, Patuzzi R, Johnstone BM: Measurements of basilar membrane motion in the guinea pig using the Mössbauer technique. J Acoust Soc Am 72:131, 1982
3. Davis H: A model for transducer action in the cochlea, Cold Spring Harbor Symposium. Quant Biol 30:181, 1965
4. Flock A, Bretscher A, Weber K: Immunohistochemical localization of several cytoskeletal proteins in inner ear sensory and supporting cells. Hear Res 7:75, 1982
5. Brownell WE, Bader CR, Bertrand D, Ribaupierre Y: Evoked mechanical responses of isolated cochlear outer hair cells. Science 227:195, 1985
6. Kemp DT: Stimulated acoustic emissions from within the human auditory system. J Acoust Soc Am 664:1386, 1978
7. Lewis RG, Huspeth AJ: Voltage and ion dependent conduction in solitary vertebrate hair cells. Nature 304:538, 1983
8. Crawford AC, Fettiplace R: An electrical tuning mechanism in turtle cochlear hair cells. J Physiol (Lond) 312:377, 1981
9. Russell IJ, Sellick PM: Tuning properties of cochlear hair cells. Nature 267:858, 1977
10. Proeschel U, Sellick PM, Johnstone BM: Measurements of endolymph flow by iontophoresis of otocis substances into scala media. p. 88. In Proceedings of the XXI Workshop on Inner Ear Biology. Taormina, Italy, 1983
11. Sykova E, Syka, J, Johnstone BM, Yates GK: Longitudinal flow of endolymph measured by distribution of tetraethylammenium and choline in scala media. Hear Res 28:161, 1987
12. Rask-Anderson H, Bredberg G, Stahle J: Structure and function of the endolymphatic duct. Menière's Disease; International Symposium, ed. Vosteen KH, Thieme-Stratton Inc. New York, 1981

## APPENDIX 7-1

For a sinusoidal sound wave in air, the pressure ($p$) and resultant velocity ($v$) of the air particles are directly proportional, that is $p = v \times z$. $z$, the constant of proportionality, is called impedance, and it is a property of the medium through which the sound wave travels. In a uniform medium of large size (compared with the wavelength of sound), the impedance is called the specific impedance. By definition the wavelength $W = c/f$, where $c$ is the velocity of sound and $f$ is the frequency. $c$ is proportional to the impedance ($z$) and inversely proportional to the density of the medium ($c = z/d$). Therefore, the denser the medium, the longer the wavelength (see Table 7-1). For a dense medium such as water, higher pressures are needed to move the molecules at a given velocity than for a less dense medium such as air. Therefore, air has a lower specific impedance than water.

Another important property of sound is the power in the wave. The power, or energy ($e$), is related to pressure and impedance by a square law, $e = p^2/z$. Note the relationships of these to the electrical case of Ohm's law, where voltage equals resistance times current, and power is equal to voltage squared over resistance. In the SI system (newtons, meters, and seconds are the units of force, length, and time, respectively), air has a specific impedance of $400\ N \cdot s/m^3$, and water is $1,580,000\ N \cdot s/m^3$, i.e., a ratio of about 4,000 times. Thus, when an airborne sound wave hits a water surface, the water hardly moves and most of the sound is reflected. The energy transmitted from air to water is $e = 4r/(r + 1)^2$, where $r$ is the ratio of the two impedances. Thus for an $r$ of 4,000, only 0.1 percent of the energy of airborne sound is transmitted into the water and 99.9 percent is reflected back.

For an ideal transformer, the power input should equal the power output. For the middle ear, this means that $(P_e)^2/Z_e = (P_s)^2/Z_s$. Subscripts e and s refer to eardrum and stapes, respectively. The pressures $P_e$ and $P_s$ are related by the transformer ratio ($T$) $P_s = T \times P_e$. Therefore, $(P_e)^2/Z_e = (T \times P_e)^2/Z_s$, or $Z_s = T^2 \times Z_e$, that is, the impedances are transformed by the square of the transformer ratio.

## APPENDIX 7-2

Any movement of fluid, ions, or other substances or molecules obeys a very simple law. Flux is proportional to force, that is, the flow of something is proportional to the force acting on it. (The force is strictly a difference in energy levels acting over a given distance to create a gradient.) This applies to electric currents, blood flow, air flow, diffusion, uncharged or charged molecules and ions, and water. The forces have different names, for electric current it is voltage; blood flow, hydrostatic pressure; uncharged molecules, concentration; water, osmotic pressure; ions, concentration plus the electric potential. In the latter case, the resultant flow is simply a sum of the two forces acting on the ion. It is possible for these two forces to be in opposition. A concentration gradient and the electric gradient could oppose each other so that the ion is balanced between them and there is no net ion flow. This occurs when the concentration gradient, $C1 : C2$ and the electrical gradient, $E1 : E2$, obey the Nernst equation, that is, $(E1 - E2) = 58 \log C1/C2$ ($E1$ and $E2$ are in mV). This means the concentration gradient force can be calculated in terms of an equivalent electric force and vice versa. When the two forces are not equal, then the ion will move, and the total flux of the ion will be proportional to $(E1 - E2) - (58 \log C1/C2)$. It is important to note that each ion species is an independent entity, and the preceding equations apply to each ion species separately.

When an ion moves down its concentration gradient, it causes charge separation and so generates a potential. Consider a membrane separating two solutions of potassium chloride. Side 1 contains 100 mM, and side 2 contains 10 mM, and the membrane is mainly permeable to potassium. Potassium starts to diffuse from side 1 to side 2, causing a charge separation as it leaves behind the impermeable chloride and so gives rise to a potential difference. This potential will finally be exactly sufficient to prevent further $K^+$ movement and so equal 58 $\log K1/K2 = 58$ mV (side 1 negative with respect to side 2). This is called a diffusion potential. If the membrane was only permeable to chloride, then the potential would be in the opposite direction. If the membrane is permeable to both, then the potential would be between $+$ or $- 58$ mV, depending on the relative permeability of potassium and chloride.

# Acoustics and Psychoacoustics  8

## Sharon M. Abel

This chapter is meant to familiarize the reader with some basic concepts relating to the measurement of sound (acoustics) and methods for characterizing the human observer's perception of an acoustic stimulus. The science of psychoacoustics, essentially the relationship between the physical (acoustic stimulus, input) and the behavioral (perception, output) lays the groundwork for the clinical specialty of audiology. This chapter presents some of the classic psychoacoustic investigations and examples of their application for the purpose of furthering both the understanding of perception in observers with hearing loss of various etiologies and the development of diagnostic procedures.

## THE PHYSICAL DIMENSIONS OF SOUND

### The Nature of Sound

Sound, the stimulus for hearing, comprises variations in air pressure. Strike a tuning fork, and the tines will vibrate in a regular fashion. These vibrations produce periodic compressions (increased pressure) and rarefactions (decreased pressure) of the surrounding air molecules. The periodic pressure variations, starting in the immediate vicinity of the tines, are transmitted through the air in all directions, like waves emanating from the impact of a small stone hitting the surface of the water. This example of simple harmonic motion is illustrated in Figure 8-1.[1] The crest of the wave corresponds to the maximum increase in pressure; the trough is the maximum decrease relative to atmospheric pressure.

### Stimulus Dimensions

The waveform shown in Figure 8-1 is known as a sine wave and is perceived as a pure tone. It can be described in terms of a number of orthogonal (i.e., independent) dimensions. In the case of a pure tone, the value for each of these dimensions will remain constant throughout the presentation. First, the frequency of the sound tells us how rapidly the pressure variations are occurring and is specified in terms of the number of cycles of pressure change per second. The unit of frequency, 1 cycle per second (cps), is known as 1 Hertz (Hz). The young normal human observer can detect frequencies between 20 and 20,000 Hz. However,

201

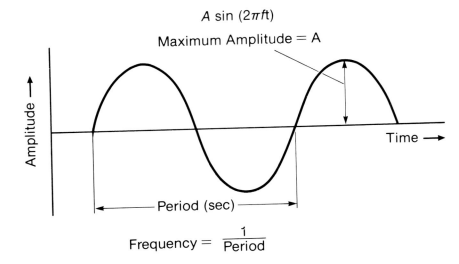

*A* sin (2π*ft*)

Maximum Amplitude = *A*

Period (sec)

$$\text{Frequency} = \frac{1}{\text{Period}}$$

**Fig. 8-1.** An example of simple harmonic motion. (From Human Information Processing: An Introduction to Psychology by P.H. Lindsay and D.A. Norman, copyright © 1972 by Harcourt Brace Jovanovich, Inc. Reprinted by permission of the publisher.)

sensitivity is not equal across this range, as shown by the curves of minimum audible pressure in Figure 8-2 from Moore,[2] based on results of Dadson and King for subjects aged 18 to 25 years. The values plotted are modes for 198 ears (164 ears at 15,000 Hz). The greatest sensitivity occurs at about 3,000 Hz (3 kHz). As shown by Hinchcliffe[3] (see Fig. 8-3) and Corso[4] the threshold of hearing increases with age at a rate dependent on the frequency. The individual's sensitivity may also depend on the type of noise he or she has been exposed to in both occupational and social settings[5,6] (Fig. 8-4).

The second dimension of measurement for sound is amplitude, which reflects the maximum excursion in pressure of the wave. In order to compress the relatively large range of amplitudes to which the normal ear can respond, a logarithmic scale is used. The measurement is not an absolute value, but rather indicates a change from a reference value. The reference commonly used is 20 μPa. The pascal is a unit of pressure in the meter-kilogram-

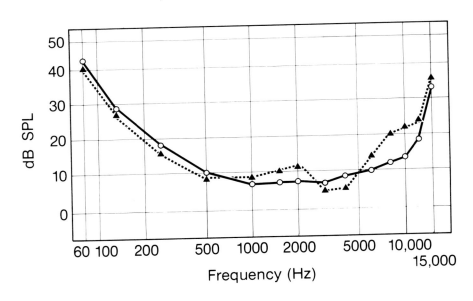

**Fig. 8-2.** Minimum audible pressure as a function of frequency at positions close to the entrance to the ear canal. (Moore BCG: An Introduction to the Psychology of Hearing. 2nd Ed. Academic press, Orlando, FL, 1982, p. 41.)

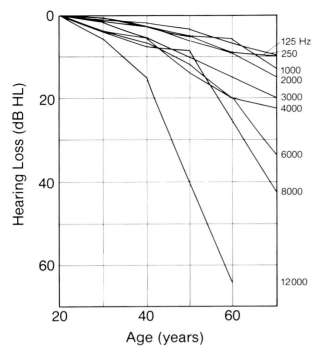

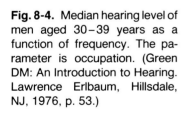

**Fig. 8-3.** Median hearing loss as a function of age in 319 clinically normal female ears. The parameter is frequency. (Hinchcliffe R: The threshold of hearing as a function of age. Acustica 9:303, 1959.)

second (mks) system equivalent to 1 N/m². A micropascal is one millionth of a pascal. The value 20 $\mu$Pa is the human observer's threshold sound pressure for hearing a 1 kHz pure tone. Let us designate this $p^2_0$. All other values are expressed in relation to this reference and are calculated in the following manner. First, the difference is computed between the logarithm of the pressure value of interest and the logarithm of the reference (i.e., log $p^2_1$ − log $p^2_0$). This is equivalent to the logarithm of their ratio (i.e., log $p^2_1/p^2_0$). A change from the reference pressure or difference of one log unit is defined as 1 bel. One-tenth of a bel is close to a discriminable change for the human observer and is referred to as a decibel (dB). Thus the number of dB is equivalent to 10 log ($p^2_1/p^2_0$) or equivalently 20 log ($p_1/p_0$). When the reference level is 20 $\mu$Pa, the term *sound pressure level* (SPL) should be affixed (e.g., 10 dB SPL). Power units may be used in preference to pressure units. Since power is equal to the square root of pressure, the formula for number of decibels is 10 log ($p_1/p_0$).

The dynamic range of the ear at 1 kHz (i.e., the distance between the threshold of hearing and the threshold of pain), is approximately 120 dB SPL, an increase in pressure of $10^6$ from the reference 20

**Fig. 8-4.** Median hearing level of men aged 30–39 years as a function of frequency. The parameter is occupation. (Green DM: An Introduction to Hearing. Lawrence Erlbaum, Hillsdale, NJ, 1976, p. 53.)

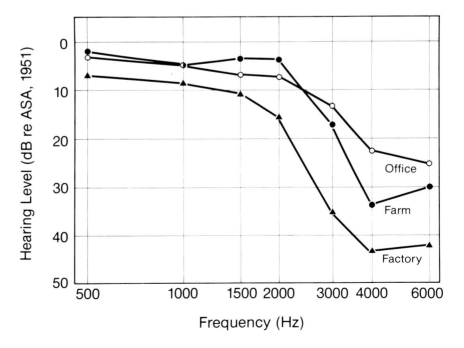

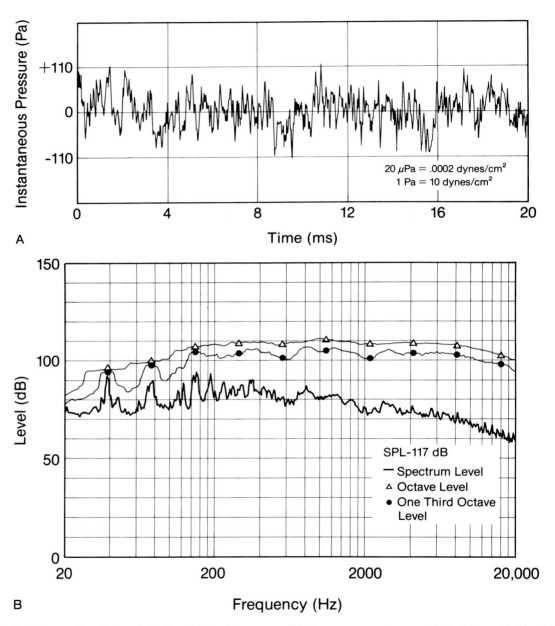

**Fig. 8-5.** A sample of industrial noise. **(a)** the time course **(b)**; the power spectrum analysis. (Kunov H, Abel SM, Pandey PC, Friedman EB: Analysis of Industrial Noise with Special Reference to Correlation Between Different Indices and Transmission of Noise Through the Middle Ear. Ontario Ministry of Labour, 113/R, Toronto, Ontario, Canada, September, 1983.)

μPa.[7] References other than 20 μPa may be used. In audiologic practice, levels are expressed relative to the average threshold for a group of normal observers. When this reference is used, the term *hearing level*, abbreviated HL, should be affixed to the number of dB (i.e., 10 dB HL). Audiometers are calibrated so that 0 dB HL at any pure-tone frequency corresponds to the threshold sound pressure level for normal listeners. Values greater than zero indicate the relative increase in amplitude necessary for the individual tested to achieve threshold performance.

The third dimension is the total duration of the stimulus from onset to termination, usually measured in milliseconds. A related but still orthogonal parameter is the rise – decay time. This refers to the time taken at the onset of stimulation for the amplitude to attain a predetermined peak value, and also for it to fall from that value at the termination of stimulation. Depending on the stimulus-generating appartus, it may also be possible to manipulate independently the shape of the rise and decay (e.g., linear or sigmoidal) and the place in the pressure cycle (Figure 8-1) at which the sound begins.

Regardless of the frequency, one complete cycle of pressure changes covers a range of phase change from 0 to 360 degrees. At 0, 180, and 360 degrees, (i.e., the beginning, middle, and end of the cycle), the amplitude is at the atmospheric level. At 90 degrees, the maximum amplitude is attained, and at 270 degrees, the minimum. For short-duration sounds, less than 20 msec, the starting phase of the stimulus may affect the power spectrum (see following discussion) of the stimulus and thus our perception of the sound.

### Problems of Measurement

Generally, the sounds we hear are more complex than pure tones. Fourier analysis is a mathematical method of describing a complex wave as a series of sine waves of different frequencies, intensities, and phases. Figure 8-5A and B[8] show the time course of a sample of industrial noise, 20 msec in duration, and its associated spectrum analysis. In Figure 8-5A the instantaneous pressure of the stimulus is plotted against time. In Figure 8-5B the level is plotted as a function of frequency in one cycle (i.e.,

spectrum level), one-third octave, and octave bands. The overall level of the stimulus is 117 dB SPL.

An important issue in investigations of auditory perception is whether the ear acts as a Fourier analyzer. Plomp[9] investigated the ability of the human observer to distinguish the fundamental tone and overtones of a complex periodic sound wave. The lowest component was varied between 44 and 2,000 Hz. Generally, the overtones could be heard as distinct sounds, if the frequency separation exceeded a critical value that changed with the frequency region, about 100 Hz in the region of 1,000 Hz and 5 Hz near 100 Hz. The supposition is that a band of frequencies that are indistinguishable correspond to the width on the basilar membrane of the stimulating pattern for a simple tone.

## THE PERCEPTION OF SOUND

### Response Dimensions

The dimensions of the sound perceived do not relate in a one-to-one fashion with the physical dimensions of the acoustic stimulus presented. The two main psychological (i.e., perceptual) correlates are pitch and loudness. Pitch is primarily determined by frequency but may change with the duration, intensity, frequency components and starting phase of the stimulus. Similarly, although loudness is influenced predominantly by the amplitude of the stimulus, it will vary with changes in the frequency of pure tones, frequency bandwidth for complex stimuli, and duration.

### Pitch

The relationship between pitch and frequency is shown in Figure 8-6. Perceived pitch is measured in mels. By definition, a tone of 1,000 Hz at 60 dB SPL has a pitch of 1,000 mels. Multiplying the frequency of the stimulus by 10 results in only a threefold increase in perceived pitch.

The minimum duration required for a sound to assume a pitch quality was studied by Doughty and

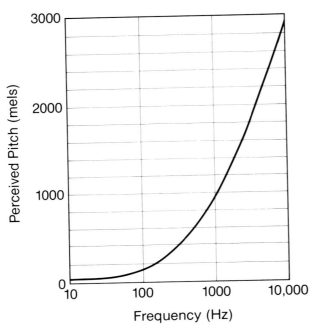

**Fig. 8-6.** The relationship between perceived pitch and frequency. (From Human Information Processing: An Introduction to Psychology by P.H. Lindsay and D.A. Norman, copyright © 1972 by Harcourt Brace Jovanovich, Inc. Reprinted by permission of the publisher.)

Garner.[10] They measured two threshold durations, one for click-pitch (i.e., the shortest duration allowing an estimation of the general frequency range of the stimulus) and one for tone-pitch (i.e., the shortest duration for which tonal quality was dominant over the perception of a click). Signal intensity was held constant at 110 dB SPL. The results are presented in Figure 8-7.

For frequencies equal to or greater than 1,000 Hz, the threshold durations for the two pitch qualities are constant at approximately 4 and 10 msec. Below 1,000 Hz, the thresholds increase as frequency decreases. In this region the number of cycles tends to remain constant. The distance between the functions is about 6 msec throughout the frequency range, indicating that duration, not number of cycles, underlies the change in percept. Figure 8-8 shows the effect of intensity of the tonepitch threshold. For 1,000 Hz, the threshold duration decreases by about 10 msec as intensity increases from 30 to 110 dB SPL.

The frequency relationship among individual components in a complex waveform will determine the nature of the sound perceived. For example, the addition of two pure tones of 1,000 Hz and 1,100 Hz will result in an overall fluctuation of

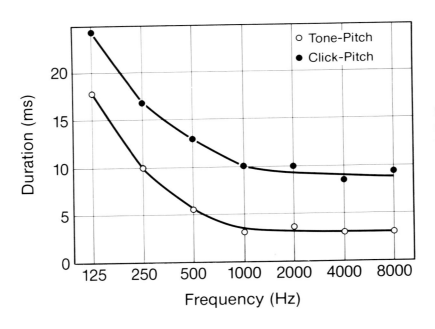

**Fig. 8-7.** The relationship between duration and frequency for the perception of two types of pitch. Each data point is the mean of 40 observations from two subjects. (Doughty JM, Garner WR: Pitch characteristics of short tones. I. Two kinds of pitch threshold. J Exp Psychol 37:351, 1947.)

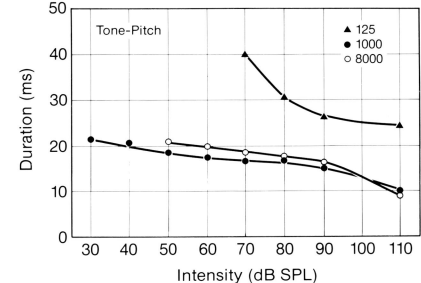

**Fig. 8-8.** The relationship between duration and intensity for the perception of tone pitch. Each data point is the mean of 16 observations from two subjects. (Doughty JM, Garner WR: Pitch characteristics of short tones. I. Two kinds of pitch thresholds. J Exp Pyschol 37:351, 1947.)

sound pressure repeating periodically every 10 msec or at the rate of 100 Hz. The observer hears this beat pattern, rather than two pure tones, even though there is no energy at the beat frequency. Similarly, a complex sound made up of frequencies from 1,000 Hz to 2,000 Hz, in steps of 200 Hz, will be matched to 200 Hz pure tone in a test of pitch matching. This result doesn't change if a low-frequency, high-amplitude masking tone is added, suggesting that perception is determined by low-frequency periodicity in the neural response of the high-frequency fibers.[11,12]

Pitch perception will also be determined by the phase of the stimulus. Ronken[13] demonstrated that listeners with normal hearing could discriminate between transient signals with the same energy spectra, but having different phase spectra. The phase spectrum of a stimulus specifies the arrival time of energy in different frequency regions. In Ronken's experiment, each stimulus consisted of a pair of clicks, that is, a pair of short-duration rectangular pulses, close enough temporally (less than 10 msec) that they would be perceived as a single event. The phase spectrum of this stimulus was manipulated by varying the amplitude ratio of the two clicks. The subject's task was to discriminate a particular click pair in which the two component clicks had different amplitudes from a pair-mate in which

the order of the amplitudes was reversed. The amplitude ratio of the two clicks necessary for 75 percent correct discrimination of pair-mates was 6 to 10 dB across observers.

In a later paper, Patterson and Green[14] delineated some of the main variables that would affect discrimination between brief stimuli with the same energy spectra. The stimulus was a pair of digital impulses passed through an all-pass digital filter. As the overall duration of the resulting waveform was decreased, the difference in arrival time of the energy in different frequency regions of the energy spectrum of the stimulus was reduced. This changed the phase spectrum but not the energy spectrum. Subjects could discriminate overall pitch differences in the waveform, as long as it was at least 10 msec in duration, signifying the ability to discriminate the temporal order of events within the waveform approximately 2.5 msec apart.

Intensity also plays a role in pitch perception. For a given pure-tone frequency, when the stimulus is small in amplitude, the response of the ear is linear and symmetric. As the intensity of the stimulus increases, the displacement for different portions of the basilar membrane will reach a constraining limit and the response will be distorted or nonlinear. Aural harmonics, or overtones, will be generated in the ear. A technique for measuring

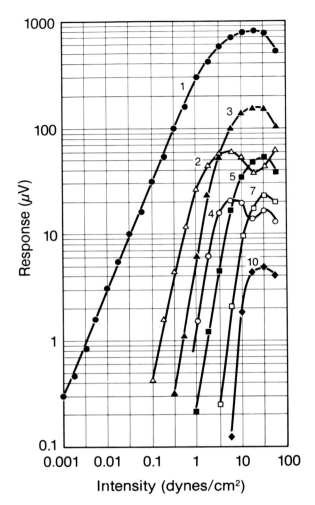

**Fig. 8-9.** The harmonics generated from stimulation of a cat's ear with a pure tone of 1,000 Hz. (Ernest Glenn Wever and Merle Lawrence, Physiological Acoustics. Princeton University Press, Princeton, NJ, 1954, p. 138. Copyright renewed by Princeton University Press. Reprinted with permission of Princeton University Press.)

distortion products was described by Wever and Lawrence.[15] Essentially, the method consisted of a wave analysis of cochlear potentials. Figure 8-9 shows the results of stimulating a cat's ear with a pure tone of 1,000 Hz, filtered to remove harmonics. Twenty intensities of the stimulating tone were presented, and the magnitudes of the fundamental and harmonics of the resulting potential were measured. The numbers on the curves plot-ted indicate frequencies in the harmonic series, "1" for 1,000 Hz, "2" for 2,000 Hz, "3" for 4,000 Hz, and so on. The limit of linearity for the fundamental is about 300 $\mu$V for a stimulus intensity of approximately 75 dB SPL. For this input, the level of the second harmonic is about 25 $\mu$V.

**Loudness**

Loudness is related to intensity by a power law. Each time the physical intensity of the stimulus is multiplied by 10, the perceived loudness is multiplied by 2. If intensity is held constant, loudness may be varied by sweeping across a range of frequencies. Pure tones near 100 Hz or 8,000 Hz will appear to be softer than tones near 3,000 Hz. Figure 8-10 shows the results of an experiment by Robinson and Dadson, reported by Lindsay and Norman.[1] A series of equal loudness contours are plotted for loudness levels ranging from 10 to 120 phons. A value of 50 phons corresponds to the perceived loudness of 1,000 Hz tone presented at 50 dB SPL. The levels (dB SPL) required to match tones of other frequencies to the 1,000 Hz standard are then determined in order to generate the 50-phon contour. The results indicate that both the dynamic range and rate of growth of loudness will depend on the frequency of the stimulus.

If both the intensity and frequency are held constant, loudness may be increased by increasing the duration of the stimulus.[16] Early experiments[17,18] investigated the change in threshold as the duration of the stimulus increased. Garner and Miller[18] found that between the limits of 12.5 and 200 msec, the threshold for detection of a pure tone presented in noise decreased at the rate of 10 dB per decade increase in duration (msec) and assumed that this was the rate of temporal integration of energy over time by the ear.

Temporal integration functions for wide-band noise, a 1,000-Hz pure tone, and a 1,000-Hz pure tone passed through a 100-Hz band-pass filter are shown in Figure 8-11.[17] The slope of the function for noise is −8 dB per log unit of time, and the slope for the unfiltered pure tone, −10 dB per log unit of time for durations equal to or greater than 8 msec. The increase in slope for durations shorter than 8 msec was attributed to an increase in the spectral spread of energy. The bandwidth of the stimulus

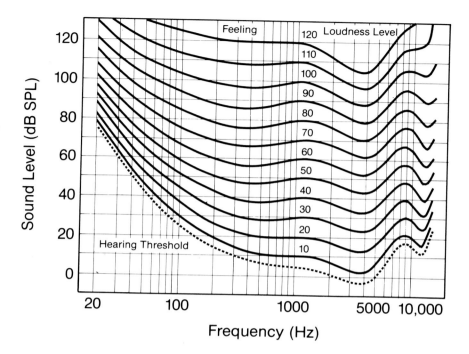

**Fig. 8-10.** Equal loudness contours. (From Human Information Processing: An Introduction to Psychology by P.H. Lindsay and D.A. Norman, copyright 1972 by Harcourt Brace Jovanovich, Inc. Reprinted by permission of the publisher.)

gets broader as the stimulus becomes shorter.[19] Since the ear can only integrate energy within a "critical band" of frequencies (see the section The Critical Band, below), a portion of the total energy of the stimulus will be lost, and the threshold will rise steeply for very short durations. The effect of a lesion in the peripheral or central auditory pathway on temporal integration is discussed in the section Temporal Resolution and Temporal Integration.

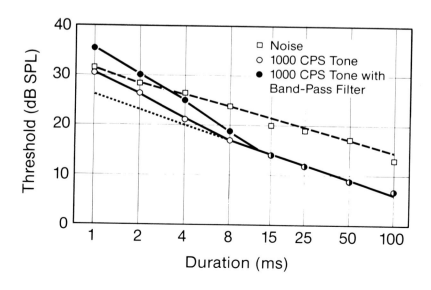

**Fig. 8-11.** The absolute threshold intensity as a function of duration for noise and pure tones of 1,000 Hz. (Garner WR: The effect of frequency spectrum on temporal integration in the ear. J Acoust Soc Am 19:808, 1947.)

## PSYCHOPHYSICAL METHODS

### Signal Detection Theory

During the late 1950s Swets and co-workers[19,20] evolved a theory of signal detection for human observers, based on statistical decision theory. The basic assumption was that the nervous system was continuously active, and therefore, an absolute threshold could not exist. The observer's task was to decide whether the activity perceived within a well-defined observation period resulted from noise alone (either internal or external) or from signal plus noise. Two parameters of this model were (1) the observer's sensitivity to the presence of a signal superimposed on the noise background and (2) the criterion or judgmental effect. With respect to the latter, it was expected that the observer's response, whether affirming or denying the presence of a stimulus, would depend on nonsensory factors such as expectations and payoffs.

The detection problem is illustrated in Figure 8-12. On a given trial, $n$, either noise alone, or signal plus noise, is presented. The observer takes a sample of "excitation" ($x$), a measure of neural activity. It is assumed that any value of $x$ will arise with specific probabilities from each of the two possible events. The probability density distributions on $x$, associated with noise alone or signal plus noise are assumed to be normal and equal in variance. The value of $x$ will tend to be greater when a signal is present. As the intensity increases the two distributions will draw further apart.

The distance between the means of the two distributions ($d'$) is a pure sensory effect. The position of a criterion value ($\beta$) for $x$ establishing the sensory cutoff for affirmative responses and negative responses is a judgmental effect. The two parameters $d'$ and $\beta$, are independent of one another. Four areas bounded by the two curves and the criterion define theoretic probabilities associated with four possible stimulus–response outcomes: (1) a hit, the probability of responding "yes" when a signal is presented; (2) a false alarm, the probability of responding "yes" for noise alone; (3) a miss, responding "no" when a signal is presented, and (4) a correct rejection, responding "no" for noise alone. These probabilities may be experimentally determined for a block of trials and used with tables of

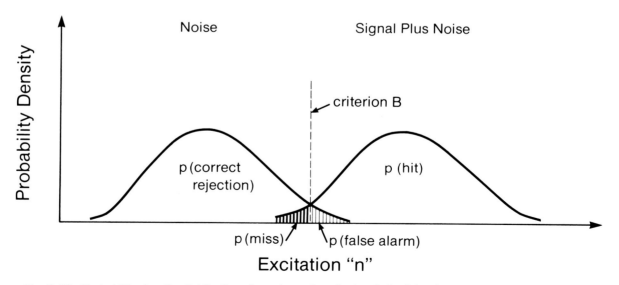

**Fig. 8-12.** Probability density distributions for values of excitation "x" arising from noise alone or signal plus noise. The criterion value of "x" is indicated, as well as four possible outcomes (hit, miss, false alarm, and correct rejection) and their associated probabilities. p (correct rejection) + p (false alarm) = 1.00; p (hit) + p miss = 1.00.

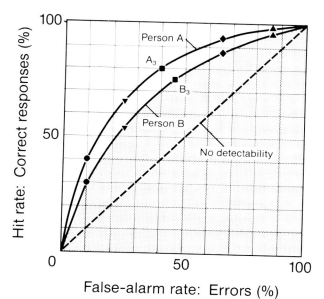

**Fig. 8-13.** Comparison of two ROC curves. person A is more sensitive than person B. (Mussen P, Rosenzweig MR (eds): Psychology: An Introduction. DC Heath, Lexington, MA, 1973, p. 550.)

normal probabilities to determine values expressed in standard normal deviates for the two theoretic parameters, $d'$ and $\beta$, for the acoustic stimulus used in the experiment.

The effects of variation in the two parameters can be seen in the plot of a receiver-operating-characteristic (ROC) curve shown in Figure 8-13.[21] The hit rate is plotted against the false alarm rate. Each curve represents a constant sensitivity, or $d'$. Points on the curve indicate changes in response bias toward decreasing caution. As the hit rate increases, so too does the false alarm rate. In Figure 8-13, person B shows less sensitivity to the presence of a signal, compared with person A.

## Experimental Methods

Psychoacoustics is the study of the relationship between the physical dimensions of the acoustic stimulus presented and the psychological dimensions of the observer's experiences. The two major problems of interest for psychoacoustics are detection: "Was that a signal?" and discrimination:

"Were those two signals the same or different?" The detection problem may be studied using either a single-interval, yes/no procedure, or a two-interval, forced-choice procedure (2IFC).

For the single-interval procedure, each trial consists of only one observation interval. Over a block of 100 or 200 trials, the signal is presented in half the observation intervals, randomly chosen. The intensity of the signal will be varied across blocks such that P(C), the probability of correct response, ranges from 0.50 (chance performance) to 1.00 (perfect detection). The values for all other stimulus dimensions are held constant. If the experimenter has an interest in studying response bias or the judgmental effect, he or she might change the a priori signal probability across blocks, while keeping intensity constant. The knowledge that signals are highly unlikely would induce greater caution in the observer, with the effect of diminishing both hits and false alarms. In Figure 8-12, the position of criterion would move to the right.

A second procedure for detection is the 2IFC paradigm. In this case, there are two observation intervals on each trial, separated by about 500 msec. The signal is presented in either interval 1 or 2, randomly determined for each trial, and the observer would be required to decide which interval contained the signal. As in the single-interval procedure, intensity would be varied across blocks. The criterion cannot be manipulated, using this procedure, and it is assumed to be midway between the means of the theoretic probability density distributions discussed previously.

Either paradigm may also be used for discrimination. A particular stimulus dimension is chosen (e.g., frequency), and a value is selected. Across blocks of trials, the comparison stimulus is varied (in frequency) so as to generate probabilities of discrimination ranging from 0.50 (chance discrimination) to 1.00 (perfect discrimination). All other stimulus dimensions are held constant. The outcome of the discrimination under investigation will, of course, be influenced by the constant values chosen for these other parameters.

The most common method of presenting the data from a psychophysical experiment is a plot of the psychometric function. Some typical results from a single observer are shown in Figure 8-14.[19] In this example, a two-interval, forced-choice detection

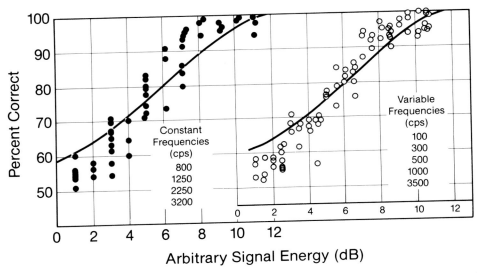

**Fig. 8-14.** The probability of a correct response as a function of signal energy for one observer. The signal frequency was varied either between blocks (constant frequencies) or from trial to trial (variable frequencies). Each point is based on 300 forced-choice trials. (Green DM, Swets JA: Signal Detection Theory and Psychophysics. John Wiley & Sons, New York, 1966, p. 221. Reprinted by permission of John Wiley & Sons Inc.)

experiment was performed. Intensity was varied across blocks of 300 trials. Thus, each data point is based on 300 observations. Replications of the experiment were conducted for four different frequencies, 800, 1,250, 2,250 and 3,200 Hz, and the results have been combined. The stimulus duration was held constant at 100 msec. By convention, the signal intensity necessary to obtain P(C) equal to 0.75 is taken as the detection threshold. The value may be interpolated using the functions best fitting the data. In the example, the detection threshold is roughly 6 dB.

## Discrimination Data

A survey of the results of several studies of the discrimination of a just noticeable change in the intensity of a 1,000 Hz pure tone is shown in Figure 8-15.[5] The ratio ($\Delta I/I$) is plotted as a function of I dB SL, where $\Delta I$ represents the discrimination threshold, and I dB sound level (SL) represents intensity measured relative to the detection threshold. As I increases, over the range of 0 to 100 dB SL, the ratio $\Delta I/I$ decreases, indicating a decrease in the relative change in intensity needed for reliable

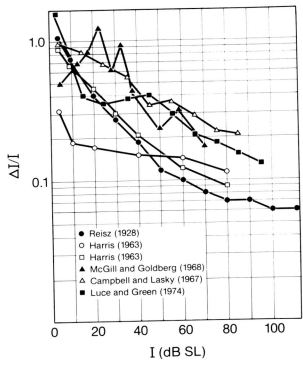

**Fig. 8-15.** The discrimination of a change in intensity as a function of absolute intensity for a pure tone of 1,000 Hz. A comparison of six studies. (Green DM: An Introduction to Hearing. Lawrence Erlbaum, Hillsdale, NJ, 1976, p. 257.)

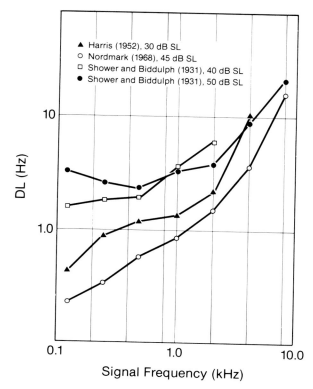

**Fig. 8-16.** The discrimination of a change in frequency as a function of frequency. A comparison of four studies. (Green DM: An Introduction to Hearing. Lawrence Erlbaum, Hillsdale, NJ, 1976, p. 262.)

discrimination of a difference. Multiplying the ratio by a factor of approximately four gives the value of $\Delta I$ in decibels. Thus, at 30 dB SL, the increment necessary for discrimination would be roughly 1.2 dB for the normal listener.

A compilation of the results of four experiments on frequency discrimination are given in Figure 8-16. The discrimination threshold ($\Delta f$) or difference limen (DL) in Hz is plotted against the signal frequency in kHz. Typically, $\Delta f$ will decrease as intensity increases. In Nordmark's[22] results for stimuli presented at 45 dB SL, at 1 kHz the discrimination threshold is about 1 to 2 Hz. Individual differences among subjects may reflect practice and musical training.

## SELECTED TOPICS IN PERCEPTION WITH SPECIAL REFERENCE TO HEARING LOSS

### Frequency Selectivity

The ability of the ear to analyze frequency has been studied psychoacoustically by means of masking experiments, which test the observer's detection of individual components of a complex sound. Masking occurs when selectivity has broken down.[23] The first quantitative investigation of frequency selectivity was conducted by Wegel and Lane,[24] and essentially consisted of measurements of the change in detectability of a pure tone (the test stimulus) in the presence of a pure tone of another frequency (the masker). Figure 8-17 shows the masking effect of a pure tone of 1,200 Hz at three intensities, 160, 1,000, and 10,000 times its minimum audible pressure value on test tones ranging from 400 to 4,000 Hz. These functions are referred to as psychoacoustic tuning curves.

The ordinate indicates the masking effect, defined as the ratio $p_2/p_1$, where $p_1$ is the minimum audible pressure of the test tone in quiet, and $p_2$, the minimum audible pressure in the presence of the masker. For the lowest intensity of the 1,200-Hz masker, the masking effect gradually decreases, as the test stimulus moves farther away, on either side of the masking tone. As the masking frequency is approached, beats will be perceived and detection will improve, accounting for the dip in the curve at 1,200 Hz. At higher intensities of the masker, we see that higher tones are relatively more easily masked than lower tones. Dips in the functions occur in the regions of the harmonics of the masker. The dashed functions indicate the level of the perceived beat in these regions.

A number of more recent investigations have compared psychophysiocal tuning curves for normal and hearing-impaired listeners.[23,25–29] Wightman and co-workers[23] used two different paradigms. In the first, similar to that of Wegel and Lane,[24] a 20-msec pure-tone signal and a 200-msec masker were presented simultaneously; and in the

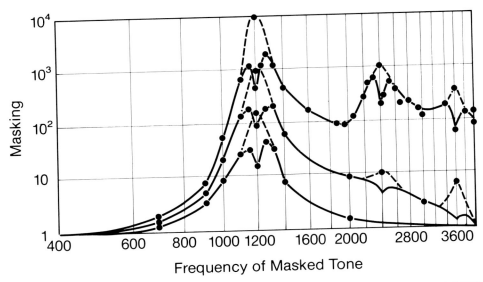

**Fig. 8-17.** The intensity of a pure tone of 1,200 Hz required to mask tones ranging from 400 to 4,000 Hz. (Wegel RL, Lane CE: 1924. The auditory masking of one pure tone by another and its probable relation to the dynamics of the inner ear. Physiol Rev 23:266, 1924.)

second, a forward-masking condition, the onset of the signal was coincident with the termination of the masker. The authors contended that the forward-masking paradigm would preclude the generation of combination tones and suppression of the signal by the masker due to nonlinear interaction of the two stimuli.

The forward-masked tuning curves for three normal listeners are shown in Figure 8-18 for test frequencies of 300, 1,000 and 3,000 Hz. In each case, the test tone was presented at 10 dB SL (i.e., 10 dB above the detection threshold value). The frequency of the masking tone is shown on the abscissa. The masker level plotted for each masking

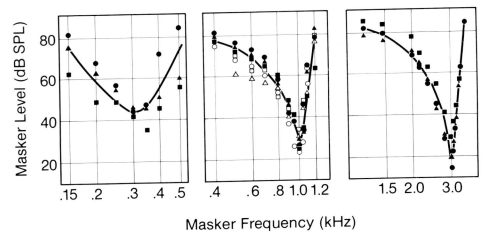

**Fig. 8-18.** Tuning curves for three normal subjects obtained using a forward-masking paradigm. The test frequencies were 300 Hz (left panel), 1,000 Hz (middle panel), and 3,000 Hz (right panel). (Evans EF, Wilson JP (eds): Psychophysics and Physiology of Hearing. Academic Press, Orlando, FL, 1977, p. 299.)

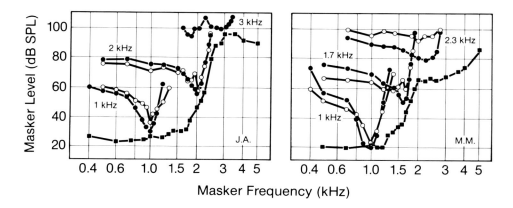

**Fig. 8-19.** Tuning curves for two hearing-impaired subjects. (Evans EF, Wilson JP (eds): Psychophysics and Physiology of Hearing. Academic Press, Orlando, FL, 1977, p. 302.)

tone is the value required for 75 percent correct detections of the test tone in a two-interval, forced-choice procedure. A method of characterizing the tuning curve is in terms of its bandwidth. One measure, $Q_{10\,dB}$, equivalent to the frequency of the probe divided by the bandwidth of the curve 10 dB above the minimum, gives values of 2.1, 9.2, and 13.5 for the three test frequencies, respectively. The values are higher, i.e., the tuning curve is sharper, for the forward as compared with simultaneous masking.

The data obtained using forward and simultaneous masking for two subjects with hearing impairment, presumed due to cochlear lesions, are shown in Figure 8-19.[30] The absolute threshold for the 20-msec probe at frequencies between 400 and 5,000 Hz are included; a value of 23 dB SPL is normal. Tuning curves were obtained at three frequencies — one in the low-frequency region of normal hearing, one in the region of the steep slope of the audiograms, and one in the high-frequency plateau region. In regions of both normal and raised thresholds, the tuning curves were broader for impaired as compared with normal listeners. There was much less difference due to the masking paradigm in the impaired. The authors contend that between-subject differences were not due to the high SPL levels (for 10 dB SL) for the impaired

listeners. In normal listeners, the value of $Q_{10\,dB}$ of the tuning curve did not vary systematically with changes in the probe level.

Florentine et al.[25] compared frequency selectivity in normal hearing listeners and those with hearing impairment described as conductive (otitis media, ruptured tympanic membrane, and cerominal occlusion), otosclerotic, noise induced (exposure to gunfire or industrial noise) and hereditary-degenerative (including presbycusis). Two test tones were used, 500 and 4,000 Hz. Masking tones were 215, 390, 460, 540, 615, and 740 Hz, for the former, and 1,720, 3,120, 3,680, 4,320, 4,920, and 5,920 Hz for the latter. The data for 4,000 Hz presented in Figure 8-20 indicate broader tuning curves in subjects with cochlear impairment, as compared with subjects with normal hearing or middle ear dysfunction. There were no significant differences at 500 Hz, where individuals in each of the groups had audiometric thresholds close to normal.

## The Critical Band

The concept of the critical band originated with Fletcher.[31] In contrast to Wegel and Lane,[24] Fletcher used noise rather than pure tones to mask

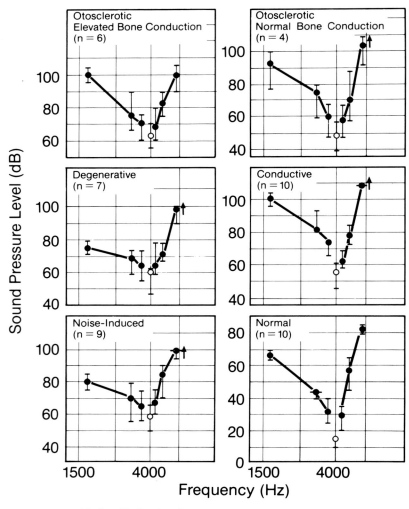

**Fig. 8-20.** Tuning curves for six groups of observers. The test frequency was 4,000 Hz. Masking frequencies ranged from 1,500 to 6,000 Hz. (Florentine M, Buus S, Scharf B, Zwicker E: Frequency selectivity in normally hearing and hearing impaired observers. J Speech Hear Res 23:646, 1980. © 1980, the American Speech-Language-Hearing Association, Rockville, Maryland.)

a continuous pure-tone stimulus and investigated the effect of decreasing the bandwidth of the noise on the detection of the signal. In broadband noise, the signal-to-noise ratio (i.e., the ratio of the signal power to the noise power in a one-cycle band) was about 18 dB. As the bandwidth of the noise centered on the frequency of the pure tone was decreased, detectability remained the same until a critical value was reached, at which point further decreases resulted in improvements in detection. For a signal of 1,000 Hz, this critical bandwidth

was about 60 Hz. Fletcher assumed that the ear "listened" through a narrow filter, whose limits could be approximated by the experimentally determined width of the critical band.

The results of four studies to determine the critical band at a wide range of frequencies are presented in Figure 8-21.[5] The ordinate on the right indicates the critical band and the ordinate on the left, the corresponding threshold signal-to-noise ratio. As indicated by the data, there is good agreement across experiments. The critical band in-

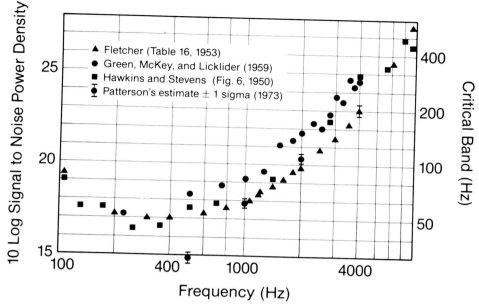

**Fig. 8-21.** The critical band plotted as a function of frequency. The data of four studies are shown. (Green DM: An Introduction to Hearing. Lawrence Erlbaum, Hillsdale, NJ, 1976, p. 140.)

creases linearly with signal frequency from about 1,000 Hz.

An experiment to investigate the change in the critical band with aging was conducted by Patterson and co-workers.[32] Patterson contended that the method used by Fletcher to determine the critical band, based effectively on a critical ratio, did not take into account the processing "efficiency" of the listener. Thus, in broadband noise, the efficient listener might require a signal-to-noise ratio of 17 dB, and the less efficient listener, 20 dB. Such differences would be interpreted in Fletcher's analysis as differences in the width of the auditory filter. The use of notched noise (e.g., Patterson[33]) with the notch centered on the stimulus to be detected allows the distinction to be made between changes in frequency selectivity and processing efficiency. In normal-hearing subjects, changing the width of the notch to infer the width of the auditory filter gives results similar to those of Fletcher (for a review see Green, 1976).[5]

In Patterson's[32] study the shape of the auditory filter was determined by masking the tone to be detected with two broad bands of noise, 40 dB/Hz SPL, one above and one below the tone. The notch

thus produced had a steep frequency roll-off on both sides and was symmetric about the tone. The detection thresholds for pure tones of 0.5, 2.0, and 4.0 kHz were determined for a range of widths of the notch. The results indicated that for all listeners, the detection threshold decreased, as the notch widened. The rate of this change decreased as age increased. While for younger listeners the threshold fell faster at 4.0 kHz than 0.5 or 2.0 kHz, this difference disappeared with age. Since the shapes of the functions were the same for all listeners, Patterson suggested that the effect of aging is a broadening of the filter (i.e., a decrease in frequency selectivity), rather than a decrease in processing efficiency.

## Temporal Resolution and Temporal Integration

Temporal resolution refers to the minimum time required between acoustic events to perceive them as separate. The gap-detection paradigm[34] measures the ability to detect a brief temporal gap between a pair of noise bursts or gated sinusoids. In listeners with normal hearing, the gap threshold is about 2 to 5 msec for practiced listeners and clearly audible acoustic events. The value will depend on other acoustic parameters, increasing as the stimulus amplitude decreases[35] and decreasing as signal frequency increases.[35,36]

A study of temporal resolution in hearing-impaired listeners is exemplified by the work of Irwin et al.[37] In their study, subjects with normal hearing and conductive, otosclerotic, and sensorineural hearing loss were presented with a brief gap in continuous broadband noise. The level of the noise was varied between 30 and 95 dB SPL. Figure 8-22 shows the gap threshold for individual subjects in two of the hearing loss groups as a function of the level of noise in comparison with the average results for six normal listeners. For all subjects the gap threshold depended on the SPL of the stimulus, ranging in normal subjects from 20.3 msec at 30 dB SPL to 3.2 msec at 80 dB SPL. The data for subjects with conductive loss are similar to those of normal subjects, but the function is displaced by about 45 dB, approximately the amount of hearing loss. By contrast, subjects with sensorineural loss show elevated thresholds even at the highest SPLs.

Temporal integration, essentially the opposite of temporal resolution, refers to the increase in the loudness of a stimulus of constant intensity as its duration increases. Studies in normal listeners, reviewed above under Response Dimensions, indicated that the detection threshold of a pure tone of 1,000 Hz decreased 10 dB per decade increase in duration (msec) over the range of durations of 12.5 to 200 msec. A number of studies have compared these data with results for hearing-impaired listeners.[38-41]

In Stephen's[41] study, 90 patients with proven or suspected cochlear nerve or central auditory pathway lesions were tested. Included were end-organ lesions (n = 20, e.g., Meniere's disease, congenital sensorineural hearing loss, post-traumatic cochlear damage, noise-induced hearing loss, and presbycusis); cochlear nerve lesions (n = 7, e.g., vascular lesions, vestibulocochlear Schwannomata, and cerebellopontine angle dermoid); vertebrobasilar artery insufficiency (n = 6); brain stem disorders (n = 37, e.g., multiple sclerosis, syringomyelia, ependymoma, malignant astrocytoma, encephalitis, and vascular lesions); temporal lobe lesions (n = 12); and diffuse disorders (n = 6). Auditory thresholds were obtained for both ears at 1,000 Hz for stimulus durations ranging from 2.4 to 327 msec. The obtained slopes of the integration function over this range were divided into three categories: "steep then normal" (abnormally large threshold difference between 2.4 and 40.1 msec, and normal difference between 40.1 and 327 msec), "steep" (abnormally large threshold differ-

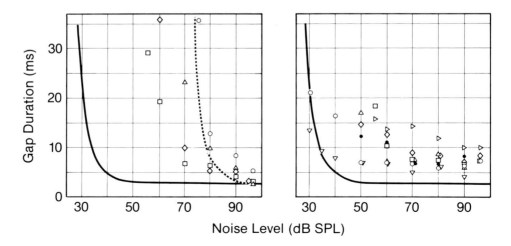

**Fig. 8-22.** Minimum detectable gap for listeners with **(A)** conductive or **(B)** sensorineural hearing loss, compared with data for normal listeners (solid function). Different symbols represent various observers. (Irwin RJ, Hinchcliffe LK, Kemp S: Temporal acuity in normal and hearing-impaired listeners. Audiology 20:234, 1981.)

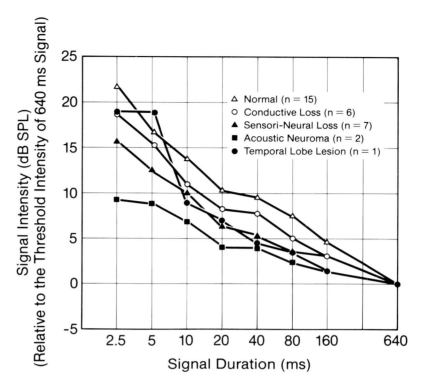

**Fig. 8-23.** A comparison of mean temporal integration functions for normal and hearing-impaired listeners for a one-third octave band centered at 4,000 Hz. The data have been normalized to 640 msec. (Papsin BC, Abel SM, Kunov H: Auditory temporal integration in normal and hearing-impaired listeners. Paper presented at the annual meeting of the Clinical Research Society of Toronto. Toronto, Ontario, Canada, March 24, 1984.)

ence in both regions), and "flat" (abnormally small threshold change over the entire range). In general, flat patterns were especially evident in patients with peripheral auditory lesions, and steep patterns, in patients with cochlear nerve and central auditory pathway lesions. To some extent the "steep then normal" pattern was indicative of a lesion in the upper central auditory pathway.

A more recent study by Papsin et al.[42] studied temporal integration for one-third octave band signals in subjects with normal hearing or hearing impairment due to middle ear dysfunction, cochlear lesions, acoustic neuroma, and temporal lobe lesions. Representative data for a noise band centered at 4 kHz are presented in Figure 8-23. For purposes of comparison, the data for individuals were normalized to their detection thresholds at 640 msec. This essentially eliminates differences due to the amount of hearing loss. In normal listeners the slope of the temporal integration function is −10 dB per decade increase in duration. Except in the case of the temporal lobe lesion, the patients show progressively flatter functions as the lesion advances from the middle to inner ear to

acoustic nerve. Statistical analysis indicated that there was no difference between the slopes of the temporal integration functions for subjects with otosclerosis and cochlear hair cell damage. However, both groups were significantly different from normal. Slopes obtained for the two subjects with acoustic neuroma were lower in magnitude than the values obtained for all but three subjects in these other groups. The one subject with the temporal lobe lesion appears to show impairment of integration only for stimulus durations less than 10 msec. Possible mechanisms underlying these between-group differences are advanced by Papsin.[43]

## DISCUSSION

The basic experiments in psychoacoustics described in this chapter generally used subjects with normal hearing. These detection and discrimination studies established the dimensions of sound to which the normal human ear is sensitive, the interrelation of these various dimensions, and acuity for a change in value along a particular dimension. Possible applications of the paradigms and problems described to observers with hearing loss due to various common causes, as well as some results, are discussed under special topics in perception. These data, collected for individuals with well-defined lesions of the peripheral or central auditory pathway, may be put to several different uses.

First, psychoacoustic information provides an index of hearing handicap. Data from frequency-selectivity experiments, for example, will indicate which frequency components in more complex signals, such as speech, are likely to be confused. The amplification of sound by means of a hearing aid will likely intensify the confusion[44] and thus be counterproductive in solving the problem of hearing loss. Second, a comparison of the performance of normal subjects and those with well-defined lesions may lead the way to new, noninvasive diagnostic test procedures for the individual whose problem is not apparent using routine audiometric evaluation. An example is sound localization ability.[45] Individuals with sensorineural loss are similar to normal in this regard, while those with small acoustic neuromas make sizeable errors in judgments of spatial position. Finally, as illustrated by Papsin et al.,[42] studies of failure of information processing in the presence of a lesion may provide important new data relating to signal encoding at different levels of the pathway in the normal system.

## ACKNOWLEDGMENTS

This research was supported in part by the National Health Research and Development Program, Health and Welfare Canada, through a National Health Research Scholar award to the author. Special thanks are due to Ms. Yasmin Nanja for her help in collecting and organizing the information presented and to Ms. Catherine Birt for her detailed editorial comments on an earlier draft of the manuscript.

## REFERENCES

1. Lindsay PH, Norman DA: An Introduction to Psychology. Academic Press, Orlando, FL, 1972
2. Moore BCJ: An Introduction to the Psychology of Hearing. 2nd Ed. Academic Press, Orlando, FL, 1972
3. Hinchcliffe R: The threshold of hearing as a function of age. Acustica 9:303, 1959
4. Corso JF: Age and sex differences in pure-tone thresholds. Arch Otolaryngol 77:385, 1963
5. Green DM: An Introduction to Hearing. Lawrence Erlbaum, Hillsdale NJ, 1976
6. Abel SM, Haythornthwaite C: The progression of noise induced hearing loss: a survey of workers in selected industries in Canada. J Otolaryngol [Suppl] 13, 1984
7. Robinson DW, Dadson RS: A redetermination of the equal-loudness relations for pure tones. Br J Appl Phys 7:166, 1956
8. Kunov H, Abel SM, Pandey PC, Friedman EB: Analysis of Industrial Noise with Special Reference to Correlation Between Different Indices and Transmission of Noise Through the Middle Ear. Ontario Ministry of Labour, 113/R, Toronto, Ontario, Canada, September 1983
9. Plomp R: The ear as a frequency analyzer. J Acoust Soc Am 36:1628, 1964
10. Doughty JM, Garner WR: Pitch characteristics of short tones. I. Two kinds of pitch threshold. J Exp Psychol 37:351, 1947
11. Patterson RD: Noise masking of a change in residue pitch. J Acoust Soc Am 45:1520, 1969
12. Bilsen FA, Ritsma RJ: Repetition pitch and its implications for hearing theory. Acustica 22:63, 1969/70
13. Ronken DA: Monaural detection of a phase difference between clicks. J Acoust Soc Am 47:1091, 1969
14. Patterson JH, Green DM: Discrimination of transient signals having identical energy spectra. J Acoust Soc Am 48:894, 1970
15. Wever EG, Lawrence M: Physiological Acoustics. Princeton University Press, Princeton, NJ, 1954
16. Green DM, Birdsall TG, Tanner WP, Jr.: Signal detection as a function of signal intensity and duration. J Acoust Soc Am 29:523, 1957
17. Garner WR: The effect of frequency spectrum on temporal integration in the ear. J Acoust Soc Am 19:808, 1947
18. Garner WR, Miller GA: The masked threshold of

pure tones as a function of duration. J Exp Psychol 37:293, 1947

19. Green DM, Swets JA: Signal Detection Theory and Psychophysics. Wiley, New York, 1966
20. Swets JA, Tanner WP, Jr., Birdsall TG: Decision processes in perception. p. 3. In Swets JA (ed): Signal Detection and Recognition by Human Observers. John Wiley, New York, 1964
21. Mussen P, Rosenzweig MR (eds): Psychology: An Introduction. DC Heath, Lexington, MA, 1973
22. Nordmark JO: Mechanisms of frequency discrimination. J Acoust Soc Am 44:1553, 1968
23. Wightman FL, McGee T, Kramer M: Factors influencing frequency selectivity in normal and hearing impaired listeners. p. 295. In Evans EF, Wilson JP (eds): Psychophysics and Physiology of Hearing. Academic Press, Orlando, FL, 1977
24. Wegel RL, Lane CE: The auditory masking of one pure tone by another and its probable relation to the dynamics of the inner ear. Physiol Rev 23:266, 1924
25. Florentine M, Buus S, Scharf B, Zwicker E: Frequency selectivity in normally-hearing and hearing impaired observers. J Speech Hear Res 23:646, 1980
26. Hoekstra A, Ritsma RJ: Perceptive hearing loss and frequency selectivity. p. 263. In Evans EF, Wilson JP (eds): Psychophysics and Physiology of Hearing. Academic Press, Orlando, FL, 1977
27. Margolis RH, Goldberg SM: Auditory frequency selectivity in normal and presbyacusis subjects. J Speech Hear Res 23:603, 1980
28. Pick GF, Evans EF, Wilson JP: Frequency resolution in patients with hearing loss of cochlear origin. p. 273. In Evans EF, Wilson JP (eds): Psychophysics and Physiology of Hearing. Academic Press, Orlando, FL, 1977
29. Zwicker E, Schorn K: Psychoacoustical tuning curves in audiology. Audiology 17:120, 1978
30. Evans EF, Wilson JP (eds): Psychophysics and Physiology of Hearing. Academic Press, Orlando, FL, 1977
31. Fletcher H: Auditory patterns. Rev Mod Phys 12:47, 1940
32. Patterson RD, Nimmo-Smith I, Weber DL, Milroy R: The deterioration of hearing with age: frequency selectivity, the critical ratio, the audiogram, and speech threshold. J Acoust Soc Am 72:1788, 1982
33. Patterson RD: Auditory filter shapes derived with noise stimuli. J Acoust Soc Am 59:640, 1976
34. Abel SM: Discrimination of temporal gaps. J Acoust Soc Am 52:519, 1972
35. Fitzgibbons PJ: Temporal gap resolution in narrowband noises with center frequencies from 6000–14000 Hz. J Acout Soc Am 75:566, 1984
36. Fitzgibbons PJ: Temporal gap detection in noise as a function of frequency, bandwidth and level. J Acoust Soc Am 74:67, 1983
37. Irwin RJ, Hinchcliffe LK, Kemp S: Temporal acuity in normal and hearing-impaired listeners. Audiology 20:234, 1981
38. Gengel RW, Watson CS: Temporal integration: I. Clinical implications of a laboratory study. II. Additional data from hearing-impaired subjects. J Speech Hear Disord 36:213, 1971
39. Hall JW, Fernandez MA: Temporal integration, frequency resolution, and off-frequency listening in normal-hearing and cochlear-impaired listeners. J Acoust Soc Am 74:1172, 1983
40. Miskolczy-Fodor F: Monaural loudness balance test and determination of recruitment degree with short sound impulses. Acta Otolaryngol (Stockh) 43:573, 1953
41. Stephens SDG: Auditory temporal summation in patients with central nervous system lesions. p. 231. In Stephens SDG (ed): Disorders of Auditory Function. Vol. 2. Academic Press, Orlando, FL, 1976
42. Papsin BC, Abel SM, Kunov H: Auditory temporal integration in normal and hearing-impaired listeners. Paper presented at the annual meeting of the Clinical Research Society of Toronto. Toronto, Ontario, Canada, March 24, 1984
43. Papsin BC: Auditory Temporal Acuity in Normal and Hearing-Impaired Listeners. Unpublished Masters thesis, University of Toronto, 1985
44. Plomp R: Auditory handicap of hearing impairment and the limited benefit of hearing aids. J Acoust Soc Am 63:533, 1978
45. Abel SM, Birt BD, McLean JAG: Sound localization in hearing-impaired listeners. p. 207. In Gatehouse RW (ed): Localization of Sound. Amphora, Groton, CT, 1982

# Physiology of the Vestibular System

9

Dennis P. O'Leary

## INTRODUCTION

The human vestibular labyrinth contains three semicircular canals, the utricle, and the saccule. The canals sense head rotational acceleration in three mutually perpendicular planes, whereas the utricle and saccule sense linear acceleration and static head position in a gravitational field. This sensory system provides information to sophisticated central control systems that govern many of our daily movements.

A modern conceptual framework for the vestibular system is biologic inertial navigation, analogous to the guidance system of rockets or ships. Although there are vast differences in the detailed mechanisms of biologic versus rocket guidance systems, a common language can be used to describe the overall operational characteristics of both. Consider a rocket traveling along a programmed trajectory that is suddenly perturbed by a disturbance that threatens to send if off course. On-board sensors detect the disturbance and send this information to a computer, which predicts the necessary compensatory control signals for the motor actuators to keep the vessel on course. A

human who trips while walking an intended trajectory undergoes a similar control systems adjustment. Sensors in the inner ear detect the sudden pitching forward of the head, and peripheral nerves project this information to the brain. The necessary compensatory control signals are then computed and sent to the neuromuscular system for regaining upright posture and continuing on the intended course.

The common feature of these two diverse examples is that of a control system guiding an intended trajectory. Because the two main purposes of vestibular information are the control of posture and coordinated motion, our knowledge of modern vestibular physiology is often expressed in terminology borrowed from systems and control theory, a language common to all control systems.[1-3]

Central vestibular control systems are more sophisticated than was thought previously. Researchers during the past 2 decades have shown the importance of the integration of vestibular, visual, and somatosensory systems for the control of movement. In addition, the vestibulo-ocular system exhibits a remarkable plasticity in its ability to adapt to external and internal changes. The communication among "classic" vestibular reflex pathways,

223

the cerebellum, and other brain centers is now better understood, as a result of extensive experimental and modeling investigations of these systems.

This chapter surveys current topics in vestibular physiology from a biologic control systems perspective. The physiological and control bases for modern vestibular testing are presented and illustrated by examples from recent physiological research.

## GENERAL VESTIBULAR CONTROL PRINCIPLES

Vestibular control systems are often studied by first determining their input–output characteristics and then fitting an equivalent model to them. In the laboratory, a physiologic stimulus such as rota-

tion or tilt is delivered to an animal in a controlled manner, and the response from one or more system outputs is recorded. The system *gain* is defined as the output magnitude divided by the input magnitude. Gain is dependent on the frequency of the input (analogous to an audiogram), but it can also depend on the time after stimulus onset (e.g., "adaptation"), whether or not repetitive stimuli have occurred ("habituation"), and the presence or absence of other inputs to that system. The system *phase lag* is defined as the time delay of the output relative to the input. It too is frequency dependent, and is expressed quantitatively in degrees, with 360 degrees defining one period. Certain systems lag the input sufficiently that, for convenience, they are said to exhibit a phase lead of m degrees. This merely means that they actually lag the stimulus by $n = (360 - m)$ degrees. These system characteristics are illustrated in Figure 9-1, which shows head and eye velocity trajectories during one sec-

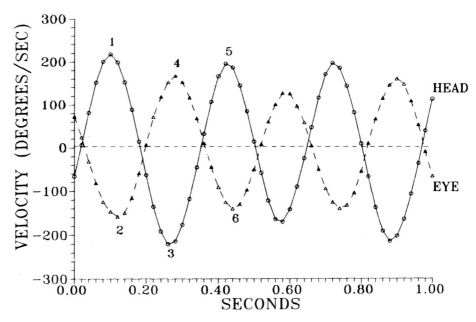

**Fig. 9-1.** Trajectories of head (solid line) and eye (dashed line) velocities sampled at the points shown during 1 second of active human horizontal head movement. For $A_i$ = the amplitude of the *i*th peak, and $t_i$ = its time of occurrence, estimated system characteristics are: *Period* = $(t_5 - t_1)$ sec, *frequency* = 1/period, *gain* = $(A_4/A_3)$, and *phase* = $([(t_4 - t_4)/(t_5 - t_1)] \times 360$ degrees). Average *frequency* is slightly greater than 3 Hz (cps) because three complete periods occurred within a 1-sec time epoch. Average gain is less than one, because peak eye amplitudes are less than the adjacent (reversed polarity) peak head amplitudes within each period. Average phase lag is greater than 180 degrees, because eye peaks lag head peaks of the same polarity by slightly more than half the period between head peaks of the same polarity.

ond of active horizontal head shaking. In Figure 9-1, active head movements produced "compensatory" (i.e., opposite polarity) eye movements. The average gain and phase could be estimated by measuring the relative amplitudes and times of occurrence of the head and eye peaks, as described in the figure legend. In practice, these quantities are often estimated by computers using Fourier analysis programs.

The gain is often transformed to decibels by multiplying by $20 \log_{10}$, and plotting decibels versus $\log_{10} f$, where $f$ is the stimulus frequency. Phase is usually plotted linearly in degrees versus $\log_{10} f$. These are defined as *Bode plots* of a system. It is now common to characterize both normal and pathologic vestibular subsystems by Bode plots.

Bode plots are often fitted with particular classes of equations, which are either time or frequency dependent. Transfer functions are frequency dependent descriptors of linear systems, defined approximately as systems in which doubling the input magnitude results in doubling the output magnitude. Because many vestibular subsystems are linear to a good approximation, they are often characterized in this manner. Transfer functions are used also to describe the frequency characteristics of electrical *filters* (i.e., networks of resistors, capacitors, and inductors). Therefore, a transfer function of a vestibular subsystem is, in effect, an *equivalent filter model* of that system, expressed in terms of quantitative, frequency-dependent parameters. Transfer functions are considered *parametric models*, because they characterize a system by only a few (less than seven) parameters. These parameters can be readily transformed to time-dependent rate constants, for direct comparison with experimental data. Differences in subsystem states (e.g., normal versus pathologic) can be tested by statistical comparisons of model parameters.[4]

---

## LABYRINTHINE RECEPTORS

### Role of the Semicircular Canal Cupula

The ampulla is an enlargement of the semicircular canal, which contains hair cells in a sensory epi-thelium, with cilia extending into a gelatinous diaphragm called the cupula. The cupula appears to be attached around the entire internal perimeter of the ampulla. The membranous labyrinth is fixed to the skull, so that head angular acceleration causes an inertial lag of endolymph within the membranous canals. The inertial lag exerts pressure on the cupula in a direction opposite to that of head rotation. This pressure causes a maximal displacement near the center of the cupula (Fig. 9-2). This phenomenon was demonstrated by Hillman and McLaren[5] via high-speed film of the stained cupula of the frog posterior canal during sinusoidal accelerations.

An earlier concept, that the cupula is normally detached and can be displaced similar to a swinging gate[6,7] is now considered unlikely, at least during physiologic stimulation. This concept derived from films of cupular preparations in the pike that were most likely damaged through overstimulation.[8]

A "torsion pendulum" equation was formulated by Egmond et al.[9] to model the angular deflection of the cupula as hypothesized by Steinhausen.[6,7] This model was a second-order differential equation with constant coefficients given by the endolymph moment of inertia, the viscous friction, and the elastic restoring force. Wilson and Melvill Jones[10] reformulated and derived the equation from physical principles on the basis of fluid motion inside a torus, with a spring-restoring force acting on a piston, simulating a watertight, elastic cupula.[10] The equation follows:

$$\ddot{q} = \ddot{\theta} + (B/I)\dot{\theta} + (K/I)\theta$$

where

$\ddot{q}$ = angular acceleration of the canal; $\theta$, $\dot{\theta}$, $\ddot{\theta}$ are angular position, velocity, and acceleration, respectively, of fluid inside the canal; $B$ = moment of viscous friction per relative angular velocity of fluid flow; $K$ = spring-restoring force per relative angular fluid displacement; $I$ = moment of inertia of a unit volume of fluid. Wilson and Melvill Jones[10] described in detail the interpretation of these quantities in terms of available experimental data. Equation 1 is valuable as a linear system approximation of endolymph–cupula hydromechanics in spite of recent revisions of the particular mode of cupular displacement during physiologic stimulation.[11]

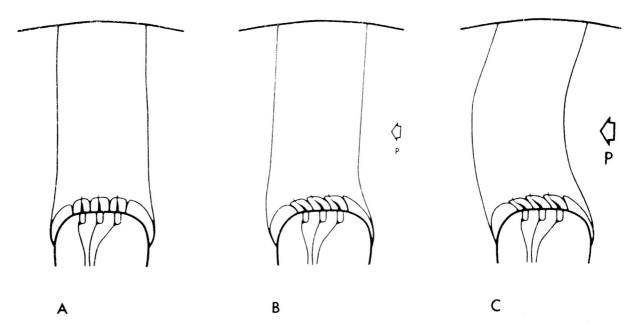

**Fig. 9-2.** A cupula displacement model. The cupula extends from the elevated crista to the opposite ampullary wall in **(A)** its resting position so that the cilia tuft essentially projects from the crista to the cupula where the kinocilium is embedded. **(B)** With slight pressures or initial endolymph displacement, the base of the cupula shifts with shearing in the subcupular space. This displacement causes a bowing of only the basal parts of the cupula. **(C)** Increased pressure (P) on the endolymph displaces broad areas of the cupula so that the maximum displacement shifts toward the center of the cupula. (Reprinted with permission from Neuroscience 4:1989: Hillman DE, McLaren JW: Displacement configuration of semicircular canal cupulae. Copyright 1979, Pergamon Journal, Ltd.)

## Receptor-Generator Mechanisms

Trincker[12] described a static potential gradient in the guinea pig semicircular canal ampulla, with the endolymph positive relative to the more negative crista. In the horizontal canal, the gradient was increased by ampullofugal and decreased by ampullopetal, cupula deflection, respectively. This directionality was reversed in the vertical canals. It persisted in the absence of nerve potentials and even after chronic nerve degeneration,[13] implying that its origin is in the hair cells but not the nerve terminals.

The ampullar generator potential is evidence for a mechanoelectrical transducer process in the hair cell, which results in transmission of a neurotransmitter at hair cell-to-afferent synapses. Our present knowledge concerning cellular and subcellular mechanisms of mechanoelectric transduc-

tion are described separately in Chapter 6. Postsynaptic potentials in afferents synapsing on the hair cells are thought to modulate the neural impulse activity in the first-order afferents.

## Neural Response Dynamics

### Semicircular Canals

The torsion pendulum model of Equation 1 was fitted to semicircular canal averaged afferent response characteristics of the thornback ray.[14] Although canals are sensitive to angular acceleration, the averaged responses were proportional to head velocity. Viscous damping and/or other processes in the receptor was therefore thought to "integrate" (in a mathematic sense) head movement accelerations to approximate head velocity. The view that the semicircular canal was a simple integrator

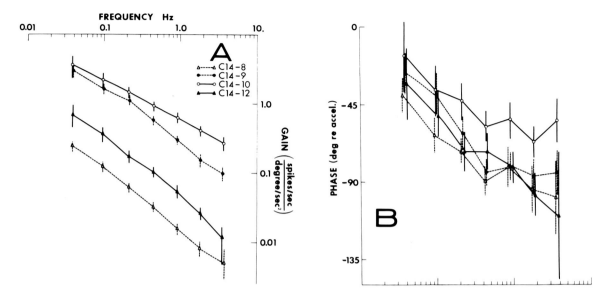

**Fig. 9-3.** Gain and phase plots showing comparative dynamic response properties of six cells. **(A)** Gain curves of five cells showing differences in gain functions. **(B)** Phase curves of three cells showing the wide variation in phase. Brackets indicate 95 percent confidence intervals and were extremely narrow on points without brackets. (Tomko DL, Peterka RJ, Schor RH, O'Leary DP: Response dynamics of horizontal canal afferents in barbituate-anesthetized cats. J Neurophysiol 45:376, 1981.)

persisted until the 1970s, when additional studies suggested a reexamination of this hypothesis.

Individual afferents were found to differ widely in their linear system response characteristics (Fig. 9-3).[15-18] Fernandez and Goldberg[15] recorded sinusoidal responses of semicircular canal afferent neurons from the squirrel monkey and modeled the responses with linear system transfer functions that were more complex than that of the simple torsion pendulum model. Parameters of the new model were used to suggest underlying receptor mechanisms. In other studies, pseudorandom binary noise rotations were used for determining linear system characteristics from semicircular canal neurons of guitarfish[19] and cats.[18] Linear system gain and phase estimates were fitted with low-order linear transfer functions, containing both integral and fractional exponents.[17,18] The results showed a wide range of system parameters that are thought to reflect a head movement frequency selectivity. Subtle differences in system parameters can cause major response differences, particularly

when predicted responses to natural stimuli were compared.[18]

The isolated horizontal canal of the guitarfish showed a topographic organization of afferent response type with location of innervation in the crista. Afferents innervating the crest region of the crista exhibited an initial maximum response amplitude followed by a rapid decay, whereas afferents innervating the crista slopes showed an initial rise up to a low-amplitude maximum followed by a slower decay.[16] Fish have only one hair cell type (type II). The observed response differences could reflect mechanoelectrical transduction properties in different receptor regions, or different filtering mechanisms operating at the cellular or synaptic levels. Figure 9-4 shows a spatiotemporal identification of afferent activity in the semicircular canal nerve of the guitarfish immediately following a sudden head movement, based on results from O'Leary and co-workers.[16]

Hartmann and Klinke[20] described transfer functions to "phase-locked" afferent responses by fit-

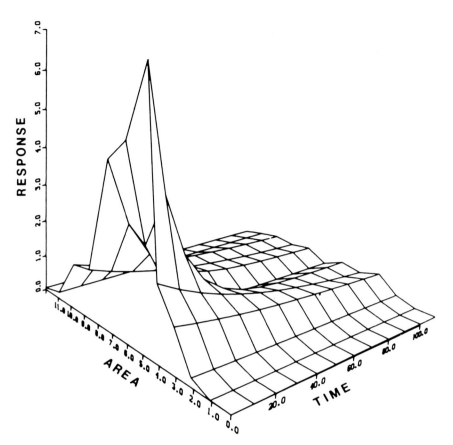

**Fig. 9-4.** A three-dimensional representation of experimental neural impulse activity from the guitarfish horizontal semicircular canal following onset of a sudden movement. Response, in units of (impulses/sec)/(degrees/sec), differs symmetrically in different areas of the nerve near the receptor during a time epoch of 100 msec. A sharp burst of nerve activity occurs from central nerve areas immediately after onset of the movement. (O'Leary DP, Dunn, RF: Multiple information channels in guitarfish vestibular receptors. Histologia Medica 1[Suppl]:27, 1985.)

ting gain and phase characteristics obtained through linearization of sinusoidal responses. Nonlinear effects resulting in phase locking could occur in the afferent membrane encoder mechanisms.[21-23]

### Utricle and Saccule

The morphology of the macular receptors supports the hypothesis that acceleration forces on the otoliths result in a shearing displacement of the gelatinous mass overlying the hair cells. This shearing causes displacement of hair cell cilia in a resultant direction determined by a summation of net forces due to linear acceleration and gravity.

Each afferent innervating the macular receptors responds preferentially to a certain direction of net forces. This results from innervation of specific regions of hair cells that are morphologically oriented in similar directions. Regional mappings of hair cell orientation within each macula therefore provide an effective guide to net directional sensitivity to regional stimulating forces. A net depolarization will occur in certain regions of the macula during stimulation in a given force direction, and activity in afferents innervating those regions will be increased. Mappings of such "functional polarization vectors" were determined from single afferent recordings in animal studies.[24]

Macular afferents are spontaneously active, with stable activity rates that vary as a function of position of the head. Thus, stationary head positions appear to be encoded in the firing rates of macular afferents. In addition to signaling static head positions by their spontaneous discharge rates, macular afferents also exhibit dynamic characteristics during head movements. Those innervating fields of greatest hair cell depolarization at a particular head position will be most active at that moment. But tilting the head by only a few degrees to a new position will significantly alter the firing rates of macular afferents. Fernandez and Goldberg[24-26] determined "polarization vector" (i.e., direction of greatest sensitivity) mappings from both superior and inferior branches of the vestibular nerve of squirrel monkeys that were thought to derive from the utricular and saccular maculae, respectively (Fig. 9-5).

Fernandez and Goldberg[26] used a sinusoidal input–output analysis to study squirrel monkey macular afferent dynamics by first determining an afferent's polarization vector and then aligning the animal's head so that the vector lay along a radius of a horizontal rotation platform. A centrifugal force was created in the labyrinth by rotating the platform with the animal's head displaced from the rotational center. The force vector was modulated by sinusoidally varying the turntable speed. Differ-

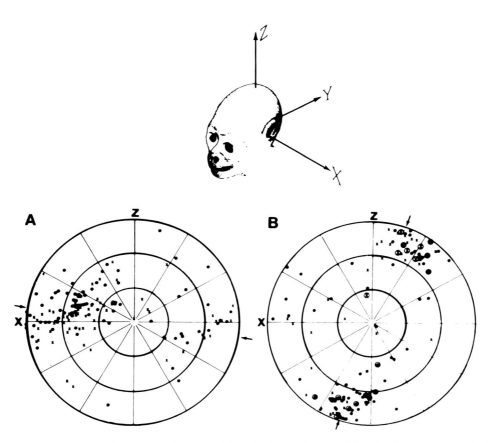

**Fig. 9-5.** Functional polarization vectors from **(A)** 142 units identified as originating from the superior (SN) and **(B)** 115 units from the inferior (IN) branch of the squirrel monkey vestibular nerve. X and Z directions correspond with those of the inset monkey's head. Both radial and circular lines demonstrate 30 degrees angular separations, the former in the plane of the page, the latter in directions extending toward (●) and away from (✕) the reader. Each point depicts one unit's vector, although the magnitude of the vectors is not represented in these diagrams, only their directions. Small arrows denote median angles of vectors of SN and IN units. Circled points denote units obtained after superior nerve section. (Fernandez C, Goldberg JM: Physiology of peripheral neurons innervating otolith organs of the squirrel monkey. I. Response to static tilts and to long-duration centrifugal force. J Neurophysiol 39:996, 1976.)

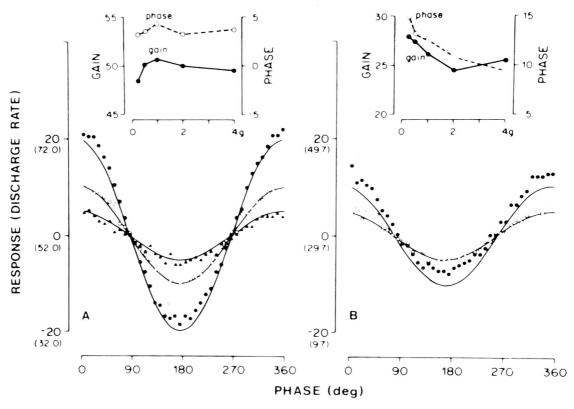

**Fig. 9-6.** Response to sinusoidal stimulation with the biased centrifugal force oriented in **(A)** excitatory and **(B)** inhibitory directions. Stimulus frequency is 0.1 Hz. Ordinate gives both change from resting discharge and (in parentheses) actual discharge frequency. The three stimulus amplitudes were 0.4 (●), 0.2 (○), and 0.1 (▲) g. Curves are best-fit sine waves centered around the resting discharge. Insets give gain (spikes per second per gravity) and phase relations, which are nearly flat. (Fernandez C, Goldberg JM: Physiology of peripheral neurons innervating otolith organs of the squirrel monkey. III. Response dynamics. J Neurophysiol 39:996, 1976.)

ences were found in "inhibitory" versus "excitatory" stimulation along the afferents' polarization vectors (Fig. 9-6). Bode plots and transfer functions from these units provided important insights into the information processing of these receptors. Both utricular and saccular afferents showed similar static and dynamic response characteristics, but with orthogonally oriented sensitivity vectors. This reinforces the concept that both the utricle and saccule incorporate similar physiologic mechanisms to produce similar information concerning head movement in their respective planes of orientation. However, the information-processing significance of the "morphologic polarization" (and associated polarization vectors of the neural re-

sponses) or the macular receptors remain poorly understood at this time. A better understanding of these receptors is a likely prerequisite for accurate future models of vestibular control, particularly in extraterrestrial environments such as manned space stations of the future.

## Efferent Innervation

Electrical activation of the efferent vestibular system inhibited afferent responses in lower vertebrates[27] but had either minimal[28] or even excitatory influences in mammals.[29] Highstein and Baker[30] recorded from identified efferent neurons that were grouped separately in the toadfish posterior canal nerve, and showed that most efferents were briskly activated by behavioral arousal but with variable decay time constant of the responses. They hypothesized that activation of the efferent system prior to impending motion can extend the dynamic range of the semicircular canals by avoiding inhibitory silencing that might be caused by rotation in the "off" direction of the canals.[30] Further studies of efferent effects on vestibular information processing are important for determining specific mechanisms of closed-loop, feedback control from central nuclei.

## CENTRAL VESTIBULAR NEUROPHYSIOLOGY

### Labyrinthine Input to the Vestibular Nuclei

The four vestibular nuclei receive projections from all labyrinthine receptors, but the input is organized in specific ways. In some regions, afferent terminations are found from only certain receptors. Other regions share overlapping termination zones of afferents from different canals, or between canal and macular afferents.[31,32] But it is important to realize that the vestibular nuclei are receiving areas for other sensory modalities as well, particularly somatosensory and visual information. Therefore, in addition to their role in relaying vestibular information, the vestibular nuclei are important centers for coordination of multisensory inputs.

Both anatomic studies, reviewed by Brodal[33] and results from natural and electrical stimulation[34,35] have provided a wealth of information concerning the nature of afferent responses in various regions of the nuclei. Electrical stimulation of afferents from specific receptors have shown detailed patterns of electrical activity (e.g., field potentials, mono- and polysynaptic convergence) arising from the various receptors.

Deiters nucleus exhibits more prominent ventral than dorsal monosynaptic field potentials evoked by stimulation of the whole vestibular nerve.[36]

Utricular and saccular afferents terminate in this nucleus,[32] and both electrical activity[37] and sensitivity to tilt[38] show evidence that this nucleus is an important projection area for the macular receptors. However, Deiters nucleus also receives afferents from all three semicircular canals,[32] indicating its lesser importance as a rotational receiving area as well.

The medial nucleus receives a strong input from all three semicircular canals in its rostral regions.[31,32] In addition, tilt-sensitive neurons are found throughout the nucleus, but with much smaller mean response amplitudes than the those of ventral Deiters nucleus.[39] Some medial nucleus cells respond to both angular acceleration and tilt.[40] In general, the second-order neurons receiving canal input predominate in the rostral parts of the nucleus, whereas tilt-sensitive neurons are concentrated in the caudal regions.

The descending nucleus receives significant utricular input[31] in addition to saccular input[32] in its rostral regions.

The superior nucleus apparently receives input only from canals,[31,32] on the basis of anatomic evidence. Within its subdivisions, superior canal responses are found laterally, and posterior canal units medially. Natural stimulation indicates relatively few horizontal canal neurons in this nucleus.[41] The major projection of the superior nucleus is to the extraocular motor nuclei.

### Responses to Natural Stimulation

Central neurons responding in the same directional sense as first-order afferents are type I, those responding in the opposite sense are type II. Others responding in both directions with increasing activity are type III, and with decreasing activity are type IV.[42] On the basis of vestibular nerve stimulation, type I responses were further categorized as "tonic" and "kinetic," on the basis of differing spontaneous and dynamic response characteristics.[34,35] However, their dynamic responses to sinusoidal rotational acceleration were similar in awake monkey[43] and decerebrate cat.[44,45] Variations in spontaneous activity in central vestibular neurons affect the degree of modulation that occurs in response to periodic rotational acceleration. An example is shown in Figure 9-7.

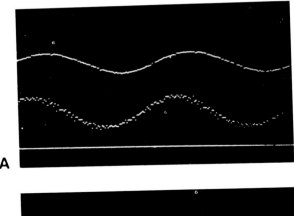

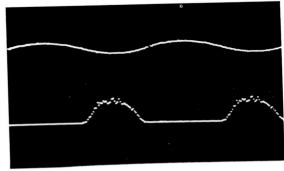

**Fig. 9-7.** Canal-dependent responses in central vestibular neurons during horizontal sinusoidal rotational stimulation. **(A)** All-round pattern seen in a type I unit, average of 14 stimulus periods. **(B)** Cutoff pattern seen in a type I spontaneously silent unit. In each set, top trace is head angular velocity, next trace is averaged discharge rate, and straight horizontal line is zero firing frequency. (A from Melvill Jones G, Milsum JH: Characteristics of neural transmission from the semicircular canal to the vestibular nuclei of cats. J Physiol (Lond) 209:295, 1970. B from Melvill Jones G, Milsum JH: Frequency response analysis of central vestibular unit activity resulting from rotation stimulation of the semicircular canals. J Physiol (Lond) 219:191, 1971.)

A different view of dynamic responses is apparent when other rotational stimuli are used. Figure 9-8 illustrates the effects of a sudden stopping of constant rotation. The resulting "pulse" of acceleration results in an exponentially related rise or decay of the neuronal response.[46] These authors noted the importance of a detectable delay in central neural responses, which reflected the extent of central processing of the projected information from the periphery.

## Commissural Activity

The vestibular nuclei communicate via commissural activity. In the cat, commissural influence is inhibitory to type I neurons from the semicircular canals.[47] This influences the spontaneous activity that is commonly found in vestibular afferents. Following unilateral labyrinthectomy, type I responses are observed on the affected side after compensation has taken place, although no input occurs from the ipsilateral labyrinth. The resulting modulation to rotational stimulation is due to changes in commissural inhibition, thus demonstrating its potentially powerful influence in compensation.[48]

Stimulation of specific canal nerve branches shows an interesting organization related to natural planes of rotational specificity. Neurons activated from stimulating the ipsilateral horizontal nerve are selectively inhibited by stimulation of the contralateral horizontal nerve. Neurons innervating the anterior and posterior canals are inhibited by stimulation of the posterior and anterior nerves, respectively.[49]

## The Vestibulospinal System

Early descriptions of vestibulospinal physiology focused on postural reflexes that are elicited behaviorally when an animal is placed in various positions relative to the gravitational vector.[50] A modern description must include the fact that man is now venturing into microgravity ("weightless") environments, in the absence of a gravitational references. Therefore, physiological control descriptions of vestibulospinal effectors should now include a dynamic component that operates effectively even in the absence of the familiar postural adjustments that occur on earth. This expanded view of vestibulospinal dynamics is now being recognized and studied with the aid of physiological control theory.

Vestibulospinal information in mammals is transmitted primarily via three tracts: the *lateral vestibulospinal tract* (LVST), the *medial vestibulospinal tract* (MLF), and the *reticulospinal tract* (RST). Physiological influences of these tracts have been studied by applying natural or electrical stimulation and recording intracellular synaptic potentials

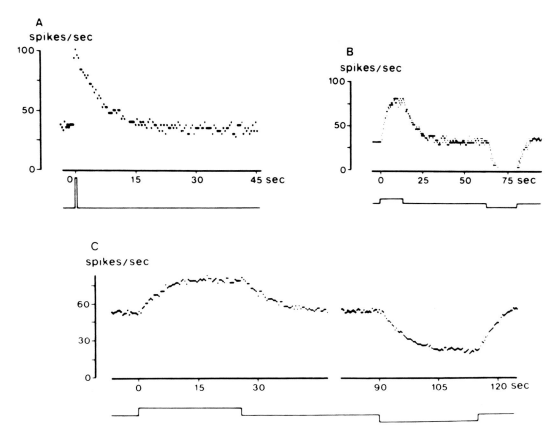

**Fig. 9-8.** Averaged transient responses of type I vestibular nuclear neurons to horizontal rotation stimuli in decerebrate cat. **(A)** Response to sudden stopping of a contralateral rotation of 60 degrees/sec. **(B,C)** Responses to extended periods of angular acceleration-steady velocity-deceleration at accelerations of 8 degrees/sec and 5 degrees/sec for **B** and **C,** respectively. Bottom traces: acceleration profiles. (Shinoda Y, Yoshida K: Dynamic characteristics of responses to horizontal head angular acceleration in the vestibulo-ocular pathway in the cat. J Neurophysiol 37:653, 1974.)

and afferent impulses evoked in motoneurons of the projected pathways.

## The Lateral Vestibulospinal Tract

Extensive work on the LVST[39–53] has shown that it regulates motor activity in $\alpha$- and $\gamma$-motoneurons through both monosynaptic and polysynaptic connections, and also by synapses on interneurons in segmental reflex pathways. The precision control of this regulation is illustrated by the following experimental result. When Deiters nucleus was stimulated during different phases of the step cycle in thalamic cats walking on a treadmill, there was strong facilitation of gastrocnemius activity when the stimuli were delivered during the extension but not during the flexion phase of the step.[54] This lack of facilitation during flexion is thought to be due to opposing influences of interneurons.

The LVST relays information from utricular, saccular, and canal afferents, as shown by exclusion in careful experiments that combined electrical and natural stimulation with selective transections of labyrinthine afferents.[51,55,56] But ablation studies show that the LVST relays information from other systems also, particularly somatosensory information via the cerebellum.[57–59]

The LVST is instrumental in a control system that modulates somatosensory excitatory inputs to Deiters nucleus from cerebellar Purkinje cells and fastigial neurons. Modulation influences from the labyrinth are less evident in dorsal than ventral regions of this nucleus. It is likely that inputs from other systems are integrated also at various stages of this control system.

### The Medial Vestibulospinal Tract

The MVST receives monosynaptic and polysynaptic input from labyrinthine receptors projecting to the medial, descending, Deiters nuclei. All three semicircular canals project second-order information to the MVST via the medial nucleus,[38,60,61] with relatively few cells that are higher than second order. Indirect evidence suggests that at least a small number of MVST neurons receive spinal excitation evoked from proximal limb joints[62] or stimulation of the spinal cord in C1 to C3 regions.[63,64]

In contrast with the LVST, the MVST projects both inhibitory and excitatory information directly to upper cervical and thoracic motoneuron, but apparently not to limb motoneurons.[61,63] The main control function of the MVST is to relay labyrinthine information, which is then integrated with other inputs in the tract neurons.

### Reticulospinal Tracts

Vestibular influences on the RSTs are less understood than those on the other two tracts. However, reticulospinal neurons are excited by stimulation of either the ipsilateral or contralateral vestibular nerves.[65] Reticulospinal axons were shown to exert monosynaptic, inhibitory[66] or excitatory[67] influences on motoneurons.

### Vestibulospinal Control

Short latency control mechanisms were studied extensively by selective stimulation of vestibular

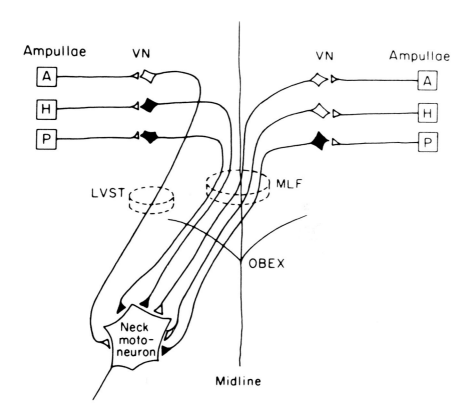

**Fig. 9-9.** Connections between ipsilateral and contralateral ampullae and neck motoneurons. Inhibitory neurons and their terminals are shown in black, excitatory in white. A, H, P, anterior, horizontal, and posterior ampullae, respectively; VN, vestibular nuclei. (Wilson VJ, Maeda M: Connections between semicircular canals and neck motoneurons in the cat. J Neurophysiol 37:346, 1974.)

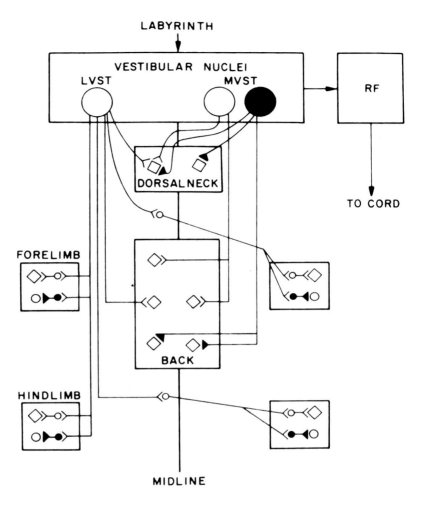

**Fig. 9-10.** Connections between labyrinth, vestibulospinal tracts, and motoneurons at different spinal cord levels. Data were obtained by stimulating the whole vestibular nerve, its canal branches, or the vestibular nuclei. ◇, Extensor motoneurons; ○, flexor motoneurons; ∞, interneurons; filled symbols, inhibitory neurons. (Wilson VJ, Melvill Jones G: Mammalian Vestibular Physiology. Plenum Press, New York, 1979.)

nerves with evoked responses recorded from motoneurons innervating the neck muscles.[56,68] These studies provided detailed information concerning patterns of excitatory postsynaptic potentials (EPSPs) and inhibitory postsynaptic potentials (IPSPs) evoked from each labyrinthine receptor as relayed via the above tracts. An example is shown in Figure 9-9. Connections between labyrinyth, vestibulospinal tracts, and motoneurons at different spinal cord levels are shown as a composite diagram in Figure 9-10.

## Control of Body Movement

The dynamic control of body movement is difficult to model from the limited data on cellular and reflex modification previously described. One reason is our limited knowledge of information processing that occurs during body movements,[69] as opposed to postural adjustments of body position. This modeling limitation is compounded by the fact that stimuli to the vestibular receptors are constantly changing during head and body movements. The changing information from those receptors is projected to the centers and tracts described above during body movements, requiring sophisticated control modeling of even simple behavioral movements.

A simulation of changing vestibular information during complex movement was described for the righting reflex of the freely falling cat[70] as shown in Figures 9-11 and 9-12. Movements of the cat's

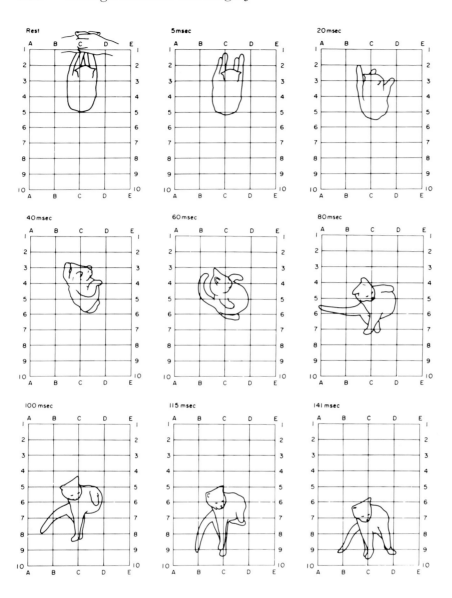

**Fig. 9-11.** Drawings of righting reflex of a cat initially at rest (upper left) and then freely falling at postrelease times indicated in milliseconds above each panel. Each drawing is from a selected frame from a high-speed film (1,000 pictures/sec) during a 30-cm fall. Dimensions of each grid division: horizontal, 5.9 cm; vertical, 3.8 cm. First landing contact (tail and one rear foot) occurred at 115 msec, and all four feet were on landing surface at 160 msec. (O'Leary DP, Ravasio MJ: Simulation of vestibular semicircular canal responses during righting movements of a freely falling cat. Biol Cybern 50:1, 1984.)

head during free fall were filmed at high speed. These movements were used as simulated imputs to transfer function models of semicircular canal afferent activity obtained previously.[18] The predicted outputs showed new, unexpected periodicities (Fig. 9-12), suggesting possible use of phase locking of semicircular canal afferents during dynamic control of fast body movements.[70]

## The Vestibulo-ocular Reflex

Movements of the eyes are due to the actions of six extraocular muscles attached to each eye. The neural signals controlling them derive from different control systems that act together as the *oculomotor system* to command voluntary and involuntary motions of the eyes. The vestibulo-ocular

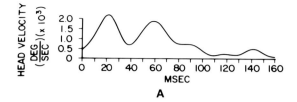

$$H_c(s) = \frac{1.7(1.3s + 1)(0.059s + 1)}{(14s + 1)(1.7s + 1)(0.025s + 1)},$$

**B**

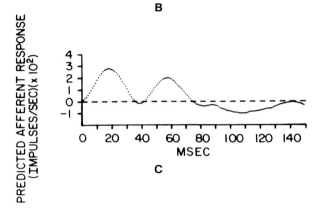

**Fig. 9-12.** A prediction of semicircular canal afferent responses during righting movements of a falling cat. **(A)** Head rotational velocity trajectory is shown during the fall. **(B)** Transfer function of a cat semicircular canal afferent determined from a white noise analysis of Tomko et al.[18] **(C)** Simulated response of the same afferent to the head velocity of **A,** as determined through linear prediction from the transfer function of **B.** (O'Leary DP, Ravasio MJ: Simulation of vestibular semicircular canal response during righting movements of a freely falling cat. Biol Cybern 50:1, 1984.)

reflex (VOR) acts to stabilize foveal fixation of the eyes during head movements by causing a counter rotation of the eyes in order to compensate for rotational movements of the head. This prevents visual images from moving across the retina during head movements, providing a stable view of the environment during locomotion. The major VOR structures and information pathways that control this process are shown in Figure 9-13.

## Central VOR Information Processing

The classic "three-neuron reflex arc" is indicated in Figure 9-13 by numerals I to III, which indicate the origins of the three neuronal tracts. Nerves from the vestibular semicircular canals generally represent head angular velocity information and not position. Therefore, a mathematic integration must occur in the central pathways of the VOR to convert head velocity information to position of the head. A "neural integrator" is assumed to be present, acting in parallel with head velocity information relayed via the VOR, to result in precise compensatory movements of the eyes in response to head movements. This integration is thought to occur via polysynaptic "side arcs" in the reticular formation, which then convey head position information to the oculomotor nuclei. The neural integrator would prolong the normal response time of the VOR and result in prolonged neural activity that sustains compensatory eye movements.

## Control Theory Modeling

Modeling of the VOR and its associated neural integration is based on application of control theory. A transfer function from the semicircular canals can be assigned to neural pathways carrying head velocity information that enter the vestibular nuclei in the brain stem. Outputs from this center then project directly to the oculomotor nuclei.[8] However, there are additional projections to the hypothesized "neural integrator." Longer time constants in vestibular nuclei neurons are thought to be due to a feedback loop with a longer time constant than are contained in the receptor transfer functions.

An overall transfer function describing VOR-controlled eye movements can be assigned, which serves as an effective parametric model of the VOR.[71-73] The specific substages of Figure 9-13 have been modeled with transfer functions that are based on observed neural activity from those substages.[74]

Although the location and structure of a neural integrator in the VOR are presently unknown, the identification of its operational characteristics is useful for testing hypotheses of neural function. For example, such an integration could be performed through actions of a multiple neural circuit,

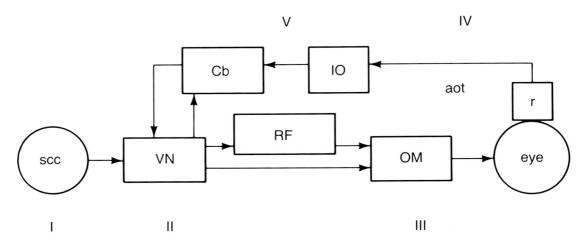

**Fig. 9-13.** Diagram of major vestibulo-ocular reflex information pathways. Roman numerals indicate the following approximate information signals occurring at adjacent system substages: *I,* head acceleration; *II,* head velocity; *III,* head velocity and position; *IV,* error signal due to unequal eye and head velocities; *V,* adaptive compensation control signals attempting to correct the error signal in *IV. aot,* accessory optic tract; *Cb,* vestibulo-cerebellum; *eye,* ocular globe; *r:* retina, *IO,* inferior olive; *OM,* oculomotor nuclei; *RF,* reticular formation; *scc,* semicircular canal; *VN, vestibular nuclei.*

in which a single impulse at the input of a chain of neurons can set up a prolonged train of impulses.[8]

Effective modeling of the VOR must include interactions with the visual system. "Optokinetic" movements of the eye occur in response to apparent motion of the visual surround. Young[75] hypothesized that the brain receives an "efference copy" of eye velocity, which when added to head velocity information from the VOR, results in the velocity of the environment with respect to the head. Robinson[74] constructed a model of these interacting systems, and he showed that a multiloop model of this type can be tested by subjecting it to specific conditions, such as rotation at constant velocity in the light versus the same rotation in the dark.

### Adaptive Control in the Oculomotor System

Robinson[76] observed that modeling of the oculomotor system offers the great advantage that the purposes of its various subsystems are assumed to be known, leaving only the question, *how* is this done? This is in contrast to most areas of neurophysiology in which the question is still *what* is being done? The answer to how a complex brain

function operates is often best approached by modeling. This is illustrated by new advances in oculomotor physiology during the 1970s, which resulted in an adaptive control model of the VOR.

The VOR was thought previously to be a machinelike, three-neuron reflex arc that operated to move the eyes in the opposite direction of the head in order to maintain a stable visual field during motion. Moving the head 10 degrees to the right caused the eyes to counter-rotate 10 degrees to the left. But reversal of the visual field, resulting from human subjects wearing left–right reversing prism goggles, was found to result in extreme changes in the manner in which eye movements responded to head motion.[77,78] This change is shown in Figure 9-14. It was characterized by tracking the gain and phase of vestibular-induced eye motion with respect to head motion. After the subjects donned the reversing prism goggles, the eye movement gain and phase changed with a characteristic time course of about 2 weeks, resulting in the eyes moving in the same direction as the head! When measured at this time, movement of the head 10 degrees to the right caused the eyes to move nearly 20 degrees to the right, such that the subjects could then compensate for the new visual conditions cre-

**Fig. 9-14. (A)** Normal and **(B)** fully adapted nystagmoid responses obtained during test stimuli in the dark from one human subject exposed to continuous vision reversal. The adapted response, which was recorded after 14 days of reversed vision, approximates a reversed replica of the normal one. Both records of eye movement are correctly phase related to the lower record **(C)** of stimulus angular velocity. (Melvill Jones G: Plasticity in the adult vestibulo-ocular reflex arc. Philos Trans R Soc Lond [Biol] 278:319, 1977.)

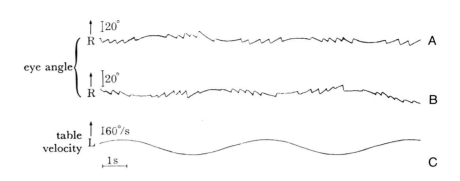

ated by wearing reversing prism glasses. Moreover, this new condition persisted even in darkness, indicating that major changes had occurred in brain processing in response to the reversed visual field, that is a phenomenon known as "neural plasticity."[78] The time course of these changes is shown in Figure 9-15.

How is this accomplished? Extensive work in multiple laboratories, summarized by Ito,[8] demonstrated additional pathways interacting with the VOR, such that an "error signal" was sent from the retina to the brain stem and cerebellum, with information that head movement caused a "blurring" of vision. This suggested an "adaptive control" model of the VOR, in which adjustment of the conventional VOR control parameters was possible in order to minimize the error signal.[79] Figure 9-13 indicates a control systems interaction model of visual (optokinetic) and vestibular information, in which the "error signal" described above is carried by neural activity in the nucleus of the accessory optic tract.

**Fig. 9-15.** VOR phase (lower curve) and normalized gain (upper curve) from one human subject exposed to continuous vision reversal for 27 days (●) and during readaptation after return to normal vision (○). Circled points ⊙ are mean control values obtained just before donning the reversing prisms. Phase is registered relative to that associated with perfect compensation using normal vision. (Melvill Jones G: Plasticity in the adult vestibulo-ocular reflex arc. Philos Trans R Soc Lond [Biol] 278:319, 1977.)

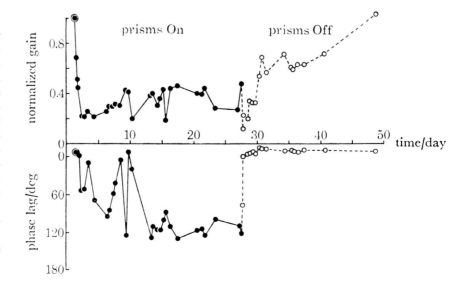

Adaptation of the VOR also occurred when the apparent visual world increased or decreased in size, resulting from the wearing of telescopic lenses.[80,81] The VOR gain of monkeys wearing 2× telescopic lenses increased by 0.4 in about 3 days.[82] Similar effects were found to occur from combined visual-vestibular stimulation that resulted in apparent movement of the visual field.

In the above studies of VOR adaptive control, linear systems modeling provided nonparametric system characteristics (gain and phase Bode plots), which allowed tracking of system changes during the 2-week period leading to reversed eye movements. Transfer function parameters of various substages of ocular control models of the VOR provided useful predictions that were tested by neurophysiological recordings from brain centers.

## Vision during Head Movements

In addition to the VOR, another neural control system stabilizes vision of the environment during head movement. The pursuit reflex is a closed-loop system that uses information from the retina to control eye movements for tracking moving objects. Benson and Barnes[83] reviewed dynamic modeling of both pursuit and VOR control systems, concluding that the relative importance of each system for visual stabilization depended on the frequency range of head motion. The pursuit system was most important below angular head motion of about 1 Hz, whereas stabilization at higher frequencies was determined primarily by the VOR. But is visual stabilization the goal of oculomotor control? Skavenski and co-workers[84] monitored small-amplitude, two-dimensional head and eye rotations during natural and artificial body rotations, concluding that the degree of compensatory oculomotor response was actively adjusted to ensure an appropriate degree of retinal image motion to prevent perceptual fading during small head movements, and to prevent perceptual blurring of images during active body movements. They suggested that the goal of oculomotor compensation is not retinal image stabilization, but rather controlled retinal image motion, which is adjusted to be optimal for visual processing over the full range of natural body movements.

## Importance of the Cerebellum

Cerebellar modeling is integral to modern interpretations of the VOR. The cerebellum has been the subject of important modeling studies for at least 2 decades, in attempts to organize the wealth of accumulated experimental data from this structure.[85] Marr[86] proposed a "learning principle" for cerebellar cortex, based on cellular organization, in which Purkinje cells were able to learn various motor skill contexts through neural modification of synaptic transmission. He considered the modification to be an enhancement of synaptic activity. Albus[87] proposed a cerebellar learning model in which depression of synaptic activity was predicted. Since both models were based on cooperative action of two different types of afferents projecting to the cortex, they could be considered spatial pattern classifiers with learning capabilities based on synaptic plasticity of cortical nerve-net structures.[88] Fujita[89] reformulated the Marr-Albus model with linear system analysis, which resulted in an adaptive linear filter model. The model predicts that a Purkinje cell output converges to a "desired response" through minimization of the mean square performance error. Fujita[90] extended this linear control model to include a phase lead or lag compensator with learning capability. Under the assumption that the cerebellar flocculus accounts for adaptive modification of the VOR dynamic characteristics, a simulation study of the Marr-Albus-Fujita model of the cerebellum was in good agreement with experimental data of human VOR adaptive control dynamics.[88,90]

Pellionicz and Llinàs[91] proposed a model of cerebellar coordination, in which no learning was assumed to occur in the cerebellar network. Alternatively, the brain was considered as a set of tensorial systems that communicate through vectorial channels (neural pathways). The cerebellum was therefore represented in multidimensional space. Cerebellar coordination of ballistic movement was described as guiding the movement onto "wired-in" trajectories of a vector field composed of the set of all such trajectories. Learning was substituted in this model by a continuum of preexisting movement trajectories.[92]

## Lesion Investigations of VOR Adaptation

Ablation studies in animals showed that the flocculus of the vestibulocerebellum was necessary for the establishment and maintainance of VOR adaptation.[79,93] This suggested two possibilities. (1) The flocculus may itself be the site of "adaptive VOR control," or (2) additional "extracerebellar" structure with inputs to the flocculus may be the command centers for VOR adaptation.

Further investigations showed that lesioning the dorsal cap of the inferior olive abolished VOR adaptation, but did not affect the gain.[94] Similarly, harmaline injections reduced VOR adaptation capabilities in monkeys, apparently by producing abnormal activity in olivary neurons.[95]

## Cellular Control Hypotheses

Investigation of cellular cerebellar control mechanisms for VOR gain adaptation led to the suggestion that it is induced by a shift of dominance between the two populations of floccular Purkinje cells, one in-phase modulating and the other out-of-phase modulating.[96] This would be expected to depress or enhance the VOR gain as the dominance shifted toward out-of-phase or in-phase populations, respectively.[8]

An alternative hypothesis places a strong influence on the commissural crossing fibers for regulating VOR adaptive control. Galiana and Outerbridge[97] modeled the VOR by including bilateral commissural connections between the vestibular nuclei on each side. The model predicted alternative mechanisms for certain mathematic operations of the VOR, on the basis of positive-feedback loops for signals across the midline. Vestibular compensation, and possible influences on VOR gain plasticity, was predicted to be strongly influenced by modulation of information in transmidline coupling pathways.[98]

## Habituation of the VOR

Repeated or prolonged application of vestibular stimuli causes a gradual decline of VOR gain.[99] This was especially pronounced following low frequency (0.002 Hz) sinusoidal stimulation of monkeys.[100] The resulting VOR phase advance and gain decline lasted for months. Slow potentials evoked in folium and tuber vermis regions of the cerebellum decreased in amplitude during VOR habituation to vestibular stimulation.[101]

## Compensation of Unilateral Lesions

Plugging one horizontal semicircular canal in monkeys caused an immediate decrease of VOR gain.[102] However, the gain recovered to about 80 percent of normal within 1 month. But this recovery did not occur either when the monkeys were prevented from moving their heads or when kept in the dark. This suggests that motion and/or visual–vestibular interaction play an essential role in VOR compensation for unilateral lesions.

# ROTATIONAL TESTING OF THE VOR

## Input–Output Analysis

Since rotational acceleration is the physiologic stimulus to the semicircular canals during natural movements of the head, it has been used for vestibular testing since the pioneering work of Barany.[103] In Barany's original design, subjects are seated in a chair that can be rotated by hand about a vertical axis, with the head secured against a headrest. After spinning for at least 30 seconds, the chair is suddenly stopped, and the resulting nystagmus is observed visually for abnormal patterns.

In rotational testing, motion of the chair is transmitted to the head and to the horizontal semicircular canals, which can be considered fixed to the skull. It is important that the input movements are carefully timed and coordinated with the observation of the resulting eye movement responses, in order to achieve accurate and reproducible results.

The control and timing of the stimulus motion has taken different forms. Initially, the Barany chair was controlled by spinning the chair by hand, a method still in use today. In this method, the subject is rotated at approximately constant velocity for at least 30 seconds. A constant rotational velocity does not stimulate the canals, but only one that changes velocity through acceleration or deceleration. Therefore, at the start of the stimulus motion, the semicircular canals undergo an initial stimulation due to the acceleration from rest, but the subsequent 30-second period of constant velocity allows the cupula-endolymph system to return to its resting configuration. A sudden stopping of the chair then acts as a strong stimulus, causing a counter rotation of the endolymph in the opposite direction.

The torsion swing utilizes an angular pendulum as the driving force for seated subject. The subject is seated in a chair suspended by springs. After an initial displacement resulting from twisting the chair, the subsequent motion is oscillatory from side-to-side at a frequency that is determined by the suspension characteristics of the chair. This oscillation is damped by friction in the system so that the subject undergoes an ever-decreasing amplitude.

The servocontrolled motor-driven chair was developed during the past 2 decades, utilizing components and concepts derived from navigational systems. The subject is seated at the center of a platform mounted on the motor shaft. The chair is controlled by a velocity servo-controller that "follows" a voltage waveform so that the resulting chair motion reproduces the commanded velocity profile. Recent implementations of this approach have included a digital computer that generates the waveform used to drive the servo-controller. The computer is often programmed for additional functions such as storage of the resulting eye movement responses and computation of specific input–output characteristics.

## Types of Motion

Two stimulus profiles that have been used recently under computer control are a sinusoidal velocity, with selectable frequency and amplitude, and a pseudorandom rotational acceleration, with a mixture of frequencies and selectable amplitude. A comparison of sinusoidal and pseudorandom stimulus waveforms is shown in Figure 9-16.

The sinusoidal stimulus differs from that generated by the torsion swing in two important aspects.

It has a constant amplitude, as opposed to one that decays due to friction, and it has an adjustable frequency, as opposed to one that is fixed. In practice, four or more periods of each frequency are delivered. The sequential use of a range of frequencies provides a useful comparison of eye movement response characteristics across that range.

The pseudorandom acceleration profile can be viewed as a mixture of many individual sinusoidal frequencies, delivered simultaneously as a combined stimulus. It is generated by a computer program that ensures specific characteristics, such as equal amplitude, for each of the combined frequencies. Advantages of this approach include its efficiency and unpredictability. It is efficient in the sense that all stimulus frequencies can be delivered in the same time required to deliver only the lowest frequency when individual sinusoids are used. Moreover, the subject cannot predict the pseudorandom profile due to its irregular nature, which eliminates the possibility that conscious prediction could bias the results.

## Eye Movement Response Patterns to Rotational Stimuli

Eye movements resulting from rotational testing are composed of slow and fast phases of nystagmus. The slow phase is under command of the vestibuloocular system, whereas the fast phase is commanded by the paramedian pontine reticular formation, a brain stem center that is also responsible for the generation of saccadic eye movements. The periodic stimulus profile results in frequent changes in the direction of nystagmus, in contrast to the nystagmus "beating" occurring in caloric testing, which can be unidirectional over relatively long time epochs. These directional changes require a specialized form of analysis so that the eye movement responses can be properly related to the input stimuli. In general, it is necessary to identify the beginning and end of fast phases in order that their occurrence can be "ignored" by the subsequent analysis. The slow phases are then "reconstructed" by repositioning to produce "cumulative eye position" in the absence of fast phases. Figure 9-17B shows slow-phase position as reconstructed from the eye position from the eye position record-

**Fig. 9-16.** Acceleration and velocity profiles for one complete period of **(A,B)** a sinusoidal and **(C,D)** a pseudorandom binary sequence (PRBS) stimulus. **(A)** One sinusoidal velocity period, frequency = 0.0078 Hz, amplitude = ± 318 degrees/sec. **(B)** Acceleration corresponding to **A.** **(C)** PRBS velocity profile of 255 sequence states (state duration = 0.5 sec), with amplitude = ± 16 degrees/sec². **(D)** Acceleration profile corresponding to **C;** The bandwidth of this profile is 0.0078 to 0.66 Hz. (Furman JM, O'Leary DP, Wolfe JW: Application of linear system analysis to the horizontal vestibulo-ocular reflex fo the alert rhesus monkey using pseudorandom binary sequence and single frequency sinusoidal stimulation. Biol Cybern 33:159, 1979.)

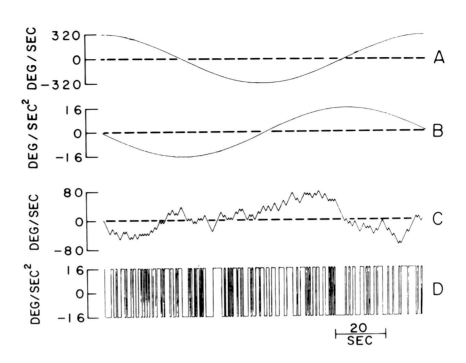

**Fig. 9-17.** Method of reconstructing nystagmus slow-phase cumulative eye position (CEP) by identifying and removing fast phases. **(A)** Eye position responses obtained from an alert rhesus monkey during PRBS rotational acceleration. **(B)** Slow-phase CEP following identification and removal of fast phases and reconstruction of the waveform with a computer algorithm. (Furman JM, O'Leary DP, Wolfe JW: Application of linear system analysis to the horizontal vestibulo-ocular reflex of the alert rhesus monkey using pseudorandom binary sequence and single frequency sinusoidal stimulation. Biol Cybern 33:159, 1979.)

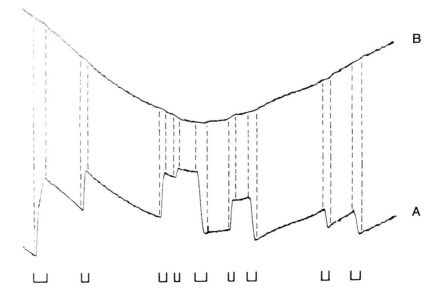

ing of Figure 9-17A. The resulting reconstructed waveform contains only information derived from the vestibular-commanded slow-phase components.

### Gain and Phase Analysis

Linear systems analysis of the VOR cumulative eye position results in relatively accurate gain and phase descriptors, because of the apparent linearity of this system over a wide physiological range. However, for practical reasons, different frequency ranges have been used for different purposes. Low-frequency testing includes a frequency range from 0.01 to 0.2 Hz, approximately. Phase changes in this range are used frequently for testing patients with vestibular disorders.[104–106]

Most passive rotational chairs have a practical limit of about 2 Hz. But recent studies have tested the human VOR at higher frequency ranges. The use of both higher power chair systems[107–109] and also active head movements[110–112] have provided VOR gain and phase data over extended ranges. Figure 9-18 shows one example of head velocity, eye position, and eye velocity information from the horizontal VOR of a human subject resulting from active head movements which linearly increased in frequency over an 18-second test epoch.[112] Although relatively new, testing the VOR above 2 Hz has certain practical advantages. (1) The smooth-pursuit tracking system does not operate at these frequencies, and therefore it does not corrupt the resulting eye movements with visually induced responses. (2) Natural head motions occur frequently in this range. (3) Fast phases do not occur, at least for small-amplitude head motions. These factors appear useful in new approaches to practical VOR testing, which include accurate monitoring of active head movements.[112]

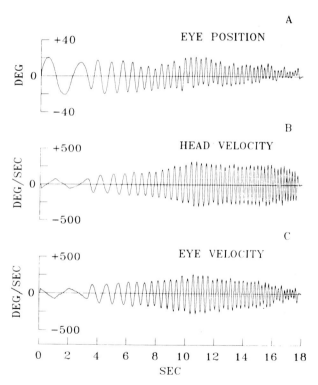

**Fig. 9-18. (A)** Eye position, **(B)** head velocity, **(C)** eye velocity responses from one human subject undergoing active horizontal head shaking for 18 seconds at linearly increasing frequencies from 0.5 to about 6 Hz. VOR responses past 6 seconds were faster than 2 Hz, which is above the range of visual tracking and therefore were not influenced by visual oculomotor systems. Note the absence of nystagmic fast phases at these frequencies.

## PHYSIOLOGICAL BASIS OF THE CALORIC TEST

The caloric test is used widely for diagnostic screening of unilateral peripheral vestibular disorders. In practice, the ear canal is perfused with air or water that is either warmer or cooler than body temperature, with the patient reclining with head positioned so that the lateral canal is in the vertical plane. After a short time, nystagmic eye movements can be observed in healthy subjects, with the direction of the fast phase toward the warm side. Why should this occur? The commonly accepted explanation is based on the action of convection currents in the endolymph of the semicircular canals. This process is shown in Figure 9-19.

Warm water in the ear canal results in gradual warming of the surrounding regions. As a region of the temporal bone slowly heats up, an adjacent part

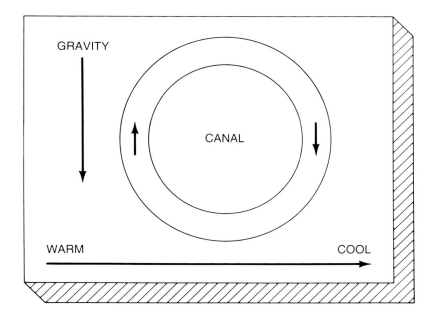

**Fig. 9-19.** Convection hypothesis of caloric stimulation of the semicircular canal. The canal is shown in the presence of a thermal gradient in the temporal bone, which causes one limb of the canal to become warmer than the other. Fluid in the warm limb becomes less dense, and therefore lighter, than fluid in the cooler limb. When the canal is oriented in the vertical plane, gravity causes the cooler fluid to sink, and the warmer fluid to rise, which results in a unilateral pressure on the cupula from the warmer to the cooler side.

of the lateral semicircular canal becomes a fraction of a degree warmer than the more medial regions of that receptor. This results in endolymph in the warmer region becoming less dense (and therefore lighter) than endolymph in the opposite, more medial region. With the plane of the canal oriented vertically, the cooler fluid tends to sink, under the influence of the gravitational pull on the heavier endolymph. The result of this action is a tendency for the endolymph to rotate inside the membranous walls of the canal and to exert pressure on the cupula. This acts as a strong unilateral stimulus, without an accompanying stimulus on the contralateral side.

Central processing of vestibular information is based on the normal occurrence of bilateral stimulation during head rotations. Therefore, a strong unilateral stimulus results in central vestibular activity that is strongly weighted in an unusual manner, and the subsequent processing of neural signals causes the observed pattern of nystagmus.

Caloric testing is widely used for diagnostic screening for peripheral vestibular pathology. In its most common use, caloric-induced nystagmus is amplified and displayed on a chart recorder (electronystagmography, ENG). The resulting patterns of nystagmus are then scanned visually and/or

measured numerically and then compared with patterns obtained from patients with known pathologic conditions.

## POSTURAL CONTROL MECHANISMS

Human bipedal motion is based on a restabilization of upright position with each step, and a moment-to-moment stabilization while standing. Effective stabilization of various parts of the body are due to the labyrinthine tonic (or static) reflexes. A change of head position induces systemic changes in postural reflexes that govern the limbs, trunk, and neck. Tonic labyrinthine reflex controlling position of the neck is considered to be a closed-loop control for holding head position, but the tonic labyrinthine reflexes operating on the trunk and limbs are thought to be under open-loop control because the labyrinthine receptors are not necessarily affected by immediate postural changes in the trunk and limbs.[8]

Effects of vestibular lesions on body equilibrium function of squirrel monkeys indicated a minimal effect after a unilateral saccular macula ablation.[113] This suggested that the utricular input (along with canal contributions) was more important than that of the saccule for maintaining body equilibrium.

Postural responses were studied in cats by measuring the forces applied by each limb to bring the animal to various supporting stances.[114] Similarly, the variability of postural "reflexes" in humans was analyzed by recording electromyographic (EMG)

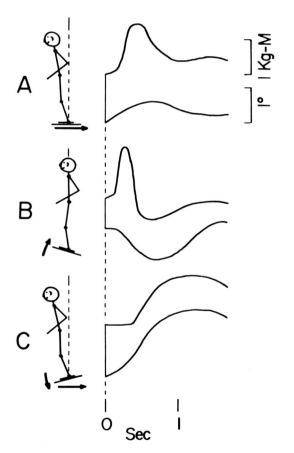

**Fig. 9-20.** *Left:* three methods for postural stimulation with a moving platform to achieve: **(A)** anteroposterior sway, **(B)** ankle rotation, **(C)** ankle stabilization by platform rotation proportional to the angle of induced anteroposterior sway. *Right:* time course of ankle reaction torque on platform base and the anteroposterior sway angle are shown for each mode of stimulation. (Nashner LM: Fixed patterns of rapid postural responses among leg muscles during stance. Exp Brain Res 30:13, 1977.)

responses of subjects standing on a force-measuring plaform.[115] The platform could be rotated in pitch around an axis aligned with the subject's ankle joint. Tilting the platform toe-up while leaning backward led to an increase of the latency of stabilizing responses from triceps surae muscle and to a decrease of response latency in the anterior tibial muscle. These latency changes, which functionally destabilize posture, can be suppressed or compensated for by reflexive cocontractions of antagonists.

Nashner[116] showed evidence that rapid postural responses among human leg muscles during stance are activated according to fixed patterns, by using a moving force platform (Fig. 9-20). Extensions to other induced motions reinforced the concept that the resulting patterns of EMG activity were highly specific for each kind of displacement and that subjects could reorganize the activity patterns from one form to another even following unexpected stimulus changes.[117]

Vision is an important sensory input in the dynamics of postural control. A moving visual surround during maintenance of upright posture on either a stationary platform[118] or on a moving cart[119] caused changes in body posture, under controlled conditions of relative motion of the subject and the visual surround. This effect is a result of the familiar perceptual illusion of translation while remaining stationary in the presence of a moving visual surround (railroad illusion). Prolonged optical reversal of vision resulted in marked decrease in the ability of human subjects to maintain balance while standing or walking on flat wooden rails, with eyes open or closed.[120] Results showed systematic pattern of adaptive changes in postural control, with the plastic nature of these changes indicated by their long-term retention and complete reversibility. Qualitative observations resembled clinical complaints: marked nausea, erroneous movements of the visual scene on rotating the head, and strange sensations of movement when lying down with eyes closed.

The above postural control elements are the basis for a recent method of computerized vestibulospinal testing[121] using two or more vertical force sensors to measure the dynamics of sway during standing. This test resembles that of Romberg,[122] updated with quantitative methods of determining direction, amplitude, and frequency of sway.

In addition to modeling with neural control elements, recent mathematic modeling of posturography[123] is based on simplified, biped-robot, linked models of human postural adjustments,[124] and these models are used to analyze types of feedback networks that can stabilize such robots. Models that combine both neural control elements and also robotic biped models will undoubtedly be a dominant direction in future descriptions of the vestibular physiology of posture and coordinated motion.

---

# REFERENCES

1. Wiener N: Cybernetics. MIT Press, Cambridge, MA, 1948
2. Marmarelis PZ, Marmarelis VZ: Analysis of Physiological Systems. Plenum Press, New York, 1978
3. O'Leary DP: Identification of sensory systems and neuronal systems. p. 77. In Barker, HA, Young, PC (eds): Identification and System Parameter Estimation. International Federation of Automatic Control 7th Symp. Pergamon Press, New York, 1985
4. O'Leary DP, Black FO, Wall C, Traini C: Distributed computer system for hierarchical control of a clinical vestibular laboratory. J Med Syst 4:227, 1980
5. Hillman DE, McLaren JW: Displacement configuration of semicircular canal cupulae. Neuroscience 4:1989, 1979
6. Steinhausen W: Uber den nachweis der bewegung der cupula in der intakten bogengangsampulle des labyrinthes bei der naturlichen rotatorischen and calorischen reizung. Pflugers Arch Ges Physiol 228:322, 1931
7. Steinhausen W: Uber die beobachtung der cupula in den bogengangsampullen des labyrinths des lebenden hechts. Pflugers Arch Ges Physiol 232:500, 1933
8. Ito M: The Cerebellum and Neural Control. Raven Press, New York, 1984
9. Egmond AAJ, Groen JJ, Jongkees BWL: The mechanics of the semicircular canal. J Physiol (Lond) 110:1, 1949
10. Wilson VJ, Melvill Jones G: Mammalian Vestibular Physiology, Plenum Press, New York, 1979
11. McLaren JW, Hillman, DE: Displacement of the semicircular canal cupula during sinusoidal rotation. Neuroscience 4:1989, 2001
12. Trincker D: Electrophysiological studies of the labyrinth of the guinea pig. Ann Otol Rhinol Laryngol 68:145, 1959
13. Valli P, Zucca G: The origin of slow potentials in semicircular canals of the frog. Acta Otolaryngol (Stockh) 81:395, 1976
14. Groen JJ, Lowenstein O, Vendrik AJH: The mechanical analysis of the responses from the end organs of the horizontal semi-circular canal of the isolated elasmobranch labyrinth. J Physiol (Lond) 117:329, 1952
15. Fernandez C, Goldberg JM: Physiology of peripheral neurons innervating semicircular canals of the squirrel monkey, II. Response to sinusoidal stimulation and dynamics of peripheral vestibular system. J Neurophysiol 34:661, 1971
16. O'Leary DP, Dunn RF, Honrubia V: Analysis of afferent responses from isolated semicircular canal of the guitarfish using rotational acceleration white-noise inputs. I,II. J Neurophysiol 39:631, 1976
17. Anastasio TJ, Correia MJ, Perachio AA: Spontaneous and driven responses of semicircular canal primary afferents in the unanesthetized pigeon. J Neurophysiol 54:335, 1985
18. Tomko DL, Peterka RJ, Schor RH, O'Leary DP: Response dynamics of horizontal canal afferents in barbiturate-anesthetized cats. J Neurophysiol 45:376, 1981
19. O'Leary DP, Honrubia V: On-line identification of sensory systems using pseudorandom binary noise perturbations. Biophys J 15:505, 1975
20. Hartmann R, Klinke R: Discharge properties of afferent fibres of the goldfish semicircular canal with high frequency stimulation. Pflugers Arch 388:111, 1980
21. Precht W, Llinas R, Clarke M: Physiological responses of frog vestibular fibers to horizontal angular rotation. Exp Brain Res 13:378, 1971
22. Segal BN, Outerbridge JS: A nonlinear model of semicircular canal primary afferents in bullfrog. J Neurophysiol 47:563, 1982
23. O'Leary DP, Wall C, III: Analysis of nonlinear afferent response properties from the guitarfish semicircular canal. Adv Otorhinolaryngol 25:66, 1979
24. Fernandez C, Goldberg JM: Physiology of peripheral neurons innervating otolith organs of the squirrel monkey. I. Response to static tilts and to long-duration centrifugal force. J Neurophysiol 39:970, 1976
25. Fernandez C, Goldberg JM: Physiology of peripheral neurons innervating otolith organs of the squirrel monkey. II. Directional selectivity and

force-response relations. J Neurophysiol 39:985, 1976

26. Fernandez C, Goldberg JM: Physiology of peripheral neurons innervating otolith organs of the squirrel monkey. III. Response dynamics. J Neurophysiol 39:996, 1976

27. Sala O: The efferent vestibular system: Electrophysiological research. Acta Otolaryngol [Suppl] (Stockh) 197:1, 1965

28. Dieringer N, Blanks RHI, Precht W: Cat efferent vestibular system: Weak suppression of primary afferent activity. Neurosci Lett 5:285, 1977

29. Goldberg JM, Fernandez C: Efferent vestibular system in the squirrel monkey: anatomical location and influence on afferent activity. J Neurophysiol 43:986, 1980

30. Highstein SM, Baker R: Action of the efferent vestibular system on primary afferent in the toadfish, *Opsanus tau.* J Neurophysiol 54:370, 1985

31. Stein BM, Carpenter MB: Central projections of portions of the vestibular ganglia innervating specific parts of the labyrinth in the Rhesus monkey. Am J Anat 120:281, 1976

32. Gacek RR: The course and central termination of first order neurons supplying vestibular endorgans in the cat. Acta Otolaryngol [Suppl] (Stockh) 254:1, 1969

33. Brodal A: Anatomy of the vestibular nuclei and their connections. p. 239. In Kornhuber HH (ed): Handbook of Sensory Physiology. Vol. 6. Vestibular System. Springer-Verlag, New York, 1974

34. Precht W, Shimazu H: Functional connections of tonic and kinetic vestibular neurons with primary vestibular afferents. J Neurophysiol 28:1014, 1965

35. Shimazu H, Precht W: Tonic and kinetic responses of cat's vestibular neurons to horizontal angular acceleration. J Neurophysiol 28:991, 1965

36. Ito M, Hongo T, Okada Y: Vestibular-evoked postsynaptic potentials in Deiters' neurones. Exp Brain Res 7:214, 1969

37. Hwang JC, Poon WF: An electrophysiological study of the sacculo-ocular pathways in cats. Jpn J Physiol 25:241, 1975

38. Shimazu H, Smith CM: Cerebellar and labyrinthine influence on single vestibular neurons identified by natural stimuli. J Neurophysiol 34:493, 1971

39. Peterson BW: Distribution of neural responses to tilting within vestibular nuclei of the cat. J Neurophysiol 33:1421, 1970

40. Curthoys IS, Markham CH: Convergence of labyrinthine influences on units in the vestibular nuclei of the cat. I. Natural stimulation. Brain Res 35:469, 1971

41. Abend WK: Functional organization of the superior vestibular nucleus of the squirrel monkey. Brain Res 132:65, 1977

42. Adrian ED: Discharges from vestibular receptors in the cat. J Physiol (Lond) 101:389, 1943

43. Fuchs A, Kimm J: Unit activity in vestibular nucleus of the alert monkey during horizontal angular acceleration and eye movement. J Neurophysiol 38:1140, 1975

44. Melvill Jones G, Milsum JH: Frequency response analysis of central vestibular unit activity resulting from rotation stimulation of the semicircular canals. J Physiol (Lond) 219:191, 1971

45. Melvill Jones G, Milsum JH: Characteristics of neural transmission from the semicircular canal to the vestibular nuclei of cats. J Physiol (Lond) 209:295, 1970

46. Shinoda Y, Yoshida K: Dynamic characteristics of responses to horizontal head angular acceleration in the vestibulo-ocular pathway in the cat. J Neurophysiol 37:653, 1974

47. Shimazu H, Precht W: Inhibition of central vestibular neurons from the contralateral labyrinth and its mediting pathway. J Neurophysiol 29:467, 1966

48. Precht W, Shimazu H, Markham CH: A mechanism of central compensation of vestibular function following hemilabyrinthectomy. J Neurophysiol 29:996, 1966

49. Kasahara M, Uchino Y: Bilateral semicircular canal inputs to neurons in cat vestibular nuclei. Exp Brain Res 20:285, 1974

50. Camis M: The physiology of the vestibular apparatus. Clarendon Press, Oxford, 1930

51. Wilson VJ, Kato M, Peterson BW, Wylie RM: A single-unit analysis of the organization of Deiters' nucleus. J Neurophysiol 30:603, 1967

52. Abzug C, Maeda M, Peterson BW, Wilson VJ: Cervical branching of lumbar vestibulospinal axons. J Physiol (Lond) 243:499, 1974

53. Ito M, Hongo T, Yoshida M, et al: Antidromic and transsynaptic activation of Deiters' neurones induced from the spinal cord. Jpn J Physiol 14:638, 1964

54. Orlovsky GN, Pavlova GA: Response of Deiters' neurons to tilt during locomotion. Brain Res 42:212, 1972

55. Rapoport S, Susswein A, Uchino Y, Wilson VJ: Properties of vestibular neurones projecting to neck segment of the cat spinal cord. J Physiol (Lond) 268:493, 1977

56. Akaike T, Fanardjian VV, Ito M, Nakajima H: Cerebellar control of vestibulospinal tract cells in rabbit. Exp Brain Res 18:446, 1973

57. Pompeiano O, Brodal A: The origin of vestibulospinal fibers in the cat. An experimental-anatomical study, with comments on the descending medial longitudinal fasciculus. Arch Ital Biol 95:166, 1957

58. Ito M, Kawai M, Udo M, Mano N: Axon reflex activation of deiters' neurons from the cerebellar cortex through collaterals of the cerebellar afferents. Exp Brain Res 8:249, 1969

59. Mori S, Mikami A: Excitation of Deiters' neurones by stimulation of the nerves to neck extensor muscles. Brain Res 56:331, 1973

60. Precht W, Grippo J, Wagner A: Contribution of different types of central vestibular neurons to the vestibulospinal system. Brain Res 4:119, 1967

61. Wilson VJ, Maeda M: Connections between semicircular canals and neck motoneurons in the cat. J Neurophysiol 37:346, 1974

62. Fredrickson JM, Schwarz D: Multisensory influence upon single units in the vestibular nucleus. p. 203. In Graybiel A (ed): The Role of the Vestibular Organs in Space Exploration. NASA SP-187, Washington DC, 1970

63. Akaike T, Fanardjian VV, Ito M, Ohno T: Electrophysiological analysis of the vestibulospinal reflex pathway of rabbit. II. Synaptic actions upon spinal neurones. Exp Brain Res 17:497, 1973

64. Wilson VJ, Wylie RM, Marco LA: Synaptic inputs to cells in the medial vestibular nucleus. J Neurophysiol 31:176, 1968

65. Peterson BW, Filion M, Felpel LP, Abzug C: Responses of medial reticular neurons to stimulation of the vestibular nerve. Exp Brain Res 22:335, 1975

66. Ito M, Udo M, Mano N: Long inhibitory and excitatory pathways converging onto cat reticular and Deiters' neurones and their relevance to reticulofugal axons. J Neurophysiol 33:210, 1970

67. Grillner S, Lund S: The origin of a descending pathway with monosynaptic action on flexor motoneurones. Acta Physiol Scand 74:274, 1968

68. Wilson VJ, Yoshida M: Bilateral connections between labyrinths and neck motoneurons. Brain Res 13:603, 1969

69. Anderson JH, Soechting JF, Terzuolo CA: Dynamic relations between natural vestibular inputs and activity of forelimb extensor muscles in the decerebrate cat. I. Motor output during sinusoidal linear accelerations. Brain Res 120:1, 1977

70. O'Leary DP, Ravasio MJ: Simulation of vestibular semicircular canal responses during righting movements of a freely falling cat. Biol Cybern 50:1, 1984

71. Furman JM, O'Leary DP, Wolfe JW: Application of linear system analysis to the horizontal vestibuloocular reflex of the alert rhesus monkey using pseudorandom binary sequence and single frequency sinusoidal stimulation. Biol Cybern 33:159, 1979

72. O'Leary DP, Furman JM, Wolfe JW: Use of pseudorandom angular acceleration in the evaluation of vestibuloocular function. p. 107. In Honrubia V, Brazier MAB (eds): Nystagmus and Vertigo. Academic Press, Orlando, FL, 1982

73. Correia MJ, Perachio AA, Eden AR: The monkey vertical vestibulo-ocular response: A frequency domain study. J Neurophysiol 54:532, 1985

74. Robinson DA: The use of control systems analysis in the neurophysiology of eye movements. Annu Rev Neurosci 4:463, 1981

75. Young LR: Pursuit eye tracking movements. p. 429. In Bach-y-Rita P, Collins CC (eds): Control of Eye Movements. Academic Press, Orlando, FL, 1971

76. Robinson DA: Vestibular and optokinetic symbiosis: an example of explaining by modelling. p. 49. In Baker R, Berthoz A (eds): Control of Gaze by Brian Stem Neurons. Elsevier, New York, 1977

77. Gonshor AG, Melvill Jones G: Extreme vestibuloocular adaptation induced by prolonged optical reversal of vision. J Physiol (Lond) 26:381, 1976

78. Melvill Jones G: Plasticity in the adult vestibuloocular reflex arc. Philos Trans R Soc Lond [Biol] 278:319, 1977

79. Robinson DA: Adaptive gain control of the vestibuloocular reflex by the cerebellum. J Neurophysiol 39:954, 1976

80. Miles FA, Fuller JH: Adaptive plasticity in the vestibuloocular responses of the rhesus monkey. Brain Res 80:512, 1974

81. Gauthier GM, Robinson DA: Adaptation of the human vestibuloocular reflex to magnifying lenses. Brain Res 92:331, 1975

82. Miles FA, Eighmy BB: Long-term adaptive changes in primate vestibuloocular reflex. I. Behavioral observations. J Neurophysiol 43:1406, 1980

83. Benson AJ, Barnes GR: Vision during angular oscillation: the dynamic interaction of visual and vestibular mechanisms. Aviat Space Environ Med 49:340, 1978

84. Skavenski AA, Hansen RM, Steinman RM, Winterson BM: Quality of retinal image stabilization dur-

ing small natural and artificial body rotations in man. Vision Res 19:675, 1979

85. Eccles JC, Ito M, Szentagothai J: The Cerebellum as a Neuronal Machine. Springer-Verlag, New York, 1967

86. Marr D: A theory of cerebellar cortex. J Physiol (Lond) 202:437, 1969

87. Albus JS: A theory of cerebellar function. Math Biosciences 10:25, 1971

88. Ito M: Questions in modeling the cerebellum. J Theor Biol 99:81, 1982

89. Fujita M: Adaptive filter model of the cerebellum. Biol Cybern 45:195, 1982

90. Fujita M: Simulation of adaptive modification of the vestibulo-ocular reflex with an adaptive filter model of the cerebellum. Biol Cybern 45:207, 1982

91. Pellionicz A, Llinàs R: The tensor concept of brain functin: A theory of the cerebellum. p. 394. In Amari S, Arbib MA (eds): Competition and Cooperation in Neural Nets. Springer-Verlag, New York, 1982

92. Pellionicz A, Llinàs R: Brain modeling by tensor network theory and computer simulation. The cerebellum: distributed processor for predictive coordination. Neuroscience 4:323, 1979

93. Ito M, Shiida N, Yagi N, Yamamoto M: The cerebellar modification of rabbit's horizontal vestibulo-ocular reflex induced by sustained head rotation combined with visual stimulation. Proc Jpn Acad 50:85, 1974

94. Haddad GM, Demer JL, Robinson DA: The effect of lesions of the dorsal cap of the inferior olive and the vestibulo-ocular and optokinetic systems of the cat. Brain Res 185:265, 1980

95. Gauthier GM, Marchetti E, Pellet J: Cerebellar control of vestibulo-ocular reflex (VOR) studied with injection of harmaline in the trained baboon. Arch Ital Biol 121:19, 1983

96. Ito M, Nisimaru N, Yamamoto M: Pathways for the vestibulo-ocular reflex excitation arising from semicircular canals of rabbits. Exp Brain Res 24:257, 1976

97. Galiana HL, Outerbridge JS: A bilateral model for central neural pathways in vestibuloocular reflex. J Neurophysiol 51:210, 1984

98. Galiana HL, Flohr H, Melville Jones G: A reevaluation of intervestibular nuclear coupling: its role in vestibular compensation. J Neurophysiol 51:242, 1984

99. Crampton GH: Habituation of ocular nystagmus of vestibular origin. p. 337. In Bender MB (ed): The

Oculomotor System. Harper & Row, New York, 1964

100. Jager J, Henn V: Habituation of the vestibul-ocular reflex (VOR) in the monkey during sinusoidal rotation in the dark. Exp Brain Res 41:108, 1981

101. Wolfe JW: Evidence for control of nystagmic habituation by folium-tuber vermis and fastigial nuclei. Acta Otolaryngol [suppl] (Stockh) 231:1, 1968

102. Paige GD: Vestibuloocular reflex and its interactions with visual following mechanisms in the squirrel monkey. II. Response characteristics and plasticity following unilateral inactivation of horizontal canal. J Neurophysiol 49:152, 1983

103. Barany R: Augenbewegungen, durch Thoraxbewegungen ausgelost. Zentralbl Physiol 20:298, 1906

104. Wolfe JW, Engelken EJ, Olson FE: Low-frequency harmonic acceleration in the evaluation of patients with peripheral labyrinthine disorders. p. 95. In Honrubia V, Brazier MAB (eds): Nystagmus and Vertigo. Academic Press, Orlando, FL, 1982

105. Hess K, Baloh RW, Honrubia V: Rotational testing in patients with bilateral peripheral vestibular disease. Laryngoscope 95:95, 1985

106. Yee RD, Jenkins HA, Baloh RW, et al: Vestibular-optokinetic interaction in normal subjects and in patients with peripheral vestibular disfunction. J Otolaryngol 7:310, 1978

107. Istl YE, Hyden D, Schwarz DWF: Quantification and localization of vestibular loss in unilaterally labyrinthectomized patients using a precise rotatory test. Acta Otolaryngol (Stockh) 96:437, 1983

108. Hyden D, Istl YE, Schwarz DWF: Human visuo-vestibular interaction as a basis for quantitative clinical diagnostics. Acta Otolaryngol (Stockh) 94:53, 1982

109. Hyden D, Larsby B, Schwarz DWF, Odkvist LM: Quantification of slow compensatory eye movements in patients with bilateral vestibular loss. Acta Otolaryngol (Stockh) 96:199, 1983

110. Takahashi M, Uemura T, Fujishior T: Studies of the visual-vestibular interactions during active head movements. Acta Otolaryngol (Stockh) 90:115, 1980

111. Tomlinson RD, Saunders GE, Schwarz DWF: Analysis of human vestibuloocular reflex during active head movements. Acta Otolaryngol (Stockh) 90:184, 1980

112. Fineberg R, O'Leary DP, Davis LL: Use of active head movements for computerized vestibular testing. Archive Otolaryngol (in press)

113. Igarashi M, Kato Y: Effect of different vestibular

lesions upon body equilibrium function in squirrel monkeys. Acta Otolaryngol [Suppl] (Stockh) 330:91, 1975

114. Coulmance M, Gahery Y, Massion J, Swett JE: The placing reaction in the standing cat: a model for the study of posture and movement. Exp Brain Res 37:265, 1979

115. Diener HC, Bootz F, Dichgans J, Bruzek W: Variability of postural "reflexes" in humans. Exp Brain Res 52:423, 1983

116. Nashner LM: Fixed patterns of rapid postural responses among leg muscles during stance. Exp Brain Res 30:13, 1977

117. Nashner LM, Woollacott M, Tuma G: Organization of rapid responses to postural and locomotor-like perturbation of standing man. Exp Brain Res 35:463, 1979

118. Lestienne F, Soechting J, Berthoz A: Postural readjustments induced by linear motion of visual scenes. Exp Brain Res 28:363, 1977

119. Soechting JF, Berthoz A: Dynamic role of vision in the control of posture in man. Exp Brain Res 36:551, 1979

120. Gonshor A, Melvill Jones G: Postural adaptation to prolonged optical reversal of vision in man. Brain Res 192:239, 1980

121. Black FO, Wall C, III, O'Leary DP: Computerized screening of the human vestibulospinal system. Ann Otol Rhinol Laryngol 87:853, 1978

122. Romberg, MH: In Manual of the Nervous Diseases of Man, 2:396 Sydenham Society (London), 1853

123. Kodde L, Caberg HB, Mol JMF, Massen CH: An application of mathematical models in posturography. J Biomed Eng 4:44, 1982

124. Hemami H, Weimer FC, Robinson CS, et al: Biped stability consideration with vestibular models. IEEE Trans Autom Control AC-23:1074, 1978

# Section 2

# EVALUATION AND ASSESSMENT

# Temporal Bone Imaging: Conventional and Computed Tomography

# 10

Arnold M. Noyek
Edward E. Kassel

Diagnostic imaging is an integral component of the overall clinical evaluation of the temporal bone. Not all suspected temporal bone disease requires diagnostic imaging; however, many management decisions depend on effective radiologic evaluations. These examinations encompass conventional radiographic studies as well as high-technology studies such as computed tomography (CT) and magnetic resonance imaging (MRI).

The advent of CT[1] has made conventional temporal bone radiology[2-6] obsolete in many parts of the world. However, otologic disease affects the entire world's population, irrespective of the diagnostic facilities available, so it is still important to be able to obtain maximum information by conventional plain film temporal bone radiographs.

This and the following chapters provide a conceptual approach to temporal bone imaging, accepting such realities. These chapters are organized as follows:

1. A concept of radiographic interpretation in temporal bone evaluation
2. A discussion of the imaging modalities
3. The current role of diagnostic imaging in temporal bone disease

## A CONCEPT OF RADIOGRAPHIC INTERPRETATION IN TEMPORAL BONE EVALUATION

Radiologic examinations are particularly applicable to the temporal bone, where structural abnormalities may lie beyond the range of the otoscope (and microscope), and many physiological abnormalities cannot be assessed by audiometric and vestibular tests. A valid working diagnosis must deal with both qualitative and quantitative parameters; diagnostic imaging can contribute substantially in both these areas.

The complex anatomy of the temporal bone does not exist in isolation; it is in immediate relation to other structures about the petrous apex—the middle cranial fossa, the posterior cranial fossa, and the adjacent skull base. The temporal bone may also be affected by systemic disorders; involvement of the temporal bone may result in complications, both of the disease itself and of its surgical/medical treatment.

Radiographic imaging rarely provides such a specific working diagnosis as, for example, the recognition of a fracture line or the thickened bone of

255

Paget's disease. More commonly, the radiologist suggests a "group disorder" diagnosis, which nevertheless is very management-directive. Bone-destructive disease for example, often implies surgical disease; suspected vascular disease implies its own set of interventional diagnostic directions.

Radiographic imaging can contribute in its major role to quantitative diagnosis; mass lesions can be quantified in all three dimensions, in both soft tissue and bony imaging modes, and extension of disease beyond definable intratemporal and extratemporal boundaries can be recognized. Intracranial extension of inflammatory temporal bone disease, for example, is easily recognized when high-technology imaging with CT or MRI is used. Temporal bone disease may be still further quantified by the recognition of specific anatomic abnormalities (e.g., cholesteatomatous erosion of the labyrinth, cerebrospinal fluid leak) and the recognition of specific physiological activity (e.g. biologic staging of osteomyelitis as active, effectively/ineffectively treated, healed, etc.). Radionuclide scans (bone and gallium scans) provide this physiological information. Finally, diagnostic imaging may permit the identification of focal temporal bone disease as a manifestation of a systemic disorder, or it may contribute to the recognition of primary temporal bone pathology disseminated beyond its origin. Close collaboration between otologist and radiologist is essential if full use is to be obtained from imaging and if mistakes are to be avoided.

The major radiologic signs are morphologic in nature and are based on alteration of normal bone (or other tissue) configuration and/or density. In conventional studies (plain films, complex motion tomography) the human eye is capable of, and limited to, recognizing differentials of 16 shades of gray, permitting the detection of structural bony abnormality. In CT, digitization of the information extends the gray scale dramatically, thereby demonstrating additional soft tissue and bony abnormalities. All these imaging studies, however, depend on the precise recognition of the normal air spaces of the middle ear cleft and its adnexae (attic, antrum, mastoid air cells). These delicate, mucosa-lined spaces do not, in a healthy person, provide radiologically recognizable soft tissue abnormali-

ties. Only when the air spaces are filled with fluid, mucosal thickening, or mass lesions are the air spaces obliterated and radiologically identifiable. The residual air spaces may, however, profile soft tissue masses (tumor, cholesteatoma), and allow their better quantification.

Magnetic resonance imaging has the complementary ability to delineate soft tissue abnormalities through $T_1$- and $T_2$-weighted images; it does not recognize bone, by virtue of the fact that it does not image cortical bone, but it effectively images fatty marrow spaces. It also images nerves which may be transmitted through bone (in canals and through foramina).

The temporal bone and its bony subunits (tympanic, styloid, mastoid, petrous, squamous) lends itself readily to imaging by conventional plain films, complex motion tomography, and CT with extended bone numbers. The varying bone densities of the temporal bone, from the thin septate cellular air cell system to the densest of bone in the petrosa, are ideally studied by radiographic examinations. Bone density may be decreased or increased, either focally or diffusely. Each of these radiographic findings has its own specific possibility for interpretation.

The temporal bone may require selective assessment of specific components including the ossicles and a variety of foraminal and canalicular relationships. These fine anatomic structures can be studied with thin section slices.

Cranial nerves V through XII all pass into or close to the temporal bone. Each of their conducting foramina can be studied en face or in specific section using high-resolution imaging with CT bone windows. MRI permits actual imaging of individual nerves (and brain relationships). CT permits axial and coronal display; MRI permits display in all three planes, including the elusive sagittal plane. Complex motion tomography permits study of fine bony structures, in the plane of section, to a thickness of 1.0 mm; this permits effective blurring of other anatomic structures both before and beyond the plane. Bony detail may be quite dramatic at times, but generally CT offers more effective bone imaging; complex motion tomography offers minimal soft tissue information and is not an effective imaging modality for such observation.

Contrast agents can be used for specific diagnostic purposes: nonionic, intrathecal contrast agents (Iohexol, Iopamidal) may be given to identify a cerebrospinal fluid (CSF) leak by thin-section CT temporal bone examination; iodinated contrast demonstrates the vascular margination about a brain abscess on CT.

Intrathecal air in small amounts (approximately 3.0 cc) provides an excellent CT contrast for studying the contents of the internal auditory canal, specifically in the search for small intracanalicular acoustic neuromas. Formerly, Pantopaque was used intrathecally (with conventional plain film or tomographic studies) to reveal obstruction to entry of contrast medium from the subarachnoid space into the internal auditory canal itself. Now, in the late 1980s, MRI is becoming the definitive imaging modality for detecting acoustic neuromas, regardless of their size or location. It certainly allows definitive assessment of the internal auditory canal and its contents. Mass lesions can be outlined prolapsing through the porus acusticus into the cerebellopontine angle itself.

The vascular structures of the temporal bone are of interest. Currently, angiographic methods using superselective catheterization allow definitive study of the vascular anatomy of the temporal bone (arterial and venous). Intravenous digital subtraction angiography is the screening examination for preliminary assessment of suspected major vascular abnormalities greater than 1.0 cm. Digitized arterial studies permit increasingly effective imaging, particularly in the anatomic distribution of the ascending pharyngeal artery and its terminal inferior tympanic branch (the feeding arterial branch to the glomus tympanicum and the glomus jugulare tumors). Many arteriovenous malformations (AVM) have their distribution within the range of the occipital artery. Early venous filling suggests the rapid shunting of AV fistulae and high-flow malformations.

The successful interpretation of radiologic signs requires a clear knowledge of anatomy, physiology, and pathology as they affect the temporal bone.

## THE IMAGING MODALITIES

Imaging of the temporal bone will be discussed under the following subsections in this and the next two chapters:

Conventional plain films
Complex-motion tomography
Computed tomography (CT)
Magnetic resonance imaging (MRI)
Angiography
Radionuclide scanning

### Conventional Plain Films

Technical advances in skull film radiology, such as commercially available skull units, have enhanced plain film capabilities.[2-6] Such skull units permit proper centering and coning of the central ray to the area of particular interest. Here as elsewhere, familiarity and expertise in temporal bone imaging are important. Knowledge of the otologist's clinical concern and the patient's history is crucial to proper adjustments in technique.

The conventional film continues to give the best overview of the temporal bone. It remains the most universally available imaging modality and the least expensive. Such studies may be totally adequate to provide the anatomic information sought. For instance, a plain film of the mastoid air cells will confirm a clinical impression of mastoiditis.

The choice and number of projections[5,6] may be determined by the clinical history and availability of complementary studies (CT, MRI, conventional tomography).

Basic projections used vary from institution to institution. The development of various projections arose from the need to demonstrate various components of the temporal bone to best advantage.[1] This especially reflected the need to demonstrate the temporal bone in at least two radiographic planes (a basic radiologic principle applicable to all parts of the body); these two planes are preferably perpendicular to each other,

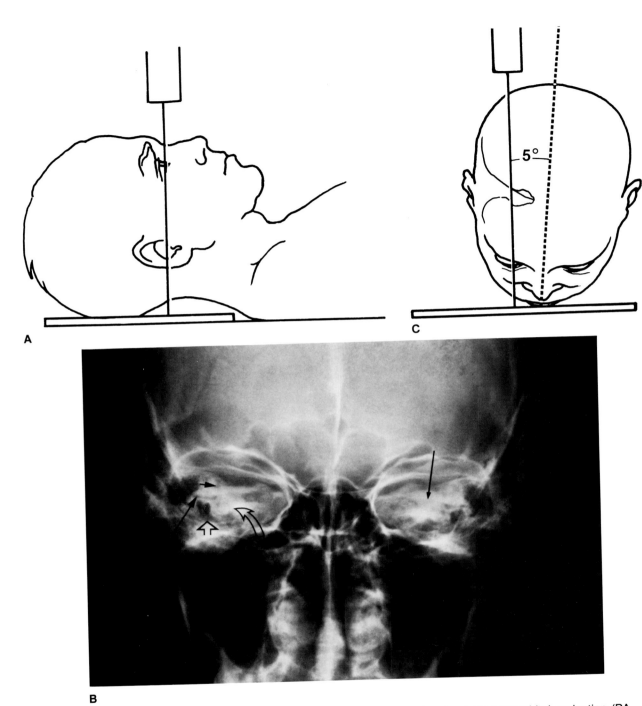

**Fig. 10-1.** Transorbital projections of temporal bones. **(A)** Lateral sketch of AP transorbital projection (PA projection may be used to reduce radiation to lens). **(B)** On radiograph, petrous bones are projected through orbits to reduce superimposition of shadows. Internal auditory canal (vertical arrow), SSCC (horizontal arrow), LSCC (oblique arrow), aerated tympanic cavity (open arrow), and cochlea (open curved arrow) are all well seen (bilateral petrous projection). **(C)** Guillen projection viewed from above. Incident beam (PA projection) is directed through ipsilateral orbit rather than through midline as for transorbital view. Sagittal plane rotated 5 to 15 degrees to ipsilateral such that tympanic cavity perpendicular to incident beam and ossicles are thrown clear of the medial tympanic wall (unilateral petrous projection).

and one should be perpendicular to the axis of the structure of maximal interest. Some projections will demonstrate both petrosa on a single film; other projections will be centered to the side of interest (with contralateral views for comparison). Projections may be classified as unilateral or bilateral, rotated or nonrotated. Projections may also be subclassified as to the anatomic area of maximal interest (mastoid views, views of the petrous bone in general, specific views for the attic-aditus-antrum, ossicles and middle ear, or petrous apex and internal auditory canals). The reader is referred to radiographic texts for more detailed discussion.[3,4,6,7]

The projections presented here are the frontal projection views, oblique frontal projection view, basal view, lateral, and lateral oblique views.

### Frontal Projection Views

**Transorbital, Anteroposterior or Posteroanterior.** The petrous bone is projected through the midportion of the orbit to offer the least amount of bone superimposition from the anterior aspect of the skull and facial bones (Fig. 10-1). The film is exposed to allow proper penetration of the dense bony labyrinth. The central ray is centered between the two orbits angled approximately 5 degrees caudally to the orbito-meatal line. This is a nonrotated projection with both sides seen simultaneously on a single film.

The transorbital projection is the premier plain film for demonstrating the internal auditory canals (IAC). Any measurements to assess the length and height of the IAC should be taken from this projection. The medial portions of the temporal bone have less superimposition of the mastoid air cells and therefore are more clearly demonstrated. The more medial portion of the external auditory canal (EAC) including the scutum is well seen. The lateral EAC, the floor of the EAC, and mastoid antrum tend to be obscured by the overlying mastoid air cells.

The anteroposterior (AP) projection is technically superior to the posteroanterior (PA) projection, offering greater detail and less magnification of the temporal bone. However, at our institutions,

we limit the use of this projection to older patients, since the radiation dose to the lens of the eye is six times that from a transorbital PA projection. The increase in detail must be balanced against the hazards of increased orbital radiation dosage.

**Transorbital (Guillen) View.** This projection differs from the "straight" transorbital skull projection by lateral rotation of the head. Only the ipsilateral petrous bone is imaged (Fig. 10-1C). This projection also is performed in the PA axis to decrease the radiation dose to the lens. The angulation of the central ray relative to the orbitomeatal line remains the same as for the more conventional transorbital view. The head (sagittal plane) is rotated 5 to 15 degrees to the ipsilateral side so that the ossicles are more clearly separated from the medial wall of the tympanic cavity. More specifically, the ossicles are thrown clear of the bone prominence of the lateral semicircular canal. The IAC is slightly foreshortened in this projection. The more medial projection of the mastoid air cells tend to obscure further details about the EAC and lateral aspects of the tympanic cavity.

This projection is favored for frontal tomography to demonstrate the ossicles and middle ear.

**Chaussé III Projection.** The patient remains in the same orbitomeatal position as for the transorbital and Guillen projections but the sagittal plane is rotated 5 to 10 degrees to the contralateral side (Fig. 10-2). The central ray again passes through the EAC; however, it will pass lateral to the outer canthus and lateral orbital rim, projecting the middle ear structures through the thinner portion of the greater wing of the sphenoid bone lateral to the orbit.

This projection is used to display the ossicles and tympanic cavity. The contralateral rotation displays the medial wall more "en face" than the conventional transorbital or Guillen projections; it may better assess some bony changes about the oval and round windows. As with the Guillen projections, the facial canal and lateral semicircular canal are well visualized. The sagittal rotation will result in the more posterior portion of the prominence overlying the lateral semicircular canal being projected tangential to the incident beam. The ossicles however, may be superimposed upon

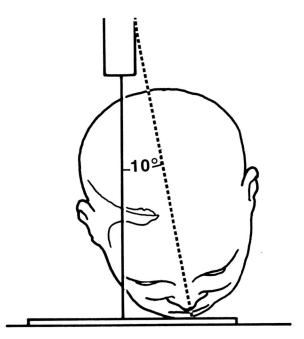

**Fig. 10-2.** Chaussé III projection viewed from above. The incident ray is directed through ipsilateral petrous bone, and the sagittal plane is rotated 5 to 10 degrees to the contralateral side. The incident beam passes through thin portion of the greater wing of the sphenoid, lateral to orbit. The relation of the incident beam to the orbital meatal line is the same as in the transorbital and Guillen projections (see Fig. 10-1A) (unilateral petrous projection).

the lateral semicircular canal, in contrast to the Guillen projection.

The 5 to 10 degrees of sagittal rotation projects the more posterior located mastoid air cells more laterally relative to the more anteriorly positioned tympanic cavity and EAC. More lateral portions of the tympanic cavity and EAC (e.g., the scutum) may be better seen on this projection, with less superimposition of the mastoid air cells than on the transorbital or Guillen projections.

**Towne Projection (30 Degree Frontal-Occipital or Half Axial Projection).** The Towne projection (Fig. 10-3) is a non-rotated view, displaying both sides simultaneously. The incident beam is angled caudally 30 degrees to the orbitomeatal line directed toward the occiput, through the level of the

EAC. If detail on one side only is required, the central ray may be centered through that petrous bone with coning restricted to that side for better resolution.

This projection is excellent for displaying the petrous ridge, mastoid antrum, and aditus ad antrum. The increased angulation (30 degree) from the orbitomeatal axis projects the antrum and aditus more en face and therefore more tangentially than the transorbital views, which partially superimpose the mastoid antrum upon the tympanic cavity as well as the mastoid air cells. The basal view, while having the advantage of greater angulation through the mastoid antrum, projects the mastoid antrum upon denser petrous structures more inferiorly as well as upon the tissues of the neck and shoulders.

The cochlea and IAC may be well displayed in this projection, but not as well as in the transorbital projection.

As with the other frontal projection studies, the PA or "reverse Towne" view is utilized in young patients to reduce the radiation dose to the lens. Unfortunately, this reverse projection is more difficult to obtain, and displays greater distortion and magnification of the petrous structures. To maximize resolution by reducing scatter radiation, the beam is coned using a slit diaphragm. If only one side is of interest, further coning may be used.

### Frontal Oblique Projection

The head is rotated 35 degrees to the sagittal plane, toward the contralateral side (oblique PA) in the so-called Stenver's projection (parallel projection of petrous ridge) (Fig. 10-4). This sagittal rotation brings the long axis of the petrous bone perpendicular to the incident beam, that is, the petrous bone to be studied lies in the transverse plane. This therefore gives an undistorted projection of the entire length of the petrous ridge. No foreshortening or superimposition of the mediolateral components upon each other is noted. The Stenver's projection is the best for assessing the integrity or continuity of the entire length of the petrous ridge. The petrous apex will be well displayed, including both the superior and inferior margins.

**Fig. 10-3.** Towne projection. **(A)** Lateral sketch of AP technique. Incident beam is angled 30 degrees to orbitomeatal line through occiput. **(B)** Petrous ridge (P, arrow) is well demonstrated. EAC (eac), IAC (iac), cochlea (c), and vestibule (v) are identified. Semicircular canals, projected superior to vestibule, are visualized but not labeled. Aditus ad antrum (a) and mastoid antrum (A) are projected more en face than for other frontal projections. M, mastoid air cells.

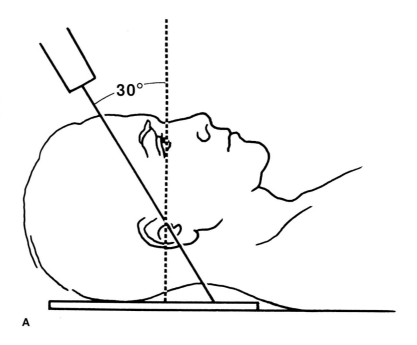

A

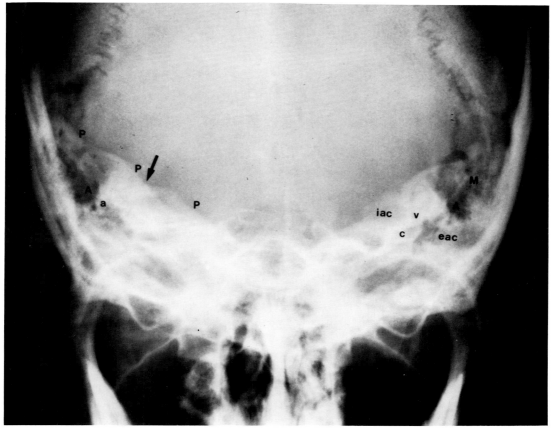

B

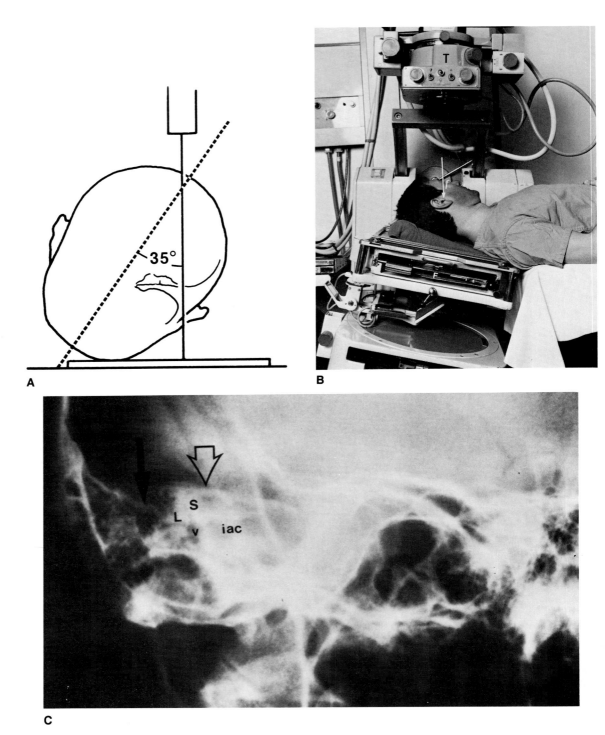

**Fig. 10-4.** Frontal oblique (Stenver's) projection: **(A)** Stenver's PA projection (viewed from above). The sagittal plane is rotated 35 degrees to the contralateral side. The long axis of the petrous bone is parallel to the film and perpendicular to the incident beam. **(B)** Positioning viewed from the side shows the slight (12 degrees) angulation caudally of the incident beam (arrow) relative to the orbitomeatal line (will be 12 degrees craniad in PA-directed study). **(C)** Radiograph. Head rotated to contralateral side displays the long axis of the ipsilateral petrous bone. The IAC, vestibule (v), SSCC (S), and LSCC (L) are well visualized. The mastoid antrum (solid arrow) and tegmen (open arrow) are also well seen. Mastoid air cells are partially obscured by superimposed occipital bone.

The IAC is well seen but foreshortened. The posterior lip of the meatus tends to be well seen. The vestibule, lateral semicircular canal (LSCC), and superior semicircular canal (SSCC) are also well displayed, with the vertical axis of the superior semicircular canal and the horizontal axis of the lateral semicircular canal perpendicular to the incident beam.

The head (sagittal plane) may be tilted 15 degrees away from the mastoid to be studied to prevent the shadow of the occipital bone from overlying the mastoid bone. The mastoid tip is well visualized without superimposed petrous bone. However, different exposure factors are required, with greater exposure (higher kilovoltage) needed to assess the petrous bone and decreased exposure (lower kilovoltage) if the mastoid tip is to be assessed.

This projection also is a favorite for conventional tomography, especially for assessing fractures through the petrous temporal bone.

### Submentovertex (Axial or Basal) Projection

In the classic position, the baseline (orbitomeatal line) is parallel to the film, with the incident ray centered midway between the angles of the mandible (Fig. 10-5).

To improve film quality, the temporal bone can be examined individually with the incident beam centered through the EAC. The views, however, are projected onto a single film to facilitate comparison and allow simultaneous development under identical conditions; this permits maximal comparison of the two sides, without differences due to processing techniques.

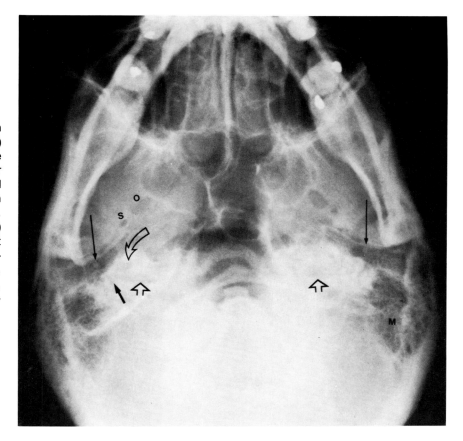

**Fig. 10-5.** Basal projection shows ossicles (long thin arrow) bilaterally as a "conglomerate density" surrounded by air within tympanic cavity. Internal auditory canals (short open arrows) are seen bilaterally. Cochlea (curved open arrow) and vestibular apparatus (short black arrow) are also seen. Mastoid air cells (M) are well aerated, with septae clearly visualized. O, foramen ovale: S, foramen spinosum.

This projection demonstrates the IAC and EAC, and middle ear cleft with the head of the malleus and body of the incus visible. The eustachian canal and lateral sinus, the cochlea, and mastoid antrum should also be visualized. This basal projection demonstrates the extent of air content within the middle ear cavity.

## Lateral Projection

On a true lateral skull film the temporal bones and mastoid processes, symmetrically located on either side of the skull, are superimposed over each other, obscuring detail. Lateral temporal bone projections in which the incident ray is angled in a

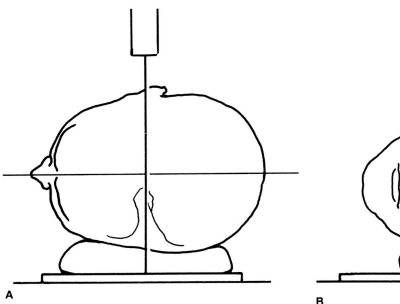

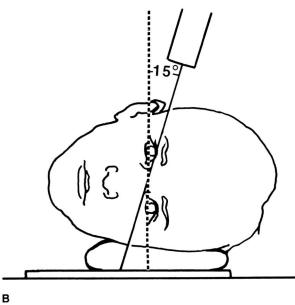

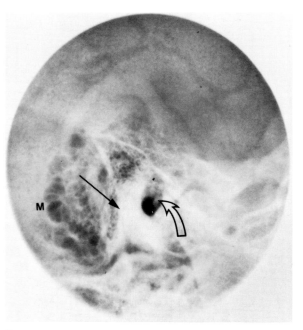

Fig. 10-6. Schuller's projection. **(A)** Viewed from above, temporal bones appear superimposed as for lateral skull film. **(B)** Viewed from the front, the 15 to 25 degree caudal angulation of incident beam separates the two temporal bones; however, superimposition of structures along long axis of viewed petrous bones (e.g., internal and external auditory canals) persists. **(C)** Radiograph. Schuller's projection is excellent for displaying pneumatization of mastoid air cells (M), the relationship of the tegmen and sigmoid sinus "plate" (thin arrow) to the mastoid air cells, and the distance from the EAC to the sigmoid sinus "plate." The IAC and EAC are superimposed with the ossicles (open arrow) partially visualized in tympanic cavity. Lateral rotation would lessen the degree of superimposition of petrous and mastoid structures.

craniocaudad direction, with or without rotation of the sagittal plane, will lessen superimposition of one petrous bone upon the other, and also control the degree of superimposition of mastoid air cells and petrous bone components from the ipsilateral side.

**Schuller's Projection.** Schuller's lateral projection (Fig. 10-6) separates the two petrous bones by an-

gling the incident ray 15 to 25 degrees caudally. (The greater the angulation, the less the superimposition but the greater the distortion.) Since the incident ray passes along the long axis of petrous bone, superimposition of the IAC and EAC, as well as the petrous bone on the mastoid air cells, is present. The antrum and epitympanic recess are usually projected clear of the bony labyrinthine structures. This projection assesses the degree of

**Fig. 10-7.** Lateral oblique projections. **(A)** Law's projection viewed from above: sagittal axis is rotated 15 degrees to side of study (next to film). This angulation or rotation in conjunction with caudal angulation (same as for Schuller's projection in Fig. 10-6B) gives lateral oblique projection with less superimposition of petrous structures on mastoid bone. **(B,C)** Mayer-Owens projection viewed from in front **(B)** and above **(C)**. Double angulations are more pronounced (45 degrees) than on Law's projection. Mastoid antrum, attic, and ossicles are better seen due to less superimposition of adjacent petrous structures.

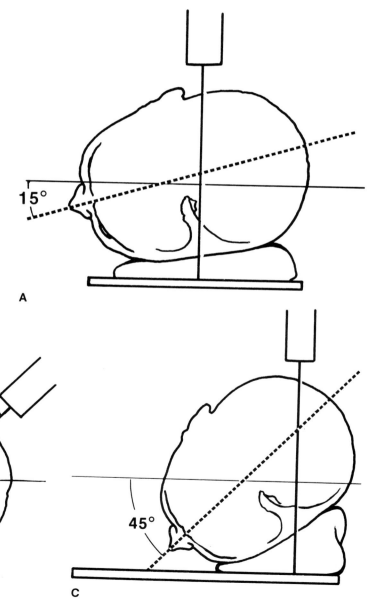

pneumatization or opacification of the mastoid air cells, the relationship of the tegmen tympani and lateral (transverse) sinus to the mastoid air cells, as well as the distance from the EAC to the transverse sinus.

### Lateral Oblique Projection: Law's and Mayer-Owens Projections

In addition to the craniocaudad angulation, a second angulation results by rotating the sagittal axis of the head (to the side of assessment) such that the petrous bone projects anterior to the mastoid antrum and air cells. The two projections differ by their degree of angulation. The Law's projection (Fig. 10-7A) uses 15 degrees of angulation craniocaudally and sagittal oblique, and the Mayer-Owen projection (Fig. 10-7B,C) uses a more pronounced angulation of 30 to 45 degrees for the double angulation. The mastoid antrum, attic, and aditus are better visualized than on the Schuller's projection. The Law's projection best demonstrates the lateral sinus plate, while the Mayer-Owens, with its greater degree of caudal angulation, better displays the attic and ossicles and is therefore used as the lateral projection to assess cholesteatoma. The Schuller's and Law's projections inadequately display the middle ear; the Mayer-Owens projection is better but still of limited value.

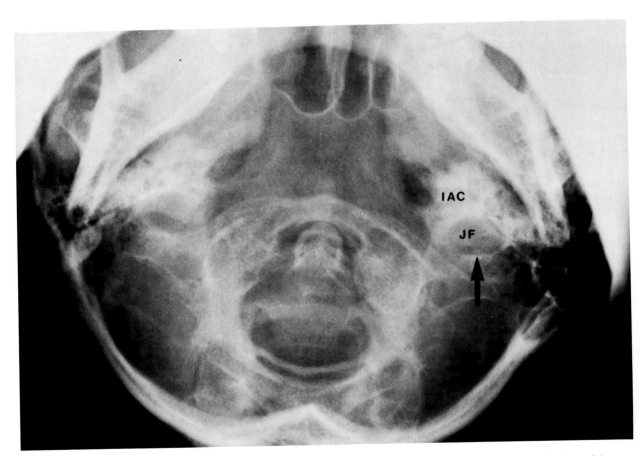

**Fig. 10-8.** Jugular foramen projection. The positioning of the face is similar to that for a Water's projection of the sinuses but the x-ray beam is centered more inferiorly. The jugular foramen (JF) is well shown with sharp corticated margins (arrow) projected just posterior to internal auditory canals (IAC).

## Jugular Foramen Projection

The skull base in the vicinity of the jugular foramen may be better displayed by placing the patient in the PA position with the orbitomeatal line elevated 45 degrees (Fig. 10-8). The central ray is directed along the midsagittal plane at the level of the EAM so that the jugular fossae are projected through the open mouth. The radiographic positioning, therefore, is very similar to that of a Water's projection of the paranasal sinuses, with more inferior centering of the incident ray.

The Chaussé II projection will also demonstrate the jugular foramen and posterior portion of the temporal bone.

## Summary of Plain Film Use

Most of the special projections to display specific anatomic segments of the temporal bone have been replaced by conventional tomographic and CT studies. Plain films remain useful to offer an overview of the temporal bone and adjacent bony structures. Such studies may be the most practical, cost-effective, and informative in specific clinical conditions (e.g., acute mastoiditis when informa-

**Table 10-2. Temporal Bone Screening Survey (Plain Film) Relative to Area of Interest**

| Area of Interest | Suggested Projections |
|---|---|
| General survey (petrous and mastoid) | Schuller's (lateral)<br>Law's (lateral oblique)<br>Stenver's (frontal oblique)<br>Transorbital (frontal)<br>Basal |
| Petrous apex (including IAC) | Transorbital<br>Stenver's<br>Basal<br>Towne |
| Tympanic cavity (including ossicles) | Guillen (frontal)<br>Chaussé III (frontal)<br>Towne<br>Basal<br>Mayer Owens (lateral oblique) |

tion regarding opacification of contained air cells is required). Lack of fine bone detail or information about adjacent soft tissue is a major disadvantage of conventional imaging. However, knowledge of the views discussed will allow a practical approach in the use of plain films either as a definitive study when the other modalities are not available, or as a guide to further studies (Table 10-1).

If plain films will be the main diagnostic modality, three or four projections will usually be required to assess adequately the region of interest (Table 10-2). If CT or MRI is to be used, two projections (frontal and lateral subtypes) may be satisfactory to offer a preliminary overview and further assist the technical direction of the advanced imaging studies. Knowledge of specific projections will also be helpful in selecting conventional tomographic planes for further assessment of the petrous temporal bone (Table 10-3).

## Complex-Motion Tomography

The temporal bone is very well suited to further investigation by conventional tomography (Figs. 10-9 through 10-11). Refinement of multidirectional (pluridirectional) tomography in the early 1960s, and the introduction of the Philips Electronics Ltd, Scarborough, Ontario, Canada Polytome, revolutionized the radiologic investigation

**Table 10-1. Overview of Temporal Bone Projections**

| Projection | Primary Structures to be Assessed |
|---|---|
| **Frontal** | |
| Transorbital | Labyrinth, IAC, scutum, petrous apex |
| Guillen | Middle ear cavity, ossicles, LSCC, facial canal (horizontal) |
| Chaussé III | Tympanic cavity, oval, round windows, scutum, EAC |
| Towne | Petrous ridge, tegmen, mastoid antrum, aditus, IAC, petrous apex |
| **Frontal Oblique** | |
| Stenver's | Petrosa continuity, ridge and apex, labryinth, mastoid tip |
| Chaussé II | Jugular bulb |
| **Basal** | Ossicles, labyrinth, IAC, tympanic cavity, EAC, mastoid antrum and air cells, petrous apex, eustachian canal, basal foramina |
| **Lateral** | |
| Schuller's | Mastoid air cells, sigmoid sinus "plate," tegmen |
| Law's | Sigmoid sinus plate, mastoid air cells, antrum |
| Mayer Owens | Mastoid antrum, aditus, attic, ossicles |

of ear pathology.[8–18] Multidirectional tomography produces radiographic slices 1 to 2 mm in thickness. Serial slices obtained every 1 to 2 mm through the temporal bone allow better recognition of structures within the bony framework. The varied path of the x-ray tube and film during the tomographic movement (usually hypocycloidal or spiral) offers significantly more detail, with more blurring of adjacent structures, yet minimal loss of sharpness in the plane of focus than that offered by linear tomography.

Complex-motion tomography remains useful in further defining pathologic changes detected on initial plain films,[7,11] or in searching for pathologic changes not seen on initial films. As with plain films of the petrous bone, specific projections may best show certain areas of temporal bone anatomy or pathologic changes.

Six basic tomographic projections have been described.[13] However, the frontal and lateral projections remain by far the most frequently used. The coronal (frontal) and sagittal (lateral) projections refer to the planes of the skull and not to the planes of the petrous pyramids. The remaining four projections refer to the axis of the petrous pyramids (Table 10-3).

### Coronal (Frontal) Projection

The coronal or frontal projection—the most frequently used projection—demonstrates all three portions of the ear (Figs. 10-9, 10-10). Slices should extend anteriorly to include the apical turn of the cochlea and posteriorly to include the posterior semicircular canal. Although five to six films are usually obtained, and seem adequate to study most petrous temporal bones, two levels in this projection tend to be more important: the cochlear plane anteriorly and the vestibular plane posteriorly.

The cochlear plane lies at the anterior aspect of the EAC. Several anatomic structures are well visualized within it. The EAC, bony spur, lateral attic wall, and ossicles are all well defined. The middle ear is visualized and should appear well aerated. The cochlea and carotid canal are easily noted with the promontory of the basal turn of the cochlea forming the inferior portion of the medial wall of the tympanic cavity. The anterior genu of the facial

**Table 10-3. Overview of Complex-Motion Tomographic Planes**

| Projections | Primary Structures to be Assessed |
| --- | --- |
| Frontal (coronal) | Labyrinth, cochlea, vestibule, LSCC, SSCC, EAC, scutum, ossicles, attic, mastoid antrum, Korner's septum, facial nerve: genu, horizontal segment, vertial segment, jugular fossa |
| Lateral (sagittal) | Ossicles, descending facial canal, carotid ridge, anterior tympanic spine, round window, SSCC |
| Guillen | Cochlear promontory, oval window, facial nerve canal: horizontal segment, prominence and associated LSCC, incudostapedial joint |
| Basal | Anterior and posterior walls of IAC and EAC; sigmoid "plate," mastoid antrum, ossicles, cochlea, petrous apex |
| Pyramidal (axial) | Cochlear turns |
| Stenver's (longitudinal) | Petrous continuity, labyrinth, petrous apex |

nerve canal may be seen as two lucencies in the bone just above and lateral to the cochlea along the superior medial aspect of the tympanic cavity. In the frontal projection, the ossicles are not recognized as individual entities but represent a superimposition of the malleus and incus, giving an appearance of a club, with the head of the club within the epitympanic recess.

The vestibular plan is 3 to 4 mm posterior to that of the cochlear plane. The EAC and bony spur are again visualized, representing the most posterior aspect of these structures. The ossicles are poorly defined in this plane. The vestibule, semicircular canals, and IAC are the basic anatomic structures assessed in the vestibular plane. The vestibule is recognized as an oval radiolucency opening into the SSCC superiorly and the LSCC laterally. The oval window may be visualized at the inferolateral aspect of the vestibule communicating with the tympanic cavity. The facial nerve canal can be assessed as it runs just inferior to the LSCC, lateral to the oval window. The bony promontory overlies the basal turn of the cochlea, forming the inferior margin of the oval window, and the bony promontory that overlies the LSCC separating it from the mastoid antrum should be assessed.

The mastoid antrum (Fig. 10-9) is noted lateral and superior to the semicircular canals and should be seen as an irregular inverted triangle-shaped air-containing space. The mastoid antra tend to be approximately equal in size and shape. A thin bony septum (Korner's septum) should be appreciated projecting from the superior lateral wall of the mastoid antrum. This septum and the mastoid antrum may be best visualized on slices just posterior to the vestibular plane.

Radiographic alterations of bony landmarks not seen on routine films but noted on coronal tomograms led to the widespread use of such imaging. Alterations in the bony spur, destruction of the long processes of the ossicles, a soft tissue density or outline of a mass in the tympanic cavity and mastoid antrum, enlargement of one mastoid antrum compared to the contralateral side, or destruction of Korner's septum are signs of a destructive lesion, (usually cholesteatoma). The extent of a destructive lesion or of previous mastoid surgery can also be assessed by tomography.

Assessment for otosclerosis includes meticulous comparison in bone configuration, including thickness and density about the oval window. Normal studies display equal bone texture in the promontory overlying the basal turn of the cochlea to that overlying the LSCC. In the early stages of otosclerosis (hyperemic stage) the bone of the cochlear promontory may appear ill-defined and less dense, giving the impression that the oval window is enlarged. In the later stages of otosclerosis, the reverse is more apparent: the oval window may appear smaller than normal as a result of the abnormally dense, thickened or sclerotic bone of the promontory and stapedial foot plate. The bone overlying the LSCC does not tend to be involved in otosclerosis and therefore serves as a control in assessing the bone about the oval window and cochlear promotory. The footplate of the stapes, due to its oblique orientation and delicate configuration, is infrequently seen in the normal state.

Frontal tomograms are useful to assess the cochlear turns (as in the Mondini deformity [Fig. 10-10C]) or to assess the possibility of a fistula between the mastoid antrum and the lateral semicircular canal. However, more commonly, the coronal tomograms are used to assess the IACs, which are seen in their entirety on the vestibular plane section.

The IACs should appear symmetrical in their size and configuration[9] (Fig. 10-9). The average vertical height is 4 mm and length from vestibule to posterior meatal wall is 8 mm. The falciform crest dividing the fundal portion of the IAC into a smaller superior and larger inferior compartment is also visualized. Acoustic nerve tumors cause erosion of the walls of the IAC and porus, resulting in increased height of the canal or shortening of the canal.[10] Displacement or erosion of the falciform crest may also be noted.

The jugular fossa lies in the same plane as the vestibule. Significant variation and asymmetry in size and configuration of the jugular fossa may be noted. Destruction of adjacent bony margins should be present before a large fossa is judged abnormal.

Structures of the occipital bone (the jugular tubercle, occipital condyle, and the intervening hypoglossal canal) may be assessed on coronal tomography. These structures will be separated from the petrous pyramid by the petrooccipital fissure. Glomus tumors and metastatic disease are the most frequent pathologic entities involving the jugular tubercle.

## Lateral (Sagittal) Tomography

Lateral tomography[10,14] (Fig. 10-11) is the second most frequently used plane. The head is oriented in a true lateral position. Sections are usually obtained at 2 mm intervals through the EAC, the middle ear, and petrous pyramid. Slice selection will vary according to the site of suspected pathologic change. As with frontal tomography, slices may be obtained at 1 mm intervals for maximum detail. The length of the petrous bone precludes haphazard imaging and excessive radiation exposure.

Lateral imaging is most frequently performed to assess the ossicles, facial canal,[16] and the carotid ridge. The cross-sectional appearance of the IAC and EAC may also be assessed.

The ossicles are best seen in this projection on sections through the middle ear cavity, which are usually 2.5 to 3.0 cm deep to the skin surface. The

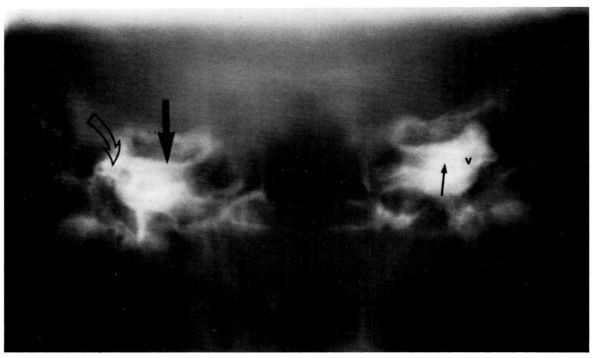

**A**

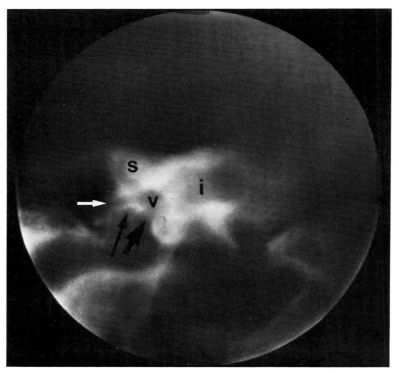

**B**

**Fig. 10-9.** Complex-motion tomography: normal frontal anatomy. **(A)** Frontal tomography through IAC plane bilaterally. IAC (large vertical black arrow), crista falciformis (small vertical arrow), vestibule (v), and horizontal semicircular canal (open arrow) are well seen. Finer detail may be obtained by coning to a single petrous bone, but if bilateral information is desired, coning will decrease the radiation exposure. **(B,C)** Complex motion collimated images — frontal projection. **(B)** Frontal plane through vestibule (v), IAC (i), SSCC (S), LSCC (horizontal arrow), groove of facial nerve canal (thin black arrow), and oval window (thick arrow). *(Figure continues.)*

**Fig. 10-9** *(continued).* **(C)** Cochlear plane: turns of cochlea (open arrow), facial nerve canal (fine arrows) just posterior to anterior genu, bony spur (s), and ossicles within epitympanic recess (E) are well seen. **(D)** Slice just posterior to vestibular plane demonstrates antrum (A, arrow).

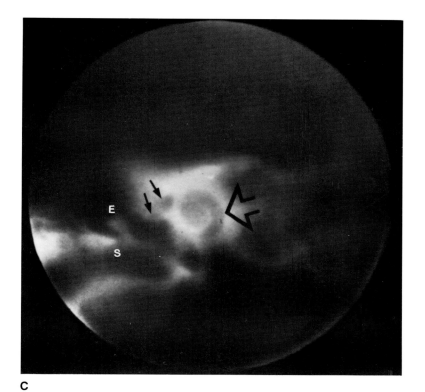

C

D

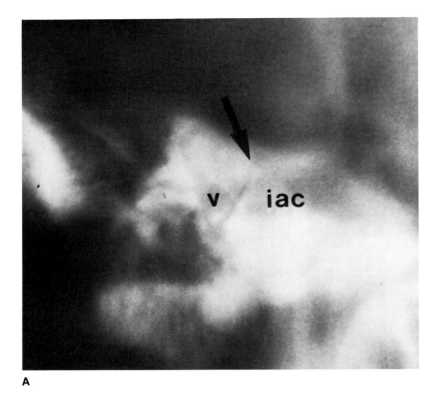

**A**

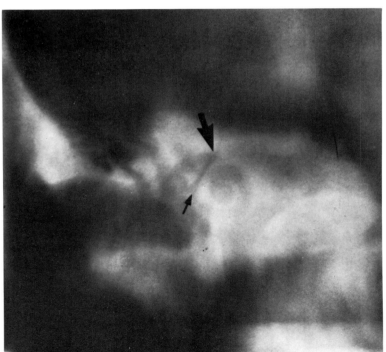

**B**

**Fig. 10-10.** Complex-motion tomography showing pathologic change. **(A,B)** Transverse fracture of right petrous bone. **(A)** Fracture line (arrow) can be seen extending vertically through the lateral aspect of the internal auditory canal (iac) just medial to vestibule (v). **(B)** More anterior slice shows fracture lateral to cochlea (heavy arrow) but extending into genu of facial nerve canal (thin arrow). *(Figure continues.)*

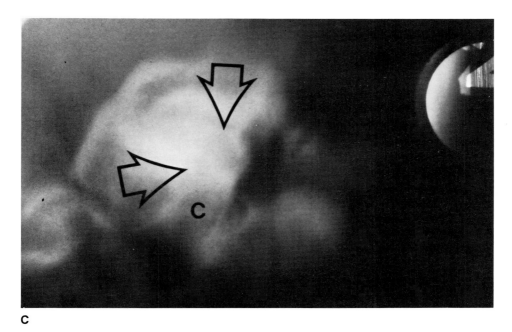

C

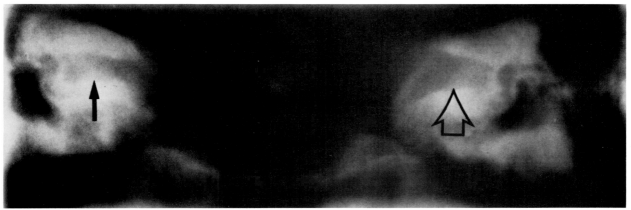

D

**Fig. 10-10** *(continued).* **(C)** Mondini deformity: AP tomogram shows deformity of left cochlea (open arrows) with loss of normal convolutions. C, carotid canal. **(D)** Left acoustic neuroma: AP tomogram shows widened, flared, and shortened left IAC (open arrow) compared to normal right IAC (solid arrow).

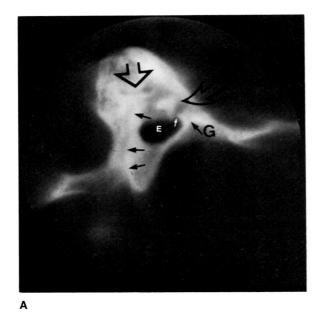

**A**

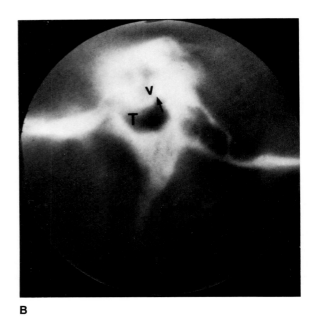

**B**

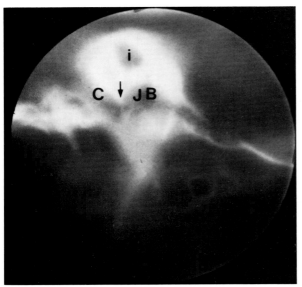

**C**

**Fig. 10-11.** Lateral (sagittal) complex-motion tomography. **(A)** "Molar tooth" appearance of anterior malleus and posterior incus is well seen (open curved arrow). Facial nerve canal (fine arrows) and LSCC (open arrow) are visible. Anterior tympanic spine (white arrow) is seen just anterior to the ossicles. E, external auditory canal; G, Glasserian fissure. **(B)** Slice through vestibule (v) displays the most medial aspect of tympanic cavity (T) and round window (arrow). Segments of the PSCC and SSCC are visualized. **(C)** Slice through IAC (i) with carotid ridge and caroticojugular spur (arrow) separating carotid canal (C) from jugular bulb (JB).

anteriorly located malleus and the posteriorly located incus resemble a typical molar tooth, with the crown of the tooth formed by the head of the malleus and body of the incus. The handle of the malleus and the long process of the incus, which should be parallel to each other, form the roots. The crown of the tooth should appear as a solid shadow. Any separation of the two components or malalignment of the crown or roots suggests dislocation.

The facial canal in its descending or mastoid portion is also best visualized on sections through the tympanic cavity in the same plane that demonstrates the ossicles. The descending canal lies in a vertical axis just posterior to the tympanic cavity and extends to the stylomastoid foramen. At its more superior portion the vertical segment bends anteriorly to form the most posterior portion of the horizontal segment of the facial nerve canal. This anterior bend, associated with the longer vertical component, gives the appearance of a cane. This cane lies just inferior to the lateral semicircular canal. The posterior portion of the horizontal facial canal lies just superior to the recess for the stapedius muscle, situated in the posterior wall of the tympanic cavity.

At the plane of the ossicles, just anterior to the "molar tooth," a thin, linear radiolucency may be visualized extending from the tympanic cavity anteriorly into the mandibular fossa. This line represents the petrotympanic fissure through which the chorda tympani nerve passes; it should not be mistaken for a fracture. The anterior tympanic spine is noted anterior to the handle of the malleus, just inferior to the posterior aspect of the petrotympanic fissure. Erosion of this spine is frequently noted in patients with cholesteatoma.

At a more medial level, 4 to 5 cm deep to the skin surface, the inferior margin of the petrous pyramid will be represented by a ridge of bone extending inferiorly. This "V-shaped" projection represents the carotid ridge and is bordered by the carotid canal anteriorly and the internal jugular vein and jugular bulb posteriorly. Destruction of the carotid ridge is highly suggestive of a glomus jugulare tumor. The IAC will be seen more superiorly in this tomographic plane. Occasionally, assessment of the walls of the IAC in this projection will confirm the diagnosis of acoustic neuroma, which would be questionable in other planes.

Lateral tomography may also be used to assess the superior and posterior semicircular canals as well as the round window. These structures will be visualized on slices just medial to the ossicles.

## Semiaxial (Guillen) Projection

The semiaxial position corresponds to the Guillen projection on conventional radiographs, which places the medial wall of the tympanic cavity tangential to the x-ray beam. This allows better assessment of the structures of the medial wall of the tympanic cavity, such as the cochlear promontory, the oval window, the horizontal portion of the facial canal, and the LSCC. Subtle changes about the oval window, such as otosclerosis involving the stapedial footplate, or fracture dislocation of the incudostapedial joint, which are difficult to demon-

strate, may occasionally be better seen on this projection.

## Basal (Hertz or Horizontal) Projection

The basal projection is obtained in the submentovertex direction, which unfortunately is uncomfortable for the patient. The IAC, especially the posterior lip of the porus acusticus, may be well assessed. This projection demonstrates the sigmoid plate well, and may be used to assess whether this structure has been penetrated by inflammation or tumor. The basal projection is ideal for visualizing the incudomallear joint, if ossicular chain dislocation is suspected.

Hemorrhage or scar formation about the ossicles may obscure fine bone detail. The cochlear turns, the promontory over the basal cochlear turn, the bone overlying the lateral semicircular canal, and the anterior genu of the facial canal are all well assessed by basal tomography. The mastoid air cells, lateral attic wall, and petrous apex are other structures well seen (but this method is essentially replaced by axial CT, which displays such structures in the identical plane).

## Axial (Pyramidal) View

For the axial view, the head is rotated 45 degrees to the side of interest, as for the Mayer's view, such that the posterior surface of the petrous pyramid (the long axis of the petrous bone) is parallel to the x-ray source and perpendicular to the x-ray film. This projection is primarily used to study the cochlear turns, with the projection parallel to the long axis of the modiolus and with contiguous sections displaying the individual coils of the cochlea.

## Longitudinal (Stenver's) Tomographic Projection

The longitudinal projection is obtained with the patient supine and the head rotated 45 degrees away from the side of interest so that the posterior wall of the petrous pyramid (the long axis of the petrous pyramid), is parallel to the plane of the film and perpendicular to the x-ray source. This projection therefore displays the entire length of the petrous bone and is useful to assess continuity of the petrous pyramid, especially if fractures of the pet-

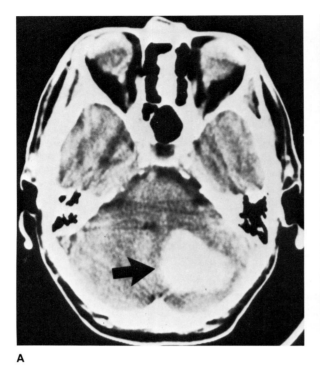

A

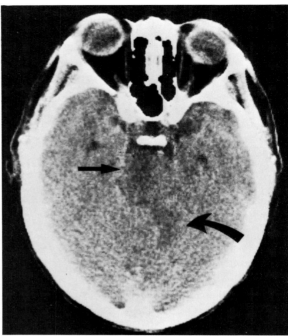

B

C

**Fig. 10-12.** Soft tissues of the posterior fossa—pathologic change. CT and MRI are the modalities of choice to visualize directly the soft tissues of the posterior fossa. Patients presented here had ataxia. **(A)** Cerebellar hemorrhage: unenhanced axial CT displays area of increased density (80 Hu) suggestive of hemorrhage (arrow). Use of contrast enhancement alone may be confusing if hemorrhage is to be considered. The 4th ventricle is displaced anteriorly and to right. **(B,C)** Infarct of brain stem and cerebellum. Unenhanced CT **(B)** displays low-density right pons (straight arrow) and left cerebellum (curved arrow). Configuration of density alteration is very suggestive of infarction. Contrast-enhanced CT **(C)** shows peripheral enhancement of right pontine (straight arrow) and left cerebellar (curved arrow) lesions. The 4th ventricle (thin arrow) not significantly displaced or compressed, further suggesting vascular insult. Neurovascular peripheral perfusion of recent infarct may resemble a neoplastic or inflammatory lesion.

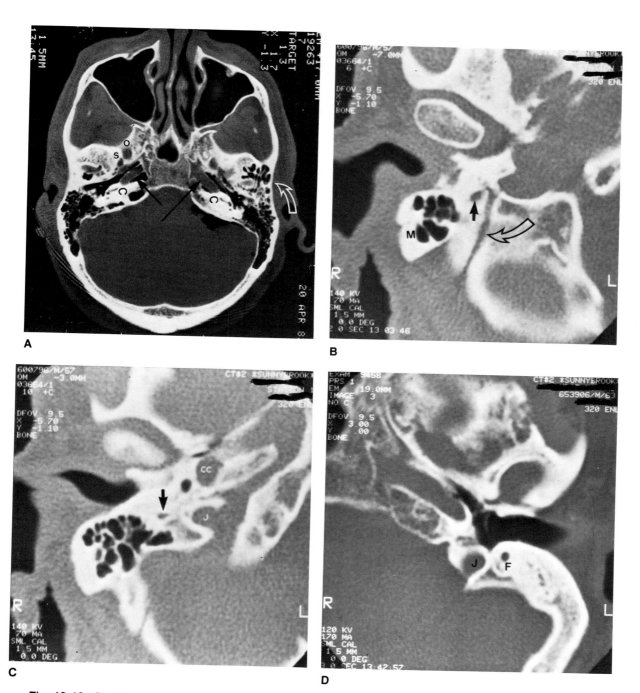

**Fig. 10-13.** Skull base and carotid canal: normal axial CT findings. **(A)** Axial CT demonstrates carotid canals (solid arrows) outlined bilaterally by petrous apex air cells medially and eustachian canal laterally. Mastoid air cells may be seen extending anteriorly (open arrow) into the left squamous temporal bone. Right foramen ovale (O) and foramen spinosum (S) are well seen. C, petrous apex. **(B)** Level of mastoid process (m): facial canal (solid arrow) appears just medial to occipitomastoid suture (open arrow). **(C)** Level of TM joint and inferior aspect of EAC: Carotid canal (cc), jugular bulb (J), and facial canal (arrow) are well seen just medial to mastoid air cells. The caroticojugular spur of bone seen here between carotid and jugular vessels is not seen on the more inferior slice in **B**. **(D)** Air extending from tympanic cavity anteriorly into bony eustachian canal, just lateral to carotid canal. Facial canal (F) is noted just lateral to jugular bulb (J).

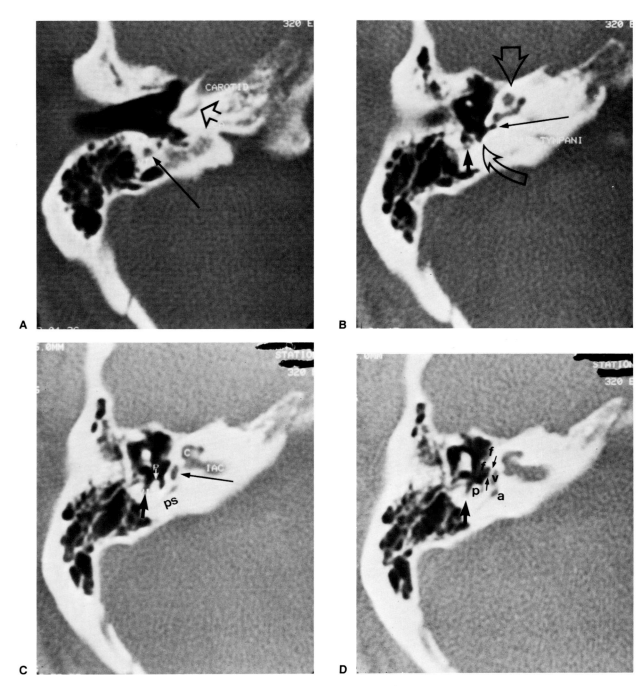

**Fig. 10-14.** Cochlea, vestibule, and tympanic cavity — normal axial CT using thin 1.5 mm slices progressing superiorly by 1 or 2 mm increments. **(A)** Slice through EAC shows anterior and posterior bony walls, inferior aspect of cochlea (open arrow), and carotid canal anterior to cochlea. Facial canal (thin arrow) may be difficult to distinguish from clouded mastoid air cells. **(B)** Inferior cochlear level: turns of cochlea are better appreciated (straight open arrow). Round window (thin arrow) is well seen just posterior to cochlea. Sinus tympani (curved arrow) and facial nerve recess (short arrow) are noted posteriorly. Long processes of ossicles are seen in well-aerated tympanic cavity. **(C)** Superior cochlear level (c): inferior aspect of IAC and vestibule (thin arrow) can be seen. Pyramidal eminence (P), to which the stapedius muscle attaches, separates the sinus tympani (just medial to P) from the facial recess (short arrow) just laterally located. The PSCC (ps) and ossicles are also noted. **(D)** Oval window (thin arrows) is seen just lateral to vestibule (v). PSCC with its ampulla (a) and pyramidal eminence (p) are still present. The facial nerve (f), seen as a faint soft tissue density, passes medial to ossicles toward facial recess (heavy arrow). *(Figure continues.)*

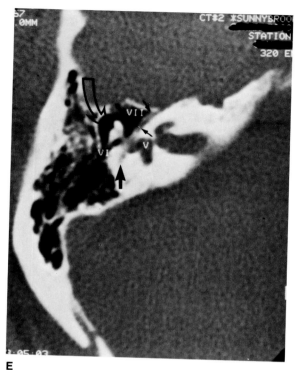

**E**

**Fig. 10-14** *(continued)*. **(E)** Head of malleus (anteriorly), body of incus (posteriorly), and articulation (open arrow) are well visualized in epitympanic recess. The facial nerve is still seen as a soft tissue density (small arrows) coursing along medial wall of tympanic cavity toward facial recess (vertical arrow). v, vestibule.

rous pyramid are suspected. Lesions of the petrous apex are well displayed in this projection. Inner ear structures, such as the posterior semicircular canal, round window, cochlea, and carotid canal may also be assessed with this projection.

## Computed Tomography

Alterations in soft tissues not detectable by conventional modalities can be imaged by CT, which remains the primary modality for displaying the cerebral tissues, including posterior fossa structures (Fig. 10-12).[19-34] Advances in technology have allowed further imaging capabilities beyond "routine" imaging of the soft tissues.

Currently available machines, for example, utilize bone algorithms and thin slices (1.0 to 1.5 mm thickness) to display high-resolution bone images of the petrosa (see Figs. 10-13 to 10-20) surpassing in detail those offered by complex-motion tomography. When appropriate, image data may be used to maximum advantage to display separately bone and soft tissue detail. Image data may also be manipulated to display enlarged images of a restricted region of interest.

Enlargement of gantry apertures allows for easier imaging of the petrous bones, skull base, and posterior fossa in the direct coronal, sagittal or oblique positions (Figs. 10-17 to 10-20). When axial scanning only is possible, images in other axes may be reformatted from the axial image data obtained (Fig. 10-21). Increased quality of reformatted images is inversely related to the thickness of the CT slices and directly to the patient's ability to lie motionless while the axial study is being performed.

Preliminary digital radiographs may be performed before the CT study to offer a radiographic overview from which slice locations and angulation may be chosen. Significantly reduced scanning times (2 seconds per slice) and increased capabilities of the x-ray tube allow for studies to be performed more quickly, allowing greater patient acceptance and less motion artifact. A rapid series of slices at a specific location (dynamic CT) utilized in conjunction with a time-coordinated intravenous injection of contrast medium allows a graphic display of tissue vascularity, which may be useful to further assess mass lesions, thus differentiating vascular tumors such as glomus jugulare from neuroma, or aneurysms from enhancing masses.

The level of sophistication required from the CT study will be influenced by the goals of patient management and effective communication between the clinician and radiologist. Further discussion of CT here will be directed to specific anatomic regions that favor bone (petrous) or soft tissue (posterior fossa and cerebellopontine angle) detail.

### Bone

In discussion of petrous bone imaging, appropriate emphasis will be placed on high resolution[11,13,33] bone imaging, illustrated by normal anatomy in both axial and coronal planes. This

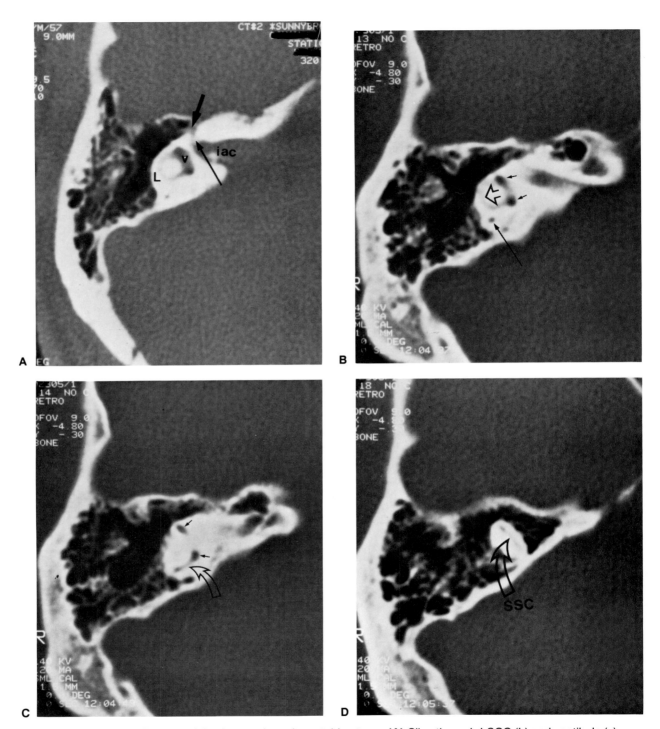

**Fig. 10-15.** Axial CT—semicircular canals and mastoid antrum. **(A)** Slice through LSCC (L) and vestibule (v). The labyrinthine (thin arrow) segment of the facial nerve exiting from the lateral aspect of the IAC is seen, as well as the geniculate segment (thicker arrow) as the facial nerve turns to form the tympanic or horizontal segment. **(B)** Anterior and posterior limbs of the SSCC (short arrows) are seen as well as the LSCC (open arrow) limbs. Posterior segment of PSCC is visible (thin arrow). **(C)** Superior limb of the PSCC (open arrow), anterior and posterior limbs of the SSCC (small arrows) are seen, and the relationship between the PSCC and posterior SSCC limb is well demonstrated. **(D)** The superior aspect of the SSCC (open arrow) is seen just inferior to the tegmen. *(Figure continues.)*

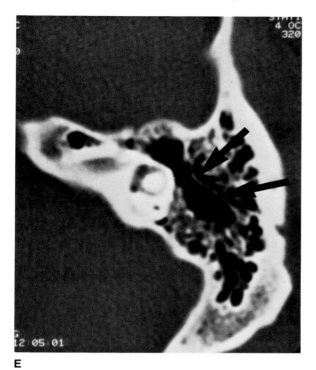

**Fig. 10-15** *(continued).* **(E)** Korner's septum (arrows) may be seen as a cortical bony structure in the lateral aspect of the aditus and mastoid antrum.

allows appreciation of the impact that proper manipulation of CT bone images has had on the display capabilities of bone detail (Figs. 10-13 to 10-22).

Imaging of petrous bone pathology will significantly differ from techniques utilized to study cerebellopontine angle (CPA) pathology. The CT assessment of fine bony structures demands high-resolution magnified images utilizing a bone algorithm. Fine detail with minimal volume averaging is a prerequisite for diagnostic studies. Thin slices (1 to 1.5 mm) are required. Density resolution becomes less important than with soft tissue assessment since the wide window display utilized to assess bony detail will obscure even moderate density changes. Technology in 1987 permits spatial resolution of the bony structures approaching 0.5 mm or less in an inherently high-contrast region such as the petrous bone. Compared to soft tissue imaging, less density contrast detail is required, owing to the very high inherent contrast of

the petrous bone surrounded by air within the EAC, tympanic cavity, and mastoid air cells, thereby allowing images to be obtained with less radiation exposure and without loss of detail.[21,30]

Low-contrast resolution is sacrificed; therefore soft tissue detail adjacent to the petrous bones will be poorly imaged. If there is any question about adjacent soft tissues, a preliminary survey of the temporal bone and posterior cranial fossa is advised utilizing a soft tissue algorithm to display optimal low-contrast discrimination. High-resolution bone imaging may then be performed in the region of special interest. Soft tissue masses in the middle ear may be assessed using the high spatial resolution achieved with the bone algorithm.

At our institutions, we do not routinely use intravenous contrast agents. If the anatomic site can be well assessed using high-resolution bone images, without the need for any imaging at a soft tissue mode, use of wide window settings in the bone algorithm negates the purpose of contrast agents. Intravenous contrast is used, however, if a vascular abnormality is suspected, and images are obtained at both bone and soft tissue mode.

For high-resolution studies, maximum quality is achieved by obtaining contiguous, thin (1.5 mm) slices in the shortest time interval so that there is minimal patient motion. Such studies may be preprogrammed with 12 to 15 slices required.

Coronal studies are performed after the axial images have been viewed. If all the information required is available on the axial slices, the examination is then terminated. Coronal CT, however, is usually complementary and not redundant when assessing the finer structures, especially of the bony labyrinth, middle ear, or facial nerve. Similarly, abnormalities of the external ear are usually assessed in both the axial and coronal plane.

Monitoring during the actual scanning is imperative to assess that the study has included all regions of interest. For symptoms or signs suggestive of vascular causes, the axial study is extended inferiorly so that the jugular foramen region is adequately visualized and that the soft tissues immediately inferior to the skull are studied at a soft tissue mode.

Pathologic change limited to a single petrous bone is usually studied at a greater magnification value (approximately 3 to 3.5 times magnification)

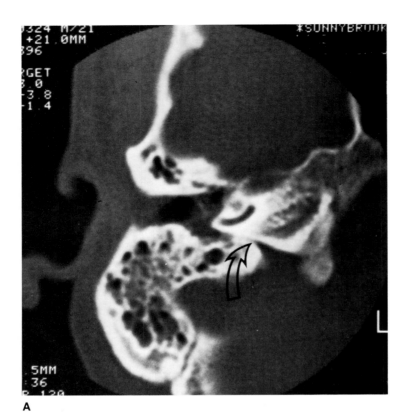

**A**

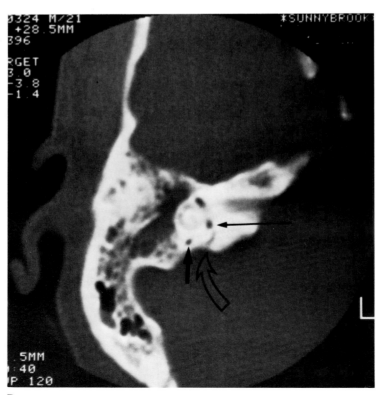

**B**

**Fig. 10-16.** Axial CT of vestibular and cochlear aqueducts. **(A)** The long, tapering cochlear aqueduct (open arrow) is seen extending from posterior petrous surface toward cochlea, is typically funnel-shaped in its more posterior aspect. It lies in the same axis as the IAC (see Fig. 10-14E) but in a more inferior location, and should not be mistaken for the IAC. **(B)** Vestibular aqueduct (open arrow) with its typical wider posterior termination is seen opening onto the posterior surface of the petrous bone. The aqueduct is directed toward its anterior communication with the common crus of the PSCC and SSCC (horizontal arrow). The aqueduct passes between the PSCC (vertical arrow) and the posterior petrous surface.

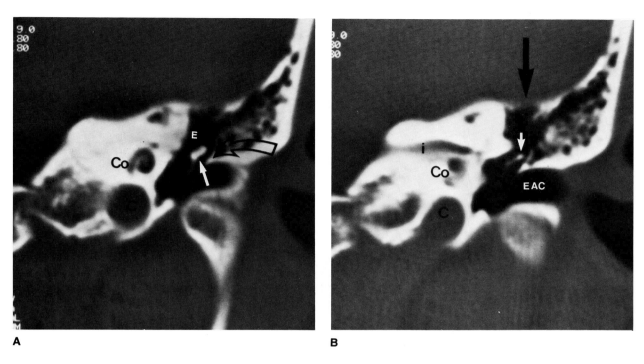

A

B

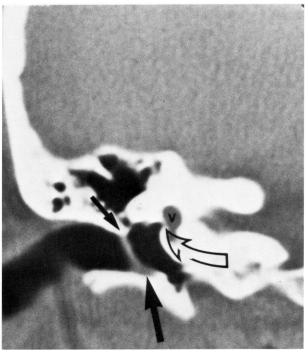

**Fig. 10-17.** Coronal CT of cochlea, carotid canal, EAC, bony spur, tympanic cavity, and attic. **(A)** anterior slice through cochlea (Co) shows carotid canal (C), bony spur (open arrow), malleus (white arrow), and epitympanic recess (E). **(B)** Slightly more posterior, cochlea (Co) and carotid canal (C) are still visualized. External auditory canal (EAC) and bony spur remain well visualized. The incus is now seen, including its long process (white arrow). The IAC (i) is just starting to be visualized, as are the LSCC and SSCC. The epitympanic recess and tegmen are well shown (black arrow). Horizontally oriented structures (i.e., tegmen, scutum) are best seen in this axis. **(C)** Image viewed at higher brightness displays slightly thickened tympanic membrane (solid arrows). Vestibule (V) and oval window (open arrow) opening into tympanic cavity are also noted.

C

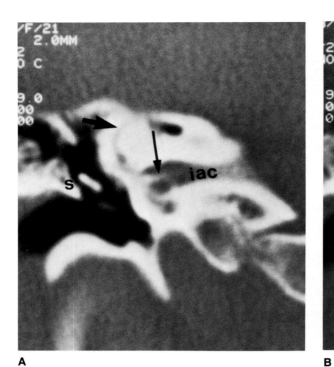

**A**

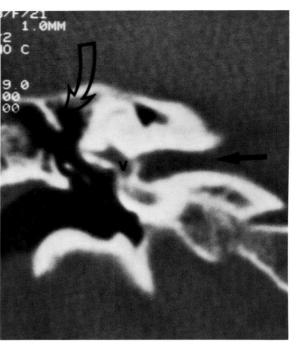

**B**

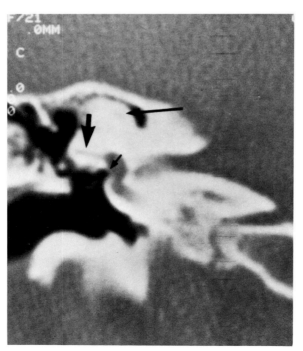

**C**

**Fig. 10-18.** Coronal CT of IAC, vestibule, oval window, and semicircular canals: progressively posterior slices on same patient. **(A)** Slice through anterior portion of IAC (iac) shows crista falciformis (vertical arrow), anterior limb of SSCC (horizontal arrow), and bony spur (s). Portion of basal turn of cochlea is seen inferior to the IAC. **(B)** The IAC (horizontal arrow) is seen at its maximum diameter; roof and floor are best assessed in this projection. The relationship of the vestibule (v) to IAC, SSCC, and LSCC is well shown. Körner's septum (open arrow) is visible projecting into the mastoid antrum. **(C)** The oval window (small arrow) is best visualized in this slice, and the anterior limb of the LSCC and overlying bony promontory are visible (vertical arrow). The SSCC is seen between its anterior and posterior limb segments (horizontal arrow) just inferior to the tegmen. The ossicle at the mouth of the oval window is faintly seen.

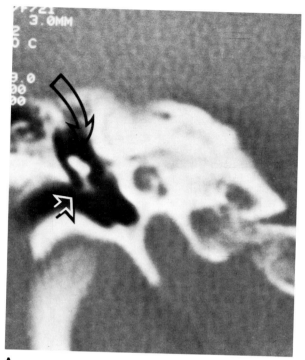

**A**

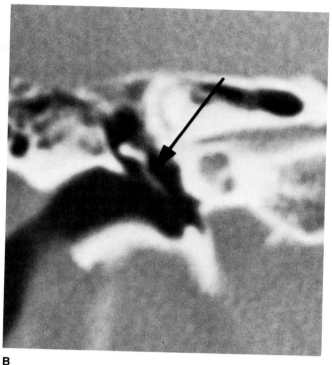

**B**

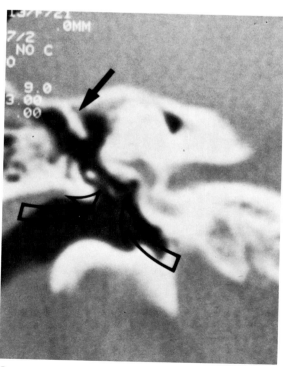

**C**

**Fig. 10-19.** Coronal CT of ossicles. **(A)** Malleus is seen more anteriorly within tympanic cavity (cochlea is visible); the head (curved arrow) and handle can be seen. The handle is fixed to the tympanic membrane by a small bony attachment (open arrow). **(B)** Body and long process of incus are well seen (arrow). The long process lies parallel and medial to the handle of malleus. **(C)** Incus and stapes (open arrows) are seen approaching the oval window. A thin slice viewed at higher brightness is required to demonstrate finer structures. Korner's septum remains well visible (solid arrow).

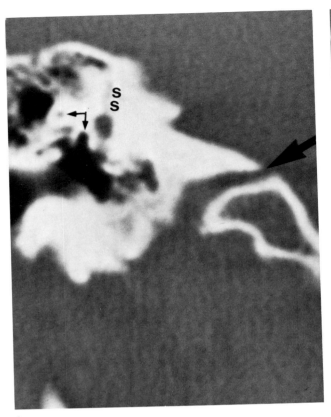

**A**

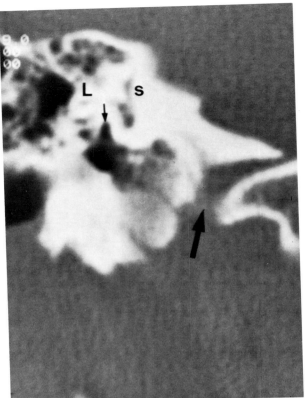

**B**

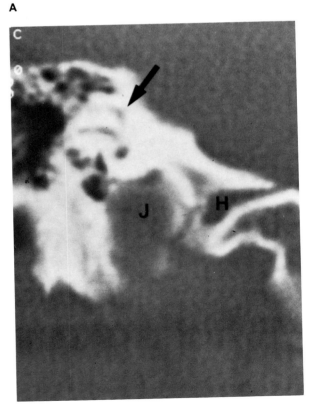

**C**

**Fig. 10-20.** Coronal CT of hypoglossal canal, facial canal, and semicircular canals. **(A–C)** Progressively posterior slices on the same patient. **(A)** Posterior limb of SSCC (SS) and lateral aspect LSCC (horizontal arrow) are seen. Horizontal portion of facial canal seen as groove (vertical arrow) just inferior to LSCC. Hypoglossal canal (larger arrow) is now visible. **(B)** Posterior limbs of SSCC (s) and LSCC (L) are seen. Facial nerve canal (small arrow) and hypoglossal canal (large arrow) are visible. **(C)** PSCC segment (arrow) is seen just posterior and lateral to posterior limb of SSCC **(B)**, and posterosuperior to LSCC. The close relationship of hypoglossal canal (H) and jugular bulb (J) can be seen. *(Figure continues.)*

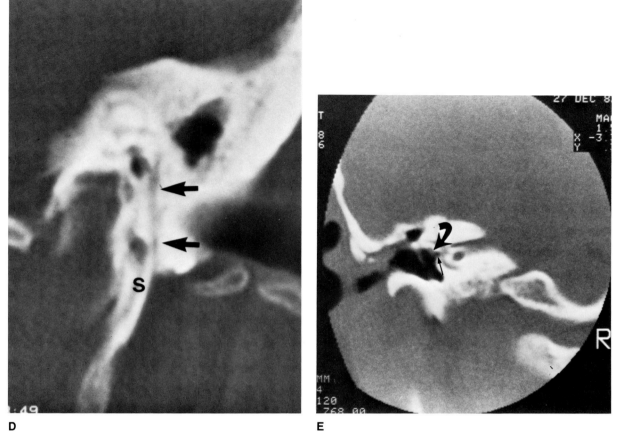

**D**    **E**

**Fig. 10-20** *(continued).* **(D)** Direct coronal CT demonstrates entire length of descending portion of facial nerve canal (arrows) exiting as stylomastoid foramen just lateral to styloid process (s). **(E)** Coronal CT shows facial tissue density (curved arrow) just lateral to oval window (straight arrow). The density represents a dehiscent facial nerve canal with lack of bony covering. (E courtesy of Dr. Joel D. Swartz, Medical College of Pennsylvania, Philadelphia.)

to offer maximum detail of the fine structures. For those studies in which both petrous bones are to be visualized, a smaller magnification factor of 1.75 to 2.0 will allow simultaneous visualization of the two bones. Coronal imaging may be performed initially if radiation exposure to the lens is to be avoided, with axial imaging performed only if required.

Since high-resolution CT became available in the early 1980s, clinical application and experience have demonstrated resolution to be equal or superior to that of conventional tomography. Pathologic changes noted on CT appear easier to identify than with conventional tomography. Knowledge of

CT petrosal anatomy has assumed increasing importance in the evaluation of petrous bone disease.

Various projections may be utilized to best demonstrate specific anatomic features within the petrous bone. As with other radiographic modalities, structures passing obliquely through the tissue plane may have their margins or density distorted. Bony surfaces are usually best visualized in a plane perpendicular to the axis of that surface. For example, the tegmen tympani, scutum, and stapes are best seen in the coronal plane while the anterior and posterior walls of the tympanic cavity are better seen in the axial plane. Structures oriented in a sagittal plane are well seen in both axial and coronal planes, (such as, the medial wall of the tympanic cavity).

For coronal imaging, a projection approximately 90 degrees to the axial plane is usually the most complementary. The occasional limitation to coronal positioning is the patient's inability to hyperextend or hyperflex the neck to allow the required gantry angulation and slice positioning through the petrous bones.

### External Ear and External Auditory Canal

The EAC (Figs. 10-14, 10-17) is seen as an air-filled structure with a thin cutaneoperiosteal lining. The tympanic membrane may be seen on coronal images paralleling the long process of the malleus. The scutum should be well visualized with no erosion of its medial lip. The attachment of the tympanic membrane at the posterosuperior aspect of the tympanic rim results in a bony protrusion — the posterior tympanic spine — well seen on axial CT and should not be mistaken for a pathologic displacement or bony reaction. The axial and coronal planes define the tympanic ring (bony walls) of the EAC and its intimate relationship to the glenoid fossa anteriorly and the mastoid air cells posteriorly. The fibrocartilaginous lateral portion of the EAC is well visualized by CT. Extension of disease processes to involve the pinna or scalp may be better studied utilizing a soft tissue mode.

### The Middle Ear

Although the middle ear cavity is complex in shape, it tends to be clearly outlined as a high-contrast structure because of the contained air (Figs. 10-14, 10-15, 10-17 to 10-19). Although its medial wall is somewhat irregular, the tympanic cavity is essentially a flattened rectangular chamber lying between the tympanic membrane and EAC laterally and the inner ear medially. This structure becomes less intimidating if one develops a systematic approach to visualizing the component parts by assessing the structure as separate subcompartments.

In a vertical axis, the middle ear is divided into three segments. The tympanic cavity proper or mesotympanum is that segment in direct contact with the tympanic membrane. The epitympanum (or epitympanic recess) lies superior to the EAC

and tympanic membrane while the hypotympanum is inferior to the tympanic membrane and EAC. As a rectangular chamber, the tympanic cavity can then be systematically studied by assessing each of its four walls (anterior, posterior, medial, and lateral) separately.[29] The floor and roof are best assessed by coronal CT, the anterior and posterior walls by axial CT, while the medial and lateral walls are well seen on both projections.

The ossicles lie within the epitympanic recess and mesotympanum. The greater proportion of the ossicles (head of malleus and body of incus) will be noted to lie in the epitympanum, with the handle of the malleus and long process of the incus extending inferiorly into the tympanum. The hypotympanum, the smallest subcompartment, is empty and the least complex.

**Anterior Wall.**   The carotid canal (Fig. 10-13) will be noted at the most medial aspect of the hypotympanum anteriorly, close to the cochlea. There are two openings in the anterior wall — the eustachian tube and the semicanal for the tensor tympani — both parallel to the carotid canal to which the semicanal is almost contiguous. The eustachian canal lies just lateral to the semicanal and is separated from it by a bony septum protruding posteriorly and partly surrounding the tensor tympani muscle. The bony eustachian tube will usually be air filled for 2 to 3 cm. The cartilaginous portion is usually collapsed and not visualized due to the lack of air content. The anterior wall of the middle ear is funnel-shaped because of its continuation into the air-filled eustachian tube.

The semicanal extends more posteriorly than the eustachian tube and passes inferior to the anterior genu of the facial nerve to end slightly anterior to the oval window. Extending laterally from the posterior termination of the semicanal is the cochleariform process, housing the tendon of the tensor tympani, which may be seen crossing the mesotympanum at a 90 degree angle to the muscle, to attach to the neck of the malleus.

**Lateral Wall.**   The EAC and tympanic membrane represent the lateral boundary of the mesotympanum (Fig. 10-14). The scutum or drum spur, which represents the medial lip of the roof of the EAC, forms the lateral wall of the epitympanic recess, and projects inferiorly for the attachment of the tympanic membrane (tympanic incisura). Coronal studies should be performed if there is any suggestion of abnormality of the scutum, which should appear pointed and well defined with no evidence of erosion in this projection. The inferior tympanic ring forms the lateral wall of the hypotympanum.

**Posterior Wall.** The posterior wall of the tympanic cavity (Fig. 10-14) appears to be a complicated structure because of the presence of several ridges and depressions. Inferomedially, the mesotympanum indents the labyrinthine capsule and mastoid as three depressions. They are separated by two bony prominences. The most medial depression represents the round window niche and is separated from the middle depression, the sinus tympani, by a bony prominence, the subiculum promontorii. The most lateral depression is the facial recess, which is separated from the sinus tympani by a bony ridge directed superiorly and anteriorly: the pyramidal eminence. The sinus tympani therefore lies between the posterior semicircular canal and the descending portion of the facial nerve canal. Assessment of the sinus tympani is extremely important by CT since the more lateral pyramidal eminence obscures the sinus from clinical examination.

The pyramidal eminence has a beaklike appearance, pointing medially toward the sinus tympani, due to the insertion of the stapedius muscle, which extends posteriorly from the stapes to this site. There is considerable variation in the configuration of these depressions and ridges, ranging from short and flat to deep and round. The facial nerve leaves the tympanic cavity by penetrating the posterior wall just superior and slightly lateral to the pyramidal eminence before turning 90 degrees inferiorly (the pyramidal turn) to enter the descending facial canal, remaining lateral to the pyramidal eminence.

More superiorly, the epitympanic space communicates with the mastoid antrum posteriorly through a narrowed communication, the aditus ad antrum. On axial CT, the air spaces at this level therefore have an hourglass configuration. Multiple small mastoid air cells representing discrete sharply defined air spaces are contiguous with the mastoid antrum and should be assessed on these slices.

**Medial Wall.** The medial wall of the tympanic cavity (Figs. 10-14, 10-18) shares common anatomic landmarks with the lateral boundaries of the labyrinth. Anteriorly, the medial wall is formed by the promontory, that is, the part of the labyrinthine capsule covering the basal turn of the cochlea. The promontory extends posteriorly to two important landmarks, the oval and round windows, before diverging into a superior and inferior ridge of bone (the ponticulus and subiculum respectively), which form the anterior margin of the sinus tympani. The oval and round windows, although located more posteriorly, are positioned between anterior and posterior prominences of the medial wall. The subiculum forms the posterior aspect of the round window niche. The round window can be seen on axial CT as a sharp deep bony depression posterior to the basal turn of the cochlea (promontory).

The oval window is superior and slightly anterior to the round window. Because it is small, the oval window may be difficult to demonstrate on axial CT and is more easily seen on coronal CT. It will be noted as a bony dehiscence just lateral to the vestibule. The stapes may be demonstrated on most high-resolution coronal images as a faint bony structure within the middle ear lateral to and abutting the oval window (Fig. 10-8G).

More superiorly, the prominence of the lateral semicircular canal forms the medial superior border of the sinus tympani. The tympanic (second or horizontal) portion of the facial nerve crosses the tympanic cavity from anterior to posterior along the medial wall of the epitympanic space. The enclosing bony canal is usually thin and may be partly deficient, especially adjacent to the oval window and cochleariform process.[17] Inferiorly, the hypotympanum is represented medially by a thin bony wall separating the jugular fossa from the middle ear.

**Roof.** The tegmen tympani forms the thin bony roof of the epitympanic recess (Fig. 10-17). The tegmen mastoideum, a posterior extension of the tegmen tympani, forms the roof of the aditus ad antrum and mastoid antrum. Coronal CT best displays the tegmen, the overlying temporal lobe, and the characteristic inverted triangular configuration of the epitympanic recess, with the tegmen representing the base of the triangle. Korner's septum is also best visualized in the coronal plane.

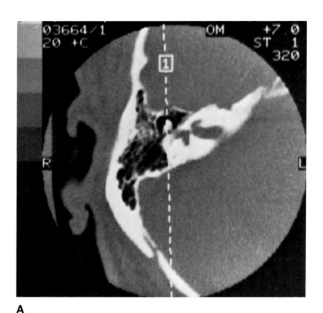

**A**

**Fig. 10-21.** Reformatted CT images. **(A)** Axial high-resolution CT with axis (dashed line) for sagittal reformatting. **(B)** Sagittal reformatted image from 1.5 mm thick axial slices. Ossicular "molar tooth" sign, formed by malleus (m) and incus (i), and vertical segment facial canal (arrow) descending to stylomastoid foramen are well demonstrated. **(C)** Sagittal oblique reformatting along long axis of ossicles better demonstrates long processes of ossicles (white arrows). More inferiorly, the caroticojugular spine (S) separates the carotid (C) and jugular (J) vessels from the hypotympanum. *(Figure continues.)*

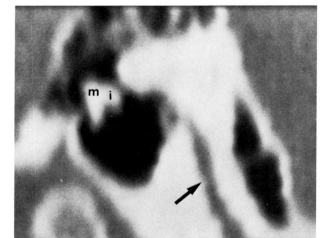

**B**

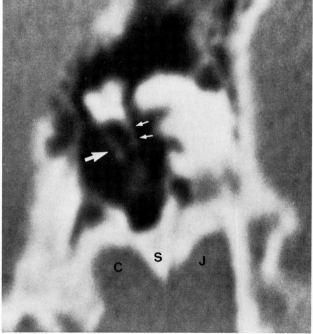

**C**

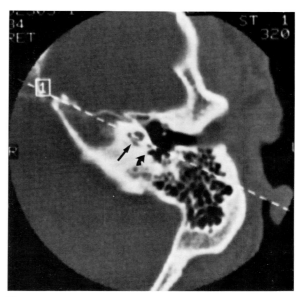

Fig. 10-21 *(continued)*. **(D)** Axial CT for oblique reformatting (dashed line) through cochlea (arrow) just anterior to round window (curved arrow) **(E)** Coronal oblique reformatting demonstrates turns of cochlea and basal promontory (arrow), tegmen (T) forming the roof of the aditus ad antrum are seen well in this projection.

D

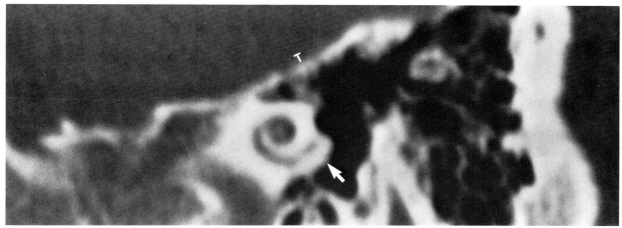

E

**Floor.** The thin bony floor (Figs. 10-21, 10-22) extends as an inverted triangle-shaped bony wedge, the caroticojugular spine, separating the hypotympanum from the more anterior internal carotid artery (carotid canal) and posterior jugular bulb. The bony projection extending inferiorly between these vascular structures may be seen on axial CT but is typically recognized on sagittal reformatting.

**Ossicles.** The handle of the malleus extending inferiorly into the mesotympanum is fixed to the tympanic membrane. The head of the malleus, which appears as a round density within the epitympanic recess, may be seen to articulate with the body of the incus. The anterior process of the malleus, providing an attachment for the anterior malleal ligament, is not visualized.

The long process of the incus extends inferiorly into the mesotympanum, parallel to, but posterior and medial to, the long process of the malleus. The most inferior extension (lenticular process) of the long process of the incus articulates with the head of the stapes. The anterior and posterior crura form the crural arch or suprastructure of the stapes, attaching anteriorly and posteriorly to the thin (0.2 mm thickness) stapes footplate.

The superoinferior axis of the ossicles can be evaluated by contiguous axial slices (Fig. 10-14). More superiorly at the level of the epitympanic recess, the head of the malleus will normally be positioned in the anterior epitympanum, presenting the well described "scoop of ice cream lying on the cone" represented just posteriorly by the body and short process of the incus. The incudomalleal articulation can be seen at this level. At the level of the EAC, the long processes of the malleus and incus will be seen as slightly oval densities due to their inferomedial angulation. The long process of the malleus is lateral to the cochlear promontory, while that of the incus is slightly more posterior and directed toward the oval window.

More inferiorly, the stapes suprastructure, because it lies in the axial plane, may occasionally be visualized in its entirety. More frequently, partial volume effect related to the adjacent horizontal facial canal obscures visualization of the crura. The neck of the stapes may infrequently be noted as a short linear density, in line with the lenticular process of the incus, directed medially toward the oval window. The incudostapedial joint is frequently seen on axial projection. It may also be seen on coronal imaging just medial to the L-shaped configuration representing the juncture of the vertically directed incus and horizontal lenticular extension. The footplate however, is too fine to detect.

Seventy degree coronal imaging (Fig. 10-19) may demonstrate the malleus along its entire length since the long process is angled slightly posteriorly. The insertion of the long process to the tympanic membrane is best appreciated in this plane. The incus will have the configuration of an inverted teardrop, representing the body superiorly and the inferomedially projected long process. The relationship between the malleus and incus is poorly demonstrated on coronal CT. However, the incudostapedial joint is best shown in this axis. The familiar lateral tomographic appearance,[14] (i.e., the molar tooth configuration formed by the malleus and incus) is well seen in reformatted images (Fig. 10-21). The axis of reformation will be approximately 15 degrees to the midsagittal plane. The coronal 105 degree angulation may demon-

strate the stapes as a faint density extending laterally from the oval window. On axial and coronal CT the ossicles should always appear well defined and surrounded by air within the tympanic cavity. Loss of definition or adjacent soft tissue density signifies pathologic changes. Attachments to the ossicles that may be visualized include the tensor tympani muscle and tendon, and the stapedius muscle and tendon. Supportive ligaments such as the superior malleal ligament and posterior incudal ligaments may be identified on axial CT.[29]

## The Cochlea and Round Window

The spiral cochlea (Figs. 10-14, 10-16, 10-17), which contains the sensory organs responsible for hearing, normally has two and three quarter turns, the basal, the middle, and apical turns. The basal turn is the largest and best defined. A bony prominence, the promontory, overlies the protruding basal turn and separates it from the middle ear cavity. The modiolus is the central bony core or inner wall of the cochlear tube. Around this central axis and projecting outward is the osseous spiral lamina, resembling the flanged thread of a screw, (representing the outer bony surface of the cochlear tube). The base of the cochlea measures 9 mm while its axial height is 5 mm. The cochlea, therefore, is easily seen on CT. The axis of the spiral is perpendicular to the posterior wall of the temporal bone with the plane of the basal turn of the cochlea noted to be parallel to this wall.

The round window (cochlear fenestra) is noted as a bony opening within the posterior lateral aspect of the basal turn of the cochlea projecting laterally and inferiorly into the middle ear (see discussion of medial wall and middle ear) just anterior to the subiculum and sinus tympani.

The CT appearance of the cochlea will vary depending on the plane of scanning. The zero degree (parallel to anthropologic baseline) axial scan parallels the modiolus or axis of the cochlea and, therefore, best demonstrates the appearance of contiguous rings from base to apex. The basal turn is well displayed; however, the middle and apical turns may be difficult to differentiate. The round window is well displayed on axial images as a niche protruding posteriorly and laterally from the basal turn. On coronal CT, portions of the contiguous turns are seen, usually as parallel arcs due to the obliquity of the coronal plane relative to the axis of the cochlea. Sagittal oblique reformatted images along the plane of the individual turns may help display the size and configuration of the cochlear turns. We tend to use such reformations when assessing patients for cochlear implantation if there is any concern based on the axial images.

The cochlear aqueduct connects the perilymphatic space of the scala tympani with the subarachnoid space. On CT, a long tapering canal parallel to and just below the IAC will be noted to penetrate the posterior petrous wall just superior to the medial margin of the jugular fossa. The aqueduct is usually best seen at the level of the carotid canal and eustachian tube. Care should be taken not to confuse it with the IAC (which lies 3 to 4 mm more superiorly) because of the tendency to have a funnel-shaped opening at its intracranial end (Fig. 10-16).

### The Vestibule and Oval Window

The vestibule (Figs. 10-14, 10-16, 10-17) is the central bony fossa or chamber within the bony labyrinth, just lateral to the fundus of the IAC. The chamber is 4 mm in diameter and is the most capacious part of the labyrinth. It is easily noted as a central landmark for the bony labyrinth on high-resolution CT; anteroinferiorly the vestibule will be noted to communicate with the cochlea (the membranous labyrinth of the cochlea is continuous with the vestibule) while posterosuperiorly the vestibule communicates with the semicircular canals.

The oval window on coronal CT is seen just inferior and medial to the horizontal portion of the facial nerve canal. The relationship of the vestibule to the semicircular canals is well visualized on the axial and coronal images. The vestibule appears, on axial images, more ovoid inferior to the semicircular canals. Superiorly, the vestibule has a triangular configuration with focal peripheral bulges at the sites of communication with the semicircular canals.

The vestibular aqueduct, seen as a bony channel, begins at the common crus of the superior and posterior semicircular canals. The channel resembles a hockey stick, extending from the common crus and

vestibule to pass between the posterior semicircular canal and posterior wall of the petrous bone to penetrate the posterior wall just above the jugular fossa. The ventral arm of the aqueduct is not visualized, but the larger posterior arm may be detected. At its termination, the aqueduct widens to accomodate the endolymphatic sac and merges with the foveate impression, which is a small plateau along the posterior surface of the petrous bone.

### Semicircular Canals

The three semicircular canals—lateral (horizontal), posterior, and superior—are perpendicular to each other and communicate with the superior posterior aspect of the vestibule (Figs. 10-15, 10-17, 10-18).

The lateral semicircular canal is essentially horizontal in orientation. Its more lateral aspect projects into the medial portion of the epitympanic space forming the medial wall of the aditus ad antrum. The axial 30 degree plane parallels the lateral semicircular canal and CT displays superbly the entire semicircular canal lucency and its cortical bony margin with visualization far superior to that seen by conventional tomography. The coronal axis complements the axial study, especially if there is any question of bony destruction or erosion to suggest fistula formation. The relationship of the lateral semicircular canal to the facial nerve is better noted on coronal CT.

The posterior semicircular canal lies parallel to the posterior wall of the petrous base while the axis of the superior semicircular canal is perpendicular to the posterior wall. These two canals are vertically oriented and therefore will be seen as portions of their respective arcs on contiguous axial slices. Similarly, coronal CT will only display segments of each canal on contiguous slices. Reformations along the plane of the specific semicircular canal are possible but seldom required. The semicircular canals tend to be easily identified based on knowledge of their locations. The posterior and superior semicircular canals will be noted to share a common limb: the common crus. The vestibular aqueduct passing between the posterior semicircular canal and the posterior surface of the petrous bone should not be mistaken for a semicircular canal.

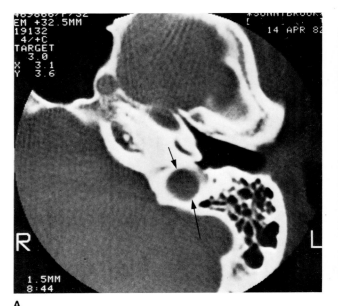

A

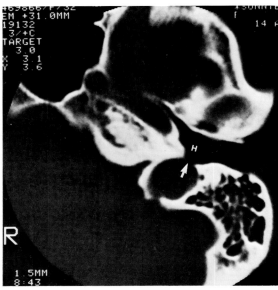

B

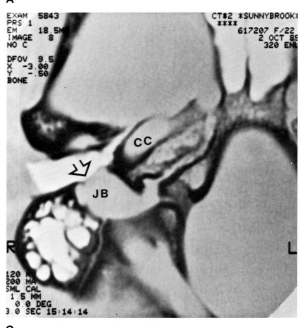

C

**Fig. 10-22.** Axial CT of high jugular bulb. **(A)** High jugular bulb (arrows): note characteristic smooth, well-corticated margin to jugular defect posterior to cochlea at level of tympanic cavity. **(B)** One slice more inferiorly: jugular bulb (arrows) is separated from hypotympanum (H) by a fine rim of bone. **(C)** Reverse image to accentuate bone detail. Dehiscent jugular bulb (JB) is eroding into posterior aspect of hypotympanum (arrow). There is no bony wall between jugular bulb and hypotympanum. CC, carotid canal.

## The Internal Auditory Canal

The IAC (Figs. 10-14, 10-18) parallels the coronal plane, slightly superior to the level of the EAC. Most patients will demonstrate a tubular configuration with the walls roughly parallel or minimally convex to each other. Varying degrees of flaring or funnel-like configurations at the porus acusticus may be noted. Symmetry of the canals is important and is best assessed if the two sides are positioned identically on the same slice levels. On coronal slices the crista falciformis is seen as a small bony spine extending medially into the fundus of the canal, to separate the IAC into a superior compartment for the facial nerve anteriorly and the superior division of the vestibular nerve posteriorly.

The inferior compartment contains the cochlear nerve anteriorly and the inferior division of the vestibular nerve posteriorly. Axial CT demonstrates the exit foramina at the fundus, producing a Y-like configuration of the most lateral aspect of the bony canal. The anteriorly directed canal for the cochlear nerve can be seen directed toward the modiolus of the cochlea just inferior to the foramen of the facial nerve canal (fallopian canal). The vestibular foramina are noted posteriorly. Air CT-cisternography allows the nerves exiting toward their respective foramina to be seen.

## Facial Nerve Canal

The facial nerve (Figs. 10-13, 10-14, 10-20) has an intimate connection with the temporal bone. High-resolution imaging, in both axial and coronal planes, augmented by reformations along the sagittal axis, has become the primary mode of study for assessment of the facial nerve canal. Because of the complex course of the facial nerve, it is best identified and assessed in segments or divisions, with the adjacent anatomic segments of the petrous bone that act as landmarks for that specific segment of the facial nerve.

The facial nerve and nervus intermedius leave the brain stem (lower pons), crossing the CPA cistern to enter the porus acusticus of the IAC. The facial nerve continues laterally within the anterior superior portion of the IAC, lying superior to the cochlear division and anterior to the superior and inferior vestibular portion of the divisions of the 8th cranial nerve to reach the fundus of the IAC. The CT assessment of this portion of the facial nerve usually commences with an intravenous enhanced CT, with 5 mm slices through the brainstem and CPA. Slices 1.5 mm thick, a soft tissue mode, and magnified images through the level of the IAC, may help detect a small intracanalicular facial nerve tumor and obviate the need for more invasive studies.

Air CT-cisternography may be used to assess the facial nerve as it travels between the brain stem and fundus of the IAC. Smaller intracanalicular masses may be well "capped" or outlined by air[33] within the IAC, or as they protrude slightly into the CPA cistern. Such masses are usually nonspecific in their appearance and difficult to differentiate from other soft tissue tumors, such as intracanalicular meningioma or the more common acoustic neuroma. Clinical correlation is essential to suggest the proper diagnosis. Larger tumors of the facial nerve, with more extension into the CPA cistern, may result in poor definition of the medial boundaries of the mass, and its relationship to the brain stem and adjacent cisterns. Larger tumors may be associated with multiple cranial nerve palsies and be difficult to distinguish from other CPA masses (see discussion of acoustic neuroma and CPA masses). Since the introduction of high-resolution CT imaging and air CT-cisternography techniques, the need for intrathecal posterior fossa myelography, with or without CT, has almost totally disappeared. If the intravenous enhanced preliminary study is unremarkable, high-resolution CT assessement of the petrous bone should be performed. However, if clinical conditions indicate the pathologic site within a particular portion of the petrous bone, assessment may, in fact, be initiated with high-resolution bone imaging.

Soft tissue imaging may be needed to complement the bone imaging detail. Magnetic resonance imaging has made significant impact on the investigation of CPA masses, including intracanalicular tumors. However, the fine bone detail available with high resolution CT petrous imaging remains unchallenged by currently available MRI.

The facial nerve canal,[19] the longest bony nerve canal in the body, begins its course at the fundus of the IAC and terminates at the stylomastoid foramen. Because of the length and complexity of the facial canal, its assessment will be described in segments.

At the lateral aspect of the IAC, the facial nerve turns anteriorly to enter the facial canal via a foramen at the anterior-superior aspect of the IAC fundus. This short anterolateral course, representing the labyrinthine segment, is well seen on axial CT, extending from the IAC fundus to the fossa of the geniculate ganglion. This portion of the facial nerve and the ganglion lies just superior to the cochlea. At the geniculate ganglion, the facial nerve makes a hairpin turn to run posterolaterally along the medial wall of the tympanic cavity, remaining on the same horizontal plane as the labyrinthine and geniculate segments. These segments are therefore considered the horizontal segments of the facial nerve canal. On the 30 degree axial CT, which parallels this portion of the facial nerve, the facial canal is seen as an inverted "V" with the geniculate ganglion at its apex, the labyrinthine segment forming the shorter but better defined medial limb, and the horizontal tympanic segment forming the longer but less well defined lateral (distal) limb. The apex of the inverted "V," at the geniculate ganglion, represents the anterior genu of the facial nerve canal. On coronal CT, the anterior genu may be seen as two small canals approximately in the horizontal plane (with the proximal limb slightly more superior) approaching each other and appearing as "snakes" or "owl's eyes," just superior and lateral to the mid- and apical cochlear turns, anterior to the plane of the IAC. A groove in the medial wall of the tympanic cavity for the semicanal of the tensor tympani muscle will be seen more anteriorly, just inferior to the distal limb. At the apex of the genu, the canal has a single, slightly oval, configuration.

The tympanic portion of the horizontal segment extends from the anterior or geniculate genu along the length of the medial wall of the tympanic cavity to the posterior genu, located just posterior to the pyramidal eminence, at which point the facial canal turns sharply inferiorly toward the stylomastoid foramen. This horizontal portion has a thickened medial wall, representing the medial wall of the tympanic cavity as well as a thick superior wall related to the prominence overlying the lateral semicircular canal. The lateral-inferior bony wall is thinner or may be dehiscent at specific regions along its course, most notably adjacent to the cochleariform process and oval window.[17] The degree of development of the lateral bony wall determines how well this portion of the distal limb is defined on axial CT. The axial CT demonstrates the facial nerve passing medial to the ossicles in the epitympanic recess, superior to the oval window. More posteriorly the nerve is seen to pass lateral to the pyramidal eminence and sinus tympani to reach the posterior genu. Even when the lateral inferior bony wall is poorly formed, the facial nerve tends to be imaged, since the soft tissue structure remains outlined by air within the tympanic cavity. Coronal

images tend to display the facial nerve better than axial slices in such circumstances. Rather than a canal, the coronal image may then display the facial nerve within a shallow groove just inferior to the lateral semicircular canal, and immediately above the oval window. Partial volume effect of the obliquely directed bony wall of the lateral semicircular canal obscures the facial canal on axial CT but not on coronal imaging.

The vertical (descending or mastoid) portion of the facial canal begins at the posterior genu just lateral to the pyramidal eminence and sinus tympani. It maintains this relationship in its more superior aspect. More inferiorly, the descending portion passes lateral to the jugular fossa to reach the stylomastoid foramen. The vertical canal will be visualized on axial CT, posterior to the EAC and tympanic cavity and anterior to the mastoid air cells as a round channel. The canal can usually be identified from adjacent or surrounding air cells by its tendency to have a thicker cortical bony wall. In young children, or in adults with obliteration or lack of development of the mastoid air cells, the facial nerve canal will be easier to identify. On coronal images, the vertical canal is usually seen as a thin, parallel-walled linear channel, bending medially and anteriorly at its superior aspect to resemble an upside-down hockey stick. A 105 degree coronal axis is required to see the vertical canal parallel to the plane of scan. Sagittal reformations may be used to demonstrate the posterior genu and descending facial canal, and offer an excellent overview of the vertical canal and adjacent structures (Fig. 21B).

Scanning of the soft tissues just inferior to the skull base, between the mastoid tip and the styloid process or more anteriorly and inferiorly through the region of the parotid gland, may be required to assess further the distribution of the facial nerve.

## The Carotid Canal

The internal carotid artery (ICA) (Fig. 10-13) courses through the temporal bone. Entering the petrous bone just inferolateral to the cochlea, the ICA turns from its superior orientation sharply medially and anteriorly in the carotid canal to exit from the petrous bone at the petrous apex, just posterior to the lateral wall of the body of the sphenoid bone and cavernous portion of the ICA.

As the ICA enters the petrous bone at the skull base, it lies immediately anterior to the jugular fossa, separated from it by a bony septum, the caroticojugular spine. The temporomandibular joint will be lateral and the hypotympanum medial to the ICA. At this more inferior level the carotid canal will have a round configuration because of the vertical or superior direction of the ICA. The zero degree axial slices demonstrate the basal foramina, vascular channels, and their relations optimally. As the ICA turns 90 degrees anteromedially to run in a more horizontal axis along the longitudinal axis of the petrous bone, the artery passes immediately anterior to the cochlea, directed from inferolateral to anteromedial. The eustachian tube, filled with air in its posterior bony segment, parallels the superior lateral margin of the carotid canal. The semicanal for the tensor tympani muscle lies between and superolateral to the carotid canal and just superior to the eustachian tube. As with the other basal skull landmarks, it is best seen on the axial zero degree scan. The foramina ovale and spinosum will be easily identified anterolateral to the carotid canal, just anterior to the anterior portion of the tympanic cavity.

The relationship of the carotid canal to the eustachian tube and semicanal may be further assessed by coronal imaging, which better demonstrates the more superior position of the semicanal.

## Jugular Bulb and Internal Jugular Vein

The jugular fossa (Figs. 10-13, 10-21, 10-22) is complex in configuration and therefore not as clearly defined as the carotid canal. More inferiorly, the fossa is circular, separated from the carotid canal by the thin crescent of bone, the caroticojugular spine. The dome of the bulb normally reaches the level of the hypotympanum, forming its medial posterior margin. It normally remains inferior to the level of the IAC and cochlea. The configuration of the fossa may be distorted by a broad communication with the sigmoid sinus, which empties into the medial inferior aspect of the bulb. The jugular fossa tends to have an "open" posteromedial border, formed by dura rather than bone, although a thin bony plate may separate this

venous structure from the posterior cranial fossa contents. A prominent jugular bulb may encroach upon the space of the tympanic cavity. Abnormality of the anterior bony wall, such as dehiscence, shows only a membranous border between the jugular bulb and the hypotympanum with varying degrees of bulging of the jugular bulb into the tympanic cavity.

The sigmoid sinus is formed in part by an overhanging lip of the posterior wall of the petrous bone. The sigmoid sinus is recognized as a semicircular impression or scalloped margin at the posterior lateral aspect of the temporal bone, lateral and superior to the jugular fossa. Because of this scalloped effect on the more lateral aspect of the posterior margin, a broad projection of bone more medially separates the sigmoid sinus from the jugular fossa. Mastoid air cells form the lateral wall of the sigmoid sinus while the medial wall is formed by dura, with no bony component present. The sigmoid sinus is best demonstrated by intravenous contrast enhancement if definition of the sinus, and especially its medial wall, is required.

The jugular bulb lies between the descending facial nerve canal laterally and the occipital condyle medially. Just superior to the occipital condyle, the hypoglossal canal is visualized extending anteriorly, posteromedial to the jugular fossa. On coronal images, the hypoglossal canal appears as a wider canal extending inferiorly and medially, medial to the jugular bulb between the jugular tubercle above and the occipital condyle below (Fig. 10-8H). The petro-occipital suture, separating the petrous bone anterolaterally from the occipital bone posteromedially, is noted medial to the jugular bulb and extends superiorly and medially to pass superior to the hypoglossal canal and jugular tubercle and extends anteriorly, medial to the carotid canal.

Considerable asymmetry of the jugular fossae may be noted, whether in size or configuration. Diverticula of the jugular bulb represent a common normal variant; if projected superiorly they form a high jugular bulb. The cortex of the margins of the jugular bulb, despite variation of size or configuration, should always be sharp and well-defined. Loss of this cortex is an early pathologic change in vascular tumors of the jugular bulb.

The 9th, 10th, and 11th cranial nerves exit from

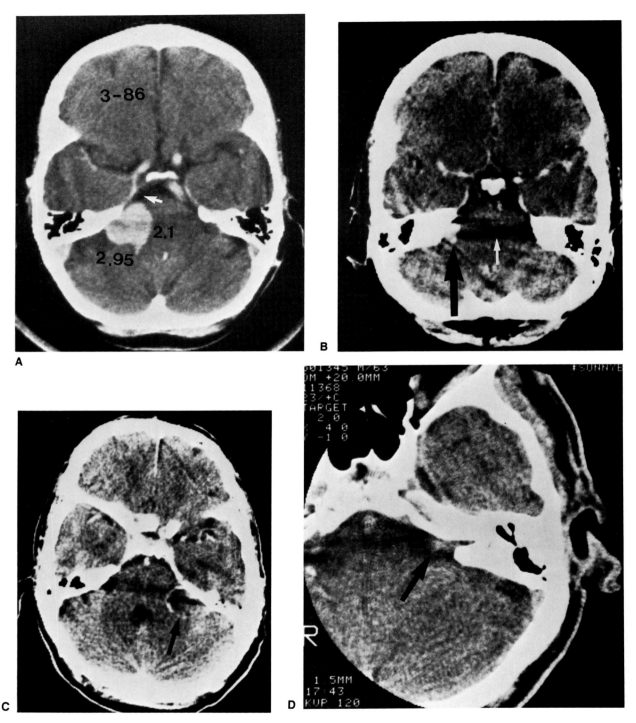

**Fig. 10-23.** Acoustic neuroma: intravenous contrast-enhanced CT. **(A)** Typical enhancement of right acoustic neuroma with anteroposterior and mediolateral dimensions given in centimeters. Brain stem is displaced to left with widening of right CPA cistern (arrow). **(B)** Small irregular-shaped enhancement defines right acoustic neuroma (dark arrow). Note streak artifact (white arrow) between petrous bones, which limits image quality and brain stem detail. **(C)** Acoustic neuroma presenting as a mass at left CPA (arrow). Only peripheral enhancement about the mass lesion is seen; there is no significant central enhancement. **(D)** Slice thick 1.5 mm through left IAC shows abnormal enhancement (arrow) of acoustic neuroma extending from porus (5 mm thick slices performed initially were normal). Additional thinner slices through IAC at time of initial enhanced 5 mm study may obviate need for air CT or MRI. An artifact may occasionally simulate a small mass at the porus.

the skull through the jugular foramen. Although not directly visualized, clinical signs or symptoms may suggest that the radiologic assessment be directed to the jugular fossa region. The adjacent 12th cranial nerve may also be involved by pathologic entities at this site.

**Soft Tissue**

When patients are referred to us for investigation of brain stem, cerebellar, or CPA symptoms, we obtain 5 mm thick axial slices of the posterior cranial fossa (PCF)[19,23,24,30,32] (Fig. 10-23; see also Figs. 12-7 through 12-11). Such studies use contiguous slices at 5 mm intervals (necessary to show the anatomic landmarks, e.g., 4th ventricle), and are continued inferiorly until the foramen magnum or inferior margin of the cerebellar tonsils is identified. Five mm slices are similarly continued superiorly to visualize the entire brain stem, cerebellum, and petrous ridges. Supratentorial structures may be assessed at 10 mm intervals, with particular attention paid to ventricular size. Such initial scanning should display the brain stem and adjacent cisterns, the cerebellum, and fourth ventricle. The CPA, cistern, and IAC may not be readily recognized at the soft tissue mode and with 5 mm slices. However, visualization of the petrous bone at an extended window will identify the slice level and bone detail of the IAC, thereby assessing flaring or shortening of this canal.

Such flaring remains the single most important sign in differentiating acoustic neuroma from other CPA masses. Even if no mass is seen on initial CT, the suggestion of flaring is supportive of an intracanalicular mass that requires further study. If the study using 5 mm slices through the posterior fossa does not show a mass lesion, or if there is a question of volume averaging that makes interpretation of a mass or density abnormality questionable, further assessment is performed at the time of initial study, by supplementing the examination using 1.5 mm thin slices through the IAC, either bilaterally or on the affected side only, depending on clinical history and individual preferences. Retrospective images to assess bone detail of the IAC may also be obtained, especially if there are any unusual features of the soft tissue mass. Occasionally, findings from such bone images may suggest pathologic changes other than acoustic neuroma, such as meningioma, epidermoid tumor, or vascular lesion.

Detection of an intracanalicular tumor by the use of thinner slices spares the patient more invasive alternatives.

Degrees of invasiveness must be balanced with diagnostic efficiency and practicality. Although an unenhanced CT scan is least invasive, the decreased diagnostic yield (60 percent detection),[19] as well as additional radiation exposure if the slices need to be repeated with contrast enhancement, suggest that for the great majority of patients the low risk of contrast media reactions is justified by the significantly increased diagnostic yield. The availability of newer, less hyperosmolar, vascular contrast media will further reduce the low risk of complications. The use of nonenhanced CT in the investigation of CPA mass is reserved for demonstration or assessment of tissue density (e.g., calcification or hemorrhage obscured by intravenous enhancement) or to rule out large masses in those patients known to be at higher risk if contrast media is used (e.g., those with allergy to contrast media). Coronal CT is infrequently used in our investigation of CPA mass lesions since such masses are usually adequately demonstrated on axial images. Occasionally, the coronal axis is useful to define better the extent of such tumors, especially their relationship to the tentorial edge.

In those patients whose CT study remains normal or questionable and clinical findings or treatment objectives demand further investigation, the next step in our protocol is an air CT-cisternogram.[33] This study must be considered more invasive and has the side effects of the lumbar puncture required for the instillation of a few cubic centimeters of a gaseous contrast medium, usually filtered room air or carbon dioxide, which, with proper patient positioning, can be manipulated to the CPA cistern. Axial slices, usually performed in conjunction with a high-resolution 1.5 mm thickness scan in magnified bone mode, will be obtained with the patient placed in the lateral decubitus position such that the air rises to the CPA cistern of concern and normally readily enters the IAC. The 7th and 8th nerves are frequently outlined and followed more laterally within the IAC.[19,23,30,31] It is usual to perform such studies bilaterally. After the side of major concern (e.g., hearing loss) is studied, the patient may be rotated to the opposite decubitus position for study of the remaining IAC and CPA. Knowledge of whether the patient has unilateral or bilateral acoustic neuromas is invaluable for further discussion and long-term treatment planning, especially in the very young patient who may have neurofibromatosis.

Since early diagnosis of acoustic neuroma is becoming more frequent, the value of further assessment beyond routine 5 mm slices of the posterior fossa is therefore stressed. Small tumors only partially filling the IAC tend to be at the more lateral portion of the canal, or more posteriorly along the usual path of the neurovascular structures. They are visualized as a filling defect in the column of air used as the contrast agent. Slightly larger masses will be seen to fill the IAC with mild bulging into the CPA. Flaring may be present and is more significant when present unilaterally; bilateral flaring usually represents a normal variant. As with CPA masses, such flaring remains the single most useful sign in distinguishing intracanalicular acoustic neuromas from other causes of soft tissue densities within the IAC. Intracanalicular meningiomas, adhesive arachnoiditis, and 7th nerve neuromas are other causes of a nonfilled (with air) IAC. Arachnoid adhesions tend to present a flat or concave surface, in contrast to the usual convex medial surface noted with acoustic neuroma or meningioma. However, acoustic neuromas have been noted to appear identical to arachnoiditis. Further efforts to move the air as far laterally as possible (fine shaking of head in lateral decubitus position) may be helpful in demonstrating fine amounts of air entering spaces within the soft tissues of the nonfilled canal, signifying arachnoid changes.

Vascular loops of the anterior-inferior cerebellar artery may occasionally be confused with nonfilling of the IAC. The configuration of the loop is usually characteristic. If further assessment is required, intravenous contrast infusion during the air CT-cisternogram may help. Occasionally, arteriography may be useful to confirm the presence of such loops.

## ACKNOWLEDGMENTS

This work was supported by the Saul A. Silverman Family Foundation, Toronto, Ontario.

The authors gratefully acknowledge Suzanne Petrevski and Rosemarie McGuire for manuscript preparation and Patsy Cunningham and Samantha Kassel for the illustrations. We appreciate the efforts of the Departments of Instructional Media at Mount Sinai Hospital and Sunnybrook Medical Centre.

## REFERENCES

1. Noyek AM, Zizmor J: The evolution of diagnostic radiology of the temporal bone. J Otolaryngol 6 [Suppl 3]:1, 1977
2. Brunner S, Jensen G, Hespersen C: Value of different projections in diagnosing cholesteatoma. Acta Radiol 54:177, 1960
3. Pendergrass EP, Schaeffer JP: The Head and Neck in Roentgen Diagnosis. Charles C Thomas, Springfield, Illinois, 1956
4. Compere WE, Radiographic Atlas of the Temporal Bone, vol. 1. American Academy of Ophthalmology and Otolaryngology, Rochester, 1964
5. Laszlo I, Conventional radiography of the temporal bone. Otolaryngol Clin North Am 6(2):323, 1973
6. Ballinger PW: Merrill's Atlas of Radiographic Positions and Radiologic Procedures, 5th ed, vol 2. CV Mosby, St. Louis, 1982
7. Phelps PD, Lloyd GAS: Radiology of the Ear. Blackwell Scientific Publications, Oxford, England, 1983
8. Brunner S, Petersen O, Stoksted P: Laminagraphy of the temporal bone. Am J Roentgenol 86:281, 1961
9. Valvassori GE, Pierce RH: The normal internal auditory canal. Am J Roentgenol 92:1232, 1964
10. Valvassori GE: The abnormal internal auditory canal: the diagnosis of acoustic neuroma. Radiology 92:449, 1969
11. Wright J Jr, Taylor CC: Polytomography of the Temporal Bone. Warren H. Green, St Louis, 1973
12. Zizmor J, Noyek AM: The protean radiologic manifestations of acquired temporal bone cholesteatoma. J Otolaryngol 10 (suppl 8):1, 1981
13. Valvassori GE, Buckingham RA: Tomography and Cross Sections of the Ear. WB Saunders, Philadelphia, 1975
14. Potter GD: The lateral projection in tomography of the petrous pyramid. Am J Roentgenol 104:194, 1968
15. Petasnick JP: Congential malformations of the ear. Otolaryngol Clin North Am 6 (2):413, 1973

16. Ericson S, Liliequist B: Tomographic examination of the vertical segment of the facial canal. Acta Radiol (Diagn) 14:673, 1973

17. Wilbrand HF, Bergstron B: Multidirectional tomography of defects of the facial canal. Acta Radiol (Diagn) 16:223, 1975

18. Hanafee WN, Gussen R: Correlation of basal projection tomography in clinical problems. Radiol Clin North Am 12:419, 1974

19. Bergeron RT, Osborn AG, Som PM (eds): Head and Neck Imaging Excluding the Brain. CV Mosby, St Louis, 1984

20. Mafee MF: Dynamic CT and its application to otolaryngology — head and neck surgery. J Otolaryngol 11:307, 1982

21. Chakares DW: CT of ear structures: a tailored approach. Radiol Clin North Am 22 (1):3, 1984

22. Swartz JD: Cholesteatomas of the middle ear: diagnosis, etiology and complications. Radiol Clin North Am 22 (1):15, 1984

23. Swartz JD: Imaging of the Temporal Bone. Thieme, New York, 1986

24. Mafee MF, Kumar A, Valvassori GE, et al: CT in the evaluation of the vestibulocochlear nerves and their central pathways; evaluations of neurotologic disorders. Radiol Clin North Am 22 (1)45, 1984

25. Damsa H, deGroot JAM, Zonneveld FW, et al: CT of cochlear otosclerosis (otospongiosis). Radiol Clin North Am 22 (1):37, 1984

26. Zonneveld FW: The technique of direct multiplanar high resolution CT of the temporal bone. Neurosurg Rev 8:5, 1985

27. Mancuso AA, Hanafee WN: Computed Tomography and Magnetic Resonance Imaging of the Head and Neck, 2nd ed. Williams & Wilkins, Baltimore, 1985

28. Shaffer KA, Haughten VM, Wilson CR: High resolution computed tomography of the temporal bone. Radiology 134:409, 1980

29. Virapongse C, Rothman SLG, Kier EL, Sarwar M: Computed tomographic anatomy of the temporal bone. Am J Neuroradiol 3:379, 1982

30. Taylor S: The petrous temporal bone (including the cerebellopontine angle). Radiol Clin North Am 20:67, 1982

31. Curtin HD: CT of acoustic neuroma and other tumors of the ear. Radiol Clin North Am 22 (1):77, 1984

32. Johnson DW: CT of the postsurgical ear. Radiol Clin North Am 22:67, 1984

33. Kricheff II, Pinto RS, Bergeron RT, Cohen N: Air-CT cisternography and canalography for small acoustic neuromas. Am J Neuroradiol 1:57, 1980

# Temporal Bone Imaging: Magnetic Resonance, Angiography, Radionuclide Scans

# 11

Edward E. Kassel
Arnold M. Noyek

## MAGNETIC RESONANCE IMAGING

Magnetic resonance imaging[1-6] (MRI) is the most recent, most complex, and most exciting of the new imaging modalities (Figs. 11-1 to 11-6). It is a noninvasive technique, performed without the use of ionizing radiation and with no known adverse biologic effects. It is used to evaluate normal and pathologic anatomy of the brain and skull base. Its greater sensitivity to soft tissue contrast has allowed earlier detection of neoplasm, edema, demyelination, contusion, and hemorrhage, which surpasses state-of-the-art computed tomography (CT).

MRI has a significant advantage over CT for providing anatomic information in that it may be displayed directly in any plane without changing the patient's position. For example, sagittal or coronal MR images are obtainable with the patient remaining supine, in contrast to the often awkward positioning required for similar planes of study by CT. The spatial resolution and anatomic detail in these various MR planes are superior to those of reformatted CT images. Use of intravenous contrast enhancement is not required as part of the routine study (in contrast to CT). However, in the future, the full potential of MRI may be better realized by the selected administration of various MR "contrast agents" (affecting proton imaging).

### Principles

Three basic physical components are required for MRI: magnetic moment, a magnetic field of significant strength, and radiofrequency waves.[2,3]

#### Nuclear Magnetic Moment

Every atomic nucleus contains neutrons and protons (nucleons). Nuclei with an odd number of protons or neutrons have an electric charge. Because all nuclei spin, those nuclei possessing an electric charge will have a magnetic moment. Under normal conditions, nuclei spin about axes that point in random directions; the vector sum of their magnetic moment is zero. However, the magnetic moments of such nuclei can be influenced by interaction with an externally applied powerful magnetic field and radiofrequency waves. The analysis of these interactions forms the basis of MRI.

The hydrogen nucleus is ideal for MRI. It has a strong magnetic moment because of its relatively high charge compared to its low mass. Also, it is the most abundant element in the body. Thus, MRI has

303

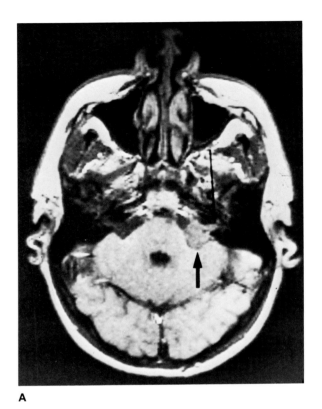

**A**

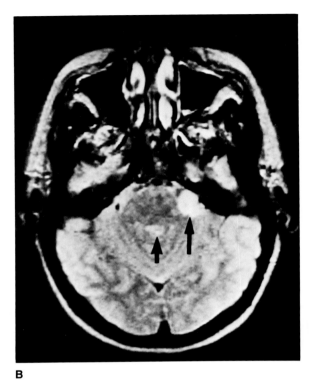

**B**

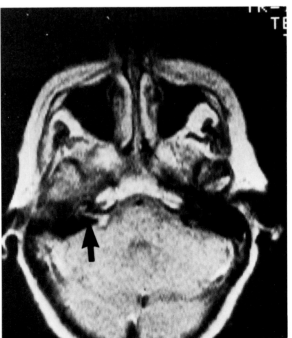

**C**

**Fig. 11-1.** Acoustic neuroma—axial MRI. **(A)** 0.5 T T$_1$-weighted image displays left acoustic neuroma (arrows) as mass lesion extending into left cerebellopontine angle (CPA) from internal auditory canal (IAC). Anatomic detail is well imaged. **(B)** 0.5 T T$_2$-weighted image accentuates pathologic characteristics of left acoustic neuroma (long arrow). Anatomic detail, however, is inferior to T$_1$ image **(A)**. T$_2$-weighted images often are used as screening mode and are generally more informative in assessing pathology. Note increased signal intensity of CSF with T$_2$ weighted studies—e.g., 4th ventricle (short arrow). **(C)** 0.35 T axial late T$_2$-weighted image shows mild thickening of 8th cranial nerve (acoustic neuroma) (arrow) with no increase in signal intensity on delayed echo (different patient with small right acoustic neuroma). A, B (courtesy of Picker International, Highland Heights, OH.)

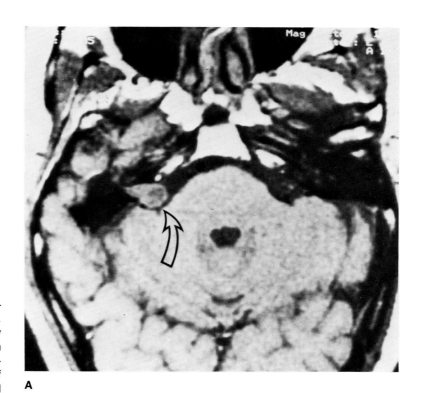

A

**Fig. 11-2.** Axial MRI of acoustic neuroma: current resolution capabilities. **(A)**T$_1$-weighted axial image superbly displays right acoustic neuroma (open arrow) within IAC, bulging into CPA cistern. **(B)** 1.5 T T$_2$-weighted image of patient with neurofibromatosis and bilateral acoustic neuromas (large arrows). Left acoustic neuroma extends significantly into CPA cistern. Faint signals from right cochlea and vestibule also seen (small arrows). *(Figure continues.)*

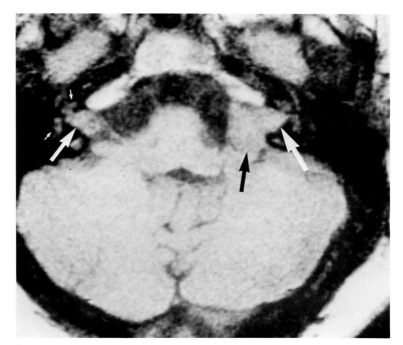

B

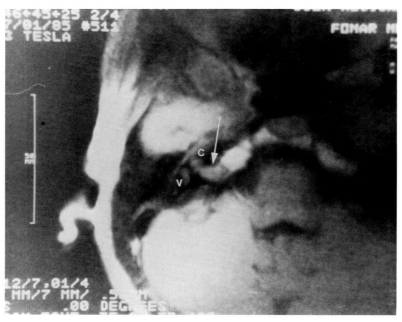

C

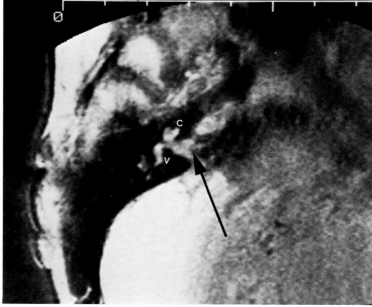

D

**Fig. 11-2** *(Continued).* **(C)** 0.3 T T$_1$-weighted image obtained using surface coil, clearly demonstrates a right acoustic neuroma (arrow) within the IAC. The bright signal adjacent and medial to the tumor is fatty marrow in the petrous apex. Faint increased signal of cochlea (c) and vestibule (v) are visible. **(D)** T$_1$-weighted, 15 cm field diameter surface coil axial study of right acoustic neuroma (arrow). Cochlea (c) and vestibular apparatus (v) are well defined in low-signal petrous bone. (A courtesy of Dr. Walter Kucharczyk, Toronto General Hospital, Toronto, Canada; B courtesy of Dr. Donald Chakares, Ohio Station University, Columbus, OH; C courtesy of Dr. William Hanafee, University of California, Los Angeles, CA; D courtesy Picker International MR, Highland Heights, OH.)

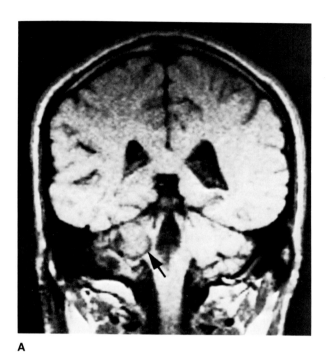

**A**

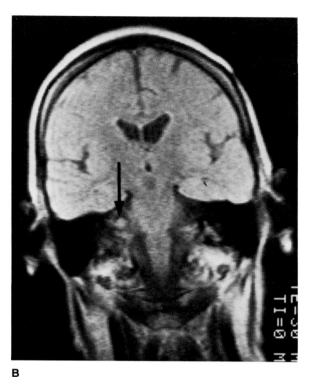

**B**

**Fig. 11-3.** Coronal MRI of acoustic neuroma. **(A)** Coronal $T_1$ image of right acoustic neuroma (arrow). Interface of tumor with brain stem is well demonstrated. There is minimal alteration in tissue intensity from adjacent tissues. **(B)** Coronal $T_2$-weighted image displays small mass (arrow) at right CPA. **(C)** Coronal $T_1$-weighted image displays right acoustic neuroma (arrow) throughout its length in the IAC. On $T_1$ images the low-signal CSF acts as an excellent contrast to outline the medial aspect of the tumor. (A courtesy of Picker International, Highland Heights, OH; B courtesy of Dr. Walter Kucharczyk, Toronto General Hospital, Toronto, Canada.)

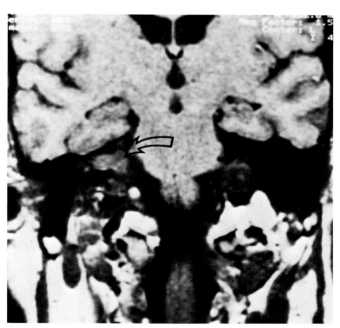

**C**

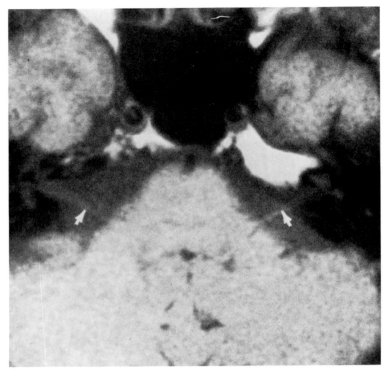

**A**

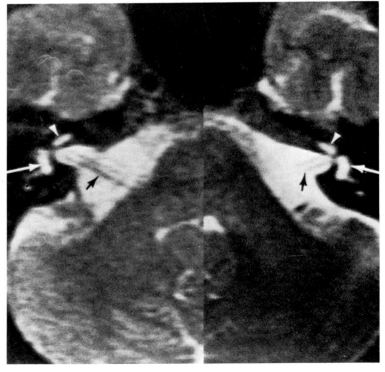

**B**

**Fig. 11-4.** MR intensity changes—
relationship of relaxation times. Normal
MR study one patient. **(A)** Axial $T_1$-
weighted image demonstrates 7th and
8th cranial nerves (short arrows) bilaterally. **(B)** Axial $T_2$-weighted image better demonstrates the cranial nerves
(dark arrows) as lower-intensity signal
relative to the increased signal of CSF.
Such manipulation of signal intensity
for CSF pathways reduces the need
for intrathecal contrast media. Cochlea
(arrowhead) and vestibule (long arrows) also seen as increased signal.
(Courtesy of Dr. Emanual Kanal, Pittsburgh MRI Institute; Dr. Hugh Curtin,
Pittsburgh Eye and Ear Hospital; and
General Electric Medical Systems, Mil-
waukee, WI.)

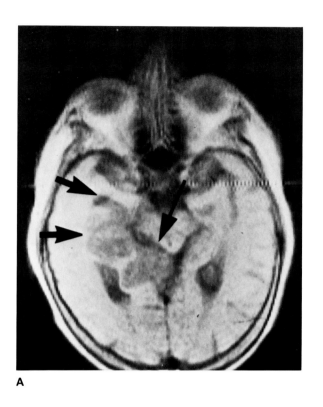

**A**

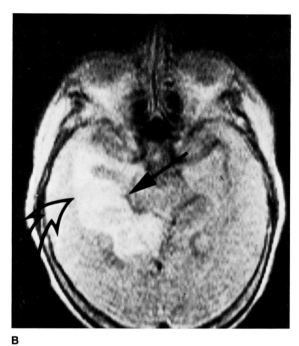

**B**

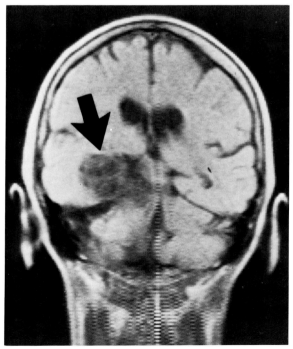

**C**

**Fig. 11-5.** Meningioma — signal intensity characteristics in relation to relaxation times. In meningioma of the posterior cranial fossa (PCF), delayed (late $T_2$) spin echo images show increased signal due to greater $T_2$ weighting compared to initial spin echo (early $T_2$). Early spin echo, however, has better anatomic resolution. **(A)** Early $T_2$-weighted axial image shows mass of decreased signal intensity (arrows) extending into medial aspect of middle cranial fossa (MCF) and superior extension into tentorial notch. **(B)** Late $T_2$-weighted axial image. Abnormal increased signal (arrows) are now seen from PCF mass involving right cerebellum, pons, and temporal lobe (MCF). **(C)** Early $T_2$-weighted coronal image displays significant superior extension of the low-intensity mass (arrow).

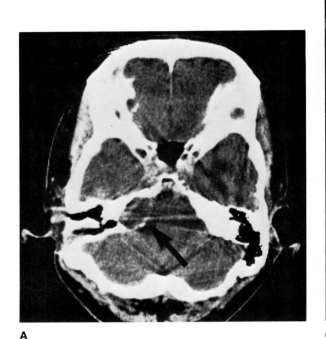

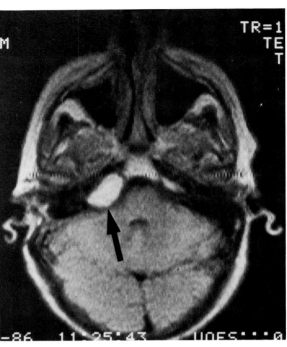

A                                                    C

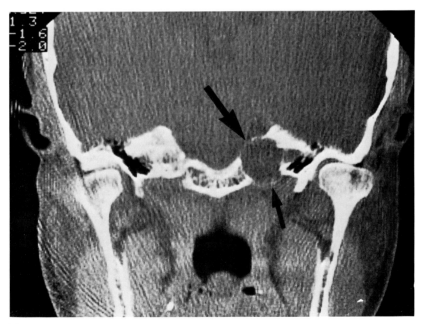

**Fig. 11-6.** MRI tissue characterization —comparison with CT in a patient with right hearing loss and 7th and 5th cranial nerve deficits. **(A)** Axial CT (enhanced to show soft tissues) displays defect in right petrous apex, with inner cortex displaced medially (arrow). No significant enhancement is noted. **(B)** Coronal CT better displays expanding nature (arrows) of well-defined lesion. Pattern of bone involvement suggests benign pathology. **(C–E)** MRI features may suggest tissue characterization to greater advantage than CT. **(C)** Early $T_1$ axial image shows increased $T_1$ signal (arrow) from the intrapetrous mass. Such signal intensity suggests stagnant blood or fat. *(Figure continues.)*

B

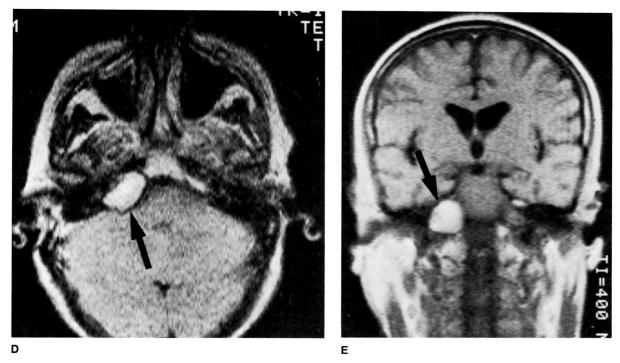

**D**                                          **E**

**Fig. 11-6.** *(Continued).*  **(D)** Late $T_1$ axial image shows persistent increased $T_1$ signal (arrow) suggesting that the lesion is vascular (slow flow). Fat tissue should have decreased in signal ($T_1$) intensity in later phase. **(E)** Coronal MRI ($T_1$ weighted) shows the increased signal intensity within petrous bone (arrow). Spatial resolution and bone detail are inferior to that of high-resolution CT but may not be required to display pathology. CT and MRI are frequently complementary in assessment of petrous bone. Diagnosis: cavernous hemangioma.

essentially, in the initial stages, been based on the hydrogen nucleus. Other nuclei are being researched for potential use. Unfortunately, their magnetic moments and their abundance are low.

## Magnetic Field

Alignment of the randomly directed magnetic axes of the spinning hydrogen protons is achieved by placing the body in a strong magnetic field. The individual nuclei align themselves along the direction of this static magnetic field. The strength of the magnetic field is expressed in terms of Tesla (T) (1 Tesla = 10 kilogauss).

## Radiofrequency Waves

For an MR signal to be produced, excitation of the aligned nuclei (e.g., hydrogen protons) within the strong magnetic field must occur. The nuclei are stimulated by radiofrequency (RF) pulsations emitted from an RF transmitter coil lying within the magnetic field. The strength of the applied magnetic field and the properties of the nucleus determine at which specific frequency excitation of the nuclei occurs. This frequency is termed the "Larmor frequency." On absorbing this RF pulse, the nuclei flip and align themselves against the static magnetic field. The protons therefore may be changed from the low-energy to high-energy state by supplying energy with a radiofrequency pulse of the appropriate frequency. The Larmor frequency is linearly proportional to the field strength. Similarly, the energy difference between low- and high-energy states is greater when the magnetic field is more powerful.

The spinning nucleus behaves like a spinning top in the magnetic field. If displaced from this vertical rotation axis it wobbles or "precesses." The angle between the axis of the primary magnetic field and the new axis of rotation is called the "precession angle." If a radiofrequency pulse at the Larmor frequency is applied, energy is absorbed by the proton from the RF pulse and the protons precess coherently and the precession angle progressively increases. This is a resonant phenomenon that only occurs at the Larmor frequency. For simplicity, the RF pulse is defined by the precession angle change that it causes (e.g., 90 degree pulse, 180 degree pulse).

When the RF pulse is terminated, the nuclei flip back to their original alignment in the fixed magnetic field. During this alignment they emit radiowaves of the same frequency as the initial RF pulse. This is the magnetic resonance signal. Nuclear magnetic resonance is therefore the spontaneous emission of energy in the form of radiosignals by nuclei that have been excited by RF waves of the appropriate Larmor frequency. The period of time during which the excess of absorbed energy is released, as the nuclei return to their initial position within the static magnetic field, is the "relaxation period." This released energy is in the form of a radiosignal and is detected by a RF receiver coil.

The effect of any RF pulse is to tilt the proton magnetization away from its alignment or equilibrium with respect to the static magnetic field (z axis). During such pulsations, nuclei are excited from a low energy to a higher energy level. Once the RF pulse has been turned off, the protons, whether flipped 90 or 180 degrees, will start to relax and realign themselves within the static magnetic field. The weak radiowaves emitted from the relaxing nuclei are received by the RF receiver coil, which transfers all data to a computer. The amplitude, frequency, and phase of the collected radiowaves are analyzed through a complex process to yield the MR images.

## Tissue Parameters

The intrinsic magnetic resonance properties of the examined tissue in large part determine signal intensity. These parameters include $T_1$ and $T_2$ relaxation times, proton density, and hydrogen motion.

### Relaxation Times

$T_1$ relaxation time is an exponential rate proportional to the time required for the net bulk magnetization to realign itself along the original z axis of the static magnetic field. Images that display differences in $T_1$, that is, $T_1$-weighted images, tend to display anatomic or spatial resolution to a better degree.

$T_2$ relaxation time is an exponential rate dependent on loss of coherence (among spins in the XY plane). Variations in $T_2$ will be noted within the same tissues, depending upon whether such tissue is healthy or diseased. Understanding $T_1$ and $T_2$ relaxation times allows one to appreciate tissue properties affecting signal intensity (Table 11-1) and allows tissue characterization (Table 11-2).

### Proton Density

Proton density (the number of protons per unit in volume) has a direct linear relationship to the overall intensity of the emitted MR signal. Those tissues with greater proton density (e.g., fat) demonstrate more intensity, while those tissues with less hydrogen proton density (e.g., compact bone) show relatively less intensity.

### Motion of Hydrogen

Although blood has a high proton density, rapidly moving protons (e.g., blood flow) return relatively little signal. Flow applications may, in the future, allow purposeful MR imaging of vascular structures.

## Operator Variables

Just as kilovoltage (kV) and milliamperage (mA) are the control variables in conventional radiogra-

**Table 11-1. Tissue Properties Affecting Signal Intensity**

Properties increasing relative signal intensity
    High hydrogen density
    Short $T_1$
    Long $T_2$

Properties decreasing relative signal intensity
    Low hydrogen density
    Long $T_1$
    Short $T_2$

° Courtesy of Dr. Walter Kucharczyk, Toronto General Hospital, Toronto, Canada.)

#### Table 11-2. Tissue Characterization

| Gray Scale[a] | | $T_1$-Weighted Image | $T_2$-Weighted Image |
|---|---|---|---|
| White | Increased signal intensity | Fat<br>Hemorrhage > 48 hrs<br>Colloid cysts | Hemorrhage (all ages)<br>Cerebral edema (nonspecific as<br>  per $T_1$)<br>CSF |
| Light gray | | White matter<br>Gray matter<br>Cerebral edema (tumor, infarct<br>  demyelination, inflammation)<br>Hemorrhage < 48 hrs | Fat<br>Colloid cysts<br>White matter<br>Gray matter |
| Dark gray | | CSF | Hemorrhage[b] |
| Black | Decreased signal intensity | Calcium<br>Blood vessels<br>Air | Calcium<br>Blood vessels<br>Air |

[a] The actual shade of gray observed will depend on the strength of the magnetic field, the window width and level, and the exact TR (repetition time or time between RF pulses) and TE (echo time or time at which signal sampled after RF pulse) of the imaging sequence.

[b] Acute hemorrhage (<24 hrs) and chronic hematomas may be dark gray-black on $T_2$-weighted images, due to apparent $T_2$ shortening caused by materials (deoxyhemoglobin and hemosiderin) within these hemorrhages that in turn create local inhomogeneities in the magnetic field. (Courtesy of Dr. Walter Kucharczyk, Toronto General Hospital, Toronto, Canada.)

phy, RF pulse sequences are operator-controlled (contrast) variables in MR. The various types of pulse sequences utilized affect the measurable MR signal.

### Spatial Localization of Signal

When a magnetic gradient is introduced into the static magnetic field, positional variations in field strength result. The frequency emitted by the excited protons will thus vary with their position along the gradient. Analysis of the frequency of RF emission permits spatial localization of the signal. Such "frequency encoding" of the signal source is the basis of MR data transference into an image format, whether onto film or display screen.

### MR Correlations

The otologist does not need to understand imaging physics, but must appreciate that the appearance of every magnetic resonance image depends on the physical characteristics of the tissue (spin density, relaxation time, hydrogen motion), as well as operator-selected imaging parameters (RF pulses).[1,4-6] MRI is a relatively new and still evolving technique. The use of surface coils as receivers

has significantly upgraded images because of better signal detection by the closer approximation of the detector to the source of the emitted radiowave. Further developments in MRI have affected the imaging of both soft tissue and bony structures. Slice thicknesses of 3 mm are now routinely available, with spatial resolution capabilities approaching 0.8 mm. This has allowed MRI to assess extremely small lesions in the cerebellopontine angle and internal auditory canal, especially in the diagnosis of intracanalicular acoustic neuromas.

### Clinical Applications

MRI has been used as a primary mode of investigation of posterior fossa and craniovertebral abnormalities (Figs. 11-1 through 11-6). The contents of the posterior fossa are better demonstrated by MRI than by CT. The sagittal demonstration of the skull base and brain stem is exquisite for craniovertebral abnormalities, including the soft tissue structures of the brain stem. Displacement of neural structures in the superior-inferior axis (such as the inferior displacement of the tonsils in Arnold-Chiari malformation) are ideally visualized using the sagittal images.

MRI may be helpful to assess those patients in whom there is clinical suspicion of disease but who appear normal by contrast-enhanced CT studies. Lesions that are isodense or low-grade on CT may be well displayed by MRI. MRI has become the preferred modality for studying the brain lesions of patients with multiple sclerosis. Where available, MRI has proven a helpful adjunct in the examination of any lesion that might be inconspicuous or confusing on CT.

For assessment of large masses in the cerebellopontine angle, MRI is as good as CT. MRI, however, has shown a definite superiority in displaying intracanalicular tumors that previously required air cisternography. Better images of the skull base and bony structures of the petrosa appear to be obtained using higher magnetic fields (superconductive) than with lower field strength resistive magnetic machines. On $T_1$ images acoustic neuromas are of higher intensity than the surrounding cerebrospinal fluid (CSF) or brain tissue (Figs. 11-1 to 11-3).

MRI now has practical advantages over conventional radiography and CT for visualizing tumors and nerves in and about the temporal bone. Since the surrounding bone and CSF have negligible signal, soft tissues in the internal auditory canal, facial nerve canal, cochlea, and vestibule are demonstrated in MR images with little artifact. The facial and vestibulocochlear nerves are effectively demonstrated in the $T_1$-weighted images and are seen as bright signals against the surrounding darker bone.

By contrast, $T_2$-weighted images demonstrate the CSF to be of increased signal intensity, with the 7th and 8th nerves outlined. Therefore, small extra-axial abnormalities within the internal auditory canal may be directly visualized as an increased signal on the $T_1$-weighted images, or as a decreased signal within the normal high-intensity CSF, suggesting that normal CSF has been displaced on the $T_2$-weighted images. The capability of the $T_2$-weighted image to show CSF as an increased signal intensity replaces and obviates the need for intrathecal CSF enhancement (Fig. 11-4).

The anatomy of bone is displayed less well by MRI than the adjacent soft tissue structures (posterior fossa and cerebral hemispheres). However, neural components or soft tissue abnormalities within the petrous bone, such as cholesteatoma or intratympanic masses, are effectively shown as areas of increased intensity within the low signal of the bony structures. At present CT remains the technique of choice to display bone configuration and detail.

Excellent MR imaging of the facial nerve, in the intracanalicular, horizontal, and descending portions of its course through the temporal bone, has been achieved using surface coil techniques. The facial nerve is well highlighted as a gray signal against the surrounding low-intensity bone.

The use of MR "contrast agents" to assess tumors further has demonstrated excellent enhancement on $T_1$-weighted images of the tumors, enabling high-resolution, high-contrast MRI studies to be obtained in less than half the time previously required. Fast scanning techniques allow data acquisition in approximately 5 minutes. This significantly lessens the degree of motion artifact, and allows a significant increase in the number of studies that can be performed per day.

MRI has become the obvious modality of choice in those patients who are at increased risk of idiosyncratic or allergic reactions to iodinated contrast media.

Pathologic features to date are often nonspecific. However, with further imaging experience, possibly supplemented with in vivo spectroscopy, MRI may provide more definitive tissue diagnoses than are currently available by CT. Vascular structures, with intraluminal flowing blood, appear as tubular structures with a low internal signal intensity. This feature improves visualization of such structures within the soft tissues of the posterior fossa or skull base and occasionally can predict the vascular nature of the petrous mass. MRI may be used to assess flow rate and hence signify vessel stenosis or occlusion. Because of the lack of signal intensity from cortical bone, MRI at present does not have a significant role in the assessment of bone trauma or changes. However, the lack of signal may act as contrast to surrounding soft tissues and allow many lesions, such as small subdural or epidural hematomas, to be visualized better. Recently, bone tumors and inflammation have been assessed by MRI. Although CT delineates the bone detail better, MRI has demonstrated changes within bone or in the surrounding tissues, indicative of infiltration not visualized by CT. Therefore, the presence of signal in the region of cortical bone suggests pathologic changes with invasion of bone. Normal bone marrow, with its high fat content, gives a strong signal on MRI in contrast to cortical bone. Abnormalities or replacement of marrow (due to tumor or osteomyelitis) is demonstrated by reduction in marrow signal intensity. Such changes have been seen in leukemia, metastases, and osteomyelitis, even when other imaging modalities, including radionuclide bone scans, are normal. MRI may prove to be most valuable in detecting the early changes of mastoiditis or petrositis.

## Limitations

Disadvantages or limitations of MRI have been noted. The thin sections currently available in CT are not yet available in MRI and therefore to some extent limit the fine detail of anatomically intricate structures within the petrous bone. Bone detail therefore is currently best assessed by CT. Tissue calcification, which may be helpful in suggesting a diagnosis, is not detectable by MRI. Some artifact or blurring may be created by CSF or vascular pulsations. Similarly motion artifact, caused by movement of the patient during data acquisition, degrades the image. Although MRI allows direct coronal and sagittal imaging, such imaging must be specified and programmed prior to data acquisition for most currently available MR systems. Retrospective reconstruction in alternate planes, as for CT, however, should be available in future software updates.

The patient undergoing MRI is placed upon a table top and positioned into a gantry (similar to CT); some patients find the close apposition of the magnetic coil used for head imaging claustrophobic and intolerable. Approximately 2 percent of MRI studies are cancelled because of patients' claustrophobia.

The time required for data accumulation is still longer than for CT. The patient therefore must be able to cooperate and lie still for a longer period of time. Accordingly, the volume of work or number of patients put through an MRI unit is relatively low compared to CT.

Not all patients are suitable for MRI. Magnetic field interactions with cardiac pacemakers, some prosthetic cardiac valves, ferromagnetic prostheses, and some surgical clips (particular vascular clips) have been documented. Currently, patients with such devices should be excluded from MRI. Care should be taken to enquire about metallic foreign bodies in the eye, which are also a relative contraindication to the examination. Patients unable to lie still or requiring mechanical life support are also not acceptable candidates. Radiofrequency deposition, a nonionizing radiation effect that causes slight heating of body tissues due to radiofrequency waves, does not appear to be a limiting factor in patient selection.

Metallic foreign bodies may be a significant limiting factor. Anteroposterior and lateral skull films may be helpful to determine their presence if there is clinical suspicion. Aneurysm clips have been seen to shift position during the course of an MRI study.

Until MRI becomes more available, studies of the posterior fossa and cerebellopontine angle using MRI as the primary mode will generally be restricted to major referral centers. At other centers, request for MRI studies of the posterior fossa or petrosa will follow initial assessment by CT. Only those patients for whom clinical assessment demands further investigation will have access to MRI because of limited accessibility. Patients with signs of craniovertebral junction pathology (e.g., Arnold-Chiari malformation), with allergy to contrast media and requiring enhancement, or those patients in whom an MRI study would obviate a more invasive and less informative study (e.g., posterior fossa or craniocervical myelography combined with CT) should be referred for MRI as the primary mode of imaging wherever possible.

## ANGIOGRAPHY

Before the advent of CT and MRI, invasive angiographic studies of the temporal bone and brain were the primary diagnostic imaging techniques for intracranial masses such as tumors or otogenic brain abscesses. These masses can now be directly and exactly imaged by CT or MRI (Figs. 11-7 to 11-10). Although indications for angiography per-

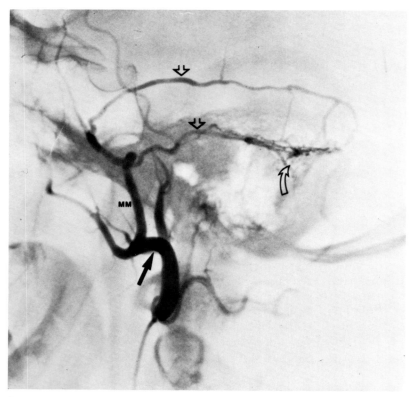

**A**

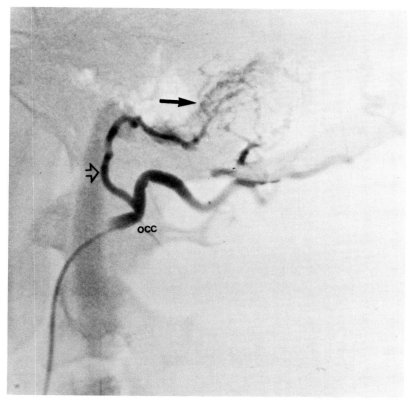

**B**

**Fig. 11-7.** Angiography of vascular malformations: conventional imaging and selective vessel catheterization in a 29 year-old man with 3-month history of left pulsatile tinnitus. Dural AVM with normal enhanced CT. **(A)** Left internal maxillary study (solid arrow). Very prominent middle mengingeal (mm) branches (open arrows) can be seen to site of malformation (curved arrow) in left petrous region. **(B)** Selective left occipital injection (OCC) with enlarged branches feeding malformation (solid arrow) are noted. Hypoglossal branch of ascending pharyngeal artery (open arrow) arises from the occipital artery. *(Figure continues.)*

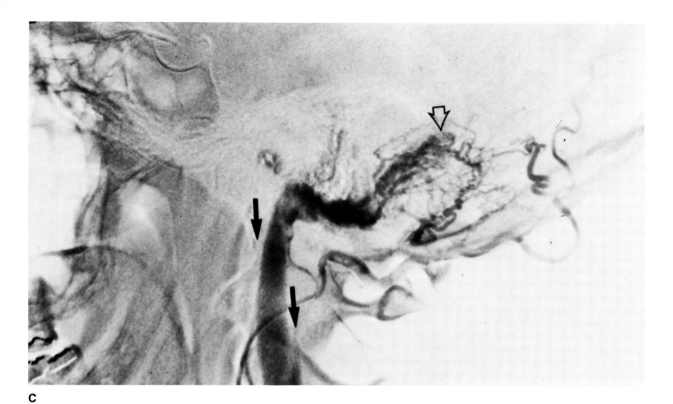

C

D

**Fig. 11-7.** *(Continued).* **(C)** One film later, marked early venous drainage into sigmoid sinus and internal jugular vein (vertical arrows) from vascular malformation (open arrow) is visible. **(D)** Left internal carotid study displays prominent meningohypophyseal artery (arrows) supplying vascular malformation. Internal carotid supply increases risk for embolization. *(Figure continues.)*

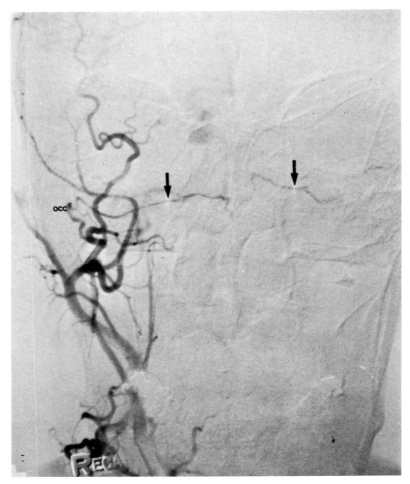

E

**Fig. 11-7** *(Continued).* **(E)** Right external carotid arteriogram demonstrates feeding by contralateral right occipital artery via meningeal branches (right arrow) to region of malformation (left arrow); this study emphasizes the tendency of such lesions to parasitize regional vascularity and demonstrates the need for extensive angiographic assessment.

sist, in order to justify utilization of an invasive procedure the yield must be great. Vertebral basilar insufficiency, aneurysms of the vertebral-basilar circulation, and pulsatile tinnitus (due to suspected tumor or arteriovenous malformation) remain the most common indications for angiography[7-10].

## Conventional Angiography

Diagnostic arteriography[7-10] remains the essential and most definitive modality for assessing vascular pathologic change. Determination of exact vessel morphology may require high-resolution angiographic mapping. Collateral pathways, especially those involving the posterior circulation, are only assessible by angiography.

Conventional arteriography has improved over the past decade. Technical improvements (fine focal spot x-ray tubes, magnification and subtraction techniques[11]) allow one to resolve finer radiographic vascular detail. Better angiographic techniques and catheter materials allow selective catheterization of the vertebral, internal, or external carotid arterial systems (via a retrograde femoral approach). Superselective catheterization of the branches of the external carotid artery is essential for proper assessment of skull base vascular lesions. Only rarely, when a femoral approach is impossible, are direct carotid punctures or retrograde brachial techniques utilized.

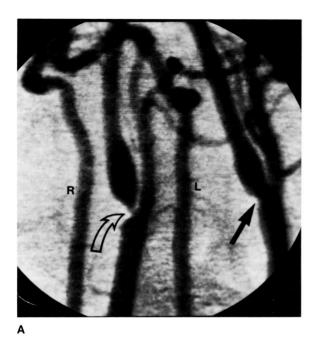

**A**

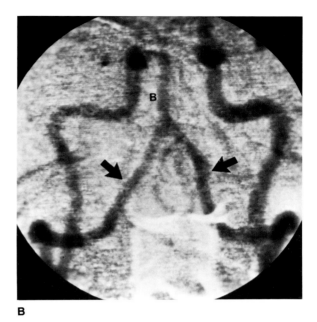

**B**

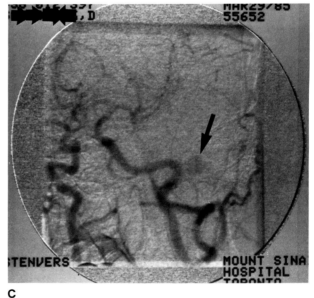

**C**

**Fig. 11-8.** Digital subtraction arteriography—intravenous approach as screening assessment. Venous studies are less selective, with superimposition of vessels; however, information available may be satisfactory for clinical needs. **(A)** Patient with pulsatile tinnitus; **(B)** patient with suspected vertebrobasilar insufficiency producing vertigo. **(A)** AP oblique projection of neck. Right (R) and left vertebral (L) arteries are well visualized. Significant stenosis is present at the origin of the right internal carotid artery (open arrow), and mild stenosis at the origin of the left ICA (solid arrow). **(B)** AP projection of head displays superior aspect of vertebral arteries (arrows) and basilar artery (B), ruling out vertebrobasilar insufficiency. Carotid arteries are noted laterally. **(C)** Patient with left glumus jugulare. Tumor stain (arrow) of left glomus jugulare is shown although feeding vessels are not recognized. *(Figure continues.)*

Embolization of vascular lesions in and about the temporal bone may be used for primary treatment or as an adjunctive procedure to reduce vascularity prior to surgery. Angiographers now understand the need to assess vascular compartmentalization[8,10] (single or multiple) and venous drainage patterns if appropriate embolization is to be successful.

The surgeon may plan the approach to vascular lesions based on the size and location of feeding and draining vessels and knowledge of intracranial and extracranial tumor extent.

Anatomic variants, such as aberrant internal carotid artery or high jugular bulb, which may clinically simulate an intratympanic vascular tumor, can be diagnosed by angiography.

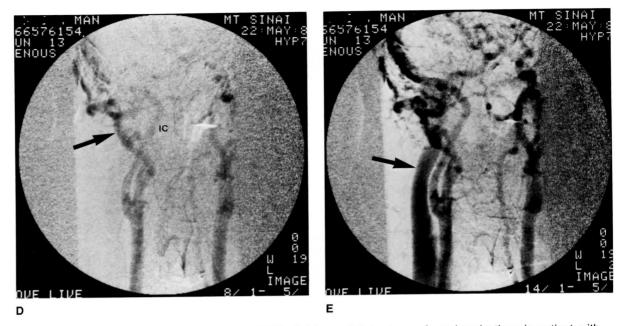

**Fig. 11-8** *(Continued).*   **(D, E)** Transdural AVM of right occipital artery—frontal projections in patient with pulsatile tinnitus. **(D)** Early film shows abnormally prominent right occipital artery (arrow) filling to greater degree than right internal carotid artery (IC). **(E)** Abnormal early filling of right internal jugular vein is noted (arrow). AVM was diagnosed using the less invasive modality. Resolution is inferior to that of conventional angiography.

Posttraumatic vascular complications (small intimal dissections, secondary embolic phenomena, occlusions, aneurysms or AV fistulae) are best assessed, and frequently only diagnosable, by angiography. While embolization of paragangliomas is usually performed as a presurgical procedure, embolization alone may be used as the definitive treatment for arteriovenous (AV) fistulae, AV malformations, and capillary hemangiomas.

## Digital Subtraction Angiography

Digital subtraction angiography (DSA) is a computer technique that allows vascular patterns to be displayed and photographed in real time in the subtracted mode (spontaneous removal of any superimposed bone or soft tissue structures) such that only the vascular system is visualized[9] (Figs. 11-8 through 11-10). Smaller amounts of intravascular contrast media are used because of the increased sensitivity of the computed image.

### Intravenous Approach

The intravenous (IV) placement of a needle peripherally or a catheter centrally represents the least dangerous of the angiographic techniques.[9] Such studies are routinely done as outpatient procedures. This avoids the risks and complications of intra-arterial catheter manipulation. However, IV studies are the least selective; there is maximal superimposition of vascularity, and reduced detail (Fig. 11-8). For each projection 40 to 50 ml of IV contrast medium must be injected. Usually a minimum of four to five projections are required to visualize the carotid and vertebral vessels (when both cervical and intracranial components are studied). Thus, a significant total volume of contrast medium is injected, which is a limiting factor in the number of projections selected in the elderly patient, or those with renal or cardiovascular disease.

Even with motion or swallowing artifact, as well as superimposition of vessels, a DSA-IV may be

**Fig. 11-9.** Digital subtraction arteriography: intra-arterial approach. Arterial approach allows for more selective catheterization and less superimposition of vessels. **(A)** Patient with vertigo due to vascular insufficiency. Aortic arch study shows origin of great vessels. Complete occlusion of brachiocephalic (open arrow) and left subclavian (closed arrow) arteries is noted, with the left common carotid artery (LCC) as the sole vascular supply to the head and neck. **(B)** Towne projection, right vertebral arterial study. Posterior cerebral (p), superior cerebellar (s), anterior inferior cerebellar (vertical arrow), and posterior inferior cerebellar (pi) arteries are seen. Reflux into left vertebral (LV) artery is noted. Normal study in a different patient with suspected vertebrobasilar insufficiency. *(Figure continues.)*

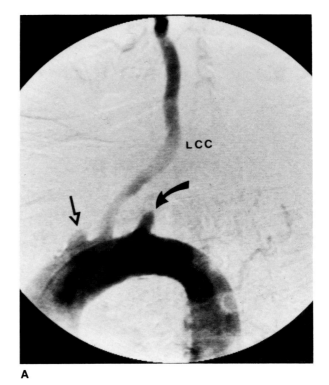

A

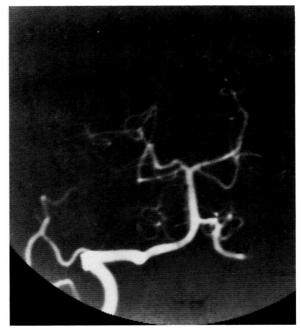

B

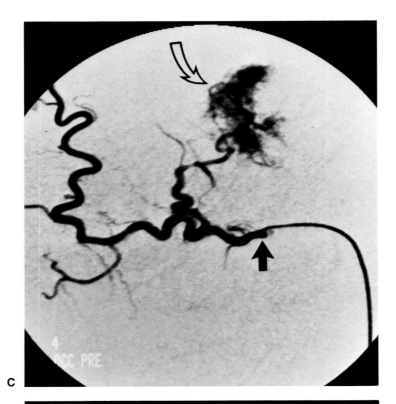

C

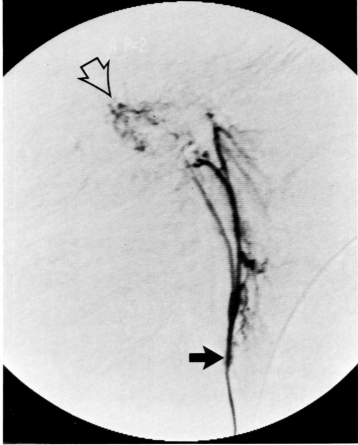

D

Fig. 11-9 *(Continued).* **(C,D)** Use of DSA-IA selectively to catheterize and compartmentalize vascular masses in the pretreatment assessment for surgery or embolization (glomus jugulare tumor). **(C)** Lateral projection of occiptal artery catheterization (solid arrow) shows vascular mass (open arrow) in right petrous region. **(D)** Lateral projection: ascending pharyngeal arterial catheterization (solid arrow) with tumor blush (open arrow) anterior to that seen from occipital arterial source **(C)**.

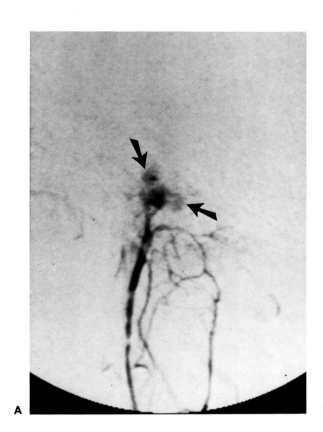

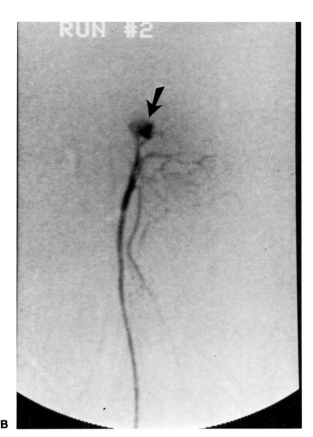

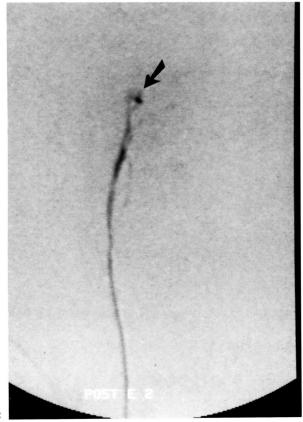

**Fig. 11-10.** Intra-arterial embolization: DSA-IA monitoring. Selective ascending pharyngeal arterial catheterization and DSA-IA were used to monitor embolization of vascular tumor (left glomus jugulare). **(A)**Pre-embolization study shows vascular blush (arrows), which decreases in size **(B)** following partial embolization (arrow). **(C)** Final arteriogram following further embolization shows obliteration of the tumor blush (arrow). Polyvinyl alcohol (PVA) microspheres were used as the embolizing agent.

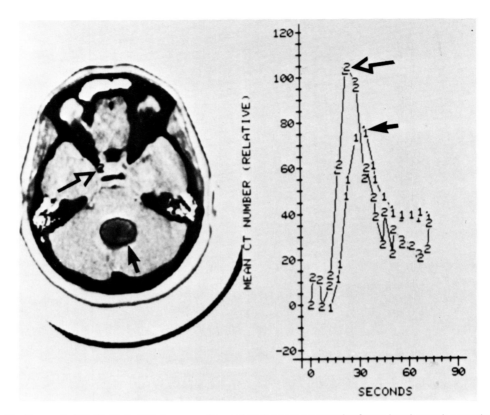

**Fig. 11-11.** Dynamic CT. Multiple CT slices, performed at the same posterior fossa level, may be used to assess the vascularity of a recognized mass, in this case in a patient being investigated for pathologic nystagmus. Sequential slices 6 sec apart showed alteration in density of posterior cranial fossa (PCF) mass during rapid introduction of contrast medium. The PCF mass (solid arrow) is shown on reverse-mode image. Density/time graph (right side of image) obtained from axial study compares vascularity of mass (arrow) to that of right internal carotid artery (2, open arrow). Sharp peak is characteristic of vascular mass. Diagnosis was hemangioblastoma. Dynamic CT may be used to assess vascularity when a less invasive test than angiography is desired as a screening procedure.

adequate to delineate the internal carotid artery or the extent of vascular tumor (glomus) in the region of the jugular bulb. Usually, however, in assessing the arterial structures, such a test must be considered a screening procedure only; the patient is advised that a further study using an arterial approach may be required. However, the intracranial venous drainage (especially the major dural sinuses) is best visualized when there is nonselective bilateral filling of the intracranial arterial supply. Such visualization of the jugular bulb and internal jugular vein has obviated any need in recent years for jugular venography to assess invasion or compression by glomus jugulare tumor.

**Intra-Arterial Approach**

Intra-arterial DSA (DSA-IA) is safer than conventional angiography, despite the need to manipulate the intra-arterial catheters, because smaller volumes and lower concentrations of contrast are injected. Tissue concentrations are approximately one-fourth those of conventional techniques. The immediate display of the subtracted image allows rapid evaluation of each projection and appropriate decision-making before moving to the next angiographic step. The duration of such studies (multiple-vessel, superselective, with embolization) is considerably shortened and complications significantly decreased.

Although fine detail and spatial resolution of the arterial structures remains inferior to that detected by conventional angiography, most vascular lesions (tumors and insufficiencies) may be adequately studied by DSA-IA (Figs. 11-9, 11-10). Tumor blush in the capillary phase (not seen on conventional imaging) may be detected on DSA-IA due to the superior contrast resolution of the digital system.

The "trade-off" between increased ease of procedure and shorter duration of study on the one hand and fine image detail (e.g., subtle vasculitis, small aneurysm) must be weighed when one decides whether to use DSA-IA or conventional angiography. Such decisions must be based on individual preferences and patients' requirements.

### Retrograde Jugular Venography

Assessment of mass lesions of the temporal bone or the skull base may include assessment of the patency of the jugular bulb and internal jugular vein. The proper programming of a conventional angiogram to include the venous phase will frequently allow proper visualization of the venous structures. If inadequate visualization results, the venous structures may be demonstrated by digital arteriography, which assesses whether the jugular bulb and internal jugular vein are patent, compressed, or invaded.

If doubt persists, or if digital angiography is unavailable, retrograde jugular venography may be performed. A fine catheter is passed retrograde from a femoral venous approach to enter the internal jugular vein on the side of interest. Such studies are performed on an outpatient basis; they previously augmented information that was not achieved by conventional arteriography. The need for such studies has been significantly reduced with the use of high-resolution CT of the skull base, contrast-enhanced and dynamic CT (Fig. 11-11) to study the vascular structures of the skull base, and

with the use of digital arteriography followed through to the venous phase.

## RADIONUCLIDE SCANS

The decay of an unstable atomic nucleus results in radioactivity that can be detected by gamma cameras. When radioactive tracers are introduced into biologic systems, the radioactive tags serve to label specific metabolites. These agents can then be studied, in physiological terms primarily, as they reflect normal and altered function within various organ systems. Radionuclide scans therefore permit the recording of physiological changes (accumulation, distribution, excretion) of radiopharmaceuticals since physiological changes precede morphologic changes, both in the evolution of disease and its healing[12,13] (Fig. 11-12).

Radionuclides that emit gamma radiation are easily detected and relatively safe to use. Images can be recorded to a resolution of 1.0 cm (or slightly less) anatomically; these images can be enhanced somewhat by computer. Radionuclide scans are highly sensitive but lack specificity. For example, the increased osteoblastic response of the "hot" bone scan (detected site of increased emission of gamma radiation) represents the focal deposition of bone due to infection, dysplasia, healing fracture, and tumor. Clinical correlation must be introduced in order to define the significance of this positive imaging finding. However, the detection of this osteoblastic response is highly sensitive. Whereas a 30 to 50 percent demineralization of bone is required for detection by conventional x-ray studies, the constant osteoblastic response about this lysis can be detected by the bone scan, which is sensitive to but a 5 to 10 percent increase in osteoblastic activity and increased bony deposition. In contrast, a 30 percent increase in bony activity (increased density) is required for such recognition by conventional x-ray studies. The reader is referred to the treatise of Noyek[12] for full details on the general concepts and specific details of bone scanning.

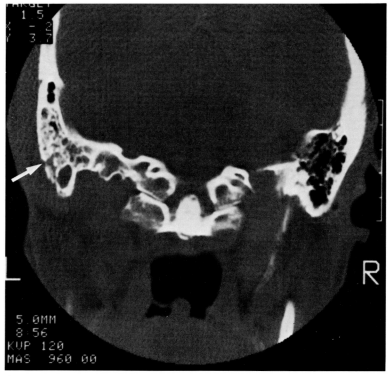

**A**

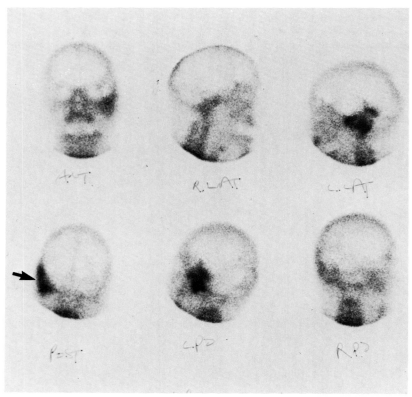

**B**

**Fig. 11-12.** Osteomyelitis (malignant external otitis) of the left temporal bone in a 55 year-old diabetic man. **(A)** Coronal CT with opacification of the left mastoid air cells. Loss of bony cortex laterally (arrow) with overlying soft tissue swelling. **(B)** Pretreatment $^{99m}$Tc methylene diphosphonate (MDP) bone scan — delayed phase. Increased activity "hot" scan allows diagnosis of osteomyelitis (multiple images). The hot bone scan images the osteoblastic response around the infective focus; arrow indicates increased activity on posterior view. *(Figure continues.)*

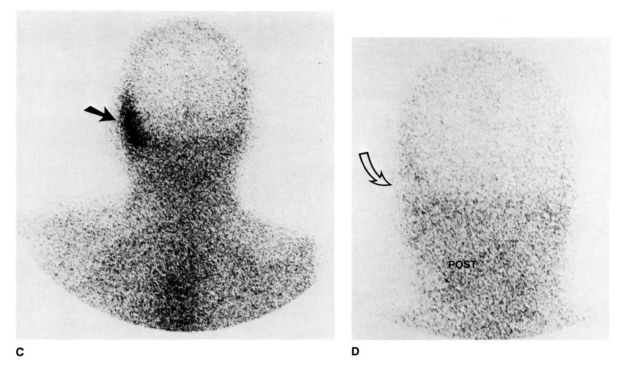

**Fig. 11-12** *(Continued).* **(C)** Pretreatment gallium scan ($^{67}$Ga citrate). Posterior image at 72 hours after radionuclide administration shows increased activity of infective focus within left petrous bone (arrow). **(D)** Post-treatment gallium scan, posterior image, also obtained at 72 hours. Infective focus has been eradicated. Normal gallium scan indicates effectiveness of antibiotic therapy.

The radiation hazard from radionuclide studies (bone scans, gallium scans) is acceptable, and can be quantified with conventional radiographic evaluations. Radionuclide scanning should be avoided during pregnancy and lactation.

The two types of radionuclide scan[13] that have significant clinical application to the evaluation of the temporal bone are the bone scan and the gallium scan. In combination, their main value is in the diagnosis of osteomyelitis of the temporal bone (malignant external otitis); the diagnosis is suggested by the increased osteoblastic activity detected on the bone scan and is confirmed by the gallium scan. The success of antibiotic therapy can also be evaluated by the follow-up gallium scan.

When osteomyelitis is suspected clinically, the technetium 99m methylene diphosphonate bone scan may allow the diagnosis of osteomyelitis as early as 12 to 24 hours into the infective process[12,13]. Conventional radiographs, including complex motion tomography and CT, may not detect the developing bone destruction for up to 10 days. The bone scan demonstrates the osteoblastic response to the infective insult and will demonstrate healing long before conventional radiographs or CT scans can.

Gallium 67 citrate is taken up by actively dividing cells (white blood cells) and will revert to normal (excluding the minor inherent osteogenic activity of gallium citrate) when successful treatment is completed. It images the inflammatory focus, hence osteomyelitis may be staged biologically by using combined bone and gallium scanning.

When local views of the temporal bone are to be recorded with the methylene diphosphonate (MDP) bone scan agent, immediate flow phase images are recorded for low-resolution vascular display in one of many positions. Blood pool images (which can show hyperemia in the plane of the image) are recorded over the next 20 minutes or so in a number of positions. Computer enhancement is used for temporal bone image recording; magnification is also possible. Whole body imaging in the delayed bone phase may be helpful if the petrous bone involvement is suspected of representing a component of systemic disease (e.g., Paget's disease, metastatic disease, or eosinophilic granuloma).

In suspected osteomyelitis, when a diagnostic "hot" bone scan has been recorded, the patient is then given the $^{67}$Ga-citrate scan agent. The patient is returned to the unit in 72 hours for large field of view gamma camera imaging (both for whole body studies and for head-temporal bone imaging).

There is little need currently for other radionuclide scans, such as brain and CSF scans. CT and MRI have superior qualities in imaging the central nervous system and its relationships.

# ACKNOWLEDGMENTS

This work was supported by the Saul A. Silverman Family Foundation, Toronto, Ontario. The authors gratefully acknowledge Suzanne Petrevski and Rosemarie McGuire for manuscript preparation. We also thank Dr. Walter Kucharczyk for his gracious help in manuscript review. We appreciate the efforts of the Departments of Instructional Media at Mount Sinai Hospital and Sunnybrook Medical Centre.

# REFERENCES

1. Mancuso AA, Hanafee WN, Computed Tomography and Magnetic Resonance Imaging of the Head and Neck, 2nd ed. Williams & Wilkins, Baltimore, 1985
2. Young SW: Nuclear Magnetic Resonance Imaging: Basic Principles. Raven Press, New York, 1984
3. Tuddenham WJ (ed): Nuclear magnetic resonance: RadioGraphics 4 (special edition), 1984
4. McGinnis BD, Brady TJ, New PFJ, et al: Nuclear magnetic resonance (NMR) imaging of tumors in the posterior fossa. J Comput Assist Tomogr 7:575, 1983
5. Young IR, Bydder GM, Hall AS, et al: The role of NMR imaging in the diagnosis and management of acoustic neuroma. Am J Neuroradiol 4:223, 1983
6. Daniels DL, Herfkins R, Kochler PR, et al: Magnetic resonance imaging of the internal auditory canal. Radiology 151:10, 1984
7. Hesselink JR, Davis KR, Taveras JM: Selective arteriography of glomus tympanicum and juglare tumors: techniques, normal and pathologic arterial anatomy. Am J Neuroradiol 2:289, 1981
8. Lasjaunias P: Craniofacial and Upper Cervical Arteries: Functional, Chemical and Angiographic Aspects. Williams & Wilkins, Baltimore, 1981
9. Carmody RF, Smith JRL, Seeger JF, et al: Intracranial applications of digital intravenous subtraction angiography. Radiology 144:529, 1982
10. Bergeron RT, Osborn AG, Som PM (eds): Head and Neck Imaging Excluding the Brain. CV Mosby, St Louis, 1984
11. Ziedses des Plantes BG: Subtraktion. Thieme, Stuttgart, 1961
12. Noyek AM: Bone scanning in otolaryngology. Laryngoscope 89(9) suppl 18:1, 1979
13. Noyek AM, Kirsh JC, Greyson ND, et al: The clinical significance of radionuclide bone and gallium scanning in osteomyelitis of the head and neck. Laryngoscope 94(5) suppl 34:1, 1984

# Current Role of Diagnostic Imaging in Temporal Bone Disease 12

Arnold M. Noyek
Edward E. Kassel

## CURRENT ROLE OF DIAGNOSTIC IMAGING IN TEMPORAL BONE DISEASE

To correlate the imaging modalities and offer a perspective on their relative values, some remarks concerning more specific imaging of various disease processes may be helpful. These are discussed as follows:

Inflammatory lesions
   Mastoiditis
   Osteomyelitis
   Cholesteatoma
Cerebellopontine angle and internal auditory canal (IAC) lesions
Vascular tumors and malformations (pulsatile tinnitus)
Temporal bone tumors
Congenital disorders
Trauma
Craniovertebral junction
Miscellaneous

## INFLAMMATORY LESIONS AND THEIR COMPLICATIONS

Referrals for temporal bone imaging of inflammatory lesions most frequently involve further evaluation of clinically suspected mastoiditis, cholesteatoma, or osteomyelitis.[1–5]

### Mastoiditis

In acute mastoiditis, conventional mastoid views display not only the opacification of the middle ear cleft and mastoid air cells, but also the destruction of bony septa resulting in coalescent mastoiditis (Fig. 12-1). Focal bone destruction of periantral cells leads to enlargement of the mastoid antrum. Increase in antral dimensions (maximum 1.0 cm in height and anteroposterior diameter [depth]; maximum 0.5 cm in medial-lateral dimension [width]), and contralateral comparison may help in the detection of early coalescent mastoiditis and development of an empyemic cavity. Complex motion to-

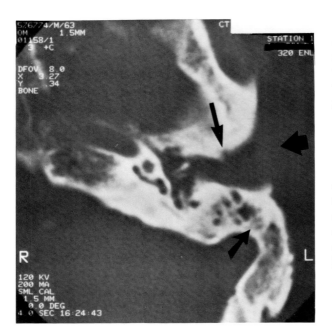

**Fig. 12-1.** Acute purulent mastoiditis without coalescence associated with osteomyelitis of the tympanic bone. Axial CT slice through the external auditory canal (EAC) shows irregularity of the anterior wall (vertical arrow) and soft tissue mass filling the tympanic cavity and EAC. Swelling of soft tissues external to the ear (horizontal arrow) is better seen on soft tissue mode. Clouded mastoid cells (oblique arrow) are due to purulent secretions and thickened mucosa; however, air cell walls are preserved without coalescence.

mography, especially in the sagittal plane, may augment initial plain film studies by displaying the mastoid antrum and air cell system.

If further information is required computed tomography (CT) using the bone mode and 1.5 to 5 mm thickness slices will display mastoid cellular detail superbly. The presence of coalescence and localization of such processes relative to the cortical and periosteal boundaries of the mastoid region may further direct attention to potential clinical complications. Sigmoid sinus "plate" involvement may be assessed by soft tissue CT imaging, with further angiographic investigation (e.g., intravenous digital subtraction angiography to visualize the venous drainage) if indicated. CT of the brain should be performed whenever inflammatory complications of the brain (abscess, cerebritis, in-

farction secondary to meningitis) are a possibility. Similarly, CT imaging of the neck may confirm inferior tracking and penetration of the inferior bony wall of the mastoid, with secondary soft tissue involvement, deep to the sternomastoid muscle, suggestive of Bezold's abscess.

## Osteomyelitis

Temporal bone osteomyelitis[5] may occur secondary to aggressive middle ear or mastoid infections (Figs. 12-1, 12-2; Fig. 11-12). Diabetics, and occasionally, the immune suppressed patient, may experience "malignant external otitis," an acute osteolytic osteomyelitis that almost universally begins as a *pseudomonas* infection of the deep ex-

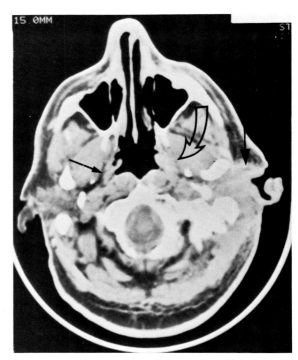

**Fig. 12-2.** Osteomyelitis of temporal bone with skull base and parapharyngeal space extension. Axial CT at level of eustachian tube using soft tissue mode shows loss of soft tissue fat planes (open arrow) due to extension of infection. Soft tissue involvement obliterates the EAC and extends anteriorly (vertical arrow). Intact fat plane marginating the parapharyngeal space is present on the right side (oblique arrow).

ternal auditory canal, ultimately invading the tympanic ring and beyond. Strong clinical suspicion of this entity is critical for early diagnosis when radiologic changes may be nonspecific.

Conventional imaging is not helpful in the early stages. When the osteomyelitic process has extended beyond the tympanic ring (usually postero-inferiorly), plain films and conventional tomography may be helpful to define the extent of involvement. Computed tomography (CT), however, is the preferred modality to demonstrate morphologic changes. Such studies allow early de-

tection of tympanic ring destructive changes. Both bone and soft tissue imaging is necessary to demonstrate the extent of disease, either within the temporal bone itself (thin slices required) or adjacent soft tissues including the brain. Radiologic changes of bone destruction are nonspecific, resembling primary carcinoma of the external canal. However, the diagnosis of malignant external otitis should be considered whenever a destructive process involving the tympanic ring is noted.

A clinical suspicion of temporal bone osteomyelitis may be confirmed in its early stages by radio-

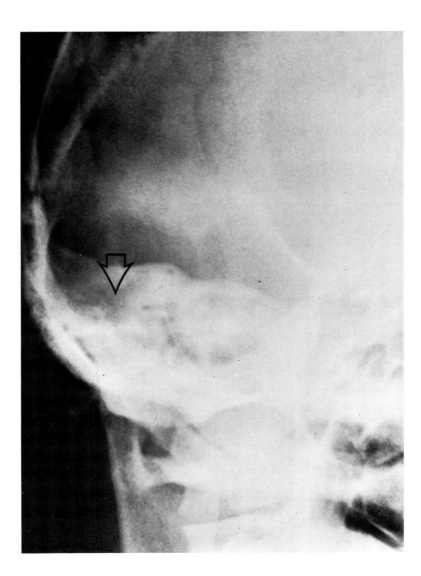

**Fig. 12-3.** Cholesteatoma, mastoid antrum. Stenver's projection of right petrous bone. Mastoid bone is sclerotic and poorly aerated. Mastoid antrum is expanded (open arrow) and both antrum and tympanic cavity are opacified due to cholesteatoma.

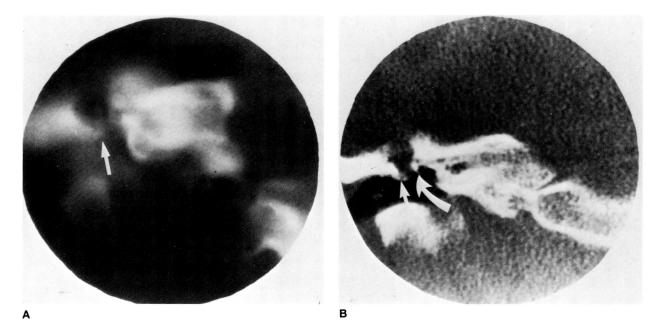

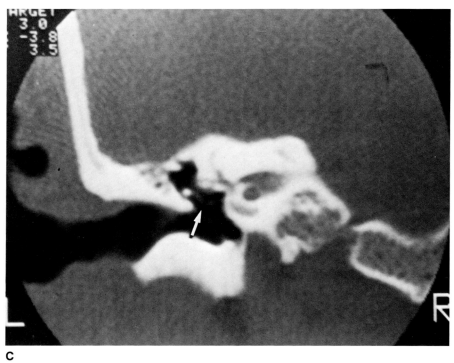

**Fig. 12-4.** Cholesteatoma with ossicular involvement. **(A)** Frontal tomogram demonstrates blunting of scutum (arrow) and poor definition of ossicles. **(B)** Corresponding coronal CT demonstrates erosion of the bony spur (straight arrow) as well as soft tissue mass in attic displacing ossicles (curved arrow) medially. **(C)** Coronal CT in another patient displays focal erosion of long process of incus (arrow) and mild blunting of bony spur. (A, B courtesy of Dr. Carmen Guirado, Barcelona, Spain; C courtesy of Dr. Joel D. Swartz, Medical College of Pennsylvania, Philadelphia, PA.)

nuclide scanning.[5] The bone scan is usually positive within 24 hours of onset of osteomyelitis.

The positive bone scan is nonspecific and reflects the marginating reparative osteoblastic response about the osteomyelitic focus. The positive gallium scan identifies the infective focus. The bone scan therefore demonstrates bone response to the infective "insult;" the gallium scan demonstrates the "insult" itself, with the radioisotope activity limited to the site of devitalized bone (in contrast to the wider extent of increased activity of the bone scan, whose "cooler" central component within the temporal bone corresponds to the area of increased activity noted on the gallium scan). The gallium scan is of value in determining efficacy of antibiotic therapy; findings revert to normal when therapy has been effective. The bone scan is of no practical value in defining duration of treatment since such scans demonstrate well some increased

activity of bone healing for 6 to 12 (or more) months after the eradication of infection.

## Primary Acquired Cholesteatoma

Plain film or CT assessment[1-9] will demonstrate varying degrees of temporal bone pneumatization. Reduction or absence of pneumatization may be related to infantile epitympanic obstruction. Adenexal air cell tracts (zygomatic root, petrous apex) usually fail to develop, allowing these portions of the temporal bone to remain diploic. Sclerosis, not normally present, occurs as a marginating osteoblastic response secondary to either the mechanical pressure of the bony erosive process or some chemical phenomenon. Radiographic findings of a dense, hypocellular contracted mastoid with closer than normal approximation of the sig-

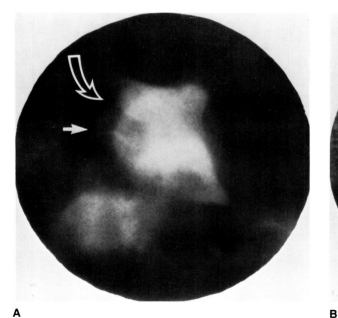
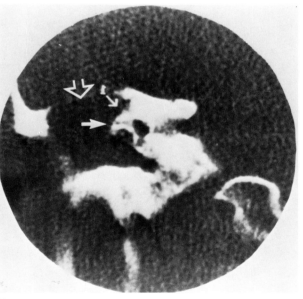

**A**          **B**

**Fig. 12-5.** Large primary acquired cholesteatoma with labyrinthine fistula. **(A)** Conventional AP tomogram shows large destructive lesion destroying the lateral aspect of the tympanic cavity and extending superiorly to destroy the tegmen. Bone overlying the lateral semicircular canal is destroyed (closed arrow); there is poor visualization of the superior semicircular canal with a large bone defect (open arrow). **(B)** Corresponding coronal CT better demonstrates bone destruction and fistula of lateral and superior semicircular canals (closed arrows); a soft tissue mass fills the tympanic cavity and mastoid antrum and destroys the tegmen (open arrow). (Courtesy of Dr. Carmen Guirado, Barcelona, Spain.)

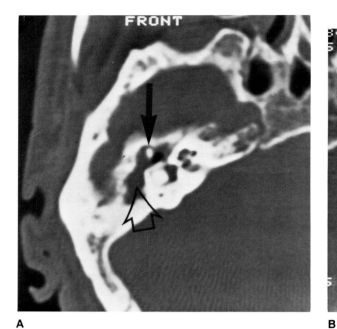

A

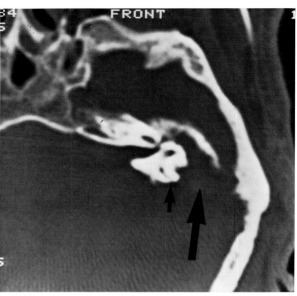

B

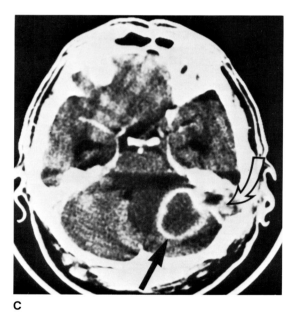

C

**Fig. 12-6.** Bilateral cholesteatomas with brain abscess. **(A)** Axial CT of right petrous bone. Soft tissue density filling mastoid antrum, aditus, and tympanic cavity (open arrow). Only the malleus is visualized (solid arrow); incus is destroyed by the soft tissue mass. Sclerotic mastoid process. **(B)** Axial slice of left petrous bone displays soft tissue mass filling tympanic cavity and mastoid antrum, destroying the ossicles and tegmen (large arrow). Fistula of the posterior semicircular canal is also present (small arrow). **(C)** Enhancing mass on left cerebellar hemisphere (solid arrow) indicates brain abscess secondary to cholesteatoma (open arrow).

moid plate to the posterior external auditory canal and narrowing of the sinodural angle represent the usual plain film background (Fig. 12-3) of which further studies (CT) to define the cholesteatomatous sac are required. Acquired cholesteatoma only rarely is found in a healthy pneumatized mastoid.

In the usual development of acquired cholesteatoma, certain features may be sought. Erosion of the scutum tends to be the first bone defect identifiable. Presence of a soft tissue mass, due either to the cholesteatoma itself or to polypoid granulation tissue (induced by the cholesteatoma), may be initially profiled by air within the tympanic cavity. Further extension of soft tissue mass leads to opacification of the middle ear cleft and inability to define soft tissue contours. Displacement or destruction of the ossicles may be noted (Fig. 12-4). Cholesteatoma enlarged beyond direct clinical assessment requires radiologic assessment prior to treatment planning. Specific attention to the facial nerve canal, especially if facial paralysis is present, is essential. CT usually performed in both axial and coronal plane, utilizing thin high resolution bone images, has replaced complex-motion tomography in the assessment of cholesteatoma. Occasionally, lateral tomography may help in assessment of the vertical segment of the facial canal, if it is inadequately seen on reformatted CT and direct sagittal CT is not deemed feasible. More recently magnetic resonance imaging (MRI) has allowed direct identification of the facial nerve, independent of its bony canal.

CT remains the primary modality to assess fistula formation (Fig. 12-5), most commonly involving the lateral semicircular canal prominence. Less commonly, erosion of the superior and/or posterior semicircular canals and the oval or round window is noted. Inferior extension may involve the carotid canal and petrous apex while posterior inferior extension may involve the jugular bulb. Superior extension causing dehiscence of the tegmen is best displayed by coronal CT bone imaging. Intracranial complications, such as brain abscess (Fig. 12-6), require soft tissue imaging by either CT or MRI.

Radiologic studies may assist postsurgical evaluation in the demonstration of recurrent secondary cholesteatoma. Morphologic defects arising from a surgical procedure alone (no remaining disease) tend to be irregular in nature, inciting minimal osteoblastic response over time (3 to 9 months). Secondary cholesteatoma defects, within a mastoidectomy cavity, conversely, tend to be smooth and erosive, inciting an osteoblastic response for years following the original surgical procedure. The isotope bone scan therefore may be of clinical use in differentiating the dense bone following surgery or healed osteomyelitis, which may be biologically inert (presenting only a volume effect on bone scan), from the increased osteoblastic response of active bone deposition induced by the cholesteatoma.

Congenital cholesteatoma represents a focal sequestering of ectoderm in lines of skull fusion developmental. Such lesions tend to involve the skull base, especially the petrous apex, and should not be confused with acquired cholesteatomas. Congenital cholesteatomas tend to be cystic in appearance, slowly expansile, with mild osteoblastic margination.

## MASS LESIONS OF THE CEREBELLOPONTINE ANGLE AND INTERNAL AUDITORY CANAL

Current techniques can outline not only the larger cerebellopontine angle (CPA) tumors, but also tumors confined within the internal auditory canal itself.[10-13]

Morphologically recognized CPA masses usually (80 to 90%) prove to be schwannomas of the 8th nerve (see Fig. 10-23) (commonly termed "acoustic neuroma"). This lesion almost invariably arises within the internal auditory canal on the vestibular portion of the 8th nerve. Other neurogenic lesions, such as the meningioma (Fig. 12-7), may mimic its presentation in many ways. These and other mass lesions (Figs. 12-8, 12-9) such as subarachnoid cysts, dermoid tumors, hemangiomas, metastases, and aneurysms produce their major effects physiologically by the compression of the 8th nerve and other adjacent nerves (cranial nerves 5 and 7). Medial extension of these tumor masses may produce brain stem compression.

The major screening examination currently used for assessing the possibility of a CPA tumor is intravenous iodinated contrast-enhanced CT scanning. This technique demonstrates the presence of enhancing mass lesions (1 cm or greater diameter). An acoustic neuroma usually pouts from the internal auditory canal when it extends through the porus; it therefore creates sharp angulation against the profile of the adjacent temporal bone. Bone window manipulation may demonstrate adjacent bone erosion or destruction. Acoustic neuromas usually enhance, indicating their basic vascularity, but they may be avascular (with or without a vascular rim) and resemble a cyst, either dermoid or ar-

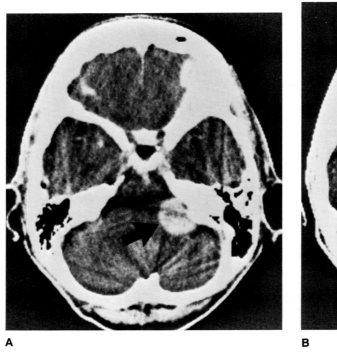

A

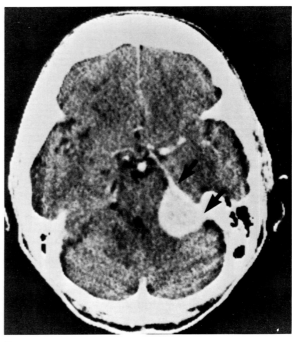

B

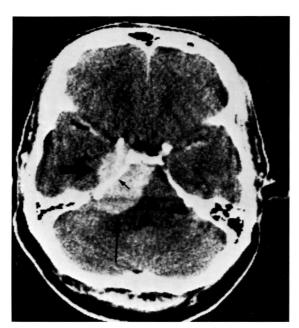

C

**Fig. 12-7.** CPA masses — meningioma. **(A)** Homogeneous enhancing mass (arrow) resembles acoustic neuroma at this level. **(B)** More superior slice of broad-based mass along tentorium and petrous ridge (arrows) indicates meningioma. **(C)** Anterior extension of enhancing mass in the middle cranial fossa (wide arrow) as well as broad base along tentorium (short arrow) defines meningioma. Vertical arrow indicates posterior extent.

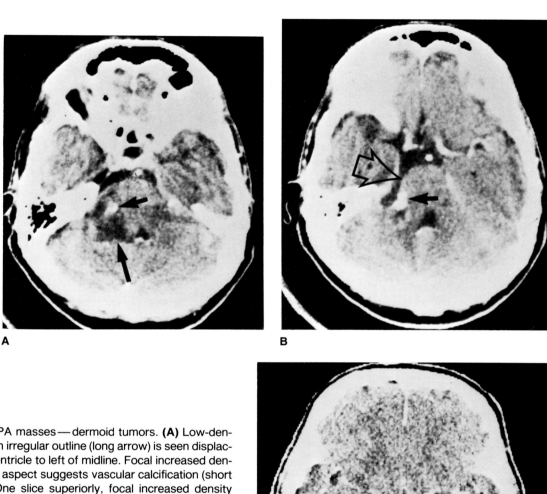

**Fig. 12-8.** CPA masses—dermoid tumors. **(A)** Low-density mass with irregular outline (long arrow) is seen displacing the 4th ventricle to left of midline. Focal increased density at medial aspect suggests vascular calcification (short arrow). **(B)** One slice superiorly, focal increased density (solid arrow) no longer has vascular configuration; it is longitudinally oriented and densely solid (bone windows). This is a tooth at the medial aspect of dermoid tumor. Note widened right CPA cistern (open arrow) suggestive of extra-axial mass. **(C)** Low-density mass with well-defined margins (open arrow) at left CPA in another patient displaces the fourth ventricle to the right (solid arrow) and is a dermoid tumor. Arachnoid cyst may have mass effect and appear identical.

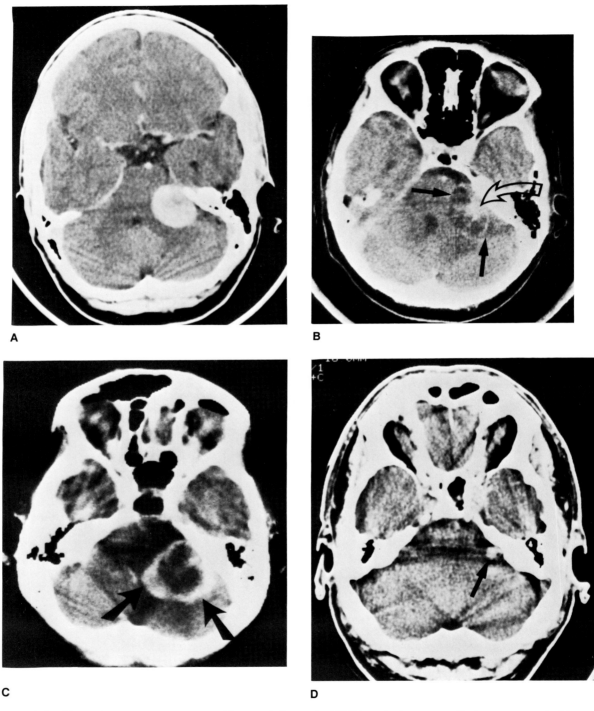

**Fig. 12-9.** CPA lesions — other lesions in differential diagnosis. **(A)** Trigeminal neuroma. Patient presented with sensory loss of the left 5th nerve. Homogeneous mass is well defined in the left CPA. Radiologic clue to diagnosis is the more superior location of the tumor relative to IAC as well as lack of IAC flaring. **(B)** Patient presented with left facial nerve signs. Mass in left CPA with central enhancement (open arrow) and surrounding hypodense mass effect (solid arrows) is a 7th nerve neuroma. **(C)** A 73-year-old woman presented with left 7th and 8th cranial nerve symptoms. Axial CT demonstrates large CPA mass with central necrosis — metastatic lung carcinoma. **(D)** Small enhancing mass (arrow) appears discrete from temporal bone on axial CT. *(Figure continues.)*

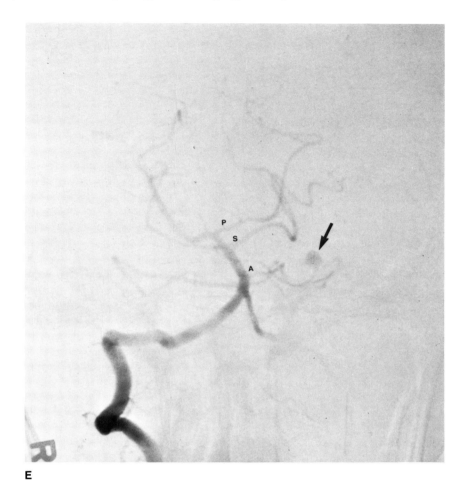

**Fig. 12-9** *(Continued).* **(E)** In same patient, right vertebral angiogram demonstrates aneurysm of peripheral left AICA (arrow).

E

achnoid in appearance. The presence of bilateral CPA masses is very suggestive of neurofibromatosis. Such masses, while almost invariably representing bilateral acoustic neuromas, occasionally are meningiomata.

The importance of the CT study is in recognizing the presence of a CPA mass lesion that, by itself, may be nonspecific in diagnostic features. A normal CT scan with contrast enhancement (in the nonallergic patient) does not eliminate the possibility of a small neurogenic tumor in the CPA or internal auditory canal. When the appropriate index of suspicion still exists, an air CT-cisternogram is usually the next diagnostic step (intrathecal small dosage [2 to 5 cc] of air via lumbar puncture) to assess the intracanalicular portion of the 8th cranial nerve (Figs. 12-10, 12-11).

The actual surface of the mass lesion can be silhouetted by the air, as can be the nerves coursing between the brain stem and the internal auditory canal.[13] A mass lesion, either within the canal or just at the porus, usually presents as a convex bulge towards the brain stem. The presence of a concave obstructive configuration to meatal air entry should suggest arachnoid adhesions or a finding other than tumor.

Valvassori studied complex-motion tomographic findings in acoustic neuroma and carefully noted the dimensions of the internal auditory canal and porus acusticus.[10,14,15] Today these findings are largely of historic interest. Screening conventional views have a variable yield. Small intracanalicular tumors will remain unrecognizable. Large tumors may insinuate themselves along the entire canal

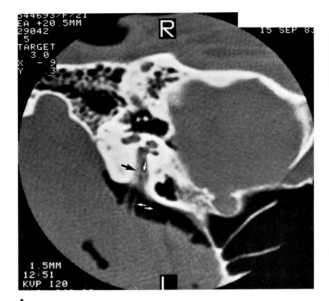

**A**

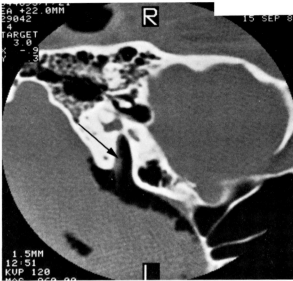

**B**

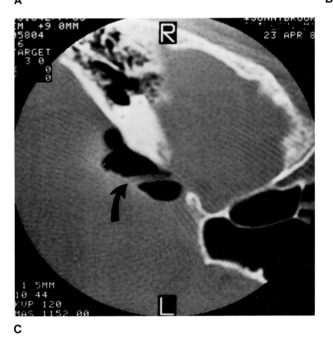

**C**

**Fig. 12-10.** Air CT-cisternography landmarks. **(A)** Normal study: combined 7th and 8th nerve bundles (arrow) typically noted along posterior portion of IAC; IAC and CPA cistern are filled with air. **(B)** One slice inferior to **A** shows loop of anterior-inferior cerebellar artery (white arrows) just anterior to 7th and 8th cranial nerves (dark arrow) and extending into IAC. **(C)** Normal trigeminal nerve (arrow), outlined by air, coursing from brain stem to petrous apex at level just superior to IAC.

and grow significantly into the CPA before beginning to erode the bony canal and porus. In general, the larger the tumor, the more likely the predilection for bone destruction, especially the posterior lip of the porus acusticus. Transorbital views, such as plain films and complex-motion tomography, comparatively demonstrating both internal audi-

tory canals are of screening benefit if CT and MRI are not yet available.

Iophendylate contrast studies of the CPA have always been effective, utilizing conventional imaging in multiple positions. These contrast studies are used infrequently now, but may remain useful (Fig. 12-12) for clinicians who do not have access to cur-

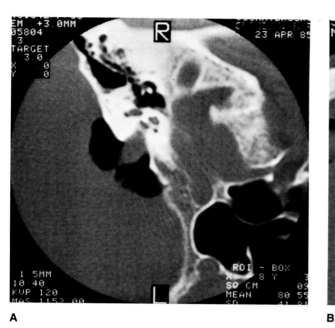

**A**

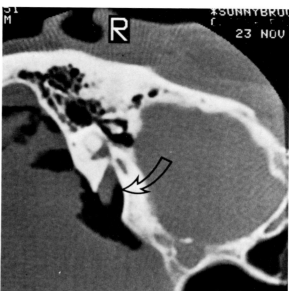

**B**

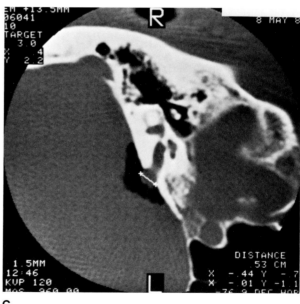

**C**

**Fig. 12-11.** Air CT-cisternography showing small acoustic neuromas. **(A)** Air "capping" soft tissue mass that fills IAC and bulges into CPA cistern. **(B)** Intracanalicular acoustic neuroma (arrow) is outlined by air. Note flaring of IAC in this patient despite limited size of tumor. Patient had symmetrical bilateral flaring on plain films as a normal anatomic variant. **(C)** Acoustic neuroma, 5 mm diameter, bulging into the CPA cistern without flaring of IAC (normal plain films and normal enhanced CT).

rent-generation CT scanners. Air profiling of such masses may also be combined with complex-motion tomography with reasonable effectiveness.

Magnetic resonance imaging is undoubtedly the most effective means of assessing any of the neurogenic tumors including acoustic neuroma[16,17] (see Figs. 11-1 to 11-3). It allows for precise definition of cranial nerves from their brain stem exit to their temporal bone or distant terminations. MRI obviates the need for CT studies and the latter's relative invasiveness due to intravenous contrast enhancement or intrathecal placement of air. Unfortunately, MRI is not universally available.

Meningiomas (Fig. 12-7) arise focally or en

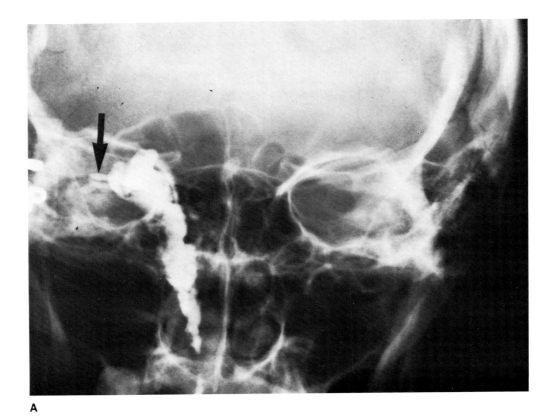

A

B

**Fig. 12-12.** Positive contrast conventional cisternography for assessment of CPA and IAC. Oil-based (Iophen-dylate) conventional cisternography. **(A)** Transorbital projection with patient in lateral decubitus position. A few ml of iophendylate are manipulated into the CPA cistern after intrathecal injection. Contrast enters right IAC (arrow), ruling out acoustic neuroma. **(B)** Basal projection similarly shows contrast medium entering left IAC (arrow). No CPA mass is seen. *(Figure continues.)*

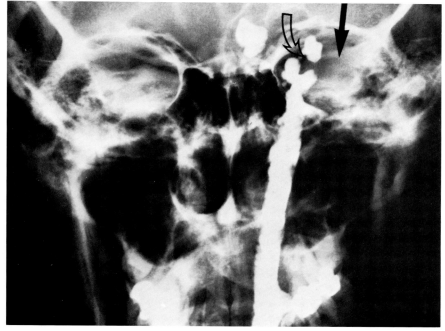

C

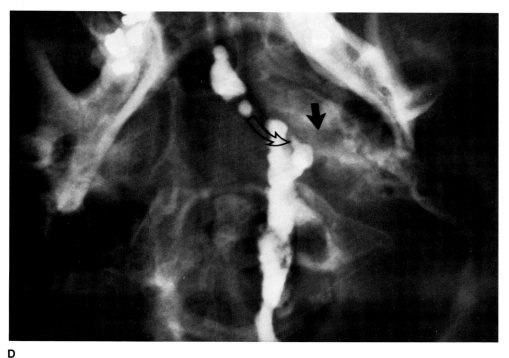

D

**Fig. 12-12** *(Continued).*    **(C,D)** Patient with left acoustic neuroma. Films were obtained with patient in left lateral decubitus position, to allow contrast medium to "fall" into IAC, but are displayed in upright position for ease of viewing. **(C)** Transorbital projection and **(D)** basal projection display the IAC (solid arrow) with the oil-based contrast agent remaining within the CPA cistern and not entering IAC. Small filling defect at the medial aspect of the canal and projecting into the contrast collection (open arrow) demonstrates extension of acoustic neuroma into the CPA cistern.

plaque about the region of the porus acusticus. In contrast to acoustic neuromas, meningiomas usually have a sessile or broad-based enhancing pattern, reflecting their attachment to the meninges of the temporal bone or adjacent tentorium. The meningioma tends to be intensely vascular, demonstrating homogeneous enhancement. Anterior extension into the middle fossa, passing beneath the tentorium, is frequently seen with meningioma, but may rarely be imitated by large acoustic neuromas. Calcification, either psammomatous or flocculent, detected on CT is strongly suggestive of meningioma. If CT is unavailable, angiography may be used to demonstrate the abnormal meningeal vessels and tumor blush of meningioma and differentiate such masses from the relatively avascular acoustic neuroma. The meningioma, when of sufficient size (greater than 2 cm), may be visualized by radionuclide brain or bone scans usually performed for other diagnostic indications.

Dermoid (and epidermoid) tumors (Fig. 12-8) usually can be diagnosed by their characteristic central low attenuation appearance, due to fat content; fat is seen as a negative density on the CT scan. Occasionally, an epidermoid tumor may appear isodense or of homogeneous increased density resembling acoustic neuroma. Unless infected, these tumors do not tend to enhance. Curtin[12] has noted that epidermoids contained within the internal auditory canal (IAC) cause considerable bone erosion and may extend laterally into the middle ear.

Fifth nerve neuromas (Fig. 12-9A) tend to be more anteriorly and superiorly located because of the course of the 5th cranial nerve relative to the IAC. Such masses may cause involvement of the petrous apex or Meckel's cave and be specifically diagnosed by such CT appearances. The 7th and 8th cranial nerve symptoms are due to secondary compression of these nerves. Larger tumors, however, may have similar appearances, whether originating from the 5th or 8th cranial nerves with the bulk of the mass extending through the CPA cistern and displacing the brain stem. A lack of flaring of the IAC is of significant importance in distinguishing these cranial nerve neuromas; flaring is present in the great majority of acoustic neuromas and only exceptionally with larger trigeminal neuromas. The trigeminal nerve, with its larger diameter than the 7th or 8th nerves, may be demonstrated easily by the use of intrathecal contrast media; oil-based myelographic contrast media was used previously and CT combined with water-soluble low-toxicity myelographic contrast media or room air has been used more recently.

Facial nerve neuromas may resemble acoustic neuromas (Fig. 12-9B) when they arise more medially or within the IAC. They may arise from any portion of the facial nerve. The 7th cranial nerve may be visualized in its more central portion passing from the pontomedullary junction through the CPA cistern to the lateral aspect of the IAC with air CT-cisternography (Fig. 12-10A) or, more recently, MRI (see Fig. 11-4). Such studies are occasionally performed to detect whether a tumor originating in the geniculate region has spread into the intracanalicular portion.

Complex motion tomography in multiple projections may identify bone erosion about the facial nerve canal, with a presumed diagnosis of facial nerve schwannoma; this study most readily recognizes the tumor when it arises on the vertical or mastoid segment by the saccular deformity of the otherwise fine tubular bony canal. CT scanning allows a more precise tracking of the entire facial nerve canal and detection of bony/soft tissue abnormalities. Tumors of the geniculate region can usually be recognized, when small, by their extension into the middle fossa and/or into the middle ear air space.

Occasionally, vascular masses, whether aneurysms (Fig. 12-9D,E) of the anterior inferior cerebellar artery (AICA) or posterior inferior cerebellar artery or dolichoectasia (arteriosclerotic elongation and tortuosity) of the vertebral artery may present as CPA masses. Calcification within the walls of the dilated tortuous vertebral artery can usually be detected in dolichoectasia. Aneurysm may be more difficult to diagnose if it is localized to the CPA adjacent to the porus acusticus. Angiography remains the definitive diagnostic modality for vascular abnormalities (Fig. 12-9E). The AICA may be seen looping into the IAC on air CT-cisternography (Fig. 12-10B).

Metastases may appear identical to acoustic neuroma (Fig. 12-9C) and should always be considered, especially if there is a history of primary neoplasm elsewhere in the body. More rapid progression of symptoms and growth of the tumor may suggest this diagnosis.

## VASCULAR TUMORS AND MALFORMATIONS (PULSATILE TINNITUS)

Vascular lesions of the temporal bone[18-22] are readily imaged if larger than 1 cm. The indications for radiologic assessment are suggested by the degree of subjective disturbance caused by pulsatile tinnitus, the objective presence of vascular bruit, or the otoscopic findings of a vascular mass involving the tympanic cavity. Degrees of clinical suspicion, whether a mass is present or not, as well as clinical impression of the mass size will have a direct effect on modalities of investigation. As a general rule, less invasive tests (CT with enhancement, or dynamic CT[21] [see Fig. 11-11]) will be performed before more invasive tests (angiography).

For small tumors (glomus tympanicum), CT assessment tends to be more valuable than angiographic assessment (Fig. 12-13). High-resolution CT using thin slices (1.5 mm thickness), a bone algorithm, and wide window to display soft tissues within the tympanic cavity will show the soft tissue mass well outlined by residual air. Assessment of the bony margins of the tympanic cavity and jugular bulb, usually performed in both axial and coronal planes, will demonstrate the mass to be limited to the tympanic cavity. The appearance and location of the soft tissue mass are characteristic and diagnostic of glomus tympanicum. Such tumors do not tend to be well visualized angiographically, with neither the feeding vessels nor tumor blush demonstrated. Angiography may be performed to assess the presence of other paragangliomas; however, enhanced axial CT may be used to assess the skull base and soft tissues of the neck, including the carotid body or bifurcation region. CT readily differentiates normal anatomic variants, such as high jugular bulb, dehiscent jugular bulb or aberrant internal carotid artery from pathologic states.

For larger tumors (glomus jugulare), enhanced axial CT will outline the extent and location of the vascular mass (Fig. 12-14). Such scanning should include the soft tissues of the upper neck, as well as the skull base and cerebral hemispheres. High-resolution bone images through the skull base will assess jugular bulb and tympanic cavity involvement. Clincally visualized large masses may be adequately studied with slice thicknesses of 3 to 5 mm, in contrast to the thin slices required for assessment of glomus tympanicum. Angiography is subsequently used to define the vascular compartments, including feeding and draining vessels.[19] Such definitive assessment is required to evaluate alternative treatment modalities and involves superselective arterial catheterization.

Angiography offers information about jugular venous outflow (i.e., whether tumor invasion or obstruction is present) that is not available by CT. Such information, which is of significant surgical importance, is assessed in the venous phase of the arteriogram, with digital subtraction techniques displaying venous channels to marked advantage and obviating the need for retrograde jugular venography.

Plain films may offer an initial overview of the jugular fossa and adjacent petrous bones. Their use is otherwise of limited value in the presence of available CT. In the absence of CT, complex motion tomography may be useful to assess bony destruction of the jugular bulb (frontal tomography) or caroticojugular ridge (lateral tomography); however, angiography, if available, tends to be more informative as the primary mode of assessment in such a clinical setting.

Arteriovenous malformations (AVM) have a predilection for the external carotid; such lesions in the region of the temporal bone produce pulsatile tinnitus and tend to arise from the occipital artery (see Fig. 11-7). Enhanced CT is the usual screening procedure performed to assess the skull base and cerebral tissues. Such studies are used to rule out the possibility of glomus tumors as well as other masses of the temporal bone. Arteriovenous malformations of the posterior fossa or cerebral tissues are generally well demonstrated by CT. Dural AVMs, however, may be poorly assessed by CT, with findings frequently being normal. The presence of prominent venous channels, however, due to transdural shunting of the vascular malforma-

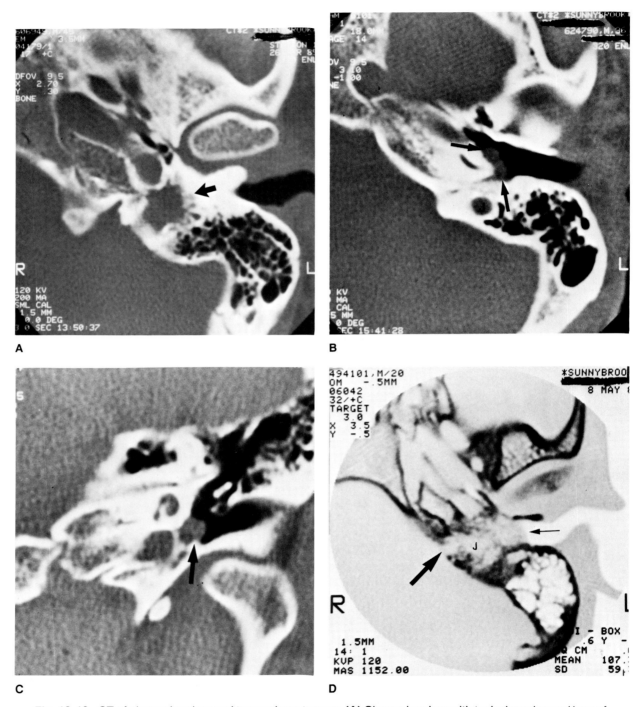

**Fig. 12-13.** CT of glomus jugulare and tympanicum tumors. **(A)** Glomus jugulare with typical erosion and loss of cortical margin of jugular bulb (arrow). **(B,C)** Glomus tympanicum. Small soft tissue density confined to hypotympanum (arrows) on axial **(B)** and coronal **(C)** CT; wall of jugular bulb (J) is intact. **(D)** Reverse image axial CT displays bone destruction (heavy arrow) and mass extending into hypotympanum (thin arrow). Jugular bulb (J) is destroyed by the glomus jugulare.

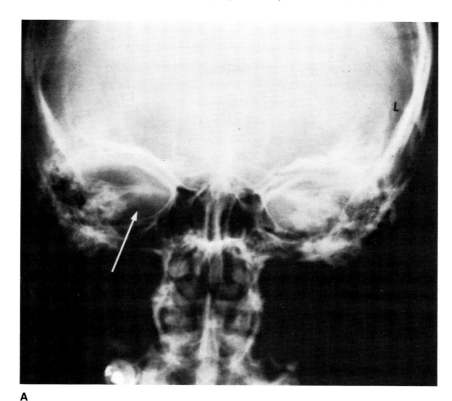

**A**

**Fig. 12-14.** Destruction of petrous apex by glomus jugulare; plain film/CT correlation. **(A)** Transorbital PA film, showing petrous bones projected through orbits. Destruction of right petrous apex and floor of right IAC (arrow) is clearly visible. **(B)** Coned down basal view demonstrates destruction and expansion (arrows) of right petrous apex. *(Figure continues.)*

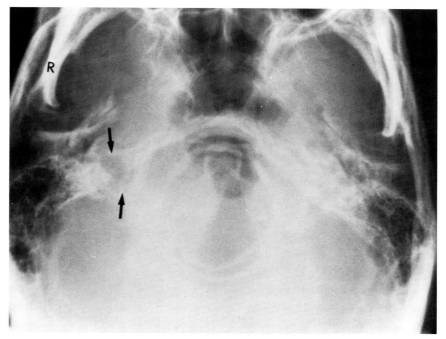

**B**

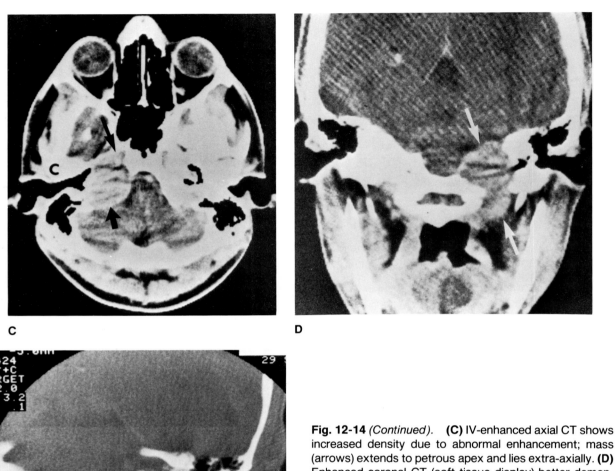

**C**

**D**

**E**

**Fig. 12-14** *(Continued).* **(C)** IV-enhanced axial CT shows increased density due to abnormal enhancement; mass (arrows) extends to petrous apex and lies extra-axially. **(D)** Enhanced coronal CT (soft tissue display) better demonstrates superoinferior extent of tumor (arrows); its inferior extension is into the upper part of the parapharyngeal space. **(E)** Coronal CT using bone algorithm better displays destruction of petrous apex (horizontal arrows) and floor of right IAC (vertical arrow). Note loss of soft tissue resolution at extended bone window.

tion, may be diagnostic and suggest the need for angiographic assessment. Although intravenous digital subtraction angiography (Fig. 11-8D,E) may grossly display or confirm the malformation and venous shunting,[20] supraselective intra-arterial angiography, as with glomus tumors, is essential to define vascular compartments and assess the feasibility of intra-arterial embolization as an alternative or adjunctive treatment.

Angiography may be used to display extratemporal causes of pulsatile tinnitus, whether intraluminal vascular pathology such as carotid stenoses

(Fig. 11-8A) or vascular tumors such as carotid tumors or glomus vagale (Fig. 11-8C).

MRI may allow the diagnosis of vascular pathology of the temporal bone (Fig. 11-6), which is suggested by tissue characteristics and blood flow assessment. Such capabilities may alter protocols for the investigation of pulsatile tinnitus in the future.

## TEMPORAL BONE TUMORS

A variety of benign (Fig. 12-15) and malignant tumors (Figs. 12-16, 12-17) may affect the temporal bone.[2,9,22] Paragangliomas, vascular malfor-

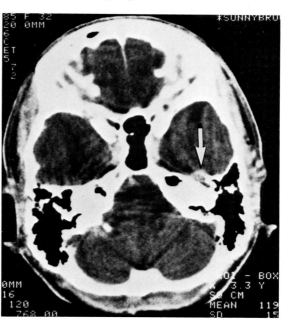

**Fig. 12-15.** Facial nerve schwannoma. **(A)** Enhanced axial CT (soft tissue mode) displays abnormal enhancement extending anteriorly (arrow) from geniculate region of left facial nerve. Mastoid air cells and epitympanum appear grossly normal. This is an isolated neuroma or schwannoma of the facial nerve. **(B)** Geniculate neuroma (open arrow) has destroyed bone in the adjacent middle fossa. Ossicles are displaced somewhat laterally by intratympanic extension. Air cisternography of left CPA shows no evidence of extension into IAC (solid arrow). **(C)** Coronal CT displays mass (thin arrows) inferior to lateral semicircular canal. Mass lies within tympanic cavity medially and is centered about course of facial nerve canal (horizontal segment). This soft tissue finding indicates posterior extension of geniculate tumor. Body and long process of incus are displaced laterally (curved arrow).

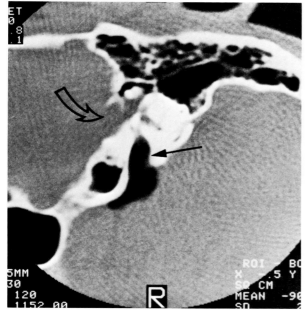

**B**

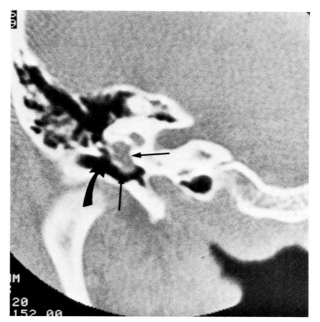

**C**

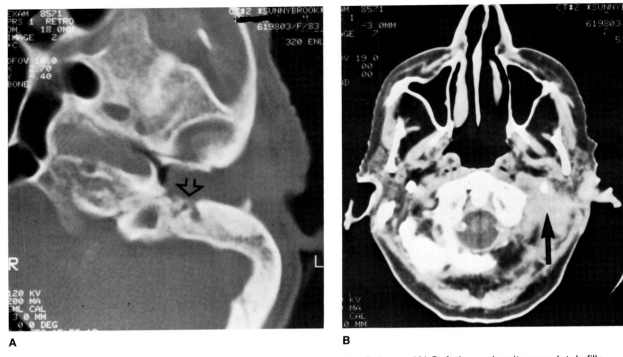

**Fig. 12-16.** Carcinoma of the EAC with extension to bone and soft tissue. **(A)** Soft tissue density completely fills EAC; the posterior bony wall has an irregular, partially destroyed appearance (arrow). **(B)** Loss of soft tissue planes (arrow) due to extension of tumor inferior to skull base.

mations, and those tumors arising in the CPA cistern have been discussed. Despite various anatomic locations of different types of tumors involving the temporal bone, CT in general is the imaging modality of choice; complementary modalities are occasionally useful. The presence or absence of bone destruction, mass lesions, and extent of disease is well assessed by CT. The enhanced mode is usually chosen to display degrees of vascularity and better display soft tissue involvement of the brain and skull base. Studies concurrently, if extended inferiorly to include the neck, can assess the presence of lymphatic spread and metastatic disease.

Although radiologic signs often will be relatively nonspecific, patterns of bone destruction, invasion, or expansion frequently allow description and prediction of benign or malignant lesions. Benign lesions may however be mimicked by malignant disease. Squamous cell carcinoma (Fig. 12-16) or basal cell carcinoma of the external ear canal may appear identical to malignant otitis externa. Osteomyelitis of the petrous apex may resemble an aggressive neoplastic process. Conversely, some malignant tumors such as myeloma may appear well defined and be mistaken for benign entities. Mastoid opacification secondary to obstruction with or without inflammatory changes may resemble tumor infiltration into the air spaces. Many tumors do not have typical presentations, but have a variety of appearances. Myeloma, leukemia, and lymphoma, for instance, may present as either focal or diffuse permeative lesions.

More specific diagnosis may occasionally be made, such as facial neuroma (Fig. 12-15). Mesenchymal tumors, such as osteoma, chondroma, or osteosarcoma and chondrosarcoma, may present with more characteristic appearances with calcification or ossification noted; however, the differentiation between benign and malignant tumors may

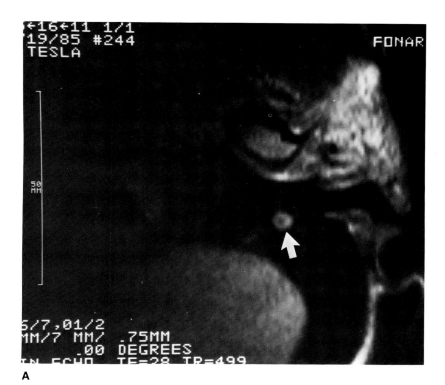

**Fig. 12-17.** Perineural extension of parotid adenocarcinoma involving vertical segment of left facial nerve. Axial **(A)** and sagittal **(B)** $T_1$-weighted MR images show increased caliber and intensity of vertical component facial nerve (white arrow) in sharp contrast to absence of signal intensity in adjacent petrous bone, tympanic cavity, and EAC. Sagittal image also shows mass in left parotid gland (black arrows) anterior to stylomastoid foramen. (Courtesy of Dr. William Hanafee, University of California at Los Angeles, Los Angeles, CA.)

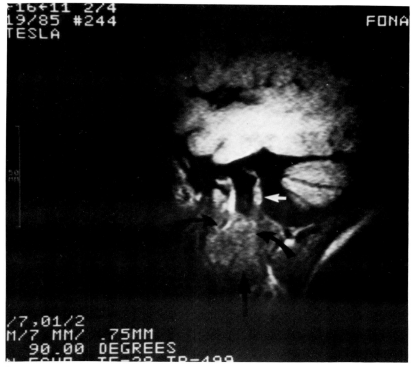

be difficult. The presence of bone destruction or associated soft tissue mass suggests malignant degeneration.

Osteoblastic lesions may suggest prostatic metastases, especially if multiple. Paget's disease may need to be differentiated. Sclerosis from chronic inflammatory reaction should not be confused.

Plain skull films may still be useful and offer an overview. Metastatic lesions to the cranial vault may not be visualized routinely on CT, yet are seen very readily on a skull film, which allows proper diagnosis of the temporal bone lesion. With high-resolution imaging, the tendency to focus total attention on a small anatomic site may be misleading, resulting in a delay in diagnosis and subsequent treatment.

Radionuclide studies may be helpful; radionuclide methylene diphosphonate bone scans are performed to assess biological activity of inflammatory or neoplastic conditions, such as osteoma. Extent of bone disease may be better defined in early stages of bone involvement and complement the CT findings. Survey for skeletal metastases may also be helpful in assessing the true nature of a temporal bone lesion. Occasionally gallium scans may be used to stage or assess lymphoma or malignant melanoma involvement of the temporal bone.

Angiography may occasionally be indicated to assess vascular compromise (internal carotid artery, internal jugular vein) by adjacent mass lesions. MRI may play a more significant role in the future, especially as more experience in tissue characterization is gained (Fig. 12-17).

## CONGENITAL DISORDERS

Congenital abnormalities of the temporal bone are difficult but important to image.[2,15,22,23] Assessment of anatomic components such as the labyrinth or ossicular chain demands high-resolution detail. CT, the primary mode of investigation, is performed utilizing thin slices and bone algorithms including the coronal plane, since most anomalies will be bone related. (Fig. 12-18). If such images cannot be obtained by CT, complex motion tomog-

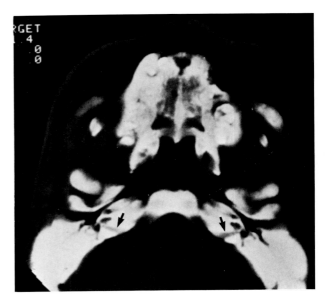

**Fig. 12-18.** Osteopetrosis. Marked density of skull base limited plain film and tomographic findings in a patient who was both blind and deaf. Axial CT demonstrates marked stenosis of the IAC bilaterally (arrows). EAC, cochlea, and vestibule are intact.

raphy (coronal) may be very adequate especially since for most such anomalies it is more important to visualize bone detail than the associated soft tissues.

The congenital anomalies most often noted are microtia and atresia involving any combination of the pinna, external auditory canal, and middle ear cleft. Treatment decisions demand display of the external auditory canal, to differentiate soft tissue from bony atresia (Figs. 12-19, 12-20). Involvement of the middle ear, whether deformity of the ossicles or obliteration of the middle ear cleft itself, is of surgical importance. The position of the facial nerve and canal (Fig. 12-19) must be defined in the presence of anomalies to avoid surgical injury. Presence or absence of bony closure of the round or oval window must also be determined before a surgical approach is decided upon. Structural abnormalities of the labyrinth (cochlea) and IAC may similarly be assessed.

Reformatted images in sagittal or oblique planes may show anatomic structures to advantage. MRI is of value to display the brain and cranial nerves if

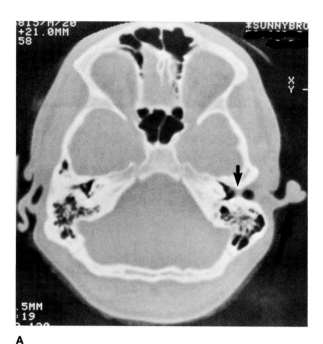

A

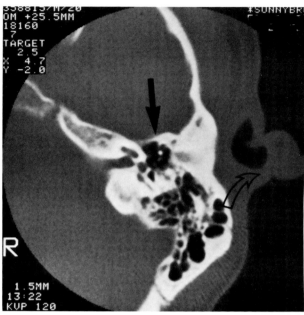

B

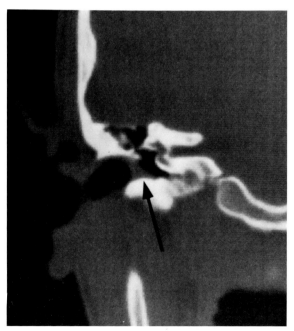

C

**Fig. 12-19.** Congenital microtia and atresia of external auditory canal; CT utilized for assessment of middle and inner ear. **(A–C)** External auditory canal atresia and normal middle ear. **(A)** Axial CT demonstrates microtic deformity of left pinna (large solid arrow); compare to normal contralateral ear. Obstructive deformity in EAC is of soft tissue density (small arrow). Aeration of tympanic cavity is normal. **(B)** High-resolution CT (axial) displays normal tympanic cavity (heavy arrow), ossicles, and inner ear. Cochlea, vestibule, IAC, and segment of posterior semicircular are all seen on this slice. Open arrow points to microtia. **(C)** Coronal CT shows soft tissue obstruction of EAC (arrow). Normal bony spur and middle and inner ear structures are well shown by CT. *(Figure continues.)*

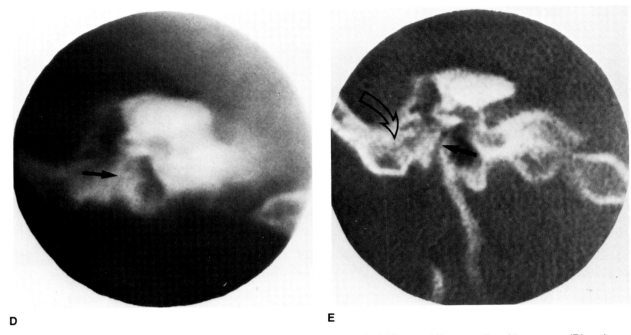

**D**  **E**

**Fig. 12-19** *(Continued).* **(D,E)** Congenital atresia of external and middle ear. AP conventional tomogram **(D)** and corresponding coronal CT **(E)** show lack of development (open arrow) of EAC and ossicular chain. Normal inner ear structures, including vestibule, semicircular canals, and IAC are visualized. Vertical portion of facial canal (solid arrow) is seen; its lateral deviation is related to external ear atresia. **(D,E** courtesy of Dr. Carmen Guirado, Barcelona, Spain.)

associated defects are suspected. Direct visualization of the facial nerve may prove to be of clinical use, especially if the facial canal cannot be demonstrated by conventional or CT imaging.

## TRAUMA

Trauma of the temporal bone may be isolated or in conjunction with other major skull and intracranial injury.[9,22] In complex major trauma of the skull, CT imaging of the brain will be performed first to assess whether immediate neurosurgical intervention is required. In the great majority of patients, imaging can then be extended inferiorly to include the skull base and petrosa, with such images displayed at both bone and soft tissue mode.

If time and the patient's clinical condition permit, contiguous thinner slices (1.5 to 5.0 mm) through the petrous bone are preferred to the thicker (10 mm) slices used routinely to scan the head. Coronal CT imaging is usually contraindicated in the acute trauma patient until the possibility of cervical injury has been ruled out, and the patient's condition has stabilized. Such images, however, can be obtained in those patients with isolated temporal bone injury. Coronal or sagittal reformations may be performed in those patients in whom high-resolution thin axial slices have been obtained.

Associated linear fractures of the cranial vault are better detected on plain skull films. CT is used, however, to display the relationship of fractures (Fig. 12-21) (whether transverse or longitudinal) to the otic capsule, ossicles, and facial nerve canal. Displacements of bone fragments or ossicles may also be noted (Fig. 12-22). Detection of fractures may explain the presence of cerebrospinal fluid

**Fig. 12-20.** Congenital obstruction of the EAC in a 17-year-old patient with congenital decreased hearing in the right ear. The otologist was unable to examine the EAC because of a bony mass at the lateral aspect. Sinus tract was suspected superiorly. **(A)** Coronal CT demonstrates bony mass (horizontal arrow) at lateral aspect of EAC. Tiny opening of EAC is seen just superior to bony mass. Soft tissue density (vertical arrows) within canal represented cerumen accumulation. **(B)** Axial CT shows origin of bony mass (horizontal arrow) arising from tympanic plate at lateral aspect of EAC. Bony walls of EAC are intact. Soft tissue density of retained cerumen (vertical arrows) cannot be differentiated from other soft tissue masses.

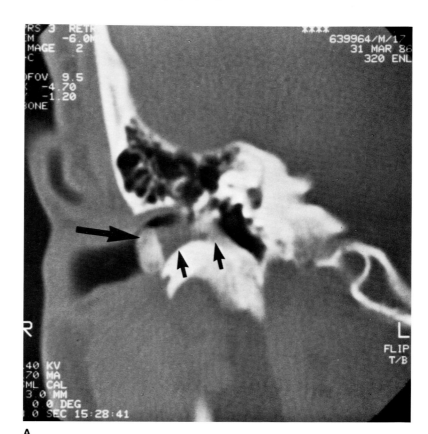

**A**

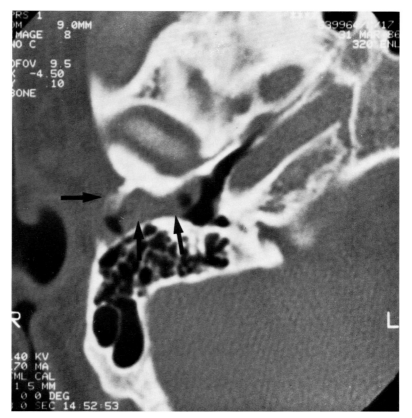

**B**

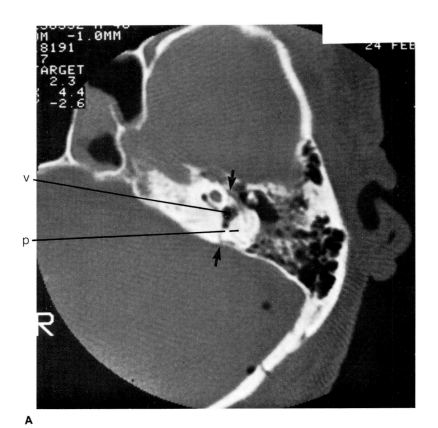

**A**

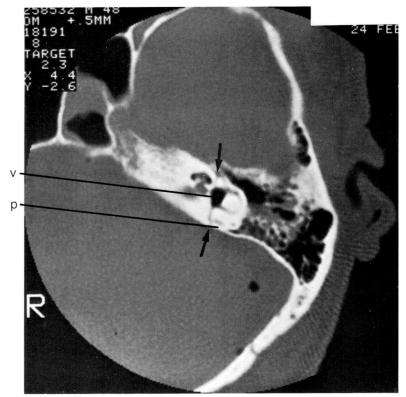

**B**

**Fig. 12-21.** Temporal bone fractures assessed by high-resolution CT (bone algorithm) **(A)** Relation of fracture line to bony labyrinth is readily visualized. Transverse fracture (arrows) extends through vestibule (v), lateral to cochlea, medial to posterior semicircular canal (p). **(B)** One slice superior to **(A)**, fracture (arrows) through vestibule is (v) better demonstrated; it extends posteriorly just medial to posterior semicircular canal (PSCC) (p). Lateral semicircular canal (LSCC) is intact. *(Figure continues.)*

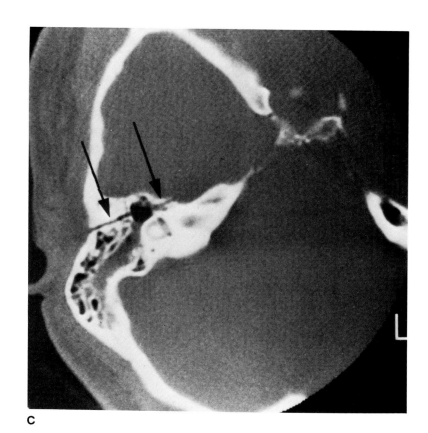

C

**Fig. 12-21** *(Continued).* **(C)** Different patient with longitudinal fracture (arrows) through tympanic cavity; LSCC and SSCC are intact. Fluid (blood, effusion, or CSF) is present in mastoid air cells. **(D)** Slice at level of IAC, in the same patient shows ossicles intact and not displaced despite fracture through the tympanic cavity (thin arrows); clouded mastoid air cells are visible (heavy arrow).

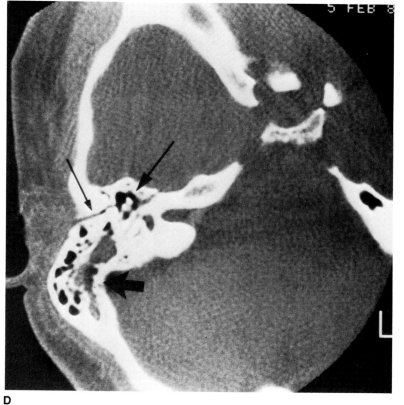

D

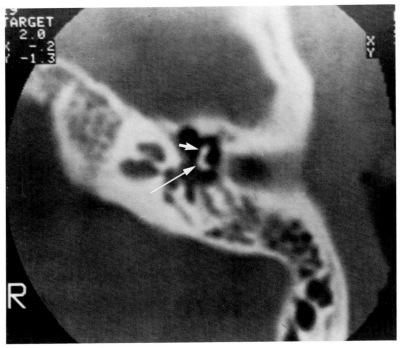

A

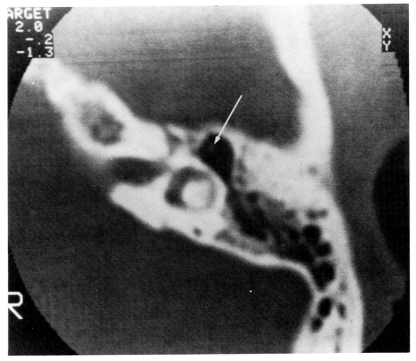

B

**Fig. 12-22.** Ossicular dislocations. **(A)** Dislocated incus (long arrow) lies in a more horizontal position with an abnormal relationship to the malleus (short arrow). **(B)** One slice more superiorly, the head of the malleus (arrow) is seen to be positioned too far anteriorly within the epitympanic space (anterior dislocation). High-resolution 1.5 mm slices are required for such detail. (Courtesy of Dr. Joel D. Swartz, Medical College of Pennsylvania, Philadelphia, PA.)

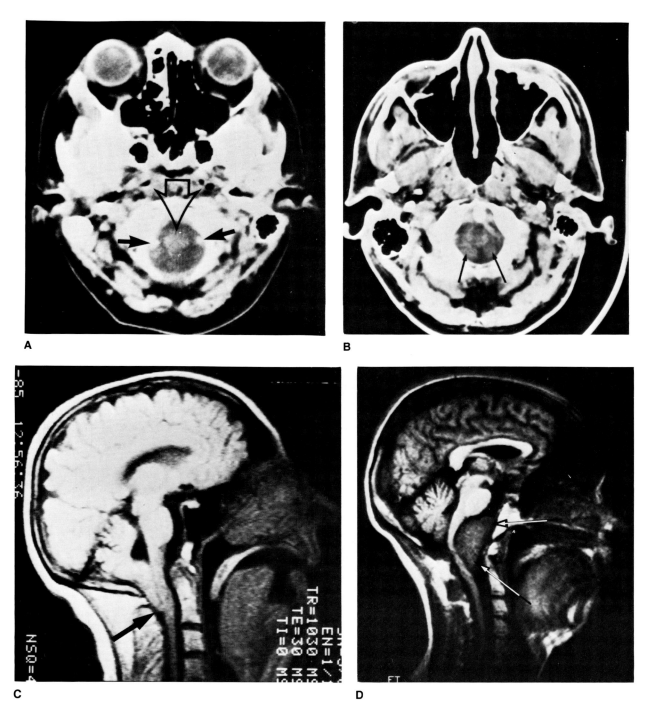

**Fig. 12-23.** Craniovertebral junction. **(A)** Normal relationships at craniovertebral junction are shown by enhanced axial CT at level of foramen magnum. Normal medulla (open arrow) is seen; tonsils are not visualized. Vertebral arteries are noted bilaterally within the foramen (solid arrows). **(B)** Enhanced axial CT at level of foramen magnum shows cerebellar tonsils (arrows) lying in inferior position, consistent with Arnold-Chiari malformation. **(C)** Sagittal MRI displays central nervous system tissues and CSF spaces directly. Inferiorly located cerebellar tonsils (arrow) are noted displaced into the cervical spinal canal in patient with Arnold-Chiari malformation. **(D)** Sagittal MRI superbly shows displacement of brainstem posteriorly by clival meningioma (arrows). (D courtesy of Picker International, Highland Heights, OH.)

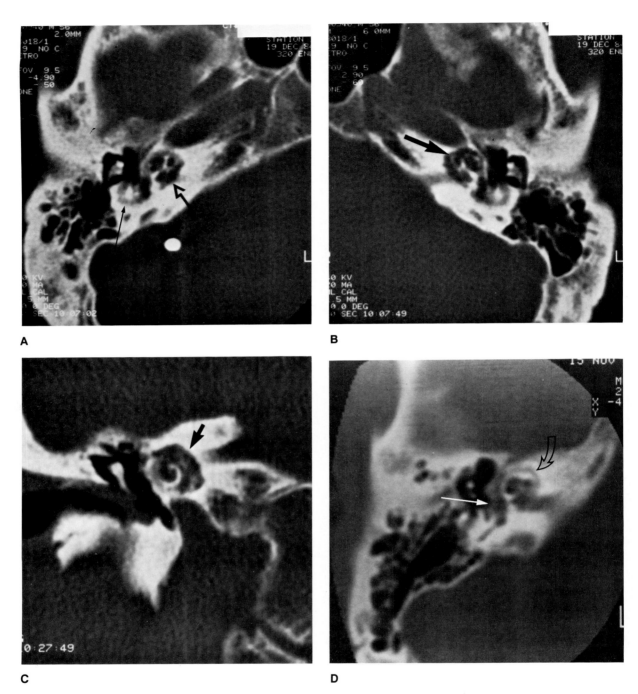

**A**

**B**

**C**

**D**

**Fig. 12-24.** Otosclerosis. **(A–C)** CT assessment of patient with bilateral otosclerosis. CT findings are not always uniform or predictable, and CT examination is rarely indicated. **(A)** Axial CT of right temporal bone shows loss of typical bone cortex about cochlear turns (open arrow). Similar loss of sharp definition of the bony labyrinth is seen about vestibule and LSCC (solid arrow). **(B)** Axial CT of left temporal bone displays scalloping of basal turn of cochlea which appears abnormally wide. Gross irregularity of cochlea is evident (arrow). **(C)** Coronal CT of right petrous bone further demonstrates the scalloped appearance of the outer bony wall and demineralization of the inner wall of the modiolus due to cochlear otosclerosis. **(D)** Axial CT of right petrous bone shows "mixed" otosclerosis with otic capsule displaying increased and decreased densities surrounding cochlea medially (open arrow). More laterally, bone of decreased density is present anterior and posterior to the oval window (thin arrow), including area of fissula ante fenestrum. (D courtesy of Dr. Joel D. Swartz, Medical College of Pennsylvania, Philadelphia, PA.)

360

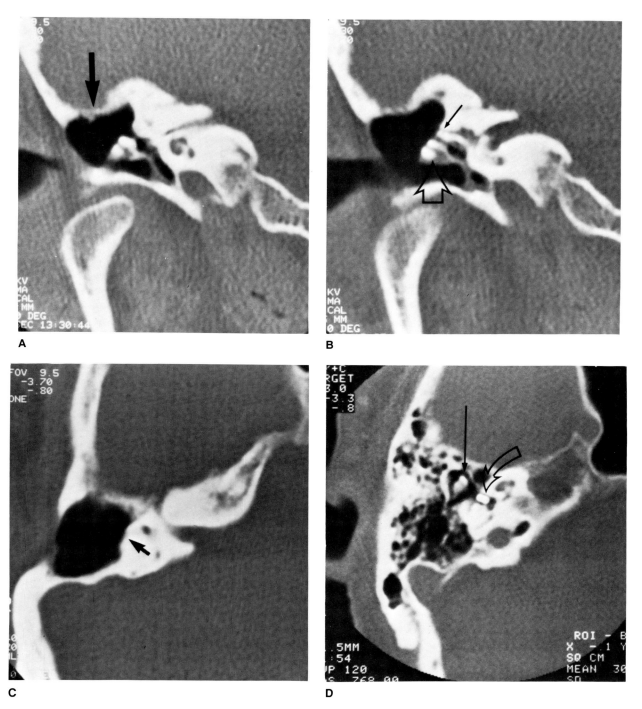

**Fig. 12-25.** CT assessment of postsurgical status. **(A–C)** Assessment of post-mastoidectomy patient who presented with vertigo due to fistula of LSCC. **(A)** Coronal CT shows evidence of previous mastoidectomy. Ossicles are present, tegmen is demineralized (arrow). **(B)** More posterior coronal slice demonstrates fistula between mastoid cavity and LSCC (small arrow). Soft tissue density about ossicles (open arrow) may represent residual adhesions, secretions, or granulation tissue. **(C)** Axial CT demonstrates discontinuity of bony labyrinth overlying LSCC (arrow). **(D)** Poststapedectomy patient with vertigo. Stapes prosthesis (open arrow) extends through oval window and into vestibule. Malleus and incus appear intact (thin arrow).

(CSF) otorrhea or rhinorrhea. Occasionally radionuclide tracer or intrathecal water-soluble contrast media in conjunction with CT may be required to localize the site of CSF leak. Conventional tomography (especially in the coronal plane) may be helpful to display the bone fractures if CT is not available.

## CRANIOVERTEBRAL JUNCTION

Pathologic changes occurring at the craniovertebral junction may occasionally simulate disease of the temporal bone or CPA. For this reason, we include the foramen magnum region on routine axial CT studies to visualize the level of the cerebellar tonsils (Fig. 12-23A,B). The lateral skull film offers an excellent overview of the craniovertebral region and should be utilized if an abnormality of this region is suspected. Lateral tomography may further define such relationships if indicated or better define bony landmarks and anomalies. Frontal projection conventional studies may be complementary but, since the availability of CT, offer minimal additional information. The availability of MRI has significantly altered the role of CT. Direct sagittal MRI has become the modality of choice to visualize the posterior cranial fossa (PCF) and upper cervical region (Fig. 12-23C,D). Water-soluble intrathecal myelographic contrast media, in combination with CT, to assess the cerebellar tonsils, cisternal spaces, syringomyelia, or mass lesions of the craniovertebral junction, has been replaced by the more informative noninvasive MRI. Enhanced CT of the posterior fossa and upper cervical spine will likewise be replaced as the primary screening modality as MRI becomes more universally available.

## MISCELLANEOUS

The temporal bone may be the focus of a variety of bone diseases and dysplasias, some with a systemic basis. Paget's disease, the most common dysplasia to affect the temporal bone, may be considered and differentiated from other pathologic change associated with increased activity on the radionuclide bone scan. The hyperemic vascular nature of the bony abnormality, due to arteriovenous shunting, may be noted in the blood pool phase of the bone scan.[24]

Whole body bone scanning may demonstrate that the temporal bone involvement represents an isolated entity or part of systemic Paget's disease. Morphologic changes of the thickened softer bone with changes in contour and encroachment of foramina may be noted on conventional imaging or CT.

Histiocytosis (eosinophilic granuloma, Hand-Schuller-Christian syndrome, Letterer-Siwe syndrome), which is primarily a disease of infants and children, may involve the temporal bone in isolation or, more frequently, as a focal manifestation of systemic disease. An index of suspicion may prevent such lesions from being confused with infective or neoplastic lesions. Bone scanning may be helpful in defining systemic involvement and local extent; the bone scan may also show bony healing of lesions after treatment. Nonspecific findings of bone destruction and opacification of air cells are seen in Wegener's granulomatosis.

Radiologic evaluation is rarely required in otosclerosis. However, morphologic changes (Fig. 12-24) about the otic capsule may be seen occasionally in otosclerosis (otospongiosis). The loss of definition of the normal otic capsule, seen on CT or complex-motion tomography, should not be confused with an osteomyelitic process.

Finally, postsurgical assessment[25] (fistulae, ossicular status, other bone defects) is best imaged with thin section high-resolution CT (Fig. 12-25).

## ACKNOWLEDGMENTS

This work was supported by The Saul A. Silverman Family Foundation, Toronto, Ontario. The authors gratefully acknowledge Suzanne Petrevski and Rosemarie McGuire for manuscript preparation. We appreciate the efforts of the Departments of Instructional Media at Mount Sinai Hospital and Sunnybrook Medical Centre.

# REFERENCES

1. Brunner S, Jensen G, Hespersen C: Value of different projections in diagnosing cholesteatoma. Acta Radiol 54:177, 1960
2. Phelps PD, Lloyd GAS: Radiology of the Ear. Blackwell Scientific Publications, Oxford, 1983
3. Zizmor J, Noyek AM: Inflammatory diseases of the temporal bone. Radiol Clin North Am 12 (3):491, 1974
4. Zizmor J, Noyek AM: The protean radiologic manifestations of acquired temporal bone cholesteatoma. J Otolaryngol 10 [suppl 8]:1, 1981
5. Noyek AM, Kirsh JC, Greyson ND, et al: The clinical significance of radionuclide bone and gallium scanning in osteomyelitis of the head and neck. Laryngoscope 94(4) suppl 34:1, 1984
6. Chakares DW: CT of ear structures: a tailored approach. Radiol Clin North Am 22 (1):3, 1984
7. Swartz JD: Cholesteatomas of the middle ear: diagnosis, etiology and complications. Radiol Clin North Am 22 (1):15, 1984
8. Swartz JD: Imaging of the Temporal Bone. Thieme, New York, 1986
9. Mancuso AA, Hanafee WN: Computed Tomography and Magnetic Resonance Imaging of the Head and Neck, 2nd ed. Williams & Wilkins, Baltimore, 1985
10. Valvassori GE: The abnormal internal auditory canal: the diagnosis of acoustic neuroma. Radiology 92:449, 1969
11. Taylor S: The petrous temporal bone (including the cerebellopontine angle). Radiol Clin North Am 20:67, 1982
12. Curtin HD: CT of acoustic neuroma and other tumors of the ear. Radiol Clin North Am 22 (1):77, 1984
13. Kricheff II, Pinto RS, Bergeron RT, Cohen N: Air-CT cisternography and canalography for small acoustic neuromas. Am J Neuroradiol 1:57, 1980
14. Valvassori GE, Pierce RH: The normal internal auditory canal, Am J Roentgenol 92:1232, 1964
15. Valvassori GE, Buckingham RA: Tomography and Cross Sections of the Ear. WB Saunders, Philadelphia, 1975
16. Young IR, Bydder GM, Hall AS, et al: The role of NMR imaging in the diagnosis and management of acoustic neuroma. Am J Neuroradiol 4:223, 1983
17. Daniels DL, Herfkins R, Kochler PR, et al. Magnetic resonance imaging of the internal auditory canal. Radiology 151:105, 1984
18. Hesselink JR, Davis KR, Taveras JM: Selective arteriography of glomus tympanicum and jugulare tumors: techniques, normal and pathologic arterial anatomy. Am J Neuroradiol 2:289, 1981
19. Lasjaunias P: Craniofacial and Upper Cervical Arteries: Functional, Chemical and Angiographic aspects. Williams & Wilkins, Baltimore, 1981
20. Carmody RF, Smith JRL, Seeger JF, et al: Intracranial applications of digital intravenous subtraction angiography. Radiology 144:529, 1982
21. Mafee MF: Dynamic CT and its application to otolaryngology — head and neck surgery. J Otolaryngol 11:307, 1982
22. Bergeron RT, Osborn AG, Som PM (eds): Head and Neck Imaging Excluding the Brain. CV Mosby, St Louis, 1984
23. Petasnick JP: Congenital malformations of the ear. Otolaryngol Clin North Am 6 (2):413, 1973
24. Noyek AM: Bone scanning in otolaryngology. Laryngoscope 89 [suppl] 18:1, 1979
25. Johnson DW: CT of the postsurgical ear. Radiol Clin North Am 22:67, 1984

# Basic Audiologic Evaluation

# 13

## Barbara Kruger

Audiologic evaluation is the application of appropriate audiometric tests and case history information to the determination of auditory integrity for communication. The purpose of an audiologic evaluation can be diagnostic, prognostic, or hab/rehabilitative. The diagnostic audiologic evaluation not only confirms the presence or absence of hearing loss but also specifies the extent and type of hearing loss. This evaluation requires, at a minimum, basic or standard audiometric testing: puretone audiometry, speech audiometry, and impedance (or admittance) measurements. Additional differential diagnostic audiometric testing may include behavioral and electrophysiological tests for pseudohypacusis, differentiation of cochlear from retrocochlear pathologic conditions, and assessment of central auditory nervous system integrity.

This chapter describes the basic audiometric evaluation: the case history, audiometric equipment, air- and bone-conduction pure-tone audiometry, masking, and speech audiometry. Impedance measures (tympanometry and acoustic reflex) will be mentioned only as they relate to the interpretation of basic audiometric findings. This topic is discussed in greater detail in Chapter 14. It is important to remember that diagnosis extends beyond basic testing and that intervention often is nonmedical. Basic audiometry is just that, a baseline or starting point.

## CASE HISTORY

A basic audiologic evaluation consists of the following: a patient history, audiometric testing, and a summary of the audiologic findings as they relate to further audiologic evaluation or intervention. Data from each are considered independently by the audiologist in the evaluation of an individual's hearing and communication ability.

Of primary concern for an adult patient is a description of the history, course, and current status of the hearing loss and/or communication problem, such as the clarity of speech heard and any changes in vocal quality or speech production. In addition to the patient's personal hearing history, inquiry extends to the speech-language and hearing problems of family members.

Medical history particularly relevant to audiologic evaluation includes previous physicians consulted and the diagnosis or treatment; allergy history; tinnitus; dizziness or vertigo; facial numbness; headaches; head trauma; childhood and adult diseases (meningitis, measles, mumps, syphilis, multiple sclerosis, diabetes); genetic history of hearing loss; and exposure to ototoxic agents (e.g., medications and noise).

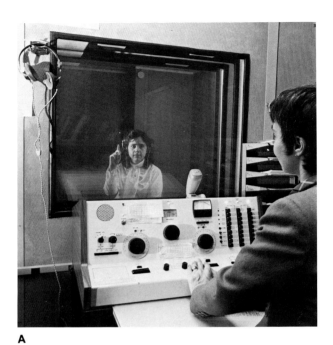

**A**

**Fig. 13-1.** Typical equipment used in an audiometric evaluation. **(A)** Two-room sound-treated audiometric test booth and an audiologist evaluating a patient. **(B)** Pair of standard supra-aural audiometric earphones used in audiologic testing. **(C)** Two bone vibrators: the one on the left is commonly used to evaluate sensitivity for bone-conducted signals (ANSI S3.13,1972); the one on the right is a more recent bone vibrator (ANSI S3.26,1981).

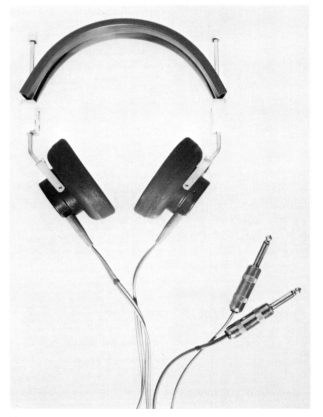

**B**

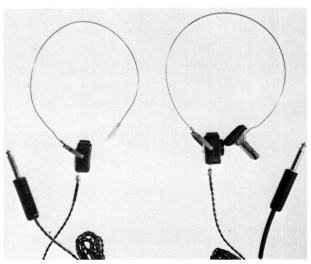

**C**

## AUDIOMETRIC EQUIPMENT AND CALIBRATION

The accuracy of the equipment used for hearing assessment is a significant variable in the validity and reliability of audiometric test results. Conclusions and recommendations drawn by the audiologist from the results of an audiologic evaluation can affect the medical diagnosis, medical or surgical treatment, and rehabilitative management. Therefore, the equipment must function properly and perform according to specifications or standards. The primary reason to calibrate is to permit the comparison of audiometric test results. Instrumentation used in an audiologic evaluation is illustrated in Figure 13-1.

Pure-tone air-conduction thresholds are assessed with standard supra-aural earphones (Telephonics TDH 39 or 49 earphones in MX41/AR or Model 51 supra-aural cushions; see Fig. 13-1B). Although some advantages for specific circumaural enclosures have been demonstrated,[1-5] the use of circumaural or other nonstandard earphone enclosures should be avoided since standards do not exist for their calibration and, therefore, do not permit clinic to clinic comparison of audiometric results.

Comparison of audiometric test results is possible only when the equipment used meets specific calibration standards. The most important and widely accepted standards for audiometry and their sources are listed in Table 13-1. The calibration equipment, their precision, and the procedures are specified in these standards and supplementary standards or guidelines.[6-9] The instrumentation and procedures necessary to calibrate audiometric equipment are discussed in Chapter 8.

The calibration should be checked at periodic intervals and whenever a problem is suspected.

The signal parameters (intensity, frequency, time, and quality) and the frequency with which each parameter should be tested[7,8] should conform to American National Standards Institute (ANSI), International Electrotechnical Commission (IEC), and International Standards Organization (ISO) standards, and American Speech–Language–Hearing Association (ASHA) guidelines. The regularity will differ according to the type of audiometric equipment, the signal, and the signal parameter.

Although periodic objective calibration is conducted on all equipment used in the audiologic evaluation, a daily biologic check of the intensity (linearity) and quality of the pure-tone signal (cross-talk, signal distortion, abnormal noise) of all transducers is extremely important. The significance of performing daily biologic listening checks can only be underscored by emphasizing the gravity of the possible outcomes when an error in equipment performance goes undetected. For example, if the signal intensity is not in calibration, the thresholds are spurious and result in an erroneous estimate of the degree of hearing loss. If the pure-tone stimulus is distorted (i.e., includes other frequencies in addition to the nominal frequency), the true audiometric configuration is not represented. The consequence of misdiagnosis that could result from not verifying accurate calibration with daily listening checks and regular electroacoustic calibration is substantial and never appropriate.

## THRESHOLD ASSESSMENT

Determination of hearing sensitivity or the threshold of audibility is one of the primary objectives of an audiologic evaluation. Hearing thresh-

**Table 13-1. Calibration Reference Standards for Audiometric Equipment**

| Equipment | Standard | Purpose |
|---|---|---|
| Audiometer and earphones | ANSI S3.6, 1969 | Ensure precise and comparable air-conducted signals |
| Audiometer and bone vibrator | ANSI S3.26, 1981 | Ensure precise and comparable bone-conducted signals |
| Audiometric test booth | ANSI S3.1, 1977 | Ensure hearing assessment is conducted in a sufficiently quiet environment |

old is defined for audiologic purposes as the minimum level at which a signal is detected 50 percent of the time. Threshold is dependent upon many measurement variables: the measurement procedure (psychophysical method), the stimulus, stimulus duration, the interstimulus interval, the response required of the listener, the motivation of the patient, the decibel step size used, the instructions, presence or absence of competing noise, and feedback given to the patient concerning accuracy of response.

Threshold methods applied in clinical audiology are derived from psychophysics.[10-12] Clinical audiometry assesses threshold with a modified method of limits procedure. The procedure is known as the modified Hughson-Westlake technique.[13] With this method, the stimulus is presented at a level above the anticipated threshold and decreased in 10 dB steps until the patient no longer hears it. The signal is then raised in 5 dB steps until the patient responds. The area of threshold is crossed in 10 dB intensity decrements and 5 dB intensity increments until a criterion response of 50 percent correct or more is achieved. In actuality, the lowest intensity level at which the patient responds to two of four or three of six stimuli is considered threshold.[14] However, because this method begins at a level above suspected threshold and familiarizes the patient with the signal and the task, variability is reduced. This technique is considered "ascending" because threshold is determined on ascending increments. This technique for manual pure-tone threshold audiometry is recommended by ASHA[15] and ANSI.[16]

## Pure-Tone Air-Conduction Audiometry

Air-conduction thresholds assess the outer, middle, and inner ear — the peripheral hearing system. Although the pure-tone signal must be transmitted to the cortex for a behavioral response to be made, lesions to the central auditory system are not easily observed in the pure-tone audiogram unless the insult is extensive. Air-conduction thresholds can be assessed under earphones or in the sound-field. Testing under earphones provides an independent evaluation of each ear whereas sound-field air-conduction assessment furnishes limited threshold information since only the better ear is evaluated.

There are various ways in which audiometric data can be presented. Two common representations are graphic (audiogram) and tabular. An audiogram is a plot of intensity in decibels hearing level (dB HL) as a function of frequency. On the audiogram, 0 dB HL is referenced to the median sound pressure level for minimum audibility under earphones obtained from a young adult population (18 to 25 years old).[17] In essence, the sound pressure levels are normalized at each frequency. An audiogram legend explains the symbol assigned to each test and each ear.[18] The audiogram can present audiometric results for both ears on a single graph (Fig. 13-2). This format is useful for diagnostic, prognostic, and rehabilitative applications since both ears are presented on a single graph. An alternative schema (Fig. 13-3) provides audiometric results for each ear on separate audiograms. This displays the hearing status of each ear independently. Another format (Fig. 13-4) depicts thresholds obtained with an automatic tracking (Békésy) audiometer. Automatic audiometry is used for site-of-lesion testing, evaluation of pseudohypacusis, and for threshold assessment in industrial settings and adult hearing screening. Finally, Figure 13-5 displays audiometric results in tabular form.

Accurate audiometric results are optimized by careful earphone placement and by careful instructions to the patient. Patients are instructed to respond when they hear something, even if it is very faint. Unless this is stressed, many patients will stop responding at suprathreshold levels and the results will not reflect threshold values. Thresholds are typically assessed at 1,000 Hz, then at octave intervals at frequencies above 1,000 Hz. As a reliability check, 1,000 Hz is retested and finally 500 and 250 Hz are assessed.[16] Interoctave frequencies are measured if a 20 dB difference in threshold exists between any two adjacent frequencies.

Soundfield air-conduction audiometry requires certain cautions. The permissible ambient noise levels in the test room are less intense for the soundfield test condition than the acceptable levels for earphone testing.[19] Earphone test conditions allow higher ambient noise levels because the earphone cushions attenuate (reduce) the noise level. However, in the soundfield condition, excessive ambient levels could effectively mask the signals. The stimuli used must also be considered when testing hearing in the soundfield. Pure-tone signals are not appropriate for soundfield testing because standing waves may develop in the test booth, thereby making calibration impossible and threshold results spurious.[20] Instead, warble tones and narrow-band noise are generally used. But since calibration standards do not currently exist, threshold norms must either be developed for all stimuli in each clinic or an average of normative data can be used for calibration.[21-29] Then the sound pressures in the soundfield must be checked periodically. Warble tones are recommended for clinical soundfield testing[20] and can produce thresholds as reliable as those obtained under earphones.[30]

## Pure-Tone Bone-Conduction Audiometry

Thresholds obtained with air-conducted signals assess the entire hearing system: conductive and sensorineural components. The individual contribution of each component cannot be separated by the air-conduction threshold. On the other hand, bone-conduction thresholds evaluate the sensorineural component; however, a bone-conduction threshold is not always a pure estimate of sensorineural integrity. Because bone-conducted signals stimulate the auditory system by vibrating the skull, the measured threshold can also reflect external and middle ear state. For example, a decrease in sensorineural sensitivity can be observed in patients with otosclerosis. These individuals often demonstrate an elevation in bone-conduction thresholds around 2,000 Hz. This elevation in the bone-conduction audiogram was first described by Carhart;[31] hence it is known as Carhart's notch.

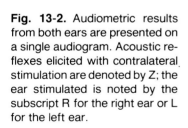

**Fig. 13-2.** Audiometric results from both ears are presented on a single audiogram. Acoustic reflexes elicited with contralateral stimulation are denoted by Z; the ear stimulated is noted by the subscript R for the right ear or L for the left ear.

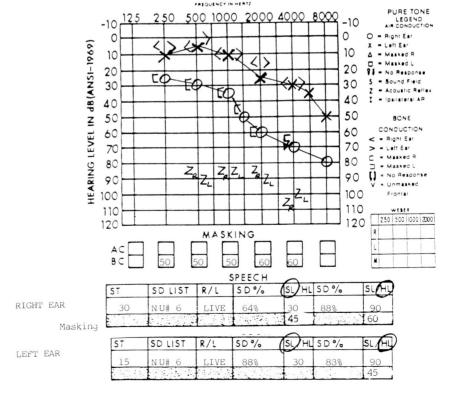

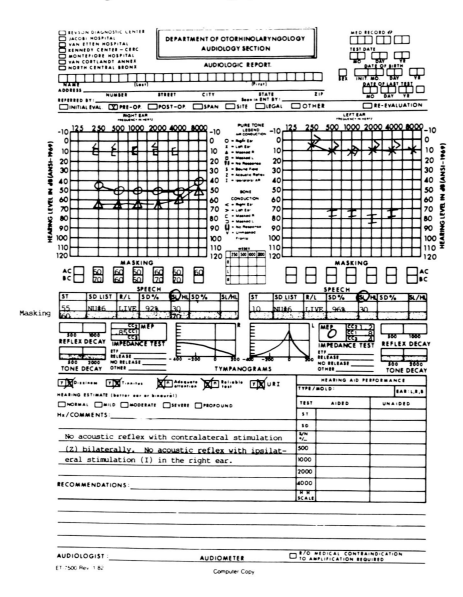

**Fig. 13-3.** Audiometric test results for individual ears are presented on separate audiograms. Acoustic reflexes elicited with ipsilateral stimulation are denoted by I.

Therefore, interpretation of pure-tone thresholds in conductive losses can be confounded by the fact that bone-conduction thresholds have an air-conduction component.[32,33] The osseotympanic and inertial bone-conduction routes (outer and middle ear pathways) can account for shifts in bone-conduction threshold with conductive hearing losses, as well as for bone-conduction thresholds that are slightly depressed relative to normal bone-conduction thresholds (suggesting a smaller air-bone gap).

The placement site of the bone-conduction oscil-lator (see Fig. 13-1C) can also influence the degree to which the external and/or middle ear systems affect bone-conduction thresholds. Bone-conduction thresholds are measured with a bone vibrator placed on the mastoid process or on the forehead (or frontal bone). Regardless of vibrator placement site, vibration of the skull results in stimulation of both inner ears. Thresholds obtained with a mastoid placement site are generally obtained at lower (better) intensity levels because less power is required to stimulate the cochlea from this site than

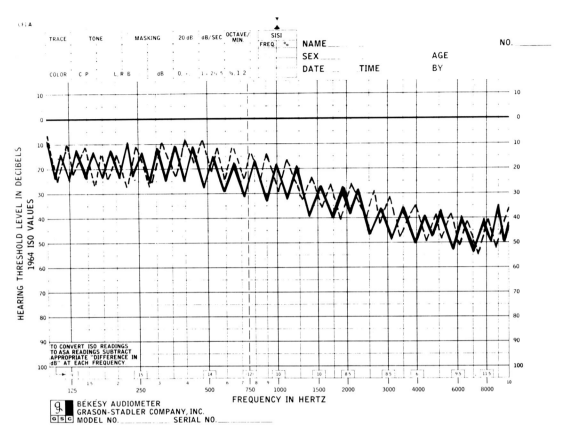

**Fig. 13-4.** The results from automatic or Bekesy audiometry. The solid lines represent thresholds obtained with a continuous tone signal; dashed lines are the results for intermittent or pulsed tones.

| RIGHT EAR | 250 | 500 | 750 | 1000 | 1500 | 2000 | 3000 | 4000 | 6000 | 8000 |
|---|---|---|---|---|---|---|---|---|---|---|
| Air Conduction | 30 | 25 | | 25 | | 20 | | 15 | | 5 |
| -- -- -- -- -- -- -- -- -- -- -- -- -- -- -- -- -- -- -- -- -- -- -- -- -- -- | | | | | | | | | | |
| Bone Conduction | 5 | 5 | | 0 | | 5 | | 0 | | |

| LEFT EAR | 250 | 500 | 750 | 1000 | 1500 | 2000 | 3000 | 4000 | 6000 | 8000 |
|---|---|---|---|---|---|---|---|---|---|---|
| Air Conduction | 20 | 15 | | 15 | | 10 | | 10 | | 0 |
| -- -- -- -- -- -- -- -- -- -- -- -- -- -- -- -- -- -- -- -- -- -- -- -- -- -- | | | | | | | | | | |
| Bone Conduction | 0 | 0 | | 5 | | 0 | | 0 | | |

**Fig. 13-5.** Audiometric findings are presented in tabular form.

with forehead placement. This is the case because there is greater contribution from the osseotympanic and inertial transmission routes of bone conduction for mastoid stimulation than is observed when the cochlea is stimulated from a forehead placement site. However, this intensive difference can be compensated for during oscillator calibration with an artificial headbone.[34,35] Thus, bone-conduction thresholds can be compared regardless of the oscillator placement site. Forehead placement is the more readily controlled bone-conduction oscillator placement area for the following reasons. First, the recommended contact force of 500 g can be easily maintained. The frontal surface is flatter than the mastoid process, hence the contact relationship of the bone-conduction vibrator to the stimulating surface is complementary. Second, the tissues of the forehead test area are more homogenous than those at the mastoid process.[36,37] Finally, testing at the frontal bone reduces the participation of the middle ear. Masking is technically necessary when testing with either bone placement whenever there is an air-bone gap, since both cochleas are stimulated due to 0 dB interaural attenuation. However, masking is generally not required unless the air-bone gap is greater than 10 dB.

Mastoid placement with the test ear unoccluded by an earphone is typically preferred in most clinical settings in North America. Reasons for this preference include control of the interaction between the air- and bone-conduction transducer headbands, less signal attenuation, and ease of masking. However, care must be taken to prevent oscillator contact with the pinna; if not, air-conducted signals may be generated. For routine bone-conduction testing, both ears remain unoccluded. When masking is indicated, however, the nontest ear must be occluded. When a normal-hearing or sensorineural-impaired ear is occluded, the intensity of bone-conducted stimuli increases due to changes in the resonance of the ear canal (osseotympanic bone conduction). This is known as the *occlusion effect.* The occlusion effect causes an increase in sensitivity for the low frequencies on the order of 20 to 30 dB at 250 Hz, 15 to 20 dB at 500 Hz, and 5 to 10 dB at 1,000 Hz.[38,39] This increase in the intensity of the bone-conducted signal results in an apparent but not real improvement in threshold, and must be taken into consideration.

The pure-tone psychophysical threshold procedure described previously for air-conduction thresholds is used to determine bone-conduction thresholds. However, the audiometer output levels and frequencies tested by bone-conduction are more limited than those of air-conduction testing due to power limitations of the bone vibrator. The audiometer's air- and bone-conduction output limits are typically noted on the audiometer.

## Extended High Frequency Audiometry

Conventional pure-tone audiometry evaluates hearing from 125 or 250 Hz through 8,000 Hz. Interest in extended high-frequency sensitivity and early detection of the effects of ototoxic agents (drugs and noise) on hearing led Rudmose[40] to develop a high-frequency audiometer. Due to transducer calibration problems, however, its clinical use was not widespread. Recently there has been renewed interest in this area of auditory sensitivity.[41-46] Berlin et al.[41] observed that some patients with severe or profound sensorineural hearing losses demonstrated unusually good speech production. Although hearing was impaired across the frequencies conventionally evaluated, these individuals had normal or good extended high-frequency hearing (8 to 16 kHz). Special experimental hearing aids are now available for patients with this type of hearing loss. With these devices, the information from the impaired listening areas is transposed to the frequency region that has normal or better sensitivity.

Both air-conduction and bone-conduction media have been used to assess extended high-frequency hearing. Most of the investigators mentioned above[41-43] used air-conducted signals transduced by circumaural earphones. However, calibration is still a problem because a standard acoustic coupler with an extended frequency response does not currently exist. As a result, each clinic must develop its own norms and incorporate special probe microphone calibrations. Other investigators[44,45] have developed special insert earphones to present extended high-frequency signals calibrated for each individual tested by a signal processing strategy. The usefulness of this system is currently being tested in clinical trials. Although extended high-frequency audiometry is still in its infancy and requires caution in both calibration and interpretation, identification and amplification of extended high-frequency islands of hearing are now possible.

### Interpretation of Pure-Tone Audiometry

Once air- and bone-conduction thresholds have been obtained, a picture of the hearing status begins to emerge. As discussed previously, air-conduction thresholds assess the entire system. Any change in sound transmission at the outer, middle, or inner ear will result in an elevation in air-conduction threshold. Bone-conduction thresholds bypass the conductive sound transmission routes and directly measure cochlear sensitivity. As a result, a pure-tone audiogram is diagnostically useful only when air- and bone-conduction thresholds are accurate. This includes the use of masking when appropriate. Although pure-tone thresholds alone do not permit a definitive diagnosis, the relationship between air- and bone-conduction thresholds

specifies the type of hearing loss: conductive, sensorineural, or mixed. A difference between the air- and bone-conduction thresholds (the air–bone gap) is attributed to a *conductive* problem (Fig. 13-3). An air–bone gap less than 10 dB is not usually considered to be significant, because of the variability of the threshold measurement (±5 dB). When sensitivity measured by air- and bone-conduction is reduced by the same degree, the type of hearing loss is called *sensorineural* (Fig. 13-2). Finally, a *mixed* hearing loss has both conductive and sensorineural components, that is, there is a conductive loss in addition to reduced sensorineural reserve (Fig. 13-6).

Hearing loss categories of mild, moderate, moderate-to-severe, severe, and profound are delineated in Table 13-2. Hearing loss is specified in terms of hearing levels according to current recommended standards.[46] However, since the medical-legal definition of hearing loss ascribes dB HL to earlier threshold references,[47] they are also included in Table 13-2 for comparison purposes only. The ANSI standards are the current reference for hearing loss categories and are used to charac-

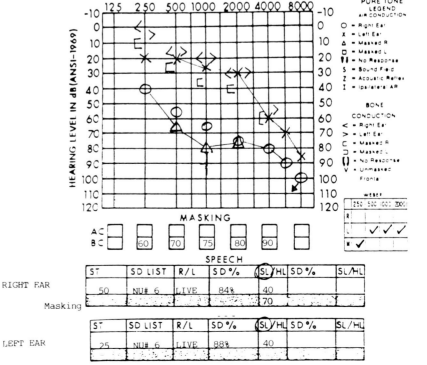

**Fig. 13-6.** Unilateral mixed hearing loss (right ear) and sensorineural hearing loss (left ear).

Table 13-2.  Hearing Loss Categories

| Degree of Hearing Loss | Hearing Level (dB HL) | |
| --- | --- | --- |
| | ASA, 1951 Reference | ANSI, 1969 Reference |
| Normal | −10−15 | −10−25 |
| Mild | 16−29 | 26−40 |
| Moderate | 30−44 | 41−55 |
| Moderate to severe | 45−59 | 56−70 |
| Severe | 60−79 | 71−90 |
| Profound | 80−limits of the audiometer | 91−limits of the audiometer |

| Frequency (Hz) | Reference Sound Pressure Level (0 dB HL) | |
| --- | --- | --- |
| | ASA, 1951 Reference | ANSI, 1969 Reference |
| 125 | 54.5 | 45.5 |
| 250 | 39.5 | 24.5 |
| 500 | 25 | 11 |
| 1,000 | 16.5 | 6.5 |
| 2,000 | 17 | 8.5 |
| 4,000 | 15 | 9 |
| 8,000 | 21 | 9.5 |

terize the hearing losses described in this chapter. Although normal hearing for adults is considered to be less than or equal to 25 dB HL, a more rigorous definition (−10 to 15 dB HL) is used to describe the region of normal hearing for children. A child whose hearing threshold is obtained at levels between 16 and 40 dB HL has a mild hearing loss. Generally, hearing thresholds for young children are obtained at less intense levels (better) than those of adults. This may be true due to limited exposure to various ototraumatic agents (e.g., noise). A more stringent cutoff for normal hearing is used for young children than for adults because reduced sensitivity is more likely to be detrimental to the developing speech and language of the child.[48] Therefore, medical and/or surgical treatment is appropriate even for conductive hearing loss of this magnitude. Audiologic intervention (i.e., amplification) is indicated for sensorineural hearing loss, even mild losses in children.

# MASKING

Masking is one of the most important aspects of clinical audiometry and one of the most frequently misunderstood. This section will explain the rationale for masking, define the terms associated with masking, describe the common masking stimuli and techniques, discuss the consequences of not masking when appropriate, and present some new approaches to the problem of signal crossover.

## Rationale and Case Discussion

The need for masking whenever there exists any possibility of cross-hearing cannot be overemphasized. The consequences of such an oversight can be deleterious, resulting in misdiagnosis and mistreatment. To highlight this point, the following cases are offered.

Figures 13-2, 13-3, 13-6, and 13-7 are representative audiograms discussed in light of the potential errors that could have occurred had masking not been used. The air-conduction thresholds in Figures 13-2 and 13-6 indicate that hearing is better in left ear than in the right ear. In both figures, attention to the unmasked bone-conduction thresholds for the right ear indicates a mild to severe conductive hearing loss in Figure 13-2 and a potentially moderate to severe mixed hearing loss in Figure 13-6. The unmasked information suggests that the patient in Figure 13-2 has a conductive problem and needs either medical or surgical intervention. The patient appears to have some

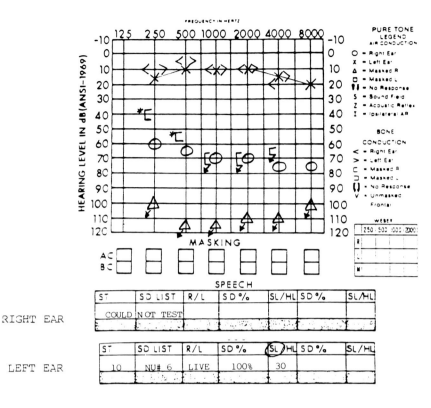

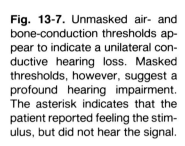

**Fig. 13-7.** Unmasked air- and bone-conduction thresholds appear to indicate a unilateral conductive hearing loss. Masked thresholds, however, suggest a profound hearing impairment. The asterisk indicates that the patient reported feeling the stimulus, but did not hear the signal.

level of conductive problem, but the true sensorineural reserve is unknown. However, when bone-conduction thresholds are reassessed with appropriate masking, the apparent right ear air-bone gap in Figure 13-2 closes and instead the true hearing status (mild-to-severe sloping sensorineural hearing loss) is identified. In Figure 13-6, masking reveals that the type, degree, and extent of hearing loss were correct, but the sensorineural reserve was overestimated.

The air-conduction thresholds for the left ear in Figures 13-3 and 13-7 indicate hearing to be within normal limits. However, hearing impairment is present in the right ears of both figures. In Figure 13-3, unmasked air- and bone-conduction thresholds suggest a mild conductive hearing loss. When masking is applied, however, the degree of hearing loss is now revealed to be moderate. Without masking, the degree of impairment was underestimated. Figure 13-7 presents the errors that can occur, both in terms of type and degree of hearing loss, when masking is not used. The unmasked air-

and bone-conduction from the right air would indicate the presence of a moderate conductive hearing impairment. However, another picture of the hearing status emerges when these thresholds are assessed with contralateral masking. The degree of impairment is profound and the type of hearing loss is sensorineural or mixed. Since bone-conduction testing has intensity output limits lower than those of air-conduction testing, only with impedance measures can we determine if a conductive pathologic condition also exists. In the case of this patient, impedance was consistent with conductive pathologic change: markedly reduced middle ear compliance, extreme negative pressure, and absent acoustic reflexes (elicited with contralateral stimulation). This would suggest a mixed hearing loss.

In conclusion, the consequences of not masking or improper masking that result from inattention to signal crossover and interaural attenuation are serious. These errors can obscure diagnosis and potentially culminate in unnecessary or inappropriate intervention, treatment, or surgery.

## Definitions

The terminology applied to masking often appears confusing and obscure. To avoid misunderstanding and to ease subsequent discussion, the common terms of masking are defined below.

Often during audiologic evaluation acoustic signals presented to the test ear are sufficiently intense that they can be perceived in the nontested ear. When the signal crosses over to and is perceived by the nontest ear, the results for the test ear are spurious. *Interaural attenuation* describes the intensity reduction between the test and nontest ear. For air-conduction assessment, interaural attenuation (IA) ranges from 45 dB at 250 Hz to 65 dB at 4,000 Hz (Table 13-3). However, individual differences exist; therefore, most clinicians consider 40 dB to be the interaural attenuation for air-conduction testing. Studebaker[49] has suggested the following "rule of thumb" to determine when masking is necessary during air-conduction evaluation: masking is needed when the air-conduction threshold for a given frequency is 40 dB greater (poorer) than the contralateral bone-conduction threshold for the same frequency. As discussed in the section on pure-tone bone-conduction testing, there is always a risk of crossover since the potential exists that both cochleas are stimulated. As a result, interaural attenuation for bone-conduction testing is considered to be 0 dB.

Should the test situation suggest that signal crossover is occurring, the nontest ear must be "occupied" or masked while the test ear is under evaluation. Masking is the elevation of signal threshold (e.g., test tone) by the presence of a second signal (masker). In the clinical situation, the audiologist presents a masking noise to the nontest ear. The presence of the noise in the nontest ear elevates its threshold for the signal presented to the test ear and eliminates nontest ear participation.

From this presentation, the question of masking appears rather straightforward. However, this area is difficult. Two dangers exist in masking: overmasking and central masking. *Overmasking* occurs when the masking signal presented to the nontest ear becomes intense enough to cross to the test ear. This will cause an elevation of the test-ear thresholds. *Central masking* is an elevation of the test-ear thresholds that results from contralateral masking, even though the masking levels are insufficient for crossover to the test ear. The phenomenon is termed central masking because the effect is believed to occur at some point along the central auditory pathways. This effect usually results in no greater than a 5 to 10 dB elevation in threshold;[36,50] but some investigators have reported threshold shifts up to 15 dB.[51] As a result, bone-conduction thresholds measured without masking in the contralateral ear may be 5 to 10 dB better than those with contralateral masking.[51,52]

## Masking Noise and Techniques

### Maskers

Selection of the appropriate masker is stimulus-dependent. Narrow-band noise is the masker of choice for masking pure tones. However, speech signals are best masked by broadband noises,[53] such as speech noise, white noise, or pink noise.

Narrowband noise is produced by selectively filtering broadband (white) noise to produce smaller bands of noise with the test frequency at the center and a bandwidth of one critical band. For example, the critical bandwidth for 1,000 Hz is approximately 64 Hz;[54] therefore, only the frequency re-

**Table 13-3. Interaural Attenuation (dB) for Two Types of Earphones: Standard Clinical Earphone (supra-aural) and Insert Phone**

| Earphone | 250 Hz | 500 Hz | 1,000 Hz | 2,000 Hz | 4,000 Hz |
|---|---|---|---|---|---|
| Supra-aural | 45–50 | 50–59 | 55–61 | 59–60 | 64–65 |
| Insert | 90 | 99 | 83 | 71 | 80 |

The given attenuation values are average data for air-conduction stimulation for the supra-aural phones (58) and one type of insert earphone (71). The results from this insert phone serve only as an example of the increased interaural attenuation that can be realized when earphone size is reduced. These data are not intended to represent all insert earphones.

gion 968 Hz to 1,032 Hz is effective for masking a 1,000 Hz tone. The narrowband noises generated by most audiometers are somewhat wider than the critical band to allow for individual differences in critical band width. Therefore, calibration of the masking noise is a required part of audiometer calibration.

Most audiometers today are calibrated in effective masking (EM) level units and referenced to dB HL. Effective masking is the amount of masking needed to make a tone of a given level inaudible or to shift its threshold by 5 dB. If the audiometer does not incorporate effective masking levels, these levels can be determined by deriving the decibel correction to 0 dB HL for 0 dB EM for 10 normal-hearing subjects. For example, if 45 dB HL is needed to mask a 30 dB, 1,000 Hz tone, 0 dB of EM is accomplished with a +15 dB correction to the dial setting. It is also possible to determine the effective masking in each narrow band of noise by measuring the overall sound pressure level (SPL) and the width of the band and calculating the level per cycle for each frequency in the band.

## Masking Techniques

There are, in general, two types of clinical masking procedures: the plateau (or Hood) method[55,56] and the minimum masking level method.[49,51,57,58] With either procedure, a masking noise presented to the nontest ear may produce a 5 dB threshold shift in the test ear due to central masking. Larger shifts in the test ear threshold indicate that the original unmasked threshold did not reflect the real test ear threshold, but rather was the nontest ear response to test signal crossover. If the masking noise presented to the nontest ear is too intense, it may cross to the test ear and elevate its threshold (overmasking). The level at which overmasking occurs describes a maximum masking level beyond which accurate masking is no longer possible.

The plateau (or Hood) method of masking introduces noise to the nontest ear at 5 dB above the pure-tone threshold for the frequency of the tone presented to the test ear. The noise is then raised in 5 dB steps until the tone in the test ear is no longer heard. At that point, the test ear threshold is determined for each 5 dB masker increment until the

minimum masking level is reached and a masked threshold is established that does not shift with further increments in masker intensity. This is the region of effective masking limited by the maximum masking level; above this level overmasking will occur.

The minimum masking level method is a computational procedure that determines the minimum and maximum effective masking levels from the air- and bone-conduction thresholds. The formula approach to masking is cumbersome because minimum and maximum levels must be determined for each individual patient at each frequency tested. In addition, the formulae assume that the maskers are calibrated in EM.

### Masking Dilemma

A masking dilemma exists when the true air-bone gap exceeds the assumed interaural attenuation: the signal presented to the test ear is of sufficient intensity that it may also be audible to the nontest ear. When a hearing loss also exists in the nontest ear, the masker must be presented to the nontest ear at high levels. Hence, the possibility exists that both cochleas may be stimulated by both the signal and the masker. Figure 13-8 is a common example of a masking dilemma. Because of the degree of conductive loss in the test ear, a high signal level is necessary. However, the conductive hearing loss in the nontest ear reduces the audibility of the masker. It is necessary to increase the masker to an audible level. Unfortunately, the masking level will exceed interaural attenuation, causing the masker to cross to the test ear and increase the test ear threshold. In Figure 13-8, the unmasked air-conduction thresholds are 55 to 65 dB HL bilaterally and the unmasked bone-conduction thresholds are 5 dB HL bilaterally. Interaural attenuation for testing via air conduction suggests that masking is indicated; however, the appropriate masking levels presented to the nontest ear could cross to the test ear and erroneously elevate the threshold.

Some viable methods can be used in an attempt to resolve a masking dilemma. The best solution is to increase interaural attenuation. One means of increasing interaural attenuation lies with the transducer used to present the signals. The smaller the earphone cushion size, the greater the inter-

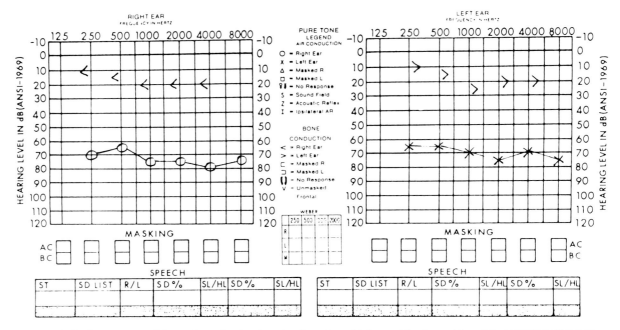

**Fig. 13-8.** An apparent bilateral conductive hearing loss for which masking is problematic: masking dilemma.

aural attenuation. This is true because less of the head area is exposed to the sound. Insert earphones contact less of the head area than the standard audiometric earphone cushions (supra-aural).[37,51,60] Until recently, insert earphones have not had wide clinical use due to calibration problems. Currently, an insert earphone (ER-3A Tubephone, see Fig. 13-9) has been developed with a frequency response similar to that of standard audiometric earphones. More importantly, it can be calibrated in accordance with standards using a standard 2 cc coupler[6] or a standard occluded-ear simulator.[60,61] This now makes the use of insert earphones practical. Proper deep insertion of the insert earphone improves interaural attenuation (Fig. 13-9). Table 13-3 also shows the amount of increase in interaural attenuation (with proper insertion) of these insert earphones.[63]

An audiometric Weber test may also aid in resolving a masking dilemma. The test is conducted by placing the bone-conduction vibrator on the patient's forehead and presenting pure tones at the frequencies where there is a masking dilemma. The signal may lateralize to the poorer-hearing ear in the case of conductive losses, to the better-hearing ear for sensorineural losses, or midline when hearing is symmetrical. Where a masking dilemma exists, the presence of bilateral primarily conductive or primarily sensorineural unilateral hearing loss may be suggested (see Fig. 13-6 and 13-10) by the audiometric Weber results. This may be useful in confirming or refuting the masked bone conduction thresholds.

The earplug procedure[63,64] is another means of assessing masking adequacy when large air-bone gaps are present. With this procedure, signal crossover for unmasked air-conduction thresholds is confirmed or ruled out. The rationale is as follows. Insertion of an earplug into the test ear is not expected to increase test ear thresholds if they were the result of the signal crossing the skull and being perceived in the nontest ear. On the other hand, if interaural attenuation or masking levels were adequate, the unmasked test ear thresholds should become elevated (minimum significant shift is $+5$ dB for a five-frequency criterion or $+15$ dB for a single-frequency criterion) when retested with the earplug inserted. This procedure can determine if

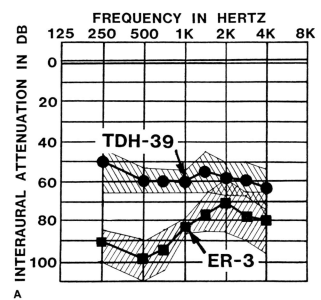

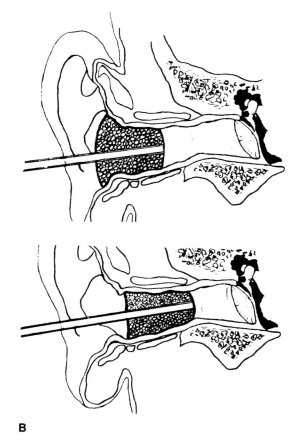

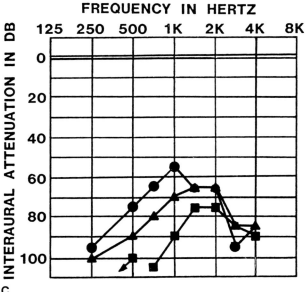

**A**

**Fig. 13-9. (A)** The range of interaural attenuation obtained from six subjects with standard supraaural audiometric earphones (TDH-39 in MX 41/AR cushions) and with an insert earphone (ER-3A Tubephone). **(B)** Shallow (top) and proper (bottom) insertion of the insert earphone. **(C)** Interaural attenuation obtained with different insert earphone insertion depths in the ear canal: ●, deep insertion in both ears; ▲, shallow insertion in dead ear only; ■, shallow insertion in both ears. (Killion MC, Wilber LA, Gudmundsen GI: Insert earphones for more interaural attenuation. Hearing Instrum 36:34, 1985.)

masking by air conduction is necessary, it can help rule out test signal cross-over in many cases of masking dilemma (Fig. 13-11, top), and it can aid in determining permissible masking levels (Fig. 13-11, bottom).

## SPEECH AUDIOMETRY

An audiologic evaluation relies on more than pure-tone audiometry for differential diagnosis. Speech audiometry (speech reception threshold and speech discrimination) provides important in-

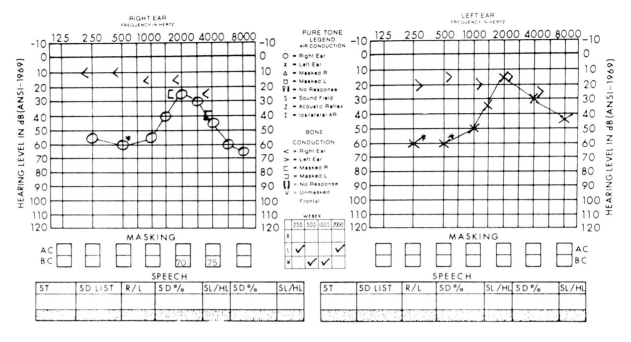

**Fig. 13-10.** Another masking dilemma is presented with the results of an audiometric Weber test. The audiogram appears to indicate bilateral mild-moderate low-frequency conductive hearing loss. However, appropriate masking cannot easily be accomplished in this situation.

* MASKING DILEMMA

formation that is necessary to formulate a complete picture of an individual s hearing loss.

### Speech Reception Threshold

The speech reception threshold (SRT) more appropriately called the speech recognition threshold [65,92] or spondee threshold (ST)[66] is a valuable part of a diagnostic audiologic evaluation primarily because it is a good indicator of pure-tone threshold accuracy. There is generally good correspondence between speech and pure-tone thresholds both for normal persons[67] and those with hearing loss.[68] Spondees (two-syllable, equal-emphasis words) are used to assess the SRT. In the clinical protocol, speech reception threshold is often determined prior to assessing pure-tone air-conduction thresholds because the task of repeating spondees is easy for most patients. In addition, SRT has apparent face validity since communication de-

pends upon listening to speech rather than pure tones.

Spondees, rather than other words or sentences, were selected to measure speech threshold since they provide homogenous audibility.[69] An SRT is obtained using a list of 36 familiar spondees (CID W-1, W-2;[70] for example: "baseball," "whitewash," "sidewalk," and "bus stop"). A number of methods have evolved from clinical practice and research to evaluate speech reception thresholds. They are similar to the manual pure-tone threshold procedure. A concise summary of the differences in the various procedures can be found in the work by Olsen and Matkin.[71] Currently no standard SRT procedure exists, but Chaiklin and Ventry's[72] protocol is commonly used and recommended. As with pure-tone threshold assessment, a modified method of limits is used to determine the SRT. Assessment begins at a level above suspected threshold to familiarize the listener with the words and

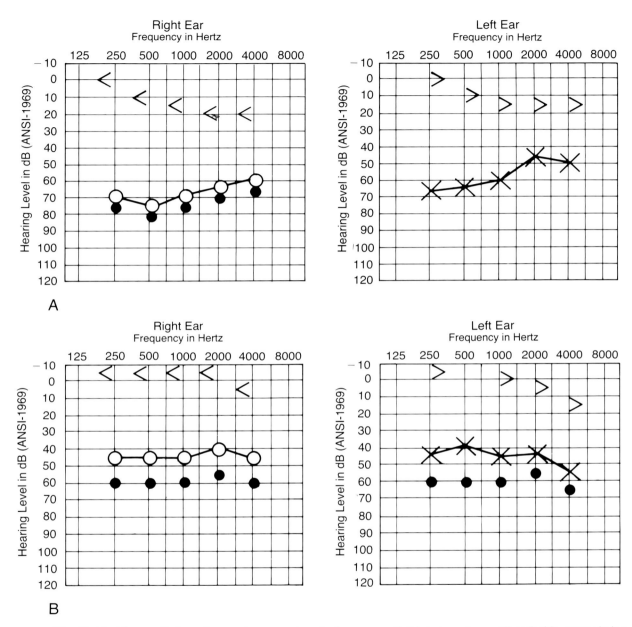

**Fig. 13-11.** The results from the earplug procedure for two cases. Solid circles, plugged thresholds; open circles and crosses, air-conduction thresholds for right and left ear, respectively; carets, unmasked bone-conduction thresholds. (Adapted from Thelin JW, Webber PT: Clinical use of the earplug procedure. Presented to the American Speech-Language-Hearing Assn, 1984.)

the task. The level is then decreased in 5 dB steps, presenting one to three words at each level decrement until a word is missed. Then the level is raised 10 dB and the threshold assessment begins. The level is lowered in 5 dB steps and raised in 10 dB increments, presenting three to six spondees at each decrement, until a level is reached where 50 percent of the spondees are correctly repeated. This is the speech reception threshold.

Spondee words can be presented to the listener as taped, phonographically recorded, or as live-voice material. Standardized taped materials are recommended for most situations, since variation due to speaker differences is reduced.[73] However, the common practice of using monitored live-voice presentation of the test materials[74] is acceptable[66,75–77] when indicated by the clinical situation, for example, in testing very young children, difficult-to-test children or adults, and some elderly patients.

The value of the SRT lies in its correspondence with pure-tone thresholds in the speech frequencies. For flat and gradually sloping losses, the agreement is best when a three-frequency pure-tone average (PTA) of the thresholds obtained at 500, 1,000, and 2,000 Hz is compared to the SRT.[67,75] With steeply sloping losses, agreement is better when the two best pure-tone thresholds are averaged and compared to the SRT.[78] However, a more recent recommendation for most audiometric configurations including very steep high-frequency losses is the average of the thresholds at 500 and 1,000 Hz minus 2 dB.[79] For example, in Figure 13-2 the three-frequency PTA for the left ear is 13 dB and the SRT is 15 dB; there is, therefore, good agreement. But when the three-frequency PTA for the right ear (42 dB) is compared to the SRT, the agreement is poor. However, the best two-frequency PTA (32 dB) and the SRT (30 dB) are in more favorable agreement.

The correspondence of the SRT and PTA is within acceptable limits if the SRT and PTA are ±6 dB of one another.[71] Results outside this region are considered pathognomonic for pseudohypacusis. They suggest that the pure-tone results are suspect and that additional testing is needed. However, a discrepancy of 10 dB or greater can be obtained from very young children or difficult-to-test adults (e.g., psychiatric or mentally retarded pa-

tients). This discrepancy is thought to result from the patient responding to the loudness of speech and does not reflect threshold for speech.[80]

It is sometimes difficult to obtain an SRT from patients with limited or unintelligible speech (e.g., young children), those with mental retardation, profoundly hearing-impaired individuals, or deaf patients. Simple modification of test procedure may be sufficient. For example, the audiologist can have the patient point to the pictures that illustrate the spoken spondee words rather than repeating the spondee heard. However, when it is impossible to determine an SRT by any means, most difficult-to-test patients will respond to the presence (or absence) of speech. This is a detection or awareness response and the measurement is termed a speech detection threshold (SDT) or a speech awareness threshold (SAT). Spondees, or simple, more familiar words, such as "go" or "mama," are used to measure SDT or SAT. In relation to the SRT, the SDT is typically elicited at a level 8 to 9 dB better (less intense) than the SRT[81–83] or PTA. Often, better agreement is found between the SDT and the 250 Hz pure-tone threshold. Either the SRT or the SDT may be used to indicate agreement with pure-tone thresholds.

The SRT or SDT described previously is most often determined with air-conducted signals. However, it is possible, and at times indicated, to determine bone-conducted speech thresholds. Bone-conducted speech can assist in confirming the presence of an air–bone gap, as well as aid in estimating the size of the air–bone gap. This provides a useful information for the medical management of the difficult-to-test patient. Bone-conducted speech thresholds correlate with either 500 to 1,000 Hz for an SRT or 250 Hz for an SDT.

## Speech Discrimination Testing

One of the primary complaints of hearing-impaired individuals, especially those with sensorineural hearing loss, is difficulty understanding speech. Although threshold information is essential for describing auditory sensitivity and quantifying hearing loss, typically we do not listen to pure tones or communicate at threshold levels. Therefore, it is also necessary to determine an individual's ability to discriminate speech signals at suprathreshold levels. Speech discrimination measures assist the audiologist in differential assessment of the site of auditory lesion (Table 13-4), serve to indicate the need for speech-related rehabilitation (lipreading, auditory training), and aid in the determination of candidacy for a hearing aid or other assistive listening aids. For the otolaryngologist, this information can yield prognostic data regarding the success of otologic surgery, as in the case of otosclerosis with concomitant cochlear involvement.

Clinical speech discrimination results provide information for quantitative evaluation of the difficulty a patient experiences with speech signals. The speech discrimination score (SDS), also referred to as a suprathreshold word recognition score (WRS),[65,92] is the percentage of words correctly identified from specified word lists (usually monosyllables). The words are presented (typically without background noise) at a suprathreshold

level selected to provide maximum intelligibility in quiet. In general, individuals with normal hearing or conductive hearing loss demonstrate excellent (90 to 100 percent) speech discrimination. However, persons with sensorineural or mixed hearing loss may exhibit speech discrimination scores that fall anywhere within the range of 0 to 100 percent, though there is a positive correlation between increasing hearing loss and decreasing word discrimination scores.[85–90]

The measurement of speech discrimination ability is influenced by many test factors. The frequency-intensity composition of the speech signal, the type and format of test material, the presentation level, the method of test administration, and the response required from the listener can affect speech discrimination test results.[91,92] The sounds of speech (consonants and vowels) vary in the frequency and intensity composition (Fig. 13-12). The effects of pure-tone threshold and audiometric configuration on speech performance[93,94] are

**Table 13-4. Hearing Loss Types as a Function of Audiologic Findings**

| Audiologic Test | Conductive Hearing Loss | Sensorineural Hearing Loss | | Mixed Hearing Loss |
|---|---|---|---|---|
| | | Cochlear | Retrocochlear | |
| Pure-tone air-conduction thresholds | Reduced sensitivity | Reduced air-conduction sensitivity | Reduced air-conduction sensitivity. With unilateral loss marked asymmetry between ears | Sensitivity reduced more by air- than bone-conduction |
| Pure-tone bone-conduction thresholds | Normal sensitivity | Bone-conduction thresholds reduced to the same extent as air-conduction thresholds | Bone-conduction thresholds reduced to the same extent as air-condition thresholds. | Reduced sensitivity |
| Speech reception threshold | Agrees with air-conduction thresholds | Agrees with air-conduction thresholds | Agrees with air-conduction thresholds | Agrees with air-conduction thresholds |
| Speech discrimination score | 90–100% | 0–100%: contingent on degree and slope of loss | 0–100%: contingent on degree and slope of loss. With unilateral retrocochlear loss, marked asymmetry between ears | 0–100%: contingent on degree and slope of the sensorineural component. |
| Impedance tympanometry | Abnormal middle-ear pressure and compliance | Normal middle-ear pressure and compliance | Normal middle-ear pressure and compliance | Abnormal middle-ear pressure and compliance |
| Acoustic reflex | Typically absent or elicited at elevated sensation levels | Elicted at reduced sensation levels | Elicted at elevated sensation levels and exhibits rapid decay, or absent | Absent |

Adapted from Ruben KJ, Kniger B: Hearing loss in the elderly. p 123. In Katzman R. Terr RD (eds): The Neurology of Aging. FA Davis, Philadelphia, 1982.

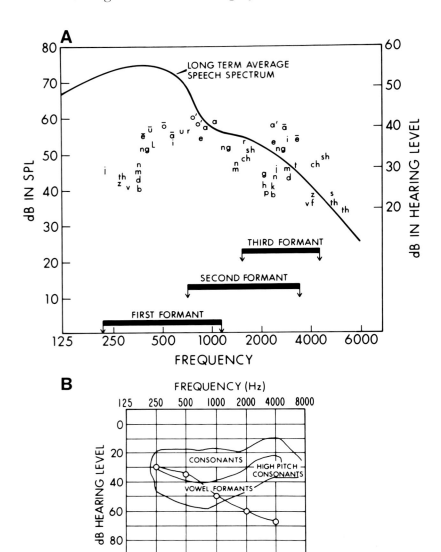

Fig. 13-12. The frequency and intensity characteristics of speech sounds are shown. **(A)** Long-term speech spectrum and the spectrum energy of speech sounds are displayed in terms of hearing level (dB HL) and sound pressure level (dB SPL). **(B)** Distribution of speech sound energy relative to audiometric levels.

clearly illustrated when the frequency and intensity characteristics are superimposed on the audiogram.

Speech discrimination performance can also be influenced by the test material. Speech materials with many contextual cues (sentences and spondee words) are easier to discriminate and, therefore, result in better discrimination scores than materials with limited (monosyllables) or no (nonsense syllables) contextual cues. The most commonly used speech discrimination materials in North America are the Central Institute for the Deaf (CID) W-22[70] and the Northwestern University (NU-6)[95] monosyllabic word lists. The words in both lists were carefully chosen to be familiar English monosyllables of similar phonetic content (or phonetic balance, PB). The words are presented in an open response set (the patient repeats or writes the word heard), rather than in a closed response set (the patient chooses from among a known set of similar discrimination words). The speech materials used for speech audiometry differ according to the nationality or language spoken.[96] There are comparable word lists for Britain (MRC lists),[96-98] Australia, Scandinavia, European and non-European languages, and Chinese.[96]

An important aspect of any test is the test-to-test reliability. In speech discrimination assessment, this is of clinical interest because a real change in speech discrimination ability signals a change in auditory integrity. For example, a difference in SDS of greater than 6 percent on the CID W-22 lists is significant for the normal-hearing ear. However, a clinically significant percentage difference depends upon various factors: the number of words (full or half list), the performance of the individual,[99,100] the difficulty of the words, and especially the degree of hearing impairment. The binomial distribution can be used to determine the reliability of a speech discrimination score since it assesses the mean and standard deviation of performance.[65,92,100] The expected standard deviations are greatest for the steepest part of the performance-intensity function (40 to 60 percent) and smallest for the extremes (90 to 100 percent and 0 to 10 percent). Therefore, as the number of words used increases/decreases, the standard deviation decreases/increases by the square root of 2.[71,100] For example, for a second SDS to be considered significantly different (within 95 percent confidence limits) from an initial SDS of 80 percent for a 50-word list, the second SDS must differ from the first by more than 12 percent. However, if the first SDS was 50 percent, the second SDS must differ from the first by more than 20 percent. If half-lists were used, the second score must differ from the first (50 percent) by 28 percent. In all examples, the expected variation in speech discrimination test scores for the normal ear were described. The variability can be substantially larger for an ear with sensorineural hearing loss.

The use of half word lists for speech discrimination testing must be considered carefully. Half-lists for speech discrimination assessment have been developed by a number of investigators.[101-106] Although these researchers have shown good agreement between half-list and whole-list SDS, the variability of speech discrimination scores increases as the word list is shortened. The evaluation time

saved by presenting 25 instead of 50 words is at the expense of the reduced confidence in SDS reliability, especially for scores between 30 and 70 percent. The use of shortened word lists is only suggested for persons with speech discrimination scores better than 90 percent or poorer than 10 percent.[71,99,100]

Another variable of the test situation that can affect speech discrimination performance is the intensity level at which the words are presented. As the intensity is increased above the speech reception threshold, speech discrimination performance typically improves. However, this is not always the case for individuals with sensorineural hearing loss. Instead, speech discrimination performance initially improves with increasing intensity level, then performance begins to deteriorate with additional increments in presentation level. Graphic representation of speech discrimination performance as a function of intensity is called a performance-intensity function or an articulation-gain function. This describes the speech audiogram or range of speech discrimination performance associated with particular cochlear and neural lesions.[96-98,107] Speech discrimination testing is typically conducted at a sensation level (the level above a given threshold, in this case the speech reception threshold) of 30 to 40 dB. This level is considered to be the level at which speech intelligibility is maximal. It is often referred to as $PB_{max}$, the level at which maximal speech performance is obtained for phonetically balanced words.[108] The term $PB_{max}$, however, may be a misnomer since the level at which maximal speech discrimination performance is observed can vary as a function of the individual and the auditory system status. This is especially typical of patients with Meniére's disease.[97]

There has been considerable discussion in the literature of the need to use a carrier phrase before the test word, the presentation with monitored live-voice versus recorded speech signals, and the evaluation of speech discrimination ability in the presence of competing noise. These factors are important in terms of potential to increase variability in SDS.[109,110]

The debate between tape-recorded or monitored live-voice presentation of test words has been a long one. Those advocating the use of recorded materials argue that different speakers introduce variability into the test situation. However, the available recorded materials used different speakers for the recordings. In addition, Carhart[111] has observed that the difference between two live-voice speakers is no greater than that found between two recordings. The situation often dictates which presentation medium should be used. For example, when testing very young children or some elderly patients, recorded materials limit the flexibility and control the audiologist needs with these individuals. The ASHA[66] advised that while both presentation methods were acceptable, recorded presentation was preferred when the clinical situation permitted. Clearly, there is no single "correct" presentation medium. The clinical situation must be evaluated on a patient-by-patient basis and the appropriate protocol selected.

Speech discrimination test stimuli are usually presented without a background noise in the test ear. Assessment of speech discrimination ability with a noise or speech babble background is a more difficult test than evaluation in quiet, but everyday communication is more often conducted in a controlled environment with some competing signal. Therefore, speech discrimination in noise can afford the audiologist additional information regarding the communication difficulties of an individual once a hearing loss has been documented.[112]

Speech discrimination tests have been modified or developed for individuals with special needs. The Phonetically Balanced-Keaster (PBK) test[113] is an open-response test designed for use with kindergarten children. For the child or adult with limited or unintelligible speech, the word identification by picture identification (WIPI) test[114,115] can be used to assess speech discrimination performance. The WIPI is a closed set of stimuli that consists of 25 plates with six pictures of similar-sounding words per plate (e.g., "rat," "cat," "bat," "hat," "mat," "pat"). The listener is asked to point to the word heard. Other speech discrimination tests include monosyllabic word tests, such as word lists comprised of high-frequency consonants,[116,117] the Modified Rhyme Test (MRT),[118,119] the California Consonant Test,[120] and the Nonsense Syllable Test (NST);[121,122] and, sentence tests, for example, the Synthetic Sentence Index (SSI)[123] and the Speech Perception in Noise (SPIN)

test.[124] The monosyllabic word tests are designed to address specific areas of speech discrimination ability, whereas the sentence discrimination tests attempt to replicate the nature of speech without its contextual cues. For additional discussion of these and other speech discrimination tests, Olsen and Matkin's chapter in Rintelmann's text[125] is recommended.

Naturally, since speech discrimination materials are presented at suprathreshold levels there is increased risk of signal crossover and overmasking compared with threshold tests. The interaural attenuation for speech is 40 dB; therefore, masking is needed when the speech signal in the test ear minus the interaural attenuation exceeds the best bone conduction threshold in the nontest ear. An adequate effective masking level of a broadband or speech noise is used.

## IMPEDANCE MEASUREMENTS

Clinical impedance measurements are an integral part of any basic audiologic evaluation. It is beyond the scope and intention of this chapter to present an indepth discussion of this topic. Chapter 14 offers a comprehensive discourse on impedance measures. However, since impedance measures are important to any basic audiologic evaluation, we will introduce impedance testing. Discussion will focus on how impedance results augment and clarify basic audiologic data.

Impedance audiometry includes assessment of middle ear pressure (tympanometry), static "compliance," and acoustic reflex thresholds. Tympanometry assesses middle ear status by measuring the sound reflected from the tympanic membrane as a function of induced change in ear canal air pressure ($+200$ to $-400$ mmH$_2$O pressure). This is plotted on a tympanogram that displays "compliance" as a function of air pressure. Although "compliance" is technically inappropriate terminology, it is commonly used to describe measurements obtained with an impedance bridge. From the tympanogram, middle pressure and ear canal volume can be found. These indices aid in the differential diagnosis of conductive pathologic change. The region of normal middle ear pressure for the adult ear[126] is between $-50$ and $+50$ mmH$_2$O. For children, the region of normal middle ear pressure extends to $-100$ mmH$_2$O.[e.g., 126–128]

Static compliance is determined in the following manner. An initial volume measurement is taken with the tympanic membrane in a position of poor compliance (i.e., extreme positive, $+200$ mmH$_2$O, or negative, $-400$ mmH$_2$O, pressure); this is CC$_1$. The normal values for CC$_1$ are 1.0 to 1.5 cc for an adult with an intact eardrum and 0.6 to 0.8 cc for a child with an intact drum.[129] A second measure is then taken with the tympanic membrane at a point of maximum compliance, CC$_2$. Static compliance is determined by this formula: CC$_2$ − CC$_1$. The normal region for adult static compliance values is 0.28 to 1.7 cc.[130] In concert with acoustic reflex findings, these metrics provide information regarding not only middle ear integrity but also peripheral auditory system integrity.

Acoustic reflex findings increase the amount of available diagnostic information. The acoustic reflex response is a bilateral response (stimulation to one ear causes a reflex reaction in both ears) of the stapedius muscle tendon to loud acoustic stimulation; its contraction stiffens the ossicular chain and eardrum. The response can be obtained and measured ipsilateral to the acoustic stimulation or contralateral to stimulation. In the normal ear, acoustic reflexes are found at 70 to 95 dB sensation level (SL) above air-conduction thresholds.[131] Acoustic reflex thresholds measured with ipsilateral stimulation are obtained at intensity levels 3 to 6 dB less intense than contralateral acoustic reflex thresholds.[132] With pathologic conditions of the cochlea, acoustic reflex thresholds are often obtained at less intense sensation levels ($<60$ dB SL). The reflex thresholds are often elevated with retrocochlear site of lesion and may demonstrate abnormal decay of the reflex. The acoustic reflex may also be absent with retrocochlear pathologic. For conductive hearing loss, the reflexes may be elevated, but more often are absent.

Reliance on pure-tone metrics alone (even with adequate masking) for differential diagnosis of conductive hearing loss is not recommended. Pure-tone audiometry provides only weak clues to the possible cause of a conductive hearing loss. Audiometric configurations associated with a conductive loss may result from stiffness disorders that present as reduced sensitivity more in the low than the high frequencies (e.g., early otosclerosis, middle-ear fluid, eardrum perforation) or mass disorders (e.g., later stages of otosclerosis and otitis media) that present as reduced sensitivity slightly more in the high frequencies than in the low frequencies. Therefore, impedance measures are necessary to complete the differential diagnosis of a conductive pathology.

## SOME EXAMPLES

Table 13-4 summarizes the expected audiologic results as a function of the type of hearing loss. This table describes the effects of conductive, sensorineural (cochlear or neural), and mixed hearing loss on each of the basic audiologic tests previously discussed.

*Conductive* losses are most often associated with an essentially flat or low-frequency elevation in air-conduction thresholds. In general, air-conduction thresholds are elevated while bone-conduction thresholds are found to be within normal limits. Occasionally (Fig. 13-13), bone-conduction thresholds will be elevated due to changes in the ear canal and/or middle ear. Only in the classic case of otosclerosis is the shift in bone-conduction thresholds maximal around 2 kHz (Carhart's notch). Air-conduction sensitivity improves with reconstructive surgery; at times, the improvement in air-conduction thresholds is to levels better than the *presurgical* bone-conduction thresholds (overclosure). However, the term *overclosure* is incorrect since the air-conduction thresholds in reality are not better than the true bone-conduction thresholds (the cochlear reserve). Rather, spongiosis of the oval window area changes the resonance characteristics of the tympanum. This results in elevation of the bone-conduction thresholds. *Postsurgical* bone-conduction thresholds reflect

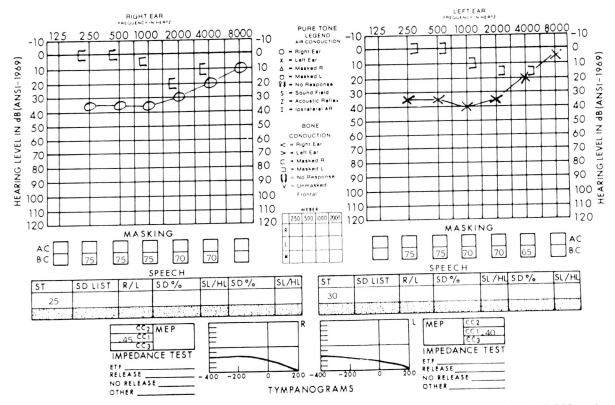

**Fig. 13-13.** Mild bilateral conductive hearing loss with elevated bone-conduction thresholds at 1,000, 2,000, and 4,000 Hz.

true cochlear reserve. This is also generally true of other middle-ear conditions; regardless of the cause, bone-conduction thresholds return to normal upon resolution of the middle ear problem (medical or surgical type of resolution).

Speech reception thresholds in the individual with conductive hearing loss are consistent with pure-tone thresholds and speech discrimination scores are excellent (90 to 100 percent). This is true because only the transmission or conduction of the signal of the cochlea is impaired; sensory and neural integrity have not been compromised. Impedance audiometry often lends important information that aids in clarifying the potential cause. For example, examine Figure 13-13. The results of impedance audiometry (reduced compliance and extreme negative pressure, a flat tympanogram) suggest otitis media; however, if the findings demonstrated shallow tympanograms with pressure

and compliance within normal limits, mallear fixation or otosclerosis may have been suggested by impedance audiometry.

Sensorineural hearing losses may present with a variety of configurations. In general, the most common configurations observed with sensorineural hearing loss are flat or predominantly high frequency (Fig. 13-2). Air- and bone-conduction thresholds are elevated to the same extent and middle ear pressure and compliance are within normal limits. The signal does not encounter difficulty in its route to the cochlea; the problem lies proximal to the middle ear. The expected speech discrimination scores will be somewhat dependent on the locus (cochlear or retrocochlear) and the degree of hearing loss. Therefore, SDS can fall anywhere along the continuum between poor and excellent.

Other configurations associated with sensorineural pathology include sharply sloping ("ski-slope"), notched, and low-frequency hearing losses. Figure 13-14 illustrates what is descriptively called a "ski-slope" configuration. Characteristic of this audiogram shape is hearing that is within normal limits below 1 to 2 kHz but dramatically drops above 1 to 2 kHz. Speech reception thresholds usually reflect the region of the audiogram within normal limits. Speech discrimination is often mildly to moderately depressed, though this is contingent upon the frequency region at which the audiogram begins to slope. In general, discrimination performance is better if less of the high-frequency region is impaired.

The high-frequency notched audiogram (Fig. 13-15) is typical of (but not exclusive to) reduced sensitivity associated with cochlear pathologic change resulting from long-term exposure to high levels of noise. However, single-incident exposures to high-intensity impulse or impact noise (such as gun fire, firecrackers, and explosions) can also induce permanent hearing loss. In Figure 13-15, the notch is broad and most impaired (moderate-to-severe) for frequencies between 3 and 6 kHz. This illustrates that the region at which hearing is maximally impaired is not always at the classic frequency, 4 kHz, but may be between 3 and 6 kHz. Noise-induced hearing loss is not always represented by a sharply notched audiogram. Therefore, it is important that interoctave frequencies be tested to document fully the extent of the impairment. Some individuals exhibit this audiometric configuration in the absence of a history of noise exposure.

The symptoms that include fluctuating flat or low-frequency sensorineural loss, rotary vertigo, nausea, vomiting, and tinnitus are associated with Meniere's syndrome (Fig. 13-16). The hearing loss has been found to be unilateral in 80 percent of the cases and accompanied by loudness recruitment. Impedance measures indicate middle-ear pressure and compliance to be within normal limits and the acoustic reflex is usually elicited at reduced sensation levels. Speech reception thresholds are con-

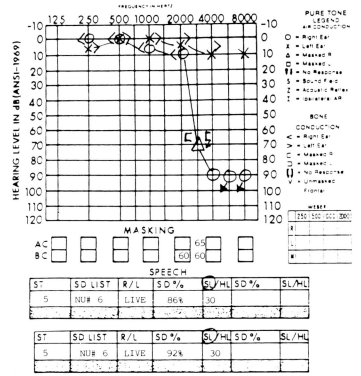

**Fig. 13-14.** Hearing for the left ear is within normal limits. In the right ear, hearing is within normal limits for the test frequencies 250 to 2,000 Hz. However, above 2,000 Hz sensitivity decreases precipitiously and there is a severe to profound sensorineural hearing loss.

RIGHT EAR

| ST | SD LIST | R/L | SD % | SL/HL | SD % | SL/HL |
|---|---|---|---|---|---|---|
| 5 | NU# 6 | LIVE | 86% | 30 | | |

LEFT EAR

| ST | SD LIST | R/L | SD % | SL/HL | SD % | SL/HL |
|---|---|---|---|---|---|---|
| 5 | NU# 6 | LIVE | 92% | 30 | | |

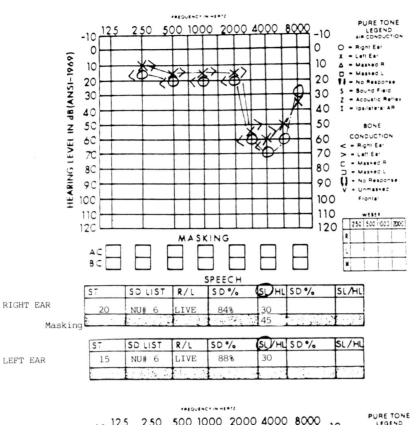

**Fig. 13-15.** Moderate, bilateral notched sensorineural hearing loss.

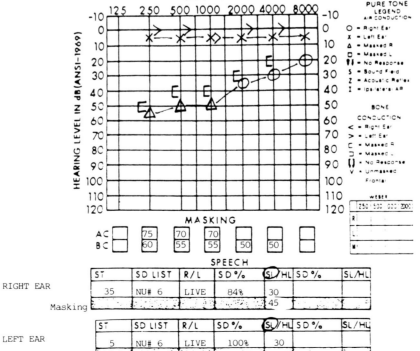

**Fig. 13-16.** Unilateral, predominantly low-frequency sensorineural hearing loss often associated with Meniére's disease.

sistent with pure-tone thresholds. Speech discrimination ability varies as a function of the progression of the disease and the degree of hearing loss.

A mixed hearing loss or impairment with a conductive overlay to a sensorineural hearing loss is seen in Figure 13-6. Speech reception thresholds are consistent with air-conduction pure-tone thresholds or slightly better. In general, speech discrimination performance is consistent with the bone-conduction rather than the air-conduction thresholds. Impedance audiometry usually suggests middle-ear conductive disorder.

## SUMMARY

In summary, the procedures discussed and cases presented in this chapter illustrate the processes surrounding the development of a clinical picture of hearing loss via audiometric testing. The information from the air- and bone-conduction pure-tone audiogram alone can only suggest possible causes, even to the best diagnostician. Speech thresholds, speech discrimination performance, and impedance measurements are needed to determine whether the hearing loss is conductive, sensorineural, or mixed. More important, these test procedures are only the initial stages in the diagnosis and assessment of prognosis and treatment of the communication deficit due to hearing impairment.

## REFERENCES

1. Villchur E: Audiometer-earphone mounting to improve intersubject and cushion-fit reliability. J Acoust Soc Am 48:1387, 1970
2. Lippman RP: MX/41AR earphone cushions versus a new circumaural mounting. J Acoust Soc Am 69:589, 1981
3. Kruger B, Solomon B, Cohen R, Newton L: Flat plate coupler calibration of circumaural audiometric and hifi earphones. J Acoust Soc Am S1:67, 111, 1980
4. Kruger B, Solomon B, Cohen R, et al: Real-ear responses of circumaural and insert earphones. J Acoust Soc Am S1:69, 1981
5. Zwislocki J, Kruger B, et al: Acoustic reliability in audiometry. Committee on Hearing Bioacoustics and Biomechanics Report Working Group 91, 1987
6. American National Standards Institute: American National Standard for Coupler Calibration of Earphones: S3.7. New York, 1973
7. Professional Services Board Manual: Accreditation of professional service programs in Speech-Language Pathology and Audiology. p.1–24. American Speech and Hearing Assn, Rockville, Maryland, October, 1978
8. Professional Services Board Accreditation Manual: American Speech- Language-Hearing Assn, Rockville, Maryland, 1984
9. Robinette MS, Barry SJ, Dybka ME, et al: Calibration of pure-tone air-conducted signals delivered via earphones. ASHA Sept: 1, 1982
10. Stevens SS: Problems and methods of psychophysics. Psychol Bull 55:177, 1958
11. Stevens SS: Mathematics, measurement, and psychophysics. p. 1. In Stevens SS (ed): Handbook of Experimental Psychology. John Wiley & Sons, New York, 1960
12. Tanner WP, Jr., Sorkin RD: The theory of signal detectability. p.63. In Tobias J (ed): Foundations of Modern Auditory Theory, Vol. II. Academic Press, New York, 1972
13. Carhart R, Jerger J: Preferred method for clinical determination of pure-tone thresholds. J Speech Hear Dis 24:330–345, 1959
14. Marshall L, Hanna T: Evaluation by computer simulation of stopping rules for audiological ascending test procedures. Presented at the 111th meeting of the Acoustical Society of America, May, 1986
15. American Speech and Hearing Association: Guidelines for manual pure-tone threshold audiometry. ASHA 19:236–240, 1977
16. American National Standards Institute: American National Standard Method for Manual Pure-Tone Threshold Audiometry: S3. 21. New York, 1978
17. American National Standards Institute: American National Standard Specification for Audiometers, S3.6. New York, 1969
18. American Speech and Hearing Association Committee on Audiometric Evaluation: Guidelines for Audiometric Symbols. ASHA 16:260–264, 1974
19. American National Standards Institute: American National Standard Criteria for Permissible Ambient Noise During Audiometric Testing: S3.1. New York, 1977

20. Dillon H, Walker G: The effect of acoustic environment on the reliability of sound field audiometry. Austral J Audiol 3:67, 1981

21. Rudmose W: Pressure vs. free field thresholds at low frequencies. Paper presented to the Fourth International Congress on Acoustics, 1962

22. Rudmose WF: The case of the missing 6 dB. J Acoust Soc Am 71:650, 1982

23. Tillman TW, Johnson RM, Olsen W: Earphone versus soundfield threshold sound pressure levels for spondee words. J Acoust Soc Am 39:125, 1966

24. Staab WJ, Rintelmann WF: Comparison of pure-tone and warble-tone thresholds. Paper presented to American Speech and Hearing Association, 1972

25. Rintelmann WF, Orchik DJ, Stephens M: A comparison of pure-tone and warble-tone thresholds. I-Effects of stimulus parameters. II-Effects of occlusion of nontest ear and changes in azimuth. Laboratory Report: Department of Audiology and Speech Sciences, Michigan State University, East Lansing, 1972

26. Morgan DE, Dirks DD: Loudness discomfort level under earphones and in the free field: the effects of calibration methods. J Acoust Soc Am 56:172, 1974

27. Stream RW, Dirks DD: Effect of loudspeaker position on differences between earphone and free-field thresholds (MAP and MAF). J Speech Hear Res 5:321, 1962

28. Robinson DO, Vaughan CR: Relative efficiency of warble-tone and conventional pure-tone testing with children. J Am Aud Soc 1:252, 1976

29. Morgan DE, Dirks DD, Bowes DR: Suggested threshold sound pressure levels for frequency-modulated (warble) tones in the soundfield. J Speech Hear Dis 27, 1979

30. Byrne D, Dillon H: Comparative reliability of warble tone thresholds under earphones and in sound field. Austral J Audiol 3:12, 1981

31. Carhart R: Clinical application of bone conduction. Arch Otolaryngol 51:789, 1950

32. Tonndorf J: Animal experiments in bone conduction: clinical conclusion. Ann Otol Rhinol Laryngol 73:659, 1964

33. Tonndorf J: Bone conduction-studies in experimental animals. Acta Otolaryngol [suppl] (Stockh) 213: 1966

34. American National Standards Institute:American National Standard for an Artificial Headbone for the Calibration of Audiometer Bone Vibrators: S3.13. New York, 1972

35. American National Standards Institute: American National Standard Reference equivalent threshold force levels for audiometric bone vibrators: S3.26. New York, 1981

36. Studebaker GA: On masking in bone-conduction testing. J Speech Hear Res 5:215, 1962

37. Dirks D: Factors related to bone conduction reliability. Arch Otolaryngol 79:551, 1964

38. Elpern B, Naunton RF: The stability of the occlusion effect. Arch Otolaryngol 77:376, 1963

39. Studebaker GA: Clinical masking. p.51. In Rintelmann WF (ed): Hearing Assessment. University Park Press, Baltimore, 1979

40. Rudmose WF: Automatic audiometry. p.30. In Jerger J (ed): Modern Developments in Audiology. Academic Press, New York, 1963

41. Berlin CI, Wexler KF, Jerger JF, et al: Superior ultraaudiometric hearing: a new type of hearing loss which correlates highly with unusually good speech in the profoundly deaf. Trans Amer Acad Opthal Otolaryngol 86:111, 1978

42. Fausti SA, Frey RH, Erickson DA, et al: A system for evaluating auditory function from 8000–20000 Hz. J Acoust Soc Am 66:1713, 1979

43. Stelmachowicz PG, Gorga MP, Cullen JK: A calibration procedure for assessment of thresholds above 8000 Hz. J Speech Hear Res 235:618, 1982

44. Green DM, Stevens KN, Berkowitz K, et al: A procedure for calibrating ear canals at high frequencies. J Soc Acoust Am 75:S11, 1984

45. Bolt, Beranek, Newman, Inc.: Development and preliminary testing of an electroacoustic device for the assessment of high-frequency hearing: Final Report Appendix A: Description and operation of a High Frequency Audiometer. NINCDS Contract No. NO1-N3-2-2394,3-85, March, 1985

46. Tonndorf J, Kurman B: High frequency audiometry. Ann Otol Rhinol Laryngol 93:576, 1984

47. American Standards Association: American Standard Specification for Audiometers for General Diagnostic Purposes: ASA Z24.5. New York, 1951

48. Northern JL, Downs MP: Hearing in Children. Williams & Wilkins, Baltimore, 1974

49. Studebaker GA: Clinical masking of the non-test ear. J Speech Hear Dis 32:360, 1967

50. Zwislocki J: Acoustic attenuation between ears. J Acoust Soc Am 25:752, 1953

51. Liden G, Nilsson G, Anderson H: Narrow band masking with white noise. Acta Otolaryngol 50:116, 1959

52. Sanders JW: Masking. p.111. In Katz J (ed): Handbook of Clinical Audiology. Williams & Wilkins, Baltimore, 1972

53. American National Standards Institute:American National Standard Psychoacoustical Terminology: S3.20. New York, 1973

54. Hawkins JE, Stevens SS: Masking of pure tones and of speech by white noise. J Acoust Soc Am 22:6, 1950

55. Hood JD: The principles and practice of bone conduction audiometry. Laryngoscope 70:1211, 1960

56. Martin FN: The masking plateau revisited. Ear Hearing 1:112, 1980

57. Studebaker GA: Clinical masking of air- and bone-conducted stimuli. J Speech Hear Res 29:23, 1964

58. Martin FN: Minimum effective masking levels in threshold audiometry. J Speech Hear Dis 39:280, 1974

59. Littler TS, Knight JJ, Strange PH; Hearing by bone conduction and the use of bone conduction hearing aids. Proc R Soc Med 45:783, 1952

60. American National Standards Institute: American National Standard For An Occluded Ear Simulator: S3.25. New York, 1979

61. International Electrotechnical Commission: Standard occluded-ear simulator for the measurement of earphones coupled to the ear by ear inserts. IEC 711:1–11, Bureau Central de la Commission Electrotechniques, Geneva, Switzerland, 1982

62. Killion MC, Wilber LA, Gudmundsen GI: Insert earphones for more interaural attenuation. Hearing Instrum 36:34, 1985

63. Thelin JW, Webber PJ: Clinical use of the earplug procedure. Presented to the American Speech-Language-Hearing Assn, 1984

64. Thelin JW, Davis WE, Khoury-Ghaffary J, et al: The earplug procedure. Otolaryngol Head Neck Surg 93:229, 1985

65. Wilson RH, Margolis RH: Measurements of auditory thresholds for speech stimuli, p 79 in Konkle DF, Rintleman WF (eds): *Principles of Speech Audiometry*, Perspectives in Audiology Series, Lyle L. Llyod (series ed). University Park Press, Baltimore, 1983.

66. American Speech and Hearing Association Committee on audiometric evaluation guidelines for determining threshold level for speech. ASHA 19:241–243, 1977

67. Fletcher H: Speech and Hearing. Van Nostrand Reinhold, Princeton, NJ, 1929

68. Hughson W, Thompson EA: Correlation of hearing acuity for speech with discrete frequency audiograms. Arch Otolaryngol 36:526, 1942

69. Hudgins CV, Hawkins JE, Jr., Karlin JE, Stevens SS: The development of recorded auditory tests for measuring hearing loss for speech. Laryngoscope 57:57, 1947

70. Hirsh IJ, Davis H, Silverman SR, et al: Development of materials for speech audiometry. J Speech Hear Dis 17:321, 1952

71. Olsen WO, Matkin ND: Speech audiometry. p. 133. In Rintelmann WF (ed): Hearing Assessment. University Park Press, Baltimore, 1979

72. Chaiklin JB, Ventry N: Spondee threshold measurement: a comparison of 2- and 5-dB methods. J Speech Hear Dis 29:47, 1964

73. Northern JL, Hattler KW: Evaluation of four speech discrimination test procedures on hearing impaired patients. J Aud Res [Suppl]1–37, 1974

74. Martin FN, Pennington CD: Current trends in audiometric practices. ASHA 13:672–677, 1971

75. Carhart R: Monitored live voice as a test of auditory acuity. J Acoust Soc Am 17:339, 1946

76. Creston JE, Gillespie M, Krahn C: Speech audiometry: taped vs live voice. Arch Otolaryngol 83:14, 1966

77. Beattie RC, Forrester PW, Ruby BK: Reliability of the Tillman-Olsen procedure for determination of spondee threshold using recorded and live voice presentations. J Am Audiol Soc 2:159, 1976

78. Fletcher H: A method of calculating hearing loss for speech from an audiogram. Acta Otolaryngol [Suppl] 90:26–37, 1950

79. Carhart R: Observations on relations between thresholds for pure tones and for speech. J Speech Hear Dis 36:476, 1971

80. Ventry IM: Pure tone-spondee threshold relationships in functional hearing loss. J Speech Hear Dis 41:16, 1976

81. Chaiklin JB: The relation among three selected auditory speech thresholds. J Speech Hear Res 2:237, 1959

82. Beattie RC, Edgerton BJ, Svihovec DV: An investigation of Auditec of St. Louis recordings of Central Institute for the Deaf spondees. J Am Aud Soc 1:97, 1975

83. Beattie RC, Svihovec DV, Edgerton BJ: Relative intelligibility of the CID spondees as presented via monitored live voice. J Speech Hear Dis 40:84, 1975

84. Ruben RJ, Kruger B: Hearing loss in the elderly. p. 123. In Katzman R, Terr RD (eds): The Neurology of Aging. FA Davis, Philadelphia, 1982

85. Quiggle RR, Glorig A, Delk JH, Summerfield AB: Predicting hearing loss for speech from pure tone audiograms. Laryngoscope 67:1, 1957

86. Elliot LL: Prediction of speech discrimination scores from other test information. J Aud Res 3:35, 1963

87. Blumfeld VG, Bergman M, Millner E: Speech discrimination in an aging population. J Speech Hear Res 12:210, 1969

88. Owens E, Benedict M, Schubert ED: Consonant phonemic errors associated with pure tone config-

urations and certain kinds of hearing impairment. J Speech Hear Res 15:308, 1972

89. Bilger RC, Wang MD: Consonant confusion in patients with sensorineural hearing loss. J Speech Hear Res 19:718, 1976

90. Hood JD: Speech Audiometry. p. 391. In Beagley HA (ed): Audiology and Audiologic Medicine. Oxford University Press, Oxford. 1982

91. Konkle DF, Rintelman WF: Principles of Speech Audiometry. p. 1. University Park Press, Baltimore, 1983

92. Kruger B, Mazor R: Speech Audiometry in the U.S.A. In Martin MC (ed): Speech Audiometry. Francis & Taylor, London, 1986

93. Skinner MW: Audibility and intelligibility of speech for listeners with sensorineural hearing losses. p.159. In Yanick P (ed): Rehabilitation Strategies for Sensorineural Hearing Loss. Grune & Stratton, Orlando, FL, 1979

94. Miller JD, Niemoeller AF, Pascoe DP, Skinner MW: Integration of the electroacoustic description of hearing aids with the audiologic description of clients. p. 355. In Studebaker GA, Hochberg I (eds): Acoustical Factors Affecting Hearing Aid Performance. University Park Press, Baltimore, 1980

95. Tillman TW, Johnson RM, Olsen W: Earphone versus soundfield threshold sound pressure levels for spondee words. J Acoust Soc Am 39:125, 1966

96. Martin MC (ed): Speech Audiometry. Francis & Taylor, London, 1986

97. Hood JD, Poole JP: Speech audiometry in conductive and sensori-neural hearing loss. Sound 5:30, 1971

98. Hood JD, Poole JP: Improving the reliability of speech audiometry. Br J Audiol 11:93, 1977

99. Hagerman B: Reliability in the determination of speech discrimination. Scand Audiol 5:219, 1976

100. Thornton A, Raffin MJM: Speech discrimination scores modeled as a binomial variable. J Speech Hear Res 21:507, 1978

101. Elpern B, Naunton RF: The stability of the occlusion effect. Arch Otolaryngol 77:376, 1963

102. Campanelli PA: A measure of intra-list stability of four PAL word lists. Aud Res 2:50, 1962

103. Campbell R: Discrimination test word difficulty. J Speech Hear Res 8:13, 1965

104. Deutsch LJ, Kruger B: The systematic selection of 25 monosyllables which predict the CID W-22 speech discrimination score. J Aud Res 11:286, 1971

105. Rintelmann WF, Schumaier DR, Jetty AJ, et al: Six experiments on speech discrimination utilizing CNC monosyllables. J Aud Res 2:1, 1974

106. Rose DE: A 10 word speech discrimination screening test. Presented to the American Speech and Hearing Assoc, 1974

107. Coles RRA: Can present day audiology really help in diagnosis? An otologist's question. J Laryngol Otol 86:191, 1972

108. Egan J: Articulation testing methods. Laryngoscope 58:955, 1948

109. Gladstone VS, Siegenthaler BM: Carrier phrase and speech intelligibility score. J Aud Res 11:101, 1971

110. Gelfand SA: Use of carrier phrase in live voice speech discrimination testing. J Aud Res 15:107, 1975

111. Carhart R: Problems in measurement of speech discrimination. Arch Otolaryngol 82:253, 1965

112. Lovrinic JH, Burgi EJ, Curry ET: A comparative evaluation of fine speech discrimination measures. J Speech Hear Res 11:372, 1968

113. Haskins M: A phonetically balanced test of speech discrimination for children. Masters thesis, Northwestern University, Evanston, IL, 1949

114. Lerman JW, Ross M, McLauchlin RM: A picture-identification test for hearing-impaired children. J Aud Res 5:273, 1965

115. Ross M, Lerman J: Picture identification test for hearing-impaired children. J Speech Hear Res 13:44, 1970

116. Gardner HJ: Application of high frequency consonant discrimination word list in hearing aid evaluation. J Speech Hear Dis 36:354, 1971

117. Pascoe DR: Frequency responses of hearing aids and their effects on the speech perception of hearing impaired subjects. Ann Otol Rhinol Laryngol [Suppl] 23:1, 1975

118. House AS, Williams CE, Necker MHL, Kryter KD: Articulation testing methods. Consonantal differentiation in a closed-response set. J Acoust Soc Am 37:158, 1965

119. Kruel EJ, Nixon JC, Kryter KD, et al: A proposed clinical test of speech discrimination. J Speech Hear Res 11:536, 1968

120. Owens E, Shubert ED: Development of the California Consonant Test. J Speech Hear Res 20:463, 1977

121. Resnick SB, Dubno JR, Hoffnung S, Levitt H: Phoneme errors on a nonsense syllable test. J Acoust Soc Am 58:S72, 1975

122. Levitt H, Resnick SB: Speech reception by the hearing impaired: methods of testing and the de-

velopment of new tests. Scand Audiol [Suppl] 6:107–130, 1978

123. Jerger J, Speaks C, Trammell J: A new approach to speech audiometry. J Speech Hear Dis 33:318, 1968

124. Kalikow DN, Stevens KN, Elliot LL: Development of a test of speech intelligibility in noise using sentence materials with controlled word predictability. J Acoust Soc Am 61:1337, 1977

125. Rintelmann WF (ed): Hearing Assessment. University Park Press, Baltimore, 1979

126. McCandless GA, Thomas GK: Impedance audiometry as a screening procedure for middle ear disease. Trans Am Acad Ophthalmol Otolaryngol 78:98, 1974

127. Jerger J: Clinical experience with impedance audiometry. Arch Otolaryngol 92:311, 1970

128. Bluestone CD, Beery QC, Paradise JL: Audiometry and tympanometry in relation to middle ear effusions in children. Laryngoscope 83:594, 1974

129. Northern JL, Grimes AM: Introduction to acoustic impedance. p.344. In Katz J (ed): Handbook of Clinical Audiology, 2nd ed. Williams & Wilkins, Baltimore, 1978

130. Feldman AS: Tympanometry. p.103. In Feldman AS, Wilber LA (eds): Acoustic Impedance and Admittance—The Measurement of Middle Ear Function. Williams & Wilkins, Baltimore, 1976

131. Metz O: Threshold of reflex contractions of the muscles of the middle ear and recruitment of loudness. Arch Otolaryngol 55:536, 1952

132. Fria T, LeBlanc J, Kristensen R, Alberti PW: Ipsilateral acoustic reflex stimulation in normal and sensori-neural impaired ears; a preliminary report. Can J Otolaryngol 4:695, 1975

# Acoustic Impedance and Auditory Reflexes    14

## Laura Ann Wilber

Acoustic immittance, or acoustic impedance, is a procedure designed to assess middle ear function. It does not directly assess hearing, although it can be used to help estimate probable hearing thresholds for patients who cannot or will not respond at their true hearing threshold. The procedure is most effective in helping to determine the state of the middle ear and in providing information about the functioning of the 7th and 8th cranial nerves.

Acoustic immittance is simply objective pneumatic otoscopy. It provides a reproducible, quantitative measure of tympanic membrane movement. It allows for more subtle evaluation than pneumatic otoscopy since immittance uses air pressures of roughly $+200$ to $-400$ daPa as opposed to $\pm 1000$ daPa. (The unit dekapascals has supplanted the older unit $mmH_2O$.) With acoustic immittance a specific pure tone is introduced into the ear canal at a preset intensity. As the tone is reflected from the eardrum, or canal wall, its intensity is measured and interpreted in terms of the air pressure (ambient, or externally introduced) in the ear canal. A machine, called an acoustic impedance audiometer or otoadmittance device, automatically measures the intensity of the reflected tone so that the clinician need only interpret the measurements. This is

a gross simplification, but basically defines the procedure. The particular device may be capable of determining not only the intensity but also the phase of the reflected signal, and thus may be capable of separating the impedance measurement into its resistive and reactive components. In this chapter, I will not go into the details of resistive and reactive measurements since they are rarely used clinically today.

This chapter will present some of the uses of acoustic immittance, both in its original primary function of assessing middle ear function and some of its secondary functions, which, in some ways, have become more important than the primary function. In addition to middle ear function, this chapter will discuss the use of acoustic immittance in screening for specific pathologic conditions, in helping to determine the presence of retrocochlear pathologic changes, and in estimating the threshold of hearing and loudness discomfort.

Before discussing how the device can be used, it is important to have some understanding of how it works. The interpretations made are limited by what the devices can do. Most of this chapter will discuss results obtained with standard clinical devices rather than those that can be obtained in the

397

laboratory and that use the same principals but much more elaborate equipment.

Acoustic immittance (previously called acoustic impedance) was originally considered a way of indirectly assessing the status of the middle ear. Since it relies on measurements made at the eardrum, it follows that the most peripheral pathologic change will be identified. The first reports of the use of acoustic immittance[1] concentrated on the relative impedance at the tympanic membrane. The measurement procedure used by Metz was intended to describe middle ear function, but because it did not take into account the size of the ear canal[2] it was really only effective in describing *change* in stiffness at the tympanic membrane. Thus it was useful in following fluctuation of pathologic change such as middle ear effusion, or progression, such as stapes fixation, but it was essentially useless in helping determine the state of a new, unknown ear. The acoustic reflex, however, did serve as a differentiator for conductive, cochlear, and retrocochlear pathologic conditions. In 1957 Zwislocki described a new type of acoustic impedance measuring device, which allowed one to compensate for the size of the canal. By using static measurements of impedance by frequency (in this case, separated into resistive and reactive components), it was possible to draw diagnostic conclusions.[2-4]

However, the Zwislocki procedure was thought to be somewhat time consuming and difficult to use clinically. It required that the size of the external auditory canal be measured precisely (which was accomplished by determining how much alcohol it took to fill the canal from the tympanic membrane to the end of a speculum), and it was not easily interpreted. The procedure did not allow compensation for differences between ambient air pressure and the pressure in the middle ear, which sometimes led to an impression of stiffness at the tympanic membrane that was misleading. However, the procedure did have the advantage of allowing one to look at impedance by frequency, and to differentiate resistive and reactive components, which was helpful in making subtle distinctions among patients and their probable pathologic conditions.

Another procedure described by Terkildsen and Nielsen[5] allowed for compensation for middle ear pressure as well as the size of the ear canal. It was initially used only at one frequency (220 Hz) and it did not allow for differentiation of resistive and reactive components. The procedure was quick and did not require physical measurement of the external auditory canal. The measurement that allowed for compensation for the size of the ear canal was done by determining the impedance in the ear canal at a high positive air pressure that had the effect of stiffening the eardrum to a point near maximum stiffness for most ears. The impedance at maximum stiffness was compared algebraically to the impedance of a 2 cc cavity, and by that comparison one could arrive at a relative ear canal volume. This measurement was *not* the same as a physical measurement[6] but was adequate for compensating for ear canal size. Assuming canal volume based on pressure comparisons is the approach most often used today. Some instruments measure acoustic impedance and some acoustic admittance (the reciprocal of impedance), so for convenience in discussion, the term (acoustic) immittance was borrowed from physics to describe either.

It was possible to assess acoustic reflexes using the Zwislocki bridge. However, it was difficult to determine ipsilateral reflexes using the original Zwislocki bridge without adding additional external filtering. (The bridge itself is obviously incapable of determining whether the increased sound in the ear canal is from the reflected sound of the probe tone or from the reflex acitivating stimulus.)

Regardless of the specific type of acoustic immittance device, certain patterns may be expected. The test is impervious to the patient's stage of sleep and it may be used with patients who are unable or unwilling to cooperate with pure-tone audiometry.

Acoustic immittance has three components: (1) static acoustic immittance; (2) tympanometry; and (3) acoustic (auditory or aural) reflexes. Today, tympanometry and the acoustic reflexes are used most often clinically, but since they are truly interrelated a short explanation of each is in order.

Static acoustic immittance refers to the compliance (or inversely, stiffness) of the eardrum either in ambient air pressure or when the air pressure in the external canal has been adjusted to be roughly equivalent to that of the middle ear. It is reported as a single number which may be in acoustic ohms, acoustic mhos, cubic centimeters, or milliliters. Although this number presumably includes the physical components of impedance (resistance and the compliant and mass components of reactance), it most often only assesses the compliant portion of reactance. In terms of stiffness, the higher the number the stiffer the eardrum, and the lower the number the more compliant the eardrum. Since acoustic immittance is measured by determining the intensity of the sound reflected from the eardrum, it follows that the pathologic condition closest to the eardrum will be the one most likely to be evident. Thus, if patient has a dislocated incus as well as a fixed stapes footplate, measurements would only reflect the dislocated incus. Also, since acoustic immittance assumes that sound has been reflected from the tympanic membrane, any rupture of that membrane makes the measurement invalid. (This is true for tympanometry and aural reflexes as well as for static measurements.) Normative values have been cited by various authors for expected results with various pathologic conditions.[7–9] However, the specific values *may* only be valid for a particular instrument calibrated in a certain way. (As of this writing, unlike audiometers, there is no American National Standards Institute [ANSI] standard for acoustic immittance devices.) Because of the variability reported for static measurements, and the difficulties encountered in taking into con-

sideration the factors that make up static acoustic immittance (for example, barometric pressure at the site where the measurements are made), it has fallen into essential disuse today. Since most devices today only allow for measurements at one frequency (226 Hz) the variation by frequency reported by Zwislocki and Feldman[10] and others[7,11] is no longer possible.

The second basic measurement is that of tympanometry. This simply refers to change in immittance as a function of variation of the ear canal pressure. The plotted shape of this change is called a tympanogram. Figures 14-1 and 14-2 show typical tympanogram for a normal ear. Note that the tympanogram may be described in terms of maximum compliance, air pressure at which the maximum compliance occured, and general shape. One may also use a classification system such as that described by Jerger.[12] The level of maximum compliance is directly related to the static impedance value. The *point* of maximum compliance on the tympanogram is also referred to as middle ear pressure (MEP). Most acoustic immittance devices, as well as tympanometric screeners, use only one frequency: this is usually 226 Hz. Recently, Shanks[13] reviewed the major effects on tympanometry of supposed ear pathologic conditions using human

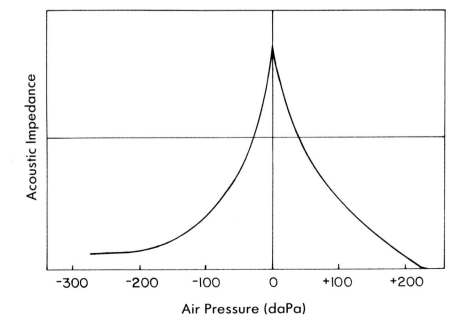

**Fig. 14-1.** Normal tympanogram in acoustic impedance.

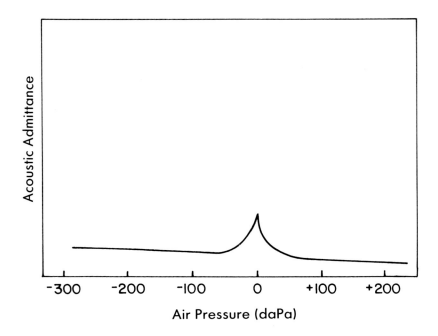

**Fig. 14-2.** Normal tympanogram in acoustic admittance.

temporal bones. She showed differences depending on the frequency, as well as with conductive versus susceptance measures. She used both 226 and 678 Hz as the test frequencies. Lilly[14] also looked at the effect of frequency on the tympanogram. Like other investigators, he found that use of a single low frequency was probably not as sensitive to specific pathologic conditions as the use of at least one more mid frequency tone near the secondary resonant frequency of the ear (somewhere around 800 Hz). Lilly quotes Berg's (1980) devising of a three-dimensional plotting system to allow one to assess the effect of frequency by air pressure by admittance. This procedure should allow finer distinctions among pathologic conditions. However, today most devices used clinically still only allow for assessment of the tympanogram at one frequency (226 Hz). In some cases, the entire tympanogram is not plotted, but the point of maximum displacement is noted. That point is assumed to be equivalent to the air pressure in the middle ear, and is, thus, called "middle ear pressure." In practice, this occurs when the minimum amount of sound is reflected from the eardrum as the air pressure in the middle ear is adjusted. Fortunately, the device makes the calculation of "minimum sound."

The acoustic reflex provides an indirect assessment of the middle ear muscle reflex. When a loud sound (above 80 dB SPL) is introduced into either ear, the sound travels through the middle ear to the cochlea; thence from the hair cells of the cochlea to the 8th nerve; from the 8th nerve to the ventral cochlear nucleus; from the ventral cochlear nucleus bilaterally to the superior olivary complex; thence to the ipsilateral and contralateral motor nuclei of the 8th nerve; and finally to the stapedius muscle.[15-17] When that happens, the stapedial muscle in *both* ears contracts.[18-20] This contraction causes a stiffening of the ossicular chain and thence of the tympanic membrane. Thus, if the system is working when a loud sound (pure-tone, white noise, or any other noise) is introduced into either ear, the acoustic impedance will increase. Typically the reflex is first reported as present or absent in the test ear. (The test ear is the ear into which the *probe* is inserted.) If it is present the levels needed to elicit the reflex with various stimuli in either the test (ipsi) or contralateral ear are usually reported. Finally the length of time before the reflex begins to decay (as indicated by a lowering of impedance over time), or decays to 50 percent of its maximum level, may also be reported. This is referred to, more properly, as "reflex adaptation."

Although the above tests are clearly interrelated,

each looks at middle ear function in a slightly different way. Together they make up the acoustic immittance test battery. How that battery is used for delineation of possible auditory pathologic change is discussed below.

## SCREENING

Use of acoustic immittance to screen for possible middle ear pathologic change has been recommended by numerous authors.[21-27]

The usefulness of this procedure depends, of course, on the same factors that influence any screening procedure. Specifically, one must ask: (1) Is the disease for which one is screening prevalent or potentially life-threatening? (2) Will screening enable one to identify the disease earlier? (3) Are there accepted methods of treatment for the disease? (4) Is the procedure cost effective?

Acoustic immittance as a screening procedure appears to be most effective for two types of auditory conditions: middle ear effusion and diseases of the 8th cranial nerve. In both it is important to assess *both* tympanometry and the acoustic reflex. The advantages of acoustic immittance as a screening tool are that it is quick, it does not require very expensive equipment, it is noninvasive, and it is easy to administer and interpret.

The procedure has been used most often as screening for middle ear effusion. The probe is inserted into the test ear and, if a seal is obtained, a tympanogram is plotted. Without removing the probe, one checks for the presence or absence of an acoustic reflex. (This can be done either ipsilaterally or contralaterally.) For screening it is usually sufficient to check the reflex using only a broadband white noise (BBN), a narrow band noise, or a single pure tone. Exactly the same procedure is used when screening for the possible 8th nerve pathologic conditions. However, in middle ear effusion one looks for an abnormal tympanogram and an absent acoustic reflex, and in 8th nerve pathologic conditions one expects to find a *normal* tympanogram in association with an absent or elevated acoustic reflex.

Although there is some question as to when to refer and when to retest, it is generally accepted that for middle ear effusion the pass criteria is middle ear pressure at ± 100 dPa and a present acoustic reflex. The American Speech Language Hearing Association[28] recommended that fail criteria be middle ear pressure greater than − 100 and an absent acoustic reflex. If middle ear pressure is abnormal but the acoustic reflex is present, or if middle ear pressure is normal and the acoustic reflex is absent, it is recommended that the patient be retested. The question that is not completely resolved is whether to refer or retest if the patient fails a single screening test. In our experience, if the ear is examined otoscopically by an experienced otolaryngologist at the time of failure it is usually found to have middle ear effusion. However, if the patient is not examined for several days following the immittance screening there is often no visible sign of pathologic change. This, of course, is commensurate with the normal course of middle ear effusion. For this reason, it is often recommended that if the patient's result is questionable *or* fails, he or she should be retested before referral to the physician. Stool[29] describes a series of tympanometric functions that might be found with various middle ear effusion and air pressure configurations. He recommends use of otoscopy and the acoustic immittance battery to evaluate children with suspected middle ear effusion.

Immittance screening is most often carried out in well-baby clinics, in Head Start programs, and in school programs (especially in classes for the hearing impaired). Although hearing testing is mandatory in most states, acoustic immittance screening is not. It is advisable to screen certain special populations routinely, specifically (1) children with severe to profound sensorineural hearing loss; (2) children with cleft palates or other orofacial anomalies; (3) native American children; and (4) mentally retarded children. In the first and last case the reason for screening is that these children do not normally present the other signs (loss of hearing, ear pain or discomfort, feeling of fullness) of middle ear effusion to their families and are thus less likely to be brought to the physician for examination and treatment. There is evidence that children with clefts are more prone to middle ear effusion than those in the normal population,[30,31] and although it is not clear whether there is a genetic or an environmental difference between native Americans and others, that population also appears to have a higher than normal incidence of middle ear effusion.[31] Obviously the purpose of any screening is to separate those children who are likely to have the disease from those who are not.

Unfortunately, partly because of the disease, partly because of the equipment, and partly because of the interpretation, acoustic immittance has a fairly high false-positive rate for identification of middle ear effusion. Therefore, it is important to determine in advance whether it is more advisable to refer all of those who fail the screening after their first failure and risk overreferral, or whether it is more advisable to retest all who fail before referring them, thus possibly either missing patients who are not rechecked or allowing the disease to go untreated for a longer period of time.

---

## DIAGNOSTIC USE OF ACOUSTIC IMMITTANCE

In addition to its screening capabilities, the acoustic immittance battery may also be used as a diagnostic tool to help in the specific diagnosis of ear conditions. Although the battery is most useful in differentiating middle ear pathologic conditions, it can be used effectively to help in the assessment and differentiation of cochlear and retrocochlear conditions.

### Conductive Pathologic Conditions

Acoustic immittance measurements have probably been used most effectively for differentiating conductive disorders. At the time these measurements were first introduced there were numerous problems with bone conduction (calibration, masking, etc.) that made it necessary to have another test of probable middle ear function. Although immittance measurements cannot determine the extent of the air-bone gap with any degree of accuracy, they can point to the probability of middle ear

pathologic conditions and their possible site within the middle ear cleft.

Expected acoustic immittance findings with various conductive pathologic conditions will be discussed here. From the outset it must be clear, however, that if the condition does not intrude on the ossicular chain or the tympanic membrane it will *not* be reflected in acoustic immittance measurements. For example, an attic cholesteotoma that does not impinge on the ossicular chain or tympanic membrane will simply be invisible to immittance measurements. In addition, the procedure is also incapable of determining the precise condition although it may identify the site. For example, one may be able to tell whether or not there is ossicular fixation, but the immittance procedure will not reveal whether that fixation is due to otosclerotic growth, fibrous tissue, or a congenital malformation.

Immittance measurements can be most helpful in monitoring the course of a disease, such as middle ear effusion, or Bell's palsy. In the former case, one may monitor the change in middle ear air pressure and the change in the shape of the tympanogram as they occur over time. (In the latter case, one monitors the return of the acoustic reflex over time.) Figure 14-3 shows a case with subsequently surgically confirmed serous otitis media. In this case note that the static impedance is high, the tympanograms are rounded in both ears, and the acoustic reflex is absent in both ears. Figure 14-4 shows another case with otitis media in which there was no visible fluid, but in which the eardrum was found to be retracted under otoscopic examination. Clinically it is noted that as the middle ear space fills with fluid the tympanogram becomes more and more rounded. If the fluid becomes very thick, the tympanogram may be completely flat. Experimentally it has not been possible to achieve significant correlations between the amount of fluid and its viscosity and the height of the tympanogram. Thus one may not be able to make a precise statement about the amount or the viscosity of fluid in a given individual, but one can monitor the course of the condition by repeated tympanograms.[29,32] Acoustic immittance measurements will be more sensitive to the presence of pathologic conditions in middle ear effusion than will pure-tone audiometry because many children have thresholds *below* "0"

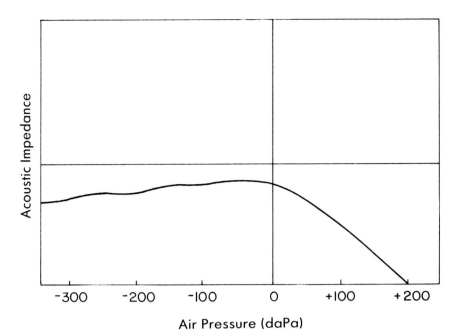

**Fig. 14-3.** Rounded tympanogram classically associated with middle ear effusion.

dB HL, and thus a shift in hearing from − 10 HL to "0" HL or from "0" HL to 20 dB HL would yield results within the normal range. In other words, the child might have a loss of hearing (relative to *his or her own norm*) of greater than 20 dB without hav-ing a loss relative to the accepted range of "normal hearing" for the population. It is often impossible to assess bone conduction thresholds at levels less than 0 dB HL when air conduction is close to "0" dB HL because of the ambient room noise in the

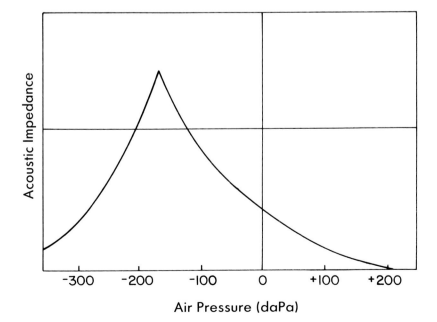

**Fig. 14-4.** Retracted tympanogram classically associated with otitis media.

test booth. In addition, since both air conduction and bone conduction may be expected to have a ±10 dB test variation, small air bone gaps may be obscured because of this normal variability. Regardless of whether the physician wishes to treat the disease in the absence of demonstrable hearing loss, certainly it is important to be able to detect its presence for further monitoring.

Feldman[32] reports that in the early stages of middle ear effusion the air pressure may be positive; it then becomes negative. Again in the early stages the shape of the tympanogram may be normal, but the air pressure at which maximum eardrum compliance is reached may be quite negative as was shown in Figure 14-4. In the very earliest stage of the pathologic condition, the acoustic reflex may be present (e.g., if air pressure is positive or only slightly negative and the fluid level does not reach above the manubrium). As the fluid level rises and the tympanic membrane becomes stiffer, it becomes more difficult for the stapedius muscle contractions to override the stiffness at the tympanic membrane, and thus the acoustic reflex will be absent.

In summary, with middle ear effusion, the classic acoustic immittance battery reveals a high static value, a negative middle ear pressure (greater than −100 daPa), a rounded tympanogram, and an absent acoustic reflex.

When the middle ear effusion is treated using myringotomy and tympanostomy tubes, acoustic immittance can be an invaluable help in monitoring the condition of the tube (see discussion of other uses of acoustic immittance).

Other types of middle ear pathologic conditions are not always as clear cut as middle ear effusion. In ossicular fixation we expect to find elevated static measurements; normal middle ear pressure; normal, albeit shallow, tympanometric shape; and an absent acoustic reflex. It was hoped initially that acoustic impedance would allow the clinician to differentiate between various types of ossicular fixation (i.e., malleus vs. stapes); however the variability in normal impedance at low frequencies has made this virtually impossible. With groups of subjects using reactance and resistance measurements at several frequencies, one can clearly differentiate among those with malleal fixation, stapes fixation, fibrotic fixation of the ossicular chain, and normal

middle ears.[7] However, the variability among groups is so great that in any given case this distinction may not be accurately made. Figure 14-5 shows the expected configuration for ossicular fixation using current instrumentation. Feldman[8,9] has pointed out that when the tympanic membrane is scarred the immittance measurements may reflect that scarring and thus yield static measures within the normal range, as well as tympanograms that are normal at 256 Hz because of the confounding factor of the elasticity of a scar or neomembrane.

Although one cannot differentiate among types of ossicular fixation at the present time, one can clearly differentiate between middle ear effusion and ossicular fixation by the shape of the tympanogram. Both problems present with high static acoustic immittance and absent acoustic reflexes, but the tympanograms are clearly different. In the

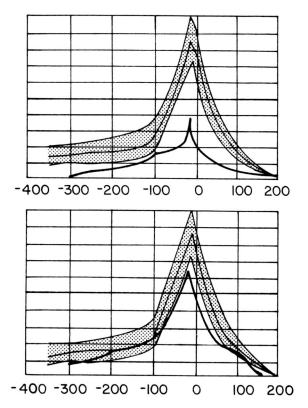

**Fig. 14-5.** Expected tympanometric results for two types of ossicular fixation (top with malleal fixation, bottom with stapes fixation).

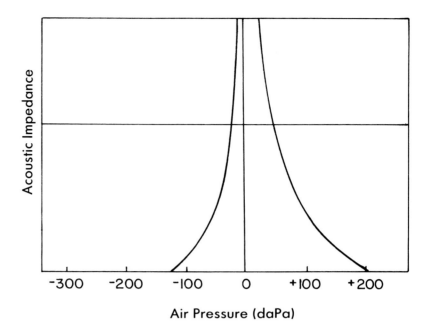

**Fig. 14-6.** Expected tympanometric results for classic (open-ended) ossicular discontinuity.

former the shape is either rounded or the pressure point is moved toward negative pressure. In fixation, the pressure point is almost always at ambient pressure (0 daPa) and the shape is normal or shallow.

In ossicular discontinuity, however, the static impedance is low and the tympanograms tend to be open ended (Fig. 14-6) or "W"-shaped (Fig. 14-7). A very steeply rising tympanometric peak (Fig. 14-8) *can* be indicative of an ossicular discontinuity, but it appears to be more often found with neomembranes.[9] The "W" configuration and the open-ended tympanogram may also be found with neomembranes when using a 660 Hz probe tone (instead of 220 or 226 Hz). The acoustic reflex will be absent *unless* the discontinuity is central to the neck of the stapes. Since the stapes tendon is attached peripheral to the crura, obviously any discontinuity of the stapes crura will not impede the reflex contraction. Fortunately this type of discontinuity is rarely seen. (It was most often seen in post-stapes mobilization patients,—who are rare today.)

As with cholesteotomas, any tumor or growth that invades the middle ear space will not affect acoustic immittance or measurements unless it impinges on the tympanic membrane or ossicular chain. Even in those cases it may not affect the measurements unless the ossicular chain is eroded or immobilized, or unless the tympanic membrane is perforated or stiffened by the presence of the growth. If a growth is present and is pressing

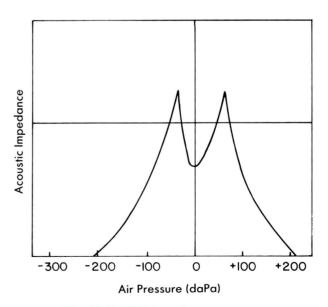

**Fig. 14-7.** "W"shaped tympanogram.

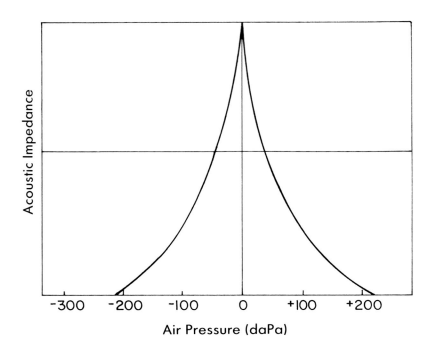

**Fig. 14-8.** Sharp, pointed tympanogram (seen with discontinuity, neomembranes, and neonates).

against the tympanic membrane, one would expect a rounded tympanogram. If a growth has eroded away the incudostapedial joint, the tympanogram would reflect the discontinuity.

In one interesting case, a cholesteotoma was found to be filling the middle ear space, having eroded part of the ossicular chain. The resultant tympanogram had some of the characteristics of anormal shape, but was broader than normal (see Fig. 14-9). The reflex was missing, and tympano-

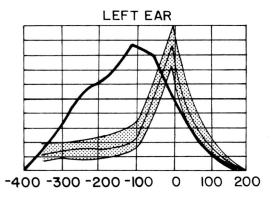

**Fig. 14-9.** Acoustic impedance results for a surgically confirmed cholesteotoma.

grams using the 660 Hz probe tone were clearly abnormal (Fig. 14-10).

## Cochlear and Retrocochlear Pathologic Conditions

Acoustic immittance can also be of help in differentiating between cochlear and retrocochlear pathologic changes. Although neither static impedance measurements nor tympanometry is helpful in this regard, they should be assessed first to *rule out* middle ear diseases. It is also essential to use a tool such as tympanometry before using such test procedures as auditory brainstem response (ABR) to rule out middle ear pathologic conditions since both retrocochlear and middle ear diseases show increased latencies.

Although immittance measures *cannot* indicate the cause of the condition, they can help point to the probable site of the lesion. In the case of cochlear conditions, for example, one expects to find normal static impedance, normal tympanograms, and acoustic reflexes at reduced (less than 60 dB) sensation levels.[33-35] The presence of an acoustic reflex is sometimes called the "Metz recruitment

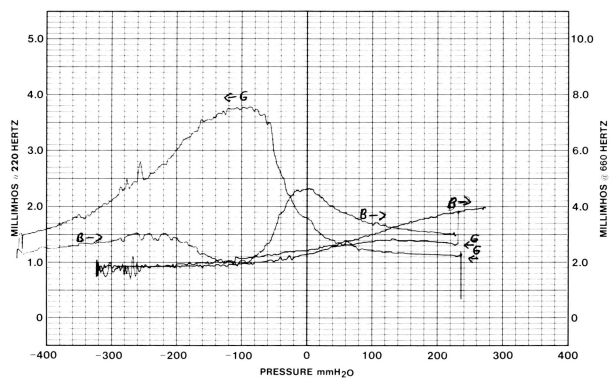

**Fig. 14-10.** Acoustic admittance results for a surgically confirmed cholesteotoma.

test," and although the reflex is certainly not a direct test of recruitment (after all, it cannot make a "loudness" judgement), it is strongly *correlated* with recruitment tests. Thus the patient who yields reflexes at sensation levels of 20 dB is much more likely to complain of other recruitment symptoms than the patient whose reflexes are at a sensation level of 60 dB or higher. Because of its high correlation with loudness recruitment, some investigators have proposed using the reflex to help determine the level at which the maximum power output of a hearing aid should be set.[36-38] However, more recent work by Greenfield et al.[39] was unable to demonstrate a predictable relationship between loudness discomfort levels and the acoustic reflex for normal hearing persons.

Thus, while static and tympanometric measurements will be the same as those for the normal ear, for both retrocochlear and cochlear pathologic conditions the reflex will yield different results. The acoustic reflex for pure tones for cochlear conditions will normally be at sensation levels less than 60 dB. However, the acoustic reflex for BBN will generally be at close to the same HL levels as for the normal ear. One word of caution, however; if the patient has a cochlear hearing loss that *exceeds* 60 dB HL, the acoustic reflex may be absent because an intensity sufficient to elicit it cannot be generated. (Few audiometers generate intensities above 110 dB HL.)

On the other hand, in retrocochlear diseases at the level of the brainstem or below, the acoustic reflex for pure tones generally will be absent or be present at elevated intensity levels. In some cases the acoustic reflex will reveal a decaying pattern. This reflex decay pattern was first reported by Anderson et al.[40,41] It should be noted that normal ears will sometimes present a decay pattern at 4,000 Hz and occasionally at 2,000 Hz, but rarely at lower frequencies. For example, Wilson et al.[42] looked at acoustic reflex adaptation (decay) for 35 normal-hearing subjects. They found very little change for frequencies below 1,000 Hz, but they did find a curvilinear function in frequencies at and above 2,000 Hz. For the frequencies of 3,000 and above decay had reached a half gain level in approximately 10 seconds. They also report that preliminary data from patients with Meniére's disease lie below the normal curve at all frequencies. However, this was not as severe as that found for 8th nerve pathologic conditions.

Fowler and Wilson[43] also reviewed some of the major studies of reflex adaptation in normal ears as well as in the problems associated with cochlear (specifically Meniére's disease) decay. Some of these cochlear pathologic conditions are different than normal and not unlike the 8th nerve lesions. They emphasized that the three possible outcomes of acoustic reflex testing in 8th nerve pathologic conditions may be (1) no reflex, (2) elevated reflex, and (3) abnormal decay (or adaptation). Most authors report that using the single criteria of decay is not sufficient in 8th nerve pathologic conditions. In addition, although the retrocochlear ear may show reflex decay at all frequencies, because normal hearing people and some with cochlear conditions present decay at higher frequencies it is suggested that reflex decay be assessed at only 500 and 1,000 Hz.

Since the reflex activation involves the 7th and 8th cranial nerves, it follows that lesions above the brainstem area (such as those in the auditory cortex) will *not* show any type of abnormal acoustic reflex. Those lesions that only affect the 8th cranial nerve are expected to show an abnormal acoustic reflex pattern with ipsilateral stimulation, but not with contralateral stimulation. (That is, if the lesion is in the right 8th cranial nerve, acoustic stimulus presented to the right ear will yield an abnormal pattern, for either ipsi- or contralateral monitoring.) If, on the other hand, the lesion is affecting the 7th cranial nerve, the acoustic reflex is expected to yield an abnormal pattern with either ipsilateral or contralateral stimulus when the *probe* is placed in the ear on the side of the lesion.

The acoustic reflex has been shown to be an extremely useful tool in early identification of 8th nerve pathologic conditions since it is noninvasive, quick, and has a high hit rate.[44] It has also been reported that the acoustic reflex is less likely to identify ears as abnormal when they are, in fact,

normal than more sophisticated auditory tests such as ABR. Sanders et al.[45] reported about 77 percent correct identification of retrocochlear lesions using the acoustic reflex, while Olsen et al.[44] reported about 95 percent correct identification of the patients with retrocochlear pathologic conditions.

The acoustic reflex has also been used to help identify the site of lesion in 7th nerve pathologic conditions as well. Generally, when there is facial paralysis, or other indication of 7th nerve pathologic conditions, the acoustic reflex is one of a battery of tests (including taste, electromyographic function, etc.) used to help pinpoint the site of damage. As mentioned above, in persons who have Bell's palsy, for example, one may sometimes track the course of the disease by regular monitoring of the acoustic reflex.[46,47] The reflex can be an early indicator of recovery from this condition. By using the reflex in conjunction with other clinical tests (such as taste and smell), the clinician can often pinpoint quite precisely the probable site of the 7th nerve lesion.

## OTHER USES OF ACOUSTIC IMMITTANCE

In addition to its use to help determine the site of lesion, the acoustic reflex has been used to estimate hearing threshold, especially when the patient cannot or will not cooperate. In 1974, Niemeyer and Sesterhenn reported that the acoustic reflex could be used to predict threshold of hearing.[48] They determined that the average difference between the acoustic reflex threshold for tone and BBN was 17 dB and that this relationship decreased linearly as the pure-tone threshold level increased. In addition, they reported that the difference between the acoustic reflex threshold and the threshold of hearing for tones also decreased. Niemeyer and Sesterhenn plotted the relationship of these two difference scores and achieved a slope factor of 2.5 dB. Thus, they reasoned, one could determine the difference between a subjects threshold for the acoustic reflex for tones and for BBN: multiply that difference by 2.5 dB and subtract it from the pure-tone average for the reflex. The resultant number would be the person's average threshold for hearing.

Later, Jerger et al.[49] modified the procedure outlined by Niemeyer and Sesterhenn and included a way of estimating the probable slope of the auditory function as well. (They looked at the difference for reflexes at low and high frequencies.) They did not try to determine specifically the level of hearing, but they made a categorical statement of normal hearing compared with mild, moderate, severe, or profound loss.

Keith asserted that one could make a gross prediction of threshold of hearing by using BBN only.[50] If the infant responds at a level of 85 dB, one assumes that the hearing is probably normal. If there is no response, one assumes a hearing loss. His data showed a false-negative rate of 3 percent and a false-positive rate of 13 percent.

Subsequently, Popelka and co-workers demonstrated differences in acoustic reflex thresholds depending on the bandwidth of the activating stimulus.[51-53] They also looked at differences in reflex thresholds for persons with sensorineural hearing loss and those with normal hearing by varying the bandwidth of the reflex-activating stimulus. This observation led to the notion of the bivariate plot, which can be used to help predict hearing level by frequency.

Acoustic immittance measurements have also been used to help assess eustachian tube funtion.[54-56] Holmquist advocated use of a swallow test monitored using the acoustic immittance meter to help determine the patency of the eustachian tube. If the eustachian tube is performing normally, an air pressure of approximately 200 daPa in the external canal will force the tube open so that one sees an immediate loss of pressure. Conversely, the patient may be asked to swallow (dry or preferably with fluid) and one determines how many swallows are necessary to release pressure. The need for more than two to three swallows indicates probable problems. This is a "quick and dirty" test that is most helpful clinically.

Similar to the procedure used above, the state of the tympanostomy tube may be monitored using acoustic immittance. When the tube is in place and functioning properly, the pressure should release at approximately 200 daPa. If the eustachian tube is still not functioning well but the tympanostomy tube is open, the tympanogram will be flat, the calculated volume of the ear canal will be larger than normal for age, and the acoustic reflex will be absent. If the tympanostomy tube is blocked, the volume will be normal and the tympanogram may be normal (although it might also be rounded or retracted as in the case of serous otitis media), and the reflex might be present. Again, this is a simple test that helps determine whether the tympanostomy tube is functioning properly or not. Although visual inspection will show whether it is in place, only a measure such as acoustic immittance will indicate whether the ventilating tube is *functioning*.

Finally, since it has been shown that the acoustic reflex can be used to estimate threshold of hearing in adult subjects,[48,49] it is tempting to use the procedure with neonates who have a high probability of hearing loss to learn whether or not hearing is normal. The problem is that an absent acoustic reflex in the absence of overt clinical signs for otologic pathologic changes is a neonate may not mean severe to profound hearing loss, as it usually does in an adult. In an adult one can screen for middle ear pathologic change using tympanometry and/or otoscopy. In the neonate the absence of a fully formed osseous canal may obscure the presence of a middle ear condition or of unabsorbed tissue in the middle ear. The drum is difficult, at best, to visualize and pneumatic otoscopy may not be possible or reliable. In addition, the infant obviously cannot report other clinical signs (i.e., dizziness, feeling of fullness in the ear) that might indicate other types of conditions. Another problem, exemplified in an older population of children by Fitz-Zaland and Zink,[57] is that the reflex may be absent for no discernable reason. These authors screened 3,510 children for hearing and acoustic immittance findings, and reported that 30 percent of the children deemed to be normal had no acoustic reflex. Finally, the acoustic reflex may be absent simply because we are using the wrong stimuli and test procedures. Thus, while early investigators showed that it was certainly possible to obtain an acoustic reflex in neonates,[58] other authors[59,60] reported very low incidence figures for the reflex in neonates.

Recent studies[61-63] have demonstrated that use

of 660 Hz probe tone can enhance the detection of the acoustic reflex in neonates. The authors were very careful to control for equipment artifact, which can easily contaminate results, and they looked for the reflex with both ipsilateral and contralateral stimuli. Sprague et al.[62] found acoustic reflexes in 88 percent of their neonates with use of one or another stimulus. (They found reflexes in 83 percent of their subjects using broadband noise and a 660 Hz probe tone.) McMillan et al.[63] were able to detect acoustic reflexes in approximately 83 percent of their neonates using a 660 Hz probe tone and pure-tone ipsilateral reflex activators. When one corrects for the intensity at the ear drum (because of the smaller volume ear canal in the case of neonates), the level of the stimulus needed to activate the reflex is essentially the same for neonates and adults in these studies. In addition, when both pure-tones and noise were used, it took less intensity to activate the reflex using broad band noise than using pure tones. Thus, it will probably be possible to adapt the techniques used for predicting thresholds for adults for use with neonates. When using these techniques one must be extremely careful to avoid equipment artifact since the procedure used for detection of a reflex is the increased intensity in the ear canal. Any leakage of sound, abnormal crossover, or a synchronous burst of reflex activator stimulus with probe tone may result in an apparent increase in intensity, and thus a false interpretation of the reflex.

The use of tympanometry has also been suggested for evaluating middle ear function in neonates. However, studies by Paradise et al.,[64] Zarnoch and Balkany,[65] and Reichert et al.[66] have demonstrated potential problems with the procedure. Specifically, these investigators variously found lack of reliability, lack of interpretability of the tympanograms, and lack of agreement with otoscopic and/or surgical findings.

Sprague et al.[62] showed that tympanometric patterns can be highly repeatable with this population if care is taken with the instrumentation. They also showed that a majority of their tympanograms were notched ("W") using a 220 Hz probe, while a few at that frequency, and most of those at 66 Hz, were flat or had a normal shape. McMillan et al.[63] also observed notched patterns for their normal neonates. They found that when using a 220 Hz

probe tone when the tympanogram appeared to be flat, pulling the ear and thus straightening the canal tended to change the shape from flat to notched. However, these authors did not do correlative studies with otoscopy or surgical exploration, and thus it is not clear whether or not middle ear function was truly normal in these neonates. It is likely that tympanometric measurements can be misleading in the case of neonates. One may find tympanograms that are normal in appearance in the presence of middle ear effusion, and, conversely, one may find flat tympanograms when the middle ear function is normal. It is probable that the normal shape of neonatal tympanograms is notched using a 220 Hz probe tone, but more complete interpretations of the tympanograms cannot be made at this time. It is not possible to do static measurements with neonates since one cannot assume that their ear canals resemble the hard-walled cavity that is necessary as a first step in calibrating the device. From the above, it is clear that although acoustic immittance may provide useful information in the case of neonates, results must be interpreted with caution, and whenever possible should be confirmed with other test procedures. The most promising immittance test for neonates is the acoustic reflex, but further work still needs to be done to confirm the usefulness of this procedure for infants at risk.

## SUMMARY

Although acoustic immittance testing can be a valuable tool for the clinician, like any tool it can be misused and the subsequent results can be misleading. As with all electronic equipment, it must be calibrated at regular intervals to make certain that it is still functioning properly. Ambient air pressure reading should be made on a daily basis since a barometric pressure change may cause immittance readings to indicate improperly the middle ear pressure in a given patient.

Another source of potential error in interpretation occurs when there are mixed pathologic changes. In these cases, the results will be commensurate with the most peripheral lesion. For example, if a patient has any conductive pathologic condition, it is useless to use the acoustic reflex to differentiate between cochlear and retrocochlear conditions. As mentioned above, if the patient has a severe to profound sensorineural hearing loss, the acoustic reflex may be absent. The lack of reflex in these cases is due to insufficient intensity to elicit the reflex.

If care is taken to avoid the above errors, acoustic immittance can be an extremely valuable tool in the hands of the clinician. It requires minimal cooperation from patients (simply that they not jerk the probe out of the ear), it can be used when the patient is conscious or under medication, it is noninvasive, and it is quick. It provides a repeatable (numerically quantifiable) measurement that can be used during the initial diagnostic work-up or over time to monitor the course of a specific condition. For these reasons the wise clinician will use the acoustic immittance battery as part of his or her aural work-up.

# REFERENCES

1. Metz O: The acoustic impedance measured on normal and pathological ears. Acta Otolaryngol Suppl 63, 1946
2. Zwislocki J: Some measurements of the impedance of the eardrum. J Acoustic Soc Am 29:349, 1957
3. Zwislocki J: Acoustic measurement of the middle ear function. Ann Otol Rhinol Laryng. 70:599, 1961
4. Zwislocki J: An acoustic method for clinical examination of the ear. J Speech Hear Res 6:303, 1963
5. Terkildsen K, Nielsen S: An electroacoustic impedance measuring bridge for clinical use. Arch Otolaryngol 72:339, 1960
6. Shanks JE, Lilly DJ: An evaluation of tympanometric estimates of ear canal volume. J Speech Hear Res 24:557, 1981
7. Wilber LA: Static acoustic impedance measurements in differential diagnosis of auditory disorders. Presented at the 1972 ASHA Convention, San Francisco
8. Feldman AS: Eardrum abnormality and the measurement of middle ear function. Arch Otolaryngol 99:211, 1974
9. Jerger J, Anthony L, Jerger S, Mauldin L: Studies in impedance audiometry III, middle ear disorders. Arch Otolaryngol 99:165, 1974
10. Zwislocki J, Feldman A: Acoustic impedance of pathological ears. ASHA Monogr 15: 1970
11. Wilber LA, Goodhill V, Hogue AC: Diagnostic implication of acoustic impedance measurements. Presented at the 1969 ASHA Convention, Chicago
12. Jerger J: Clinical experience with impedance audiometry. Arch Otolaryngol 92:311, 1970
13. Shanks JE: Tympanometry. Ear Hearing 5:268, 1984
14. Lilly DV: Multiple frequency, multiple component tympanometry: new approaches to an old diagnostic problem. Ear Hearing 5:300, 1984
15. Borg E: On the neuronal organization of the acoustic middle ear reflex. A physiological and anatomical study. Brain Res 49:101, 1973
16. Borg E: Dynamic characteristics of the intra-aural muscle reflex. p. 236. In Feldman A, Wilber L: Acoustic Impedance and Admittance—The Measurement of Middle Ear Function. Williams & Wilkins, Baltimore, 1976
17. Lyon M: The central location of the motor neurons to the stapedius muscle in the cat. Brain Res 143:437, 1978
18. Jepsen O: Middle ear muscle reflexes in man. p. 193. In Jerger J (ed): Modern Developments in Audiology. Academic Press, New York, 1963
19. Dallos P: Dynamics of the acoustic reflex: phenomenological aspects. J Acoustic Soc Am 36:2175, 1964
20. Djupesland G: Electromyography of the tympanic muscles in man. Int Aud 4:33, 1965
21. Renval V, Liden G, Jungert S, Nilsson E: Impedance audiometry as a screening method in school children. Scand Audiom 2:133, 1973
22. McCandless GA, Thomas GK: Impedance audiometry as a screening procedure for middle ear disease. Trans Acad Ophthalmol Otolaryngol 78:98, 1974
23. Harker L, vonWagoner R: Application of impedance audiometry as a screening instrument. Acta Otolaryngol 77:198, 1974
24. Harford E, Bess FH, Bluestone CD, Klein JO: Impedance Screening for Middle Ear Disease in Children. Grune & Stratton, Orlando, FL, 1978
25. Bess FH: Impedance screening for children: a need for more research. Ann Otol Rhinol Laryngol Suppl 68 89:229, 1980
26. Northern J: Impedance screening: an integral part of hearing screening. Ann Otol Rhinol Laryngol Suppl 68 89:233, 1980
27. Roeser R, Northern J: Screening for hearing loss and middle ear disorders. p. 120. In Roser R, Downs M

(eds): Auditory Disorders in School Children. Thieme-Stratton, New York, 1981

28. American Speech-Language-Hearing Association: Guidelines for acoustic immittance screening of middle ear function. ASHA 21:283, 1978

29. Stool S: Medical relevancy of immittance measurements. Ear Hearing 5:309, 1984

30. Brooks D, Wooley H, Kanjilal GC: Hearing loss and middle ear disorders in patients with Down's syndrome (mongolism). J Ment Defic Res 16:21, 1972

31. Northern JL: Impedance screening in special populations, state of the art. In Harford ER, Bess FH, Bluestone CD, Klein J (eds): Impedance Screening for Middle Ear Disease in Children. Grune & Stratton, Orlando, FL, 1978

32. Feldman AS: Tympanometry — procedures, interpretations and variables. p. 103. In Feldman A, Wilber LA (eds): Acoustic Impedance and Admittance — The Measurement of Middle Ear Function. Williams & Wilkins, Baltimore, 1976

33. Metz O: Threshold of reflex contractions of muscles of the middle ear and recruitment of loudness. Arch Otolaryngol 55:536, 1952

34. Alberti P: The stapedial reflex estimation and the loudness recruitment phenomenon. Mayo Foundation Impedance Symposium (Zenith Hearing Inst. Corp., Chicago), 1972, pp. 269–281 1972

35. Wilber LA: Acoustic reflex measurement procedures, interpretations and variables. p. 197. In Feldman A, Wilber LA (eds): Acoustic Impedance and Admittance — The Measurement of Middle Ear Function. Williams & Wilkins, Baltimore, 1976

36. McCandless GA, Miller DL: Loudness discomfort in hearing aids. Nat Hearing Aid J 25:7, 1972

37. Esser G, Schunicht R: Kinder audiologische diagnostik zur anpassung von Horgeraten. *Hals Nasen Ohr* 21:369, 1973

38. Snow T, McCandless GA: The use of impedance measures in hearing aid selection. Nat Hearing Aid J 29:7, 1976

39. Greenfield DG, Wiley TL, Block MG: Acoustic-reflex dynamics and the loudness-discomfort level. J Speech Hear Dis 50:14, 1985

40. Anderson H, Barr B, Wedenberg E: Intra-aural reflexes in retrocochlear lesions. p. 48. In Hamburger CA, Wersall J (eds): Nobel Symposium 10, Disorders of the Skull Base Region. Almqvist and Wiksell, Stockholm, 1969

41. Anderson H, Barr B, Wedenberg E: Early diagnosis of VIIIth nerve tumors by acoustic reflex tests. Acta Otolaryngol 262:232, 1970

42. Wilson RH, McCullough JK, Lilly DJ: Acoustic-reflex adaptation: morphology and half-life data for subjects with normal hearing. J Speech Hear Res 27:586, 1984

43. Fowler CG, Wilson RH: Adaptation of the acoustic reflex. Ear Hearing 5:282, 1984

44. Olsen W, Stach B, Kurdziel S: Acoustic reflex decay in 10 second and 5 seconds for Meniere's disease patients and for VIIIth nerve tumor patients. Ear Hearing 2:180, 1981

45. Sanders J, Josey A, Glasscock M, Jackson C: The acoustic reflex test in cochlear and eighth nerve pathology ears. Laryngoscope 91:787, 1981

46. Jeppsen O: Studies on the acoustic stapedius reflex in man. Thesis, University of Aarhus, Denmark, 1955

47. McCandless GA, Allred PL: Tympanometry and emergence of the acoustic reflex in infants. In Harford ER, Bess FH, Bluestone CD, Klein JO (eds): Impedance Screening for Middle Ear Disease in Children. Grune & Stratton, Orlando, FL, 1978

48. Niemeyer W, Sesterhenn G: Calculating the hearing threshold from the stapedius reflex threshold for different sound stimuli. Audiology 13:421, 1974

49. Jerger J, Burney P, Mauldin L, Crump B: Predicting hearing loss from the acoustic reflex. J Speech Hear Dis 39:11, 1974

50. Keith R: An evaluation of predicting hearing loss from the acoustic reflex. Arch Otolaryngol 103:419, 1977

51. Popelka G, Margolis R, Wiley T: The effect of activating stimulus bandwidth on acoustic reflex thresholds. J Acoust Soc Am 59:153, 1976

52. Margolis R, Fox S, Lilly D, et al: The bivariate plotting procedure for hearing assessment with acoustic-reflex threshold measure. In Popelka GR (ed): Hearing Assessment with the Acoustic Reflex. Grune & Stratton, Orlando, FL, 1981

53. Popelka GR: Hearing Assessment with the Acoustic Reflex. Grune & Stratton, Orlando, FL, 1981

54. Bluestone CD: Assessment of eustachian tube function. p. 127. In Jerger J (ed): Handbook of Clinical Impedance Audiometry. American Electromedics, Dobbs Ferry, NY 1975

55. Holmquist J: Eustachian tube evaluation. p. 156. In Feldman A, Wilber LA (eds): Acoustic Impedance and Admittance — The Measurement of Middle Ear Function. Williams & Wilkins, Baltimore, 1976

56. Givens GD, Seidemann MF: Acoustic immittance testing of the eustachian tube. Ear Hearing 5:297, 1984

57. FitzZaland RE, Zink GD: A comparative study of hearing screening procedures. Ear Hearing 5: 205, 1984

58. McCandless GA, Allred PL: Tympanometry and

emergence of the acoustic reflex in infants. In Harford ER, Bess FH, Bluestone CD, Klein JO (eds): Impedance Screening for Middle Ear Disease in Children. Grune & Stratton, Orlando, FL, 1978

59. Bennett MJ: Acoustic impedance bridge measurements with the neonate. Br J Aud 9:117, 1978
60. Keith R, Bench RJ: Stapedial reflex in neonates. Scand Aud 7:187, 1978
61. Bennett MJ, Weatherby LA: Newborn acoustic reflexes to noise and pure-tone signals. J. Speech Hear Res 25:383, 1982
62. Sprague B, Wiley TL, Goldstein R: Tympanometric and acoustic-reflex studies in neonates. J Speech Hear Res 28:265, 1985
63. McMillan P, Bennett MJ, Marchant CD, Shurin PA: Ipsilateral and contralateral acoustic reflexes in neonates. Ear Hearing 6:320, 1985

64. Paradise JL, Smith CJ, Bluestone CD: Tympanometric detection of middle ear effusion in infants and young children. Pediatrics 58:198, 1976
65. Zarnoch JM, Balkany TJ: Tympanometric screening of a normal and intensive care unit newborns: validity and reliability. In Harford ER, Bess FH, Bluestone CD, Klein JO (eds): Impedance Screening for Middle Ear Disease in Children. Grune & Stratton, Orlando, FL, 1977
66. Reichert TJ, Cantekin EI, Riding KH, et al: Diagnosis of middle ear effusions in young infants by otoscopy and tympanometry. p. 81. In Harford ER, Bess FH, Bluestone CD, Klein JO (eds): Impedance Screening for Middle Ear Disease in Children. Grune & Stratton, Orlando, FL, 1977

# Pediatric Testing: Behavioral

# 15

## Wesley R. Wilson

Two convergent themes guide the recent interest in the early assessment of auditory function in infants. The first theme evolves from the increasing literature suggesting that even mild hearing loss during infancy and/or childhood may result in a measurable and permanent impairment, both physiological and in communication behaviors (see for example refs. 1–3). Likewise, carefully controlled research with animals has demonstrated in several species that the auditory system is modified after early auditory deprivation (see for example refs. 4–11). Although evidence of a causal relationship between brief periods of auditory deprivation (such as might be caused by otitis media) and language development is far from complete, early intervention would seem the prudent course of action *provided adequate assessment occurs.* Certainly, concern in the past has focused on procedures for early identification of hearing problems; however, the procedures developed such as neonatal screening, high-risk registry, and others have not been particularly well suited to the identification of mild loss nor have they always led to necessary and appropriate assessment with procedures that are sensitive indicators of threshold status.

The term "assessment" describes a detailed evaluation and description of abilities, and must be differentiated from "screening." The purpose of screening procedures is to define a subgroup of a total population that needs more detailed study (assessment). The more detailed study should facilitate appropriate intervention, complemented by continued assessment. The results of screening evaluations usually do not allow appropriate intervention if the best possible assessment is not completed as an intermediary step. (A case in point was the indiscriminate placement of hearing aids on infants following neonatal screening.) A corollary to this assumption is that assessment should not be limited to sensitivity measures only. In the hearing assessment of adults, the audiologist devotes substantial time to the determination of both air-conduction and bone-conduction hearing sensitivity, based on a medical model of disease. As audiologists have approached the assessment of infants in a clinical setting, the assumption has often been that the primary focus should be on hearing sensitivity. In fact, much of the literature is devoted to discussions of methodologies for determining hearing sensitivity in infants with greater precision. The point of this argument is not to minimize the information available in such assessment, but to say that a view of auditory function tied predominantly to sensitivity is totally inappropriate. We need only remind ourselves that central lesions of the auditory system may not manifest themselves in

**415**

changes in peripheral hearing sensitivity to realize one serious error in such a focus.

The second theme is that work in the past decade has demonstrated that infants possess substantially more sophisticated auditory capabilities than previously suspected or determined. In 1975, Cairns and Butterfield developed the argument that auditory assessment must recognize a new view of infants as active receptors of auditory information, who, if given the chance, will interact with and control their auditory environments.[12] In the clinical assessment of audition, historical precedent favored behavioral observation procedures without reinforcement, because of the lack of alternative methodologies. Thus, many clinicians continue to view the young infant as passively involved with the environment because the test methodology favors such a notion. Work in the last decade has demonstrated the error of this assumption. In fact, the infant has been shown to be an active receptor of auditory information, who, if given the chance, will interact with and control the auditory environment.

In addition, it has been shown that normally developing infants are evidencing learned changes in speech/sound discrimination at least as early as 6 months of age. For example, it has been shown that infants reared in Spanish-speaking environments make different discriminations at 6 months of age than infants reared in English-speaking environments, based on the linguistic rules of the respective language environment.[13] In a similar study, Werker and Tees compared the discrimination abilities of three different aged infant groups — 6 to 8 months, 8 to 10 months, and 10 to 12 months — and one adult group to nonnative speech contrasts drawn from the Hindi and Thompson languages.[14] Their results showed that 80 percent of the youngest infant group showed discrimination while only 30 percent of the adults reached criterion on the nonnative contrasts. The older infant group showed poorer performance than the younger infants and better performance than the adults. Werker et al. compared discrimination abilities of English-speaking adults, Hindi-speaking adults, and 6- to 7-month-old English-learning infants on two Hindi speech contrasts.[15] The Hindi adults and the English-learning infants were successful in discriminating both Hindi contrasts;

however, only a small number of the English-speaking adult subjects could make one of the Hindi discriminations and only 1 of 20 could make the second Hindi discrimination. Collectively, the results of these studies are consistent with an assumption that infants must certainly come into the world with the abilities to perceive salient cues in any language (since they do not have information immediately as to which language they will be learning), and then begin a perceptual reorganization during the first year of life based on their language environment. Evidence of this type suggests that substantial learned responses are occurring during very early childhood. Thus, in cases of suspected hearing loss, we can no longer assume that we have a "free" interval during which auditory input makes little difference in later learning.

Based on the above themes, recent advances in behavioral audiometry for children have centered on improved assessment procedures for infants. Before about 1970, it generally was believed that only gross behavioral hearing tests could be obtained on infants 2 years of age and younger. Refinements in methodology over the past few years have dramatically altered this view, as well as allowing us to understand better the auditory abilities of infants. It is now becoming possible to obtain complete behavioral assessment of auditory function in infants 6 months through 2 years of age.

Behavioral assessment of infants' auditory thresholds is based on observation of overt responses to controlled auditory signals. Two general approaches have been used clinically. They can be differentiated by whether or not reinforcement is used. When no reinforcement is used, the procedure is usually called behavior observation audiometry (BOA). As the name implies, this is a passive approach. The examiner observes changes in behavior (responses) that are time-locked to auditory signals, but does not assume an active "teaching" role. As an estimator of hearing sensitivity, the BOA procedure has inherent limitations because infant responses are not brought under stimulus control by the examiner. For neonates, suprathreshold stimulation is required to elicit reflexive responses such as startle or eye widening. Older infants demonstrate "awareness" or spontaneous head-turn responses at reasonably low intensity levels,[16-18] but the probability of obtaining a response is dependent on the nature of the auditory stimulus,[18-21] response habituation is likely,[22] and variability is high.[23] Even though BOA lacks precision as an indicator of hearing status, it is the only available behavioral procedure for some profoundly retarded children, or very young infants who cannot be conditioned to respond to auditory signals. In such cases, alternative electrophysiologic procedures must be considered.

When reinforcement is used, the testing approach is a form of operant conditioning in which the auditory signal (discriminative stimulus) cues the availability of reinforcement following the desired response behavior. Among conditioning procedures for infants, visual reinforcement audiometry (VRA) has emerged as a successful assessment tool for infants 6 months through 2 years of age. In this procedure, head turns toward a sound source are reinforced by an attractive visual stimulus (animated toy). Another reinforcement procedure makes use of a bar-press response coupled with either edible reinforcement or visual reinforcement and is called tangible reinforcement operant conditioning audiometry (TROCA).

The remaining sections of this chapter will explore the following: (1) the results of studies of infant audition that have used BOA or nonreinforced behavioral procedures; (2) comparisons of conjugate and operant reinforcement procedures; (3) effects of reinforcement on infant response behaviors; behavioral threshold testing; (4) behavioral suprathreshold testing; and (5) applications to clinical populations.

## BEHAVIOR OBSERVATION AUDIOMETRY

### Neonates

The use of BOA with neonates and very young infants requires attention to a number of factors. Eisenberg[19] has provided an excellent review. First, the state of the infant has a major effect on responsiveness. For example, in rating sleep in stages from deep sleep to fully awake, it has been demonstrated that the middle states allow the highest response ratios. In terms of signal factors, Eisenberg[19] reports that band-pass signals are better than pure tones; that low-frequency signals soothe the infant, whereas high-frequency signals distress the infant; that the response ratio of the infant increases with signal duration; and that rapid rise-time signals produce defense reflexes, whereas slow rise-time signals produce orienting responses. The factors used in determining a response are generally reflexive behaviors, for example, eye widening, blink, and arousal. Because a wide variety of response behaviors are monitored, one major difficulty is that the tester may be influenced by preinformation bias, that is, the examiner's expectations of the outcome of the test. For example, if an infant is seen whose history includes a normal Apgar score and normal pregnancy and family history, the expectation of the examiner is somewhat different than in the case of an infant born to deaf parents. Likewise, when the examiner is aware of the sound stimuli presentations, he or she adopts a different criterion in defining infant responses than in test protocols in which the examiner does not know when sound is presented, and in which "blind" control (no-sound) intervals are included. The potential effects of these forms of preinformation bias have been discussed.[24-27] Goldstein and Tait[24] and Weber[26] suggest procedural approaches that may reduce or remove the effects of these types of bias. One difficulty that remains, however, is that the signal levels used in BOA testing with neonates would, at best, identify only those infants with severe to profound losses. The testing does not provide results that allow adequate description of an infant's auditory function, nor any substantial information concerning habilitative needs.

### Infants and Young Children

A number of sources have described the application of BOA procedures to the developing infant. The procedures generally are discussed in terms of effectiveness of different signal types, the "development" of responses in infants, and the signal levels necessary to produce a response. A major emphasis is often placed on the "development" of the auditory response as a function of the signal level necessary to elicit a response. An example of this approach is illustrated by Northern and Downs.[28] They report that between the newborn period and 4 months of age, the normal infant is aroused from sleep by sound signals of 90 dB sound pressure level (SPL) in a noisy environment and 50 to 70 dB SPL in a quiet environment. They indicate that at approximately 3 to 4 months of age the normal infant begins to make a rudimentary head turn toward a sound signal of 50 to 60 dB SPL. From 4 to 7 months, the infant turns directly to the side of signal presentation at a level of 40 to 50 dB SPL. From 7 to 9 months, the infant directly locates a sound source of 30 to 40 dB to the side and below. From 9 to 13 months, the infant locates a sound source of 25 to 35 dB SPL to the side and below. From 13 to 16 months, the infant localizes sound signals of 25 to 30 dB SPL to the side, below, and indirectly above, and from 16 months to 21 months, the vertical localization improves. As can be seen in this sequence, the infant is depicted as showing a development of the localization response, as well as a marked shift in the level of signal necessary to produce the response.[28] This has led many practitioners to talk in terms of a pronounced development of auditory sensitivity in the first few years of life.

Another example of similar information is provided by Sweitzer,[29] and is shown in Figure 15-1. The minimal response level for speech is depicted as shifting from 70 dB SPL for a neonate, to 45 dB SPL for a 6-month-old infant, and finally reaching a response level similar to adults at 24 months of age. Put another way, the minimal response level for speech is shown to shift approximately 45 to 50 dB during the first 2 years of life. Again, this finding has sometimes been overinterpreted to mean that the infant's hearing sensitivity is shifting by this amount during the 2 years of infancy.

With reference to the issue of development of localization, Muir and Field and colleagues have presented an interesting series of studies demonstrating that neonates consistently will turn their heads toward a sound source.[30–33] Their experimental procedure involved the use of video scoring and other controls for potential observer bias. In most cases, the latency of the neonates' responses was long: 2.5 seconds to the beginning of the head-

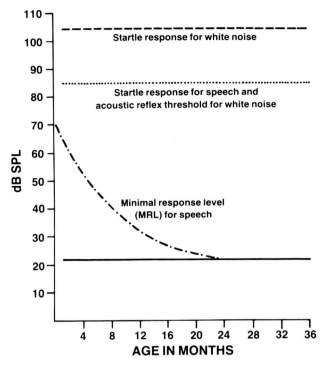

**Fig. 15-1.** Response levels for speech as a function of age. ( Sweitzer RS: Audiologic evaluation of the infant and young child. In Jaffe BF (ed): Hearing Loss in Children. © 1977 The Williams & Wilkins Co., Baltimore.)

turn response and 5.5 seconds to the end of the response. Another finding of interest in their longitudinal study of infants was that the localization responses tended to decline at 2 to 3 months of age and return strongly at 4 months. Comparing these collective findings of Muir and colleagues to the literature in pediatric audiology, one is struck by the fact that our ideas about the development of localization responses may have seriously underestimated the actual abilities of infants. No clinical application of the work of Muir et al. has been undertaken yet, and it is to be emphasized that their studies were for the purpose of studying the localization behavior of infants. The findings remain provocative, however.

Another major theme in the BOA literature is the relative effectiveness of different signals, again as a function of age. Table 15-1 from Northern and Downs,[28] provides one summary of this type of information. Observe, for example, the 4 to 7-month

**Table 15-1. Response Levels as a Function of Signal and Age**

| Age | Noisemakers (Approx. SPL, in dB) | Warbled Pure Tones (Re Audiometric Zero) | Speech (Re: Audiometric Zero) |
| --- | --- | --- | --- |
| 0–6 weeks | 50–70 | 78 dB (SD = 6 dB) | 40–60 dB |
| 6 weeks–4 months | 50–60 | 70 dB (SD = 10 dB) | 47 dB (SD = 2 dB) |
| 4–7 months | 40–50 | 51 dB (SD = 9 dB) | 21 dB (SD = 8 dB) |
| 7–9 months | 30–40 | 45 dB (SD = 15 dB) | 15 dB (SD = 7 dB) |
| 9–13 months | 25–35 | 38 dB (SD = 8 dB) | 8 dB (SD = 7 dB) |
| 13–16 months | 25–30 | 32 dB (SD = 10 dB) | 5 dB (SD = 5 dB) |
| 16–21 months | 25 | 25 dB (SD = 10 dB) | 5 dB (SD = 1 dB) |
| 21–24 months | 25 | 26 dB (SD = 10 dB) | 3 dB (SD = 2 dB) |

(Northern JL, Downs MP: Hearing in Children. © 1978, The Williams & Wilkins Co., Baltimore.)

age frame, and note that an infant will respond to speech at 21 dB relative to normal adult thresholds, while responding to warbled pure tones at 51 dB relative to audiometric zero. This difference of 30 dB is an indication of the relative inefficiency of warbled pure tones for producing appropriate auditory thresholds using a BOA approach. Table 15-1 illustrates again the marked changes in signal intensities necessary to produce responses over the first 2 years of life using the BOA procedure. Using warbled pure tones as an example, the shift is 52 dB. This shift has sometimes been discussed from the point of view of "auditory development." Data from test procedures using reinforcement would suggest an interpretation showing the major portion of this shift as a function of test methodology, and not of marked changes in true hearing sensitivity.

In another study on the relative effectiveness of different test stimuli with infants, Thompson and Thompson compared a speech signal, filtered speech signal, white noise, filtered white noise, and a 3,000 Hz pure tone.[18] As is evident in Figure 15-2, the speech signal produced the highest percentage of responses in infants 7 to 12 months of age, with the pure tone producing the fewest responses. For the most part, the signals showed similar efficiency regardless of the presentation level of the signal. Note, however, that in this BOA procedure the most efficient signal, speech, produced fewer than 50 percent responses at an HL of 15 dB in infants aged 7 to 12 months. Looking at results from the same study with older infants in Figure 15-3, one again finds a clear difference in the effectiveness of various signals, with speech producing the highest percentage of responses and the 3,000 Hz pure tone producing the fewest responses. For

the older infants, the overall percentage of response is increased for all signals compared to the younger infants. Note, however, that for even the most efficient signals, the response rate remains at a level of 65 to 75 percent for signals at 15 dB hearing level (HL) in this unreinforced test paradigm.

Another area of concern involving the BOA procedure is intra- and intersubject variability. Thompson and Weber presented data on both topics.[23] Using a band-pass filtered complex-noise signal, they reported intrasubject variability of

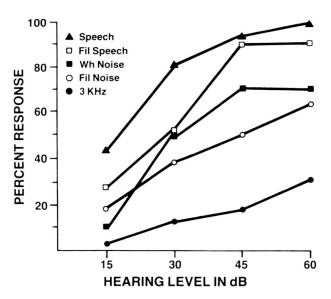

**Fig. 15-2.** Percentage response to five stimuli as a function of hearing level: 7 to 12 months of age. (Thompson M, Thompson G: Response of infants and young children as a function of auditory stimuli and test methods. J Speech Hear Res 15:699, 1972.)

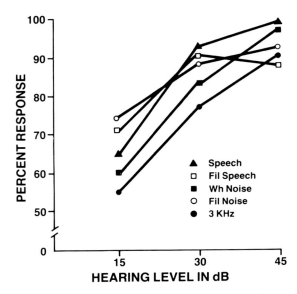

**Fig. 15-3.** Percentage response to five stimuli as a function of hearing level: 22 to 36 months of age. (Thompson M, Thompson G: Response of infants and young children as a function of auditory stimuli and test methods. J Speech Hear Res 15:699, 1972.)

more than 20 dB for three signal presentations in one-third of their subjects, ranging in age from 3 months through 5 years. Generally, trial 1 produced the best threshold, with succeedingly poorer (higher) thresholds in trials 2 and 3. The clinical import of this finding is that use of the BOA procedure allows one a very limited number of responses for answering clinical questions. Furthermore, the wide intrasubject variability makes it difficult to consider test-retest situations, for example, in monitoring the effectiveness of drug therapy in treatment of middle-ear problems.

In terms of intersubject variability, the same study illustrated a wide spread in obtained BOA "thresholds" from infants and young children of similar ages with presumed normal hearing.[23] For example, in infants 3 to 5 months, the dispersion between the 10th and 90th percentile is on the order of 65 dB, as can be seen in Figure 15-4. From 6 through 18 months, the dispersion remains substantial. This wide intersubject variability is one of the major limiting factors in the use of BOA. If a population of normally developing infants yields a range of responses that encompasses nearly the total measurement range used in hearing assessment, it is impossible to define hearing loss as a change or deviation from this "norm." That is, the essence of hearing assessment is to find a procedure and signal that yield a very tight grouping of scores for a normal population, with a wide range available for defining abnormal scores. The BOA procedure does not meet this goal. As Thompson and Weber point out in their study[23]:

> BOA thresholds may well tend to underestimate the extent of a child's hearing. That is, the child who does not respond below 50 dB HL may well have a "true threshold" somewhat below this

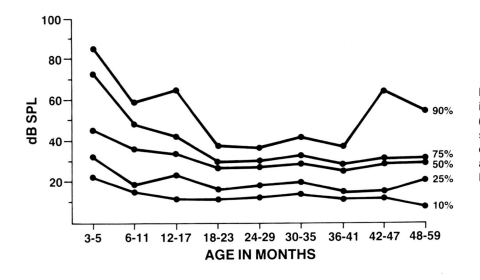

**Fig. 15-4.** Intersubject variability in BOA as a function of age. (Thompson G, Weber BA: Responses of infants and young children to behavior observation audiometry (BOA). J Speech Hear Dis 39:140, 1974.)

level. Unfortunately, there is no way to determine an appropriate correction factor for an individual child. Put in proper perspective, BOA is probably best viewed as a screening assessment procedure.

Finally, the problem of observer bias again manifests itself with clinical populations of older children. Gans and Flexer studied observer bias in the BOA testing of profoundly involved multiply handicapped children and reported clear bias effects in the testing of 85 percent of the children as a function of the examiners being aware of the stimulus type and intensity.[34] They suggest that the effects of this particular form of bias can be reduced by using a video-scoring procedure in which the examiners are unaware of stimulus events.

Interpretations of previous behavioral data, generated through use of the BOA procedure, allow us to make the following summary statements:

1. The potential for observer bias in judging responses complicates the task.
2. The obtained thresholds improve substantially as a function of age.
3. The obtained thresholds vary substantially as a function of signal used: pure tones are not an effective signal.
4. Infants and young children habituate to the test stimulus, which results in large intrasubject variability in a substantial number of cases.
5. A substantial variability in threshold estimates occurs across infants; this variability makes it difficult to establish "norms" using the BOA procedure.

## OPERANT CONDITIONING

Among the difficulties that occur as a result of use of BOA, two stand out. The first is that a variety of responses are used, making response judgment problematic. The second is that any pediatric audiometric test procedure is dependent upon the infant continuing to show consistent responses to sound over a number of presentations. In the BOA procedure it is apparent that sound is not a highly motivating signal for continued or consistent re-

sponse behavior. First, the infant does not necessarily respond at or near threshold and, second, the infant quickly habituates to repeated signal presentations.

To overcome these shortcomings, one can consider the selection of a single response coupled with reinforcement to increase the number of responses. Two operant conditioning approaches have been used for this purpose: conjugate procedures and operant discrimination procedures. In conjugate procedures, the stimulus follows the response as a consequence and is the reinforcer. Conversely, in an operant discrimination paradigm, the stimulus is used to cue the infant that a response will produce reinforcement. Any reinforcer may be used.

### Conjugate Procedures

An example of application of the conjugate procedure is contained in a study by Eisele and colleagues.[35] They connected a nonnutritive nipple (pacifier), used as a pressure transducer, to a Bekesy-type audiometer so that the sucking behavior of the infant would control the intensity of the pulsed pure-tone signals. The signal was delivered through a loudspeaker positioned over the infant's crib. This conjugate procedure allowed the intensity of a continuously available reinforcing stimulus to vary as a function of the sucking-response rate. Sucking rates equal to or higher than baseline rates resulted in a 5 dB/sec intensity increase; cessation of sucking resulted in an intensity decrease. Figure 15-5 shows a tracing from a 36-hour-old infant, which demonstrates five reversals or cessations of sucking;[35] the arrows correspond to behavioral responses scored by observers as a means of a validity judgment. Certain infants were also seen 24 hours later and produced comparable results. It is interesting to note that although this procedure was described in 1975, the results have not been replicated to my knowledge, and it has not been adapted as a procedure for clinical evaluation of neonates. Friedlander also has described the application of conjugate procedures in what he calls "the playtest for selective listening."[36,37]

A major drawback of conjugate procedures for threshold determination is that the sound stimuli used for assessment are not particularly reinforcing

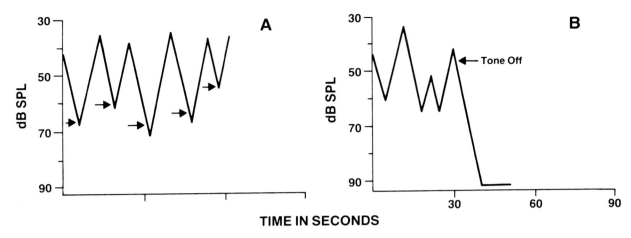

**Fig. 15-5.** Békésy tracings from sucking behavior of a 36-hour-old infant. Arrows indicate behavioral responses. ( Eisele WA, Berry RC, Shriner TH: Infant sucking response patterns as a conjugate function of changes in the sound pressure level of auditory stimuli. J Speech Hear Res 18:296, 1975.)

for normally developing infants. Since conjugate procedures require that the stimulus serve as a reinforcer, this may be considered a fatal drawback in terms of their usefulness as a clinical test of auditory threshold. However, the conjugate procedures might have considerable application to tasks of auditory preference carried out at suprathreshold levels.

### Operant Discrimination Procedures

As noted above, in this category of procedures the stimulus is independent of the reinforcer; the stimulus cues the infant that a response will immediately produce reinforcement. One is free to select the most potent reinforcer for the particular age of infant being tested. In selecting a response to use with the procedure, one obviously must consider the neuromuscular development of the infant to be tested. Among the response repertoire available, the leg swing can be used with very young infants; a head turn is a natural response mode for infants aged 4 to 6 months and older (see, however, the previous comments on auditory localization); and the bar-press response has been used with infants as young as 7 to 8 months and older. The leg-swing response has not been used extensively,

nor does it, at present, seem applicable in the clinical process because a substantial number of training sessions are required to bring the response under stimulus control.

The head-turn response has been used extensively. Figures 15-6A through 15-6C illustrate a common use of this in the VRA task. In Figure 15-6A, the assistant holds the infant's attention at midline. When the infant is in a response-ready state, a sound is introduced, in this case through a loudspeaker to the left of the infant at an angle of approximately 45 degrees from the midline position. Figure 15-6B shows the head-turn response followed by the visual reinforcer in Figure 15-6C.

Use of the bar-press procedure, coupled with food reinforcement, is illustrated in Figures 15-7A through 15-7D. In Figure 15-7A, the sound stimulus has been presented, and the infant responds by pressing the manipulandum. The correct response coupled to the stimulus presentation results in reinforcement: Figure 15-7B. The reinforcement includes a light to draw the infant's attention to the area where the food is presented, and then the food bit. Figures 15-7C and 15-7D show completion of the process. In Figure 15-8, the bar-press response is shown coupled with a visual reinforcer. In this case, a correct response (hit) provides a short duration of visual reinforcement.

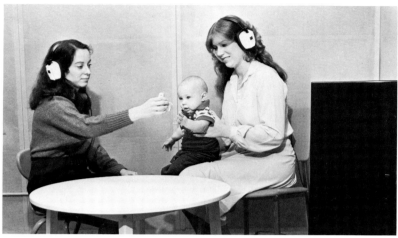

A

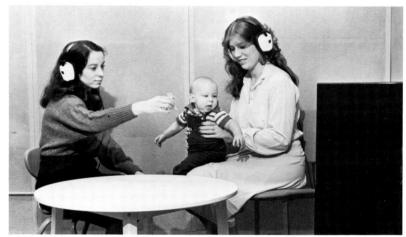

B

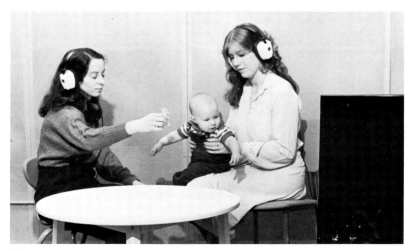

C

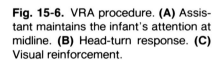

**Fig. 15-6.** VRA procedure. **(A)** Assistant maintains the infant's attention at midline. **(B)** Head-turn response. **(C)** Visual reinforcement.

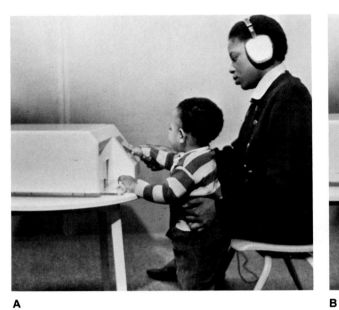

A

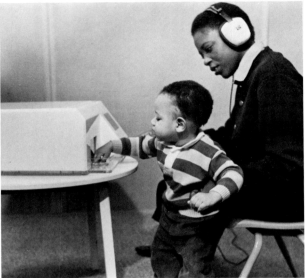

B

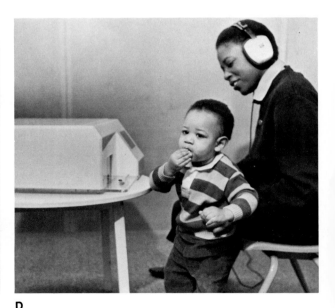

C

D

**Fig. 15-7.** TROCA procedure. **(A)** Infant presses manipulandum. **(B)** Food reinforcement. **(C, D)** Infant completes task.

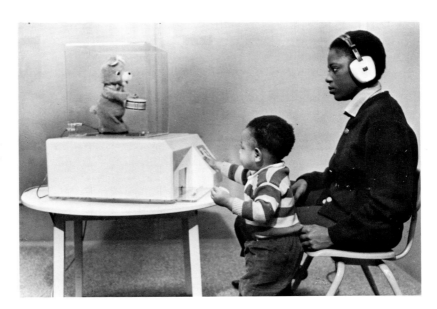

**Fig. 15-8.** VROCA procedure: bar-press response with visual reinforcement.

## VISUAL REINFORCEMENT AUDIOMETRY

### Historical Perspective

Normally developing infants make head turns toward a sound source in the first few months of life. The localization response represents a behavioral "window" through which many aspects of auditory behavior can be studied. If an infant's localization behavior deviates markedly from the normal developmental pattern, there is strong reason to suspect either hearing loss or other problems, such as mental retardation. While there is a decided tendency for infants to turn initially toward "interesting" or "novel" auditory stimuli, there is a limit to the number of times head turns will occur to repeated stimuli.[22,38] From a hearing-assessment standpoint, habituation of response to repeated stimulus presentations is undesirable because it reduces the number of stimulus trials available for threshold determination.

Suzuki and Ogiba[39,40] were the first to report on a conditioning procedure involving the localization response. The procedure was called *conditioned orientation reflex (COR)* audiometry and was based on the observation that infants will reflexively turn their heads toward a strange auditory or visual stimulus. In the initial stages of conditioning, a pure tone was presented through a loudspeaker at an intensity level estimated to be 30 to 40 dB above the infant's threshold. One second later a visual stimulus (illuminated doll) was presented from the same location. The combined tone and light stimulus lasted for about 4 seconds. After a few conditioning trials, the timing sequence was changed so that the visual stimulus followed the auditory stimulus and was presented only if the child had first responded to the tone. It was presumed that the visual stimulus served to reinforce head-turn responses leading to successful threshold estimates for over 80 percent of children in the 1- to 3-year age category. The success rate was less than 50 percent for infants under 1 year of age.

Liden and Kankkunen were the first to use the term VRA to describe a modified COR procedure they developed.[41] Since they accepted any type of response behavior that could be judged (at least for young infants), and always provided "reinforcement," their procedure differed markedly from that described by Suzuki and Ogiba. Even though Liden and Kankkunen used the term VRA to describe a specific test protocol, the term has come to be used in a generic sense to describe a class of procedures involving the use of visual stimuli as reinforcers. We believe that the term VRA is more appropriate than COR for describing this general category of tests because we have been able to use the head-turn response and visual reinforcement with some infants and older retarded children who did not initially show an orienting-localization response to sound, but could be taught this response.

A number of other authors have also reported on the use of VRA procedures for assessment of hearing sensitivity in infants and young children.[42,43] Generally, these studies suggest that the lower age limit for widespread use of this procedure is 12 months, although Haug and colleagues reported clinical success with a small number of infants in the 5- to 12-month range.

### Effectiveness of Visual Reinforcement

While the above-mentioned studies provided support for the use of VRA, there remained doubt as to the specific reinforcing value of the visual stimulus because control (no reinforcement) groups were not included for comparison. Also, it was not clear if the type of visual stimulus used had any bearing on its effectiveness as a reinforcer. Moore et al. studied auditory localization behavior as a function of four reinforcement conditions: (1) no reinforcement; (2) social reinforcement (a smile, verbal praise, and/or a pat on the shoulder); (3) simple visual reinforcement (a blinking red light); and (4) complex visual reinforcement (a colorful, animated toy bear that danced in place and beat a drum when activated).[22] The subjects were 48 normal infants between 12 and 18 months of age. They were classified into groups of 12 and assigned to one of the four reinforcement conditions. Each subject sat on the parent's lap in the center of the test room. A test-room examiner kept the infant's attention focused to the front by means of soft, colorful toys. Each subject received 30 complex-noise stimulus presentations at 70 dB SPL from a loudspeaker at a 45 degree angle from the

infant's front line of vision. Following each appropriate head-turn response, subjects in the experimental groups received social or visual reinforcement. The control group received no reinforcement. Interspersed among the 30 test trials were 10 control trials, during which the test-room and control-room examiners recorded whether or not the infant turned toward the loudspeaker in the absence of an auditory stimulus.

Results of test trials are shown in Figure 15-9. The mean number of responses for the complex visual reinforcement, simple visual reinforcement, social reinforcement, and no reinforcement groups was 27.3, 20.5, 15.2, and 9.7, respectively, all of which are significantly different from each other. It should be noted that among the reinforcement groups, the complex reinforcement group in particular continued to show a high rate of response, averaging 8 responses during the last 10 stimulus presentations. In contrast, the control group habituated rapidly and showed only a few responses during the last 15 trials. The range of responses for

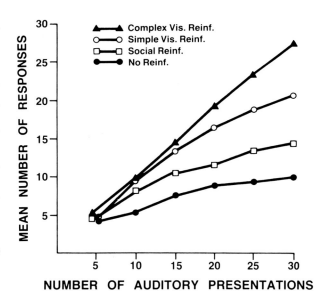

**Fig. 15-9.** Cumulative mean head-turn responses in blocks of stimulus trials as a function of reinforcement condition in 48 infants 12 to 18 months of age. (Moore JM, Thompson G, Thompson M: Auditory localization of infants as a function of reinforcement conditions. J Speech Hearing Dis 40:29, 1975.)

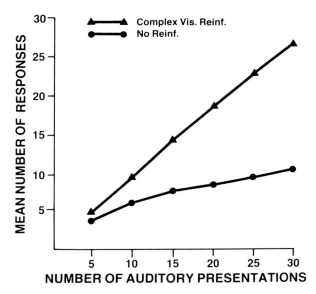

**Fig. 15-10.** Cumulative mean head-turn responses in blocks of stimulus trials as a function of reinforcement condition in 20 infants 7 to 11 months of age. (Moore JM, Wilson WR, Thompson G: Visual reinforcement of head-turn responses in infants under 12 months of age. J Speech Hear Dis 42:328, 1977.)

the complex reinforcement group was from 13 to 30, as contrasted to a range of 5 to 16 for the no reinforcement group. Subjects randomly looked toward the sound source only 4.8 percent of the time during the control trials, that is, when no auditory stimulus was presented. Therefore, random behavior was ruled out as a major factor accounting for the number of positive responses obtained using the various reinforcement conditions. The results of this study indicate that auditory localization behavior of 12 to 18-month-old infants is strongly influenced by reinforcement, and that the type of reinforcement used has a systematic differentiated effect on head-turn response behavior. Visual stimuli containing movement, color, and contour are more apt to be effective reinforcers than less dimensional visual stimuli.

In a follow-up study, Moore et al. used the same complex visual reinforcer (animated toy) and a similar experimental design to explore the lower-age boundary of VRA.[38] Sixty normal infants were classified into three groups based on age. Group 1 con-

tained infants 7 through 11 months of age (6 months, 16 days, through 11 months, 15 days), group 2 contained 5- and 6-month olds, and group 3 contained 4-month olds. Within each age group, there were 10 experimental subjects (visual reinforcement) and 10 control subjects (no reinforcement). Results are shown in Figures 15-10 to 15-12. Differences between the experimental and control groups were significant for 7 to 11 and 5 to 6 month-old groups. The difference between groups at 4 months of age was not significant. These data imply that a complex visual stimulus can be used to reinforce localization behavior of infants as young as 5 months of age.

Whereas the previous studies explored the relative effectiveness of reinforcement and no reinforcement conditions in a cross-sectional design, the same question can be approached in a single-subject design using a reversal paradigm. The strength of this approach rests on the fact that the subject serves as his or her own control. If reinstatement of treatment (in this case, reinforce-

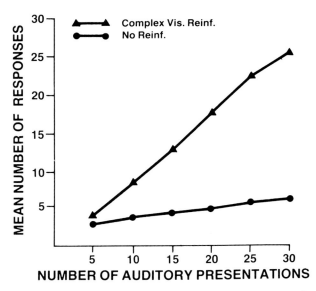

**Fig. 15-11.** Cumulative mean head-turn responses in blocks of stimulus trials as a function of reinforcement condition in 20 infants 5 and 6 months of age. (Moore JM, Wilson WR, Thompson G: Visual reinforcement of head-turn responses in infants under 12 months of age. J Speech Hear Dis 42:328, 1977.)

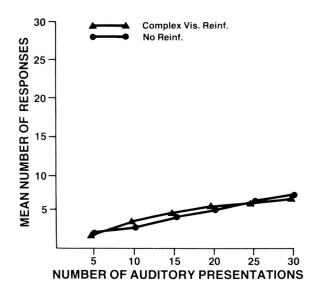

**Fig. 15-12.** Cumulative mean head-turn responses in blocks of stimulus trials as a function of reinforcement condition in 20 infants 4 months of age. (N=20) (Moore JM, Wilson WR, Thompson G: Visual reinforcement of head-turn responses in infants under 12 months of age. J Speech Hear Dis 42:328, 1977.)

ment) following habituation of the response results in an increased rate of response, one can properly assign that effect to the treatment. Two 6 month-olds served as subjects in a study using a single-subject design.[44] All conditions were identical to the previously described study, except for the distribution of reinforcement and no reinforcement trials. Each subject first received five signal presentations coupled with reinforcement for correct responses. The reinforcement contingency was then removed for the next 15 trials and, as is apparent in Figure 15-13, both infants stopped responding within that interval and their behavior stabilized in a no-response mode. On trial 21, the visual reinforcer was coupled with the auditory signal serving as a teaching trial. For the remaining nine trials, each correct response earned reinforcement and, as illustrated, both infants responded at a 100 percent rate. These data provide a powerful demonstration of the strength of this reinforcement procedure for 6-month-old infants.

Thompson and Folsom and Primus and Thompson have also studied the effectiveness of various signals in the VRA paradigm.[45,46] Both studies found that whereas stimulus characteristic plays an important role in eliciting spontaneous responses, they do not appear to influence response behavior after conditioning has been established. In contrast to BOA, the examiner may select signal type based on the clinical exigencies of the case and not be restricted because of a fear of degrading response behavior.

## Soundfield Threshold Assessment

Wilson and colleagues studied soundfield auditory thresholds using VRA.[44] Ninety normally developing infants between 5 and 18 months were classified into groups of 15, according to age. The auditory stimulus was complex noise, and threshold sampling followed a protocol of attenuating the signal 20 dB after each positive head-turn response and increasing the signal 10 dB after each failure to respond. Control intervals were included as before. All appropriate responses were visually reinforced (animated toy). Threshold was defined as the lowest presentation level at which the infant responded a minimum of three times out of a maximum of six signal presentations. Results are shown in Figure 15-14 and are reported in dB SPL. (Note: audiometric thresholds and intensity levels are reported in dB SPL, since no standard exists for converting these values into comparable HL. For comparative purposes, the modal threshold of normal hearing young adult listeners was 20 dB SPL, with a range of 10 to 20 dB SPL, under the same signal and measurement-step conditions.) As can be noted, the average response levels improved slightly with age, ranging from 21 to 29 dB SPL. The 10th and 90th percentile points were 20 and 40 dB SPL for the 5 month-olds and 20 and 30 dB SPL for the 6 to 18-month-olds. Compared to thresholds obtained by BOA for the same ages,[23] the VRA thresholds are lower. Of far greater importance is the reduced variability of response associated with the VRA procedure. For infants 6 months old and above, the range between the 10th and 90th percentile is reduced from the 45 to 50 dB reported for BOA to 10 dB (or one measurement step) for VRA.

Of further interest, from the point of view of clinical applicability, was that a total of 94 infants was tested to complete the sample reported. The data on three infants were not considered because

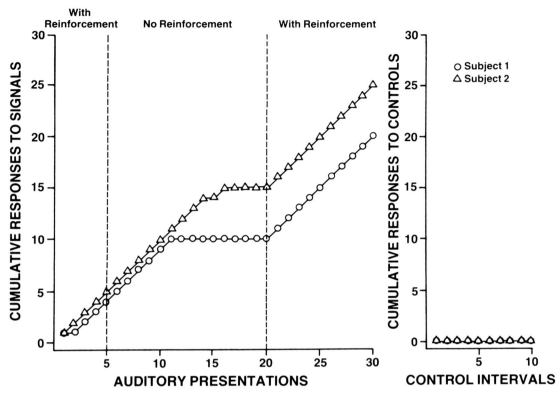

**Fig. 15-13.** Infant head-turn responses as a function of reinforcement: single subject design. (Wilson WR, Moore JM, Thompson G: Sound-field auditory thresholds of infants utilizing visual reinforcement audiometry [VRA]. Paper presented at the American Speech and Hearing Association Convention, Houston, 1976.)

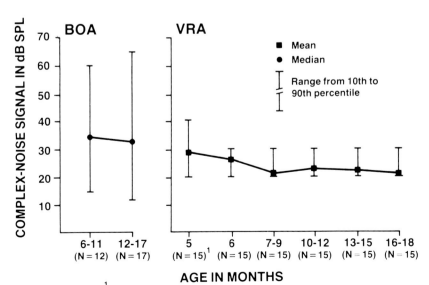

**Fig. 15-14.** Auditory thresholds of infants as obtained by BOA and VRA methods. (Wilson WR, Moore JM, Thompson G: Sound-field auditory thresholds of infants utilizing visual reinforcement audiometry [VRA]. Paper presented at the American Speech and Hearing Association Convention, Houston, 1976.)

[1] Six of the fifteen did not complete test--datum based on nine subjects

of more than one false-positive response during the control intervals. (The average number of control intervals was 4.6 and the average number of false-positive responses was 0.37.) All but one infant 6 months of age and older yielded thresholds in one visit, with the exception requiring two visits. The clinical implications of this study are substantial: (1) thresholds obtained from infants do not vary dramatically as a function of age and are elevated only slightly from those obtained from adults using the same test protocol; (2) even more importantly, the range of thresholds for the population of presumed normal-hearing infants was very small, indicating that the values obtained can serve a usable function as clinical norms, a finding in direct contrast to the very wide dispersion demonstrated for BOA procedures; and (3) the procedure is economical of time and highly applicable to infants 6 months of age and older.

Whereas the above study used a broad-band signal, Wilson and Moore investigated the use of VRA with pure-tone stimuli in a soundfield.[47] Two groups of 15 normally developing infant subjects aged 6 to 7 months and 12 to 13 months, were selected by the same criteria as in our previous studies. Pure tones of 500, 1,000, and 4,000 Hz with a 5 percent warble served as the auditory stimuli. (This study also included an earphone condition, which is described later in this chapter; the

order of the soundfield and earphone conditions was counterbalanced.) Threshold measurement involved the same protocol described previously. Figure 15-15 provides the pure-tone soundfield thresholds for the two age groups of infants. As is apparent, thresholds do not vary systematically as a function of age, at least, given the 10-dB step size used in this experiment. The results obtained for the two groups of infants were collapsed and compared to a group (N = 10) of young adults, tested with the same protocol and step size, as shown in Figure 15-16. The difference in obtained thresholds is from 5 to 12 dB, depending on frequency, with the range of responses similar between the two groups. This study demonstrates that a pure-tone signal can be used successfully with infants and that the obtained thresholds do not vary dramatically from those of adults. The differences between these findings and those of earlier studies using BOA, with reference to the use of pure-tone stimuli, demonstrate the important effect of methodology.

In a study similar to that of Wilson and Moore, accomplished in a different laboratory, Goldman also used VRA with infants 6 to 12 months of age.[48] His test protocol was similar to that used by Wilson and Moore, including the use of control trials. Warbled (5 percent) pure-tone signals of 500, 1,000, 2,000, and 4,000 Hz were presented in a sound-

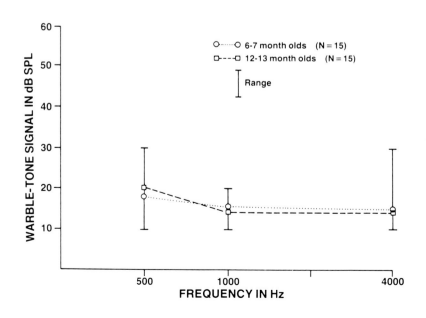

**Fig. 15-15.** VRA pure-tone soundfield thresholds in infant groups. (Wilson WR, Moore JM: Pure-tone earphone thresholds of infants utilizing visual reinforcement audiometry [VRA]. Paper presented at the American Speech and Hearing Association Convention, San Francisco, 1978.)

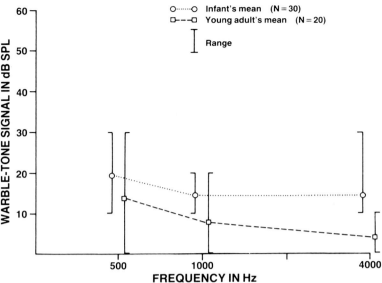

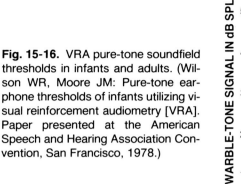

**Fig. 15-16.** VRA pure-tone soundfield thresholds in infants and adults. (Wilson WR, Moore JM: Pure-tone earphone thresholds of infants utilizing visual reinforcement audiometry [VRA]. Paper presented at the American Speech and Hearing Association Convention, San Francisco, 1978.)

field test environment. Of the 29 infants studied, 23 were tested successfully at all four frequencies in one visit. For the remaining six subjects, two yielded thresholds at three test frequencies, two provided thresholds at two frequencies, one at a single frequency, and one gave no thresholds. The mean thresholds were 17 dB SPL at 500 Hz, 14 dB SPL at 1,000 Hz, 17 dB SPL at 2,000 Hz, and 15 dB SPL at 4,000 Hz. Figure 15-17 provides a compari-

son of the Goldman and Wilson and Moore data, with both data sets plotted relative to young adult thresholds for the same signal and protocol conditions.[47,48] As can be noted, there is excellent agreement across studies accomplished in two different settings by two independent research groups, which lends support to the validity of the findings.

These soundfield studies used a test paradigm modeled on the clinical protocol used with adults

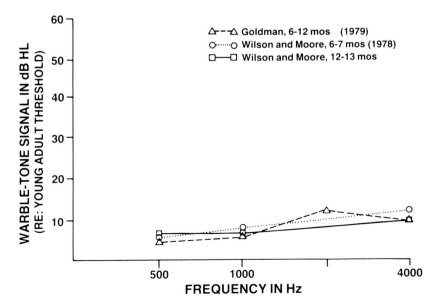

**Fig. 15-17.** VRA pure-tone soundfield threshold agreement across studies using a clinical protocol. (Data from Wilson WR, Moore JM: Pure-tone earphone thresholds of infants utilizing visual reinforcement audiometry [VRA]. Paper presented at the American Speech and Hearing Association Convention, San Francisco, 1978; Goldman TM: Response of infants to warble-tone signals presented in soundfield using visual reinforcement audiometry. Master's thesis, University of Cincinnati, 1979.)

and had as their main purpose the development of clinical procedures for infant auditory assessment. A modification of the VRA procedure described above has been developed by Trehub and colleagues for studying basic auditory function in infants.[49-51] Instead of using the fixed-interval discrimination task, as developed in our lab, they use a turn-left/turn-right localization task with unlimited duration stimulus intervals. Specifically, when the infant is looking directly ahead, a sound is presented from one of two loudspeakers located 45 degrees to each side of the infant. The sound is terminated when the infant turns his or her head 45 degrees to either side. If the head turn is correct (to the side of the sound) the response is reinforced. They describe the procedure as a two-alternative forced-choice signal detection task and use group data to plot psychometric functions for infant auditory thresholds.

Using half-octave and octave bands of noise as signals, Schneider et al. have used their procedure to chart infant hearing sensitivity from 200 through 19,000 Hz.[50,51] Figure 15-18 provides a comparison of various data, as well as illustrating the overall pattern of the infant's sensitivity curve as developed by Trehub and colleagues.[47,48,51] In comparing the infant results to those of adults in the same procedure, Schneider and colleagues report the greatest infant/adult differences in the low frequencies, with the infant thresholds equaling adult

thresholds at the highest frequencies they studied.[50,51] They postulate that the course of development in infant auditory sensitivity may be occurring primarily in the low frequencies.

Several caveats should be considered relative to this interpretation, however. First, this presumes that the adult sensitivity has not declined in the high frequencies. Recent work with pure-tone frequencies through 20,000 Hz suggests this is not true.[52] Next, use of localization judgments for each signal presentation, as in the Trehub-Schneider procedure, may be problematic. Localization cues are frequency dependent, with interaural time differences predominating in the low frequencies and intensity differences in the high frequencies. Thus, results obtained with this procedure may reflect different infant abilities in the two areas of time and intensity resolution. It also should be noted that the use of a soundfield procedure that requires localization to both the right and left would be difficult for many clinical cases. For example, cases of unilateral loss or differences in sensitivity between the two ears would present difficulties.

Another example of an operant conditioning paradigm makes use of a bar-press response coupled with edible reinforcement and is called TROCA. In 1968, Lloyd and co-workers described the use of TROCA with three normally developing infants 7, 15, and 18 months of age.[53] Fulton et al., using pure tones and earphone presentation, stud-

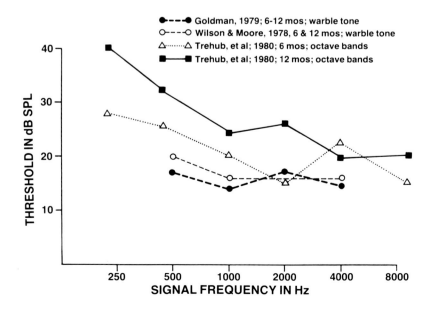

**Fig. 15-18.** VRA soundfield thresholds across studies with differing methodologies. (Data from Wilson WR, Moore JM: Pure-tone earphone thresholds of infants utilizing visual reinforcement audiometry [VRA]. Paper presented at the American Speech and Hearing Association Convention, San Francisco, 1978; Goldman TM: Response of infants to warble-tone signals presented in soundfield using visual reinforcement audiometry. Master's thesis, University of Cincinnati, 1979; Trehub SE, Schneider BA, Endman M: Developmental changes in infants' sensitivity to octave-band noises. J Exp Child Psychol 29:282, 1980.)

ied 12 children between 9 and 25 months of age with a median age of 12 months and found the procedure to be successful with 7 of the children.[54] Of the remaining five, two were withdrawn by their parents and three did not demonstrate stimulus control. All of the subjects who successfully completed the task were 12 months of age or older. A second study using TROCA and VROCA (bar-press response coupled with visual reinforcement) evaluated 32 infants between the ages of 7 and 20 months.[55] Threshold was determined by a bracketing procedure using 10-dB measurement steps. The signals were warbled pure tones of 0.5, 1.0, 2.0, and 4.0 kHz, presented in a soundfield. The procedure was successful with 64 percent of the infants under 12 months of age, and with 82 percent of those 13 to 20 months of age. Multiple test sessions were required.

### Earphone Threshold Assessment

Since many clinical and research questions involving auditory sensitivity and perceptual abilities of infants demand individual ear data as well as greater signal specificity, Moore et al. developed a headband/harness made of elastic and Velcro to hold a standard TDH-39 earphone and MX 41-AR cushion in place.[56] Twenty infants between 6 and 8 months of age were selected, as in the previous studies. The auditory signal was the same complex broadband noise and the threshold protocol remained the same. Thresholds were obtained for both ears and soundfield: mean thresholds were 35 dB SPL for earphones and 28.5 dB SPL for the soundfield. When the infant results were compared to a small sample of young, normal-hearing adults, using the same signal and test protocol, the adult thresholds were approximately 10 dB better than the infant thresholds for each condition. The difference between the minimum audible field (MAF) and minimum audible pressure (MAP) values was the same: 6 dB for both groups.

Wilson and Moore investigated the use of VRA with pure-tone stimuli under earphones.[47] Two groups of normal infant subjects, 6 to 7 months of age and 12 to 13 months, were selected, with 15 infants in each group. The auditory stimuli were 5 percent warbled pure tones of 500, 1,000, and 4,000 Hz. The headband/harness made of elastic and Velcro, or a modified child's headset, held a standard TDH-39 earphone and MX 41-AR cushion in place on the left ear of each subject. Thresholds were determined using the same testing procedure as described above. On the average, two 15-minute sessions were required to obtain thresholds for the three pure-tone stimuli. Average thresholds were approximately 33 dB SPL at 500 Hz and approximately 24 dB SPL at 1,000 and 4,000 Hz. Figure 15-19 shows the results. At 1,000 and 4,000 Hz, no systematic threshold differences

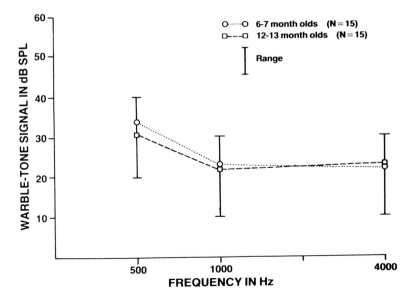

**Fig. 15-19.** VRA pure-tone earphone thresholds in infant groups. (Wilson WR, Moore JM: Pure-tone earphone thresholds of infants utilizing visual reinforcement audiometry [VRA]. Paper presented at the American Speech and Hearing Association Convention, San Francisco, 1978.)

between the two age groups are observed. At 500 Hz, the younger infants are set apart from the older infants with poorer mean thresholds. Figure 15-20 groups the infant data and provides a comparison with a group of normal-hearing young adults tested under the same conditions, including the 10-dB step size. Whereas the infant/adult soundfield differences were 5 dB at 500 Hz and 12 dB at 4,000 Hz in the same study, the infant/adult earphone differences were on the order of 16 dB at 500 Hz and 11 dB at 4,000 Hz. Likewise, a comparison of the threshold curves in the soundfield condition (Fig. 15-18) as compared to the threshold curves in the earphone condition (Fig. 15-20) demonstrates an exaggerated rise in the low frequencies with use of the infant earphones. These findings first led us to question the possible effect of leakage around the earphone cushion as one cause of the elevated low-frequency earphone thresholds for the infants. However, a study by Hesketh in our lab utilized a subminiature microphone mounted in the MX-41/AR cushion to record acoustic energy in the canal during testing of infants, children, and young adults.[57] Her results do not support a finding of differential energy in the canal. In a recent study, Berg and Smith reported pure-tone threshold values quite similar to those of Wilson and Moore, including elevated low-frequency thresholds for infants tested with an earphone.[47,58] Further study

is needed to determine the cause of these apparent differences.

Nozza and Wilson, as a part of a study on critical ratios in infants, used a computer-controlled adaptive procedure to develop auditory thresholds in quiet and in noise.[59] This procedure used a 5-dB step size with threshold defined as the mean of the intensity levels of the last eight turn-around points. Of interest here is that the infants were able to accomplish this psychophysical procedure and yielded pure-tone thresholds in quiet of 19 dB at 1,000 Hz and 15 dB at 4,000 Hz under earphones. Nozza and Wilson's results, accomplished in the same lab, may be compared to the Wilson and Moore earphone data using the clinical test paradigm (Fig. 15-21). As is apparent, the use of the 5-dB step size and the adaptive procedure reduces the thresholds by 5 to 9 dB, as contrasted to those obtained with the 10-dB step size and clinical procedure. One other factor that also may account for some of the difference is that Nozza and Wilson used an impedance screen in addition to the oral history/screen used by Wilson and Moore, and excluded any infants with negative middle-ear pressure in excess of $-100$ mmH$_2$O at the time of the test.

Throughout the discussions of the recent studies of auditory thresholds of infants, we have provided comparisons between results in adults and infants.

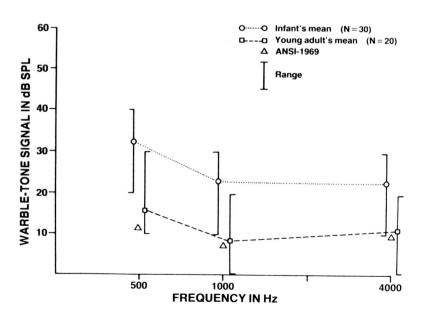

**Fig. 15-20.** VRA pure-tone earphone thresholds in infants and adults. (Wilson WR, Moore JM: Pure-tone earphone thresholds of infants utilizing visual reinforcement audiometry [VRA]. Paper presented at the American Speech and Hearing Association Convention, San Francisco, 1978.)

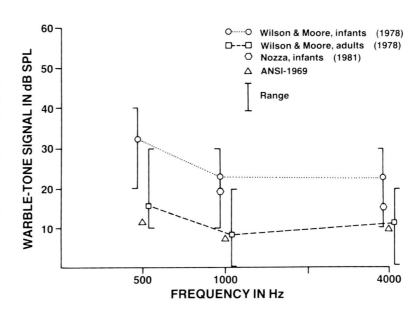

**Fig. 15-21.** Comparison of VRA pure-tone earphone thresholds as a function of test protocol. (Data from Wilson WR, Moore JM: Pure-tone earphone thresholds of infants utilizing visual reinforcement audiometry [VRA]. Paper presented at the American Speech and Hearing Association Convention, San Francisco, 1978; Nozza RJ, Wilson WR: Mashed and unmashed pure-tone thresholds of infants and adults: development of auditory frequency selectivity and sensitivity. J Speech Hear Res 27:613, 1984.)

The reasons for the comparisons are two. First, as noted above, an underlying theme in this literature is an interest in understanding the developmental course of auditory sensitivity. Second, the clinician needs to know the adult/infant threshold relationships so as to assign "normal" threshold to obtained results as a function of age. Specific to this point, however, is that although the studies reported provide very tight groupings of obtained threshold values, caution must be exercised in generalizing these values to other clinics. Differences in signal, soundfield test environments, and **VRA** test protocol may lead to differences in individual clinic normative values. Each clinic should see a small sample of normally developing infants to establish normative data for its setting. The sample need not be large, based on the findings that infant dispersion data in these procedures are equal to that of young adults in the same procedures.

Finally, we do not take the infant/adult differences to indicate that infants' thresholds are *necessarily* less sensitive than adults'. The task expected of the infant involves responding to a low-level signal while being visually distracted with toys, in order to maintain the infant's attention toward a midline position. It is quite possible that a slightly higher level signal is required to overcome the attention directed toward visual stimulation as the infant is being "entertained" during the test procedure. No such visual distraction exists for adult testing. This question should be amenable to experimental manipulation and would be a fruitful area for further investigation.

A question of interest relates to how accurately early behavioral audiograms predict degree of hearing loss as determined by later testing. Talbott recently reported a very interesting study in which she evaluated 25 moderately to profoundly hearing impaired infants and found that differences in serial audiograms were no greater than 15 dB at any single frequency and most typically were on the order of 0 to 5 dB.[60] VRA was used as the first test procedure and the results were very predictive of later test results at 3, 4, and 5 years of age, using play and standard audiometry.

In terms of clinical utility, it has been our experience that the VRA procedure is as robust as the TROCA/VROCA procedure and far less time consuming. Normally developing infants turn their head toward a sound source in the first few months of life. The localization response represents a behavioral "window" through which many aspects of auditory behavior can be studied. If an infant's localization behavior deviates markedly from the normal developmental pattern, there is strong reason to suspect either hearing loss or other problems, such as mental retardation. While there is a decided tendency for infants to turn initially toward "interesting" or "novel" auditory stimuli, there is a limit to the number of times head turns will occur to repeated stimuli.[22,38] Proper use of operant conditioning procedures greatly reduces this habituation of response.

## Assessment of Suprathreshold Auditory Abilities

The VRA test procedure is an operant discrimination paradigm in which detection of a change in signal state coupled with a correct response allows reinforcement. Whereas the VRA threshold task involves detection of the presence or absence of signal, suprathreshold tasks involve detection of a change in signal. Initial work involving suprathreshold stimulation has been reported in the area of speech-sound discrimination. Eilers and colleagues developed a procedure called the visually reinforced infant speech discrimination (VRISD) paradigm to study developmental changes in discrimination as a function of age.[61] All details of the VRA paradigm remained the same, except that one syllable of a recorded contrastive pair was presented at a repetition rate of one syllable per second at 50 dB SPL. While the infant was entertained at midline, the syllable was changed during a 4-second interval, with the temporal pattern of repetitions held constant. The infant was reinforced for a head turn to the change in signal by the activation of an animated toy. Initially, the *figure* (change) stimulus was presented at a higher intensity than the *ground* (background) stimulus. Once the infant had demonstrated responses to the intensity and/or speech-sound difference, the intensities were equated. Each infant was then presented with three change and three control (no-change) trials; to reach significance, the infant had to respond appropriately five out of six times.

Three studies using the VRISD procedure have shown that a high percentage of infants 6 to 14 months of age can be tested for discrimination of subtle speech contrasts.[13,61,62] Furthermore, it has been demonstrated that the VRISD paradigm can provide data on individual infants on a repeated basis, in order to obtain information concerning discrimination of a variety of contrasts over time. Some infants have been tested on as many as 10

speech contrasts in as few as three 20-minute sessions. Since the original description of the VRISD procedure,[61] a number of researchers have used variations of the procedure to study different aspects of infant speech perception. Although the primary focus of this work to date has been on theoretical issues in the area of infant speech perception, the possibilities for applying this procedure to disordered populations are exciting. For example, since this discrimination procedure does not require receptive language abilities, as other tests of auditory discrimination for children do, testing of discrimination function can occur at a very early age. Further, as more information about the discrimination abilities of normal infants becomes available, a normative guide will be available against which to compare performance of developmentally delayed youngsters. Resnick et al. have described the results of preliminary work in this direction.[63]

Diefendorf made use of the basic VRISD paradigm to study binaural fusion in infants 6 to 8-months old.[64] Binaural fusion is the capacity of the auditory system to integrate separate inputs to the two ears into a single auditory percept. When the two ears are stimulated by dichotic speech signals (signals differing with respect to each other in one or more signal parameters), a listener perceives one central image and is incapable of separating the individual speech signals. When the left or right ear only is stimulated, no centrally fused subjective image is formed. Diefendorf used two computer-generated speech-like vowels made up of a high and low passband each.[64] The four waveforms (two vowels × two passbands) could be instrumentally presented with the low passband of vowel one combined with the high passband of either vowel one or vowel two. Likewise, the low passband of vowel two could be combined with the high passband of either vowel two or vowel one. The resultant four signals could be presented in diotic or dichotic mix. If one of the "vowel" sounds was discriminated from the second "vowel" sound, four possible explanations could account for this behavior. First, it is possible that the dichotic presentations fused, and the infant discriminated one vowel sound from the other vowel sound, diotic or dichotic. A second, and equally plausible, explanation is that the infants simply memorized which individual vowel sounds were reinforced and which were not. With only four items, an infant might remember which two vowel sounds were reinforced and which two were not. Finally, it is possible that the infants discriminated the two vowels by paying attention to either the high or the low pitch of the two-formant vowel. Since the high and low formant of each vowel have different pitches, simply by listening to or perceiving the high or low pitch of each vowel the infant could discriminate one from the other, regardless of whether the vowel was presented diotically or dichotically. Therefore, four experiments were run with four separate groups of infants and four different signal combinations to address each of the possible outcomes: (1) binaural fusion; (2) memory; (3) high-formant discrimination; and (4) low-formant discrimination.

The results showed that the infants in the fusion group maintained a perception of the two vowels regardless of whether the presentation was diotic or dichotic. The other infants were not able to resolve the task by memorizing two of four stimuli or by discriminating on the basis of low- or high-formant information only. Thus, the results of this study suggest that 6 to 8-month-old infants demonstrate fusion of auditory information in the central auditory system.

The literature reports that binaural fusion has been utilized as a test of central auditory function with children as young as 5 years of age.[65] Additionally, Willeford suggested that this ability seems to be age related, showing a "maturational pattern" from age 5 through 9. The mean scores on Willeford's norms do improve with age. However, the wide dispersion of scores, at any single age, raises questions about task variables as contrasted to developmental or maturational factors in binaural fusion. The data from Diefendorf would suggest that binaural fusion may not be strongly age related, since infants at 6 months of age demonstrated success on a binaural fusion task.[64] In most previous fusion tasks, words or sentences have been used as stimuli. With adults and older children, this may not affect the outcome. However, with young children, one would expect language to be a critical factor. In addition, the clinical populations of interest in many cases are those with demonstrated language/learning difficulties. Instructions, memory, and response task can also play a role in the outcome of a binaural fusion task. If the task requires oral and/or written instruction, its use will again be restricted in terms of the age and language level of persons for whom it will be appropriate. Memory and response task interact in that certain responses (e.g., "point to the picture") place additional memory constraints on the task, as well as introducing visual-motor components to the procedure. We believe that the approach used in the VRISD procedure overcomes many of these problems and can be applied to other studies of central auditory function in normal children, and eventually in the clinic.

Three studies have explored the topic of masking with infants using head-turn procedures.[59,66,67] Masking studies provide information not only relative to the effect of noise (or other masking signals) on thresholds but also on the basic frequency selectivity of the ear. Masking is a consequence of the ear's limited frequency selectivity; as the energy in a masking stimulus approaches a test stimulus in frequency, there is an increase in the masking effect. Bull and co-workers used the turn-right/turn-left unlimited-response-interval procedure to study the effects of broad-band noise on a 4,000 Hz center frequency octave band[66] and on a speech phrase.[68] Subjects were 6-, 12-, 18-, and 24-month-old infants and adults. Increases in masking levels produced comparable threshold shifts for all age groups. Nozza and Wilson, using the fixed-interval unidirection head-turn procedure with 6- and 12-month-old infants and adults, found similar results for pure-tone stimuli and a broadband masker.[59] Collectively these studies suggest that the use of a masking signal in a clinical paradigm should produce similar results in infants and adults. In terms of frequency selectivity, the work of Nozza and Wilson demonstrated that the critical ratios (inferred auditory-filter-bandwidth estimates) are proportional for all ages. The actual critical ratios of infants are larger than those of adults. However, the infant/adult difference results from elevated infant thresholds in the detection-in-noise condition. The reader will recall a systematic infant/adult difference in threshold estimates. Nozza and Wilson argue that the consistent relationship between infant and adult thresholds across studies may point to the effect of attention/motivational factors. This work is important in providing initial information in the area of frequency selectivity in infants and suggests that more direct measures such as band-limiting experiments may be possible.

In the area of frequency discrimination, Olsho et al. used the fixed-interval unidirection head-turn procedure with 5 to 8-month-old infants.[69] The signal was a repeating background tone (1,000, 2,000, and 3,000 Hz pure tones) which was contrasted to a variable target tone. Their results suggested that infants could detect a 2 percent change in frequency, whereas adults detected changes of 1 percent or less. The data from infants showed considerable variability, however. Continued work in the area of frequency and intensity discrimination is underway in several labs. As the results of these normative studies describe the developmental course in each area, clinical applications should become possible.

### Application to Developmentally Disabled Populations

Greenberg and colleagues investigated the effectiveness of VRA with infants and young children with Down's syndrome.[70] There were 41 subjects between 6 months and 6 years of age. Twenty-five of the subjects were also administered the *Bayley Scales of Infant Development (BSID)*. VRA soundfield threshold test procedures, as previously described, were used. Each subject was required to respond to two out of three presentations (complex noise) at either a 50 or 70 dB SPL conditioning level. If a subject failed to satisfy this initial conditioning criterion, an attempt was made to teach the turning response by pairing the auditory and visual stimulus. If consistent responses occurred within a maximum of 10 teaching trials, the original test procedure was again attempted. Results were as follows: (1) 28 (68 percent) of the subjects spontaneously oriented toward the source of the auditory stimulus; (2) only a few of the subjects who did not initially orient could be taught to respond; (3) of the children who initially oriented or were taught to respond, thresholds were obtained on a large number (81 percent) in one visit; and (4) a system-

atic relationship was demonstrated between consistency of response using the VRA technique and *BSID* mental age equivalent, with 10 months being the critical age for determining the potential success of the procedure. The threshold values ranged from 30 to 60 dB SPL with a mean of 38.4 dB SPL. These results can be compared to those obtained on 75 normal infants between 6 and 18 months of age, whose thresholds ranged from 10 to 40 dB SPL with a mean of 22.5 dB SPL.[44]

Interpretation of these threshold data as fundamental indicators of hearing sensitivity is complicated by the possibility that some subjects may have been experiencing mild middle ear involvement at the time of testing. Both studies attempted to minimize the effects of middle-ear involvement through subject selection procedures.[44,70] These included no cold on the test day and no recent history of middle ear problems. Tympanometry results were not reported, however, which leaves open the possibility that the average threshold data for the subjects with Down's syndrome, in particular, may have been slightly inflated above true sensorineural hearing status, since this population has been shown to have a high incidence of middle ear involvement.[71-73]

In regard to the age at which children with Down's syndrome can be satisfactorily tested with VRA, Greenberg's study suggested that a mental-age equivalent (i.e., a functioning level) of 10 months was required.[70] A follow-up study supported this finding.[74] In view of this, it is of interest that in recent months we have seen clinically a few infants with Down's syndrome who have performed VRA satisfactorily at a *chronologic* age of approximately 10 months. Each of these particular infants demonstrated hearing thresholds at about 20 dB HL, had normal tympanograms, had *never* experienced middle ear involvement (according to parental report), and were involved in a formal infant-stimulation program in an educational setting. One hesitates to place undue emphasis on a few clinical cases; still, it is tempting to speculate on the developmental advantage that may accrue to infants with Down's syndrome who have been free of middle ear involvement since birth and who have been involved in programs designed to maximize communication skills.

## SUMMARY

Over the past decade major methodologic advances have occurred in the behavioral assessment of auditory function in infants. Procedures that capitalize on the infant's willingness to interact with his or her auditory environment have provided new insights into the auditory abilities of infants; they have shown themselves to be reliable responders able to answer sophisticated psychophysical questions. As a result, it is now possible to chart hearing sensitivity as well as measure certain suprathreshold abilities including speech-sound discrimination. In many comparisons, infants demonstrate reliability equivalent to adult patients. The task before us is to bring this new view of infant auditory function into clearer focus for many practitioners; they continue to be guided by outdated information.

Certainly, we have just begun to learn about the development of auditory function. However, we can no longer accept the broadly held notion that during the first year of life hearing sensitivity is resolving dramatically. Instead, infants are teaching us that the development is much more sophisticated than we had imagined.

## ACKNOWLEDGMENT

The research accomplished at the Child Development and Mental Retardation Center, University of Washington, has been supported in part by grants from The Deafness Research Foundation; The National Foundation–March of Dimes; Maternal and Child Health Services; and National Institute of Child Health and Human Development. The work reported by this author is the work of many; I wish to acknowledge particularly my colleague Gary Thompson, whose work has been instrumental in our progress throughout the years, and the late K. Lee, who provided most of the instrumentation for the projects.

## REFERENCES

1. Goetzinger CP, Harrison C, Baer CJ: Small perceptive hearing loss: its effect in school-age children. Volta Rev 63:124, 1964
2. Holm VA, Kunze LH: Effect of chronic otitis media on language and speech development. Pediatrics 43:833, 1969
3. Sak RJ, Ruben RJ: Recurrent middle ear effusion in childhood: implications of temporary auditory deprivation for language and learning. Ann Otol 90:546, 1981
4. Batkin S, Groth H, Watson JR, Ansberry M: Effects of auditory deprivation on the development of auditory sensitivity in albino rats. Electroencephalogr Clin Neurol 28:351, 1970
5. Clopton BM: Neurophysiology of auditory deprivation. Birth Defects 16:271, 1980
6. Gray L, Smith Z, Rubel EW: Developmental and experiential changes in dendritic symmetry in n. laminaris of the chick. Brain Res 244:360, 1982
7. Smith ZDF, Gray L, Rubel EW: Afferent influences on brainstem nuclei of the chicken: n. laminaris dendritic length following monaural conductive hearing loss. J Comp Neurol 220:199, 1983
8. Silverman MS, Clopton BM: Plasticity of binaural interaction. I. Effect of early auditory deprivation. J Neurophysiol 40:1266, 1977
9. Webster DB: Auditory neuronal sizes after a unilateral conductive hearing loss. Exp Neurol 79:130, 1983
10. Webster DB, Webster M: Neonatal sound deprivation affects brainstem auditory nuclei. Arch Otolaryngol 103:392, 1977
11. Webster DB, Webster M: Effects of neonatal conductive hearing loss on brainstem auditory nuclei. Ann Otol 88:684,1979
12. Cairns GF, Butterfield EC: Assessing infants' auditory functioning. In Friedlander BZ, Sterritt GM, Kirk GE (eds): Exceptional Infant, vol. III. Brunner/Mazel, New York, 1975
13. Eilers RE, Gavin W, Wilson WR: Linguistic experience and phonemic perception in infancy: a cross-linguistic study. Child Dev 50:14, 1979
14. Werker JF, Tees RC: Cross-language speech perception: evidence for perceptual reorganization during the first year of life. Infant Behav Dev 7:49, 1984
15. Werker JF, Gilbert JHV, Humphrey K, Tees RC:

Developmental aspects of cross-language speech perception. Child Dev 52:349, 1981

16. Downs MP, Sterritt GM: A guide to newborn and infant hearing screening programs. Arch Otolaryngol 85:15, 1967

17. Suzuki T, Sato I: Free field startle response audiometry. Ann Otorhinolaryngol 70:998, 1961

18. Thompson M, Thompson G: Response of infants and young children as a function of auditory stimuli and test methods. J Speech Hear Res 15:699, 1972

19. Eisenberg RB: Auditory Competence in Early Life —The Roots of Communicative Behavior. University Park Press, Baltimore, 1976

20. Hoversten G, Moncur J: Stimuli and intensity factors in testing infants. J Speech Hear Res 12:687, 1969

21. Ling D, Ling AH, Doehring DG: Stimulus response and observer variables in the auditory screening of newborn infants. J Speech Hear Res 13:9, 1970

22. Moore JM, Thompson G, Thompson M: Auditory localization of infants as a function of reinforcement conditions. J Speech Hear Dis 40:29, 1975

23. Thompson G, Weber BA: Responses of infants and young children to behavior observation audiometry (BOA). J Speech Hear Dis 39:140, 1974

24. Goldstein R, Tait C: Critique of neonatal hearing evaluation. J Speech Hear Dis 36:3, 1971

25. Moncur JP: Judge reliability in infant testing. J Speech Hear Res 11:348, 1968

26. Weber BA: Validation of observer judgments in behavioral observation audiometry. J Speech Hear Dis 34:350, 1969

27. Weber BA: Comparison of two approaches to behavioral observation audiometry. J Speech Hear Res 13:823, 1970

28. Northern JL, Downs MP: Hearing in Children. Williams & Wilkins, Baltimore, 1978

29. Sweitzer RS: Audiologic evaluation of the infant and young child. In Jaffe BF (ed): Hearing Loss in Children. University Park Press, Baltimore, 1977

30. Field J, DiFranco D, Dodwell P, Muir D: Auditory-visual coordination in two and one-half-month-old infants. Infant Behav Dev 2:113, 1979

31. Field J, Muir D, Pilon R, Sinclair M, Dodwell P: Infants' orientation to lateral sounds from birth to three months. Child Dev 51:295, 1980

32. Muir D, Abraham W, Forbes B, Harris L: The ontogenesis of an auditory localization response from birth to four months of age. Can J Psychol 33:320, 1979

33. Muir D, Field J: Newborn infants orient to sounds. Child Dev 50:431, 1979

34. Gans DP, Flexer C: Observer bias in the hearing testing of profoundly involved multiply handicapped children. Ear Hearing 3:309, 1982

35. Eisele WA, Berry RC, Shriner TH: Infant sucking response patterns as a conjugate function of changes in the sound pressure level of auditory stimuli. J Speech Hear Res 18:296, 1975

36. Friedlander BZ: Automated playtest systems for evaluating infant's and young children's selective listening to natural sounds and language. Scientific Exhibit, American Speech and Hearing Association Convention, Chicago, 1969

37. Friedlander BZ: Receptive language development in infancy: Issues and problems. Merrill-Palmer Q 16:7, 1970

38. Moore JM, Wilson WR, Thompson G: Visual reinforcement of head-turn responses in infants under 12 months of age. J Speech Hear Dis 42:328, 1977

39. Suzuki T, Ogiba Y: A technique of pure-tone audiometry for children under three years of age: conditioned orientation reflex (COR) audiometry. Rev Laryngol 81:33, 1960

40. Suzuki T, Ogiba Y: Conditioned orientation reflex audiometry. Arch Otolaryngol 74:192, 1961

41. Liden G, Kankkunen A: Visual reinforcement audiometry. Acta Otolaryngol 67:281, 1969

42. Haug O, Baccaro P, Guilford FR: A pure-tone audiogram on the infant: the PIWI technique. Arch Otolaryngol 86:435, 1967

43. Motta G, Facchini GM, D'Auria E: Objective conditioned-reflex audiometry in children. Acta Otolaryngol [Suppl] 273:l, 1970

44. Wilson WR, Moore JM, Thompson G: Sound-field auditory thresholds of infants utilizing visual reinforcement audiometry (VRA). Paper presented at the American Speech and Hearing Association Convention, Houston, 1976

45. Thompson G, Folsom RC: A comparison of two conditioning procedures in the use of visual reinforcement audiometry (VRA). J Speech Hear Dis 49:241, 1984

46. Primus MA, Thompson G: Response strength of young children in operant audiometry. J Speech Hear Res 28:539, 1985

47. Wilson WR, Moore JM: Pure-tone earphone thresholds of infants utilizing visual reinforcement audiometry (VRA). Paper presented at the American Speech and Hearing Association Convention, San Francisco, 1978

48. Goldman TM: Response of infants to warble-tone signals presented in soundfield using visual reinforcement audiometry. Master's thesis, University of Cincinnati, 1979

49. Schneider BA, Trehub SE, Bull D: The development of basic auditory processes in infants. Can J Psychol 33:306, 1979

50. Schneider BA, Trehub SE, Bull D: High-frequency sensitivity in infants. Science 207:1003, 1980

51. Trehub SE, Schneider BA, Endman M: Developmental changes in infants' sensitivity to octave-band noises. J Exp Child Psychol 29:282, 1980

52. Fausti SA, Erickson DA, Frey RH, et al: The effects of noise upon human hearing sensitivity from 8000 to 20000 Hz. J Acoust Soc Am 69:1343, 1981

53. Lloyd LL, Spradlin JE, Reid MJ: An operant audiometric procedure for difficult-to-test patients. J Speech Hear Dis 33:236, 1968

54. Fulton R.T, Gorzycki PA, Hull WL: Hearing assessment with young children. J Speech Hear Dis 40:397, 1975

55. Wilson WR, Decker NT: Auditory thresholds of infants using operant audiometry with tangible and/or visual reinforcement. Paper presented at the American Association of Mental Deficiency Convention, Chicago, 1976

56. Moore JM, Wilson WR, Lillis KE, Talbott SA: Earphone audiometry thresholds of infants utilizing visual reinforcement audiometry (VRA). Paper presented at the American Speech and Hearing Association Convention, Houston, 1976

57. Hesketh LJ: Pure-tone thresholds and ear-canal pressure levels in infants, young children and adults. Master's thesis, University of Washington, 1983

58. Berg KM, Smith MC: Behavioral thresholds for tones during infancy. J Exp Child Psychol 35:409, 1983

59. Nozza RJ, Wilson WR: Masked and unmasked pure-tone thresholds of infants and adults: development of auditory frequency selectivity and sensitivity. J Speech Hear Res 27:613, 1984

60. Talbott CB: A longitudinal study comparing responses of hearing impaired infants to pure tones using visual reinforcement and play audiometry. Paper presented at Audiology Update, Newport, Rhode Island, 1984

61. Eilers RE, Wilson WR, Moore JM: Developmental changes in speech discrimination in infants. J Speech Hear Res 20:766, 1977

62. Eilers RE, Wilson WR, Moore JM: Speech discrimination in the language-innocent and the language-wise: a study in the perception of voice onset time. J Child Language 6:1, 1979

63. Resnick SB, Bookstein EW, Talkin D: Clinical measurement of nonsense syllable discrimination in infants. Paper presented at the American Speech-Language-Hearing Association Convention, Toronto, 1982

64. Diefendorf AO: An investigation of one aspect of central auditory function in an infant population utilizing a binaural resynthesis (fusion) task. Doctoral dissertation, University of Washington, 1981

65. Willeford JA: Assessing central auditory behavior in children: A test battery approach. In Keith RW (ed): Central Auditory Dysfunction. Grune & Stratton, Orlando, FL, 1977

66. Bull D, Schneider BA, Trehub SE: The masking of octave-band noise by broad-spectrum noise: a comparison of infant and adult thresholds. Percept Psychophys 30:101, 1981

67. Trehub SE, Bull D, Schneider BA: Infants' detection of speech and noise. J Speech Hear Res 24:202, 1981

68. Trehub SE, Schneider BA, Bull D: Effect of reinforcement on infants' performance in an auditory detection task. Dev Psych 17:872, 1981

69. Olsho LW, Schoon C, Sakai R, et al: Preliminary data on frequency discrimination in infancy. J Acoust Soc Am 71:509, 1982

70. Greenberg DB, Wilson WR, Moore JM, Thompson G: Visual reinforcement audiometry (VRA) with young Down's syndrome children. J Speech Hear Dis 43:448, 1978

71. Balkany T, Downs MP, Jafek BW, Krajicek MJ: Hearing loss in Down's syndrome. Clin Pediatr 18:116, 1979

72. Brooks DN, Wooley H, Kanjilal GC: Hearing loss and middle ear disorders in patients with Down's syndrome (Mongolism). J Ment Defic Res 16:21, 1972

73. Schwartz DM, Schwartz RH: Acoustic impedance and otoscopic findings in young children with Down's syndrome. Arch Otolaryngol 104:652, 1978

74. Thompson G, Wilson WR, Moore JM: Application of visual reinforcement audiometry (VRA) to low-functioning children. J Speech Hear Dis 44:80, 1979

# Auditory Evoked Potentials

# 16

## Martyn L. Hyde

### GOALS AND HISTORY

In the last 20 years, auditory evoked potentials (AEPs) have had a strong impact on audiologic and otoneurologic assessment. They are now an essential part of the clinical armamentarium. Their most important uses are to estimate hearing thresholds in patients for whom behavioral audiometry is inadequate or impossible, and to detect retrocochlear lesions. The importance of AEP tests will continue to increase, due to technical advances, intensive research, and accumulation of clinical experience. For these tests to be selected and interpreted properly, the otolaryngologist should understand thoroughly their role and significance, and should grasp their theoretical and practical basis.

This chapter offers an overview of AEPs and some insight into important points governing their effective use. The phenomena are inherently complex, and many technical and pathophysiologic factors must be taken into account. The field is dynamic, current knowledge is limited, and some aspects are matters of opinion. Thus, a cookbook approach is inappropriate. Some technical gruel is unavoidable before clinical delicacies can be appreciated.

There are many AEPs, many factors affecting them, and several clinical uses. Complete coverage of all tests is not feasible here, so there are omissions and liberal references to other reviews and specialized texts. The material can be organized by AEP, or by topics that cross AEP boundaries; the latter method is used, reducing repetition and emphasizing trends, but with the result that material on the auditory brainstem response (ABR), for example, is distributed through the chapter. However, there are several good books on the ABR.[1,2]

Early AEP history was reviewed by Hallowell Davis,[3] the father of this field. Accumulation of knowledge about AEPs followed naturally from study of electrical brain activity, and development of auditory electrophysiology. The seminal discoveries were Caton's[4] demonstration in 1875 of both evoked and spontaneous electrical activity in the rabbit brain, and the report by Wever and Bray[5] in 1930 concerning encoding of speech frequency components in cat auditory nerve impulse volleys. Subsequent developments in both auditory electrophysiology and electroencephalography converged in Davis' 1939 report[6] of human scalp AEPs to single sounds. Postwar microelectrode exploration of the electrical activity of the cochlea and auditory nerve was very productive,[7] but there was little advance in study of scalp AEPs until the development of the electronic averager by Dawson, reported in 1954.[8] This device extracts the minute AEPs from the much larger spontaneous EEG activity, by summating the responses to many repeated stimuli.

The "averaging computer" precipitated massive research into the properties and applications of averaged evoked potentials, which continues to this day. In 1960, Geisler's MIT thesis[9] described click-evoked average AEPs from the human scalp, and sparked a major controversy about their neurogenic or myogenic origin; we know now that both types occur. In 1963, a symposium in New York assembled investigators of auditory, somatosensory, and visual EPs.[10] In 1964, a Toronto symposium on the deaf child yielded a major report on the audiometric application of scalp AEPs arising from the cerebral cortex.[11]

The 1960s saw rapid and diverse development. Aran and LeBert,[12] Ruben,[13] Sohmer and Feinmesser,[14] Yoshie et al.,[15] and many others applied averaging to the potentials of the cochlea and auditory nerve, and introduced electrocochleography as a clinical tool. Other workers continued to explore the audiometric uses of responses from higher parts of the auditory system.[16,17] Also, the first reports appeared of long-latency EPs related to cognitive processes such as expectancy and decision-making.[18,19]

The major event of the 1970s was the definitive description by Jewett and Williston[20] in 1971 of the ABR. Some of the curious history of the ABR was reviewed by Jewett.[2] The first ABR uses for audiometry were described by Hecox and Galambos[21] in 1974. Applications to the differential diagnosis of acoustic tumor were described in a large-sample study by Selters and Brackmann[22] in 1979. By the 1980s, a wide variety of ABR applications in neurology had emerged.[23,24] The ABR has also achieved prominence as a tool for audiometric assessment of infants.[24,25]

The modern history of AEPs suggests at least two points of perspective: first, hindsight continually indicates that practices of even only a year ago may have involved unwarranted assumptions or simplistic interpretations; the AEP field is still in infancy and is evolving rapidly. Second, innovations lead to bandwagon effects and uncritical acceptance of new fashions. For example, the advent of the ABR tended to eclipse other AEPs. In fact, no AEP is "best" for all purposes, and many AEPs may contribute to a given clinical goal. AEPs have spawned not a test but an entire class of tests, each with its own strengths and weaknesses. It is important to grasp the commonalities and distinctions between tests, and the strategy of selection and combination.

## AEP CLASSIFICATION AND TERMINOLOGY

A sound may elicit a vast set of bioelectric events, some of which are recordable by electrodes in the ear or on the scalp. This type of recording registers a summation of minute electric events in many active cells; the resulting AEPs are "gross" or "compound," as distinct from microelectrode recordings from single cells or small groups. The key to development of gross potentials at recording sites "remote" from their sources is the *synchrony* of a sufficiently large number of underlying electrical events. These events must have waveforms and timing such that they can summate constructively at the recording site. Figure 16-1 shows schematically some of these principles.

Gross AEPs arise from many parts of the auditory pathway, from the cochlea to the cerebral cortex. There are so many AEPs that it is helpful to classify them. Important attributes that can be used for this are physiologic source, relationship to the stimulus, latency, and anatomic source.

### Physiologic Source

*Neurogenic* AEPs come from neurons and *myogenic* AEPs from muscle fibers. The former are far more important and widely used, but the many myogenic AEPs cannot be ignored, because they may contaminate recordings of neurogenic responses. Myogenic AEPs occur in response to loud sounds, and tend to be spatially localized over the active muscle, for example, frontalis, temporalis,

SOURCES                     RESULTANT

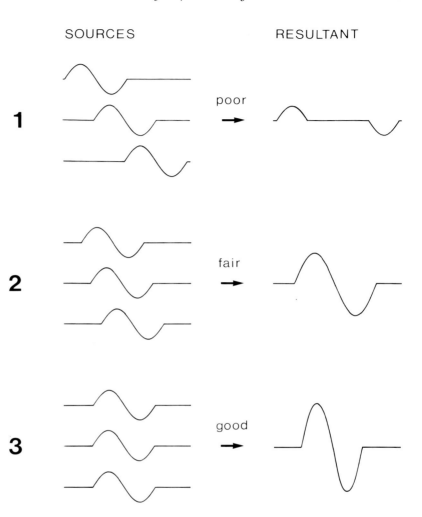

**Fig. 16-1.** Effects of source synchrony on the resultant gross AEP. Gross AEPs are a summation at the recording electrodes of the net effect of many underlying elementary potentials. As the synchrony in time of these source potentials varies, so do the size and waveform of the resultant. In case (1), with poor synchrony, a low-amplitude resultant bears little relationship to the source waveform. In case (2), with fair synchrony, the resultant has moderate amplitude but is broader than the source. In case (3), with good synchrony, the resultant closely resembles the sources and has greatest amplitude. Only three source waveforms are shown here; in the real situation with thousands of sources, the effects of synchrony are much more marked, but follow these general principles.

and postauricular myogenic (PAM, "sonomotor") responses.[3,26] They vary greatly between individuals, and with electrode site, tonus, and head position. Thus, myogenic responses have very limited audiometric or otoneurologic use.

In the large neurogenic group, a distinction is sometimes drawn between potentials from the cochlear hair cells and those from higher parts of the auditory pathways. The hair cell is the primary receptor of audition and potentials associated with this action may be termed *receptor potentials*. Some caution is needed in interpreting these, since it is not clear whether these cochlear potentials are causative of audition or are merely epiphenomena of stimulus transduction.[27]

Two important types of cellular activity that underlie neurogenic AEPs are action potentials (APs) and postsynaptic (dendritic) potentials (PSPs).[3,28] APs are large, rapidly propagated all-or-none phenomena, whereas PSPs are small, localized, and graded potentials associated with synaptic transmission. An example of this distinction is the term *compound action potential* (CAP) in reference to the gross neurogenic AEP from the cochlear nerve, indicating that this AEP is made up of summated APs. For some AEPs, such as the ABR, the relative contributions of APs and PSPs are unclear.[29] For AEPs from higher parts of the auditory pathways (e.g., cerebral cortex), PSPs are probably the major source.[3]

## Relationship to the Stimulus

Figure 16-2 outlines various classes of neurogenic AEP, as determined by their stimulus reltions. If the basic properties of an AEP such as its size and shape are governed by physical stimulus parameters such as intensity and frequency, it is *exogenous*. This class includes all AEPs commonly used in audiology and otoneurology, and this chapter will concentrate upon them. If psychological factors such as attention or stimulus "significance" influence the AEP strongly, it is *endogenous*. This is so for certain cortical AEPs described as "perceptual" or "cognitive," examples of which are the so-called $P_{300}$ and the contingent negative variation (CNV). These AEPs may become increasingly relevant to auditory perceptual assessment, and good reviews of their use are available.[30,31] They will not be discussed further here.

An important distinction that applies to exogenous responses is between *sustained* and *transient* AEPs. A sustained AEP lasts for about as long as the stimulus, whereas a transient AEP is associated with some particular stimulus feature, such as its onset or offset. *Onset* and *offset* responses are types of transient AEP, and the onset responses are by far the most common in clinical applications. Normally, onset AEPs are recorded using trains of stimuli sufficiently far apart that there is no overlap of the responses to successive stimuli; these might be termed *discrete* AEPs. When the stimuli are presented so rapidly that the AEPs overlap to form a quasicontinuous response, the result is called a *steady-state* AEP.[32] Myogenic AEPs are usually of the transient onset type, and are not included in Figure 16-2.

## Latency

*Latency* describes the time interval between a response feature (usually a waveform peak or trough) and a reference point on the stimulus (usually its onset), which serves as time zero. The entire span of latency can be divided into ranges such as those shown in Table 16-1. These ranges are a useful but not infallible guide; they refer to the response latency for a normal adult, using click stimuli at moderate intensity. The actual latency of any particular AEP depends on many features of the stimulus, the recording conditions, and the patient. For example, for low-intensity, low-frequency stimuli in infants, it is possible to see part of the ABR (a "fast" AEP) at latencies in the "middle" range. Most myogenic AEPs, not shown in Table 16-1, occur in the middle latency range, where they may overlap with the neurogenic middle-latency responses.

## Anatomic Source

For the majority of AEPs, the detailed anatomic sites of origin are uncertain. However, when there is reasonable evidence of the generator site, it is

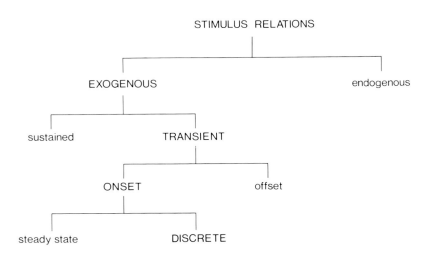

**Fig. 16-2.** A classification of neurogenic AEPs based on their relationship to the properties of the stimulus. Potentials in upper case are discussed in detail in the text.

**Table 16-1. Classification of Gross Neurogenic AEPs by Latency of AEP Onset**

| Stimulus-Relations Class | Onset-Latency Class | AEP Name |
|---|---|---|
| Sustained | First (0–1 msec) | Cochlear microphonic potential |
| | | Cochlear summating potential |
| | Fast (1–10 msec) | Frequency-following response |
| | Middle (10–75 msec) | None |
| | Slow (75–300 msec) | Sustained cortical potential |
| Transient | First (0–1 msec) | None |
| | Fast (1–10 msec) | Compound action potential |
| | | Auditory brainstem response |
| | Middle (10–75 msec) | Middle-latency response |
| | Slow (75–300 msec) | Slow vertex response |

used in reference, for example, cochlear microphonic potential (CM), cochlear summating potential (SP), ABR, cortical response. Many of these terms are less than ideal. For example, the ABR includes components (wave I, at least) that do not arise from the brain stem, and the term *cortical response* is nonspecific because there are many AEPs thought to be of cortical origin but that have quite different properties.[3] In general, it is simplistic to assume a one-to-one correspondence between AEPs and specific anatomic sites. The various component waves of any AEP may have different sources; furthermore, the complexity of the ascending auditory pathways makes it probable that even a single AEP wave may have multiple sources which are activated concurrently, for example, for the ABR.[29]

Table 16-2 lists AEPs of prime concern here, their common abbreviations, and their physiologic and anatomic sources. Much of Table 16-2 is still open to debate, especially for ABR[29,33,34] and SVR[3,35] origins.

## Other Classifications

There are many viewpoints about AEP classification. The reader should note significant differences between this development and comparable classifications.[3,36,37] Such attempts to impose apparent order upon apparent chaos will continue to evolve.

**Table 16-2. AEP Nomenclature and Sources**

| AEP | Abbreviation | Anatomic and Physiologic Sources |
|---|---|---|
| **Sustained Type** | | |
| Cochlear microphonic | CM | Hair cells, AC receptor potential |
| Summating potential | SP | Hair cells, DC receptor potential |
| Frequency-following response | FFR | Caudal brain stem, APs[a](?) |
| Sustained cortical potential | SCP | Cerebral cortex, PSPs[b] |
| | | |
| **Transient Type** | | |
| Compound action potential | CAP | Cochlear nerve, APs |
| Auditory brain stem response | ABR | |
|   Wave I | | Cochlear nerve, APs |
|   Wave II | | Cochlear nerve(?), APs(?) |
|   Wave III | | Cochlear nucleus(?), APs(?) |
|   Wave IV | | Superior olivary complex(?), APs(?) |
|   Wave V | | Lateral lemniscus(?), APs(?) |
|   Waves, VI, VII | | Inferior colliculus(?), APs(?) |
| Middle-latency response | MLR | Thalamus(?), primary cortex(?), PSPs |
| Slow vertex response | SVR | Primary cortex(?), PSPs |

[a] Action potential
[b] Postsynaptic potential
?, Uncertain

## Wave Nomenclature

Figure 16-3 illustrates some AEP waveforms for the neurogenic class. For the transient group, in each latency range there may be a complex waveform with many peaks and troughs. Several wave labeling systems have arisen, and often they reflect the preferences of their progenitors; Figure 16-3 shows the most commonly used nomenclature. The labels usually reflect wave order within a latency category. This, again, contains assumptions about stimuli, recording conditions, and patients. For example, in various situations, ABR wave V might be the first, or third, or sixth wave actually observed, yet it remains wave V.

The use of the symbols N or P to denote wave polarity can be both helpful and confusing. For example, ABR wave V is scalp-positive, but was designated by some as wave $N_4$. This is due to a matter of recording technique, which is discussed later. Furthermore, wave V is also known as $P_6$, reflecting a "typical" latency of 6 msec. In fact, depending on the conditions, wave $P_6$ can occur at latencies from about 5 to 15 msec. Overall, there is no satisfactory and standard nomenclature, which can frustrate an understanding of published reports unless authors give clear definitions. Often, they do not. The final straw is that some authors plot positivity upwards, others do it downwards, and some do not bother to say which way it is plotted. Debates about up or down are interminable. Electrophysiologists are weaned on negative up, but the much more pervasive classic Cartesian approach is positive up, which will be used here unless the contrary is stated.

## Jargon

Already, it will be apparent that a barrage of jargon is encountered in the AEP field. No apology is made for its use here, because it is terse and inescapable in publications. Frequently, many terms are in use for any given AEP. For example, the ABR has myriad other names, including brain stem auditory evoked potential (BAEP), brain stem evoked response (BSER), and others. A related AEP is the $SN_{10}$ of Davis and Hirsh,[38] (a Slow [sic] vertex-Negative wave with typical latency of *10* msec); it is probably a variant of ABR wave V, its appearance being dictated primarily by technical factors of the recording.[39,40] The slow cortical response was originally dubbed the vertex potential (V-potential) by Davis,[3] due to its broad vertex-maximal scalp topography. Many AEPs are now known to have roughly this topography, so the term slow vertex response (SVR) is more specific in terms of latency.

The general term event-related potential (ERP) is not specific to auditory EPs, but is encountered for the so-called 40 Hz ERP reported by Galambos et al.[41] This steady-state AEP is mainly a variant of the middle latency response (MLR), obtained by using such a high stimulus repetition rate (about 40/sec) that the MLRs to successive stimuli overlap. The terms 40 Hz MLR or just 40 Hz response are also used. For sustained AEPs, the terms CM, SP, and FFR are well-established; here, the term FFR refers to a response of brainstem origin, though some authors use the term more generically and include the CM as a particular case. The sustained cortical potential (SCP) is also known as the cortical DC potential.

One must name not only AEPs but the tests based upon them. Many AEPs are applied audiometrically, and a common term for this is *electric response audiometry* (ERA). This is better than the earlier term evoked response audiometry (also ERA), because all response is evoked. Audiometry with the ABR is sometimes called brain stem electric response audiometry (BERA), though the obvious possibility, adopted here, is to append audiometry to the abbreviation for the response, yielding ABRA, MLRA, SVRA. As mentioned, cortical audiometry is not specific enough, nor is electrophysiologic audiometry. The term objective audiometry is both vague and misleading. It is arguable that some AEP applications, such as the use of the ABR to detect neurologic disease, are not audiometry, but if one considers that all AEPs reflect some aspect of auditory function, all AEP applications are ERA of a kind.

The term *electrocochleography* is well entrenched, with reference to the recording of the CM, SP or compound action potential (CAP), using an intra-auricular electrode. Electrocochleography is one particular type of ERA. There is lingering debate (confined to North America) about whether this technique should be abbreviated as ECochG or ECoG, yet the latter term is already used for electrocorticography. ECochG will be used here. Finally, one meets the terms

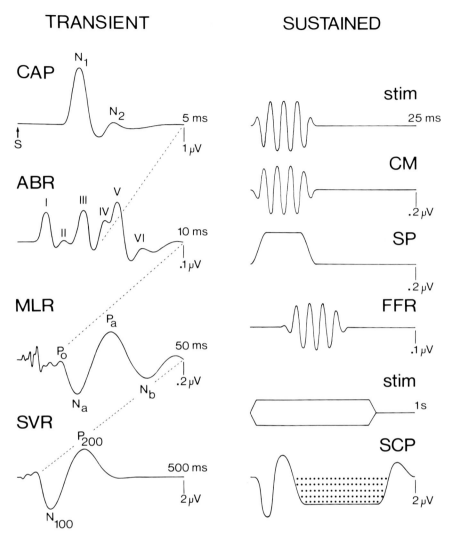

**Fig. 16-3.** Waveforms (idealized) and wave nomenclature for some important AEPs. In the transient neurogenic class, the stimulus is a click of moderate intensity, and waveforms are typical for a normal adult. For the CAP, a transtympanic needle electrode is used, whereas for the ABR, MLR, and SVR a vertex to mastoid scalp electrode placement is used; an upward deflection indicates vertex positivity or ear/mastoid negativity. The CAP is plotted upward to emphasize its relationship to the early part of the ABR. See text and Figure 16-10 for discussion of differential recording and its effects on apparent AEP polarity. For the sustained class, stimulus waveforms are included for clarity. The CM and SP are as recorded transtympanically; the SP is upward for consistency with the CAP as shown. The FFR and SCP are as recorded with a vertex to mastoid electrode placement, vertex positive up. For all potentials, note carefully the time and amplitude scales.

near-field and far-field in descriptions of responses or techniques, relating to whether the recording electrodes are near or far from the response generator sites. There are engineering definitions of what constitutes near or far, but these are of little practical consequence; the only point of substance is that in near-field recording the AEP is more sensitive to small changes in electrode position than in far-field recording. ECochG is the only near-field technique considered here.

## BASIC STIMULATION AND RECORDING TECHNIQUES

### Outline

The most commonly used stimuli are acoustical transients such as clicks or brief tones, usually delivered monaurally by earphone. The stimulation is synchronized with the recording of bioelectric activity. The major problem in AEP recording is that most of what is picked up by the electrodes is not AEP but spontaneous bioelectric noise. At the scalp, this is essentially a single-channel electroencephalogram (EEG), a random signal that may include classic rhythms (alpha, etc.) and much electrical activity arising in cranial musculature. This noise is usually much larger than the minute AEPs, and several techniques must be used to render the AEP detectable and measurable. Stimulation and recording methods are detailed elsewhere,[3,42-45] and only the most important points will be reviewed here.

Figure 16-4 shows a block diagram of the major functions required for AEP measurements. These are implemented in most commercial AEP instrumentation. Most systems can do all the AEP tests described here, but there is a trade-off of cost, flexibility, and ease of use. In the past, systems that were the easiest to use clinically lacked the range of functions desirable for clinical research. The latest systems make much use of digital technology, including microprocessors, and are programmable for a wide range of performance.

### Stimuli

The stimulus waveform can be viewed on a duration axis, with the click at one end and a long toneburst at the other. It is also useful to consider the frequency distribution of stimulus energy, that is,

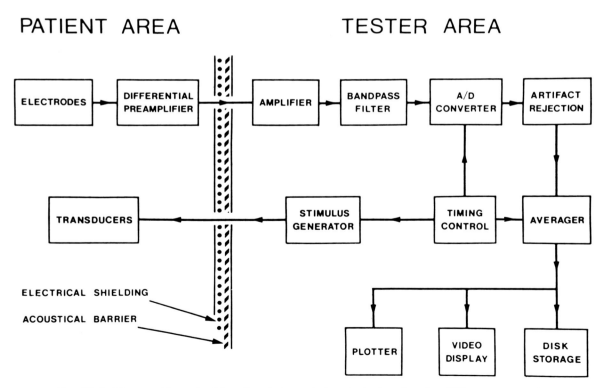

**Fig. 16-4.** The most important functional elements in a typical system for AEP measurements.

its frequency spectrum. The waveform in time and the spectrum are alternative representations that are mathematically interconvertible. A result of the formulae relating them is that stimulus duration is inversely related to the width of the spectrum. Thus, the briefer a stimulus, the larger is its bandwidth, and vice versa.

Some stimulus waveforms are shown in Figure 16-5. The click is often produced by exciting the earphone with a rectangular voltage pulse of typical duration 0.1 msec. The resulting acoustic pressure waveform at the tympanic membrane depends on the frequency response of the earphone and ear canal. The excitation produced by the click has the most rapid onset possible, is very brief, and has a wide bandwidth. Filtered clicks used to be generated by passing a voltage pulse through an electronic filter, whereas the tonepip or toneburst was produced by electronic modulation (shaping) of a sinusoid. Sometimes, filtered clicks are referred to as tonepips. It is common to specify the tonepip or toneburst envelope rise, plateau, and fall times in

**Fig. 16-5.** Common stimuli used in AEP measurement. The click is a highly damped oscillation produced by driving the headphone with a rectangular voltage pulse, usually of duration 100 microseconds (msec). The filtered click was produced by exciting (ringing) a narrow bandpass filter with a click; the filter passband center was at 500 Hz. Note the asymmetrical envelope of the oscillation. The tonepip was produced by electronic "shaping" of a 500 Hz sinusoid; note the trapezoidal envelope with linear rise, plateau, and fall segments. For the toneburst, only the envelope is shown; in this example, the rise and fall were shaped nonlinearly by a cosine wave. In the most modern AEP instrumentation, these waveforms are produced entirely by digital synthesis; many other possible shapes may be used in an attempt to optimize both AEP clarity and the stimulus frequency-specificity.

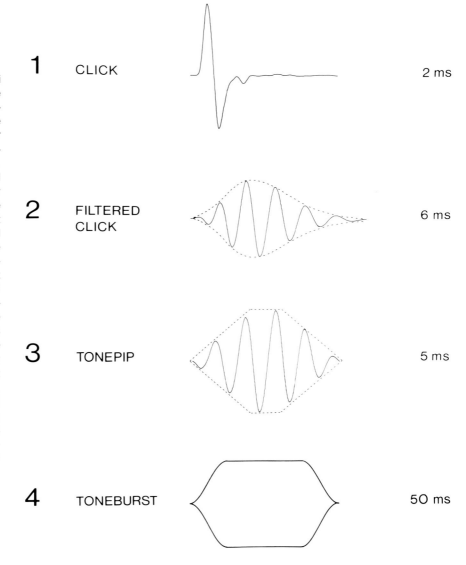

1 CLICK — 2 ms

2 FILTERED CLICK — 6 ms

3 TONEPIP — 5 ms

4 TONEBURST — 50 ms

milliseconds or in terms of the number of cycles of the sinusoid. There is no formal distinction between the pip and burst, but a duration of about 10 msec might be a reasonable division. Nowadays, these various types of stimulus are often generated digitally.

Filtered clicks, tonepips, and tonebursts have narrower bandwidth than the click, the bandwidth being governed by the duration and the rise/fall times. For example, long tonebursts have small bandwidth, energy being concentrated at the "nominal" burst frequency. However, if the burst starts and stops abruptly, there is energy spread, which is audible as a click percept. This is reduced by using gradual onset and offset, as is obligatory for the stimuli used in conventional puretone audiometry.

The choice of stimulus depends mainly on the test objective. To probe the functional integrity of the cochlear nerve or brain stem, it seems at least superficially reasonable to try and elicit the clearest AEPs. Because gross AEP development depends on neural synchrony, the click is a logical choice; its rapid onset and wide bandwidth excite the cochlea in a broad and synchronized way, giving a strong volley of nerve impulses to more rostral structures. The click is by far the most common stimulus used to explore neural function with the CAP or the ABR. On the other hand, if the goal is to estimate audiometric sensitivity, the click is widely used but has significant limitations because it is not frequency-specific. Here, it is desirable to use stimuli with narrower bandwidth, in order to approximate the puretone audiogram.[46]

## Recording Electrodes

Needle electrodes are rarely used, except for investigation of the CM, SP, or CAP by ECochG. Transtympanic ECochG involves a needle electrode through the tympanum onto the middle-ear promontory.[47] In endomeatal ECochG, the electrode is usually a silver ball within the ear canal.[44]

Most AEPs are recorded using disc or cup EEG electrodes on the scalp.[48] Scalp electrodes are often of silver, coated with chloride to reduce electrical artifacts due to polarization. Conductive paste or gel lies between the electrode and the skin, and mechanical adhesion is achieved either by the paste or by adhesive disks or tape. The skin is previously cleaned with alcohol and lightly abraded. A mechanically and electrically adequate connection is essential, more practical problems being caused by bad electrode contact than by any other technical matters. The electrical resistance or, more correctly, the impedance of the electrode-patient contact is expressed in kilohms; a value of under 5 kilohms is usually considered adequate in scalp recording.

Electrode position is governed primarily by the distribution of the AEP over the head. At any instant, this can be visualized as a contour map of potential, analogous to a geographical survey map. Most AEP recordings are done using a *differential* technique, which measures potential differences between two electrode sites. To maximize the recorded AEP, one electrode is placed near the point of highest potential and the other near a point of minimum potential. The brainstem and cortical potentials of interest have broad topographies, developing maxima in the region of the scalp vertex. Thus, one electrode is placed near the vertex; the other is conveniently placed on an earlobe or mastoid. Other placements are possible but the vertex-mastoid derivation, or an approximation, is the most common.[3]

## Differential Preamplification

AEPs are in the microvolt range or less, and typical preamplifier gains are 10,000 to 50,000. The differential action involves subtracting the activity at one electrode from that at another, to eliminate activity common to both sites. This is critical for enhancing the AEP relative to the noise, much of which is similar over the head; examples are noise due to electromagnetic pickup from radio stations or from power cables, and from major physiological sources such as the heart. One electrode is called noninverting and the other, which provides the activity that is subtracted, is the inverting electrode. Use of the old terminology of active and reference is discouraged because often both electrodes register part of the AEP. A third electrode is a kind of electrical ground, often placed on the other earlobe or mastoid.

The rejection of common activity is imperfect and is expressed by the common-mode rejection ratio (CMRR), which is the ratio of gain for activity at one input versus that for the same activity at both inputs. A typical CMRR is 80 dB (i.e., a factor of 10,000). High CMRR is essential for AEP enhancement, and a loss of only a few dB can degrade the AEP record. CMRR is reduced by large or asymmetrical electrode impedances. Note that the ratio only applies to activity that is identical at the differential electrodes; even slight differences will be amplified by the regular gain.

## Filtering

Filtering (filtration) is the next step in AEP enhancement. It is best thought of in the frequency domain, the goal being to suppress those frequency components containing most noise energy, but to pass unchanged the components containing most AEP energy. Basic concepts are shown in Figure 16-6. The simplest elements are high-pass and low-pass filters; these terms are very descriptive: high-pass filters pass high-frequency energy but block low-frequency energy. Low-pass filters have the converse action. Equipment manufacturers often complicate the matter with spurious terms such as high filter in reference to the low-pass filter. More complex filters, such as band-pass and band-stop (band-reject, notch) filters can be thought of as combinations of high-pass and low-pass units. Real filters do not stop energy perfectly but, rather, progressively. Filters vary in the steepness of this cut-off slope, often expressed in multiples of 6dB attenuation per octave of frequency. There are many filter designs, for example, the Bessel and Butterworth types.

AEP and noise spectra differ greatly for various AEPs, so the filter requirements also differ. In general, the more rostral the AEP source the "slower" the AEP voltage fluctuation, and the spectral concentration moves to lower frequency. A rough idea of filter requirements is gained by inspection of the AEP waveform. For example, the ABR to a high-intensity click looks like an oscillation at about 1 kHz (see Fig. 16-3); its spectrum has a great deal of energy at that frequency, so the filter should include 1 kHz in its passband. SVR energy, on the other hand, occurs at a much lower frequency, about 5 Hz or so, and the filter for SVR work should pass that frequency. Filtering works best if the AEP and noise spectra are dissimilar, but often there is much spectral overlap, so filtering usually achieves limited but important gains in AEP clarity.

Most filters are boxes of electronics that operate on input signals that vary continuously; these are "analog" filters. It is also possible to filter using calculations operating upon bioelectric data that have been captured and stored as streams of digits in a computer memory; this is called digital filtering. It is more flexible and powerful than analog filtering, and is becoming widely used in the most modern AEP instrumentation systems.

## Analog to Digital Conversion

Conversion of the amplifier/filter output into a sequence of numbers for computer processing is achieved by rapid, periodic sampling. The *sampling rate* must be at least twice the highest frequency component in the signal; for example, if there is energy up to 2 kHz, the rate must be at least 4,000/sec. Failure to achieve at least this *Nyquist* rate causes a distortion known as aliasing, which is a shifting of high-frequency energy to low frequencies. It is usually possible to sample much faster than the Nyquist rate.

Another factor is analog to digital (A/D) *resolution.* One meets descriptions such as "10-bit A/D conversion." A bit is a binary digit, which can be zero or unity. Digital computers store numbers in words, which are strings of bits. Arithmetic shows that a 1-bit word can take two values, a 2-bit word four values, etc. In general, a k-bit word can take $2^k$ distinct values. A/D resolution is the number of bits in the word generated at each sampling instant. Thus, a 10-bit converter forces its input voltage range into $2^{10}$ (1,024) values; this causes small errors (quantization errors) when the input does not match a possible output value exactly. In practice, such errors are rarely important, and a 10-bit conversion is quite adequate; in fact, one can get away with much less.

For each stimulus, a time-locked activity segment is digitized. Segments are "sweeps" or "windows." Typical sweeps include 256 data points, the

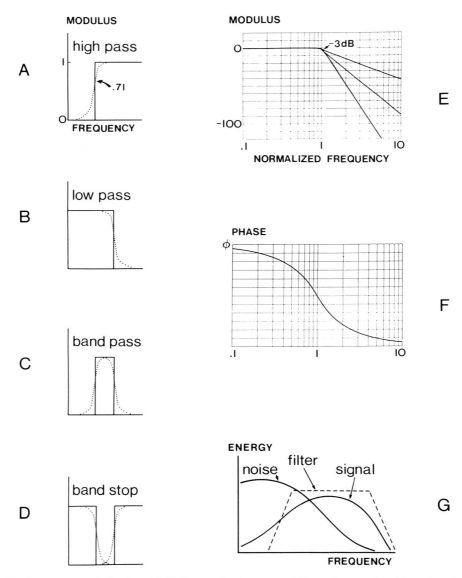

**Fig. 16-6.** Basic concepts of filtering. **(A-D)** Some simple types of filter, showing ideal (solid) and real (dotted) filter moduli. The modulus is the filter output magnitude divided by the input magnitude, and varies between zero (perfect stop) and unity (perfect pass). **(E)** Various low-pass filter moduli in a common format, using a modulus scale in dB of attenuation, and a logarithmic frequency scale "normalized" by dividing all frequencies by the "cut-off" frequency. The cut-off frequency is the frequency at which the modulus is 0.71, or 3 dB smaller than unity. On a dB scale, the filter "roll-off" is linear, and various common slopes that are multiples of 6 dB per octave (doubling) of frequency are shown. **(F)** The way in which filters alter not only the magnitude of an input signal but also its phase, and the amount of phase shift is shown as a function of normalized frequency. The absolute amount of phase shift increases with the roll-off slope. See later text for a discussion of AEP distortion due to phase shift. **(G)** The frequency spectra of the AEP and the bioelectric noise are often broad and overlapping; a choice of filter will focus upon the main AEP energy but will inevitably affect some of that energy, as well as passing some of the noise.

power of two being a mere technicality. For example, in ABR measurement, 256 points sampled at 20 kHz gives a 12.8 msec window, suitable for otoneurologic studies. For the SVR, on the other hand, a window of at least 500 msec is required; 256 points at a rate of 250 Hz would give a window of 1.024 seconds, which is quite suitable. This much lower sampling rate is sufficient because whereas the ABR has energy up to about 2 kHz, the SVR has little energy above 20 Hz.

## Summation or Averaging

The next step in AEP enhancement is summation, or averaging, of the sweeps in a columnwise fashion, corresponding points of each sweep being added to produce a sum or average array of the same length as each sweep. We will define the AEP as the signal and the spontaneous activity as noise. The activity in each sweep is modeled as the sum of signal and noise, with the assumption that they are statistically independent, that is, the noise is as it would have been in the absence of signal, and vice versa. Another important assumption is that the signal (AEP) occurs at exactly the same time, with identical waveform, for all stimuli.

The key to summation or averaging is that the AEP is constant, but the noise is random and partially cancels itself over the set of sweeps. A useful concept is the *signal-to-noise ratio* (SNR), which is the ratio of AEP amplitude to noise standard deviation (SD). For example, if a typical ABR amplitude is $0.25 \mu V$, and typical noise in a single sweep has an SD of $5 \mu V$, the SNR is roughly 0.05, so we cannot see the ABR. After summing $n$ sweeps, the ABR increases by a factor $n$, and statistical theory reveals that the noise SD in the sum increases by only $\sqrt{n}$. Thus, the SNR in the sum is $\sqrt{n}$ times the single-sweep SNR. This result is unchanged, whether we deal with sums or averages; the statistical argument differs, as does the appearance of the process on the computer display screen, but the result is the same. Figure 16-7 illustrates the process of averaging.

Several points follow from the $\sqrt{n}$ law. First, noise is never abolished: part of the sum or average record *may* be real AEP, and part of it *will* be noise.

Second, averaging yields diminishing returns of SNR enhancement per unit time. For example, if the starting SNR is $x$, it takes 100 sweeps to achieve $10x$, and 10,000 sweeps to increase it by a further factor of 10. Whatever the rate, 10,000 sweeps take 100 times longer than 100 sweeps. Third, the $\sqrt{n}$ law allows the required number of sweeps to be estimated, if AEP size and noise SD are known approximately. When observers look at an average, they are confident of genuine response if they see activity at some point at least about twice the size of the fluctuations in the rest of the record. Thus, they need an SNR of about two, or more. For the ABR, for example, if the initial SNR is 0.05 and the target SNR after $n$ sweeps is at least 2, $\sqrt{n}$ must be at least 40, so $n$ must be at least 1,600. This is in the right ballpark, averages of 2,000 or more sweeps being typical. For the SVR, the typical initial SNR is more like 0.5, which implies a need to average only about 16 sweeps, and indeed the typical number is in the 20 to 50 range.

## Artifact Rejection

The $\sqrt{n}$ law assumes that the noise has constant statistical properties over time, that it is *stationary*. Often, however, the activity contains large voltage transients due to sporadic myogenic activity or movement of the electrode/skin interface. These transients are not governed by the $\sqrt{n}$ law. For example, one of $200 \mu V$ will have a size of $0.2 \mu V$ after 1,000 sweeps, which is about as big as an ABR. These artifacts can simulate, distort, or abolish real AEPs. A method of reducing this problem is to acquire each sweep to a temporary "buffer," test the buffer for large values, and discard it if an artifact is found. Most commercial AEP systems have this artifact rejection facility, and it can be very helpful in obtaining good AEP estimates under poor conditions.

## After Averaging

Most AEP systems permit simultaneous display of several averages, and this is helpful when superimposing them to assess response reproducibility, or for examining trends of response change over

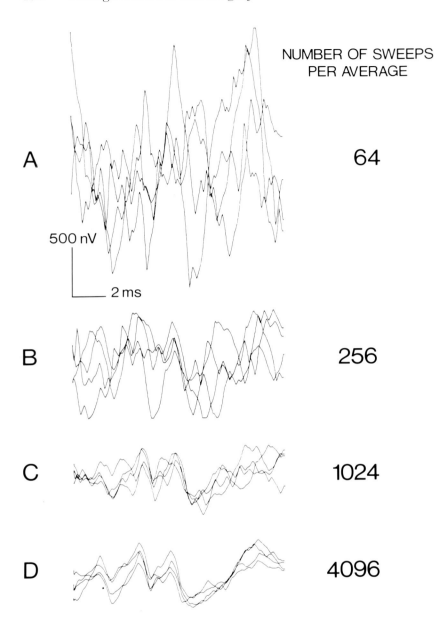

NUMBER OF SWEEPS
PER AVERAGE

A          64

500 nV

2 ms

B         256

C        1024

D        4096

**Fig. 16-7.** The effects of averaging on signal to noise ratio (SNR). For each group, four independent traces are superimposed, each having the number of sweeps indicated. The sweep numbers are chosen so that the SNR doubles each time (**A–D**), according to the square root law (see text). Note how the averaging causes progressive convergence due to noise cancellation (all traces have the same amplitude and time scales), and how there is residual noise even after 4,096 sweeps.

several stimulus conditions. Particular response features can be picked by cursor control, and read-outs of amplitude and latency obtained. There is often a digital smoothing option, and the ability to add or subtract averages from one another. Waveforms are usually plotted on a hard copy device (printer or plotter), and some systems allow digital storage of waveforms, together with information about the patient and test conditions.

## IMPORTANT VARIABLES UNDERLYING CLINICAL AEP TESTS

Clinical applications depend upon AEP amplitude, latency, and morphology. These characteristics in turn depend on many physical and psychophysiological variables. Thus, an understanding of the most important effects is essential for appreciation of the rationale and pitfalls of clinical testing. The main variables fall into three classes: stimulus, recording, and patient-related factors. Some of these have comparable effects on many AEPs, whereas for others there may be large differences in susceptibility. Within each class, there may be several important factors, and these may interact strongly. In many cases, the truth is as yet far from clear. Only the main points will be dealt with here; more detailed descriptions are available for ECochG,[47] the ABR,[29,49] the MLR,[50] and the SVR.[3,51]

## Effects of Stimulus Parameters

### Input-Output Functions

An *input-output* (I-O) function is a curve relating a stimulus parameter, plotted on the x axis, to a response parameter, plotted on the y axis. Examples are the intensity-latency function (also known less logically as the latency-intensity function), the rate-amplitude function, among others. Such functions influence test protocols strongly.

### Intensity

The units of intensity are the audiometric standard dB hearing level (HL) for long tone bursts, but for brief stimuli there are no such standards. Accordingly, it is common to refer intensity to the average threshold for a group of subjects with normal hearing, which defines the dBnHL scale (dB normal hearing level). One can also use purely physical measures such as dB peak-equivalent sound pressure level (dB peSPL), or measures relating to the behavioral threshold of the individual (dB sensation level, dB SL).[42]

Typical intensity-amplitude and intensity-latency functions are illustrated in Figure 16-8. In general, as stimulus intensity increases, AEP amplitude increases and latency decreases. The intensity below which the response is not detectable is the AEP threshold. Usually, amplitude thereafter increases steadily with intensity, with saturation or even reversal at the highest intensities. For "peripheral" AEPs (e.g., CM, SP, and CAP) there is a rough correspondence between stimulus and re-

sponse amplitude, at least for the lower part of the intensity range. Intensity is measured logarithmically, in dB, so the intensity-amplitude function will be roughly linear when amplitude is plotted on a *logarithmic* scale. For AEPs from more rostral sites, the pattern of roughly linear growth, with saturation, is observed when amplitude is plotted on a *linear* scale, as for the ABR in Figure 16-8. These lesser rates of response growth are presumably attributable to transformations effected by the chain of neurons now interposed between the cochlea and the site of AEP generation. In general, for the transient responses, the increase in amplitude is attributable to increasing numbers of responding neurons, and probably to increasing neural synchrony as well.

Intensity-amplitude curves do not convey the general impression of change in an entire group of waves, such as the ABR or MLR. An "intensity series" for the ABR is also shown in Figure 16-8. There is an impression of increasing AEP complexity as the various waves develop, above their respective thresholds.

The latency of the cochlear potentials CM and SP is almost zero for all stimulus intensities. For most other exogenous neurogenic AEPs, the latency is greatest close to threshold intensity, and thereafter decreases smoothly. The rate of decrease is usually largest close to threshold and tapers off at high intensities, though the form of the curve may vary. The mechanisms governing the decrease in latency as intensity increases are not very well understood, and differ across AEPs. Some possibilities include shift of the cochlear sites of AEP initiation towards the basal (high-frequency) regions, increase in the population of neurons activated, and increased rate of postsynaptic summation and excitation. While the curves of Figure 16-8 are typical, the exact intensity functions usually depend strongly upon other stimulus features, such as its frequency or repetition rate. Thus, the effects of these variables *interact*.

### Frequency

All other stimulus variables being held constant, the amplitudes and latencies of neurogenic AEPs often change with the nominal frequency of the tonepip or toneburst. It is generally agreed that for

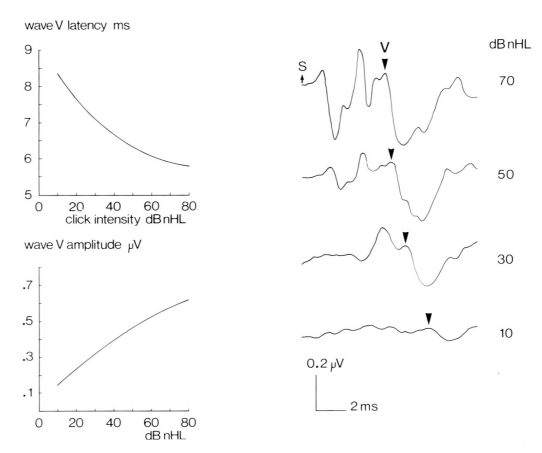

**Fig. 16-8.** Input-output functions and an intensity series for the ABR. The intensity-latency and intensity-amplitude functions for wave V are diagrammatic, derived from combination of many published studies; note that neither curve is linear over click level. In the illustrative intensity series obtained from a normal subject, only wave V remains visible at click levels near the AEP threshold.

relatively peripheral AEPs such as the CAP and ABR, increasing stimulus frequency reduces latency. Amplitude effects are more obscure, though there is a tendency towards larger amplitudes at higher frequencies. One reason for these effects is that such responses are governed by neural synchrony, and high-frequency stimuli promote better synchrony. Also, the higher the frequency, the closer to the cochlear base is the site of AEP initiation, and basal excitation tends to occur earlier than apical excitation.

For more rostral AEPs such as the MLR and SVR, increasing frequency tends to reduce response amplitude and increase latency, though there is considerable difference of opinion in the literature.

The reasons for these effects are not well-understood, but we can speculate: first, these AEPs have much larger latencies than the CAP or ABR, so any changes of the order of a millisecond related to cochlear site of initiation would be almost irrelevant. Second, the more rostral AEPs are not nearly as sensitive to neural synchrony, and are governed more by the sheer volume of afferent neural flow, which tends to be larger for low-frequency stimuli.

For the MLR and SVR, the stimuli can be tone-bursts with sufficiently long rise-fall times and durations to ensure narrow bandwidth and adequate frequency-specificity. For these situations, the concept of stimulus frequency is straightforward. On the other hand, the CAP and ABR are elicited by brief stimuli with complex spectra. Here, it is necessary to consider carefully the details of cochlear and neural excitation patterns, particularly the spread of stimulus energy over a range of frequencies, and how that spread may change with nominal frequency and intensity. This complex issue is addressed later, in relation to estimation of the audiogram.

It should be noted that lack of attention to recording parameters may give misleading results in I-O function studies. For example, it was once thought that low-frequency stimuli elicited little or no ABR; later, it was shown that there is indeed an ABR but its waveshape is much broader and later than the response to high-frequency stimuli or to clicks.[52] The use of recording filters appropriate for click ABRs was not appropriate for low-frequency ABRs, and tended to abolish them.

### Stimulus Envelope Parameters

We must recall that the transient neurogenic AEPs considered here are regarded as on-effects, meaning that their characteristics are determined largely by events during some small time interval following the start of the stimulus.[3,29,53] In general, the longer the AEP latency, the greater the length of this response-determinant epoch. For example, it appears that the CAP and ABR are governed by events in the first few milliseconds of stimulation,[29] whereas the SVR is influenced by events over a much longer epoch, up to about 25msec or so.[46] Clearly, the onset profile of the stimulus envelope will influence the response-determinant events strongly. In general, the shorter the rise time of a brief tone, the smaller the AEP latency and the larger its amplitude. These changes are especially marked for the CAP and ABR, and particularly for latency. The effects change with stimulus frequency and intensity, and the underlying mechanism is not fully understood; neural synchrony is likely to play a major role, and as rise time decreases spectral spread and neural synchrony increase.[29,46]

The study of stimulus duration effects is not straightforward; first, the rise time must not exceed the response-determinant epoch. Second, a true duration effect is only measurable within the remainder of the determinant epoch; it is remarkable how many "duration" studies have explored durations even longer than the response latency itself. Third, if the duration occupies more than about 10 percent of the interval between stimulus onsets, one is probably studying neural recovery rather than duration effects.

Duration effects on the CAP and ABR are far from clear, and the problem is complicated by interactions between stimulus shape parameters, frequency, and intensity.[29] An effect has been demonstrated for later responses, such as the SVR, the amplitude of which increases with stimulus duration up to about 30 msec.[51] This effect is analogous, at least superficially, to the so-called "temporal summation" of percepts such as loudness.[54]

### Polarity

Especially for click stimuli, it is reported that the initial polarity of the stimulus may affect CAP and ABR parameters.[29,49] Effects on later responses such as MLR and SVR are negligible. Depending on the electrical polarity of the earphone input, the initial deflection of the earphone diaphragm may cause a pressure increase (condensation) or a decrease (rarefaction). In normal-hearing persons it is reported that CAP (and ABR wave I) latency is smaller for rarefaction clicks. Stimulus polarity is known to affect discharge patterns in individual auditory nerve fibers,[54] and it is not unreasonable that these effects may be revealed in gross AEPs. An explanatory hypothesis is that primary neurons are preferentially activated by basilar membrane displacement in the direction associated with rarefaction; for the rarefaction click, this excitatory motion is immediate, but for condensation clicks the AEP initiation is delayed until the first excitatory phase of basilar membrane oscillation. This simple notion is not universally accepted, nor is there unanimous agreement that rarefaction responses are always earlier. In particular, patients with cochlear disorders might exhibit complex interactions between stimulus polarity and the mechanical and electrophysiological state of the cochlea, with unpredictable effects on AEP waveform. Certainly, polarity effects warrant caution in the interpretation of responses, particularly if click polarity has been alternated to reduce stimulus artifact in the averaged record.

## Repetition Rate

The CM and SP are not affected by stimulus repetition rate. For transient AEPs, increasing rate tends to reduce amplitude and increase latency. For fast AEPs, the mechanism is probably a matter of limited neural recovery between stimuli. For more rostral AEPs such as the SVR, it may be appropriate to talk of "habituation," which implies some active inhibitory neural mechanism.[51] Again, there are interactions between the effects of various stimulus parameters, so the rate functions may change with, for example, stimulus intensity or frequency. In general, the more rostral the response, the longer it takes to recover between stimuli. Thus, for the SVR, rates much above 1/sec depress the response strongly, whereas the CAP and ABR can withstand much higher rates; the MLR is intermediate. ABR wave V is anomalous in that it can tolerate higher rates (over 50/sec) than the earlier waves, without much loss of amplitude. The reason why is not clear.

For any AEP, how is an appropriate rate for clinical testing determined? This important choice will govern the testing time, because most of an AEP test is spent waiting for averages to accumulate. The goal is to optimize measurement efficiency. If one is interested in response detection, as in threshold ERA, the rate should optimize the response detectability achievable in a given test time. The trade-off is that the higher the rate, the smaller the response per stimulus but the more averaging is possible within the fixed test time. A useful measure is response amplitude divided by the standard deviation of the residual noise in the average; the latter decreases with the square root of the number of stimuli, which increases with increasing rate. This ratio has been called "efficiency," and the rate selection should maximize it.[56] The principle is illustrated in Figure 16-9.

For ABR and MLR recording, the rate should never be an integer multiple or submultiple of the power line frequency (e.g., 60 Hz), which would synchronize the averaging to the power line interference. This is why one sees odd rates such as 21/sec or 33/sec, in the literature. Second, for the ABR there is the problem that at high rates AEPs of longer latency, such as myogenic response or the MLR, will spill over into successive averaging windows and cause distortion.

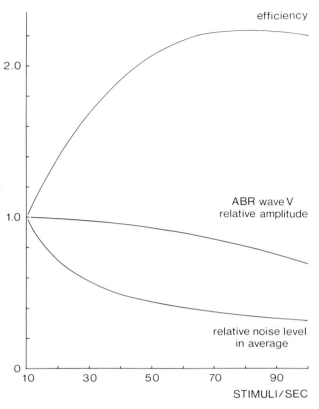

**Fig. 16-9.** Test efficiency in relation to stimulus repetition rate. The argument for selection of an optimal rate is illustrated using ABR wave V. The higher the rate, the smaller the amplitude of wave V, but the more averaging can be done within a fixed test period. Thus the noise level in the average decreases according to an inverse square root law (see Fig. 16-7), with increasing repetition rate. The "clarity" of the AEP in the average is closely related to the "efficiency", which is the ratio of response amplitude to noise standard deviation. This example indicates that low repetition rates are very inefficient for ABR wave V recording. Both amplitude and noise level are normalized to unity at a rate of 10/sec. The wave V rate-amplitude function is derived from many published studies.

## Transducers

Most earphones or bone conductors can transduce tonepips or tonebursts adequately, and there is no difficulty in using these transducers to elicit later responses such as MLR or SVR. A problem arises when using rectangular-pulse click stimuli, and this is one reason for a movement away from the use of clicks. Such a pulse produces a pressure waveform that differs between transducers, or even over time for any given transducer. This is so because the pulse excites the entire bandwidth of the transducer, so the output waveform depends on the frequency response. These differences cause changes in CAP and ABR parameters.[57] Also, there are major differences in frequency response between earphones and bone conductors, the latter having much poorer high-frequency response. This is one of the difficulties with CAP and ABR testing with bone conductors, using click stimuli, particularly if responses elicited by air and bone conduction are to be compared.[57,58]

### Masking

For the CAP recorded either transtympanically or endomeatally, the electrode montage focuses attention exclusively on response from the test ear, so contralateral masking is unnecessary. This is one of the strengths of audiometry by ECochG, which is of particular relevance in bilateral mixed losses that cause classic masking problems. For more rostral AEPs, electrode montages are such that either ear may contribute to the observed waveform, so contralateral noise masking should be used in both audiometric and otoneurologic testing. For click stimuli, fixed 50 dB HL white or pink noise masking is adequate for most purposes. For ERA with tone-pips, standard contralateral noise masking procedures as indicated for behavioral pure-tone audiometry are appropriate.

### Binaural Stimuli

Most clinical AEP testing involves monaural stimuli, but there is some interest in binaural phenomena, especially for the ABR. The ABR to binaural stimuli is almost exactly the sum of the ABR from each ear stimulated monaurally. This implies either different neural sources excited by each ear, or simple additive response of sources common to both ears, or both. This is unexpected, in view of the classical picture of bilateral activity in the ascending auditory pathway, but we understand little of the relationship between ABR and the classical auditory pathways.

Slight differences between the binaural ABR and the sum of monaural ABRs have been observed at about 6 msec latency. This might reflect activation of brainstem neurons exclusively sensitive to binaural stimulation, but another possibility is that there are indeed neurons common to both ears but their response is not linearly additive. All in all, the significance of apparent binaural interaction effects remains controversial.[29]

## Effects of Recording Variables

### Electrode Position

The placement of the differential electrode pair should optimize AEP clarity, taking account of the spatial distributions of the AEP and noise. In Figure 16-10, relationships between preamplifier inputs and outputs are illustrated, and an understanding of these is necessary for appreciation of how *observed* waveforms relate to the *actual* potentials.

To reveal the CM, SP, and the CAP, the transtympanic needle gives the clearest recordings. The position of the other electrode is not critical; often, the ipsilateral earlobe or mastoid is used. There is no problem with response cancellation at the two electrodes, because the AEP is much larger at the promontory. For endomeatal ECochG, a silver ball is more common; pressure against the meatal wall is maintained by a V-shaped plastic spring inserted in the canal under compression.[44] The best site is within a few millimeters of the tympanic annulus, in the posterior aspect. AEPs are much smaller here than from the middle ear,[59] and there is a lack of consensus about the utility of the endomeatal method; it appears that if the goal is merely to enhance the CAP so that its latency is measurable, the canal electrode is useful. For detailed measurements of CM, SP, and CAP parameters or thresholds, transtympanic recording is preferable.

Electrode placements for ABR recording are usually a compromise between clarity of the individual waves and the desire to register the complete sequence. ABR wave I (the CAP) radiates mainly to the periauricular region, as a scalp-negative wave. It appears to have the same polarity as the later vertex-positive ABR waves because either it, or they, are inverted by the differential preamplifier (see Figs. 16-3, and 16-10). Wave V has a broad, scalp-positive, vertex-maximal topography, but there is significant amplitude at the mastoid. For wave V, a vertex-neck placement may yield

DIFFERENTIAL AMPLIFICATION

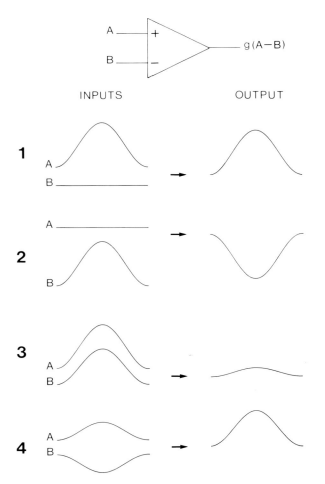

INPUTS                    OUTPUT

**Fig. 16-10.** Effects of differential amplification on AEPs. The amplifier subtracts the signal at input B (the inverting input, denoted as −) from that at input A (the noninverting input, denoted as +), and multiplies the result by the gain factor g. (1) A positive AEP at A and zero at B gives a positive result at the output. (2) if the situation is reversed, the output is now negative, even though the input AEP is positive. (3) If the AEP is similar at A and B, the output is reduced; if A and B have identical inputs, the output is zero. (4) If the AEP is positive at A and negative at B, the output is larger and positive. These examples illustrate how care is required in inferring what is happening on the scalp or in the ear from the differential amplifier output. For example, with vertex **(A)** to mastoid **(B)** recording of the ABR, wave I is the CAP that appears mainly as a negative potential at the mastoid; its polarity is reversed so that it appears as a positive wave in the same direction as wave V, which is truly a scalp-positive wave appearing mainly at the vertex. In ECochG, if the transtympanic electrode is connected to the noninverting input, the CAP and SP will appear as negative deflections, which they really are.

greater amplitude, but would not register wave I well. In the author's view, there is little difference between vertex and forehead, or between mastoid and earlobe, but there are reports that wave I is larger at the earlobe.[60] Parker[61] has provided details of ABR distribution over the scalp.

For the MLR and SVR, the scalp topographies are broad and a vertex-mastoid placement is generally best.[3] The vertex-maximal topography does not imply that the sources of these AEPs underlie the vertex; rather, it is a net result of interactions between fields from distributed cortical sources.[3,35] In general, it must be remembered that recording from a single differential pair gives only a very limited view of the potential topography, which may contain much more information than is presently accessed.

## Filtering

Filtering is used to improve the SNR and to "clean up" the AEP waveform. The choice of filter is dictated mainly by the AEP and noise spectra, as shown earlier. Unfortunately, most filters in common use distort the AEP.[62] The effects include change in amplitude and latency, introduction of spurious peaks, and AEP abolition. This can cause inefficiency and errors, both in research and clinical tests.

Filters distort AEPs in two ways: they may attenuate certain AEP frequency components, called amplitude distortion, and they may introduce time-shifts between AEP frequency components, even those that are not attenuated. This is called phase distortion because, when one is considering the sinusoidal frequency components of complex signals, time and sinusoid phase angle have a simple relationship (see Fig. 16-6). Low-pass filtering tends to smooth waveforms, reduce amplitude, and increase latency. High-pass filtering reduces latency, and tends to reduce amplitude as well, but as a result of the associated phase distortion its effects are often more difficult to anticipate. Some examples of filter effects on various AEPs are shown in Figure 16-11. The bottom line is that careful attention must be given to technical aspects of AEP recording; the literature is full of studies that take insufficient account of such matters.

Amplitude distortion is inherent in filtering, but the increasing use of digital technology in AEP systems allows much of the phase distortion problem to be avoided. Analog filters are obliged to deal with incoming signals as they happen, whereas digital filters operate on stored data. This gives much greater scope for manipulation, and zero-phase digital filters are likely to be the norm in future AEP systems.

AEP systems often include two special filters that may cause distortion. The power line notch filter is a narrow band-stop filter intended to supress 60 Hz interference. Even though this filter may not attenuate AEP energy significantly, it can still cause phase distortion and is a potentially misleading addition that should be avoided where possible. It is far better to reduce the interference at the source, and usually the problem is one of poor electrode contact or recording too close to an unshielded power cable. The other special filtering operation is digital smoothing, often a pushbutton option used repeatedly to "clean up" a waveform. This can change response amplitudes and latencies considerably, and should not be used indiscriminately.

## Patient-Related Factors

### Noise Properties and Patient's State

The bioelectric noise in which an AEP is embedded has a major effect on the feasibility of AEP

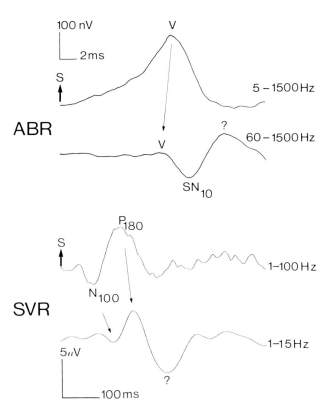

**Fig. 16-11.** Distortion of AEPs by filtering. The ABR for a low-intensity, low-frequency tonepip is frequently only a relatively "slow" vertex-positive wave V peak. Moving the high-pass filter cut-off from 5 to 60 Hz drastically alters the waveform; wave V is earlier and smaller, a new negative wave known as $SN_{10}$ (Slow Negative at about 10msec latency) is introduced, as well as a later positive peak. In this case, these new peaks are pure artifacts of filter distortion. Some of the distortion is due to the filter modulus, but much of it is due to phase shifting of the various AEP frequency components by different amounts (see text and Fig. 16-6). For the SVR, the effects of introducing strong low-pass filtering are shown; note the latency increases and, again, an artifactual peak.

measurement, the test time, and the accuracy of threshold or wave parameter estimates. For the CM, SP, and CAP recorded transtympanically, the relatively large SNR means that serious physiological noise problems are rare. ECochG is performed under general anesthesia in children, which lowers the noise levels. For all AEPs up to and including the MLR, the main physiological noise problem is electromyogenic activity, which has much of its energy in the range 50 to 250 Hz, and this may overlap strongly with the response recording passband. ABR and MLR recordings are very vulnerable; passive cooperation of the patient is mandatory, and even in cooperative patients myogenic noise levels may be high enough to preclude reliable testing. The problem is worst for threshold estimation, but even otoneurologic tests with high-level stimuli may be rendered useless by myogenic noise in tense and anxious patients. Myogenic levels are greatly improved in sleeping patients, and use of general anesthesia is better still. The ABR itself is unaffected by sleep and most sedative or anesthetic agents.[29] Depression of the MLR and 40 Hz MLR has been reported during sleep,[50] though this may be offset by the gain in clarity due to reduced myogenic noise.

SVR measurement is less affected directly by myogenic activity than the ABR and MLR, because the SVR passband is around 1 to 15 Hz. However, gross movement of the patient and of the electrode/skin interface or electrode leads can introduce large, low-frequency movement artifacts. Also, classical EEG rhythms such as alpha (8 to 13 Hz) can interfere strongly; some adults have such large alpha that SVR measurement is very difficult, but in many cases the alpha level can be reduced to acceptable values by visual attention. During natural or sedated sleep, the SVR waveform changes in a manner that reflects the spectral characteristics of the various EEG stages of sleep.[3,51] In fact, response morphology and latency change so drastically that the response should probably be considered to be a different one from that obtained in the waking state.[3] Sedative or anesthetic agents that alter the spontaneous EEG also tend to alter the SVR in a similar manner.[3,51] These changes can cause difficulty in both averaging and in response interpretation, so SVR testing during sleep or general anesthesia is widely, but not universally, considered to be unreliable.

In the awake patient, attention has negligible effects on cochlear and brainstem AEPs, a possible small effect on the MLR, and a definite effect on the SVR.[63] Having the patient pay attention to the stimuli, for example, can enhance SVR amplitude considerably.[3,51] Thus, the SVR is not entirely exogenous.

## Age

In the next few sections on effects of subject variables, it will be apparent that the clearest effects are observed for the ABR. This is probably a result of three factors: first, the ABR is generated high enough in the auditory pathway to permit expression of neurologic variables; second, the ABR is sensitive to fine changes in the volume and timing of underlying neural events; and, third, AEPs from more rostral sites exhibit much greater intrinsic variability than the ABR.

Age has a marked effect on some AEPs. We can distinguish maturational effects in the young child,[64] and degenerative effects in the elderly. The most extensive maturational data exist for the ABR,[29,49] for which massive and progressive changes in amplitude, latency, and morphology occur from birth to about 2 years of age. It is thought that most of these changes reflect development, especially myelination, in central auditory pathways, though maturational changes in cochlear function may contribute. For the MLR, there appears to be little change in response parameters with maturation, but the distribution of potential over the scalp is much more asymmetrical in the neonate than in the adult.[50] There are reports that cortical responses are smaller and later in young children than in adults, though these studies are often complicated by effects of sleep stage.[51] In the elderly there is some evidence of increased ABR latency,[57,65,66] but care is required to factor out the effects of presbycusis.

## Gender

Marked gender effects have been reported for the ABR, the latencies of waves III and V being larger in men than women by about 0.2 msec, with consequent differences in interwave intervals.[67] There is disagreement as to the maturational development of these differences. Their underlying causes are not clear, though presumably the answer lies in neuronal characteristics such as tract length, fiber diameter, and number and organization of fibers. These gender effects, though small, must be taken into account in any audiometric or otoneurologic interpretation based upon ABR latency. For other AEPs, there is little information on gender effects, which does not mean that they do not exist.

### Temperature

Later ABR waves are affected by core temperature, low temperatures causing latency increases that may resemble the effects of neurologic lesions. This is relevant in newborns, severely intoxicated or comatose patients, or during neurosurgical operative monitoring.[29,49]

### Auditory and Neurologic Disorders

The factors described above must be either controlled or accounted for in clinical AEP applications. All of the AEPs considered here are also affected in some way by hearing loss, which is the basis for their use as audiometric tools. Some AEPs are also affected by neurologic disorders, which is the basis for their use in otoneurologic assessment. Before examining these applications, it is stressed that when the clinical objective is audiometric, neurologic factors may act as confounding variables; conversely, if the intent is otoneurologic assessment, hearing impairment is a confounding variable. It is essential to be alert to all of the factors that may produce interpretive error.

---

# ELECTRIC RESPONSE AUDIOMETRY

This section deals with the use of AEPs to estimate hearing thresholds. This is valuable in patients for whom conventional behavioral audiometry is impossible, inaccurate, or suspect. The population includes neonates, infants, difficult-to-test children, multiply handicapped patients, and those suspected of functional (non-organic) hearing loss medicolegal or compensation cases. For some of these, other "objective" ways of estimating the audiogram exist; examples are respiration audiometry in infants,[68] and predictions based on acoustic reflex thresholds in older children and adults.[69] Usually ERA methods offer greater accu-

racy, but the equipment costs and expertise requirements are considerable.

## A Selection of AEPs

Many AEPs are used in threshold estimation, and test strategies may involve several of them. A selection of AEPs that are useful or promising as components of an integrated scheme includes:

1. The cochlear nerve CAP
2. The V-SN$_{10}$ complex of the ABR
3. The MLR or its 40 Hz variant
4. The SVR

Other AEPs are used audiometrically in some centers throughout the world, but in this writer's view those listed above are the major tools. Here, we are concerned with AEP properties near threshold, and these can be very different from those observed at high stimulus levels. For example, one usually thinks of the ABR as a multiwave sequence completed within about 8 msec of stimulus onset. Yet, for a shaped 500 Hz tonepip at 30 dB SL, the response may be a single vertex-positive wave with a latency of up to 15 msec.

## Comparative Assessment of Various AEP Techniques

An ERA test is usually a series of estimations of behavioral thresholds. For each type and route of stimulus, the level at which the average AEP is just detectable is determined. This is an estimate of the AEP threshold, which in turn is assumed to be related to the true perceptual threshold. Thus there are really two estimation processes, each of which is a source of error. The clinical value of many ERA procedure is governed by these errors, as well as other factors.

ERA procedures may be compared on the basis of several performance criteria.[3,70,71] Six important attributes of a clinically useful ERA method are validity, objectivity, accuracy, frequency-specificity, efficiency, and freedom from discomfort and risk. Qualities such as convenience, low cost, and simplicity are desirable but less fundamental. Inevitably, published reports reflect individual bias, and the picture will change over time. Perhaps the most important observation is that each AEP to be considered here has its own peculiar role and merits; it is a mistake to be wedded to a single method.

### Validity

The assumption that a recordable AEP implies a suprathreshold stimulus, and the converse, should be valid. This may not be so, for many reasons. The human auditory system has no functional resemblance to an EEG amplifier and averager. Because neither audition nor AEPs has a well-understood neurophysiologic basis, their relationship is obscure even in the normal case, and is so a fortiori in the presence of dysfunction.

Some AEPs, such as the ABR, may be mediated by neural pathways that are different from, or a subset of, those that mediate perceptual events. Also, the neural synchrony requirement for AEP development does not apply, at least to the same degree, for perception of sound. In patients with multiple sclerosis, for example, neuronal desynchronisation due to a demyelinating plaque may abolish the ABR, yet the puretone audiogram may be normal.[72] This can also happen in patients with acoustic tumors. Other cases of idiopathic ABR absence or depression have been reported.[73] The thresholds of high-level AEPs such as the MLR and SVR are less sensitive to neuropathy, partly because they are less dependent upon neural synchrony.

The converse situation, in which the AEP threshold is much better than the *true* behavioral threshold, is rarer. Disorders that are more rostral than the AEP source may cause hearing loss but not affect the AEP thresholds. This situation is uncommon not only because most disorders causing puretone hearing loss are peripheral to the auditory nerve but also because lesions at a high neuronal level usually do not affect puretone thresholds drastically, unless they are bilateral and severe. A good example of discrepancy between AEP and behavioral thresholds, and of the use of more than one AEP to localize a lesion within the auditory neuraxis, was reported by Ozdamar et al.;[74] the patient had bilateral temporal lobe lesions, severe behavioral puretone hearing loss, normal ABR thresholds, and absent MLR.

At present, it is wise to regard relationships between AEP and perceptual measures as serendipitous. The validity of ERA is not intrinsic but it is probabilistic, and must be established empirically through comprehensive study of threshold correlations over a wide range of normative case material. This empiricism is a fundamental limitation, and implies not only that ERA must be treated as a multi-AEP scheme but also that it should not be adopted as a stand-alone substitute for other feasible tests, if any.

Discrepancies between AEP and behavioral tests should not be dismissed lightly. When they occur, the first step is to examine each for errors, the most common problem being procedural or interpretive error in either procedure, or both. If there is no obvious error, the case must be monitored until the cause of divergence is revealed, or it resolves, or the behavioral data become indisputable. However, it is important to remember that the puretone audiogram has many limitations as a tool for diagnosis, a measure of communicative deficit, and a guide to rehabilitation. Ultimately, it is to be expected that behavioral and AEP measures will improve and diversify in a complementary fashion.

### Objectivity

A truly objective test requires, at most, the passive cooperation of the patient; none of the tests discussed here even requires that the patient attend to the stimulus. However, AEP threshold estimation can depend strongly on the tester's subjective judgement, and can require substantial skill, for both efficient testing and interpretation of averaged records. The key decisions concern presence or absence of response, and averages are often highly contaminated with residual noise or artifacts. Errors of judgment by inexperienced testers can give wildly inaccurate thresholds. Interpretation is best done on-line; clues such as the trend of response development and EEG characteristics can improve judgments and are not apparent in the final tracing. Post hoc reading of records can be unreliable, especially by persons without extensive experience.

Techniques that assist or replace subjective interpretation can improve ERA objectivity. Computer-based statistical interpretation of AEP records is an important goal.[75,76] It is possible to automate both acquisition and interpretation of ERA records, but this is not straightforward. It is easy to formulate algorithms that avoid the blatant errors committed by inexperienced testers, but difficult to imitate the performance of a skilled tester. This area is one of active research but little commercial implementation.

### Accuracy

Acceptable limits of threshold estimation error depend on the test objective; for example, the accuracy needed to define habilitation for hearing-impaired infants is less than for adult diagnostic audiometry, which in turn is less than for medicolegal or compensation evaluation.

In normative groups for which both AEP and behavioral thresholds are obtained, they are rarely equal. Many factors cause these differences to be distributed statistically over patients, so the AEP threshold is a statistical estimator of the behavioral threshold. The question is: Given an observed AEP threshold, what inference can be made about the associated behavioral threshold? Estimation theory distinguishes two components of accuracy: *bias* and *variability*. Bias is the expected average difference between a quantity and its estimates, while variability reflects random variation from estimate to estimate. These two components may behave independently.

Given an AEP threshold, the best estimate of the behavioral threshold is the AEP threshold minus the average of the appropriate normative distribution of threshold differences. This average is the bias value, as illustrated in Figure 16-12. Bias has been loosely termed "sensitivity," in the sense that a method with large positive bias will tend to produce AEP thresholds much higher (worse) than the behavioral thresholds, and is "insensitive."

The clinical impact of bias is its restrictive effect on the range of hearing losses that can be assessed. Suppose the click-evoked ABR wave I were considered as an audiometric tool. This wave disappears in the normal adult at about 50 dB nHL; that is, its bias is 50 dB. If this persists in the presence of hearing loss, then because most earphones cannot

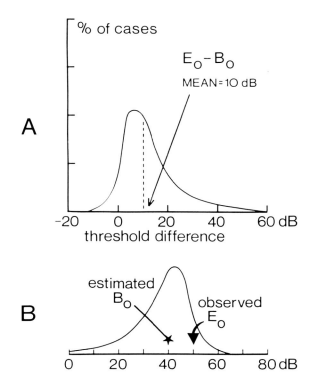

**Fig. 16-12.** The principle of audiometric threshold estimation by ERA. **(A)** A typical normative distribution, over many subjects, of differences between the true behavioral threshold $B_0$ and the AEP threshold $E_0$. Note that the mean difference (the AEP "bias") is typically positive (meaning that the AEP threshold is higher), and that the distribution is skewed towards substantial positive differences. **(B)** For a single patient in whom the behavioral threshold is to be estimated, first the AEP threshold is determined. The normative difference distribution is now used to infer the best estimate of the true behavioral threshold, and the range of uncertainty.

deliver clicks at more than 95 dB nHL, hearing losses greater than 45 dB could not be measured.

For any AEP, bias is affected by many factors such as test methodology, the type of stimulus, the amount and type of hearing loss, and patient characteristics. For example, the bias may vary with stimulus frequency, or differ between children and adults. Normative studies of bias must take into account the host of variables to be specified and controlled. Thus, while normative data are available for many AEPs, there is frequently a lack of consensus, which is probably attributable to variations in procedures and in test populations. Typically, bias is within the range of 5 to 25 dB.

Variability of ERA threshold estimates is perhaps even more important than bias. While the AEP threshold minus the bias gives the best *point* estimate of the behavioral threshold, it gives no clue as to the amount of random error (*interval* estimate). In fact, the distribution of error in the individual patient is approximated by the normative difference distribution shown in Figure 16-12. For example, suppose this distribution had a mean (bias) of 10 dB, but the differences exceeded 25 dB in 5 percent of normative cases. Given an AEP threshold estimate of 45 dB, we infer that the behavioral threshold is most probably 35 dB, but it could be better than 20 dB with 5 percent probability. If ERA results routinely included statements about reliability, there would be fewer cases of "conflict" with other tests.

In general, variability is much more difficult to quantify than bias; large sample sizes are required, and results are more prone to distortion by oddball values. Published variability norms are questionable because so many factors influence the distributions, and their use requires exact emulation of all aspects of the procedures and population to which they refer. The history of ERA reveals part of this problem: those who accumulate much experience with a specific AEP often report greater accuracy than that achieved by others in subsequent "replication" studies. An alternate AEP may be proposed, only to suffer the same sequence of events. Comparative studies, often based on limited experience in each procedure, may produce poor results on each test, and either a battery approach is proposed or all the tests are castigated. This pattern suggests that skill and experience are critical for accurate ERA, regardless of the AEP. Published norms are mere guidelines, and any clinic establishing ERA should obtain advice and training for the testers and should develop its own norms. It is easy to become complacent about one's ability to judge AEP records correctly; tester performance should be monitored with blind trials on hearing-impaired subjects with reliable behavioral thresholds.

One source of variability is lability of the AEP itself: the more unpredictable the waveform, the more difficult it is to detect. Intrinsic AEP stability

is greater for the most peripheral AEPs, such as the CAP and ABR. However, threshold variation is determined mainly by EEG noise characteristics. For example, the ABR is less variable than the SVR, but in awake adults it is easier to achieve acceptable accuracy with the SVR, given adequate skill with each; the ABR threshold is strongly affected by myogenic noise, which may vary considerably between averages and between patients.

Because several AEPs might be tried, and other options exist such as whether or not to use sedation, the actual bias and variability figures are influenced by the overall strategy. For example, the accuracy of ABR audiometry in the awake child depends on the point at which it is decided that the observed level of EEG noise is unacceptable and sedation or anasthesia must be used. The effect of these strategic decisions is to reduce the variability associated with each technique, and probably to make the variabilities more similar. The exception is transtympanic ECochG, which has lower variability due to the better SNR.

For any AEP, the typical normative difference distribution (Fig. 16-12) has a positive mean, a standard deviation of 10 dB or less, and is skewed towards large positive differences. Some possible sources of large differences were noted earlier.

### Frequency-Specificity of the AEP Threshold

The ideal ERA method should reproduce the puretone audiogram regardless of its profile. If the frequency-specificity is poor, there will be no problem with flat audiograms, but sloping or notched audiograms will not be estimated correctly. For the AEP threshold to be frequency-specific, a necessary *but not sufficient* condition is that the stimulus should be frequency-specific. This is quantifiable in terms of the shape of its spectrum; for example, if the nominal frequency of a tonepip were 2 kHz, how many dB below this is the energy at 1 kHz? As noted previously, bandwidth is related to rise/fall time and duration of the tonepip or toneburst. Errors in audiogram estimation can occur for stimuli having short rise/fall times or durations, whether the audiometric method is behavioral or AEP-based.[46]

For SVRA and MLRA, tonebursts with envelopes likely to give adequate frequency-specificity can be used; SVRA can reproduce the audiometric contour quite well, and the same is probably true for MLRA, though further validation in very steep hearing losses would not go amiss. The problem arises with the CAP and ABR, because these are onset responses with brief determinant epochs and require short stimulus rise-times to induce adequate neural synchrony. A further complication is that to excite low-frequency cochlear regions, the traveling wave must pass through basal regions where it may also elicit neural activity picked up by the recording electrode. For example, ABR latencies for low-frequency tonepips are prolonged by high-pass filtered masking noise,[77] which suggests basal spread of cochlear excitation. This problem may be compounded in patients with cochlear hearing impairment, in whom the normal ability of primary neurons to respond preferentially to a very narrow range of stimulus frequencies, known as "tuning" or "frequency selectivity," is often markedly degraded.[78] This increases the potential for contribution to the AEP from cochlear regions other than those normally associated with the nominal stimulus frequency.

The frequency-specificity problem is complex and unclear.[79,80] It might be thought that close to threshold, the cochlear region responding to a tonepip must be narrow and specific. However, AEP thresholds are usually biased, especially for tonepip stimuli, and the near-threshold stimulus might be 20 dB or 30 dB above the true threshold, which is ample to permit spread of excitation if cochlear tuning is degraded. It is probable that adequate frequency-specificity may not be achievable with the CAP and ABR, using tonepips alone. The data are conflicting, and further research is required.

It is possible to control cochlear excitation using ipsilateral masking noise. The principle is that masked cochlear regions will not be available to respond to the transient. The so-called derived response and band-stop masking methods depend on this concept, which is illustrated in Figure 16-13. These methods have been reviewed in detail by Stapells et al.[79] In the derived-response method, the stimulus is a click in high-pass filtered masking noise; the response arises from the unmasked region of the cochlea. A second determination with lower filter cutoff frequency will yield response

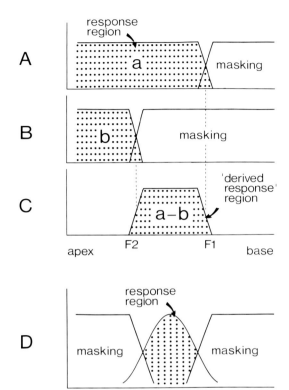

**Fig. 16-13.** Two methods of ipsilateral masking to determine frequency-specific AEPs. **(A-C)** In the "derived response" method the stimulus is a click, which excites a wide range of the cochlear partition. Masking with high-pass filtered noise at $F_1$ blocks the cochlear region basal to the site of $F_1$, so the response obtained reflects only the dotted, more apical region. A second AEP recording with the click masked at $F_2$ yields response from a smaller region. The second AEP is subtracted from the first, leaving a "derived AEP" that reflects the restricted region between $F_2$ and $F_1$. **(D)** In the "band-stop" or "notch-filtered" masking method, the stimulus is a brief tonepip. Spectral spread of tonepip energy is restricted by masking noise that has been filtered to leave a narrow unmasked region.

from a smaller region. Provided that CAP or ABR contributions from various cochlear regions are linearly additive, subtraction of the second response from the first gives the derived response from the region between the cutoff frequencies. This may be the best way to achieve frequency-specificity for the CAP and ABR, but it can be prohibitively time-consuming.

The band-stop (notch) masking method is

quicker: masking noise is filtered to remove a narrow band of energy, centered on the frequency of interest. The stimulus must excite this unmasked region, and is usually a tonepip with frequency at the center of the notch. This procedure limits the spread of activity, and may provide adequate specificity for the ABR. The method needs extra instrumentation, and its use is not yet widespread. Further research is required to clarify problems of masking spread and interactions between the masking and the stimulus.[80]

### Efficiency

Any ERA method should be efficient in terms of the time needed to obtain a given amount of data with a specified accuracy. Test time is usually constrained, and there is a trade-off between accuracy and the number of stimulus frequencies and routes. Two important factors are the number of averages and the test time per average. For a given stimulus type and route, the intensity sequence should yield progressively more exact estimates; a generally efficient approach is to select levels that bisect the current range of uncertainty about threshold. The time per average is determined mainly by the number of stimuli and their repetition rate, and the quantitative basis for selecting these parameters was outlined earlier (see Fig. 16-9). To achieve the highest efficiency requires much experience and ability to adapt protocols to the exigencies of the individual patient.

Of the methods considered here, transtympanic CAP recording is the most efficient. ABR V-SN$_{10}$, MLR, and SVR methods appear to have similar efficiencies, *when each is optimized properly*; for example, doing ABRA at repetition rates less than about 35/sec is very inefficient. Further research is required.

### Noninvasiveness and Risk

The ideal ERA method should be free of discomfort and risk. Of course, there are degrees of these to be weighed against the benefit of the information and the likelihood of obtaining it. The major issue is the use of sedation or anesthesia, if adequate recordings cannot be obtained in the waking state, and if natural sleep cannot be induced. The preferred procedure will vary with attitude and

facilities. Difficulties may include variable response to medication, and the requirement for adequate medical cover from drug administration to discharge, which can extend to a half-day or more. All in all, sedation for ERA can be costly in personnel and facilities, and a case can be made for doing the tests with the patient under light general anesthesia in the operating room. An advantage is that if the ABR or MLR results indicate the need for ECochG, it can be done immediately.

The only surgical technique considered here is transtympanic ECochG, for which the needle electrode placement should be done by an otolaryngologist. The procedure is straightforward and the patient may experience only momentary discomfort, but general anesthesia is necessary in children. The risk of complications from electrode placement is negligible.[3]

## Strategies of ERA

### General Considerations

The choice of initial ERA procedure is based upon the type of patient, the clinical question, and resources. Often, there are methodologic changes to cope with problems unique to particular types of patient; sometimes, the problems or results indicate that another ERA procedure should be tried. In most cases, the initial choice is governed by simple factors. First, if the patient is likely to be passively cooperative and alert for about an hour, SVRA is the test of choice. Any patient who is too active for SVRA will generate too much myogenic noise for waking-state ABRA or MLRA. If the patient is somnolent, ABRA is preferable to SVRA. If neither waking-state SVRA nor natural sleep is possible, sedation or anesthesia is indicated, and again ABRA is preferred on variability grounds. At present, at least in this author's view, MLRA and ECochG are reserved for cases in which SVRA and ABRA are inadequate. There are always exceptions to such rules, and many aspects of ERA remain matters of opinion. A general flow diagram reflecting this writer's view of ERA strategy is given in Figure 16-14. Various points of this strategy are covered in the following discussion of specific populations.

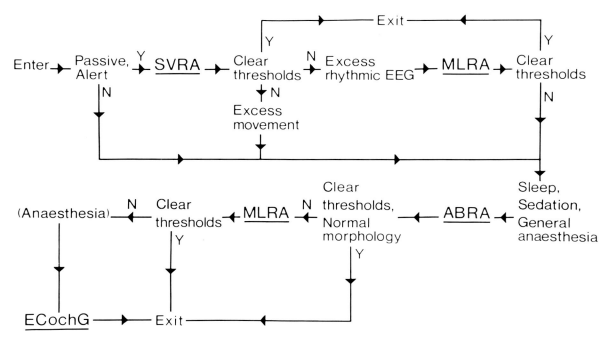

**Fig. 16-14.** A Flow diagram indicating a proposed strategy for ERA.

## Neonates and Infants

Early detection of hearing loss is an increasingly widely espoused goal.[81,82] The aim is to quantify hearing loss and initiate management at or before the age of 6 months, in order to optimize development of communication skills. There is ample evidence that detection and management of hearing loss are falling short of these goals.[83,84] Evidence is accumulating that impairments that are less than moderate-severe, or are unilateral, or purely conductive, may also warrant greater efforts at detection and management.[85,86] Furthermore, early audiometric assessment can be an important contributor to the management of the multiply handicapped infant.[87]

Behavioral screening, whether subjective or automated, is limited in sensitivity and reliability in the neonate and young infant.[88,89] ERA is considered by many to be very useful.[25,90] It is impractical to screen every live birth with ERA, and registers of high-risk factors for hearing loss, including low birth weight and severe asphyxia, are helpful in selection of the population most in need of testing,[81] though it must not be forgotten that the high-risk register has far from perfect sensitivity and specificity. Many neonates receiving intensive care are at risk for hearing loss,[25] and in some centers all infants leaving the intensive care nursery are screened.

Neonatal ERA screening during the postpartum hospital stay has the advantage of assured access to the child. Neonates spend most of their time asleep, during which excellent EEG conditions for ABRA are obtained; this test is the preferred technique and is feasible within a few hours of birth. SVRA is unreliable in this sleeping and immature population, and ECochG is unwarranted here because it is invasive and requires general anesthesia. MLRA is a possibility, but seems unlikely to challenge ABRA because both the regular MLR and the 40 Hz response are adversely affected by sleep.[50,91] ABRA screening is fairly quick and effective with click stimuli at about 40 dB,[90,92] though such a screen may miss deficits at low or high frequency.[40] Also, ABRA may be affected by acute illness or maturational delay, and hearing losses may develop or resolve,[49,93] so neonatal ERA screening failure is not a definitive result but serves as a flag for follow-up testing.

ERA is useful for detailed audiometric evaluation of infants under the age of 6 months. The target group includes those who have failed a neonatal screening, babies with risk factors associated with congenital or early-onset hearing loss, and those showing delayed development. In some centers, assessment of high-risk babies is deferred until 3 or 4 months of age, mainly on the grounds that at that time recovery from neonatal illness, maturation, resolution and expression of hearing loss are likely to give better and more relevant results.[93] Most babies under 6 months can be tested asleep by ABRA, if testing is correctly timed in relation to feeding and sleeping habits. Few older infants are untestable awake, but success requires much skill and patience. At some point, which depends upon resources and attitudes, testing under sedation or general anesthesia must be considered.

The need for efficient, progressive test protocols is particularly acute for the sleeping infant. A click-based categorization of hearing sensitivity is appropriate as a first step. Any abnormality may lead to more accurate click threshold measurements, though there is an increasing trend towards the use of more quantifiable and frequency-specific stimuli. Click ERA can miss both low- and high-frequency losses, and the detailed audiometric contour is useful diagnostically and for defining appropriate hearing aids.

Whenever ABRA is used, it is desirable to exclude significant neurologic abnormality that may affect the ABR directly and compromise the accuracy of threshold estimates.[94] Brain stem status may be inferred from the ABR waveform for clicks well above threshold; if the interpeak latency interval between waves I and V is not prolonged, neural conduction within the brainstem is normal and confidence in ABR thresholds increases. Sometimes it is difficult to confirm brainstem normality because severe, high-frequency, or mixed hearing losses may also affect the ABR waveform.[49,94] When the ABR is absent at the highest stimulus levels, the most probable cause is severe hearing loss; if anesthesia is feasible, ECochG may be useful because of its low bias. If, however, there is ABR evidence of neurologic abnormality, the value of using a more peripheral AEP is questionable, and the MLR is probably the last resort (see Fig. 16-14).

Having detected a hearing loss and excluded gross neurologic disorders, the differentiation of conductive and sensory loss by ABRA is not simple. Otomicroscopy can rule out gross middle-ear disease. Tympanometry and acoustic reflex measurements can be helpful, but a normal tympanogram or absent acoustic reflexes are not specific findings in infants under 6 months of age.[95] Bone conduction ABRA can be useful[96] but there are problems of large stimulus artifact, consistency of transducer coupling to the head, and restricted transducer frequency response.[57,58] Further research is needed to validate bone-conduction ABRA.[97]

The wave V intensity-latency function may help differentiate the lesion site, because the slope may be larger in recruiting sensorineural hearing loss.[79] However, some cochlear deficits, especially sloping high-frequency losses, do not give this effect; also, accuracy of latency measurement is an issue, and careful attention is required to age-related latency norms. Overall, the diagnostic accuracy of slope in the individual case is open to question,[98] and further research is required. The latency of wave I is helpful, in that marked prolongation that does not return to normal at high stimulus levels suggests a conductive pathologic condition. Wave I is recordable at much lower sensation levels in infants than in adults, and its latency matures and stabilizes much earlier than that of wave V.[99]

## The Difficult-to-Test Child

This population includes older children for whom behavioral testing may be problematic, such as those with multiple or neurologic deficits, developmental delays, or varying degrees of hyperkineticism or uncooperative behavior. The demand for ERA is inversely related to the availability and competence of behavioral testing, but there is a core group that is very difficult to test behaviorally. The choice of ERA procedure depends on why the child is difficult to test. Unless the child is actively uncooperative or continuously moving, SVRA should be tried. Toleration of electrodes is a sine qua non, and periods of inactivity are essential. Quiet play is acceptable. If headphones are not tolerated, sound-field SVRA is feasible but is obviously more limited in scope. The advantages of

SVRA include frequency specificity, the high level of response generation in the auditory neuraxis, and the ability to use standard contralateral masking and bone conduction procedures, where necessary.

Common causes of pediatric SVRA failure are low-frequency artifacts due to movement of the electrodes or leads, or high levels of EEG theta rhythm (5 to 8 Hz). EEG filtering can ameliorate the first problem but not the second, and commercial units may not include adequate filters. If the SVR thresholds are not well defined, confirmation by another AEP is desirable. If the cause of the problem is rhythmic EEG, and not excessive movement, MLRA is a viable alternative. ABRA in the waking state is possible, but very little electromyogenic activity can be tolerated, especially for frequency-specific testing. On the other hand, if SVRA failure is due to excessive movement, it is unlikely that waking-state MLRA or ABRA will be successful. A fortiori, if SVRA were not attempted on behavioral grounds, testing under sedation or anesthesia is the only possible route. In that case, the relative roles of MLRA, ABRA, and ECochG are the same as for the infant, except that ECochG is more readily used (see Fig. 16-14).

## Functional, Medicolegal, and Compensation Patients

Patients suspected of having functional (nonorganic) hearing loss are usually older children, or adult patients involved in compensation or medicolegal cases. There may be a functional component overlaying genuine hearing loss. Various methods of assessing functional patients have been reviewed by Alberti.[100] While a functional component may be suspected from the history, ERA is often considered after conventional audiometry has given variable or contradictory results.

ERA is useful here not only to obtain estimates of the true thresholds but also because it is disconcerting for the patient not to have to respond. This can promote better performance on subsequent conventional tests. Functional patients are often at least superficially cooperative, so they are good candidates for SVRA, and a reliable audiogram can usually be obtained. In most cases, this will be accu-

rate within 10 dB, for air and bone conduction, between 500 Hz and 4 kHz. Indeed, patients who are exaggerating hearing loss often give remarkably clear SVRs, probably because their anxiety promotes stimulus-oriented attention. This effect can be enhanced by instructing the patient specifically to ignore the stimuli, whereupon he or she may promptly begin to count them.

The SVRA should start at 500 Hz or 1 kHz, because at these frequencies the SVR is clearest and functional components are often larger, especially in compensation patients. The events following SVRA depend upon the clarity of the SVR thresholds. If the results are clear and better than the behavioral ones, exaggeration is highly likely. Here, SVR thresholds may be more consistent with conventional speech or bone conduction data, or with the clinical impression of the skilled audiologist. If SVRA is clear and consistent with conventional results, the latter are strongly supported. If SVRA thresholds are worse than the conventional audiogram, the ERA is noncontributory. As noted earlier, the relationship between conventional and AEP thresholds is one of correlation not identity. If the SVRA fails, subsequent procedures with other AEPs are similar to those for the difficult-to-test child and depend on the cause of failure (see Fig. 16-14).

Occasionally a patient may try to conceal a genuine hearing loss; the SVR thresholds will be higher than those obtained conventionally, and it is difficult to differentiate this from idiopathic SVR threshold elevation.

Where there is a persistent difference between conventional audiometry and the final outcome of the ERA scheme, every effort should be made to resolve the discrepancy and to obtain plausible behavioral data. For a unilateral functional loss, the Stenger test can be confirmatory. Acoustic reflex thresholds can be useful when discrepancies are gross, but puretone threshold prediction based upon the ART is too inaccurate to quantify most discrepancies between behavioral and ERA data.[101] Usually the competent audiologist is able to integrate the overall findings into a coherent evaluation.

In medicolegal cases the objectivity of ERA is the key. SVRA is again the method of choice. When SVRA and conventional audiometry agree, the case for their accuracy is strong, but a legal attack might focus on the subjective nature of AEP detection judgements. Thus, the ERA should be done with a demonstrable lack of foreknowledge of the behavioral audiogram. Objective response detection criteria are helpful. Scrambling and encoding records for interpretation by a third party are also possible methods.

If ERA results are better than the conventional ones, the implications are quite serious for the patient, and false-positive response detection must be scrupulously avoided. Response presence below the admitted threshold must be carefully confirmed and recorded graphically. In these cases, demonstration of discrepancy is probably of greater significance than the absolute ERA result, and testing effort should focus on accuracy rather than on complete audiometric description. Confirmation with another AEP adds credibility. If the SVRA gives higher thresholds than those given voluntarily, it is noncontributory and MLRA procedures may be more productive; a patient may give inexplicably poor results with one AEP but not with another.

For compensation evaluations, such as in claims for noise-induced hearing loss, ERA is indicated if conventional audiometry is internally inconsistent or incompatible with the noise-exposure history. High-slope audiograms are common in these patients, and the frequency-specificity of SVRA is a strong point in its favor, as is the large body of normative data. At present, no other AEP test is suitable as the initial method for such patients. Tonepip MLRA is the second option if SVRA fails to give clear thresholds, and the 40 Hz procedure is promising because the patients are awake and it is a little more efficient than regular MLRA. ABRA may not have the frequency-specificity required for this population, and is strongly affected by myogenic noise. ECochG is a last resort since it is invasive, and only the time-consuming derived-response masking method could give adequate frequency-specificity. Testing with click stimuli is inappropriate in this population, for any AEP.

A special consideration here is the need for very high accuracy. As noted earlier, comprehensive ERA is extremely time-consuming and skill-dependent; nowhere is this more true than for the compensation case, for which 5 dB intensity increments and frequent replications may be necessary. The arguments in cases of discrepancy between behavioral and ERA data are similar to those for the medicolegal case. Again, it is far better to resolve the differences than to adopt the ERA as the true audiogram. If the ERA is more than 10 dB better than the conventional audiogram, careful and repeated "reinstruction" of the patient is indicated. Smaller differences than this may be attributable to many minor factors that may be cumulative, such as random error, effects of headphone fit, and the patient's decision criterion. There is no definite point at which a high criterion for behavioral response becomes frank exaggeration, so unless discrepancies are substantial, the patient must be given the benefit of the doubt. In a few cases, there is a significant and intractable discrepancy, and ERA is the only plausible basis for compensation.

## Conclusions

ERA is certainly a major advance in audiologic technique. Electrophysiologic and behavioral testing are complementary tools in the overall assessment. Their relative roles and utility depend strongly upon expertise and facilities in each domain. ERA has an important and varied target population base, and is not a test but a scheme. To achieve reliable results, both methodology and strategy must be adapted to the exigencies and objectives in the individual case. The need for adequate training, case load, and monitoring cannot be overemphasized. Failure to recognize this can lead to results that are worse than useless clinically, and has contributed to gross misconceptions about the value of ERA. Given adequate facilities, skill, and strategy, there are few patients in whom audiometric uncertainty need be tolerated.

Much further research is needed. In particular, computer-based automatic test control and interpretive decision support will help to improve accuracy and efficiency, and to reduce the dependence of ERA utility upon individual skills. Except for SVRA, frequency-specificity requires further study, and all techniques merit further study of optimization and comparative performance.

## OTONEUROLOGIC INVESTIGATION

### Detection of Acoustic Tumors

Disorders of the axial brainstem or cerebral cortex are rare in comparison to cerebellopontine angle lesions, particularly acoustic tumors. It was noted earlier that neural synchrony is the key to AEP development. Neoplastic lesions can affect the volume and synchrony of neural excitation in several ways: by direct involvement of neural pathways, or indirectly by pressure effects, for example. Neurons may be compromised either by direct structural damage or by impairment of their metabolic supply. These changes in underlying neural activity may be reflected in waveforms of gross AEPs originating at, or rostral, to the site of action of the lesion.

Acoustic tumors usually arise in the vestibular branch of the 8th cranial nerve, either within the medial portion of the internal auditory canal or at its porus into the posterior fossa.[102] In these regions, the cochlear and vestibular branches are physically contiguous. Thus, the acoustic tumor can reduce the volume and synchrony of activity at the level of the first-order neurons. It follows that any AEP from that level or above might be modified by the lesion. The relatively high variability and long time course of cortical AEPs make them insensitive to details of neural discharge at the periphery. On the other hand, the cochlear nerve CAP and the ABR are highly sensitive to the pattern of underlying neural activity, and are the prime candidates for acoustic tumor detection. The fact that ABR testing is noninvasive has made it by far the more popular AEP for this purpose.

In the past, a barrage of audiologic tests was often used in patients suspected of having acoustic tumors. These included pure-tone audiometry, speech tests, tone decay, short-increment sensitivity index (SISI), Békésy audiometry, binaural loudness balance, and acoustic reflex tests, among others. It is clear that with the possible exception of acoustic reflex tests, each of these tests is unimpressive as a discriminator of cochlear versus retrocochlear disease.[103,104] The practice of considering the battery to be positive for tumor if at least one test is positive increases the sensitivity, but at the cost of very poor specificity.

The advent of ABR testing has radically changed the situation; both the sensitivity and the specificity of the test are very high, and this has led to considerable rationalization of the audiologic test battery.

### Grounds for ABR Testing

The motivation of screening for acoustic tumor is that early detection can facilitate surgical procedures and lead to improved outcomes.[102] Liberal ABR testing is reasonable because it is accurate and noninvasive, it causes negligible discomfort to the patient, and it is quite cheap and quick. The ABR test is by far the best audiologic screening test for acoustic tumor, and it is indicated in almost all suspected cases.

The clinical grounds for suspicion are dealt with in detail elsewhere. Briefly, there is enormous variety in signs and symptoms of acoustic tumor, and there is no truly typical presentation. An important sign is unilateral or asymmetrical neurosensory hearing loss, and ABR testing is indicated regardless of the speed of onset. Chronic tinnitus, particularly if unilateral, is also sufficient grounds for ABR testing, even in the absence of significant hearing loss. Many would argue that balance disorders also warrant ABR testing, irrespective of vestibulometry results. More subtle symptoms include unclear speech perception, or difficulty understanding on the telephone. The major problem with candidacy for ABR testing is where to draw the line. Certainly, it is dubious to make the ABR testing conditional upon the results of other audiometric tests, because none has adequate performance. To the author's knowledge, a malpractice suit on the grounds of failing to perform an ABR test has not yet arisen, but it probably will.

### Test Methodology

Test methods are described elsewhere,[1,23,24] so only the main points are reviewed here. To minimize electromyogenic noise, the patient should lie supine with eyes closed, preferably in a darkened soundroom, isolated from the tester and main instrumentation. If the patient will sleep, so much the better. Electrodes are at the vertex or high on the forehead, and on each earlobe or mastoid. Each ear is tested individually. Stimuli and masking are delivered by earphone. Clicks or more controlled stimuli such as 2 kHz single-cycle sinusoids are used most commonly. Stimulus polarity if often alternated for successive stimuli, to cancel stimulus artifact due to electromagnetic radiation to the electrodes, from the earphone and input leads. Potential problems of alternation were outlined earlier. It is possible, but not trivial, to reduce stimulus artifact by electrostatic and electromagnetic shielding of the earphone, leads, and electrodes.[105]

Stimulus intensity is important, not only because ABR parameters change with intensity but also because most patients will have some hearing loss, which also can affect the response. It is essential to excite the brainstem adequately, and also we wish to avoid or factor out effects of conductive and cochlear hearing loss, so as to give the most consistent and accurate differential diagnostic decisions. The apparently simple step of stimulating at some fixed, high sensation level (SL) is not necessarily satisfactory because of the complex relationship between ABR parameters, click threshold, and the various types, degrees, and contours of hearing loss. Also, the constant-SL strategy is limited by the maximum of about 95 dB nHL clicks, for most ERA devices. Practices vary, but it is common to use stimuli at specific dB nHL, typically in the range of 70 to 95 dB nHL. Too low a level risks poor ABR definition, especially for wave I. Too high a level can cause discomfort, which is counterproductive because of increased electromyogenic noise.

Stimulus repetition rate affects test efficiency. Rates between 10 and 90/sec are used, and again, practices vary. The most efficient rate for wave V is higher than that for wave I, because the wave V rate-amplitude function drops off more slowly at high repetition rates. One strategy is to use a rate high enough to be efficient for wave V, at least initially. The basic test tool might be a pair of averaged ABRs with at least 2,000 sweeps each, using 80 dB nHL clicks at a rate of at least 30/sec. This is done on each ear, and records are analyzed primarily in terms of absolute, interwave, and interaural

latency characteristics. If any of these is unclear, or takes a value that is unexpected, it may be necessary to lower rates to 20/sec to clarify wave I, or to increase intensities or the amount of averaging, or all of these. Rates lower than 20/sec are usually inefficient (see Fig. 16-9).

### Diagnostic Parameters

The waveform features (parameters) normally used to detect acoustic tumor are shown in Figure 16-15. It is possible to detect retrocochlear disorders quite effectively using only wave V latency. We can compare the latency in each ear to absolute norms, or examine the interaural latency difference (ILD, also known as interaural time, IT). The latter avoids some of the problems of intersubject latency variability, absolute effects of recording filters, and other factors, because the patient acts as

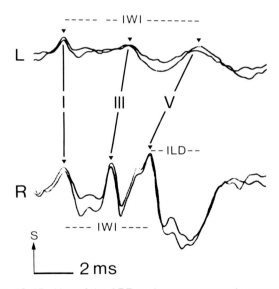

**Fig. 16-15.** Use of the ABR to detect an acoustic tumor. In the right ear, the ABR is normal. On the affected side, the latencies of waves III and V are prolonged. In more drastic cases, the entire ABR may be abolished. The common diagnostic parameters are the interaural latency difference for wave V (ILD V) and the I-V interwave (IWI). This patient had entirely normal results of puretone and speech tests, and a 1.5 cm tumor.

his or her own control. For example, absolute wave V latency is 0.21 msec smaller in female patients, but this is irrelevant if ILD is used. The main disadvantage of ILD V is that it is insensitive to bilateral retrocochlear pathologic changes, but the latter is unlikely unless the history suggests neurofibromatoses or demyelinating disease. In fact, test protocol and interpretation can depend upon the presumptive diagnoses, so the tester must know them in advance.

The ILD V has a mean of zero and an SD of about 0.2 msec in normal-hearing adults.[22] The critical value that distinguishes retrocochlear pathologic change is chosen on the basis of the false-positive and false-negative error probabilities. Suppose we adopt a criterion[106] of 0.4 msec, with larger values indicating retrocochlear disease. In most populations there would be a massive false-positive error rate because both conductive and cochlear hearing loss can increase wave V latency.[22,66,97,106] Thus, we adjust for these effects in each ear, before calculating the "corrected" ILD V. The correction is different for conductive and cochlear losses. The former is thought to cause a latency increase roughly equivalent to that due to reducing stimulus intensity by the size of the average air-bone gap in the 1 to 4 kHz region. Thus, if the stimulus is 80 dB nHL and the air-bone gap is 20 dB, the effective intensity at the cochlea is 60 dB nHL. The normal intensity-latency function[29] reveals that latency should increase by about 0.3 msec per 10 dB, so the conductive correction would be 0.6 msec. The problem is that the individual patient's intensity-latency function might not be exactly the norm, and so the correction used will be in error. In general, the larger the correction, the more possibility exists for error.

Cochlear hearing losses increase wave V latency in a more complex way.[66] The audiogram is a complicated measure and it is problematic to express its relationship to wave V latency in a simple way. Fortunately, it seems that the 4 kHz puretone threshold is a fairly good predictor of wave V latency. The slope of the hearing loss may also be influential, but this question is not resolved. The relationship between the 4kHz threshold and wave V latency is expressed schematically in Figure 16-16. The curve can be used as the latency correction function. One refinement, shown in the fig-

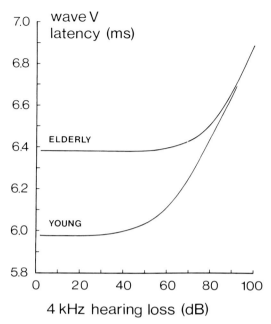

**Fig. 16-16.** Effect of cochlear hearing loss and age on the latency of ABR wave V. The diagnosis of retrocochlear lesions on the basis of wave V requires correction of the observed wave V latency for effects of hearing loss of presumed cochlear origin. If the loss is truly retrocochlear, the latency prolongation is likely to be greater than expected. Here, average wave V latency is plotted versus the behavioral puretone threshold at 4 kHz. The model is derived from over 200 cases of proven cochlear hearing loss. A complication is that the effect of hearing loss itself changes with the age of the patient; correction curves for young and elderly adults are shown.

ure, is to use different latency correction functions, depending on the age of the patient.[65,66] Another is to allow for the fact that the variability of wave V across patients increases with hearing loss severity, so the decision criterion should be adjusted if constant rates of error are the goal. There are many other possible refinements, and the achievement of controlled and consistent test accuracy is far from straightforward.

An alternative to wave V latency and ILD V, as diagnostic parameters, is the interwave interval (IWI) for waves I and V (also known as the interpeak latency, IPL). The argument in favor of this is that many of the variables that affect wave V also affect wave I in a similar manner, and so the IWI is relatively robust and invariant. Conductive hearing loss, for example, has much less effect on IWI than on wave V latency. An early impression that IWI was impervious to both conductive and cochlear hearing loss is no longer widely held.[29,49] Both conductive and cochlear losses can affect the IWI, though to a lesser extent than they affect wave V latency. The effects are not yet completely understood. The main problem with IWI is that in the typical population referred for ABR testing by the otolaryngologist, wave I will not be observable bilaterally in up to about half the patients[106] because it is vulnerable to conductive or high-frequency neurosensory hearing loss. One approach is to emphasize IWI criteria when wave I is available, and to fall back on wave V criteria when it is not. Just as for wave V, where either absolute or interaural criteria may be used, so it is for IWI. Various methods to enhance wave I have been proposed,[107] but the best enhancements are obtained by using a novel electrostatic earphone,[108] or by supplementing the ABR with either endomeatal[109] or transtympanic[110] ECochG. An example of results with endomeatal ECochG and ABR is shown in Figure 16-17. The endomeatal procedure should probably be reserved for retest in those patients who are marginally abnormal, and who would benefit from the wave I enhancement.

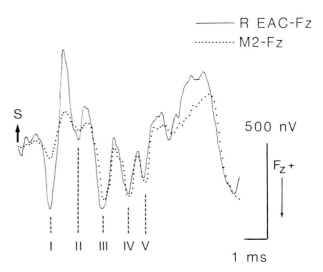

**Fig. 16-17.** Enhancement of ABR wave I (CAP) by endomeatal recording. Wave I is not apparent in many patients with high-frequency hearing loss, using a mastoid-forehead ($M_2$-$F_z$) electrode derivation. By using an electrode in the external auditory canal (EAC), wave I amplitude may be enhanced, permitting computation of the I-V IWI. Simultaneous canal-forehead and mastoid-forehead recordings are shown here; forehead-positive is down. The degree of wave I enhancement varies greatly over patients.

### Diagnostic Error Rates

In general, for all of these latency measures, departures from the norm of more than about 0.3 msec begin to suggest retrocochlear disease. Of course, there is no firm line beyond which acoustic tumor is definite or within which tumor can be categorically excluded: it is a question of balancing false-positive and false-negative error rates. As with any other statistical decision problems involving random error, these two error rates vary inversely as the decision criterion is changed. Because most patients who have ABR testing in the typical otolaryngology practice do not, in fact, have retrocochlear disease, it is feasible to estimate the false-positive rate quite accurately; for a criterion of 0.4 msec, an error rate of between 5 and 10 percent is typical. Suppose 1 percent of patients referred had an acoustic tumor, and these all had abnormal ABRs; this criterion would give between

about 1 in 5 to 1 in 10 correct tumor calls. This is a reasonable basis for the physician to take a tumor call seriously. Altering the criterion to give a 20 percent false-positive rate would begin to degrade the predictive value of a positive call, whereas altering it to cut the false-positive rate to, say, 2 percent would lead one to run the risk of missing a significant proportion of tumors.

The primary cause of false-positive ABR tests is hearing loss, for which either the correction process has failed or it has not been applied properly. On the other hand, if there were a definite ABR abnormality in the absence of severe hearing loss, further investigation would be strongly indicated. Most of those with many years' experience of ABR testing can recall such patients who have not been investigated further, and who present later with severe symptoms that turn out to be due to tumor. We hope that this situation will improve, through extended experience and education.

Certainly, a small number of patients have apparently idiopathic ABR abnormalities. In fact, certain ABR abnormalities are more positive than others. For example, a clear wave I with depressed or delayed subsequent waves is an extremely strong indicator of pathologic change and if one cannot be found, it is probably because the investigative procedures are inadequate. It must be remembered that the ABR reflects certain specific features of neural *function,* so its changes may not be associated with gross structural or behavioral changes. On the other hand, total absence of all ABR waves, with no more than moderate hearing loss, inspires first the suspicion of technical or interpretive error, such as ear canal collapse, or a fault in the stimulation or recording systems. These possibilities must be ruled out systematically, before one decides on an interpretation of retrocochlear disorder.

Estimation of the false-negative rate for acoustic tumor detection is problematic, for many reasons. First, there is no totally accurate procedure to determine tumor presence or absence, with the possible exception of surgical exploration. Even the so-called definitive radiologic procedures such as air-contrast computed tomography (CT), have finite false-positive rates. Less accurate radiologic procedures such as regular tomography or plain films, or even CT without contrast, are simply not reliable enough to act as arbiters of ABR accuracy. Of course, all of this discussion is predicated on competent ABR testing, and it is not uncommon for the training and expertise required to be grossly underestimated. Anyone who has not personally performed at least 50 ABR tests, and who is not interpreting them at a rate of at least one or two per week, would be wise to seek more qualified guidance.

The ABR test has limitations. First, some patients have corrected ABR latencies that are borderline, and the test is not contributory. Second, for ears with severe or profound hearing loss in the 2 kHz region, absence of the ABR has no diagnostic significance. If such a patient has no more than moderate hearing loss in the other ear, there is still value in the ABR test because many large acoustic tumors induce contralateral ABR abnormalities through pressure effects associated with brainstem displacement.[111] Third, acoustic tumor is not the only lesion possible. Posterior fossa meningioma, for example, does not produce ABR abnormalities as consistently as acoustic tumor, and it follows that a normal ABR is a good tool for ruling out acoustic tumor, but is not as strong a rule-out for meningioma. It must be stressed that current techniques of ABR analysis do not identify the lesion, nor can its location be specified very exactly. For example, an ABR picture typical of a small acoustic tumor is a normal wave I, and prolonged wave III and wave V latency (see Fig. 16-15). A meningioma or multiple sclerosis might produce the same picture. Thus, the correct inference is "retrocochlear lesion," as opposed to "acoustic tumor."

Finally, even for acoustic tumors, there is no well-established relationship between the degree of ABR abnormality and the size of the tumor, just as there is no strong relationship between tumor size and results of any other audiologic tests. This is scarcely surprising, particularly because tumor size is a very gross concept and tumor effect must depend on many aspects of tumor site, shape, and detailed relationships to nerve trunk and blood supply.

## MISCELLANY

### Further Otoneurologic Applications of ABR

As was intimated earlier, the ABR has a much wider range of applications to otoneurology and neurology than the mere detection of acoustic tumors. It is valuable in a wide range of neurologic disorders that may affect the central auditory pathways.[1,23,24] These include not only space-occupying lesions but also demyelinating and vascular disorders. In general, an important feature of the ABR is that it is a correlate of *functional* impairment of neurons, and as such it offers a view that is complementary, and perhaps more sensitive, than many techniques for the investigation of structural abnormality (e.g., standard radiologic techniques). In multiple sclerosis, for example, ABR abnormalities are seen frequently,[72] and the test is useful not only for establishing the diagnosis but also for monitoring the course of disease.

Other areas of great interest include intraoperative monitoring,[112] either for auditory nerve function in posterior fossa surgery, or of more general aspects of brainstem function, for example, in brain or cardiovascular surgery. Also, the ABR appears to be a valuable tool for many types of neurologic monitoring, such as for coma patients.[113]

In principle, the ABR may also provide insight into neural function in the absence of frank disease. For example, it may prove to be valuable as a correlate, or as a prognosticator, of neurologic development in the premature newborn, or it may have a role in the quantification of degenerative processes in the elderly.

In summary, it is clear that the ABR, in particular, has not only proven clinical utility at the present time but also has a much greater amount of potential utility in diverse areas. In all of this discussion, it must be remembered that we have glimpsed only the tip of the iceberg. In particular, our current methods of stimulation and response measurement are truly rudimentary, and there are clear prospects for major advances. For example, it was implied in earlier sections that the use of a single differential channel to visualize the ABR offers only a very restricted view of the true three-dimensional distribution of electrical potential. Already, there is evidence that the use of multichannel recording and sophisticated computer analyses to construct more complete images of intracranial electrical events may offer significant new insight and clinical utility.[114,115] There is some justification for regarding the present state of AEP measurement as comparable to that of radiology before the advent of computerized imaging.

## Exploration of Cochlear Dysfunction

It is clear that direct and clinically practicable electrophysiologic correlates of entities such as cochlear otosclerosis, Meniere's disease, noise-induced hearing loss, and others would be extremely helpful. To date, the contribution of gross AEPs to the detailed elucidation of cochlear disorders has not been impressive, though there are several interesting lines of inquiry.[116] It is reported, for example, that endolymphatic hydrops is associated with increased amplitude of the cochlear summating potential. The use of this measure to refine diagnosis is not widespread, but certainly there are

adequate grounds for further development and implementation.[116]

Another area of perhaps even greater interest is the investigation of cochlear frequency-selectivity.[78,116] It is painfully apparent that simple audiologic measures such as the puretone audiogram and conventional speech discrimination tests provide little insight into the nature, severity, and communicative consequences of cochlear dysfunction. Thus, there is much research aimed at the development of better audiologic tests. One important concept is that the frequency-selectivity of the cochlea is a more sensitive and meaningful function than mere sensitivity thresholds. Certainly, it is reasonable to expect that the ability of the cochlea to separate various frequency components of complex signals such as speech would be critical to communicative function. Also, while absolute sensitivity to sound and frequency-selectivity are correlated, there is some degree of independence, and frequency-selectivity may be compromised in the presence of near-normal sensitivity. The prospect is that cochlear frequency-selectivity might help to explain phenomena such as difficulty with speech discrimination in patients with little or no puretone hearing loss, and variable success with hearing aids across patients with similar audiograms. Also, frequency-selectivity might provide the means to detect incipient impairment due to noise exposure, or to differentiate pathologic conditions with more sensitivity than is possible currently.

Measurement of more sophisticated aspects of auditory function such as frequency-selectivity can be done with psychoacoustic techniques, but these are frequently tedious and too demanding to be practicable in many patients. Hence, there is a role here for AEPs, which may provide a simpler and more objective approach. It has been demonstrated that frequency-selectivity can be measured in humans, using the transtympanically recorded CAP,[116] and it also seems feasible to use endomeatal CAP or ABR techniques. This is an area of active research and considerable potential clinical benefit.

## Evoked Auditory Magnetic Fields

The ultimate sources of AEPs are movements of charged particles associated with activation of neurons. Within a conducting medium, these movements can be considered as electric currents. It is well-known, from classic physics, that a magnetic field is associated with the flow of current in a conductor, and that the field radiates perpendicularly to the direction of current flow. When the current changes, the magnetic field changes. It follows, therefore, that there is a magnetic analog to the AEP.

Exploration of evoked magnetic fields is a recent development.[117] The equipment required is far more sophisticated and expensive than that needed for AEP measurements. As yet, the technique does not have proven clinical utility, though there have been several reports dealing with the basic phenomenology. It appears that evoked magnetic fields reflect events in cerebral cortex, as opposed to events deep within the brain. The relationship between bioelectric and biomagnetic fields is such that transverse current flow in cortical layers is easiest to detect. It is reasonable to expect intensive research in this area, and the technique may prove clinically useful for evaluating cortical function and pathophysiology.

### Evoked Otoacoustic Emissions

Evoked acoustic emissions can be recorded by a microphone in the external canal of normal-hearing persons.[118] These emissions are evoked by clicks or brief tonepips, have latencies in the range of 5 to 10 msec, and usually appear as a decaying oscillatory waveform lasting about 10 msec with frequency components in the 750 to 2,000 Hz range.[119] They originate within the cochlea, and have been called cochlear echos; this may be misleading, as there is some evidence that the emissions are generated by active processes involving hair cells, rather than mere passive reflection of sound from impedance discontinuities in cochlear structures.

Cochlear emissions are not evoked potentials, but they are included here because their measurement involves many techniques in common with AEPs, such as the use of averaging. The clinical significance of evoked cochlear emissions is not yet clear. They do not occur in the presence of neurosensory hearing loss, and it follows that they might be useful for objective detection of such losses. Their mechanism is not fully understood, so it is not clear whether they have a role in exploration of

cochlear function, for example in persons with hearing difficulties but no actual hearing loss, or in assessment of susceptibility to damage or of subclinical pathophysiology. Nevertheless, the emissions are an interesting phenomenon that warrant further exploration.

## REFERENCES

1. Jacobson JT (ed): The Auditory Brainstem Response. College-Hill Press, San Diego, 1985
2. Moore EJ (ed): Bases of Auditory Brainstem Evoked Responses. Grune & Stratton, Orlando, FL, 1983
3. Davis H: Principles of Electric Response Audiometry. Ann Otol Rhinol Laryngol 85 [Suppl] 28, 1976
4. Caton R: The electric currents of the brain. Br Med J 2:278, 1875
5. Wever EG, Bray CW: The nature of acoustic response: the relation between sound frequency and frequency of impulses in the auditory nerve. J Exp Psychol 13:373, 1930
6. Davis PA: Effects of acoustic stimuli on the waking human brain. J Neurophysiol 2:494, 1939
7. Davis H: The excitatory process in the cochlea. Proc Natl Acad Sci 36:580, 1950
8. Dawson GD: A summation technique for the detection of small evoked potentials. Electroencephalogr Clin Neurophysiol 6:65, 1954
9. Geisler CD: Average responses to clicks in man recorded by scalp electrodes. Technical Report 380. Massachusetts Institute of Technology, 1960
10. Katzman R (ed): Sensory evoked response in man. Ann NY Acad Sci 112, 1964
11. Davis H: The young deaf child: identification and management. Acta Otolaryngol 206 [Suppl] 1965
12. Aran J-M, LeBert G: Les résponses nerveuses cochleaires chez l'homme, image du fonctionnement de l'oreille et nouveau test d'audiometrie objective. Rev Laryngol Otol Rhinol (Bord) 89:361, 1968
13. Ruben RJ: Cochlear potentials as a diagnostic test in deafness. In Graham AB (ed): Sensorineural Hearing Processes and Disorders. Little, Brown, Boston, 1967
14. Sohmer H, Feinmesser M: Cochlear action potentials recorded from the external ear in man. Ann Otol Rhinol Laryngol 76: 427, 1967

15. Yoshie N, Ohashi T, Suzuki T: Non-surgical recording of auditory nerve action potentials in man. Laryngoscope 77:76, 1967

16. Rapin H, Graziani LJ: Auditory-evoked responses in normal, brain-damaged, and deaf infants. Neurology 17:881, 1967

17. Mendel MI, Goldstein R: Stability of the early components of the averaged electroencephalic response. J Speech Hear Res 12:351, 1969

18. Walter WG, Cooper R, Aldridge VJ, et al: Contingent negative variation: an electric sign of sensorimotor association and expectancy in the human brain. Nature 203:380, 1964

19. Sutton M, Braren M, Zubin J, et al: Evoked potential correlates of stimulus uncertainty. Science 150:1187, 1965

20. Jewett DL, Williston JS: Auditory evoked far-fields averaged from the scalp of humans. Brain 94:681, 1971

21. Hecox K, Galambos R: Brain stem auditory evoked responses in human infants and adults. Arch Otolaryngol 99:30, 1974

22. Selters WA, Brackmann DE: Brainstem electric response audiometry in acoustic tumor detection. p. 225. In House WF, Luetje CM (eds): Acoustic Tumors, vol. I. Diagnosis. University Park Press, Baltimore, 1979

23. Stockard JJ, Stockard JE, Sharbrough FW: Brainstem auditory evoked potentials in neurology: methodology, interpretation, clinical application. p. 370. In Aminoff MJ (ed): Electrodiagnosis in Clinical Neurology. Churchill Livingstone, New York, 1980

24. Fria TJ: The Auditory Brain Stem Response: Background and Clinical Applications. Maico Monographs in Contemporary Audiology 2, 1980

25. Galambos R, Hicks GE, Wilson MJ: The auditory brainstem response reliably predicts hearing loss in graduates of a tertiary intensive care nursery. Ear Hearing 5:254, 1984

26. Picton TW, Hillyard S, Krausz H, et al: Human auditory evoked potentials. I. Evaluation of components. Electroencephalogr Clin Neurophysiol 36:179, 1974

27. Dallos P: Cochlear electrophysiology. p. 141. In Naunton RF, Fernandez C (eds): Evoked Electrical Activity in the Auditory Nervous System. Academic Press, New York, 1978

28. Tsuchitani C: Physiology of the auditory system. p. 67. In Moore EJ (ed): Bases of Auditory Brain-Stem Evoked Responses. Grune & Stratton, Orlando, FL, 1983

29. Picton TW, Stapells DR, Campbell KB: Auditory evoked potentials from the human cochlea and brainstem. J Otolaryngol 10 [Suppl] 9, 1981

30. Picton TW, Stuss DT: The component structure of the human event-related potentials. p. 17. In Kornhuber HH, Deecke L (eds): Progress in Brain Research vol. 54. Motivation, Motor and Sensory Processes of the Brain: Electrical Potentials, Behaviour and Clinical Use. Elsevier Biomedical Amsterdam, 1980

31. Callaway EC: Brain Electrical Potentials and Individual Psychological Differences. Grune & Stratton, Orlando, FL, 1975

32. Linden RD, Campbell KB, Hamel G, et al: Electrophysiological techniques in audiology and otology: human auditory steady state evoked potentials during sleep. Ear Hearing 6:167, 1985

33. Moller AR, Jannetta PJ: Neural generators of the auditory brainstem response. p. 13. In Jacobson JT (ed): The Auditory Brainstem Response. College-Hill Press, San Diego, 1985

34. Scherg M, von Cramon D: A new interpretation of the generators of BAEP waves I-V: results of a spatiotemporal dipole model. Electroencephalogr Clin Neurophysiol 62:290, 1985

35. Scherg M, von Cramon D: Two bilateral sources of the late AEP as identified by a spatio-temporal dipole model. Electroencephalogr Clin Neurophysiol 62:32, 1985

36. Owen JH, Davis H (eds): Evoked Potential Testing: Clinical Applications. Grune & Stratton, Orlando, FL, 1985

37. Picton TW, Fitzgerald PG: A general description of the human auditory evoked potentials. p. 141. In Moore EJ (ed): Bases of Auditory Brain-Stem Evoked Responses. Grune & Stratton, Orlando, FL, 1983

38. Davis H, Hirsh SK: A slow brainstem response for low frequency audiometry. Audiology 18:445, 1979

39. Stapells DR, Picton TW: Technical aspects of brainstem evoked potential audiometry using tones. Ear Hearing 2:20, 1981

40. Hyde ML: Frequency-specific BERA in infants. J Otolaryngol 14 [Suppl 14] 1985

41. Galambos R, Makeig S, Talmachoff PJ: A 40-Hz auditory potential recorded from the human scalp. Proc Natl Acad Sci 78: 2643, 1981

42. Durrant JD: Fundamentals of sound generation. p. 15. In Moore EJ (ed): Bases of Auditory Brain-Stem Evoked Responses. Grune & Stratton, Orlando, FL, 1983

43. Gorga M, Abbas PJ, Worthington DW: Stimulus calibration in ABR measurements. p. 49. In Jacob-

son JR (ed): The Auditory Brainstem Response. College-Hill Press, San Diego, 1985

44. Coats AC: Instrumentation. p. 197. In Moore EJ (ed): Bases of Auditory Brain-Stem Evoked Responses. Grune & Stratton, Orlando, FL, 1983

45. Jacobson JT, Hyde ML: An introduction to auditory evoked potentials. p. 496. In Katz J (ed): Handbook of Clinical Audiology, 3rd ed. Williams & Wilkins, Baltimore, 1985

46. Davis H, Hirsh SK, Popelka GR, et al: Frequency selectivity and thresholds of brief stimuli suitable for electric response audiometry. Audiology 23:59, 1984

47. Eggermont JJ: Electrocochleography. In Keidel WD, Neff WD (eds): Handbook of Sensory Physiology, vol V/3. Auditory Systems: Clinical and Special Topics. Springer-Verlag, Berlin, 1976

48. Kriss A: Setting up an evoked potential (EP) laboratory. p. 1. In Halliday AM (ed): Evoked Potentials in Clinical Testing. Churchill Livingstone, New York, 1982

49. Stockard JE, Stockard JJ: Recording and analyzing. p. 255. In Moore EJ (ed): Bases of Auditory Brain-Stem Evoked Responses. Grune & Stratton, Orlando, FL, 1983

50. Mendel MI, Wolf KE: Clinical applications of the middle latency responses. Audiology (J Cont Ed) VIII:141, 1983

51. Reneau JP, Hnatiow GZ: Evoked Response Audiometry. University Park Press, Baltimore, 1975

52. Suzuki T, Horiuchi K: Effect of high-pass filter on auditory brainstem responses to tone pips. Scand Audiol 6:123, 1977

53. Suzuki T, Horiuchi K: Rise-time of pure-tone stimuli in brainstem response audiometry. Audiology 20:101, 1981

54. Zwislocki JJ: Temporal summation of loudness: an analysis. J Acoust Soc Am 46:431, 1969

55. Kiang N Y-S, Watanabe T, Thomas EC et al: Discharge Patterns of Single Fibers in the Cat's Auditory Nerve. MIT Press, Cambridge, MA, 1965

56. Picton TW, Linden RD, Hamel G, et al: Aspects of averaging. Semin Hearing 4:327, 1983

57. Schwartz DM, Berry GA: Normative aspects of the ABR. p. 65. In Jacobson JT (ed): The Auditory Brainstem Response. College-Hill Press, San Diego, 1985

58. Mauldin L, Jerger J: Auditory brain stem evoked responses to bone-conducted signals. Arch Otolaryngol 105:656, 1979

59. Chatrian GE, Wirch AL, Lettich E, et al: Click-evoked human electrocochleogram. Noninvasive recording method, origin and physiologic significance. Am J EEG Technol 22:151, 1982

60. Stockard JJ, Stockard JE, Sharbrough FW: Non-pathologic factors influencing brainstem auditory evoked potentials. Am J EEG Technol 18:177, 1978

61. Parker DJ: Dependence of the auditory brainstem response on electrode location. Arch Otolaryngol 107:367, 1981

62. Doyle DJ, Hyde ML: Analogue and digital filtering of auditory brainstem potentials. Scand Audiol 10:81, 1981

63. Picton TW, Hillyard S, Krausz H, et al: Human auditory evoked potentials. II. Effects of attention. Electroencephalogr Clin Neurophysiol, 36:191, 1974

64. Eggermont JJ: Physiology of the developing auditory system. In Trehub S, Schneider B (eds): Auditory Development in Infancy. Plenum, New York, 1983

65. Otto WC, McCandless GA: Aging and the auditory brain stem response. Audiology 21:466, 1982

66. Hyde ML: The effect of cochlear lesions on the ABR. p. 133. In Jacobson JT (ed): The Auditory Brainstem Response. College-Hill Press, San Diego, 1985

67. Jerger J, Hall J: Effects of age and sex on the auditory brainstem response. Arch Otolaryngol 106:382, 1980

68. Kankkunen A: Pre-school children with impaired hearing. Acta Otolaryngol [Suppl] 391, 1982

69. Popelka GR (ed): Hearing Assessment with the Acoustic Reflex. Grune & Stratton, Orlando, FL, 1981

70. Davis H: Electric Response audiometry: past, present, and future. Ear Hearing 2:5, 1981

71. Picton TW, Woods D, Baribeau-Braun B, et al: Evoked potential audiometry. J Otolaryngol 6:90, 1977

72. Paludetti G, Ottaviani F, et al: Autitory brainstem responses (ABR) in multiple sclerosis. Scand Audiol 14:27, 1985

73. Worthington DW, Peters JF: Quantifiable hearing and no ABR: paradox or error? Ear Hearing 1:281, 1980

74. Ozdamar O, Kraus N, Curry F: Auditory brain stem and middle latency responses in a patient with cortical deafness. Electroencephalogr Clin Neurophysiol 53:224, 1982

75. Don M, Elberling C, Waring M, 1984: Objective detection of averaged auditory brainstem responses. Scand Audiol 13:219–228.

76. Fridman J, Zappulla R, et al: Application of phase

spectral analysis for brain stem auditory evoked potential detection in normal subjects and patients with posterior fossa tumors. Audiology 23:99, 1984

77. Kileny P: The frequency specificity of tone-pip evoked auditory brainstem responses. Ear Hearing 2:270, 1981

78. Salvi RJ, Henderson D, Hamernik R, et al: Neural correlates of sensorineural hearing loss. Ear Hearing 4:115, 1983

79. Stapells DR, Picton TW, Perez-Abalo M, et al: Frequency specificity in evoked potential audiometry. P. 147. In Jacobson JT (ed): The Auditory Brainstem Response. College-Hill Press, San Diego, 1985

80. Gorga M, Worthington DW: Some issues relevant to the measurement of frequency-specific auditory brainstem responses. Semin Hear 4:353, 1983

81. Joint Committee on Infant Hearing: Position statement 1982. Pediatrics 70:496, 1982

82. Northern JL, Downs MP: Hearing in Children, 3rd ed. Williams & Wilkins, Baltimore, 1984

83. Stein LK, Ozdamar O, Kraus N, et al: Follow-up of infants screened by auditory brainstem response in the neonatal intensive care unit. J Pediatr 103:447, 1983

84. Ruben RJ: Delay in diagnosis. Volta Rev 80:201, 1978

85. Ruben RJ: An inquiry into the minimal amount of auditory deprivation which results in a cognitive effect in man. Acta Otolaryngol (Stockh) [Suppl.] 414, 157–164, 1984

86. Bess FH: The minimally hearing-impaired child. Ear Hearing 6:43, 1985

87. Stein LK, Kraus N: Auditory brainstem response measures with multiply handicapped children and adults. p. 337. In Jacobson JT (ed): The Auditory Brainstem Response. College-Hill Press, San Diego, 1985

88. Parving A, Elberling C, Salomon G: ECochG and psychoacoustic tests compared in identification of hearing loss in young children. Audiology 20:365, 1981

89. Jacobson JT, Morehouse CR: A comparison of auditory brainstem response and behavioral screening in high risk and normal newborn infants. Ear Hearing 5:247, 1984

90. Murray AD, Javel E, Watson CS: Prognostic validity of auditory brainstem evoked response screening in newborn infants. Am J Otolaryngol 6:120, 1985

91. Shallop JK, Osterhammel PA: A comparative study of measurements of $SN_{10}$ and the 40/sec middle latency responses in newborns. Scand Audiol 12:91, 1983

92. Fria TJ: Identification of congenital hearing loss with the auditory brainstem response. p. 317. In Jacobson JT (ed): The Auditory Brainstem Response. College-Hill Press, San Diego, 1985

93. Alberti PW, Hyde ML, Riko K, et al: Issues in early identification of hearing loss. Laryngoscope 95:373, 1985

94. Stein LK, Ozdamar O, Schnabel M: Auditory brainstem responses (ABR) with suspected deaf-blind children. Ear Hearing 2:30, 1981

95. Paradise JL: Tympanometry. N Engl J Med 307:1074, 1982

96. Weber BA: Masking and bone conduction testing in brainstem response audiometry. Semin Hear 4:343, 1983

97. Finitzo-Hieber T, Friel-Patti S: Conductive hearing loss and the ABR. In Jacobson JT (ed): The Auditory Brainstem Response. College-Hill Press, San Diego, 1985

98. Eggermont JJ: The inadequacy of click-evoked auditory brainstem responses in audiological applications. Ann NY Acad Sci 388:707, 1982

99. Fria TJ, Doyle WJ: Maturation of the auditory brain stem response (ABR): additional perspectives. Ear Hearing 5:361, 1984

100. Alberti PW: Non-organic hearing loss in adults. p. 910. In Beagley HA (ed): Audiology and Audiological Medicine, vol. 2. Oxford University Press, Oxford, 1981

101. Hyde ML, Alberti PW, Morgan P, et al: Pure-tone threshold estimation from acoustic reflex thresholds—a myth? Acta Otolaryngol 89:345, 1980

102. House WF, Luetje CM (eds): Acoustic Tumors, vol. I. Diagnosis, vol. II. Management. University Park Press, Baltimore, 1979

103. Johnson EW: Results of auditory tests in acoustic tumor patients. p. 209. In House WF, Luetje CM (eds): Acoustic Tumors, vol. I. Diagnosis. University Park Press, Baltimore, 1979

104. Jerger S, Jerger J: Evaluation of diagnostic audiometric tests. Audiology 22:144, 1983

105. Cooper WA Jr, Parker DJ: Stimulus artefact reduction systems for the TDH-49 headphone in the recording of auditory evoked potentials. Ear Hearing 2:283, 1981

106. Hyde ML, Blair RL: The auditory brainstem response in neuro-otology: perspectives and problems. J Otolaryngol 10:117, 1981

107. Ruth RA, Hildebrand DL, Cantrell RW: A study of methods used to enhance Wave I in the auditory

brain stem response. Otolaryngol Head Neck Surg 90:635, 1982

108. Stackenburg M, Wit HP: Piezoelectric earphone for artifact-free recording of auditory brainstem responses (ABR). Scand Audiol 12:79, 1983

109. Harder H, Arlinger S: Ear-canal compared to mastoid electrode placement in ABR. Scand Audiol [Suppl.] 13, 55–57, 1981

110. Eggermont JJ, Don M, Brackmann DE: Electrocochleography and auditory brainstem electric responses in patients with pontine angle tumors. Ann Otol Rhinol Laryngol 89 [Suppl] 75, 1980

111. Musiek FE, Gollegly KM: ABR in eighth nerve and low brainstem lesions. p. 181. In Jacobson JT (ed): The Auditory Brainstem Response. College-Hill Press, San Diego, 1985

112. Kileny P, Mcintyre J: The ABR in intraoperative monitoring. p. 237. In Jacobson JT (ed): The Auditory Brainstem Response. College-Hill Press, San Diego, 1985

113. Hall III JW, Mackey-Hargadine J, Allen SJ: Monitoring neurologic status of comatose patients in the intensive care unit. p. 253. In Jacobson JT (ed): The Auditory Brainstem Response. College-Hill Press, San Diego, 1985

114. Pratt H, Har'el Z, Golos E: Three-channel Lissajous' trajectory of human auditory brain-stem evoked potentials. Electroencephalogr Clin Neurophysiol 56:682, 1983

115. Scherg M: Spatio-temporal modelling of early auditory evoked potentials. Rev Laryngol (Bord) 105:163, 1984

116. Eggermont JJ: Audiologic Disorders. p. 287. In Moore EJ (ed): Bases of Auditory Brain-Stem Evoked Responses. Grune & Stratton, Orlando, FL, 1983

117. Elberling C, Bak C, Kofoed B et al: Auditory magnetic fields: source location and 'tonotopical organisation' in the right hemisphere of the human brain. Scand Audiol 11:61, 1982

118. Kemp DT: Stimulated acoustic emissions from within the human auditory system. J Acoust Soc Am 64:1386, 1978

119. Grandori F: Nonlinear Phenomena in click- and tone-burst-evoked otoacoustic emissions from human ears. Audiology 24:71, 1985

# Vestibular Diagnostic Tests

# 17

## W.P.R. Gibson

The importance of the vestibular system is often unappreciated until the mechanism fails. During every waking hour, the vestibular system is working diligently to maintain balance, posture, and equilibrium. It works with such quiet efficiency that its role may easily be overlooked.

The heart of the vestibular systems lies in the brain stem within the vestibular nuclei. Here sensory inputs — visual, labyrinthine and proprioceptive — merge and interact; and further influences are provided by the reticular system, cerebellum, and cerebrum. The output of the vestibular nuclei pass via vestibulo-ocular pathways to maintain the stability of the vision as we move about and move our heads. The output of the vestibular nuclei also passes out along the vestibulospinal and vestibulocerebellar tracts to influence the body posture and tone and pass to the cerebrum to provide a conscious feeling of equilibrium.

Failure of the vestibular system causes unpleasant feelings of disequilibrium. They are quite unlike any usual sensations, and may be difficult for a patient to describe adequately. Severe disruption will cause difficulty in keeping the vision steady and loss of body posture.

## HISTORY

Many vestibular disorders, especially those of the peripheral vestibular system, resolve completely between attacks, so that no clinical signs exist unless the patient is examined during the acute episode. For this reason, it is well worth the inconvenience to examine the patient at the time of the attack. Certainly a clear distinction between peripheral and central dysfunction most often can be made. Nevertheless, in the majority of cases, no such examination has been undertaken and all signs have resolved, either completely or imcompletely. Under these circumstances, the clinical history is of paramount importance. Table 17-1 presents guidelines for classifying symptoms. Five critical symptoms are mentioned for five different groups of disorders.

### Labyrinthine Disorders

**True Vertigo.** Vertigo is derived from the Latin word, *vertere*, to turn. As each labyrinth is projected unilaterally onto the vestibular nuclei on each side of the brain stem, labyrinthine dysfunc-

487

**Table 17-1. History-Classification of Key Symptoms**

**Labyrinthine disorders**
    True vertigo
    Occurs in episodes
    Associated with nausea and vomiting
    Worse on head movement
    Associated with cochlear symptoms

**Eighth nerve disorders**
    Unsteadiness, especially in the dark
    Loss of speech discrimination
    Tinnitus but not bothersome
    Numbness or discomfort around ear
    Neurologic symptoms of CPA lesion

**Disorders affecting the vestibular nuclei (VBI)**
    Brief rotational vertigo
    Crumbling sensations
    Posturally induced vertigo
    Clouding or narrowing of vision
    Hypertensive treatment

**Central vestibular disorders**
    Imbalance
    Headaches worse on straining or coughing
    Vomiting without preceding nausea
    Blurred vision
    Neurologic symptoms—unconsciousness, etc.

**Psychogenic disorders**
    Vagueness of history
    Constant "dizziness"
    Reaction to crowds or enclosed spaces
    Hyperventilation/palpitations
    Receiving psychotropic drugs

tion alters the vestibular output in a manner similar to head turning. Thus, dysfunction of a labyrinth gives an impression of movement resembling that experienced on alighting from a merry-go-round; a similar sensation also occurs during caloric testing.

Patients usually describe a sensation of the environment turning around. Less often, patients feel as if their own bodies are turning. If all labyrinthine receptors are affected, the sensation is usually in a horizontal plane as the lateral semicircular canal dominates.

**Episodic Attacks.** Sudden total loss of a peripheral labyrinth causes a distressing episode of vertigo lasting several days. Usually the nystagmus and vertigo fade after 48 hours (depending on the patient's age). Afterward, the patient feels off balance, especially when tired, for several weeks until full compensation has occurred. Less catastrophic labyrinthine dysfunction, such as attacks of Men-iére's disease, causes an episode of vertigo that lasts from several minutes to several hours. In Meniére's disease it is unusual for the vertigo to have a duration of less than 10 minutes or more than 4 hours. Benign paroxysmal positional vertigo (BPPV) is characterized by vertigo lasting less than 1 minute. The vertigo associated with a perilymph leak is similar to BPPV but less severe and causes less subjective reaction. In the former three conditions, the patient has many attacks at varying intervals. Between the attacks, the patient is physically well.

**Nausea and Vomiting.** Peripheral vestibular vertigo is characteristically associated with severe nausea and often vomiting on the first episode. Patients with recurrent episodes may learn to control the vomiting but continue to become nauseated.

**Inability to Move Head.** During an attack of peripheral labyrinthine vertigo, the patient will keep the head very still, as even a slight head movement increases the vertigo and may cause vomiting. Never will the patient shake his head to "clear it." Patients suffering from an attack of Meniére's disease usually retire to bed and lie very still on their backs or with the affected ear uppermost.

BPPV is characteristically initiated by lying down suddenly on the affected side or rolling over onto the affected side in bed. Rising from the bed may also cause some vertigo, but it is less severe than when lying down quickly. Similarly, the vertigo associated with a perilymph leak may occur on lying on the affected side; it may also be provoked in some cases by suddenly raising the intratympanic pressure (by Valsalva maneuver) or, in some cases, by raising the pressure of the cerebrospinal fluid (CSF) by raising the intrathoracic pressure.

**Associated Cochlear Symptoms.** Apart from BPPV and some perilymph leaks, all other known labyrinthine disorders are associated with cochlear dysfunction. In most forms of labyrinthitis, both bacterial and viral (e.g., mumps), the cochlea is severely affected either causing a total loss of hearing or a severe high-frequency loss.

In Meniére's disease, as in other causes of endolymphatic hydrops, the cochlear symptoms may be overlooked as the patient struggles with the nausea and vertigo. Later, once the disease has become established, the cochlear symptoms persist between attacks and the presence of a sensory hearing loss and tinnitus, which may worsen with the vertiginous attacks, becomes an important part of the syndrome. Typically, endolymphatic hydrops causes a fluctuating low-frequency (below 3 kHz) hearing loss.

A perilymph leak may be associated with a high-frequency loss due to hair cell damage in the basal cochlear turn or may be associated with a fluctuating low-frequency loss, due either to loss of perilymphatic pressure or, perhaps, to secondary endolymphatic hydrops.

## Disorders of the 8th Nerve

Total disruption of the 8th cranial nerve rarely occurs, even after a severe head injury. It would lead to loss of all vestibular and cochlear function and the vestibular symptoms would mimic those of a total peripheral labyrinthine loss.

More commonly, an 8th nerve lesion results from a tumor, usually an acoustic neuroma but more rarely other tumors such as a facial neuroma, meningioma, or glioma, which so gradually destroy the neural elements that vestibular compensation can keep pace with the destruction. Thus patients with an acoustic tumor rarely suffer from an acute episode of vertigo (only 3.5 percent according to Morrison[1]), but more usually notice a gradual loss of their overall balance.

**Unsteadiness.**   Typically a patient with an acoustic tumor experiences difficult walking along a dimly lit street. Attacks of vertigo are unusual.

**Loss of Speech Discrimination.**   Commonly the patient notices an inability to hear speech over the telephone using the affected ear.

**Tinnitus.**   It is unusual for tinnitis to be bothersome. Typically it is a constant pure-tone tinnitus.

**Numbness or Discomfort Around the Affected Ear**

**Neurologic Signs.**   Neurological signs may occur once the tumor has extended into the cerebellopontine angle and is pressing on the brain stem. The trigeminal nerve is often the first affected, with loss of corneal sensation. Ominous symptoms are blurring of vision (caused by papilledema) and headaches, which worsen on coughing or straining.

## Disorders Affecting the Vestibular Nuclei

The vestibular nuclei are the pivot of the vestibular system. They are supplied by an end branch of the posterior inferior artery. This is the longest and most tortuous vessel supplying the brain stem. Thus, ischemia will affect the vestibular nuclei readily and can occur in isolation without any other brain stem symptoms or signs.

If the blood supply of the vestibular nuclei on only one side of the brain stem is suddenly compromised, the effect will be similar to sudden loss of labyrinthine or 8th nerve function; the patient experiences rotational vertigo.

Transient ischemia of the vestibular nuclei caused by postural hypotension is commonplace. Many patients receiving hypotensive drugs to lower their blood pressure will experience vertigo if they rise too quickly, especially if they have been lying down. Vertigo is not a symptom of raised blood pressure but of low blood pressure. The hypertensive patient experiences vertigo only when medication causes the blood pressure to fall too low. Furthermore, hypertensive patients experience a failure of the autonomic nervous system to adapt and adjust the blood pressure on adopting an upright posture.

**Brief Rotational Vertigo.**   The rotational associated with transient ischemia is usually less severe than labyrinthine vertigo, during which both sides are compromised in most patients. A sensation of rotation is only produced if one side is marginally more anoxic than the other. The attacks usually only last for seconds and cause little nausea. Vomiting is very rare.

A sudden catastrophic unilateral lesion, such as Wallenberg's (lateral medially) syndrome caused by thrombosis of the posterior inferior cerebellar artery, produces severe vertigo with vomiting similar to that caused by sudden loss of a labyrinth. Associated symptoms are hiccups, blurred vision, hoarseness, and swallowing difficulty. Interestingly, loss of thermal and pain sensation over the face is less often noticed, and it is rare for the patient to complain of analgesia or athermia of the opposite limbs.[2]

Slow growing tumors of the brain stem may cause

little vertigo as compensation can occur, but the patient will complain of unsteadiness similar to that caused by an acoustic neuroma.

Thirty percent of patients with multiple sclerosis suffer some episodes of vertigo due probably to demyelination affecting the vestibular pathways within the brain stem.

**Feeling of "Crumbling".** The corticospinal fibers, which carry motor instructions from the precentral gyrus to the limb muscles, pass through the pyramids of the medulla. Transient ischemia of the pyramids causes a sensation of weakness of the limbs. Typically this causes a sensation of "crumbling" and the limbs lose strength so that the patient subsides gently to the ground without loss of consciousness. Such symptoms are almost pathognomonic of brain stem ischemia.

**Posturally-Induced Vertigo.** The attacks of vertigo are induced by movements that cause a sudden drop in the blood pressure. Almost all sufferers complain that the attacks will occur if they get out of bed too quickly in the mornings and that they have to hang their legs over the edge of the bed before arising. Prolonged standing and sudden neck extension or neck turning may also cause attacks.

**Clouding or Narrowing of Vision.** The posterior cerebral arteries supply the occipital lobes and part of the temporal lobes. Anoxic changes in these areas cause a clouding of vision and some narrowing of the visual fields.

**Hypertensive Heart Disease.** The vast majority of patients are known hypertensives who are receiving treatment.

**Other Disorders.** Other causes include the subclavian steal syndrome,[3] basilar migraine, bypass surgery, and head injuries. Subclavian syndrome is caused by a diminished basilar blood flow caused by innominate stenosis or occlusion. Blood flow to the upper arm does not come from the innominate artery on that side but from a reverse flow down the ipsilateral vertebral artery and blood is "stolen" from the basilar artery and brain stem. Episodic vertigo and diplopia are commonly precipitated by exercise of the arms (e.g. carrying heavy loads).

Basilar migraine usually occurs in young adults who often have a past history of classical migraine.

A considerable proportion of postbypass surgery patients, especially those with repeated surgery, complain of dizziness, vertigo, unsteadiness, and diplopia; dizziness is the most common symptom. The cause is not clear but is probably due to impairment of the central vestibular compensatory mechanisms.

Even after seemingly mild head injuries, patients may complain of symptoms similar to those mentioned after bypass surgery. Often the symptoms are aggravated by postural change. The picture is obscured by possible compensation claims. Nevertheless it is likely that some disturbance of the central vestibular compensatory mechanism has occurred.

### Central Vestibular Dysfunction

Tumors of the posterior fossa often cause disorders of balance. In adults, the common infiltrative tumors are gliomas and metastatic tumors, usually from the lung or breast. Neuromas and meningiomas are essentially benign. In children, intracranial tumors occur most commonly in the cerebellum or pons; the tumors are often malignant gliomas, such as medullablastomas or astrocytomas.

**Imbalance with Little Subjective Vertigo.** Often a child is thought to be clumsy or an adult complains of difficulty walking or making fine hand movements.

**Headache Aggravated by Coughing or Straining.** When the intracranial pressure is raised, the resulting headache is aggravated by further rises in CSF pressure.

**Vomiting Without Preceding Nausea.** This condition occurs especially in children with posterior fossa tumors.

**Blurred Vision.** Raised intracranial pressure leads to papilledema and hence causes blurring of vision.

**Other Neurologic Symptoms.** Symptoms such as numbness or tingling of the face or tongue may alert the clinician to the possibility of a central disorder. True loss of consciousness is suggestive of epilepsy or severe vertebrobasilar insufficiency. A history of migraine from the patient or the family may alert the clinician to the possible diagnosis of basilar migraine or a migraine variant.

## Psychogenic Dizziness

Patients suffering from anxiety disorders and other psychiatric disturbances commonly complain of dizziness. In many instances it may be difficult to exclude an underlying organic cause, but the following symptoms help to make one confident that the major component is nonorganic and that treatment should be primarily aimed at the psychiatric disturbance.

**Vagueness of History.** Often the patients are unable to explain their giddiness precisely. Nevertheless the patients must be given "free rein," as direct questioning can lead to a grossly inaccurate history.

**Constant Dizziness and/or Exacerbations Lasting Several Days.** Usually the patient has a feeling of "uneasy balance," which has lasted several months.

**Reaction to Crowds and Being Enclosed.** The reaction depends on the underlying disturbance. Hysterics tend to "collapse" in front of an audience; claustrophobics may hyperventilate in an enclosed area, whereas agoraphobics hate large open supermarkets, etc.

**Hyperventilation, Palpitations, Sensations Within the Head.** Patients who become anxious may hyperventilate and this may initiate the giddiness. Often patients complain of other psychogenic symptoms such as palpitations, chest pains, banging inside the head, sleep disturbances, etc.

**On Psychotropic Drugs/Previous History of a Psychiatric Disturbance.** Almost all patients suffering from psychogenic giddiness are already receiving medication and have a history of mental disturbance. It is suggested that some unfortunate patients suffering from true peripheral vestibular disturbance have been misdiagnosed as being nonorganic, but I have found this to be true only rarely.

## CLINICAL EXAMINATION

As previously stated, patients suffering from peripheral labyrinthine lesions are often completely well between attacks. Abnormal physical signs are usually only visible during or immediately after attacks; between attacks there are no abnormal physical signs. Patients suffering from central vestibular problems may have other coexisting central nervous system (CNS) signs.

Before the patient is examined, it is helpful to have the nursing staff record the blood pressure and test the urine for protein and sugar.

### Examination of the Ears, Nose, and Throat

Chronic suppurative otitis media is a rare cause of vertigo today. If suspected, the "fistula test" should be undertaken. Wax must be removed and the status of the tympanic membranes is noted before undertaking the auditory and vestibular investigations.

### Examination of the Cranial Nerves

Each cranial nerve is assessed in turn (Table 17-2). The examination of the eye movements and the auditory and vestibular parts of the 8th nerve require detailed testing.

### Examination of the Eyes

The examination of the eyes is of paramount importance. An arcus senilis is suggestive of vascular insufficiency. The presence of any strabismus or latent nystagmus must be noted.

The fundi should be examined for papilledema especially if an 8th nerve tumor or a central disorder is suspected.

#### Assessment of Eye Movement

Many of the tests performed using electronystagmography (ENG) can be accomplished clini-

**Table 17-2.   Examination of the Cranial Nerves**

| Cranial Nerve | Examination |
|---|---|
| I Olfactory nerve | Test sense of smell with vapors; required after head injuries |
| II Optic nerve | Examine fundi, especially if raised CSF pressure suspected |
| III Oculomotor ⎫ | |
| IV Trochlear ⎬ | Examine eye movements |
| V Abducens ⎭ | |
| VI Trigeminal | Sensation in frontal, maxillary, and mandibular areas of face; corneal reflexes |
| VII Facial | Movement of face, taste sensations, lacrimation (Schirmer's test) |
| VIII Auditory Vestibular | Specialized audiometric tests; specialized vestibular tests |
| IX Glossopharyngeal | Sensation on and above each tonsil |
| X Vagus | Gag reflex, palate movements, and vocal cord movements |
| XI Accessory | Sternomastoid movement |
| XII Hypoglossal | Tongue movements |

cally, although the sensitivity using the naked eye is obviously less. The full significance of the results is discussed more fully in the section covering ENG.

The presence of nystagmus should be carefully evaluated as the detection of any pathologic nystagmus is of paramount importance.

Peripheral vestibular nystagmus is reduced by optic fixation and may not be evident until optic fixation is abolished. Clinically this can be accomplished by using Frenzel's glasses.[4] Frenzel's glasses are goggles with 20 diopter lenses and illumination within the goggles so that, although the patient cannot see clearly out of the goggles, it is easy to observe the patient's eyes under magnification. An alternative method is to use the opthalmoscope covering the nonexamined eye; the bright light of the opthalmoscope obscures vision and nystagmus is observed by movement of the retina (remembering that this movement is in a direction opposite to that of the pupil). The eyes should be observed with and without opic fixation while in straight ahead gaze and on looking 30 degrees to each side. This is approximately when the edge of the pupil meets the caruncle. The features of pathologic nystagmus are outlined in Table 17-3.

Vestibular nystagmus has a characteristic saw-toothed appearance. It is enhanced when the patient looks away from the side of the paresis.

Congenital nystagmus usually has a jelly-like quality and, despite its presence, the patient has no impairment of visual acuity. Two important features of congenital nystagmus are that it is reduced or abolished on convergence and it remains horizontal in direction on upwards gaze.

Rotatory nystagmus is especially frequent with lesions of the vestibular nuclei in the floor of the fourth ventricle.

Vertical nystagmus indicates a brain stem lesion. Lower medullary lesions (e.g. Arnold Chiari syndrome) cause a down beating nystagmus; whereas up beating nystagmus indicates a pontine lesion.

Ocular myoclonus is a pendular vertical nystagmus synchronous with oscillations of the palate, larynx, and midline structures. It is secondary to bilateral pseudohypertrophy of the inferior olivary nuclei and occurs with lesions of the contralateral dentate nucleus or ipsilateral tegmental tract.

Dissociated nystagmus indicates a midbrain lesion. Bilateral internuclear ophthalmoplegia, caused by a lesion such as a plaque of multiple sclerosis, which disrupts the medial longitudinal bun-

**Table 17-3.   Characteristics of Spontaneous Nystagmus**

| | Peripheral | Central |
|---|---|---|
| Duration; direction | Temporary; unidirectional | Permanent; may be multidirectional; may be vertical |
| Character | | May be disconjugate or dissociated |
| Effect of gaze direction | Enhanced in direction of fast component | No alteration |
| Effect of removing optic fixation | Enhanced | Unchanged |

dles, results in paresis of adduction of one eye in the presence of normal convergence and horizontal nystagmus of the abducting eye.

Nystagmus retractorius is noted when the patient looks at an optokinetic drum revolving downward. The eye beats in an irregular fashion toward the back of the orbit. It is usually associated with paralysis of upward gaze and is caused by lesions of the midbrain, especially in the region of the aqueduct of Sylvius.

Convergent nystagmus is a rare manifestation of an anterior midbrain lesion. However, it may also rarely occur in hysterics.

See-saw nystagmus is rare. It consists of one eye rising while the other falls. It occurs with lesions in the region of the optic chiasma.

### Observation of the Vestibulo-Ocular Reflex

The usual function of the labyrinths is to maintain steady gaze despite head movement. If both vestibular labyrinths are affected, the vestibulo-ocular reflex is lost and the patient suffers from oscillopsia. This can be easily examined by asking the patient to read from a book while moving the head from side to side. Normal subjects can read clearly despite moving the head at rates up to 4 Hz. Patients with bilateral labyrinthine dysfunction find the print blurs at slower rates.

### Observation of Doll's Head Movements

When a subject's head is moved while the gaze is fixed on an object, the eyes remain steady despite the head movements. Loss of doll's head movements only occurs with massive lesions of the brain stem. Doll's head movements are preserved in patients suffering from supranuclear palsies, even though they cannot voluntarily move their eyes vertically.

### Observation of Pursuit Tracking

The smooth pursuit system is responsible for maintaining gaze on a moving target. Normally smooth pursuit is possible up to speeds of 40°/sec. Clinically, the patient is asked to follow an object or a finger, which is slowly moved from side to side.

Disruptions of smooth pursuit are discussed under ENG recordings.

### Observation of Saccadic Eye Movements

The saccadic system initiates rapid eye movements so that the subject can quickly and accurately alter gaze from one object to another. Normally this is done very accurately and only a minute adjustment is needed to center the fovea on the target after the initial fast movement.

"Saccadic palsy" occurs in some patients with acute frontal cortex lesions who are unable to make saccadic eye movements to the opposite side to the lesion, even though the pursuit mechanism remains normal. Less severe abnormalities cause "dysmetria" when the initial fast eye movement either undershoots (hypodysmetria—an ocular form of dysdiadochokinesia common in cerebellar disease) or overshoots (hyperdysmetria—seen in brain stem-cerebellar disease) the target.

### Observation of Optokinetic Nystagmus (OKN)

This is the classic "carwash effect." The driver feels the car is moving, although it is the carwash moving around the car. Nature assumes the environment is static, and hence any movement is attributed to the person. Normally optokinetic signals complement the signals from the labyrinths but when the labyrinths produce signals while the head is stationary, the optokinetic signals oppose the labyrinthine signals. This is the reason why peripheral nystagmus is inhibited by optic fixation.

Clinically the patient is sometimes asked to look at a small revolving striped drum. Often this method will measure smooth pursuit mechanisms rather than optokinetic mechanisms. Barber and Stockwell[5] argue that the stimulus should be a moving visual scene that subtends the patient's entire visual field. (Further discussion of OKN appears under ENG testing). Some of the characteristics of visual ocular control mechanisms are shown in Table 17-4.[6]

### Observation for Positioning Nystagmus

Positional tests are of limited value. The patient's head position is changed slowly from erect to su-

**Table 17-4.    Characteristics of Visual Ocular Control Abnormalities**

| Location of Lesion | Saccades | Smooth Pursuit | Optokinetic Nystagmus |
|---|---|---|---|
| Unilateral peripheral vestibular | Normal | Transient contralateral impairment | Transient contralateral decreased SCV[a] |
| Cerebellopontine angle | Ipsilateral dysmetria[b] | Progressive ipsilateral or bilateral impairment | Progressive ipsilateral or bilateral decreased SCV |
| Diffuse cerebellar | Bilateral dysmetria | Bilateral impairment | Bilateral decreased SCV |
| Intrinsic brain stem | Decreased maximum velocity, increased delay time | Ipsilateral or bilateral impairment | Ipsilateral or bilateral decreased SCV, disconjugate |
| Basal ganglia | Hypometria[c] increased bilateral delay time | Bilateral impairment | Bilateral decreased SCV |
| Frontoparietal | Contralateral | Normal | Normal |
| Parieto-occipital cortex | Normal | Ipsilateral impairment | Ipsilateral decreased SCV |

[a] Slow component velocity of ENG.
[b] Under- and overshoots.
[c] Undershoots only.

pine, supine with head turned left, or left lateral, right lateral, and head hanging. Any nystagmus is recorded using ENG. Many normal subjects have horizontal nystagmus with eyes closed in one of these positions. The nystagmus is deemed to be pathologic[7] if (1) direction changes in a single position, (2) it is persistent in three or more of the five head positions, (3) it is intermittent in four or more head positions, or (4) slow phase speed (ENG) of the three strongest beats exceeds 6 degrees/sec in any head position.

Positional nystagmus with eyes open is always abnormal. If the patient is recovering from an acute peripheral lesion, then the nystagmus is direction fixed (always beats the same way), is enhanced by eye closure, and is accompanied by vertigo. Posterior fossa lesions may cause direction fixed or direction changing positional vertigo, which persists for as long as the head maintains that position, and is accompanied by little or no vertigo.

Some workers believe that cervical sensory root problems may cause a positional nystagmus,[8] but it remains a matter of conjecture.

**Positional Alcohol Nystagmus (PAN)**

Thirty minutes after ingesting large amounts of alcohol (over lg/kg body weight), subjects develop positional nystagmus, which is most prominent with the head in the left lateral and right lateral positions. This nystagmus is called **PAN I**; it beats geotropically (toward the ground) and is stronger with the eyes closed. **PAN I** lasts 3 to 4 hours. After

5 hours, positional nystagmus reappears in the opposite direction (ageotropic or away from the ground) and may last for 24 hours. This is called **PAN II**. It is thought that alcohol diffuses into the labyrinth and affects the cupulae, initially causing them to become less dense and float. The alcohol diffuses out into the endolymph, initially restoring the normal densities but later causing the cupulae to be more dense and to sink. Clinically, **PAN II** must be excluded before placing pathologic significance on the finding of positional nystagmus.

**Positioning Tests**

Positioning nystagmus was first described by Barany[9] and later by Nylen[10] and by Dix and Hallpike.[11] The method used to elicit the nystagmus was best described by Dix and Hallpike.[11]

**Procedure for Testing.** The patient sits on a couch, either wearing Frenzel's glasses or with the gaze fixed on the examiner's forehead. The examiner grasps the patient's head firmly and quickly turns it to one side and brings it down below the edge of the couch.

**Classification of Positioning Nystagmus.** The most common finding is "benign paroxysmal positional nystagmus," which is a disorder of the otolith organ. It is thought that chalky particles break off from the utricle and hamper the function of the posterior semicircular canal.[12] The striking feature is the subjective vertigo on reaching the critical position; classically, after a few seconds, the patient cries out in horror. If the head is maintained in the position, after several seconds, the vertigo subsides but if the patients sits up again too quickly, it recurs. Usually a rotational nystagmus can be observed, which appears to beat toward the ground (geotropic), although ENG studies give a conflicting result because of the rotational component moving the electrical axis of the eye.[13] The subjective sensations can outlive the disappearance of nystagmus with optic fixation and, thus, testing using Frenzel's glasses can be helpful.

Central positioning nystagmus is relatively uncommon. The nystagmus is not usually accompanied by vertigo. It does not fatigue and may occur in any direction. It is found in cerebellar and brain stem lesions due to a variety of causes, including familial cerebellar atrophy, olivopontocerebellar degeneration, multiple sclerosis (MS), intra- and extra-axial tumors, vascular disease and Arnold-Chiari malformation (Table 17-5).

## Examination of Cerebellar Function

The signs of cerebellar dysfunction vary depending on whether the cerebellar hemisphere, the vermis, or both are affected (Table 17-6).[14]

Tests for cerebellar hemisphere function are performed with the patient sitting. Asynergia is noted by getting the patient to pat the back of each hand rapidly. Dysmetria is assessed using the finger-to-nose-to-finger test. The patient touches the examiner's finger and then the patient's own nose and then the examiner's finger, and so forth. The examiner moves his finger between each trial so that the patient has to find a different target each time. Failure to hit the target consistently indicates cerebellar dysfunction. Dysdiadochokinesia is noted by asking the patient to rapidly flip the hands

**Table 17-6.   Signs of Cerebellar Dysfunction**

**Neurologic**

Cerebellar hemisphere dysfunction (nonequilibratory)
  Asynergia or dissociated movements
  Dysmetria or past pointing
  Dysdiadochokinesis
  Rebound

Midline cerebellar dysfunction (equilibratory)
  Truncal ataxia
  Wide-based gait
  Falling in any direction and unable to make sudden turns

**Neuro-otologic**

Spontaneous nystagmus
  Coarse nystagmus — may be directional (Brun's nystagmus)
  Vertical down beating nystagmus if cerebellum is compressed into foramen magnum
  Absence of subjective symptoms such as nausea

Induced nystagmus
  Atypical positional nystagmus
  Enhanced caloric responses
  Often directional preponderance to affected side
  Optokinetic responses may be deranged or broken up

Smooth pursuit
  Broken up

Saccadic movements
  Hypodysmetria and hyperdysmetria

Electronystagmography
  Abnormal saccades
  Failure to maintain gaze position or drifting of eyes in darkness
  Dysmetria
  Rebound nystagmus[14]
  Centripetal nystagmus on eye closure or in darkness

over. Rebound is noted by asking the patient to move a limb against resistance and then suddenly removing the resistance; normally the patient should be able to stop the limb abruptly; failure to do so indicates hyperdysmetria.

Midline cerebellar disease disrupts the balance and causes gross ataxia.

**Table 17-5.   Classification of Positioning Nystagmus**

|  | Benign Paroxysmal | Central |
|---|---|---|
| Latent period | 2–15 sec | None |
| Adaptation | Disappears within 50 sec | Persists |
| Fatigability | Decreases on repetition | Persists |
| Subjective reaction | Marked nystagmus | Usually none |
| Direction of nystagmus | Toward undermost ear [a] | Variable |
| Incidence | Relatively common | Rare |

[a] On ENG recordings, the direction of the nystagmus appears to be away from the undermost ear because of the effect of the electrical axis of the eye.

## Examination of Stance and Gait

Usually tests of stance and gait are performed as part of the clinical examination. Many tests have been suggested; the following are most commonly used.

**The Romberg Test.**   In the Romberg test,[15] the patient is required to stand with eyes closed, feet together and arms to the side. Originally the test was devised to detect proprioceptive instability such as that caused by tabes dorsalis.

An uncompensated peripheral vestibular lesion invariably causes body sway toward the side of the lesion. Hysterical imbalance may cause the patient to fall straight backward like a "wooden soldier," a phenomenon never encountered with organic disease.

**The Unterberger Test.**   In the Unterberger test,[16] the patient stretches the hands out in front, like a sleepwalker, and steps up and down in the same place, like a soldier marching on the spot. In studying 40 normal subjects (nurses and students), I found that 95 percent of them did not rotate by more than 15 degrees to either side within a period of 15 seconds. This test appeared more sensitive than the Romberg test. Further refinements were added by Fukuda.[17]

**Gait Testing.**   The patient is asked to walk a short distance in a straight line with eyes open and then closed. I tested 40 normal subjects and found that 95 percent were able to walk over to and touch a wall within 15 inches of a target set 15 feet in front of them with their eyes closed. Patients with unilateral uncompensated vestibular lesions will deviate toward the side of the lesion. Hysterics may walk with a bizarre gait, for example, a scissor gait.

## TESTS OF VESTIBULAR FUNCTION

Tests of vestibular function have not been standardized as adequately as the auditory tests. One problem may be the selection of a control group, as many seemingly normal individuals may have a labyrinthine deficit of which they are unaware. The recording of the nystagmus, which results from activation of the vestibulo-ocular reflex, forms the basis of most tests of vestibular function. Electronystagmography (ENG) is the most commonly used means of recording eye movements.

## Electronystagmography

The ENG records a steady potential of approximately 1 mV, known as the corneoretinal potential, the cornea being positively charged in respect to the retina (Fig. 17-1). Electrodes are placed on the skin immediately lateral to each eye and on the skin above the bridge of the nose to detect any horizontal eye movements. Electrodes may also be placed below and above the eye to detect vertical eye movements.

By convention, a movement of the eyes to the right is recorded as an upward deflection and a movement of the eyes to the left is shown as a downward deflection. On the vertical recording, the direction of the recording relates to the particular vertical eye movement.

### DC Versus AC Recordings

It is important to know the position of the eyes during ENG testing. After a unilateral labyrinthine

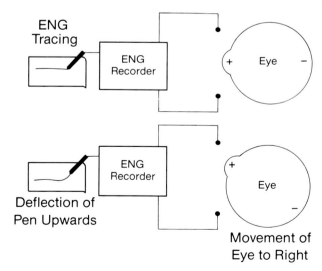

**Fig. 17-1.** A diagrammatic representation of electronystagmography.

lesion, a nystagmus occurs with the fast component beating away from the affected ear. The nystagmus has greatest amplitude looking away from the side of the lesion, and as recovery occurs, the nystagmus may not be evident on looking toward the side of the lesion. The eye in most patients will tend to drift from the midline toward the affected ear when optic fixation is removed, thus suppressing the nystagmus. The nystagmus can only be correctly interpreted if the eye position is known. DC recordings will indicate the eye position, but these recordings are demanding as other factors will cause the recording pen to drift, and the recordings are prone to electrical interference. One solution is to use the simpler AC recordings but to monitor the eye position using an infrared television system, which is relatively inexpensive.

### Effect of Eye Closure

ENG recordings are grossly inaccurate during eye closure as most subjects tend to roll their eyes upward causing fixation of the eye within the orbit (Bell's phenomenon). This can easily be observed by asking a patient with a complete facial palsy to try to close the eyes. Caloric testing performed with eyes closed is notoriously inaccurate.

### The Clinical Procedure

The subject is seated and must not have received any vestibular sedatives or alcohol within the previous 24 hours. Electrodes are carefully applied, taking care to reduce maximally the skin/electrode impedance. The machine is calibrated by asking the subject to look at colored lights placed at the center and at 30 degrees to the left and to the right; if vertical eye movements are also being recorded, a similar procedure is performed looking up and down.

### Measurements of Nystagmus

Nystagmus is shown on the ENG as a saw-toothed waveform. Figure 17-2 shows right vestibular nystagmus. The most widely accepted measure of nystagmus is the velocity of the slow phase. To make this measure the speed of paper (e.g., 1 cm/sec) is compared with the number of degrees of eye movement (e.g. 20 degrees) and the velocity is calculated (20 degrees/sec).

### The Gaze Test

The subject is seated in front of the calibration lights. Spontaneous nystagmus is sought by asking the subject to look at each of the lights in turn and then to repeat the procedure in total darkness. Recording during eye closure is of dubious validity. The position of the eyes in total darkness is monitored from DC recordings or from infrared monitors. Peripheral vestibular nystagmus may only be evident in darkness in one field of gaze.

Some normal, but typically anxious subjects, display square wave movements. If these square waves persist with the eyes open, then they are evidence of a pathologic condition; usually a cerebellar dysfunction. Normal subjects may also exhibit sinusoidal oscillations of the eyes at approximately 0.3 Hz: This indicates drowsiness and the

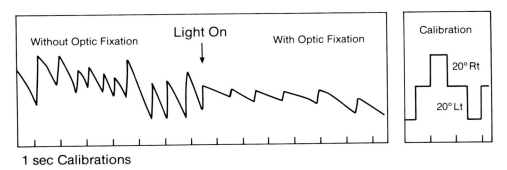

**Fig. 17-2.** A sample ENG tracing after a left labyrinthine lesion. Note that the right-beating nystagmus is diminished by optic fixation.

subject must be alerted. Normal subjects may occasionally display a horizontal nystagmus during gaze testing in the dark, which may be present in all fields but is usually strongest when looking in the direction of the fast phase. It is never present with the eyes open. The features of pathologic nystagmus were shown in Tables 17-3 and 17-4.

### The Tracking or Ocular Pursuit Test

The ENG may be used to measure the pursuit control system or ability of the eyes to follow a moving object (see *Observation of Pursuit Tracking,* above). Usually a swinging pendulum bob is used for this test. There is normally a smooth pursuit mechanism until target speeds in excess of 40 degrees/sec are reached, when saccadic movements may occur. Lesions affecting the pursuit control mechanism cause saccades superimposed upon the tracing ("cog-wheeling") at much lower speeds (Fig. 17-3).

### Optokinetic Testing

The test is performed best by moving a striped curtain around the patient during ENG recording. The small optokinetic drums have the drawback that they often measure pursuit.

Table 17-4 shows the abnormalities of optokinetic nystagmus (OKN) that can be encountered. When there is a directional preponderance (DP) revealed by caloric testing or rotational testing, the directional preponderance is often also evident on OKN testing; however, the DP is transient, disappearing when central compensation occurs. Broken up or disconjugate OKN is very suggestive of an intrinsic brain stem lesion.

A DP of OKN toward the affected side may occur with unilateral lesions deep in the parietal lobe, occipital lesions extending forward into the corpus callosum,[18] and subcortical frontal lesions.[19] Lesions affecting the connecting pathways between the occipital lobe and frontal cortex or between the frontal lobe and oculomotor nuclei selectively impair the fast component of OKN, which is easiest to detect on ENG recordings. Advanced lesions may abolish the fast phase completely so that no nystagmus is seen.

### Positional and Positioning Testing

ENG recordings of positioning testing are difficult for technical reasons as the recording has to be undertaken during head movement. It is interesting that the direction of benign positioning nystagmus on ENG recordings is usually up beating.

## Caloric Testing

This test provides a simple means of testing each labyrinth separately. The bithermal caloric test was popularized by Fitzgerald and Hallpike[20] who

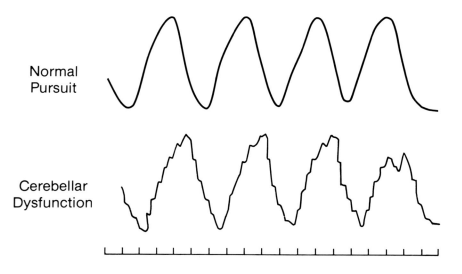

Normal
Pursuit

Cerebellar
Dysfunction

**Fig. 17-3.** The tracking test.

measured the duration of the responses, but today most clinicians prefer to record the test using ENG.

For descriptive purposes, the simpler method of recording the duration of visible nystagmus will be described first.

### The Procedure

The subject lies on a couch with the head raised at an angle of 30 degrees so that the lateral semicircular canal will lie in the vertical plane. After removing any wax, each ear in turn is irrigated with warm (44°C) and cold (30°C) water or air. Water provides a better stimulus because it conveys the temperature better.[21] Air has no advantages. If there is a perforation, the water can be delivered inside a thin rubber sleeve.

The concept, which may need some revision after the recent NASA experiments in weightlessness in the space shuttle, is that a thermal gradient is produced along the intracanalicular fluid, causing a convection current within the lateral semicircular canal. This current causes the fluid to flow toward or away from the cristae in the ampulla. This either increases or decreases the activity of the vestibular nerve and causes deviation of the eyes due to the vestibulo-ocular reflex. The slow drift of the eyes is corrected by a fast corrective movement in the opposite direction, and a sawtooth nystagmus results. A temperature either 7°C above or below body temperature is chosen because it provides a measurable response that is tolerable to the patient. If there is no response, then either water at 20°C or even at 0° can be chosen.

### Recording the Duration of Visible Nystagmus

The duration of the nystagmus is measured first with optic fixation, and when the induced nystagmus is no longer visible, the duration of nystagmus without optic fixation (using either Frenzel's glasses or an infrared viewer in darkness) is measured. With optic fixation, the nystagmus is suppressed by the optokinetic system and a clear end point is usually seen. Without optic fixation, the end point is much more difficult to measure precisely. The difference in duration of the nystagmus with and without optic fixation may be called the "fixation index." The fixation index was

originally described by Demanez and Ledoux[22] who defined it as

$$FI = \frac{\text{nystagmus magnitude in light}}{\text{nystagmus magnitude in dark}}$$

### Results of Caloric Testing

**Normal.** A normal person should have approximately the same reaction in both ears to water of the same temperature. The nystagmus is suppressed by optic fixation. Subjects vary in the amplitude of the nystagmus and in the amount of vertigo they sense, but generally the greater the duration and amplitude of the nystagmus, the greater the sensation of vertigo; most normal subjects feel some nausea.

**Canal Paresis.** The affected ear provides less nystagmus than the normal ear. Greater than 20 percent asymmetry indicates a lesion on the side of the decreased response.[23] The subject feels less vertigo when the affected ear is irrigated. If a partial canal paresis is present, when optic fixation is removed, the duration of nystagmus may equal that of the normal ear. It can be useful to note if the sensation caused by caloric stimulation is similar to that suffered during the attack.

**Directional Preponderance.** After a canal paresis has occurred, central vestibular mechanisms attempt to rebalance the subject and this results in a "directional preponderance to the opposite side to a paralytic lesion." The irritative (warm) calorics become more differentiated while the paretic (cold) calorics tend to become equalized.

It is important to stress that if a quick "clinical" test is to be done using nystagmus duration as the measure, then it must be performed with optic fixation and either using bithermal tests or hot tests but never using cold tests alone.

**Cerebellar Disease.** This may destroy the optokinetic suppression so that a coarse prolonged response is seen, which is not altered by optic fixation. Furthermore, the subject has little sensation of vertigo.[24]

**Results in Anxious Patients.** Anxious patients may have a hyperactive optokinetic suppression of the response so that little or no nystagmus is seen during optic fixation even though the subject complains bitterly of the sensation of vertigo. On removing optic fixation, a normal response is observed.

### ENG Measurement of the Caloric Test

The great advantage of using ENG recordings for caloric testing is that a permanent record is obtained. The same pitfalls mentioned for duration testing must be applied. Furthermore, some means of knowing the eye position is needed (DC recording or an infrared TV system) as there is a tendency for the eyes to drift in the direction of the slow component of the nystagmus during testing, which suppresses the nystagmus. Testing with eyes closed is forbidden because Bell's phenomenon often occurs, suppressing the nystagmus; in addition, the subject may become drowsy.

The normal results are shown in Table 17-7. The best measure appears to be the velocity of the slow phase: Measurements begin 10 seconds after finishing the irrigation and are averaged over a 10-second period.

*Canal paresis* is determined from the following formula:

$$\frac{(R30° + R44°) - (L30° + L44°)}{R30° + R44° + L30° + L44°} \times 100$$

This formula compares the left and right sides, and the upper limit of normal is 22 percent.[25]

*Directional preponderance* is determined from the following formula:

$$\frac{(R30° + L44°) - (R44° + L30°)}{R30° + L44° + R44° + L30°} \times 100$$

This formula compares the hot and cold calorics; a directional preponderance is assumed for values greater than 26 percent.[25]

*Optic fixation index* is determined from the formula:

$$\frac{\text{Average slow}}{\text{Average slow phase velocity with fixation} \times 100}{\text{Average slow phase velocity without fixation}}$$

The average visual suppression in normal subjects is $48 \pm 10$ percent.[25,26]

## Rotational Testing

The physical forces engendered by caloric testing cannot readily be measured. In contrast the physical forces applied by rotational testing can be measured precisely and can give an exact measure of the absolute sensitivity of the semicircular canal mechanism. Barany[27] introduced a chair rotated by hand; today the chair is rotated by a precision motor. The drawbacks of rotational testing are the expensive equipment needed and the fact that rotational testing stimulates both ears simultaneously.

The semicircular canals (sc) only respond to angular acceleration or deceleration, not to a constant speed. Hence, the following procedures have been adopted.

### Cupulometry

The subject is rotated at a constant velocity ranging from 2°/sec to 60°/sec and abruptly brought to rest. Observations are made on the duration of the resulting nystagmus and the sensations of vertigo.[28]

This test is time consuming and the responses are extremely variable as habituation effects often occur. It is not popular in clinical practice.

### Threshold Testing

The chair accelerates smoothly to apply a constant angular acceleration for a period of time which is just sufficient to cause a response. These threshold values are heavily dependent on the con-

**Table 17-7. Normal Values for Caloric Testing in Adults[a]**

| Parameter | With Optic Fixation (Light) | Without Fixation (Dark) |
|---|---|---|
| Duration (sec) | 90–120 (x̄107.5) | 155–240 (x̄198) |
| Maximum slow phase velocity (degrees/sec) | 1–8.5 (x̄3.2) | 8–48 (x̄23.8) |
| Beat frequency (Hz) | 1.0–3.1 (x̄2.05) | 1.3–3.3 (x̄2.43) |

[a] For 40 sec irrigations using water at 44°C and 30°C.

ditions of the test and the particular response elicited. The most sensitive method is to have the subject, while seated in darkness, view a light rotating with the chair. Extremely small accelerations will cause the illusion of movement of the light. Clark[29] found the normal threshold values for sensation alone was 0.10 degrees sec$^{-2}$ with a range of 0.05 to 0.18 degrees sec$^{-2}$. The mean threshold for a constant speed of rotation is 0.29 degrees sec$^{-2}$, which illustrates the remarkable sensitivity of the semicircular canals to angular acceleration.

Using ENG, recordings are usually made in darkness with eyes open (without optic fixation). The threshold values vary between laboratories but approximate the figures given by Clark[27] for sensation thresholds.

### Interpreting the Results

An asymmetry in rotational testing has the same significance as a directional preponderance in caloric testing. After an acute unilateral canal lesion, a clear asymmetry is observed but as the patient compensates, the asymmetry is gradually lost. Typically, although asymmetry is lost within a few months, the increased phase lead at low frequencies remains for years.[30] Rotational testing is excellent for documenting recovery after a unilateral acute labyrinthine loss.

Rotational testing is also excellent for evaluating bilateral peripheral disease such as caused by ototoxic exposure.

Rotational testing can also be used to determine the effect of (optokinetic) vestibular suppression resulting from optic fixation. The subject is rotated in darkness first without and then with a target lit.

### The Torsion Chair Test

This is a simple variant of the rotational test requiring only a chair restrained by a torsion bar, which is deviated by hand to set it into a pendular movement. The nystagmic eye movements are recorded on ENG and show reversals with each change of direction of the chair, revealing any directional preponderance. Some measure of the threshold can also be obtained. On testing patients with supranuclear lesions in whom saccadic movements may be impaired with sparing of the slow component, no nystagmus is apparent; instead, the eyes execute smooth oscillatory movements matching the movements of the chair.

### Sinusoidal Harmonic Acceleration Test

This test is performed using a computer controlled rotating chair which is commercially available (Neurokinetics Inc. Pittsburgh, PA) and has been popularized by Dr. Wallace Rubin. The subject is seated in darkness with the head bent forward 30 degrees so that the horizontal canal lies horizontally. The chair is rotated first to one side, stopped, and then rotated to the opposite side in a smooth acceleration. The time taken in seconds for each cycle is termed "frequency." Frequencies of 0.01, 0.02, 0.04, 0.08 and 0.16 Hz are tested. The commercial system records only an average of slow phase velocity. Other major drawbacks of the commercial apparatus are lack of flexibility and the fact that data is only obtained at very slow speeds of acceleration.

The following data is recorded: the chair position, chair velocity, chair acceleration and slow phase eye velocity (Fig. 17-4). Normally, when the head is displaced in one direction, the eyes deviate at the same velocity in the opposite direction. Hence, the eye movement velocity and the chair velocity are 180 degrees out of phase. A delay in the subject's ability to maintain this normal phase relationship is termed "phase lag." With visual and vestibular inputs, the movements are entirely compensatory, so the velocities equal each other but are in opposite directions (a "gain" of 1). In darkness with no visual input, the velocity of eye movement is reduced, and there is a reduction in gain. The symmetry of the eye velocity during movement in each direction can also be compared at each frequency and shown as a preponderance to one side or the other.

Thus, after each test session, two graphs are produced by the computer, which show the phase lag, preponderance, and a numerical record of gain. The normal *one* standard deviations are shown (Fig. 17-5). It has been found that phase lag has a remarkable consistent intertest reliability. Differences appear to persist for years after a unilateral canal lesion, whereas preponderance may norma-

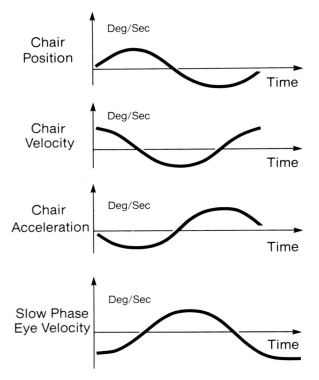

**Fig. 17-4.** Sinusoidal harmonic test (Neurokinetics, Inc., Pittsburgh, PA). Graphs showing the time relationship different chair functions and the slow phase velocity of the resulting nystagmus.

lize after a few months. Gain is a useful measure for detecting bilateral labyrinthine failure.

The drawback of using a one standard deviation normal control is that nearly one-third of normal subjects will give results that appear abnormal. A major criticism is that many patients may have been falsely labeled as having a vestibular problem using this test.

## Linear Acceleration Tests and Tests of Otolith Function

The otolith organs (utricle and saccule) detect linear movements. Testing can be performed by placing the subject on a seat attached to an arm extending 10 feet out from a central rotating point (available commercially from Servo-Med in Sweden). The subject is subjected to linear movement as well as rotation and will experience a tilting sensation similar to going around a corner on a motorcycle. The subject then controls a lever and is instructed to place it in the vertical position. The amount of tilt is recorded graphically against the acceleration of the chair.

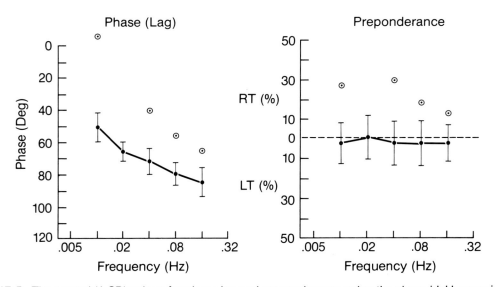

**Fig. 17-5.** The normal (1 SD) values for phase lag and preponderance using the sinusoidal harmonic test.

## Computerized Body Sway Testing

This test has been described in the past[31,32] but has recently been popularized by Owen Black.[33] Dr. Owen Black and Dr. Lewis Nashner developed and tested a computerized system which is now commercially available; the Equitest manufactured by Neurocom International Inc.

The patient stands with each foot on a special sensor plate. Sensors from each corner detect body sway and feed the data to a computer for analysis. The footplates and the wall of the booth on which the subject optically fixates can be moved ("sway-references"). Six different test conditions are investigated:

1. Eyes open, platform stable, visual field stable
2. Eyes shut, platform stable (Rhomberg test)
3. Eyes open, platform stable, visual field swayed
4. Eyes open, platform swayed, visual field stable
5. Eyes shut, platform stable
6. Eyes open, platform swayed, visual field swayed

The test relies on the hypothesis that three sensory inputs are responsible for balance; the labyrinths, proprioceptors, and vision. Test condition 1 allows inputs from all three, whereas test condition 2 only receives labyrinthine and proprioceptor inputs. When the platform sways, the ability of the visual and labyrinthine inputs to overcome this anomalous input is measured. In test conditions 5 and 6, the subject relies only on labyrinthine inputs. Even normal subjects find test conditions 5 and 6 difficult (Fig. 17-6).

Black[33] has suggested that this test can distinguish between three types of vestibular dysfunction: (1) bilaterally or unilaterally reduced labyrinthine function; (2) fluctuations in vestibular function, such as those accompanying endolymphatic hydrops or perilymph fistula; and (3) distortions of vestibular reflex function of the benign paroxysmal positional nystagmus type. The claims, particularly in regard to detection of perilymph leaks, appear promising although they have not yet been substantiated.

The main objection to Equitest is the cost of the equipment, and many research laboratories may feel they are able to construct similar equipment at a fraction of the cost.

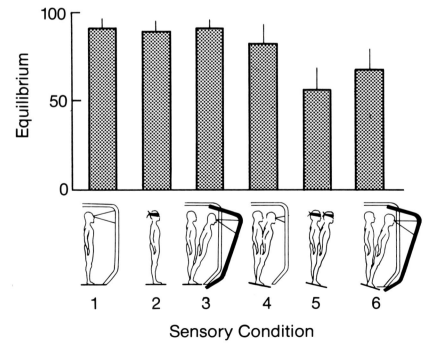

**Fig. 17-6.** The normal values of the Equitest posture platform for each of the six different test conditions. (Courtesy of Neurocom Int. Inc.)

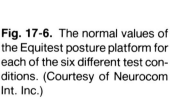

## VESTIBULAR TESTING FOR CHILDREN

Children can suffer from vertigo for many reasons: head trauma, perilymph leaks, benign paroxysmal vertigo of childhood, migraine, or tumors. Often, the history can only be obtained indirectly from the parents so in evaulating a child the caloric test is especially helpful and should be combined with the ENG if possible.[34] Rotation tests and posture platform tests can also be applied.

The typical caloric trace in a child shows a large amplitude and a relatively small slow phase velocity when compared to an adult. This has been attributed to incomplete maturation of the vestibular system. The reader is referred to Chapter 10 for additional information on this topic.

## CONCLUSIONS

The traditional methods of reaching a diagnosis of a vestibular disorder relied on the clinical history, clinical examination, and certain vestibular tests. The first two methods are still as valid today as in the past. The last method, however, has undergone dramatic changes over the last decade due to the introduction of computerized analysis. The caloric test has stood the test of time and introduction of the computer to allow a continuous reading of the slow phase velocity of the induced nystagmus will enhance its usefulness. The introduction of computerized and commercially available equipment for rotational testing and for posture testing has brought these useful tests into the reach of the busy clinician.

## REFERENCES

1. Morrison AW: Management of Sensorineural Deafness. Butterworth Publishers, London and Boston, 1975
2. Rudge P: Clinical Neuro-Otology. Churchill Livingstone, Edinburgh, 1983
3. Patel A, Toole JF: Subclavian steal syndrome—reversal of cephalic blood flow. Medicine 44:289, 1965
4. Frenzel H: Der Nachweis von Scwaachem Bei Gewohnlicher Beobachtung Nicht Sichtbarem Spontannystagmus. Klinische Wochenschrift 41:461, 1928
5. Barber HO, Stockwell CW: Manual of Electronystagmography. CV Mosby, St Louis, 1980
6. Baloh AT, Honrubia V: Clinical Neurophysiology of the Vestibular System. FA Davis, Philadelphia, 1979
7. Barber HO, Wright G: Positional nystagmus in normals. Adv Otorhinolaryngol 19:276, 1973
8. Biemond A, deJong JMBV: On cervical nystagmus and related disorders. Brain 92:437, 1969
9. Barany R: Diagnose von Krankheitserschereingen in Bereiche des Otolithenapparates. Acta Otolaryngol (Stockh) 2:434, 1921
10. Nylen CO: A clinical study on positional nystagmus in cases of brain tumour. Acta Otolaryngol [Stockh] Suppl. 15, 1931
11. Dix MR, Hallpike CS: The pathology, symptomatology and diagnosis of certain common disorders of the vestibular system. Ann Otol Rhinol Laryngol 61:987, 1952
12. Schuknecht HL: Cupulolithiasis. Arch Otolaryngol 90:765, 1969
13. Barber HO: Electronystagmographic findings in benign poaitional nystagmus. Acta Otolaryngol 6:37, 1983
14. Hood JD, Kayan A, Leech J: Rebound nystagmus. Brain 96:507, 1973
15. Romberg MH: Lehrbuch der NervenKrankheiten des Mennschen. A. Duncker, Berlin, 1846
16. Unterberger S: Neue Objectiv Registrierbare Vestibularis-Korper Dreahreaktion Erhalten Durch Treten Auf der Stelle der "tretversuch" Arch fur on u Kehlkopfheilkunde 145:478, 1938
17. Fukuda T: The stepping test. Acta Otolaryngol (Stockh) 50:95, 1959
18. Dix MR: The mechanism and clinical significance of optokinetic nystagmus. J Laryngol Otol 94:845, 1980
19. Kornhuber HH: Nystagmus and related phenomena in man. In Kornhuber HH (ed): Handbook of Sensory Physiology. Vol 6. Springer-Verlag, New York, 1974
20. Fitzgerald G, Hallpike CS: Studies in human vestibular function. Observations on the directional preponderance of caloric nystagmus resulting from cerebral lesions. Brain 65:115, 1942
21. Al-Sheikli ARJ, Gibson WPR, Oppenheimer S: A comparative study of air and water as a caloric stimu-

lus. p. 161. In Taylor IG, Markides A (eds): Disorders of Auditory Function III. Academic Press, Orlando, FL, 1980

22. Demanez JP, Ledoux A: Automatic fixation mechanisms and vestibular stimulation. Adv Otorhinolaryngol 17:90, 1970

23. Sills AW, Baloh RW, Honrubia V: Caloric testing. II. Results in normal subjects. Ann Otol Rhinol Laryngol 86[Suppl 43]:7-14, 1977

24. Gibson WPR, Oppenheimer S: The physiological significance of the abnormal caloric induced nystagmus encountered in cerebellar disorders. p. 167. In Taylor IG, Markides A (eds): Disorders of Auditory Function III. Academic Press, Orlando, FL, 1980

25. Baloh RW: The Essentials of Neurotology. FA Davis, Philadelphia, 1984

26. Takemori S, Cohen B: Loss of visual suppression of vestibular nystagmus after flocculus lesions. Brain Res 72:213, 1974

27. Barany R: Untersuchungen Uber Den Vom Vestibularapparat des Ohres Reflectorisch Ausgelosten Rhythmischen Nystagmus und Seine Begleiterscheinungen, Mschr Ohrenheilk 40:193, 1906

28. Benson AJ: Modification of the response time to angular acceleration by linear accelerations. p. 281. In Kornhuber HH (ed): Handbook of Sensory Physiology. Vol 6. Springer-Verlag, New York, 1974

29. Clark B: Some recent studies on the perception of rotation. p. 43. In Stahle J (ed): Vestibular Function on Earth and in Space. Pergamon Press, New York, 1970

30. Honrubia V, Jenkins HA, Baloh RW, Lau CGY: Evaluation of rotary tests in peripheral labyrinthine lesions. In Honrubia V, Brazier AB (eds): Nystagmus and Vertigo. Academic Press, Orlando, FL, 1982

31. Baron JB: Statokinesimetrie Kes Feullets du Practicien. 2:23, 1978

32. Booth JB, Stockwell CWA: A method for evaluating vestibular control of posture. Trans Am Acad Ophthal Otolaryngol 86:ORL93, 1978

33. Black FO: Vestibulospinal function assessment by moving platform posturography. Am J Otol 7 [Suppl]:39, 1985

34. Busis SN: Vertigo. p. 261. In Bluestone CD, Stool SE (eds): Paediatric Otolaryngology. WB Saunders, Philadelphia, 1983

# Electronystagmography and Vestibular Testing in Children

# 18

Lydia Eviatar
Abraham Eviatar

The vestibular apparatus is among the first sensory organs to develop phylogenetically and ontogenetically. In primitive animals such as the coelenterates, the vestibular system is solely responsible for orienting behavior necessary to avoid danger or acquire food. As we ascend in the phylogenetic scale, orientation in space is gradually subserved by additional sensory systems such as the visual, auditory, and proprioceptive systems, with less reliance on labyrinthine function. In spite of its diminishing role as an orienting control system, the vestibular apparatus and its connections in the brain are crucial in the development of head and postural control in the child. Embryologic studies reveal that the membranous labyrinth develops very early in embryonal life and is fully differentiated in the 30 mm embryo.[1] Functionally it becomes active by the 8th or 9th month of gestation, being responsible in part for startle responses during fetal life.[2] Between the 12th and the 24th week of gestation, the connections of the labyrinth to the oculomotor nuclei in the brain stem develop and brain stem oculomotor reflexes are initiated.[3] The vestibular nerve is the earliest cranial nerve to achieve full myelination, by the age of 16 weeks.[4] Maturation of vestibular function proceeds rapidly during the first 6 months of postnatal life, contrib-uting significantly to the development of head and postural control in the infant and to the appearance of righting reflexes that enable the child to maintain his or her balance as a result of abrupt changes in the center of gravity.

The peripheral organ of equilibrium—the labyrinth—is located in the inner ear and consists of the three semicircular canals, the utricle, and the saccule.[5] Peripheral endings of the vestibular nerve are located on the hair cells of the maculae of the utricle and saccule and in the cristae of the ampullae of the semicircular canals. The semicircular canals are primarily concerned with responses to angular acceleration of the head and body while the utricle is primarily concerned with gravitational motion and linear acceleration. Abrupt head motions in the horizontal or perpendicular plane induce movement of the endolymphatic fluid, which is transmitted via the hair cells of the macula and cristae to the peripheral nerve endings of the vestibular nerve. The information concerning the relative position of the head in space during motion is conveyed through the vestibular nerve to the vestibular nuclei in the brain stem. A few fibers of the vestibular nerve ascend directly to the cerebellum ending in the cortex of the flocculonodular lobe. Connections are made in the cerebellum with the nuclei fastigii where efferent impulses originate and exert a modulating influence on the vestibular nuclei and labyrinth via the fastigial-bulbar tract. From the vestibular nuclei labyrinthine impulses are transmitted to the motor neurons in the anterior horns of the spinal cord through the vestibulospinal tract, reinforcing local myotactic reflexes in the extensor muscles of the trunk and extremities and· producing enough extra strength to support the body against gravity and maintain an upright posture. Afferent vestibular impulses ascent through the medial longitudinal fasciculus to cranial nerves III, IV, and VI, which are directly responsible for oculomotor control. Thus, movement of endolymphatic fluid in the horizontal semicircular canals elicits vestibular impulses that are transmitted to the abducens and oculomotor nuclei inducing a slow conjugate eye deviation in the direction of motion of the endolymphatic fluid. Once the ocular muscles reach their maximum tension, the eyes will quickly return to their resting position. When the eyes move in rapid succession, as for instance during rotatory stimulation in a Baranyi chair, a nystagmus results. The direction of nystagmus is designated in accordance with the direction of the fast component (quick ocular realignment), although it is the slow component of nystagmus that represents the true result of vestibular stimulation. Recording of the oculomotor responses to peripheral labyrinthine stimulation by rotation or caloric irrigation of the ear canals is widely used as a method of investigating the integrity of the labyrinth and the labyrinthine pathways.

A comprehensive evaluation of the role of the vestibular system includes the assessment of muscle tone, head and postural control, and developmental reflexes during the various stages of human development. In the small infant, up to the age of 4 months, these consist primarily of tonic neck responses. By 6 months, righting responses can be observed, while in the fully developed nervous system of the preschool child more complex equilibrium responses are already present. The vestibular system has widespread connections throughout the brain, primarily to the reticular activating system, basal ganglia, and posterior superior temporal cortex. Damage in any one of the projection areas may produce abnormalities in vestibular responses and during vestibular testing. The paroxysmal discharges originating in the posterior temporal cortex may produce vertiginous seizures. Physiological states such as sleep or drowsiness, during which the activity of the reticular activating system is reduced, may significantly inhibit vestibular responses. Cerebellar dysfunction, primarily damage involving the flocculonodular lobe, is notoriously implicated in a variety of dysequilibrium and vertiginous syndromes.

The neurovestibular examination is classified into two major parts: the clinical evaluation of the vestibular system, and laboratory evaluation with the help of electronystagmography.

## CLINICAL EVALUATION

The clinical evaluation consists of a neurologic examination of all afferent and efferent pathways that contribute to the maintenance of equilibrium in humans (Fig. 18-1). This consists of detailed evaluation of the visual system to test extraocular motions, the presence of strabismus or spontaneous nystagmus, the presence of refraction errors, or funduscopic changes. All cranial nerves and specifically the 5th, 7th, 8th (cochlear part), 9th, 11th, and 12th are evaluated since they may be involved in diseases of the brainstem or cerebellopontine (CP) angle, in which the vestibular nerve is often affected.

The evaluation of posture and tone is supplemented by a specific and detailed evaluation of primitive reflexes in infants from birth until about 4 months of age (Figs. 18-2 to 18-6) and righting reflexes from 6 to 24 months (Figs. 18-7 to 18-10). Coordination tests are specifically adapted to the patient's age and involve manipulation of blocks in the young infant, the ability to pick up tiny objects such as raisins, the ability to stack blocks one on top of the other, and to use a pencil to scribble and reproduce designs. Position in space (kinesthesia) can be evaluated beginning at around 4 years of age. Specific tests for the clinical vestibular evalua-

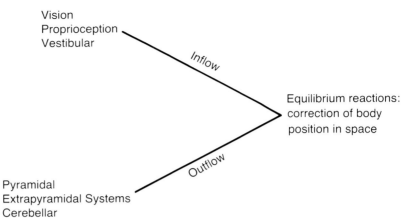

**Fig. 18-1.** Equilibrium responses.

Vision
Proprioception
Vestibular

Inflow

Equilibrium reactions:
correction of body
position in space

Outflow

Pyramidal
Extrapyramidal Systems
Cerebellar

tion involve testing for presence of spontaneous or induced nystagmus.

Spontaneous nystagmus is tested with the patient seated with the head straight up in the primary position. The child is then asked to fixate with the eyes in midposition, 30 degrees to the right, to the left, up, and down. A first-degree nystagmus is defined as a nystagmus that occurs only during lateral gaze in the direction of the fast component. The second-degree nystagmus is also present in midposition. A third degree nystagmus is present on straight gaze as well as lateral gaze both in the di-

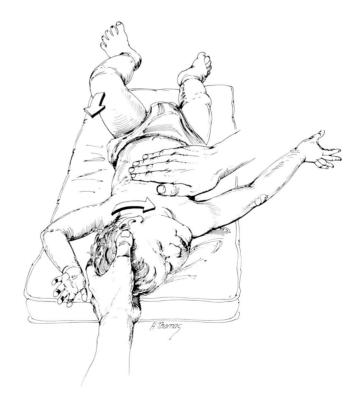

**Fig. 18-2.** Asymmetrictonic neck reflex.

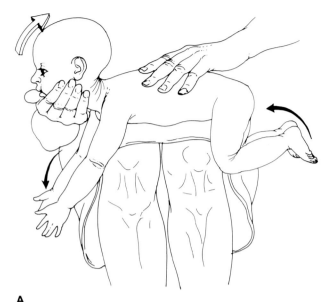

**A**

**Fig. 18-3.** Symmetrictonic neck reflex. **(A)** Head dorsiflexed. **(B)** Head ventroflexed.

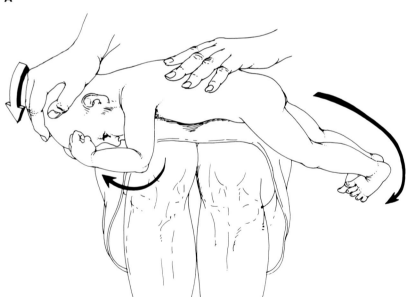

**B**

rection of the fast and the slow component. Vestibular nystagmus is usually inhibited by fixation as opposed to gaze paretic, rebound, or congenital nystagmus, which are all prominent during fixation. Electronystagmography is the ideal way to evaluate vestibular nystagmus as the test is done in the dark with the eyes closed to eliminate fixation. The differentiation between vestibular nystagmus of peripheral or central origin is difficult. Central nystagmus is more often found in conjunction with brain stem disease and other cranial nerve deficits and is not effectively inhibited by fixation. The presence of a vestibular nystagmus as an isolated finding completely suppressed by fixation is suggestive of peripheral vestibular disease.[6]

Positional nystagmus is most often seen with le-

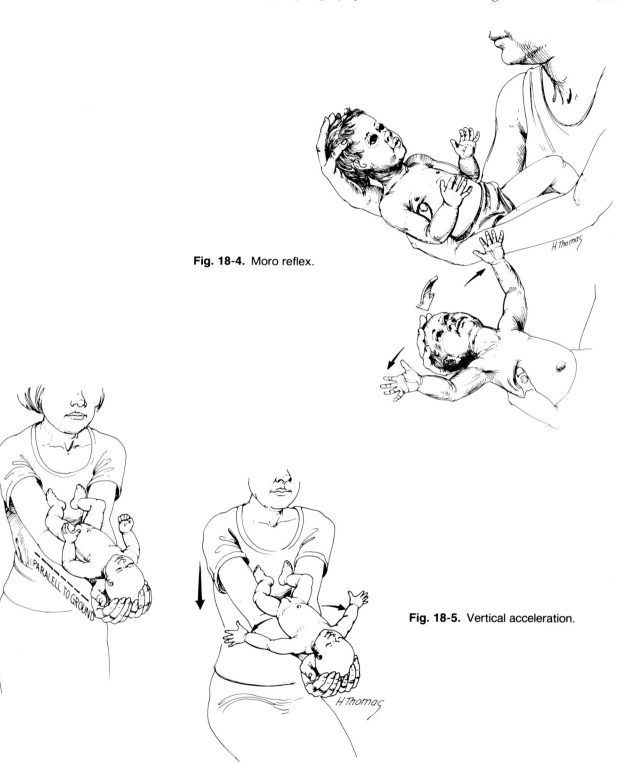

**Fig. 18-4.** Moro reflex.

**Fig. 18-5.** Vertical acceleration.

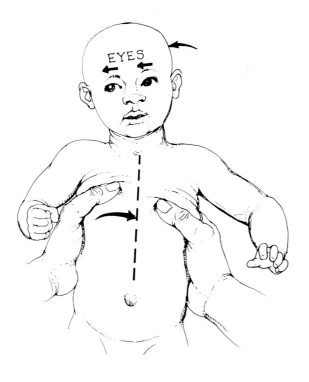

**Fig. 18-6.** Doll's eyes response.

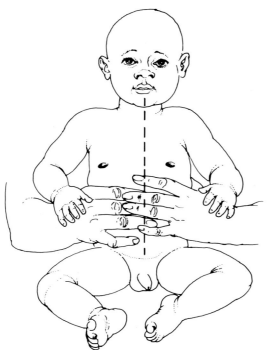

**Fig. 18-7.** Buttress reaction.

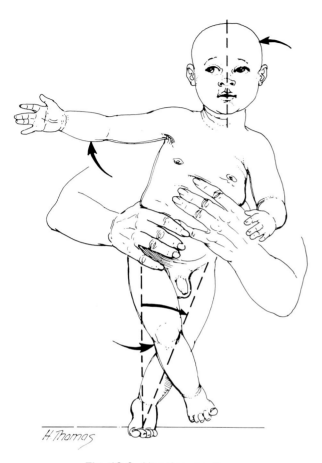

**Fig. 18-8.** Hopping reaction.

sions of the labyrinth and can also be seen in a variety of metabolic disorders affecting the specific gravity of the cupula or during intoxication by alcohol or ototoxic drugs. Head trauma affecting the labyrinth is also likely to produce positional nystagmus. A Hallpike maneuver is most commonly used to elicit paroxysmal positional nystagmus in the office. This involves moving the patient rapidly from the sitting to the head hanging position with the head 45 degrees below the horizontal and rotated 45 degrees to one side. The benign paroxysmal positional nystagmus seen with peripheral organ disease usually has a latency of 3 to 10 seconds and rarely lasts longer than 15 seconds. It is usually most marked in one head-hanging position, and the patient complains of severe vertigo with the initial positioning but with repeated positionings the vertigo and nystagmus rapidly disappear. When paroxysmal positional nystagmus is associated with unilateral caloric hypoexcitability, it is strongly suggestive of peripheral vestibular damage, such as occurs as a sequela of head injury, viral labyrinthitis, or occulusion of the vasculature to the inner ear. The paroxysmal positional nystagmus associated with brain stem or cerebellar disease is a nonfatiguing type and does not decrease in amplitude or duration with repeated positionings of the head. There is usually no clear latency and it lasts longer than 30 seconds, often for as long as the head position is maintained.

**Fig. 18-9.** Horizontal suspension in supine.

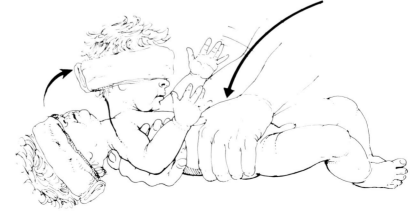

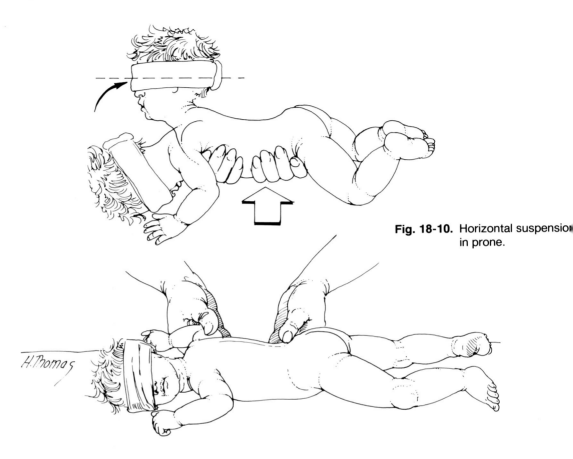

**Fig. 18-10.** Horizontal suspension in prone.

## POSTURAL REACTIONS

The evaluation is simplified by classifying the children in four groups according to age and level of maturation of the central nervous system.

### Group 1 (Birth to 4 months)

Movement and postural responses in this age group are primarily dominated by tonic neck responses, which are primitive labyrinthine reflexes integrated at the brain stem level. The tonic neck reflexes are obtained by passive or active motion of the head relative to a fixed position of the body. The afferent stimulus is provided from the endolymphatic movement in the semicircular canals as well as proprioceptive stimuli from the cervical vertebrae and muscles. The motor response, which involves the extremities and trunk, depends on the integrity of the vestibular and proprioceptive afferent pathways and the efferent motor pathways. Neck righting—head turning from the midline to the side—in a supine infant induces rolling of the whole body in the direction of the head.

### Asymmetrical Tonic Neck Reflex

Rotation of the baby's head to the side while restraining the chest in the supine position induces flexion of the extremities on the side of the occiput and extension of the extremities on the side of the face (Fig. 18-2).

### Symmetrical Tonic Neck

The baby is maintained in the horizontal prone position; the examiner's hand under the baby's trunk. Dorsiflexion of the head induces extension of the upper extremities and flexion of the lower extremities (Fig. 18-3A,B). The reverse occurs with ventroflexion of the head.

### Moro Reflex

The baby lies supine with the head ventroflexed and supported by the examiner's hand (Fig. 18-4). As the head is allowed to drop backward about 30 degrees in relation to the trunk, abduction of the arms followed by embrace occurs.

### Vertical Acceleration

The baby is maintained on the examiner's extended forearms in the supine position (Fig. 18-5). The head and trunk are aligned parallel to the ground. A rapid downward acceleration is produced to the baby's horizontal body by the examiner, who bends the knees abruptly. This vertical acceleration provides the stimulus to the utricle and the appropriate response consists of slight extension of the baby's head and abduction with extension of the arms with fanning of the hands. This reflex has the advantage over the Moro in eliminating the proprioceptive input from the neck muscles and joint.

### Doll's Eye Phenomenon

This reflex is the most primitive response to rotation obtained in full-term babies, usually for the first 2 weeks of life (Fig. 18-6). This response persists much longer in the premature baby. The reflex is obtained by holding the baby vertically and facing the examiner as the examiner's hands surround the baby's trunk and maintain the baby's head bent forward 30 degrees over the body. Rotation of the baby around the examiner's axis produces deviation of the eyes and head opposite to the direction of rotation. As the baby gets older and the vestibular response matures, the doll's eye phenomenon is substituted by nystagmus with the quick component in the direction of rotation.

## Group II (4 to 6 months)

Many normal babies in this group retain some of the primitive tonic neck reflexes while others develop righting reflexes at this early age, indicating a higher level of maturation and integration of vestibular responses.

## Group III (6 to 24 months)

Myelination of the various tracts as well as the axonodendritic synapses between the various cortical neurons proceeds rapidly. A better integration of the visual, proprioceptive, and vestibular stimuli with appropriate motor responses occurs primarily at the midbrain level, resulting in motor responses called righting reflexes. Righting reflexes are obtained by tilting the patient abruptly sideways, frontward, or backward and thus changing rapidly his or her center of gravity. The acceleration imposed on the vestibular organs elicits stimuli that bring about righting of the head and protective reactions of the extremities. It can first be elicited in the sitting position (buttress or propping reaction, Fig. 18-7) or in the standing position by 8 to 10 months (hopping reaction, Fig. 18-8). Since optical and vestibular righting responses are very similar, the tests for vestibular righting are done with the patient blindfolded. Head righting reflexes can also be obtained by lifting the patient rapidly from supine or prone position (Figs. 18-9, 18-10).

### Parachute Response

A downward vertical acceleration can be applied to the baby who is held around the chest (Fig. 18-11). Immediate extension of the arms with abduction and extension of the fingers occurs as well as righting of the head. This test, as well as the previous one, is also performed blindfolded. This response usually persists throughout life, being inhibited only by voluntary control in the older individual.

## Group IV (4 through Adult)

By age 4 most children are sufficiently cooperative to be tested for the presence of equilibrium responses and undergo a complete neurologic evaluation as outlined in Table 18-1. The child can be tested in the sitting position with the examiner pulling the child by the arms sideways. A normal response consists of righting of the head and extension with abduction of the extremities on the side

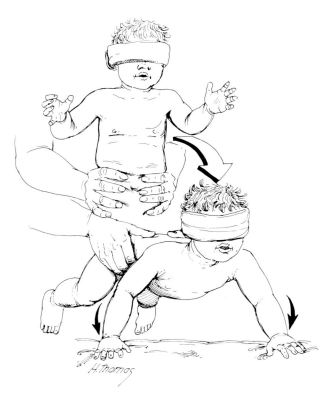

**Fig. 18-11.** Parachute reflex.

the extremities. Equilibrium and postural reactions may be significantly impaired in the presence of vestibular disease, with the patient usually falling toward the affected side. They may also be disturbed in the presence of neuromuscular disorders affecting the pyramidal or extrapyramidal tracts. Thus, before determining that one is dealing with a labyrinthine dysfunction, the possibility of neuromuscular disease should be ruled out. Individuals with a labyrinthine disease learn to compensate for the loss of labyrinthine function, especially by using visual cues. If visual cues are also eliminated, a total disorientation occurs.

Clinical tests of vestibular function are the Romberg test and tandem gait blindfolded. In cases of unilateral labyrinthine involvement, swaying toward the side of the lesion during tandem gait is observed as well as falling toward the side of the lesion during the performance of a Romberg test. A more sensitive vestibular test is the *tandem Romberg*. The patient is asked to stand with one foot in front of the other as though getting ready to walk, with the arms folded and eyes closed. Normal individuals are able to maintain this position for 6 to 7 seconds uninterrupted. In the presence of unilateral labyrinthine disease, the patient falls immediately toward the affected side. This test remains positive even in long-standing unilateral vestibular lesions and is therefore likely to detect mild vestibular abnormalities.

*The stepping test* is a modification of the old stepping test introduced by Fukuda. The patient is asked to take 60 steps on the same spot at the intersection of two perpendicular lines while the examiner records the angle of rotation as well as forward or backward displacement. The test is performed

opposite the direction of tilt (Fig. 18-12). A similar response can be obtained in the kneeling position (Fig. 18-13). Total body postural responses can be obtained using a small tilting board on which the child lies either prone (Fig. 18-14) or supine (Fig. 18-15). As the examiner tilts the board about 45 degrees sideways, there is a righting response of the head and extension with abduction reactions of

**Table 18-1.    Complete Neurologic Examination**

| Cranial Nerves | Test Procedure |
| --- | --- |
| III, IV, VI | Extraocular movement (strabismus, nystagmus, refraction) |
| II | Funduscopy |
| V – XII | Corneals, hearing responses, facial expression gag, tongue motions |
| | Audiometry adapted to patient's age |
| | Posture, tone, DTR |
| | Developmental reflexes |
| | Coordination tests ⎫ |
| | Cerebellar tests ⎬ adapted to patient's age |
| | Sensory exam (proprioception, kinesthetic) |

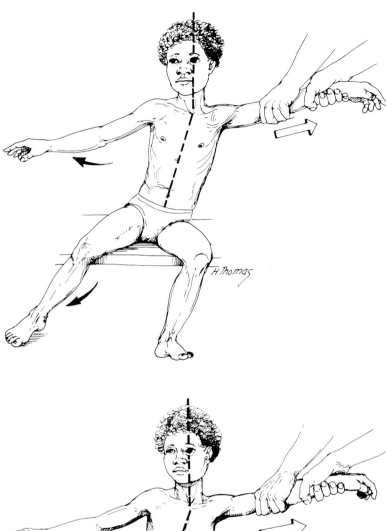

**Fig. 18-12.** Equilibrium reaction to pull in sitting.

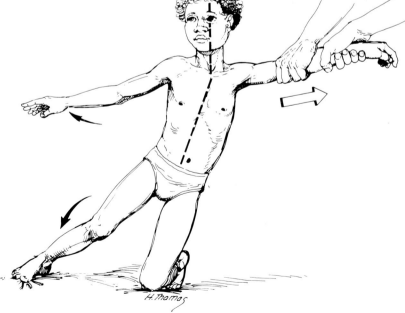

**Fig. 18-13.** Equilibrium reaction to pull in kneeling.

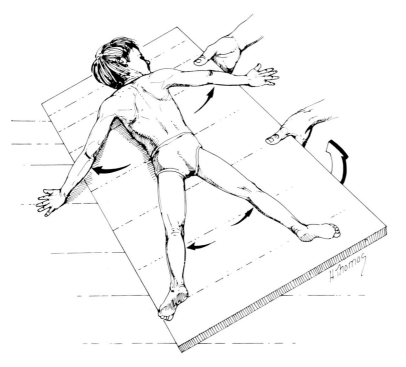

**Fig. 18-14.** Equilibrium reaction to tilt in prone.

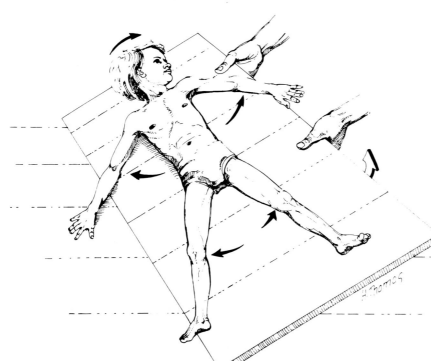

**Fig. 18-15.** Equilibrium reaction to tilt in supine.

with the patient's arms extended parallel and horizontal to the ground and the eyes closed. In the presence of labyrinthine disease there is a general tendency to rotate toward the side of the lesion by an angle larger than 45 degrees. In some bilateral lesions or in utricular lesions, forward displacement occurs.

*Past pointing* is an additional attempt to assess vestibular function clinically. The patient is asked to sit in front of the examiner with the eyes closed, arms extended forward, and the patient places an extended index finger to the vertical position and attempts to return the index finger to the examiner's. A consistent deviation to one side is called past pointing and suggests ipsilateral vestibular dysfunction.

## ELECTRONYSTAGMOGRAPHY

Electronystagmography is the recording of eye movements during visual pursuit and in response to vestibular stimulation. A recording is possible because each eyeball acts as a dipole with the cornea being electropositive and the retina electronegative. The direction of the dipole is oriented in the direction of the long axis of the eye. Changes in the magnetic field generated by eye movements are picked up by two electrodes placed bitemporally for recording of conjugate horizontal eye movements. A reference (ground electrode) is placed on the nasion. The difference in potential between the bitemporal electrodes is amplified and used to control the displacement of a pen writing recorder that provides a permanent record of the eye movements. The availability of a permanent recording of oculomotor responses to various types of stimulation presents a significant advantage both in clinical and research work. Electronystagmography is performed in a quiet and dark room; the patient should be awake and alert throughout the period of testing. A one channel AC dynograph recorder is adequate for general clinical use. A two channel recorder will permit recording of both horizontal and vertical eye movements simultaneously by placing one electrode above the orbit and one

below in the midline position. The test is started whenever possible with recording of *pathologic nystagmus*. Gaze nystagmus is recorded with the patient staring straight ahead as well as 30 degrees lateral to the right, left, up, and down for 1 minute in each position. The next step is recording for *positional nystagmus*. The recording is done with the patient in the supine, prone, and lateral positions as well as in the sitting position with the head straight and the head turned to the right and to the left, whenever the child is able to sit. During positional testing, the patient is blindfolded to inhibit fixation or visual pursuit.

## PERROTATORY STIMULATION

A commercially available torsion swing is used to provide a sinusoidal angular stimulation to the labyrinth. In young infants, the test is performed with the baby seated in the mother's lap on the torsion swing. Her right hand maintains the baby's head flexed 30 degrees over the body to align the horizontal semicircular canals parallel to the ground. During the sinusoidal rotation, the stimulus alternately deviates the cupula in ampullopetal and ampullofugal directions, producing nystagmus in opposite directions with each half cycle of rotation. The average slow component velocity of nystagmus is used to quantify the response during each half cycle. The response is then compared between the clockwise and the counterclockwise rotation in a given subject. If the number of beats in response to clockwise rotation exceeds by 25 percent the number of beats to counterclockwise rotations, the asymmetry is significant and suggests a directional preponderance. A directional preponderance is seen in the presence of a labyrinthine imbalance or in central lesions. Overall reduction in the amplitude of nystagmus may be caused by ototoxic drugs. Cerebellar or pontine lesions as well as lesions of the medial longitudinal fasciculus (MLF) may alter the waveform of the nystagmus induced by sinusoidal rotation. These abnormalities are best demonstrated by monocular recording.[6] Most full-term babies born with a weight appropriate for gestational age will show a positive nystagmus in response to perrotatory stimulation within the first months of life. In small premature infants, this response may be absent during the first 3 months.[7] Once the nystagmic response to perrotatory stimulation is present, its quality does not change significantly with maturation.[8]

# CALORIC STIMULATION

Caloric irrigation of the ear canals is performed to test each labyrinth individually. In the very young baby who cannot tolerate a prolonged period of testing, we use a 10-second cold caloric irrigation of the ear canals with the water temperature not to exceed 5°C. The baby is blindfolded and restrained in a papoose board in the supine position with the head ventroflexed at 30 degrees. The recording is started immediately and the latency period between the cessation of stimulation and onset of nystagmus is recorded. The direction of nystagmus is oppostie to the ear stimulated. As soon as a good response is obtained, the baby is turned in the prone position, and the direction of nystagmus reverses when the labyrinth is intact. As soon as this new response begins to fade, the baby is turned back to the supine position and the nystagmus is expected to revert to the initial direction, away from the ear stimulated. By doing this maneuver, we want to ensure that the response obtained from the caloric stimulation of the labyrinth is a true labyrinthine response as opposed to an intensification of a latent nystagmus that will not revert from supine to prone.[8] Ten minutes should elapse before stimulating the other ear canal with cold water. A positive nystagmic response to cold caloric stimulation is present in the vast majority of full-term babies of appropriate weight for gestational age within the first 3 months of life. Only around 20 percent of premature babies and babies born small for gestational age have a positive nystagmic response to caloric stimulation within the first 3 months. The majority will have an appropriate response after 6 months of life.[9] The quality of response is evaluated by measuring the speed of the slope of the slow component of nystagmus at culmi-

nation of response, and the responses from the right and left ear irrigations are compared. A unilaterally depressed response suggests a hypoactive labyrinth on that side. Bilaterally suppressed responses may occur during sleep and drowsiness or as a result of damage secondary to ototoxic drugs. Infection of the middle ear or mastoid air cells may produce an exaggerated caloric response. Tonic deviation of the eyes without nystagmus is seen in the immature baby (premature and small for gestational age) during the first few months of life or in the presence of a parapontine lesion if the child is fully mature at the time of testing. Normative data on the quality of nystagmus and the various parameters that can be tested for various gestational age groups and different ages at testing are presently available.[8] After 36 months of age, most children are able to tolerate the bithermal caloric irrigation. The technique is similar to the one used in adults and consists of irrigation of the external auditory canal for 30 seconds with 30°C for cold and 44°C for warm. A 10-minute interval is allowed between two consecutive irrigations. The intensity of nystagmus represented by the speed of the slow component at culmination is used for calculation. In our laboratory, Jongkee's formula is used for the determination of labyrinthine preponderance or directional preponderance (Table 18-2). The presence of directional preponderance in children and young individuals is strongly suggestive of central vestibular pathology. The presence of labyrinthine preponderance is highly correlated with the presence of peripheral organ disease or disease of the

**Table 18-2. Electronystagmography**

Positional test
Recording pathologic nystagmus
Perrotatory test (torsion swing)
Ice cold caloric irrigation for 10 seconds:
    Supine
    Prone
    Supine
Bithermal caloric irrigation for children over $3\frac{1}{2}$ yrs
Labyrinthine Preponderance:
$$\frac{(RW \& RC) - (LW \& LC)}{(RW \& RC + LW \& LC)} \times 100 > 14\%$$
Directional Preponderance:
$$\frac{(RW \& LC) - (LW \& RC)}{(RW \& LC) + (LW \& RC)} \times 100 > 18\%$$
Binaural bithermal stimulation > 6 months
Optokinetic nystagmus
Smooth pursuit
Pendulum test

8th nerve. The term labyrinthine preponderance is often used interchangeably with that of hypoactive labyrinth. When the findings are of both directional and labyrinthine preponderance in a young patient, the correlation is higher with central lesions; however, a peripheral lesion cannot be excluded.[10] When a bithermal irrigation elicits no response, the test is followed by an ice-cold caloric stimulation of the unresponsive labyrinth. This maximal stimulation will then provide evidence of whether we are dealing with a dead or a hypoactive labyrinth. Hyperactive caloric responses are sometimes seen in the presence of cerebellar disease. A dysrhythmic nystagmus pattern is also suggestive of a cerebellar involvement. Dysconjugate nystagmus (on monocular recording) suggests intrinsic brain stem disease usually affecting the MLF.

## TESTS OF VISUAL OCULAR CONTROL

The test includes a tracking response, during which the patient is asked to follow lights moving on a dark screen from right to left and left to right at various speeds.

### Pendulum Test

The patient is asked to follow a light oscillating back and forth at various speeds, 10 degrees and 20 degrees per second usually, or to follow a pendulum.

### Optokinetic Test

A filmstrip is presented moving from right to left and left to right at various speeds ranging from 4 degrees per second to 30 degrees per second. The ability of the child to follow with an adequate optokinetic nystagmus is evaluated. In older children vertical lines moving at various speeds in the horizontal and vertical planes are presented. Electronystagmographic recording of visually controlled eye movements adds significant information regarding central controls or visual pathways and their possible influence on changing the vestibulo-ocular responses. Visual fields deficits are also well identified in this objective way.

## ACKNOWLEDGMENT

This work was supported in part by the Speech and Hearing Association of the Long Island Jewish–Hillside Medical Center.

## REFERENCES

1. Dekaban A: Neurology of Early Childhood. Williams & Wilkins, Baltimore, 1970
2. Holt K: Movement and child development. In Clinics in Developmental Medicine, no. 55. JB Lippincott, Philadelphia, 1975
3. Bergstrom L: Electrical parameters of the brain during ontogeny. p. 15. In Robinson (ed): Brain and Early Behavior Development in the Fetus and Infant: CASDS Study Group on Brain Mechanisms of Early Behavior Development. Academic Press, New York, 1969
4. Gesell A, Amatrude CS: The Embryology of Behavior: The Beginning of the Human Mind. Harper, New York, 1945
5. Gatz AJ: Manter's Essentials of Clinical Neuroanatomy and Neurophysiology, FA Davis, Philadelphia, 1974
6. Baloh RW, Hourubia V: Clinical Neurophysiology of the Vestibular System, C.N.S. FA Davis, Philadelphia, 1979
7. Eviatar L, Eviatar A, Naray I: Maturation of neurovestibular responses in infants. Dev Med Child Neurol 16:435, 1974
8. Eviatar L, Eviatar A: The normal nystagmus response of infants to caloric and perrotatory stimulation. Laryngoscope 89:1036, 1979
9. Eviatar L et al: The development of nystagmus in response to vestibular stimulation. Ann Neurol 5:6, 1979
10. Eviatar A, Wassertheil S: The clinical significance of directional preponderance concluded by electro nystagmography, J Laryngol 85:355, 1971

# Facial Nerve Function and Assessment

# 19

## Jean-Jacques Dufour

## EMBRYOLOGY

In the early embryologic stages, some groups of cells separate from the neural tube to form the neural crest. From this structure will emerge the neural ganglions. These neural cells will invade the branchial arches very early to constitute the neural elements.[1] In the second branchial arch, they will form the facial or seventh nerve. The motor fibers will be joined by the sympathetic, parasympathetic, and sensory elements, also coming from the neural crest.

In the temporal bone, the facial nerve course is in close relation to the otic capsule. The facial canal is formed from a differentiation of the capsule. The canal starts as a sulcus, but the margins grow to enclose the nerve completely at 6 months. In the area of the pyramidal eminence, the facial canal comes from the Reichert's cartilage, which constitutes its tympanic boundary.[2]

## CENTRAL PATHWAYS

The central pathways extend from the cerebral cortex to the nucleus. These motor fibers originate from the motor area 4 of Brodmann, which is located on the anterior wall of the central sulcus and the adjacent portions of the precentral gyrus. The face is represented in the inferior and lateral part of the precentral gyrus. There is also participation of the premotor area (area 6 of Brodmann), situated dorsoventrally along the whole lateral aspect of the frontal lobe and continuing on the medial surface to the sulcus seguli. These areas are referred to the sulcus seguli. These areas are referred to as agranular frontal cortex. In the dominant hemisphere, the facial motor neurons are closely related to the speech area.[3]

The efferent motor fibers constitute the corticobulbar fibers, which descend through the corona radiata and become localized near the genu of the internal capsule. They pass through the basal part of the pons along with the pyramidal tract. The greater portion crosses in the caudal pons and reaches the opposite facial nucleus. Some fibers diverge towards the homolateral facial nucleus, which therefore receives innervation from both sides of the cortex. Then the superior part of the nucleus receives fibers from both cortices and the inferior part is supplemented by fibers from the contralateral cortex only.

The neurons of the upper part of the facial nucleus give innervation to the occipitofrontal muscle, the upper part of the orbicularis oculi, and the corrugator supercilii. The fibers conducting emotional facial expressions probably arise in the thalamus.[4]

other methods, they will result in a better understanding of the complex behavior of facial nerve neurophysiology.

## CENTRAL CONNECTIONS

The neurophysiology of the facial nerve is now being investigated by many authors, whose works focus particularly on the connections between the facial nerve nucleus and other nuclei in the brain stem. Panneton and Martin[5] have demonstrated, using horseradish peroxidase and autoradiographic techniques, many of the connections of the facial nucleus with different parts and/or nuclei of the brain stem. Itoh et al.[6] pointed out that the pretectofacial fibers may cause protective lid closure with certain visual stimuli. Hinrichsen et al.,[7] following injections of horseradish peroxidase, demonstrated the connections of the facial nucleus with the trigeminal nucleus, both medial vestibular nuclei, the reticular formation, the nucleus of the lateral lemniscus, and others. Petrovicky[8] demonstrated the origin, course, and precise points of origin of the reticulorubro and spinonuclear connections in the facial and trigeminal nuclei. Dom et al.[9] studied the representation of the muscles in the nucleus and its connection with other nuclei in the brain stem. Henkel et al.[10] studied the role of the superior colliculus in the control of pinna movements in the cat. The afferents of the facial nucleus have been studied by Arends et al.[11] and Takeuchi et al.[12] Strominger et al.[13] demonstrated the motor neurons to the stapedius muscle in the monkey.

The connections between vestibular nuclei and facial nucleus have been studied by Shaw and Baker,[14] who assumed that their role is the coordination of facial movements with eye and head movements. The relations between the trigeminal, facial, and hypoglossus nuclei have been demonstrated by Thomander et al.[15] Stennert et al.[16] and Holstege et al.[17,18] Using horseradish peroxidase injected in the facial muscles of a cat, Radpour[19] did not find any labeled neurons in any brain stem nuclei other than the facial nerve nucleus.

The functional significance of these studies is not yet completely understood but, combined with

## NUCLEAR ORGANIZATION

The motor nucleus of the facial nerve forms a column of multipolar neurons in the ventrolateral tegmentum, dorsal to the superior olivary nucleus and ventromedial to the spinal trigeminal nucleus.[20] Many studies have been made of the subdivisions of the nucleus.[11,19–33]

From these studies, using different techniques and animals, it has been shown that the facial nucleus is subdivided in two main portions (lateral and medial), each one being subdivided into a rostral and a caudal part. There is also an intermediate subdivision and a dorsal accessory nucleus.

The topographic representation of the different branches of the facial nerve has been studied by the same authors. There are differences in their findings but, independent of the animals used, there is general agreement that the mimetic facial muscles (orbicularis oris and oculi) are represented in the lateral part and the auricular muscles in the medial subdivision. The motor neurons supplying the stapedius muscle are located in the dorsal accessory subnucleus.[30] Lyon[34] has demonstrated that this muscle is represented in an area between the facial nucleus and the lateral superior olivary complex. The platysma and posterior belly of the digastric are represented in the medial part. The motor neurons of the frontalis are located in both the medial and lateral divisions.

## PERIPHERAL PATHWAYS

### Course of the Facial Nerve

The peripheral pathways of the facial nerve are classically divided into three major segments (Fig. 19-1). Each segment features some particular ana-

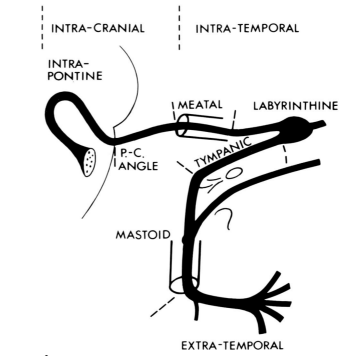

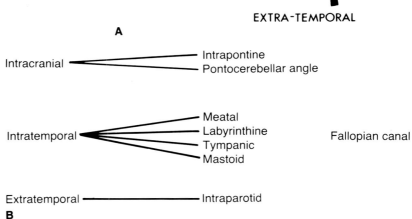

**Fig. 19-1.** Course of the facial nerve, from the pons to the face, and the nerve's different segments.

tomic landmarks, pathophysiological considerations, and surgical implications.

## Intracranial

This part of the nerve is subdivided into an intrapontine segment and the portion crossing the cerebellopontine angle.

**Intrapontine.** The nerve of the second branchial arch is a mixed nerve containing about 10,000 fibers. There are four different groups of fibers: motor, parasympathetic, taste, and sensory (Fig. 19-2).

*Motor Fibers.* From the dorsal surface of the nucleus, in the dorsolateral portion of the pons, the axons run dorsomedially toward the floor of the fourth ventricle. They pass medial to the abducens nucleus and dorsal to the medial longitudinal fasciculus, forming the internal genu of the facial nerve. Then the fibers run ventrolaterally to emerge from the lateral aspect of the brain stem in the cerebellopontine angle. There are about 6,000 motor fibers and 4,000 sensory and parasympathetic fibers.

*Parasympathetic Fibers.* The secretomotor efferent fibers originate from the superior salivatory

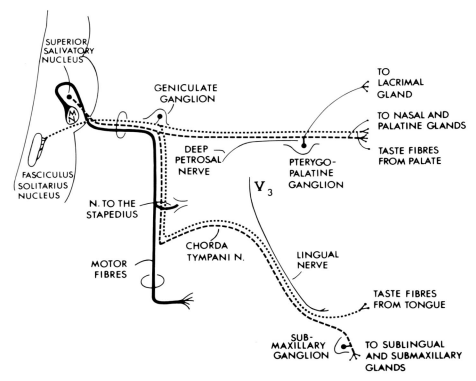

**Fig. 19-2.** Course of the facial nerve with its different components (parasympathetic and taste fibers). MN, motor nucleus.

nucleus, which is formed by a scattered group of cells in the lateral part of the reticular formation. These preganglionic fibers leave the pons ventrolaterally and constitute a part of the intermediate nerve of Wrisberg, which joins the facial nerve.

*Taste Fibers.* The afferent taste fibers carry the taste sensation from the anterior two-thirds of the tongue via the lingual nerve and chorda tympani. The axons synapse in the geniculate ganglion and the central axons pass through the intermediate nerve to the nucleus of the tractus solitarius. The facial nerve also carries taste fibers from the palate, which travel in the greater petrosal nerve to the geniculate ganglion.

*Sensory Fibers.* These afferent fibers carry the sensory innervation of the ear lobe, the concavity of the auricle, the posterior aspect of the external canal, and part of the ear drum.[35] Probably these somatosensory afferents join the facial nerve through the greater petrosal nerve and the geniculate ganglion. They travel via the intermediate

nerve to the brain stem. Their distribution is not clear. Many authors have studied these afferents: Contreras et al.,[36] Nomura et al.,[37] Hosoya et al.,[38] and Arvidsson et al.[39] According to these studies, these visceral and somatosensory afferents would terminate in different nuclei (trigeminal nucleus, nucleus of the tractus solitarius, cuneate nucleus). There are many interconnections with the sensory components of the vagus.

**Cerebellopontine Angle (about 15 mm).** From the pons, the facial nerve crosses the cerebellopontine cistern together with the vestibulocochlear nerve and the intermediate nerve of Wrisberg. It exits the brain stem 3 mm caudal and anterior to the cochlear nerve and travels anterior to the vestibulocochlear nerve.[40]

**Intratemporal**

These nerves enter the porus of the internal auditory canal. At this point starts the intratemporal course of the nerve, which is divided into four different segments[41]: meatal, labyrinthine, tympanic, and mastoid.

**Meatal Segment (about 8 mm).** In the internal auditory canal, the facial nerve travels in the anterior and superior portion (anterior to the superior vestibular nerve and over the cochlear nerve). The intermediate nerve is very close to the facial nerve, but separated from it, especially in its medial course. In the canal, the nerve is not enclosed by a sheath but surrounded by loose arachnoid tissue and bathed in cerebrospinal fluid. The dura adheres to the walls all around. The relation of the nerve to the anteroinferior cerebellar artery and the labyrinthine artery varies greatly. These variations have been studied by Boussens et al.[42] At the fundus, the facial nerve is separated from the superior vestibular nerve by the superior vestibular crest, the so-called "Bill's bar."

**Labyrinthine Segment (about 5.6 mm).** Here starts the fallopian canal which is about 30 mm long. The labyrinthine portion is formed by a short segment starting at the exit of the nerve from the internal auditory canal to the distal portion of the geniculate ganglion. Fisch[41] has demonstrated that the first segment is the narrowest portion of the facial canal (about 1.3 mm). The sheath is very thin and the nerve is in close contact with the bony wall. The labyrinthine portion curves slightly upward and anteriorly, passing in front of the superior semicircular canal. The cochlea is anterior and inferior to the nerve. The geniculate ganglion is covered by a very thin layer of bone, which is often absent. From the ganglion, the greater and lesser petrosal nerves run medially in the hiatus facialis toward the foramen lacerum.

**Tympanic Segment (about 10 mm).** From the geniculate ganglion, the nerve turns about 75 degrees backward.[43] According to Lang,[44] this angle varies from 45 to 97.5 degrees, the average being 69.1 degrees. In the first portion, anterior to the processus cochleariformis, the bony coverage is thick and perforated by cells that form the epitympanic sinus, described by Wigand et al.[45] The relations of this sinus with the facial nerve have been studied by Cheng and Wand.[46] The nerve runs over the canal of the tensor tympani muscle, the processus cochleariformis, and the oval window niche, medial to the long process of incus and under the

lateral semicircular canal up to the genu of the nerve, inferior to the lateral semicircular canal.

**Mastoid Segment (about 12 mm).** The nerve forms an angle of about 95 degrees downwards, called the genu. The mastoid or vertical segment goes down from the inferior aspect of the lateral semicircular canal to the stylomastoid foramen. Sometimes the nerve passes through the mastoid cells, where it can be injured during surgery. In this segment, the sheath gets thicker as the nerve descends.

The genu is closely related to the medial and inferior aspect of the fossa incudis. Anteriorly the nerve gives innervation to the stapes muscle in the pyramidal eminence, and lower down the chorda tympani nerve leaves the facial nerve going anteriorly through the posterior wall of the middle ear. The anterior aspect of this segment is related to the sinus tympani medially and to the facial recess laterally. The depth of the sinus and of the recess varies greatly. Inferiorly, the jugular bulb can be very close to the medial aspect of the nerve. At the stylomastoid foramen, the nerve passes anterior to the digastric ridge and goes forward out of the temporal bone. The sheath is very thick and mixed with the fibrous attachments of the digastric muscle.

### Extratemporal

Emerging from the stylomastoid foramen, the trunk runs anteriorly, lateral to the styloid process, and penetrates the parotid gland. The facial nerve does not enter the parotid substance, but passes between the two lobes of the gland, wrapped in loose connective tissue. Leaving the stylomastoid foramen, the nerve gives off two branches: a posterior auricular branch going to the muscles of the auricule and a second branch to the posterior belly of the digastric and stylohyoid muscles. There are two additional twigs, one connecting to the auricular branch of the vagus and a lingual branch.[2]

The first division usually occurs in the parotid gland. The numerous subdivisions of the nerve take on the aspect of a "goose foot" between the two lobes of the gland. There are many anastomoses between the different branches. The main subdivisions are temporal, zygomatic, buccal, mandibular, and cervical, but there is a great variation in the arrangement and anastomoses of these terminal motor branches in the face. Anson and Donaldson[2] published the six main types of subdivisions quoted from Davis et al.[47] Recently Bernstein[48] has studied precisely the anatomic landmarks of the different branches. At the extreme end, small branches cross the midline and innervate muscles of the opposite side. This contralateral innervation has been reported by Passerini[49] and Fisch[50] and has been studied by Nishimura et al.[51] Willer et al.[52] demonstrated electrophysiological evidence for crossed oligosynaptic trigeminofacial connections between branches in the face.

### Branches of the Facial Nerve

Along its course, the facial nerve separates into the following branches:

1. The greater superficial petrosal nerve
2. A twig to the tympanic plexus
3. The nerve to the stapedius muscle
4. The chorda tympani
5. Branches to the stylohyoid and posterior belly of digastric muscles
6. Finally, in the parotid gland, five main subdivisions to the muscles of the face

# ORGANIZATION OF FIBERS

The spatial orientation of fibers in the main trunk has not yet been clearly demonstrated.

The parasympathetic and sensory components of the facial nerve seem to be well localized in the trunk. The chorda tympani runs in the superolateral part of the nerve in the tympanic portion and in a posterior situation in the mastoid segment, but the organization of the motor fibers throughout the intratemporal facial nerve is not as clear.

Variation in techniques could explain the different results. Sunderland and Cossar,[53] Harris,[54] and White and Verma[55] did not find a precise spatial representation of the peripheral branches in the trunk. Thomander et al.[56] reported a diffuse distribution of horseradish peroxidase in the trunk after staining separately three different peripheral branches. Kempe[57] observed a definite and persist-

ent topical arrangement in three main fascicles. Podvinec and Pfaty[58] recognized a definite spatial orientation. May[59] demonstrated a very precise arrangement of the motor fibers and discussed the clinical applications of this organization.[60] Podvinec[61] emphasized this spatial orientation and its clinical application.

Radpour and Gacek[62] found a diffuse distribution of the peripheral motor fibers throughout the temporal course of the facial nerve. Therefore, because of this mixed arrangement, repair of the facial nerve by primary anastomosis cannot result in organized reinnervation of muscles, no matter how precisely the repair is carried out. The lateral location of the chorda tympani in a compact bundle inside the trunk is accepted by most authors. A sensory component making up 15 to 20 percent of the nerve, is scattered throughout the cross-section of the nerve trunk. According to Radpour and Gacek, each fiber contains contributions to all peripheral branches, even those in the internal auditory canal.

# PARSYMPATHETIC SECRETORY FIBERS

These secretomotor fibers originate in the superior salivatory nucleus. The preganglionic fibers leave the brain stem via the intermediate nerve of Wrisberg. These fibers are responsible for the secretion of lacrimal, nasal, sublingual and submandibular glands. They are distributed through the greater petrosal nerve and the chorda tympani.

### Greater Petrosal Nerve

The greater petrosal nerve leaves the facial nerve at the geniculate ganglion, running medially in the floor of the middle fossa in the hiatus of the facial canal. It passes through the foramen lacerum and is joined by the deep petrosal nerve, carrying sympathetic fibers from the internal carotid plexus. Then it is called the vidian nerve, which reaches the pterygopalatine ganglion via the pterygoid canal.

The postganglionic fibers join the maxillary nerve through the zygomatic branch, and then proceed to the lacrimal gland, and through the palatine branch, to the glands of the palate and nasal cavity.

## Chorda Tympani

Some parasympathetic fibers continue with the facial nerve, leaving the trunk in the mastoid segment as the chorda tympani. This nerve travels upward and anteriorly penetrating the middle ear cavity through its posterior wall, lateral to the pyramid. Running anteriorly, it passes lateral to the long process of the incus and medial to the handle of the malleus, inferior to the tendon of the tensor tympani muscle. It leaves the middle ear cavity through the canal of Hugier in the petrotympanic fissure.

The chorda tympani joins the lingual nerve. The preganglonic fibers relay in the submandibular ganglion. The very short postganglionic fibers are distributed in the submandibular and sublingual glands.

According to Chouard,[63] some fibers pass through the vestibulofacial anastomoses and are responsible for the parasympathetic innervation of the inner ear.

## TASTE FIBERS

The afferent taste fibers from the anterior two-thirds of the tongue run through the lingual nerve, the chorda tympani, and the facial nerve. The relay is in the geniculate ganglion. The central axons pass in the intermediate nerve of Wrisberg to the medulla oblongata and the nucleus of the tractus solitarius. Taste fibers from the palate travel via the greater petrosal nerve to the geniculate ganglion. Spassova[64] described two types of neurons in the geniculate ganglion: light and dark cells, but their functional meaning is not understood.

## VASCULAR SUPPLY

The intratemporal facial nerve derives its major blood supply from three sources. The portion proximal to the geniculate ganglion is supplied by branches coming from the anterior-inferior-cerebellar artery. The ganglion and the adjacent labyrinthine part receive their supply from branches of the superficial petrosal artery, which runs with the superficial petrosal nerve, emanating from the menigeal artery. These vessels form a vascular network in the horizontal segment of the fallopian canal. At the level of the oval window this network anastomoses with ramifications of the stylomastoid artery coming from the posterior auricular artery. This vessel enters the facial canal through the stylomastoid foramen and branches out extensively, forming the vascular network of the vertical portion.[65]

Apart from these major arterial supplies, many smaller vessels leave or enter the fallopian canal through the surrounding bone. All these vessels are situated in a loose connective tissue in the space between the periosteum and the epineurial sheath.

There is also an intrinsic vascular supply following the arrangement of the nerve fibers. From the larger vessels emanate some smaller arteries and capillaries penetrating between the nerve fascicles and also among the fibers. In the horizontal part, and even more in the vertical part, there are fibrous septa separating the fascicles. Larger vessels run in these septa. Between the fascicles and nerve fibers, most of the capillaries have a longitudinal course.

Veins are even more numerous and follow the same pattern. There are no lymph vessels within the neural compartment.

## STRUCTURE OF NERVE FIBER AND NERVE TRUNK

The axon is a long and slender process or prolongation of the nerve cell from which it originates Fig. 19-3[3]. It is composed of closely packed, paral-

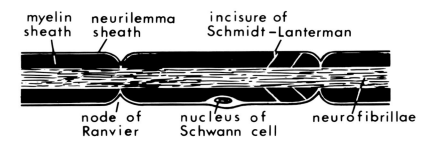

myelin sheath · neurilemma sheath · incisure of Schmidt–Lanterman · node of Ranvier · nucleus of Schwann cell · neurofibrillae

**Fig. 19-3.** Structure of a nerve fiber. (Modified from Truex RC, Carpenter MB: In Strong OS, Elwyn A (eds): Human Neuroanatomy., ©1964, The Williams & Wilkins Co., Baltimore.)

lel-running neurofibrils embedded in the axoplasm, without Nissl bodies. The axons of the facial nerve are covered by two sheaths: the myelin sheath and the neurilemma (sheath of Schwann). At regular intervals, the myelin sheath is interrupted by constrictions known as the nodes of Ranvier, where the axon is slightly constricted and traversed by a delicate membrane (quermembran), delimiting each internodal segment of the axon. Between the axon and the myelin sheath is a membrane known as the axolemma, which is part of the neuron plasma membrane. Myelin is formed by a double-layered infolding of the Schwann cell membrane, which wraps around the axon in concentric layers. The length of the internodal segments varies proportionally with the diameter of the fiber, the thicker fiber having the longer segment. The myelin sheath is perforated by clefts, called the incisures of Schmidt-Lantermann.

The Schwann cells are derived from the ectoderm of the neural crest and constitute the neurilemma. This forms a continous investment of all the fibers, known as the Schwann sheath.

The facial nerve trunk is formed by about 10,000 of these nerve fibers. The trunk itself is subdivided into funiculi and is protected by three envelopes: the endoneurium, the perineurium, and the epineurium.

The endoneurium is the framework of the interior of the funiculus.[66] It encircles each nerve fiber. The perineurium envelopes each funiculus and the epineurium enclopes the funiculi and constitutes the external sheath of the facial nerve trunk.

From the pons up to the fundus of the internal auditory canal the epineurium and the perineurium are absent. The motor fibers are arranged in parallel bundles protected only by the endoneurium. In the labyrinthine portion, the perineurium is very thin. Distally the nerve is still composed of a single bundle as far as the beginning of the mastoid segment, distal to the stapedius. The perineurium is well constituted, becoming thicker and thicker as it runs down distally, while the trunk separates into several bundles in the distal half of the mastoid segment.

## DEGENERATION AND REGENERATION

The interruption of a nerve fiber produces many changes in the axon itself and in its cell body. In the proximal segment of the axon, the retrograde degeneration extends only a short distance, depending on the nature and severity of the lesion. Usually only one or two internodes are involved. In the distal portion, the axon and its myelin sheath completely disintegrate throughout the whole length of the fiber. This is called the Wallerian degeneration. The myelin is removed by macrophages. The Schwann cells proliferate and then cytoplasm increases and later fills the entire tube.

The cell body undergoes degenerative changes. These are more severe if the lesion is closer to the cell body. Chromatolysis begins in the center of the cell, which becomes swollen, the nucleus is displaced at the periphery, and the Nissl bodies are dissolved.

Recovery of the cell is characterized by the return of the nucleus to its central position and reappearance of the Nissl bodies. The regeneration of the axon appears in the central segment and goes in a proximodistal direction. It crosses the scar tissue at the site of injury to reach the neurilemma tubes of the distal stump. The thin axon gradually enlarges and myelination occurs from the Schwann cells. The internodes are shorter and no longer proportional to the diameter of the fiber.

## Degrees of Damage

Following injury to the facial nerve, the involvement of the nerve may be classified in five degrees according to the severity of the damage.[66,67]

**First degree.** This corresponds to a physiological conduction block in which continuity of the axon is preserved. There is no Wallerian degeneration. There is some disturbance of the myelin sheath. This is the *neurapraxia.*
**Second degree.** The endoneurial sheath is kept intact but the nerve fiber undergoes Wallerian degeneration. This corresponds to the *axonotmesis.* The axon and myelin debris are removed by macrophages and the tubes are occupied by Schwann cells.
**Third degree.** The damage causes intrafunicular lesions, but the perineurium is preserved. Retrograde degeneration is more severe and there is loss of some neurons. Regeneration will result in misdirection of the axons and will produce abnormal associated movements in the face (synkinesia).
**Fourth degree.** The whole trunk is traumatized and continuity of the nerve is maintained only by the epineurium and damaged tissue.
**Fifth degree.** The nerve trunk continuity is lost with a gap between the two segments.

The fourth and fifth degrees correspond to *neurotmesis.*

## ASSESSMENT OF THE FACIAL NERVE

Evaluation of the facial nerve must be done based on an overview of the nerve itself, its connections, its adjacent structures, and the whole body function. This investigation must not be confined to the nerve itself.

This discussion of facial nerve assessment will be organized as follows:

Clinical (subjective assessment — grading)
Topographical diagnosis
    Lacrimation
    Stapedial reflex
    Salivation
    Taste
Electrophysiological testing
Radiology
Adjacent structures
    Auditory functions
    Vestibular functions
    Brain stem and other cranial nerves
Other — thermographic evaluation

## Clinical

A facial nerve problem must be first considered as any other disease. The evaluation begins with a careful history and physical examination. The clinician will assess more precisely the ear and adjacent structures and will pay more attention to the neurologic examination.

In order to make a precise diagnosis, the clinical examination must look for some important clinical signs. These will help to find the type and the site of the lesion. This subject has been discussed by Jepsen,[68] Gagnon,[69] May,[70] Alford,[71] and Miehlke.[72]. A supranuclear lesion spares the upper face, which is innervated by both cortices. In the brain stem, the lesion involving the facial nerve will cause some other neurologic impairment, pariticularly a 6th nerve palsy. In the cerebellopontine angle and in the internal auditory canal, the lesion is prone to disturb both hearing and balance. Hearing loss will be of the sensorineural type. Lacrimation, salivation, taste, and stapedial reflex may be also disturbed. At the geniculate ganglion, hearing and balance may be saved, but the parasympathetic and sensory fibers will be particularly disturbed. A lesion in the tympanic portion may be associated with conductive hearing loss. Lacrimation is normal, but salivation, taste, and stapedial reflex are still disturbed. In the mastoid segment, the manifestations depend on the site of the lesion, but they are similar to the tympanic lesion, except for hearing, which is normal. Most often extracranial lesions cause partial palsy.

During clinical testing, two other signs may be mentioned: sensory deficiency and hyperacusis. The sensory fibers of the 7th nerve can be tested by probing the posterior part of the external auditory canal and concha. Hitselberger and House[73] brought attention to this test as a reliable sign of acoustic neuroma. However, this deficiency is also found in other situations without any lesion in the internal auditory canal.

Hyperacusis is often reported by patients presenting with facial nerve palsy. This has been attributed to the impairment of the stapedial reflex, but it is probably caused by the involvement of the parasympathetic fibers crossing through the vestibulofacial anastomoses. Citron and Adour[74] have found a relation between dysacusis and multiple cranial nerve disorder, but no constant relation between acoustic reflex deficiency and the threshold of discomfort. Miehlke[72] reported that this is not hyperacusis but dysacusis, which is not a result of the impaired acoustic reflex but a recruitment phenomenon. According to May et al.,[74a] dysacusis reflects the involvement of the cochlea by the viral process and carries a poor prognosis.

At the end of the physical examination, it is necessary to assess the degree of the paralysis in order to follow its evolution. Many systems have been proposed. This subject has been a matter of discussion at the Third and Fifth International Congresses on the Facial Nerve in Zurich (1976) and Bordeaux (1985). In Bordeaux, two systems were proposed, one more clinical by J.W. House[75,76] and one more selective by N. Yanagihara.[77] The first one is gaining acceptance by many clinicians.

## Topographic

For consideration of the topographic diagnosis, the clinical evaluation must be supported by testing of the various functions of the facial nerve: lacrimation, stapedial reflex, salivation, and taste.

### Lacrimation

The Schirmer test[78] is performed using two strips of blotting paper placed in the lower conjunctival fornix. The amount of tearing is measured directly on the paper and the two sides are compared. In case of lesions of the geniculate ganglion or proximal to it, lacrimation can be diminished on the same side. Gontier[79] and Fisch[80] have presented a critical analysis of this test and demonstrated that the results are relative to the severity of the lesion.

Some variants have been described using anesthesia of the conjunctiva with cocaine[81] and stimulation of lacrimation with ammonia.[82]

### Stapedial Reflex

For reliable results, the inner and middle ears must be normal (no sensorineural or conductive hearing loss). This has been emphasized by Alford et al.[71] Most authors agree with the prognostic value of this test, if these conditions are respected. If the stapedial reflex is present in the first weeks, the prognosis is good and the recovery of the reflex indicates that the facial nerve motor function recovery will follow soon.[74,83–87] For many reasons, Hirsch[88] found a limited prognostic value and pointed out that the stapedial reflex measurements are of no value in nontraumatic cases of facial paralysis.

As a topographic indicator, the value of the stapedial reflex is recognized.[68,71,83] In any case, if the reflex is disturbed, it is reasonable to believe that the lesion is proximal to or at the exit of the nerve to the stapedius muscle, in the presence of normal hearing and normal tympanogram.

### Salivation

The parasympathetic component of the facial nerve can be assessed by measuring the salivary flow, or the pH of the saliva, and by functional scintigraphy of the salivary glands. The salivary flow measurement is the most popular method. A small tube is introduced in each Wharton's duct and, during stimulation with lemon, the number of drops are counted. The number of drops of the paralyzed side are expressed as a percentage of the normal side. Blatt[89,90] has described this method. In 1982,[91] he stated that this test appears to be 86 percent successful in accurately providing prognostic information 2 to 14 days earlier than the nerve excitability test and electrical tests in general. May[92] stated that salivary flow measurement is a more valuable guide to therapy and is a critical part of the topesthetic work-up. According to him, this test is able to predict accurately which cases will degenerate before any abnormality is detected by the nerve excitability test.

Salivary gland scanning with technetium 99m pertechnetate is a well known method of evaluating the salivary glands. So-called *sialoscintigraphy* has been used to assess the salivary function of the submaxillary glands during facial nerve paralysis. Marsan et al.[93] demonstrated the reliability of this method in relation to other tests regarding the prognosis of the paralysis in 10 cases. Thomas et al.[94] prefer this method to the standard salivation test despite a minimal exposure of the patient to radiation.

According to Saito,[95] the salivary pH reflects activity of the chorda tympani and salivary flow. The saliva is taken from Wharton's duct under stimulation with 3 percent citric acid and checked for pH and quantity. Normal values are between 6.2 and 7.6. Patients with a pH of 6.2 and lower were found to have a poor prognosis.

## Taste

The fibers of the chorda tympani and intermediate nerve can be assessed also by testing the taste. This can be done clinically with salt, sugar, and citric acid, but the results cannot give a quantitative measurement. Electrogustometry is the preferred method, as described by Krarup,[96] Harbert et al.,[97] and Peiris et al.[98] Jepsen[68] gave a good description of the technique and commented on its value as a good topographic indicator. A galvanic current producing a metallic taste is applied to the tongue. The threshold of the response is expressed in microamperes. Usually each side is stimulated several times and the results are calculated and averaged.

The results correspond to those of the salivary flow regarding prognosis. Tomita et al.[99] examined 95 cases with electrogustometry and found that this method helps to localize the lesion and to establish the prognosis of the paralysis. Diamant[100] stated that taste evaluation helps to complete the investigation and in some cases facilitates the decision regarding treatment. This technique has the disadvantage of being subjective, but it is quick and painless.

## Electrophysiological

Many techniques using electrical stimulation of the facial nerve have been described. Each one differs in its stimulus, type of response, parameters, and results. With time and experience, many refinements have been proposed. Here, we will present the following techniques: intensity-duration curve (rheobase and chronaxy), nerve excitability test, electromyography, electroneuronography, trigeminofacial reflexes and facial nerve reflex, and antidromically evoked potentials.

### Intensity-Duration Curve

To trace this curve, the examiner records the intensity necessary to evoke a just detectable contraction with an impulse of sufficient duration. This is the rheobase. The duration is varied from 0.1 to 100 msec. Duration of impulse is placed on the abscissa and intensity on the ordinate. The threshold is between 0.1 and 0.3 msec for the normal nerve. The active electrode is placed at the stylomastoid foramen and the ground electrode in the hand of the same side.

The intensity necessary to produce a contraction increases if the duration of impulse is diminished and the variations in the intensity are proportional to the severity of the nerve lesion. This test is long and time-consuming, and is now rarely used.

To make it simpler, Podvinec[61] determines two points on the curve: the rheobase and the chronaxy. This is the minimal impulse duration to elicit a contraction at double the rheobase. The normal value for rheobase at impulse duration of 1 second is 1.5 to 4 mA and the mean value for chronaxy is 2 msec. The difference between the two sides of the face should not exceed 25 percent for rheobase and 30 percent for chronaxy for a normal facial nerve.

### Nerve Excitability Test

This test is derived from the strength-duration curve. The stimulus is a square wave of 0.3 msec applied to the facial nerve at the stylomastoid foramen. The intensity is increased until a detectable contraction can be seen. This is the threshold for minimal contraction, expressed in mA. The palsied side is compared with the normal one. According to Jonkees,[101] the average difference between the two sides is 0.4 mA. In 1965, Laumans[102] postulated that a difference of 3.5 mA represented a critical value. This point has been considered as an indication for decompression surgery for many years.

### Electromyography

Electromyography is the recording of the electrical activity of the striated muscles. This is done without nerve stimulation. The recordings are monitored on an oscilloscope. According to Alford et al.,[72] the interpretation of results can be simplified as follows: if the nerve is normal, there is no activity at rest but a large number of voluntary motor units under voluntary contraction. Fibrillation potentials are seen at rest, if the nerve has undergone wallerian degeneration, after 14 to 21 days. These potentials come from spontaneous contraction of individual fibers. If the lesion is complete, no voluntary motor units will be seen. If the lesion is neurapraxic, however, no denervation potentials and no voluntary motor units will be observed.

### Electroneuronography

Electromyography can be complemented by electrical nerve stimulation with recording of the summation potentials. According to Esslen,[103] this is called electroneuronography (Fig. 19-4).

This method delivers three different sets of information: latency, speed of conduction, and quantitative determination of the proportion of blocked and degenerated nerve fibers. Stimulation is produced via bipolar surface electrodes at the stylomastoid foramen and recording is made with the same type of electrodes in the nasolabial fold. The stimulus is a rectangular impulse with an automatic frequency of 1 second. Duration of impulses is fixed at 0.2 msec. The voltage is increased until there is no further increase of amplitude of the summation potential seen on the screen (maximal stimulation). This corresponds to the maximal excitability test proposed by May.[92] To make sure that the sum of all motor units is stimulated, the maximal intensity is exceeded by 10 percent. This is a supramaximal stimulation. Of the three available parameters (latency, amplitude, and duration of potential), Esslen considers only the amplitude, which gives more concrete results. Normal amplitude lies between 4 and 5 mV. The summation potential of the palsied side is expressed in percentage of the normal side. This represents the proportion of degenerated and not degenerated fibers: a fall in amplitude of 50 percent indicates that 50 percent of the fibers are degenerated. From this statement, some criteria for management of facial nerve palsy have been established.

### Trigeminofacial Reflexes and Facial Reflex

The trigeminofacial reflexes or blink reflexes are currently used for clinical investigation of facial or trigeminal nerves lesions and of problems in the

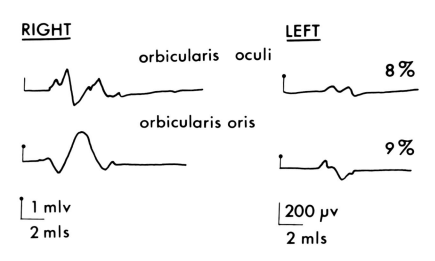

**RIGHT**          **LEFT**

orbicularis oculi          8%

orbicularis oris          9%

1 mlv
2 mls

200 μv
2 mls

**Fig. 19-4.** Electroneuronography recordings 1 week after a left Bell's palsy in a 21-year-old woman, who recovered spontaneously in 6 weeks. Note that the scale amplitude is not the same on both sides.

brain stem affecting these nerves and the reflex arc between them.

As described by Molina et al.,[104] the stimulus is a square wave of 100 to 200 msec duration at an intensity of 6 to 12 mA delivered by a bipolar electrode with the cathode close to a trigeminal branch. The response is captured by monopolar needles electrodes in the lateral part of the orbicularis oculi muscle on both sides. This response has 2 components: $R_1$ is ipsilateral with a latency of 7 to 12 msec, and $R_2$ is bilateral with a latency of 25 to 30 msec. This test allows one to investigate the afferent trigeminal pathway and the efferent facial pathway on both sides and also the reflex arc in the brain stem (Figs. 19-5, 19-6).

The facial reflex follows the same principle, but this time the facial nerve is also the afferent pathway. It is a matter of discussion whether the afferent impulses are carried out by the sensory fibers arising in the external auditory canal as a constituant of the intermediate nerve of Wrisberg. An alternative is that the impulses travel along with the muscle proprioceptive afferents accompanying the efferent motor fibers. The responses are similar to the trigeminofacial reflexes, but the latencies are shorter. This test assesses the afference as well as the efference of the facial nerve.

The results of 3,000 electrophysiological tests were presented in 1982 by Molina et al.,[105] Stennert et al.[106] discussed the conditions of the stimulation and recording, noting the importance of averaging the responses. Kimura[107] presented an excellent review of the blink reflexes in clinical testing.

### Antidromically Evoked Potentials

In the temporal bone, the testing principle of neurophysiological electrophysiology, namely

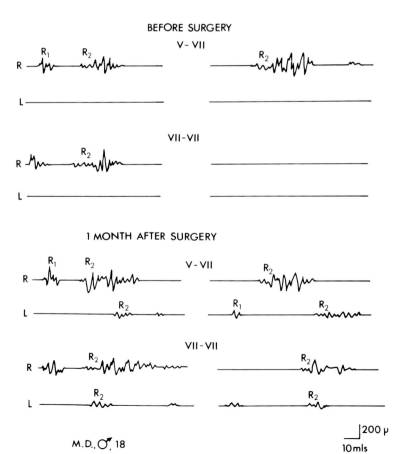

**Fig. 19-5.** Trigeminofacial (V to VII) and faciofacial (VII to VII) stimulations and recordings from a patient presenting with a left facial palsy, at the first examination and after recuperation from surgery. Left column represents the right stimulus, right column the left stimulus.

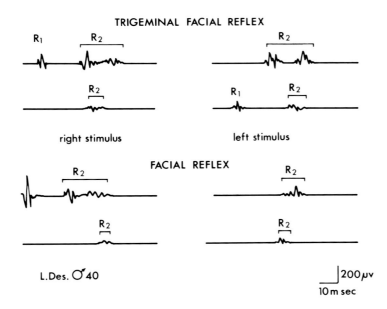

right stimulus          left stimulus

**Fig. 19-6.** Trigeminofacial reflex and faciofacial reflex from a patient presenting with a small (6 mm) left acoustic neuroma. This demonstrates the involvement of the facial nerve even with a very small lesion.

L.Des. ♂ 40

200 μv
10 m sec

stimulating the nerve proximal to the lesion and recording its activity distally, cannot be realized.[108] Therefore these authors studied the antidromic conduction of the facial nerve by distal stimulation with the recording electrode in the external auditory canal. In 1985, Zealear et al.[109] used this same principle with the recording electrode on the eardrum in animals and humans. This method has been reported also by Hanson et al.,[110] Niparko et al.,[111] and Muller-Deile et al.[112]

This method, using different sites for the recording electrodes, still leads to many difficulties in recording, but it seems mostly promising and is certainly more logical.

All these electrophysiological tests have their own merits, advantages, and limitations. The method of choice does not yet exist. Each test must be chosen for its particular merit and also according to the type or the site of the lesion to be investigated. Probably the best methods available today for complete investigation are electroneuronography and the trigeminofacial reflexes. Further developments in methods using the antidromic conduction with near-field and far-field recordings will probably give us some important answers to the major questions about the assessment of the paralyzed facial nerve. No test is yet able to give the exact prognosis of a facial nerve lesion.

## Radiologic Evaluation

Radiology is a necessary tool for assessing the facial nerve. Potter[113,114] gave a very complete overview of the radiologic evaluation of the facial nerve, but he did not discuss the use of high-resolution computed tomography or magnetic resonance imaging. There are now many radiologic techniques and each must be chosen for its particular benefits. Moreover, for any technique, the proper projection must be determined precisely to reveal what you are seeking.

Tomography, with hypocycloidal sweep, remains the basic radiologic method of investigation. Temporal bone fractures, longitudinal or transverse, can be demonstrated by tomograms in most cases. It is necessary to use anteroposterior, lateral, and skull base projections according to the type of fractures being investigated. Polytomography can demonstrate the enlargement of the internal auditory canal by an acoustic neuroma and the lateral projections reveal the mastoid segment. The publications of Valvassori[115] on this subject are very well known.

High-resolution computed tomography is the instrument of choice for assessment of the facial nerve. This is used with or without contrast medium. Valvanis et al.[116] studied the anatomy and pathology of the facial nerve using this method. They demonstrated each part of the facial nerve and related pathologic conditions. This work is the most complete and precise study of the facial nerve using this technique.

Magnetic resonance is not yet routinely used, but it is more effective for revealing neural elements and small tumors.[117]

## Adjacent Structures

The facial nerve is in close relationship with many other structures along its course. Among them are the auditory and vestibular systems. These functions are often impaired by lesions involving the facial nerve. The other cranial nerves, particularly the 5th and the 6th must be evaluated.

### Auditory Functions

Evaluation of auditory function can provide some important information about the extent, location and type of lesions involving the facial nerve. If there is hearing impairment of sensorineural type, the lesion is more likely situated before the cochlea, in the internal auditory canal or even more proximal. Auditory brain stem responses are most useful to determine the retrocochlear type of impairment, in cases of tumors, inflammatory processes such as Bell's palsy, and other types of lesions. Hendrix et al.[118] recently presented their results of hearing assessment in idiopathic facial nerve paralysis. If there is a conductive type of hearing loss, the lesion is more probably located in the middle ear cavity, causing disturbance of the tympano-ossicular system. Moreover, when surgical intervention on the facial nerve is planned, hearing assessment is necessary.

### Vestibular Function

Assessment of the vestibular function can reveal some important points in cases of facial nerve pathologic conditions. Vestibular disturbances have been demonstrated by Philipzoon,[119] Bouch et al.,[120] and Lämmli et al.[121] Mangabeira-Albernaz et al.[122] found that vestibular evaluation can provide valid information about the extent of the pathologic condition involving the facial nerve and also

its location. Brookler[123] stated that every candidate for surgical decompression should undergo vestibular evaluation and, if it reveals a reduced caloric response on the same side of the palsy, should undergo decompression proximal to the geniculate ganglion.

### Brainstem and Other Cranial Nerves

The proximity of the facial nerve nucleus to other nuclei in the brain stem emphasizes the importance of evaluating other cranial nerves. Any lesion in the brain stem can involve many nuclei or nerve pathways at the same time.

The facial nerve turns around the nucleus of the 6th nerve on the floor of the fourth ventricle. The lesions in the brain stem can cause disturbance in the abduction movement of the eye on the same side as the paralysis. The trigeminal nerve is also frequently impaired by a lesion of the facial nerve, and this can occur in the cerebellopontine angle. The trigeminal is assessed by testing the sensibility of the cornea and of the face and by the trigeminofacial reflexes. The glossopharyngeal, vagus, and hypoglossus are easily tested clinically during physical examination.

## Thermographic Evaluation

Okamura et al.[124] evaluated the thermal distributions of the face in case of facial palsy and concluded that this technique can provide no information for evaluation of the degree and prognosis of the palsy. This method can, however, demonstrate inflammatory process that could be responsible for facial nerve pathologic conditions.[125]

---

## REFERENCES

1. Giroud A, Lilièvre A: Eléments d'Embryologie. E Lefrancois, Paris, 1962
2. Anson BJ, Donaldson JA: Surgical Anatomy of the Temporal Bone and Ear. WB Saunders, Philadelphia, 1973

3. Truex RC, Carpenter MB: The internal structure of the pons, p. 283. In Strong OS, Elwyn A (eds): Human Neuroanatomy. Williams & Wilkins, Baltimore, 1964

4. Miehlke A: Anatomy of the facial nerve. p. 7. In Miehlke A (ed): Surgery of the Facial Nerve. WB Saunders, Philadelphia, 1973

5. Panneton WM, Martin GF: Brain stem projections to the facial nucleus of the opossum. A study using axonal transport techniques. Brain Res 267:19, 1983

6. Itoh K, Takada N, Yasui Y, Mizuno N: A pretectofacial projection in the cat: a possible link in the visually triggered blink reflex pathways. Brain Res 275:332, 1983

7. Hinrichsen CFL, Watson CD: Brain stem projections to the facial nucleus of the rat. Brain Behav Evol 22:153, 1983

8. Petrovicky P: Reticular, rubral and spinal afferents to the trigemino-facial motoneurons. Ata Univ Carol [Med] [Praha] 27:217, 1981

9. Dom RM, Falls W, Martin GF: The motor nucleus of the facial nerve in the opossum (*Didelphis marsupialis virginiana*). Its organization and connections. J Comp Neurol 152:373, 1973

10. Henkel CK, Edwards SB: The superior colliculus control of pinna movements in the cat: possible anatomical considerations. J Comp Neuro 182:763, 1978

11. Arends JJA, Dubbeldam JL: Exteroceptive and proprioceptive afferents of the trigeminal and facial motor nuclei in the mallard (*Anas platyrhynchos L.*). J Comp Neurol 209:313, 1982

12. Takeuchi Y, Nakano K, Uemura M, et al: Mesencephalic and pontine afferent fibre systems to the facial nucleus in the cat: a study using the horseradish peroxidase and silver impregnation techniques. Exp Neurol 66:330, 1979

13. Strominger NL, Silver SM, Truscott TC, Goldstein JC: Horseradish peroxidase demonstration of motoneurons to the stapedius muscle in the rhesus monkey. Soc Neurosci (abstr) 6:553, 1980

14. Shaw MD, Baker R: Direct projections from vestibular nuclei to facial nucleus in cats. J Neurophysiol 50:1265, 1983

15. Thomander L, Aldskogius H, Arvidsson J: Uptake and transport of exogenous macromolecules from the tongue to the facial nerve complex in the rat. Am J Otol 5:120, 1983

16. Stennert E, Limberg CH: Central connections between fifth, seventh and twelfth cranial nerves and their clinical significance. p. 57. In Graham MD, House WF (eds): Disorders of the Facial Nerve, Raven Press, New York, 1982

17. Holstege G, Kuypers HGJM, Dekker JJ: The organization of the bulbar fibre connections to the trigeminal, facial and hypoglossal motor nuclei. II. An autoradiographic tracing study in the cat. Brain 100:265, 1977

18. Holstege G, Huypers HGJM: Propriobulbar fibre connections to the trigeminal, facial and hypoglossal motor nuclei. I. An anterograde degeneration study in the cat. Brain 100:239, 1977

19. Radpour S: Facial nerve nucleus of the cat. p. 147. In Portmann M (ed): Facial Nerve. Masson, New York, 1985

20. Carpenter MB: Core Text of Neuroanatomy. Williams & Wilkins, Baltimore, 1974

21. Reighard J, Jenning HS: Anatomy of the Cat. Henry Holt, New York, 1935

22. Vraa-Jensen GF: The Motor Nucleus of the Facial Nerve with a Survey of the Efferent Innervation of the Facial Muscles. Munksgaard, Copenhagen, 1942

23. Szentagothai J: The representation of facial and scalp muscles in the facial nucleus. Comp Neuro 88:207, 1948

24. Courville J: The nucleus of the facial nerve; the relation between cellular groups and peripheral branches of the nerve. Brain I: 338, 1966

25. Berman AL: The Brain Stem of the Cat. A Cytoarchitectonic Atlas with Sterotaxic Coordinates. University of Wisconsin Press, Madison, WI, 1968

26. Chouard CH, et al: Anatomie, pathologie et Chirurgie du Nerf Facial. Masson, Paris, 1972

27. Provis J: The organization of the facial nucleus of the brush tailed possum (*Trichosurus vulpecula*). Comp Neruol 172:177, 1977

28. Watson CRR, Sakai ST: The topographic organization of the rat facial nucleus. Neurosc. Abstr 4:102, 1978

29. Radpour S, Gacek R: Facial nerve nucleus in the cat. Further study. Laryngoscope 90:685, 1980

30. Ashwell KN: The adult mouse facial nerve nucleus: morphology and musculotopic organization. J Anat 135:531, 1982

31. Szekely G, Mastesz C: The accessory motor nuclei of the trigeminal, facial, and abducens nerves in the rat. J Comp Neurol 210:258, 1982

32. Dom RM: Topographical respresentation of the peripheral nerve branches of the facial nucleus of the opossum: a study utilizing horseradish peroxidase. Brain Res 246:281, 1982

33. Radpour S: Organization of the facial nerve nucleus in the cat. Laryngoscope 87:557, 1977

34. Lyon MJ: The central location of the motor neurons to the stapedius muscle in the cat. Brain Res 143:437, 1978

35. Hollinshead WH: Anatomy for Surgeons, vol. I: The Head and Neck. Hoeber-Harper, New York, 1954

36. Contreras RJ, Beckstead RM, Norgren R: The central projections of the trigeminal, facial, glossopharyngeal and vagus nerves: an autoradiographic study in the rat. J Autonom Nerv Syst 6:303, 1982

37. Nomura S, Mizuno N: Central distribution of afferent fibres in the intermediate nerve: a transganglionic HRP study in the cat. Neurosc Letts 41:227, 1983

38. Hosoya Y, Sugiura Y: The primary afferent projection of the greater petrosal nerve to the solitary complex in the rat, revealed by transganglionic transport of HRP. Neurosci: Letts 44:13, 1984

39. Arvidsson J, Thomander L: An HRP study of the central course of sensory intermediate and vagal fibres in peripheral facial nerve branches in the cat. J comp Neurol 223:35, 1984

40. Silverstein H: Surgery for vertigo. J Otolaryngol 10:343, 1981

41. Fisch U: Surgery for Bell's Palsy. Arch Otolaryngol 107:1, 1981

42. Boussens J, Ducamin JP, Schloss MD, Midy D: Anatomical relationships between the antero-inferior auditory cerebellar artery and the stato-acoustico-facial bundle. p. 153. In Portmann M (ed): Facial Nerve. Masson, New York, 1985

43. Proctor B, Nager GT: The facial canal: normal anatomy, variations and anomalies. Ann Otol Rhinol Laryngol [Suppl.] 97:33, 1982

44. Lang J: N. facialis, preliminary remarks on anatomy. p. 3. In Portmann M (ed): Facial Nerve. Masson, New York, 1985

45. Wigand ME, Trillsch K: Surgical anatomy of the sinus epitympani. Ann Otol Rhinol Laryngol 82:378, 1973

46. Cheng HO, Wang AL: Landmark of the first elbow of the facial nerve: clinical and anatomical study of the "epitympanic sinus". p. 157. In Portmann M (ed): Facial Nerve. Masson, New York, 1985

47. Davis RA, Anson BJ, Budniger JM, Kurth LE: Surgical anatomy of the facial nerve and parotid gland based upon a study of 350 cervicofacial halves. Surg. Gynecol Obstet 102:384, 1956

48. Passerini D, Dala E, Valli G: Contralateral reinnervation in facial palsy. Electromyography 8:115, 1968

49. Bernstein L, Nelson RH: Surgical anatomy of the extraparotid distribution of the facial nerve. Arch Otolaryngol 110:177, 1984

50. Fisch U, Esslen E, Ulrich J: Zur Frage der Re-Innervation des Gesichtsmuskulatur nach Resektion des Zugehörigen Nervus Facialis. Pract Oto-Rhino-Laryngol 80:1, 1968

51. Nishimura H, Morimoto M, Yanagihara N: Contralateral innervation of the facial nerve. p. 227. In Fisch U (ed): Facial Nerve Study. Aesculapius, Birmingham, AL, 1977

52. Willer JC, Boulu P., Bratzlavsky M: Electrophysiological evidence for crossed oligosynaptic trigemino-facial connections in normal man. J Neurol Neurosurg Psychiatry 47:87, 1984

53. Sunderland S, Cossar F: The structure of the facial nerve. Anat Rec 116:147, 1953

54. Harris WD: Topography of the facial nerve. Arch Otolaryngol 88:264, 1968

55. White A, Verma PL: Spatial arrangement of facial nerve fibres, J Laryngol Otol 87:957, 1973

56. Thomander L, Aldskogius H, Grant G: Motor fibre organization in the intratemporal portion of the facial nerve in the rat. p. 75. In Graham MD, House WF (eds): Disorders of the Facial Nerve. Raven Press, New York, 1982

57. Kempe LG: Topical organization of the distal portion of the facial nerve. J Neurosurg 52:671, 1980

58. Podvinec M, Pfalty CR: Studies on the anatomy of the facial nerve. Acta Otolaryngol 81:173, 1976

59. May M: Anatomy of the facial nerve (spatial orientation of fibres in the temporal bone). Laryngoscope 83:1311, 1973

60. May M: Anatomy of cross-section of facial nerve in the temporal bone: clinical application. p. 40. In Fisch U (ed): Facial Nerve Surgery. Aesculapius, Birmingham, AL, 1977

61. Podvinec M: Facial nerve disorders: anatomical, histological and clinical aspects. Adv Otorhinolaryngol 32:124, 1984

62. Radpour S, Gacek R: Facial nerve fibre orientation. Experimental study. p. 171. In Portmann M (ed): Facial Nerve. Masson, New York, 1985

63. Chouard CH: Wrisberg intermediary nerve. p. 24. In Fisch U (ed): In Facial Nerve Surgery. Aesculapius, Birmingham, AL, 1977

64. Spassova I: Fine structure of the neurons of the geniculate ganglion of the cat. J Hirnforsch 24:123, 1983

65. Bagger-Sjöbäck D, Graham MD, Thomander L: The intratemporal vascular supply of the facial nerve: a light and electron microscopic study. p. 17. In Graham MD, House WF (eds): Disorders of the Facial Nerve. Raven Press, New York, 1982

66. Sunderland S: Some anatomical and pathophysiological data relevant to facial nerve injury and repair. p. 47. In Fisch U (ed): Facial Nerve Surgery. Aesculapius, Birmingham, AL, 1977

67. Sunderland S: Basic anatomical and pathophysio-

logical changes in facial nerve paralysis. p. 67. In Graham MD, House WF (eds): Disorders of the Facial Nerve. Raven Press, New York, 1982

68. Jepsen O: Topognosis of facial nerve lesions. Arch Otolaryngol 81:446, 1965

69. Gagnon NB: La paralysie de Bell et son traitement. Union Med Can 96:1, 1967

70. May M: Facial paralysis, peripheral type: a proposed method of reporting. Laryngoscope 80:331, 1970

71. Alford BR, Jerger JF, Coats AC, et al: Neurophysiology of facial nerve testing. Arch Otolaryngol 97:214, 1973

72. Miehlke A: Surgery of the Facial Nerve. WB Saunders, Philadelphia, 1973

73. Hitselberger WE, House WF: Acoustic neuroma diagnosis. Arch Otolaryngol 83:218, 1966

74. Citron D, Adour KK: Acoustic reflex and loudness discomfort in acute facial paralysis. Arch Otolaryngol 104:303, 1978

74A May M, Hardin WB, Jr: Facial palsy: interpretation of neurologic findings. ORL 84:710, 1977

75. House JW: Facial nerve grading systems. Laryngoscope 93:1056, 1983

76. House JW: Facial nerve grading systems. p.35. In Portmann M (ed): Facial Nerve. Masson, New York, 1985

77. Yanagihara N: Grading system for evaluation of facial palsy. p. 41. In Portmann M (ed): Facial Nerve. Masson, New York, 1985

78. Schirmer O: Studien zur Physiologie und Pathologie der Tränenabsonderung und Tränenabfuhr. Arch Ophthal (D) 56:197, 1903

79. Gontier J: Valeurs normales et signification clinique du test de Schirmer. Med Hyg 1120:1653, 1974

80. Fisch U: Lacrimation. p. 147. In Fisch U (ed): Facial Nerve Surgery. Aseculapius, Birmingham, AL, 1977

81. Gasteiger H: Ophthalmologische Operationslehre. Thieme, Leip, 1945

82. Cawthorne T: Peripheral facial paralysis, some aspects of its pathology. Laryngoscope 56:653, 1946

83. Koike Y, Hojo K, Iwasaki E: Prognosis of facial palsy based on the stapedial reflex - test. p. 159. In Fisch U (ed): Facial Nerve Surgery. Aesculapius, Birmingham, AL, 1977

84. Ralli G, Maglulo G: Study of stapedial reflex and its latency pattern in Bell's palsy, p. 384. In Portmann M (ed): Facial Nerve. Masson, New York, 1985

85. Dauman R, Negrevergne M, Cazenave M: Significance of stapedius reflex in peripheral facial palsy. p. 389. In Portmann M (ed): Facial Nerve. Masson, New York, 1985

86. Tato JM, Tato JM, Jr, Carri A, Ranieri C: Clinical value of the stapedial reflex in Bell's palsy. p. 133. In Graham MD, House WF (eds): Disorders of the facial nerve. Raven Press, New York, 1982

87. Koike Y, Ighige A: Changes in the parameters of stapedial reflex in Bell's palsy. p. 244. In Portmann M (ed): Facial Nerve. Masson, New York, 1985

88. Hirsch A: The stapedius reflex and its importance for diagnosis. p. 31. In Portmann M (ed): Facial Nerve. Masson, New York, 1985

89. Blatt IM: Submaxillary flow: a test of chorda tympani nerve function as a basis for surgical intervention in Bell's palsy: a study of 61 patients. Trans Am Acad Ophthalmol Otolaryngol 66:723, 1962

90. Blatt IM: Bell's palsy I: diagnosis and prognosis of idiopathic peripheral facial paralysis by submaxillary flow chorda tympani nerve testing: a study of 102 patients. Laryngoscope 75:1081, 1965

91. Blatt IM: The prognostic reliability of provocative sialometry in Bell's palsy: a 25 year study of 703 patients. p. 85. In Graham MD, House WF (eds): Disorders of the Facial Nerve. Raven Press, New York, 1982

92. May M, Harvey JE, Marovity WF: The prognostic accuracy of the maximal stimulation compared with that of the nerve excitability test in Bell's palsy. Laryngoscope 81:931, 1971

93. Marsan JG, Forget G, Levasseur A: La sialoscintimétrie dans les atteintes du nerf facial. J Otolaryngol 8:138, 1979

94. Thomas JP, Bertram G, Nödder G: Beurteilung des Nervus Intermedius-Funktion mit Hilfe der funktionellen Speicheldrüsenszintigraphie. HNO 30:269, 1982

95. Saito H, Higashitsuji Y, Hishimoto S, et al: Submandibular salivary pH as a diagnostic aid for prognosis of facial palsy. p. 143. In Fisch U (ed): Facial Nerve Surgery. Aesculapius, Birmingham, Alabama, 1977

96. Krarup B: Electrogustometry: a method for clinical taste examination. Acta Otolaryngol 49:294, 1958

97. Harbert F, Wagner S, Young IM: The quantitative measurement of taste function. Arch Otolaryngol 75:138, 1962

98. Peiris O, Miles DW: Galvanic stimulation of the tongue as a prognostic index in Bell's palsy. Br Med J 2:1162, 1965

99. Tomita H, Okuda Y, Tomiyama H, Hida A: Electrogustometry in facial palsy. Arch Otolaryngol 95:383, 1972

100. Diamant H: Taste examination. p. 154. In Fisch U

(ed): Facial Nerve Surgery. Aesculapius, Birmingham, AL, 1977

101. Jonkees LBW: Tests for facial nerve function. Arch. Otolaryngol 89:127, 1969

102. Laumans EPJ: Nerve excitability tests, in facial paralysis. Arch Otolaryngol 81:478, 1965

103. Esslen E: Electrodiagnosis of Facial Palsy. p. 45. In Miehlke A (ed): Surgery of the Facial Nerve. WB Saunders, Philadelphia, 1973

104. Molina-Negro P, Bertrand RA, Hardy J: The trigemino-facial reflexes. p. 107. In Fisch U (ed): Facial Nerve Surgery. Aesculapius, Birmingham, AL, 1977

105. Molina-Negro P, Bertrand RA, Dufour JJ: The trigeminal-facial reflexes. p. 105. In Graham MD, House WF (ed): Disorders of the Facial Nerve. Raven Press, New York, 1982

106. Stennert E, Frentup KP, Limberg CH: Modern recording technique of the trigemino-facial reflexes. p. 124. In Fisch U (ed): Facial Nerve Surgery. Aesculapius, Birmingham, AL, 1977

107. Kimura J: Clinical uses of the electrically elicited blink reflex. p. 773. In Desmedt JE (ed): Motor Control Mechanisms in Health and Disease. Raven Press, New York, 1983

108. Wigand ME, Bumm P, Berg M: Recording of antidromic nerve action potentials in the facial nerve. p. 101. In Fisch U (ed): Facial Nerve Surgery. Aesculapius, Birmingham, AL, 1977

109. Zealear DL, Kurago Z: Facial nerve recording from the eardrum: a possible method for evaluating idiopathic facial nerve paralysis. Otolaryngol Head Neck Surg. 93:474, 1985

110. Hanson DG, Honrubia V: Evoked responses from peripheral stimulation of the facial nerve. Am J Otolaryngol 6:98, 1985

111. Niparko JK, Kartush JM, Bledsoe SC, Graham MD: Antidromically evoked facial nerve response. Am J Otolaryngol 6:353, 1985

112. Muller-Deile J, Benz B, Bumm P: Experiences with the recording of antidromically conducted action potentials of the nervus facialis. p. 183. In Portmann M (ed): Facial Nerve. Masson, New York, 1985

113. Potter GD, Radiological assessment of the facial nerve. Otolaryngol Clin North Am 7:343, 1974

114. Potter GD: Radiological assessment of the facial nerve. p. 123. In Graham MD, House WF (eds): Disorders of the Facial Nerve. Raven Press, New York, 1982

115. Valvassori GE, Buckingham RA: Tomography and Cross Sections of the Ear. WB Saunders, Philadelphia, 1975

116. Valvanis A, Kubik S, Oguz M: Exploration of the facial nerve canal by high-resolution computed tomography: anatomy and pathology. Neuroradiology 24:139, 1983

117. Daniels DL, Herfkins R, Koehler PR, et al: Magnetic resonance imaging of the internal auditory canal. Radiology 151:105, 1984

118. Hendrix RA, Melnick W: Auditory brain stem response and audiologic tests in idiopathic facial nerve paralysis. Otolaryngol Head Neck Surg. 91:686, 1983

119. Philipszoon AJ: Nystagmus and Bell's palsy. Pract. Oto-rhino-laryngol 24:233, 1962

120. Bouche J, Frèche C, Tronche R, Ray J: L'intérêt de l'électronystagmographie dans les paralysies faciales spontanées. Ann Oto-Laryngol (Paris) 88:509, 1969

121. Lämmli K, Fisch U: Vestibular symptoms in idiopathic facial palsy. Acta Otolaryngol 78:15, 1975

122. Mangabeira-Albernaz PL, Gananca MM: Vestibular function and facial nerve paralysis. p. 400. In Portmann M (ed): Facial Nerve. Masson, New York, 1985

123. Brookler KH: Vestibular evaluation of the patient with Bell's palsy. p. 107. In Graham MD, House WF (eds): Disorders of the facial nerve. Raven Press, New York, 1982

124. Okamura H, Tamaki M: Thermodynamics in facial nerve palsy. In Graham MD, House WF (eds): Disorders of the Facial Nerve. Raven Press, New York, 1982

125. Ceresa F, Faredo C, Torossian F: Thermographic evaluation by conventional and numerised pictures of facial paralysis. p. 400. In Portmann M (ed): Facial Nerve. Masson, New York, 1985

# Physiology and Evaluation of the Eustachian Tube

# 20

Bengt Magnuson
Bernt Falk

Poor tubal function is a prominent pathogenetic factor in the development of middle ear diseases; this seems to be an obvious fact that is generally agreed upon. How to define or how to measure "good tubal function" is, however, far from evident. For many other physiological variables it is possible to carry out specific tests by which the variable can be classified as being within the normal range or to be pathologic, but not so with tubal function. There is a wide range for normal variation, and we have no good tests for discriminating between normal and abnormal function.

The widely entertained idea that tubal obstruction is the cause of negative middle ear pressure and development of middle ear disease relates back to the classic hydrops ex vacuo theory.[1-3] When the eustachian tube is obstructed, the gas trapped in the middle ear is absorbed. Negative pressure develops, which subsequently leads to effusion of fluid in the middle ear and retraction of the tympanic membrane. This concept has prevailed to our time as the principal pathophysiological theme in otology: When we think of "impaired tubal function" we usually mean that the tube is obstructed.

The eustachian tube is often described as being highly complex and difficult to understand. This probably owes to the fact that one has tried to draw conclusions regarding the physiologic function of the tube from results obtained in investigations where the tube has been studied under nonphysiologic conditions. The physiological disturbances associated with flight and diving focused attention on the function of the tube. Different tests of tubal function were designed; most were based on the application of artificial test pressures with a pump or a pressure chamber for studying the responses of the tube in simulated flight. Tubal function soon came to be defined operationally in terms of pressure equalization. When pressure was not transmitted, the tube was thought to be obstructed.

It is not difficult to understand the assumption that the tube is blocked since many diseased ears are so obviously underaerated. Perhaps one does not appreciate that the function of the tube in response to the relatively fast artificial pressure change brought about in a typical test situation constitutes a special case that does not apply for normal physiology. The two different situations were supposed to be equivalent because of the belief that the middle ear gas is constantly being absorbed, causing large spontaneous pressure changes. However, the existence of continous gas absorption is no more than a hypothetical assumption. It has not been demonstrated by experiments

543

that gas absorption does produce high negative pressure in the middle ear. The origin of negative pressure of the magnitude often found in tympanometric investigations must be explained in a different way.[4]

Thus, we have two different situations: the well studied nonphysiologic situation where artifical pressures are involved, and the physiologic situation about which fairly little is known. If these two different situations are not confused, tubal function may be easier to understand. Humans always were a land-living species, and in the physiologic environment there have been no obvious requirements for equalization of fast ambient pressure changes. Perhaps the eustachian tube evolved to deal only incidentally with those rare situations when we were exposed to fast changes of ambient pressure. The primary function of the tube may be not to equalize large fluctuations of the ambient pressure, but to make the middle ear independent of the physiologic pressure variations originating in the airways. If this is true, the physiological function of the eustachian tube can be described as being mainly protective: the normal tube should protect the middle ear from respiratory pressure variations, from the loud sounds of phonation, and from the potentially harmful bacterial flora existing in the nasopharynx. In the physiologic situation, reliable closure of the tube is of prime concern. This a priori statement was based on clinical observations in persons with healthy and diseased ears, and has later been corroborated in experimental studies.[5,6]

anism. The term "pressure regulation system" is adopted to denote a series of regulatory processes involved in the physiologic regulation of middle ear pressure. Tubal function is subordinated as an important component of this regulatory system.

There is also a difference of views with regard to malfunction of the eustachian tube. Here, the interest is focused mainly on "tubal closing failure." This term is used as a heading for different degrees of defective tubal closure. When the tube fails to close, negative middle ear pressure is often caused by direct evacuation of the ear during the act of sniffing (defined as forceful nasal inhalation). Failure of the tube to close seems to be crucial in tubal malfunction, and here the effects of two different modalities are combined in the induction of negative middle ear pressure: tubal mechanics and human behavior. Habitual sniffing behavior has long since been recognized in patients who have a patulous tube, but not until recently was a connection considered with the induction of negative intratympanic pressure, and with development of chronic ear disease.[5,7] Negative pressure is often induced in the middle ear on sniffing in subjects who do not have a patulous tube in the classic sense. In this chapter the term "patulous tube" is avoided since the meaning of the term is so deeply influenced by traditional views. In fact there is a spectrum of different manifestations of tubal closing failure; this is dealt with in Chapter 22.

## OUTLINE OF A NEW CONCEPT

Tubal opening is often though of as the single factor responsible for middle ear pressure regulation. In the following the term "tubal function" is used in a wider context than usual. First, the tubal closing and opening actions are both included as integral features of the eustachian tube function since both actions are essential for a proper regulation of the pressure in the middle ear. Second, the eustachian tube with its closing and opening actions is not treated as a detached and isolated mech-

## STRUCTURE AND MECHANICS

Comprehensive reviews of tubal anatomy have been published by Graves and Edwards and by Proctor.[8,9] Here we will give only a very brief description of the anatomy of the tube as applies to describe its function.

The eustachian tube and middle ear are formed by a dorsal slitlike extension from the pharynx: the first branchial pouch. The antomic location of the eustachian tube, connecting the middle ear with nasopharyngeal cavity, is the basis of a remarkable construction by which the ear is part of the respiratory system. The length of the cartilaginous tube is approximately 25 mm from the nasopharyngeal opening to the isthmus where the tube connects to the protympanum. Despite its name — "tuba eustachii" — the structure is very different from a simple tube. In its resting position the tube forms a closed slit. The medial wall of the slit is reinforced by the tubal cartilage and the lateral wall is constituted by a fibrous sheet. The walls are covered with a relatively thick mucosal membrane containing ciliated cells, goblet cells, and mucus glands.

## Closure

Closure of the tube is a passive process in which the force is supplied from three main sources: the spring effect of the tubal cartilage, the pressure of the surrounding tissues, and the adhesive force of the mucus blanket that covers the inner surfaces. The mucus secreted by the tubal glands is very sticky and normally keeps the medial and lateral surfaces closely approximated. Tubal closure is enforced by the venous pressure. This is seen most clearly in a case of a wide-open tube that usually closes in the recumbent body position.[10] Analogously, active muscular opening of the tube is more efficient when a person is standing or sitting than when recumbent owing to the difference in hydrostatic venous pressure.[11]

## Opening

Under physiologic conditions the tube opens during contraction of the dilator tubae muscle, which is the medial part of the tensor veli palatini muscle. This was shown clearly in 1920 by Rich, who made careful dissections in animal preparations and stimulated electrically the different muscles, isolated and in combination.[12] As the dilator tubae muscle pulled on the lateral wall of the tube, the lateral wall separated from the medial, and the tube opened. The role of the medial portion of the tensor veli palatini as the dilator tubae has later been confirmed by other investigators.[13,14] The levator veli palatini muscle elevates the palate on swallowing and is not primarily involved in tubal opening.[15] A schematic picture of the tubal muscles is seen in Figure 20-1.

The tensor tympani muscle can be seen as an extension of the tensor veli palatini muscle.[12] The three muscle portions — tensor veli palatini, dilator tubae, and tensor tympani — are all activated on swallowing, and all are probably involved in

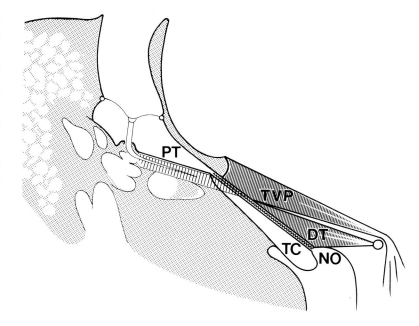

**Fig. 20-1.** Schematic picture of the tube and its muscles; left ear seen from above (oblique horizontal section). The tensor tympani tendon curves at right angles at the cochleariform process. The tensor tympani muscle (light hatching) connects anteriorly to the lateral portion of the tensor veli palatini muscle (dark hatching). The tendon of the tensor veli palatini curves round the pterygoid hamulus and inserts in the aponeurosis of the soft palate in a fan-shaped manner. The medial portion of the tensor veli palatini is attached to the hamulus and inserts along the fibrous lateral wall of the eustachian tube and the superior edge of the tubal cartilage. PT, protympanum with tubal isthmus; TC, tubal cartilage: NO, nasopharyngeal orifice of the tube; TVP, tensor veli palatini muscle, lateral portion; DT, dilator tubae muscle (medial portion of the tensor veli palatini muscle).

tubal opening. The tube may open during swallowing; the duration of the opening is only a fraction of a second (0.3 to 0.5 seconds).[16] It often opens during yawning, and some individuals can open the tube voluntarily.

## Synchronization of Tubal Opening with Swallowing

There is thus a close neuromuscular connection between the soft palate and the eustachian tube, providing for good synchronization between tubal opening and the act of swallowing. During respiratory activity the pressure in the nasopharynx varies within wide ranges and synchronization of tubal opening with the act of swallowing is essential for normal fucntion. On swallowing, as the palate elevates and closes off the nasopharyngeal cavity, there is a brief pause in respiration during which the pressure in the nasopharynx equals ambient pressure. It is essential that the tube remain closed, except during these brief intervals, in order to isolate the middle ear from the continuous pressure variations caused by normal breathing and the associated sound. Only with proper timing of the tubal opening action can the middle ear space equalize to ambient pressure.

---

# FUNCTION IN AUDITION

In order to hear air-conducted sounds we need a signal modifier. Sound is constituted by small pressure perturbations in the air that are transformed to vibratory movements. The tympanic membrane and the middle ear constitute a pressure-to-displacement transformer: The middle ear is a compressible gas pocket, and on exposure to sound the eardrum responds with pulsating movements. The vibrations of the tympanic membrane are conducted by the ossicular chain and focused at the oval window. The gas pocket enclosed by the middle ear cavity is thus an essential part of the human ear. In analogy, the hearing of water-conducted sounds is improved in certain fish species thanks to a gas-filled compressible swimbladder, which serves as a displacement amplifier.[17] The surface area of the human tympanic membrane is larger than that of the stapedial footplate, which gears down the vibration amplitude by a factor of about 20.[18] The resulting gain in force is essential for bridging the impedance gap between the environmental air and the inner ear fluid.

The eustachian tube serves the sense of hearing by maintaining stable physical (and acoustical) conditions in the gas-filled middle ear. This is accomplished by virtue of the dual mechanical action of the tube: The closed tube prevents vocalization sounds from reaching the middle ear directly through the tube. The attenuation of sound provided by the closed tube is essential for protecting the highly sensitive ear. The sound level in the nasopharynx during normal speech is over 100 dB, measured as 1 minute equivalent sound level, dBA (Magnuson B, unpublished data, 1984). For optimal hearing, the gas pressure in the middle ear should equal the atmospheric pressure. If not, the tympanic membrane will bulge outwards or inwards, and the membrane and the ossicles will be exposed to undue tension. The increased stiffness impedes low-frequency hearing by a maximum of 15 to 20 dB, depending on the actual pressure difference over the eardrum, while hearing at 2 kHz and above is changed very little.[18] Intermittent corrections of the middle ear pressure are accomplished by tubal opening. Maintenance of a correct pressure in the middle ear is also largely dependent on a reliable tubal closure that prevents respiratory pressure variations from being transmitted from the airway to the middle ear.

---

# PRESSURE-REGULATING SYSTEM

In addition to the mechanical opening and closing actions of the eustachian tube, the ear is equipped with a series of homeostatic control variables for maintaining the middle ear pressure close to the ambient pressure (see Fig. 20-2). The continual interplay between these variables constitutes a system for pressure regulation.

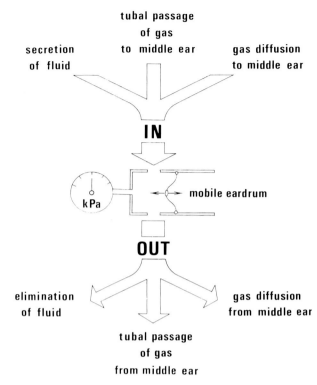

**Fig. 20-2.** Scheme to illustrate the pressure regulating system of the middle ear. The intratympanic pressure is a result of a dynamic balance between input and output of gas and fluid. The eustachian tube is an essential component in the pressure-regulating system, but not the only one.

## Eardum Mobility

A small environmental pressure change is immediately compensated in full or in part by a slight movement of the eardrum. For example, when the tympanic membrane is forced inwards by an increase of ambient pressure, the middle ear gas is compressed and the intratympanic pressure increases.

The tympanic membrane does not move like a piston, but the "mean deviation" of the eardrum needed to compensate fully a change of ambient pressure is $a = F(V/A)$; where $a$ is the mean deviation of the eardrum in mm, $F$ is the fractional pressure change, $V$ is the total volume of the middle ear and cell system in mm$^3$, and $A$ is the area of the eardrum that can be set approximately to 50 mm$^2$.

An ambient pressure change amounting to 1 kPa

(kilopascal) is equivalent to 1/100 of the atmospheric pressure, and in this case $F=0.01$. If the ambient pressure is changed by 1 kPa in an ear with a total volume of 6 ml (middle ear plus mastoid air cell system), the mean deviation of the eardrum from the neutral position needed to compensate fully for this pressure change is in the order of 1.2 mm.

There are a perplexing number of different pressure units. The SI unit kilopascal (kPa) is now recommended for general use. One pascal is defined as 1 N/m$^2$. A pressure expressed in other units given in Table 20-1 can be converted to kPa by multiplying by the conversion factor, and a pressure expressed in kPa is converted to another unit when divided by the appropriate conversion factor.

The large volume amplitude of a hypermobile, flaccid tympanic membrane, especially in combination with a small cell system, can eliminate fairly large changes of ambient pressure, meaning that no pressure difference builds up between the middle ear and the environment until the eardrum is stretched. This is of special interest in tympanometry and when studying tubal function in a pressure chamber. When the ear canal pressure or the chamber pressure is changed by a certain amount, the eardrum may not be exposed to the desired pressure differential. In Figure 20-3 this is illustrated in a model experiment.

## Tubal Mechanics

The two mechanical actions of the eustachian tube should not be seen as being opposed to each other. It is clear that a reliable closure of the eustachian tube is a most important point in the physiological pressure regulation in the middle ear, since

**Table 20-1.   Conversion Table for Pressure Units**

| Pressure Unit | Conversion Factor |
| --- | --- |
| Atmosphere | 101 |
| Bar | $10^2$ |
| mBar | $10^{-1}$ |
| Kilopound/cm$^2$ | 98.1 |
| Pounds/sq inch (psi) | 6.90 |
| Pounds/sq foot | $4.79 \times 10^{-2}$ |
| mmHg (Torr) | 0.133 |
| mmH$_2$O | $9.81 \times 10^{-3}$ |
| Dyne/cm$^2$ | $10^{-4}$ |

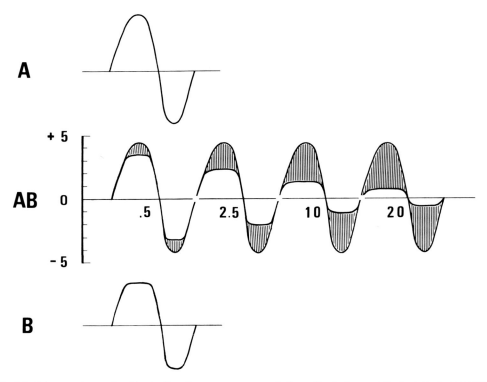

**Fig. 20-3.** Model experiment for illustrating the pressure regulating effect of a mobile tympanic membrane. The pressure differential over the eardrum caused by a change of ambient pressure is reduced by a mobile tympanic membrane. This reduction is most pronounced when the eardrum is flaccid and the gas volume enclosed in the middle ear and cell system is small. In this experiment an eardrum was simulated by a circular piece of wet temporalis fascia suspended as an airtight partition between two cavities. Such a membrane performs much like a flaccid eardrum. The diameter of the membrane was 8 mm. A sinusoid pressure sweep was applied to the "ear canal" side by a motorized pump; curve A shows one full period. The resulting pressure variation on the "middle ear" side of the model was measured (curve B). Curves A and B were superimposed (curve AB) to display the differential pressure (shaded areas). The volume of the "middle ear" cavity was changed from 0.5 ml in the first sweep to 2.5, 10 and 20 ml respectively in the following three sweeps. It is seen that the "middle ear" pressure follows the pressure applied in the ear canal until the membrane is fully stretched. The differential pressure over the membrane is a direct function of the "middle ear" volume: with a small volume the differential pressure is small, and with a large volume the differential pressure is large. It follows that the differential pressure may be very different from the pressure applied in the ear canal; this can explain irregular tympanometric curve forms often seen when the tympanic membrane is hypermobile.

it prevents unwanted respiratory pressure fluctuations in the ear. Tubal opening and closure are complementary actions and normally work together in maintaining a stable middle ear pressure. Poor closure can be compensated by good opening ability that eliminates any pressure changes in the middle ear caused, for example, by sniffing. Reduced ability to open the tube can be balanced by good closure that ensures that negative pressure is not induced.

If an ambient pressure change is greater than can be compensated for only by eardrum mobility, the eustachian tube can open and equalize the pressure difference. The ability to equalize pressue by tubal opening on swallowing differs from one individual to another and also shows variations from time to time in the same person.[19] Among factors influencing the muscular opening ability of the tube are the age of the individual, the body position, and the presence of upper respiratory infections. Adult subjects generally have better ability to equalize pressure than children.[20] Tubal opening and pressure equalization are more efficient when the subject is standing or sitting than in the recumbent position.[11] Pressure equalization ability is usually reduced in the presence of the common cold.[21]

The eustachian tube displays a certain one-way valve action in both normal and diseased ears. When the middle ear pressure is higher than the ambient pressure (positive middle ear pressure), equalization by tubal opening is usually very simple. When the middle ear pressure is lower than the ambient (negative middle ear pressure), equalization is often difficult.

## Turnover of Middle Ear Gas

The middle ear is said to contain air, or to be "aerated," but the gas composition in the middle ear is normally very different from that of air. The gas mixture is rich in carbon dioxide and fully saturated with water vapor, but the oxygen concentration is less than half that of the ambient air.[22–24]

A change of ambient pressure means that the partial pressures of oxygen and nitrogen are changed up or down. If the eustachian tube is not ready to open, the pressure difference will slowly

be reduced, and eventually eliminated, by diffusion over the middle ear mucosa. This follows from Henry's gas law, which states that the quantity of a gas physically dissolved in a liquid is directly proportional to the partial pressure of the gas in the gas phase.[25] In the present context we have different gas pressures in the middle ear and in the blood, enabling a two-way exchange of gas; the direction of gas transfer is determined by the diffusion gradient.

The effects of gas diffusion on the middle ear pressure are observed most easily with fast-diffusing gases, such as carbon dioxide and nitrous oxide. The concentration of $CO_2$ in the blood depends on the rate and depth of respiration. Hyperventilation leads to hypocapnia, and some $CO_2$ leaves the middle ear by diffusion, causing negative middle ear pressure. One example of this is seen in Figure 20-4. Relative hypoventilation, as in sleep, leads to a higher concentration of $CO_2$ and a subsequent increase of the middle ear pressure. Thus, after a night's sleep the middle ear pressure is often positive.[26–28] A spontaneous increase of the middle ear pressure during slow breathing is illustrated in Figure 20-5.

During general anesthesia when a patient is ventilated with a gas mixture containing a high propor-

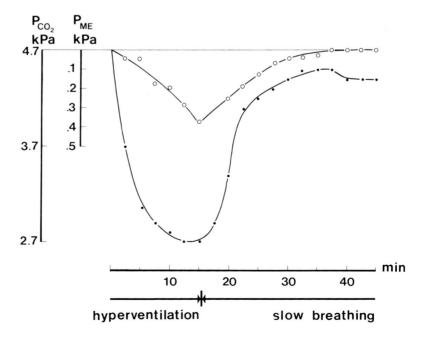

**Fig. 20-4.** The result of hyperventilation on middle ear pressure. During the first 15 minutes of this experiment the subject performed moderately forced hyperventilation, which reduced the end-expiratory $CO_2$ tension by 2 kPa (filled dots). The middle ear pressure was measured with serial tympanometry, using a slightly modified Madsen ZO 70 tympanometer equipped with more sensitive pressure meter than the original to resolve small pressure changes. The middle ear pressure decreased during hyperventilation and returned spontaneously to normal when normal breathing was resumed (open dots). Middle ear pressure ($P_{ME}$) and end-expiratory $CO_2$ pressure ($P_{CO_2}$) are given in kilopascals.

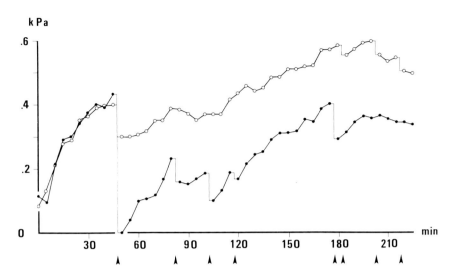

**Fig. 20-5.** Middle ear pressure recorded during slow breathing. Pressures in both of the ears were monitored by serial tympanometry (filled dots, right ear; open dots, left ear). The subject was recumbent and maintained a shallow sleep-like breathing with an end-expiratory pause. An initial rapid increase of both middle ear pressures was followed by equalization on swallowing. Total equalization occurred in the right ear, and partial equalization in the left. This was followed by a slower increase of the pressures, now and then interrupted by partial equalization in connection with swallowing (deglutitions indicated by arrowheads). The same tympanometer as in the experiment shown in Fig. 20-4 was used.

tion of nitrous oxide, the gas dissolves in the blood and diffuses to the middle ear, causing a fast increase of the intratympanic pressure.[29] At intervals the eustachian tube is forced open and some gas leaves the middle ear. When anesthesia is discontinued the $N_2O$ is rapidly ventilated out through the lungs. The partial pressure of $N_2O$ is still high in the middle ear, however, and the gas diffuses back to the blood, causing negative intratympanic pressure in the immediate postoperative period. These events take place only when there is some gas in the middle ear (a gas-to-liquid interphase must be present), and *not* when the middle ear, including the protympanum and the air cell system, is completely filled with effusion.

### Turnover of Fluid

The production of fluid by the middle ear mucosa, and the elimination of fluid through the eustachian tube by ciliary clearance, are also parts of the pressure-regulating system. A slight change of the balance between production and elimination of fluid can change the middle ear pressure and compensate for a pressure difference over the tym-

panic membrane. Small amounts of fluid are produced normally in the middle ear and the rate of secretion can increase drastically in inflammatory disorders. Fluid can also be produced by transudation when the middle ear pressure is negative; at the same time the ciliary transportation rate is supposedly impaired by negative intratympanic pressure. Increased production and reduced elimination lead to accumulation of fluid in the middle ear. The accumulated fluid occupies volume and can thus replace a volume of gas. It can be calculated that even a minute change of the thickness of the thin fluid film covering the mucosa can compensate for substantial pressure changes. For example, a change of ambient pressure of 1kPa (102 mmH$_2$O) can be compensated for by a change of the fluid film thickness in the order of 0.005 mm.

The ratio of volume to surface area is special in the ear where the volume is subdivided in small compartments in the mastoid air cell system. The change of fluid film thickness necessary to compensate fully a change of ambient pressure is: $b = F \times r/3$, where $b$ is the change of fluid film thickness in mm, $F$ is the fractional change of pressure ($F = 0.01$), and $r$ is the mean radius of an air cell in mm, the form of which is assumed to be spherical. In an ear with a total volume of 6 ml, the change of fluid film thickness necessary to compensate a pressure change of 1 kPa would be on the order of 0.04 mm if the volume were not subdivided in compartments. On the other hand, when the volume is subdivided in cells, the mean radius of which is arbitrarily assumed to be 1.5 mm in this example, the change of fluid film thickness would be in the order of 0.005 mm to compensate for the pressure change. The turnover of fluid, thus, is a most powerful regulator of middle ear pressure.

### The Mucosal Factor

A minute change of thickness of the fluid film covering the mucosa can compensate for a pressure change in the middle ear and, likewise, a slight change of the thickness of the mucosa itself can influence the middle ear pressure. "The mucosal factor" depends on the extent of vascular dilation and the amount of extracellular fluid and, in turn, these depend on the middle ear pressure. With a positive intratympanic pressure the volume of the mucosa decreases, and with a negative pressure the volume increases. Measurements in a pressure chamber have shown a linear change of mucosal volume by 1 mm$^3$/cmH$_2$O, or 10 mm$^3$/kPa within the range of ± 1.5 kPa middle ear pressure.[30]

### Summary

As emphasized above, the middle ear pressure is the result of a dynamic balance between the total input and output of gas and fluid (see Fig. 20-2). If one of the components is stretched beyond its physiologic range of variation, the other components conspire to restore the balance of the whole system. The pressure-regulating system is thus composed of several components that usually work in concert; by virtue of this process the middle ear pressure is normally very stable.

Large pressure changes are often provoked in nonphysiologic situations. A pressure change caused, for example, by flying or diving can be equalized by tubal opening. The eustachain tube can often equalize very large pressure differences but the function is not always reliable, especially when there is a fast increase of ambient pressure with resulting negative middle ear pressure. A change of ambient pressure that is not equalized by tubal opening is compensated for in part by a change of position of the eardrum. This is an immediate response, but the volume amplitude of the normal eardrum is limited, and so is the pressure range that can be compensated by eardrum mobility. The same applies for the mucosal factor; a pressure change induces a volume change of the middle ear mucosa that to some extent reduces the pressure change. Compensation of pressure differences by changes of gas diffusion rates is a time-consuming procedure that can take 1 or more hours. The turnover of fluid is a much faster process. When the pressure regulating system is severely challenged by nonphysiologic pressure strains, accumulation of fluid temporarily takes over and restores the balance. When normal conditions are re-established the fluid is eliminated spontaneously, and the system runs smoothly again.

Under physiologic conditions a reliable closure of the tube is essential for normal function. During a common cold the tube normally closes more firmly; this can be regarded as a physiologic adaptation that does not mean that the function is impaired. However, because of the enforced closure, the ability to equalize ambient pressure changes is commonly reduced during a common cold; this applies to the normal tube as well as to the malfunctioning tube.

---

## ONE-WAY CHARACTERISTICS OF TUBAL PASSAGE

The tube has limited ability to eliminate negative pressure; this valvular property of the eustachian tube makes the ear vulnerable. Flying and diving include nonphysiologic pressure strains that are potentially harmful. From sea level, the atmospheric pressure decreases exponentially with altitude. The following formula approximates the pressure as a function of altitude:

$$P = 101.3 \times 2^{-0.00018 \times c};$$

where $P$ = ambient pressure expressed in kPa, and $c$ = altitude in meters above sea level (See Table 20-1 for pressure units). At 5,500 m (18,000 feet) the pressure is half that at sea level, and at 10,300 m (34,000 feet) the ambient pressure is reduced to one quarter of the pressure at sea level.

Severe trouble with pressure equalization is unusual during ascent in an aircraft, but occurs frequently on descent. During ascent, as the ambient pressure decreases, the gas volume enclosed in the middle ear cavity and air cell system expands and the tympanic membrane bulges outwards. At intervals some of the gas passes out of the middle ear through the eustachian tube. This is facilitated by contraction of the dilator tubae and the tensor tympani muscles on swallowing. (One of the functions of the tensor tympani muscle may actually be to facilitate the elimination of positive middle ear pressure.) However, even without contraction of any of the muscles the expanding gas volume can force its way out through the tube.

Thus, when the middle ear pressure is higher than that of the environment (positive intratympanic pressure), the eustachian tube functions as a pressure valve to permit escape of gas when a certain pressure difference is reached. However, during descent, when the pressure differential is reversed (negative intratympanic pressure), no spontaneous elimination of the pressure difference occurs. When tubal opening by swallowing is not successful, active ventilation of the ears by inflation must be used to eliminate the pressure difference. In this respect the eustachian tube acts as a one-way passage permitting passage of gas out of the middle ear without much effort when the middle ear pressure is positive, while passage in the retrograde direction is more difficult.

The undersea pressure is the sum of the atmospheric pressure and the pressure of the water: $P = 101.3 \times 10d$, where $P$ = pressure expressed in kPa, and $d$ = depth in m. The water pressure thus increases linearly with depth by 10 kPa/per m, or 1 atmosphere for every 10 m water. The diver is exposed to very high rates of pressure change. This is illustrated by the following example. At 100 m above sea level the air pressure is reduced by 1% (1 kPa), but 100 m below the water surface there is a 10-fold increase of the pressure (1 MPa). A diver must have good ability to equalize pressure, and deep sea diving is reserved for those who can ventilate their ears actively by inflation. There is thus a natural selection of divers, since those who cannot ventilate their ears will experience pain in the ears and be frustrated from further diving.

## Aural Barotrauma

As a term, barotrauma is usually associated with damage to the ear by the pressure strains encountered in flying and diving. As already mentioned, the eustachian tube has limited ability to equalize negative intratympanic pressure caused by descent during flying and diving. If negative intratympanic pressure is not relieved and a large pressure difference is allowed to build up, the tube becomes locked and equalization is no longer possible.[31,32] The eardrum is progressively forced inwards, which causes pain and reduced hearing. Effusion of fluid in the middle ear and bleeding in the mucosa occur, and the eardrum may eventually rupture. However, barotrauma as a result of high differential pressure over the eardrum can also be caused, for example, by a slap on the ear. A violent pressure increase occurs in the auricular choncha and the external ear canal, which not seldom leads to rupture of the tympanic membrane. Barotrauma can also occur in connection with forced sniffing. This is a repetitive form of barotrauma that is of special interest in the development of chronic middle ear disease and will be discussed in Chapter 22.

## Delayed Barotrauma

To avoid hypoxia when flying at high altitude, military pilots and air crews breathe oxygen-enriched air through a tight-fitting orofacial mask. During flight at extremely high altitude pure oxygen is delivered by the breathing equipment at a pressure higher than that of the cabin (pressure breathing). On descent from altitude, as the cabin pressure increases, oxygen-enriched air or pure oxygen is forced up the eustachian tubes to the middle ears.

The rapid pressure change on descent may by itself lead to bartrauma, but oxygen-breathing adds the further penalty of a disturbed composition of the gas mixture contained in the middle ear and mastoid cell system. The partial pressure of oxygen is artificially increased and oxygen starts to diffuse through the middle ear mucosa to the blood. Since diffusion continues over several hours, negative pressure develops in the middle ear after the flight.[32] As mentioned, tubal opening is less efficient in the recumbent body position, and the symptoms and signs of delayed barotrauma may appear after a night's sleep: The hearing is impaired, the tympanic membrane retracted, and effusion of fluid fills the middle ear cavity.

### Prevention of Barotrauma

Barotrauma in connection with flying or diving occurs especially in subjects who are inexperienced in active ventilation of the ears. Many pilots and air crews have learnt to open the tube voluntarily by swallowings or jaw movements, but as many as 50 percent of trained air crews must inflate their ears at intervals during descent to ground level by Valsalva or Frenzel maneuvers.[33] The presence of a common cold makes the subject more prone to acute barotrauma.

The physiological disturbances induced by the low environmental pressures encountered during flight at high altitude are reduced by a pressure cabin. In military aircraft, where structural failure of the cabin is a risk due to war action, a low pressure differential is maintained. In civil aircraft, where the comfort of passengers is more important, a high pressure differential cabin is necessary. The plane may be cruising at an altitude of 12,000 m (40,000 feet), but the "cabin altitude" does not exceed 2,000 m (6,000 feet). Even though the rate of pressure change in the cabin is kept low (maximum of 1.5 kPa/min) some passengers experience ear discomfort during the descent (which is not to say that they have poor tubal function; this is a nonphysiologic situation).

Active ventilation of the ears can be learned by practice, and many cases of barotrauma could be avoided with the aid of simple instruction and some training in active ventilation. Inflation of the ears should be started at an early phase of the plane's descent and be repeated at intervals. If inflation is delayed until the person experiences severe pressure or pain in the ears, the eustachian tubes may already have become firmly locked by the pressure, and the person may no longer be able to inflate the ears. Active ventilation is described in more detail in connection with management of eustachian tube malfunction, in Chapter 22.

## TESTS OF FUNCTION

A number of different tests have been designed and modifications of test procedures abound. It is therefore difficult to compare results from different investigations. In the clinical evaluation of eustachian tube function, simple methods are preferred, while more elaborate methods requiring special equipment are reserved for research purposes. Otomicroscopic examination is now commonly used in daily office practice and the otologic microscope is an important tool in the clinical evaluation. A negative otologic history and the finding of a normal tympanic membrane provide the best evidence that the eustachian tube function is adequate.

The exactness of measurement one can obtain with modern sophisticated equipment used in some tests of eustachian tube function can give an illusory impression of the exactness and reliability of the results. In fact, measuring tubal function is much like measuring the length of an earthworm; by definition this is variable. Whatever tubal function variable we chose to study, we must keep in mind that there is a normal variation between ears, and an intraindividual variability over time is also present.[19] Tubal function is influenced by several factors, some of which have been commented upon previously. There is a considerable overlap between the results of tubal function tests in healthy and diseased ears.[34]

One important aspect of studies on tubal function is the composition of the normal reference group, because the selection of normal subjects can influence the result of comparison between healthy and diseased ears. Usually subjects with healthy ears, with no history of previous ear disease, and with no obvious difficulty in equalizing pressure, have served as a normal series. If this selection of normal subjects is carried too far it may be questioned whether the group will indeed represent a normal population. In some studies civil or military air pilots have served as a reference population. Rather than respresenting "normality," such a selected group may be an "ideal selection" from one of the tails of the normal distribution, and will always show "better" results than any other group of subjects. Thus, the result obtained in a group of subjects depends on the selection criteria and on the general design of the test, but the result in an individual ear depends on the time of the test; the response may differ qualitatively or quantitatively from one time to another.[19,34] The eustachian tube can be looked upon as having three independent physiological functions:

1. *Protection* of the middle ear from nasopharyngeal pressure variations and sounds (reliable closing action of the tube)
2. *Equalization* of middle ear pressure (adequate opening action of the tube)
3. *Drainage* of secretions from the middle ear (efficient mucociliary clearance)

The three functions are not strictly separate since points 2 and 3 both involve protection. An adequate opening action ensures that the ear is protected from pressure changes encountered in the physiologic environment, and an efficient mucociliary clearance protects the ear against ascending infection from the nasopharynx. Most tests of tubal function are designed to evaluate the ability to transmit pressure (according to point 2 above), and test pressures are applied to the ear in some way.

## Patency Tests

### Valsalva Inflation

This is a simple test of tubal patency. The subject pinches the nose and makes an effort to exhale, keeping the mouth and nose closed. If the inflation is successful the subject hears a popping sound and experiences a feeling of fullness in the ear. After instruction, about 80 percent of subjects with healthy ears can inflate their ears by the Valsalva maneuver.[35] The result can be checked by listening to the popping sound through a rubber tubing connecting the ear canal of the investigator with that of the subject. It is often more feasible to check the result of inflation with the aid of the otomicroscope; the eardrum is seen to bulge outwards as a positive result of the Valsalva inflation. However, in the presence of "tubal closing failure" the tube can often not hold any positive pressure within the middle ear. The closing force of the eustachian tube is then weak or absent, and in this case the tympanic membrane bulges outwards only *during* inflation. After inflation the eardrum may move back to its original position as the inflated air is ventilated out of the middle ear through the tube.[4,5]

### Politzer Inflation

In this test air is forced up the tube with the aid of a rubber bag equipped with a nasal tip. The tip is fitted in one nostril and the other nostril is pinched. The subject is then told to swallow, or to pronounce the letter "K" repeatedly (**KAKE**). When the soft palate elevates and closes off the nasopharynx, the Politzer bag is compressed and air is forced up the tube. At the moment of a successful inflation the subject hears a popping sound and experiences a feeling of pressure in the ear. The result can be checked with the otomicroscope but, as in the Valsalva inflation, when tubal closure is weak, the positive middle ear pressure and the bulging of the eardrum caused by the inflation are very soon released. Politzer inflation should be used with care in children because the sudden pressure change in the ear is uncomfortable; it is often frightening or even painful.

### Toynbee Test

In this test passage through the tube is provoked by swallowing while pinching the nose. As a result of the movement of the soft palate and the contraction of the superior constrictor muscle, the nasopharyngeal pressure changes during swallowing with a closed nose. An initial positive pressure caused by palatinal elevation is followed by negative pressure as the palate moves down again. This biphasic pressure change is often transmitted through the eustachian tube to the middle ear; in other cases only the positive or the negative pressure peak is transmitted.[36] To record these pressure changes accurately a perforation or a myringotomy opening must be present and a manometer must be fitted to the external ear canal. During otomicroscopy the tympanic membrane is often seen to make an in-out movement on swallowing with an *open* nose. This movement is probably caused by contraction of the tensor tympani muscle.

## Tubal Catheterization

Catheterization of the tube is performed with a curved metal cannula that is introduced through the nose and rotated so that the tip enters the pharyngeal ostium of the eustachian tube. Air can then be inflated through the cannula. Catheterization of the eustachian tube is no longer used often in clinical practice because it is difficult to perform, causes pain, and is potentially harmful.

## Sonotubometry

In this test a constant sound is presented by a loudspeaker connected to the nose by a piece of tubing. The sound intensity in the external ear canal is recorded with a microphone. When the eustachian tube opens on swallowing, sound is conducted through the tube, increasing the sound intensity in the ear canal. This method was first developed by Gyergyay.[37] Over the years many investigators have tried different frequencies of the test tone.[38] Sonotubometry appears to be an ideal method since no test pressure is applied in the ear, and the function of the tube is thus not disturbed by the measurement. However, the method is hampered to a high degree by technical difficulty in isolating the test tone from noise.

A low-frequency tone is masked by the physiologic sounds evoked by the swallowing act, and a high-frequency tone tends to radiate to the microphone by other routes than through the eustachian tube. It is also difficult to keep the intensity of the test tone constant because the airspaces in the naso- and oropharynx are altered in their form and volume during swallowing. It is therefore not possible to know with certainty that a small change of sound intensity as measured in the external ear canal during the swallowing act depends on tubal opening.[39,40]

## Estimation of Middle Ear Pressure

Just as a normal tympanic membrane indicates that the tubal function is adequate, normal middle ear pressure is also a good indicator of normal tubal function. A simple otomicroscopic examination aided by the pneumatic ear speculum can thus show evidence of normal or abnormal conditions. The otomicroscope can be used to judge whether positive, normal, or negative pressure is present in the middle ear, and the pressure can be quantified with tympanometry or manometry.

## Otomicroscopic Evaluation

During the otomicroscopic examination the position and mobility of the eardrum are checked, with special attention paid to the posterosuperior part of the drumhead. If the normal convex curvature of the membrane is flattened, or if there is frank retraction, this indicates the possiblity of negative pressure. A retracted tympanic membrane that is not adhesive can be repositioned by aspirating slightly with the pneumatic otoscope; this confirms the presence of negative pressure. (The lens of the pneumatic otoscope must be exchanged for a flat glass plate when used with the microscope.) In the presence of normal middle ear pressure, the tympanic membrane moves freely at the slightest touch on the rubber bag. The skill of judging otomicroscopically the presence of normal, negative or positive middle ear pressure can be significantly improved if a tympanometer is available in the same room for reference.

## Tympanometry

The acoustic method for estimating middle ear pressure was first developed by van Dishoeck.[41] The principle is based on the fact that sound transmission is optimal when there is no pressure differential over the tympanic membrane; hearing is thus most acute when the middle ear pressure equals that of the ambient air. Van Dishoeck's "pneumophone" included a sound source presenting a constant sound and a pressure pump connected to the external ear canal. When the pressure was changed up and down the subject reported the moment when the sound was heard most loudly; this corresponded to the moment when the pressure applied in the ear canal equaled the middle ear pressure.

The same principle was used by Metz and by Thomsen when developing the electroacoustic technique for estimating the middle ear pressure.[42,43] In tympanometry the subjective hearing of the test sound is exchanged for an objective recording of the sound intensity in the ear canal with the aid of a microphone and a chart recorder. A probe is fitted airtightly in the external ear canal. The probe is connected to a small loudspeaker that presents a test tone of constant frequency and intensity. The probe is also connected to a microphone, a pressure transducer, and a pump. The microphone signal is amplified, filtered, rectified, and fed to an indicator instrument and a chart recorder. In the "impedance bridge" the variable microphone voltage is balanced against a reference voltage. The output of the amplifier is not a function of the small absolute change of input voltage from the microphone, but is a function of the *difference* between the microphone and reference voltages. By this network the device can be made more sensitive. The tympanometer provides an indirect measure of impedance, admittance, and middle ear pressure. The sound intensity as a function of ear canal pressure is measured. Impedance is a direct function of the sound intensity; admittance is simply the inverse of impedance.

The procedure is started by applying positive pressure in the ear canal, forcing the tympanic membrane inwards. The bridge is balanced by aligning the reference voltage until the microphone signal is cancelled. The reference voltage then remains fixed during the measurement. The recorder and the pump are activated and the sound level is recorded as the pump starts to reduce the pressure in the ear canal (the pressure sweep). As the ear canal pressure approaches the actual middle ear pressure, the sound level decreases; it comes to a minimum when there is no pressure differential over the eardrum. (The tympanic membrane is more "transparent" to sound when relaxed.) The sound level increases again when the pressure in the ear canal becomes lower than that of the middle ear and the tympanic membrane is forced to bulge outwards. The recorded curve thus describes peak, and the position of the peak on the pressure scale indicates the actual middle ear pressure.

A normal tympanogram is a good indicator that the ear is healthy, but pathologic tympanograms must be interpreted with caution. It should be kept in mind that the tympanometer gives a reliable estimate of the middle ear pressure only in normal ears, and that a single tympanogram estimates the middle ear pressure only at one moment in time. Serial tympanometry is necessary to record changes of middle ear pressure. The single-peaked type of tympanogram is seen when the tympanic membrane is normal and when no major ossicular changes are present. In the presence of a highly mobile tympanic membrane (a flaccid eardrum or a mobile retraction pocket), or when the ossicular chain is broken, a broad complex curve with more than one peak is often produced. W-shaped curve forms are seen especially when the test tone is close to the resonant frequency of the middle ear (i.e., 800 Hz). A "flat curve" is seen when the middle ear is filled with effusion. In this case the tympanometer cannot be used for estimating middle ear pressure. In the presence of very high negative middle ear pressure, which exceeds the range of the pressure sweep, the tympanogram shows no peak but a "flat curve." If the tympanometer is modified so the pressure sweep is extended to higher negative pressure, the peak appears.[44]

**Measurement Errors**

The tympanometric technique is now used widely for estimation of middle ear pressure and several automatic tympanometers are available for office use. Tympanometry has the undisputable advantage that measurements are carried out in the presence of an intact tympanic membrane. However, one error is inherent in the tympanometric method. The position of the tympanic membrane is changed by the pressure sweep; this causes a change of the pressure being measured. Several factors are of importance, such as the original pressure level in the middle ear and the initial position of the tympanic membrane, the volume of the middle ear and the mobility of the eardrum, and the rate and direction of the pressure sweep. The result of measurement depends on the type of equipment used because different tympanometers have different rates of pressure change during the sweep.[45]

Thus, the tympanometric method illustrates the fact that the procedure of measurement can influence the measured variable. This is explained by the following example.

Assume that we will measure the pressure in an ear with a flaccid eardrum. The typanometric procedure starts with application of positive pressure in the ear canal. This is the first point where the measurement can go wrong. The mobile eardrum is pushed in by the positive ear canal pressure. The middle ear gas is compressed and the intratympanic pressure increases. If the closing force of the tube is weak some gas can be pressed out of the middle ear through the tube, thus reducing the amount of gas. This can happen especially when a slow pressure sweep is used. Then, as the pump of the tympanometer starts to reduce the ear canal pressure, the eardrum is moved in the outward direction. As a result, the volume of the middle ear is expanded, and the intratympanic pressure decreases. This is the second point where the accurateness of the measurement is endangered. The peak of the tympanogram is displayed when the eardrum approaches its most relaxed, intermediate positon. By that time the pressure is lower than was the original intratympanic pressure. In the worst possible case a negative intratympanic pressure that did not exist prior to the measurement is caused by the tympanometric procedure. The magnitude of this negative pressure is overestimated in numerical terms; this is especially true when a fast pressure sweep is used. The error of measurement is greatest in measuring small pressures in the presence of a flaccid eardrum and a small cell system. (The volume amplitude of the eardrum is then significant relative to the total volume of gas enclosed within the middle ear and mastoid air cell system; see also Fig. 20-3.)

## Manometry

Direct recording of the middle ear pressure can be performed when the tympanic membrane is perforated or when a ventilating tube is present. The method can be used in connection with patency tests, tests of tubal closure, and for tests of the pressure equalization ability. A pressure trans-ducer is connected to the external ear canal by a catheter and a tight-fitting earprobe, and the middle ear pressure is recorded continuously during the test. Direct measurement of the pressure is superior to conventional tympanometry because the method allows a continuous recording of pressure changes.

## Measurement Errors

Since the ear canal, the connecting catheter, and the transducer housing each add some volume of gas, a small pressure change in the middle ear "dilutes" in the total volume. The measured pressure value therefore is a numerical underestimation of the real pressure. The error depends on the ratio between middle ear volume and total volume:

$$P = P_o(Vm/Vtot)$$

where $P$ is the measured pressure, $P_o$ is the "real" pressure, $Vm$ is the volume of the middle ear, and $Vtot$ is the total volume of the ear and the measuring system. It is essential that the volume of the measuring system be minimized so that the volume is only a fraction of the volume of the ear. For example, if the volume enclosed in the measuring system is equal to the volume of the ear, the meter will show only 50 percent of the real pressure change that results after a small amount of gas has passed the tube.

The magnitude of the measurement error as indicated by the formula above is correct only when the pressure transducer is provided with a stiff membrane. The error will be greater if the membrane is highly mobile. This can be exemplified by the common U-tube often used as a simple manometer. In addition to the error introduced by the compliant volume of gas contained in the connecting tubing, the mobile column of fluid in the U-tube causes a change of volume whenever a pressure change occurs. When the pressure in a very small cavity such as the middle ear is measured, this can cause a considerable error. To measure the pressure in a fluid-filled middle ear is still more critical; here a fluid-filled measuring system is necessary for obtaining a good result, and even a small bubble of air trapped in the system can result in a considerable measurement error.

## Tests of Tubal Closure

Three different tests have been designed for evaluation of tubal closure in qualitative or quantitative terms. In these tests a flow of gas from the middle ear through the eustachian tube to the nasopharynx is provoked. The closing ability of the tube is defined as the resistance to such a flow.

### Sniff Test

In this test a physiologic pressure difference over the tube is provoked by the act of sniffing or by a reverse Valsalva maneuver. In its simplest form the test is carried out with the aid of the otomicroscope.[5] Starting with the tympanic membrane in the "out position," as confirmed with the otomicroscope after a Valsalva or Politzer inflation, the subject is told to sniff forcibly while occluding one nostril with the finger. The position of the eardrum is again checked with the microscope; if the membrane is found to be retracted, the test indicates tubal closing failure. The test is best performed in the sitting position since the tube closes more firmly when the person is lying down on an examination table. Serial tympanograms taken before and after sniffing can provide a qualitative determination of whether evacuation of the middle ear takes place.[46] Evidence for tubal closing failure is present when the first tympanogram shows positive and the second tympanogram shows negative pressure. However, a wide-open tube is not revealed in this test unless a tympanogram is taken while the subject performs a reverse Valsalva maneuver.[44]

The sniff test, using otomicroscopic judgment of the change of eardrum position or serial tympanometry, can be used only in ears with an intact tympanic membrane. In the presence of a perforation or a ventilating tube, a direct manometric measurement of middle ear pressure changes is possible. We have used three separate transducers, one connected to each ear and one connected to the nose or to the nasopharyngeal cavity (see Fig. 20-6). The pressure changes evoked by sniffing were recorded simultaneously on three channels, and the negative nasopharyngeal pressure needed to evacuate the ears could thus be determined as well as the positive pressure needed to inflate the ears

during a Valsalva maneuver.[47] Induction of negative middle ear pressure by sniffing is found in 15 to 30 percent of healthy ears, and thus is not confined to diseased ears.[4,46,48] In many diseased ears it was found that evacuation of the ears on sniffing occurred more easily than inflation during a Valsalva maneuver, which displays an exaggerated one-way valve action.[4] Evacuation of the ears was found also in cases that, according to firm tradition, were believed to have obstructed tubes, for example, cases of persistent middle ear effusion, and patients with a cleft palate.[49,50] Repeated sniffing often caused progressive evacuation of the ear with stepwise increase of the negative intratympanic pressure (see Fig. 20-7). In some cases there was positive evidence that the subject opened the tube actively by muscular contraction at the moment of sniffing, thus facilitating the evacuation of the middle ear.[4,51,52]

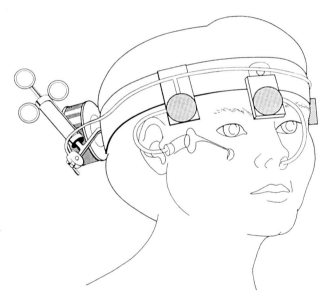

**Fig. 20-6.** Equipment for three-channel manometry. Three pressure transducers are mounted on a headpiece and connected to the ears and the nose by short catheters with rubber probes. The equipment enables simultaneous recording of pressures in the ears in response to nasopharyngeal pressure variations. (The tympanic membranes are perforated or supplied with ventilating tubes.) A glass syringe and a mechanical manometer, also shown, are used when performing forced opening tests and pressure equalization tests.

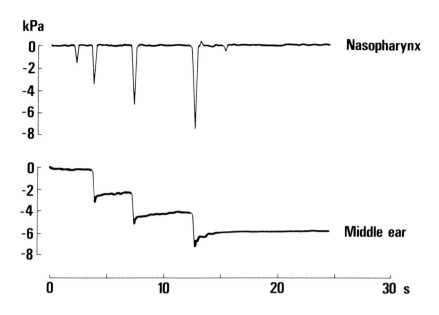

**Fig. 20-7.** Simultaneous pressure recordings from the nasopharynx and middle ear. A deep retraction of the tympanic membrane was present. The negative nasopharyngeal pressure peaks caused by sniffing (top curve) induced a progressive reduction of the middle ear pressure in a staircase pattern (bottom curve).

## Forced Opening Test

In this test a pressure difference over the tube is applied by the investigator and the subject remains passive. The middle ear pressure is recorded with a pressure transducer. Positive middle ear pressure is applied with a manually operated syringe or a pump, or positive pressure is applied during simulated flight in a pressure chamber. As the pressure is increased, the tube suddenly opens up, which causes a quick pressure drop. The sharp deflection point on the curve indicates the positive pressure needed to open the tube; this is called the "opening pressure" (or the forced opening pressure). The opening pressure depends on the applied rate of pressure increase: With a high rate the opening pressure is higher, and with a low rate the opening pressure is lower.[53]

After tubal opening has occurred the pressure does not normally drop all the way to the zero line, but some positive pressure remains in the middle ear; this is called the "closing pressure" (or the closing pressure level; see Fig. 20-8). When healthy and diseased ears are compared, a considerable overlapping of results is found, but in a group of subjects with diseased ears both the opening pressure and the closing pressure are generally low compared to findings in a group of subjects

with healthy ears.[34] In many cases the closing pressure is close to zero, meaning that once the tube is forced open it cannot hold any positive pressure within the middle ear. Results of the forced opening test show variations from time to time in the same ear, but the test shows more constant results than the sniff test.[34] However, since the test does not reflect the highly dynamic events when the subject evacuates his or her ears under natural conditions, the forced opening test can only offer supplementary information.

## Forced Response Test

In this test a constant airflow through the tube is obtained by connecting a pump to the external ear canal. (The eardrum must be perforated or equipped with a ventilating tube.) The pressure in the system as well as the airflow through the eustachian tube are recorded. During constant flow the "passive resistance" is calculated as the quotient between pressure and flow. A change of resistance as indicated by an increase or decrease of the flow occurs at the moment of swallowing and is called the "active resistance." It has been shown that the resistance usually decreases on swallowing, but in some diseased ears the resistance against airflow increases on swallowing.[54]

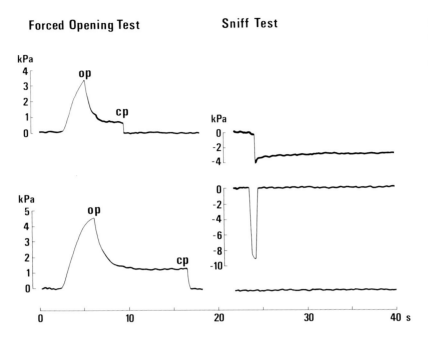

**Fig. 20-8.** Forced opening test and sniff test performed in a patient with unilateral middle ear disease. In the forced opening test the middle ear pressure is increased artificially until the tube suddenly snaps open and releases most of the positive pressure (left top and bottom). The sharp deflection point on the pressure curve indicates the opening pressure (op). After the tube has been forced open the pressure drops to a slight positive level: the closing pressure level (cp). In this case both the opening and closing pressures were lower in the diseased ear (top left) than in the healthy ear (bottom left). The sniff test is shown in the right part of the graph. A forced sniff caused a high negative pressure peak seen in the recording from the nasopharynx (center right). The diseased ear was evacuated (top right), but no pressure change occurred in the healthy ear (bottom right).

## Pressure Equalization Tests

The pressure equalization ability was first studied by Magnus, who published his observations on the influence of compressed air on the ears of caisson workers in 1864.[55] Interest in pressure equalization was increased during World War II when transportation of troops by air was undertaken on a large scale. Pressure chambers for simulating the pressure conditions encountered in flight and diving were constructed at centers of aviation and naval medicine for training and research purposes. Pressure equalization tests have verified the one-way characteristics of the tubal passage displayed in flight and diving: positive middle ear pressure is mostly equalized without much difficulty, while negative middle ear pressure is often difficult to equalize by swallowing. Zöllner investigated a large number of fighter pilots, and developed a clinical test based on graded inflation of the ears.[56] He observed the movement of the eardrum with a microscope while inflating the ear with a graded pressure applied to the nose by a pump. Ingelstedt et al. found that inflation of the ear from the nasopharynx was not truly physiologic and developed

the "aspiration-deflation" test.[36] In ears with perforation a positive or negative test pressure was applied directly, and the ability to reduce or eliminate the test pressure by swallowing was studied. A "microflow technique" was developed by Ingelstedt et al. for studying the pressure equalization ability in ears with an intact tympanic membrane.[57] In this method test pressures were applied with the aid of a pressure chamber, and the movement of the eardrum was recorded by a flowmeter connected to the external ear canal. Very small volume changes (on the order of a few mm³) could be determined after integration with time. (A flow meter is a pressure transducer that measures the pressure differential over a mechanical resistance introduced in the airstream, the pressure difference being proportional to the flow.) After these pioneering investigations a number of modifications of the pressure equalization test have been developed.

Holmquist induced positive or negative pressure in the middle ear with a pump connected to the nose.[58] Tubal passage was induced by asking the subject to swallow. The pressure induced in the middle ear was measured tympanometrically, and then the ability to eliminate the test pressure by swallowing was determined. In another modification the tympanometer is used during the whole procedure.[59] After an initial tympanogram has been taken, positive or negative pressure is applied in the external ear canal, making the eardrum bulge in or out. This causes a change of the intratympanic pressure. The subject is asked to swallow, and if tubal passage occurs a second tympanogram will indicate a pressure that differs from the first.

Different criteria have been used for selecting test subjects and for interpreting the results of tubal function tests. Different investigators use different magnitudes and modes of application of test pressures; there are differences in the measuring techniques, and the procedures vary, for example, as to the number of swallows and whether wet or dry swallowing is used. In some cases only a few deglutions are used, and in other cases the subject is allowed to swallow and to make mandibular movements during the course of 10 minutes.[60] Because of all these metholdologic differences it is difficult to compare the results from different investigations.

Elner classified his material into four function groups[35]:

1. Ears able to equalize both negative and positive test pressure
2. Ears able to equalize positive pressure, but which showed incomplete equalization of negative pressure (a residual pressure remained)
3. Ears able to equalize only positive pressure
4. Ears unable to equalize pressure

In Elner's material very few normal subjects were unable to equalize pressure but, depending on selection criteria and methods, other investigations have shown that inability to equalize pressure in the test situation is not unusual and cannot be judged as being abnormal.[4,61]

### Tests of Mucociliary Function

These tests have little value in the clinical setting. A substance is placed in the middle ear and the time elapsed until the substance can be traced in the nasopharynx is determined. The simplest method is to place a substance with a distinct taste in the middle ear, for example, saccharin.[62] Other investigators have used radiopaque contrast media instilled directly in the middle ear or in a retrograde fashion from the nasopharynx.[63] Fluorescent dye and methylene blue have also been used as tracer substances.[64] Finally, saline solution marked with a radioisotope has been used; here the scintigraphic method has served to detect the substance.[65]

## SUMMARY AND CLOSING COMMENTS

Eustachian tube physiology, as a science, is about 100 years old. The knowledge might be expected to be well established by now, and the basic facts all lined up. However, this is not so. All over the world a few groups are working with eustachian tube physiology, and all deeply involved and fascinated by the problem of the tube. The fascination grows from the fact that the story of the eustachian tube is not complete: the picture is changing in front of our eyes. We should remember that we are not dealing with hard facts but with conceptual models. Facts can be interpreted differently depending upon what line of thought we are using. As in many other developing areas, progress is powered by divergence of opinions and thought models. If one of these models is right, the others are not necessarily wrong.

The ability to equalize pressure is exploited on a large scale in modern transportation technology, which is associated with fast and extensive pressure changes. Naturally, it is important for pilots and divers to be able to equalize pressure by swallowing or Valsalva maneuvers, but this does not necessarily carry over to the physiologic situation. Despite the fact that the ambient pressure shows relatively small fluctuations under normal physiologic conditions, it was previously assumed that pressure equalization is an important physiological function of the eustachian tube. Most methods that have been used for studying the tube are based on the tacit acceptance of a nonphysiologic test situation and use artificial test pressures. This is a questionable approach. The difficulty of carrying out measurements, without seriously disturbing the measured system, is highlighted by the tubal function tests in current use. In the ideal case a measuring method should not influence the measured variable.

The central theme in the present chapter is that the traditional firm adherence to the "ex vacuo" theory should be abandoned. We have seen the physiologic pressure regulation in the middle ear as the effect of a dynamic balance between input and output of gas and fluid. Balance is accomplished by a series of coordinated and mutually interdependent processes, such as gas diffusion over the middle ear mucosa in a two-way fashion, and production and elimination of fluid. The functions of the eustachian tube (including the opening and closing actions, as well as the mucociliary action) are integral parts of the pressure-regulating system. We have stressed the importance of a reliable closure of the eustachian tube in maintaining normal conditions in the middle ear. The protective function is a leading principle in the physiologic function of the eustachian tube, and failure of protection is equally important in tubal malfunction.

In future research on eustachian tube function the emphasis on acute experiments and the use of artificial test pressures will probably be reduced. New measuring techniques focusing on spontaneous pressure changes in the middle ear will be developed. By monitoring the middle ear pressure under natural conditions during longer periods of time, we hope to learn more about physiologic pressure regulation in the middle ear.

---

# REFERENCES

1. Politzer A: Diagnose und Therapie der Annsammlung seröser Flüssigkeit in der Trommenhöhle. Wien Med Wochenschr 17:244, 1867
2. Zaufal E: Uber das Vorkommen seröser Flüsigkeit in der Paukenhöhle. Arch Ohrenheilk 5:38, 1870
3. Bezold F: Die Verschliessung der Tuba Eustachi, ihre physikalische Diagnose und Einwirkung auf die Function des Ohres. Berl Klin Wochenschr 36:551, 1883
4. Magnuson B: On the origin of the high negative pressure in the middle ear space. Am J Otolaryngol 2:1, 1981
5. Magnuson B: Tubal closing failure in retraction type cholesteatoma and adhesive middle ear lesions. Acta Otolaryngol 86:408, 1978
6. Falk B, Magnuson B: Evacuation of the middle ear by sniffing: a cause of high negative pressure and development of middle ear disease. Otolaryngol Head Neck Surg 92:313, 1984
7. Brunner G: Aetiologie und Symptomatologie der sog. Autophonie. Zschr Ohrenheilk 12:268, 1883
8. Graves G, Edwards L: The eustachian tube. Arch Otolaryngol 39:359, 1944
9. Proctor B: Embryology and anatomy of the eustachian tube. Arch Otolaryngol 86:503, 1967
10. Perlman HB: The eustachian tube: abnormal patency and normal physiologic state. Arch Otolaryngol 30:212, 1939
11. Rundcrantz H: Posture and eustachian tube function. Acta Otolaryngol 68:279, 1969
12. Rich AR: A physiological study of the eustachian and its related muscles. Bull Johns Hopkins Hosp 31:206, 1920
13. Rood SR, Doyle WJ: Morphology of tensor veli palatini, tensor tympani, and dilator tubae muscles. Ann Otol Rhinol Laryngol 87:202, 1978
14. Honjo I, Okazaki N, Kumazawa T: Experimental study of the eustachian tube function with regard to its related muscles. Acta Otolaryngol 87:84, 1979
15. Cantekin EI, Doyle WJ, Reichert TJ, et al: Dilation of the eustachian tube by electrical stimulation of the mandibular nerve. Ann Otol Rhinol Laryngol 88:40, 1979
16. Flisberg K: Ventilatory studies on the eustachian tube, a clinical investigation of cases with intact eardrums. Acta Otolaryngol [Suppl] 219:1, 1966
17. Sand O, Enger S: Function of the swimbladder in fish hearing. p. 893. In Møller AR (ed): Basic Mechanics in Hearing. Academic Press, New York, 1973
18. Møller AR: Function of the middle ear. p. 491. In Autrum H, Jung R, Loewenstein WR, et al (eds): Handbook of Sensory Physiology. Springer Verlag, Berlin, 1974
19. Falk B, Magnuson B: Test-retest variability of eustachian tube responses in children with persistent middle ear effusion. Arch Otorhinolaryngol 240:145, 1984
20. Bylander A, Ivarsson A, Tjernström Ö: Eustachian

tube function in normal children and adults. Acta Otolaryngol 92:481, 1981

21. Bylander A: Upper respiratory tract infection and eustachian tube function in children. Acta Otolaryngol 97:343, 1984

22. Matsumura H: Studies on the composition of air in the tympanic cavity. Acta Otolaryngol 61:220, 1955

23. Riu R, Flottes L, Bouche J, LeDen R: La Physiologie de la Trompe d'Eustache. Librairie Anette, Paris, 1966

24. Ostfeldt E: Middle ear gas composition. Ann Otol Laryngol [Suppl] 120:32, 1985.

25. Ruch TC, Patton HD: Physiology and Biophysics. WB Saunders, Philadelphia, 1965

26. Buckingham RA, Stewart DR, Girgis SJ, et al: Experimental evidence against middle ear oxygen absorption. Laryngoscope 95:437, 1985.

27. Hergils L, Magnuson B: Morning pressure in the middle ear. Arch Otolaryngol 111:86, 1985

28. Bylander A, Ivarsson A, Tjernström Ö, et al: Middle ear pressure variations during 24 hours in children. Ann Otol Laryngol [Suppl] 120:33, 1985.

29. Thomsen KA, Terkildsen K, Arnfred J: Middle ear pressure variations during anesthesia. Arch Otolaryngol 82:609, 1965

30. Andréasson L, Ingelstedt S, Ivarsson A, et al: Pressure dependent variations in volume of mucosal lining of the middle ear. Acta Otolaryngol 81:442, 1976

31. Flisberg K, Ingelstedt S, Örtegren U: The valve and "locking" mechanism of the eustachian tube. Acta Otolaryngol [Suppl] 182:57, 1963

32. King PF: The eustachian tube and its signficance in flight. J Laryngol Otol 93:659, 1979

33. Dhenin G (ed): Aviation Medicine. Physiology and Human Factors. Tre-Med Books, London, 1978

34. Magnuson B: Tubal opening and closing ability in unilateral middle ear disease. Am J Otolaryngol 2:199, 1981

35. Elner Å, Ingelstedt S, Ivarsson A: The normal function of the eustachian tube: a study of 102 cases. Acta Otolaryngol 72:320, 1971

36. Ingelstedt S, Örtegren U: Qualitative testing of the eustachian tube function. Acta Otolaryngol [Suppl] 182:7, 1963

37. Gyergyay A: Neue Wege zur Erkennung der Physiologie und Patologie der Orhtrumpete. Monatschr Ohrenheilk 66:769, 1932

38. Virtanen H: Sonotubometry: An acoustical method for objective measurement of auditory tubal opening. Acta Otolaryngol 86:93, 1978

39. Lildholdt T, Brask T, Hvidegaard T: Intepretation of sonotubometry. Acta Otolaryngol 98:250, 1984

40. Andréasson L, Ivarsson A, Luttrup S: Eustachian tube function measured as pressure equalization and sound transmission capacity. A comparison in healthy ears. ORL 46:74, 1984

41. Dishoeck HA: Das Pneumophone. Ein Apparat zur Druckbestimmung im Mittelohr. Arch Ohren Nasen Kehlkopfheilk. 144:53, 1938

42. Metz O: The acoustic impedance measured in normal and pathological ears. Acta Otolaryngol [Suppl] 63:1, 1946

43. Thomsen KA: Eustachian tube function tested by employment of impedance measuring. Acta Otolaryngol 45:252, 1955

44. Falk B: Variability of the tympanogram due to eustachian tube closing failure. Scand Audiol [Suppl] 17:11, 1983

45. Feldman RM, Fria TJ, Palfrey CC, Dellecker CM: Effects of rate of air pressure change on tympanometry. Ear Hearing 5:91, 1984

46. Falk B: Negative middle ear pressure induced by sniffing. A tympanometric study in persons with healthy ears. J Otolaryngol 10:299, 1981

47. Magnuson B, Falk B: New techniques for measuring eustachian tube response. p. 49. In Lim DJ, Bluestone CD, Klein JO, Nelson JD (eds): Recent Advances in Otitis Media with Effusion. BC Decker Inc., Philadelphia, Toronto, 1983

48. Bylander A, Tjernström Ö, Ivarsson A: Pressure opening and closing functions of the eustachian tube by inflation and deflation in children and adults with normal ears. Acta Otolaryngol 96:255, 1983

49. Falk B, Magnuson B: Eustachian tube closing failure in children with persistent middle ear effusion. Int J Pediatr Otorhinolaryngol 7:97, 1984

50. Falk B, Magnuson B: Eustachian tube closing failure, occurrence in patients with cleft palate and middle ear disease. Arch Otolaryngol 110:10, 1984

51. Magnuson B: Eustachian tube pathophysiology. Am J Otolaryngol 4:123, 1983

52. Magnuson B: Tympanoplasty and recurrent disease. Am J Otolaryngol 2:277, 1981

53. Cantekin EI, Bluestone CD, Saez C, et al: Normal and abnormal middle ear ventilation. Ann Otol Rhinol Laryngol 86 [Suppl] 41:1, 1977

54. Cantekin EI, Saez C, Bluestone CD, Bern S: Airflow through the eustachian tube. Ann Otol Rhinol Laryngol 88:603, 1979

55. Magnus A: Werhalten des Gehörorgan in komprimirter Luft. Arch Ohren 1:269, 1864

56. Zöllner F: Wiederstandsmessung an der Ohrtrumpete zur Prufung ihrer Wegsamkeit. Arch Ohren Nasen Kehlkopfheilk 140:137, 1936

57. Ingelstedt S, Ivarsson A, Jonson B: Mechanics of the

human middle ear; pressure regulating in aviation and diving: a nontraumatic method. Acta Otolaryngol [Suppl] 228:5, 1967

58. Holmquist J: Eustachian tube function assessed with tympanometry. A new testing procedure in ears with intact tympanic membranes. Acta Otolaryngol 68:501, 1969

59. Williams P: A tympanometric swallow-test for assessment of eustachian tube function. Ann Otol Rhinol Laryngol 84:339, 1975

60. Bylander A, Ivarsson A, Tjernström Ö: Eustachian tube function in normal children and adults. Acta Otolaryngol 92:481, 1981

61. Siedentop K: Eustachian tube function assessed with tympanometry. Ann Otol Rhinol Laryngol 97:163, 1978

62. Elbrönd O, Larsen E: Mucociliary function of the eustachian tube. Arch Otolaryngol 102:539, 1976

63. Bluestone CD: Eustachian tube obstruction in the infant with cleft palate. Ann Otol Rhinol Laryngol 80:1, 1971

64. Rogers RL, Kirchner FR, Proud GO: The evaluation of eustachian tubal function by fluorescent dye studies. Laryngoscope 72:456, 1962

65. LaFaye M, Gaillard de Collogny L, Jourde H, et al: Etude de la perméabilite de la trompe d'eustache par les radioisotopes. Ann Otolaryngol Chir Cervicofac 91:665, 1974

Section 3

# PATHOLOGY AND PATHOPHYSIOLOGY

# Clinical Epidemiology of Hearing Loss

# 21

## John Chong

## BASIC PRINCIPLES OF CLINICAL EPIDEMIOLOGY

### What Is Clinical Epidemiology?

Clinicians are faced daily by four main challenges: reaching the correct diagnosis, understanding the relationship of the problem with possible causative factors, selecting the management that does more good than harm, and keeping up to date with useful advances in their disciplines. These important acts require the application, to the individual patient, of our prior experiences with groups of similar patients. For example, the rational evaluation of a symptom, sign, or laboratory test result of a patient demands critical appraisal of how this clinical finding has behaved previously among groups of patients with the same differential diagnosis. Many chronic diseases, such as sensorineural hearing loss, have a multifactorial etiology that necessitates consideration of the evidence linking putative factors and the disease. The rational selection of a treatment for today's patient requires an evaluation of how similar patients have fared on various treatments in the past. If, on average, they enjoyed better clinical outcomes and fewer side effects on one treatment than on others,

that regimen would likely be prescribed for the patient.[1,2]

In everyday clinical practice, clinicians ask themselves or patients ask them the following basic questions:

*Frequency:* How often does a disease occur?
*Diagnosis:* How accurate are diagnostic tests or strategies used to find a disease?
*Normality/abnormality:* Is a person sick or well? What abnormalities are associated with having a disease?
*Risk:* What factors are associated with an increased likelihood of disease?
*Cause:* What conditions result in disease? What is the pathogenetic mechanism of disease?
*Prognosis:* What are the consequences of having a disease?
*Treatment:* How does treatment change the future course of a disease?[3]

If rational clinical practice requires the projection of diagnostic findings, causative factors, prognoses, and therapeutic responses from groups of patients to the individual patient, the strategic tactics used to understand groups of patients should be useful to the clinician. It should be possible to take a set of epidemiologic and biostatistical strategies developed to study the distribution and determinants of disease in groups and populations, recast them in a clinical perspective, and use them to improve clinical performance.[4,5] The basic science of clinical epidemiology gives the practicing otologist fundamental tools with which to answer these questions in a rigorous fashion when applying critical appraisal skills to the scientific literature. The basic mission of clinical epidemiology is to develop and apply methods of clinical observation which will lead to valid clinical conclusions.[6,7]

A framework for assembling the specific subset of health information that is most likely to tell us how to reduce the burden of both morbidity (symptoms; physical, emotional, and social functional impairment) and mortality has been proposed.[8,9] This is accomplished by subdividing the spectrum of health information into groups that constitute a logical progression from accurately quantifying the burden of disease, through identifying its likely causes, to validating interventions that prevent or ameliorate it and evaluating their efficiency, to monitoring the application of these interventions and determining whether the burden of disease has been reduced.[10] Each of the seven

steps in the measurement loop (Fig. 21-1) poses a different type of research or evaluation question, and new information is required for a different set of methods. This approach offers not only methods of understanding and improving quality of care, but a systematic algorithm for a critical appraisal of the need, benefits, and costs of health interventions as well. The reduction or alleviation of the burden of illness from hearing loss is the primary goal of clinical otologists through preventative, therapeutic, rehabilitative, and supportive interventions.[11]

For example, it would be important for otologists to know the burden of illness of the various types of hearing disorders in the community in which they practice; the causes of these particular hearing disorders, such as whether these factors were avoidable or unavoidable; what types of interventions would be effective in treating the disorders of interest; whether the treatment programs in the practice were efficient in terms of health care costs and health improvement gained; and how to monitor the progress or quality of care in a practice to evaluate the total impact on the burden of illness from hearing disorders in the community.

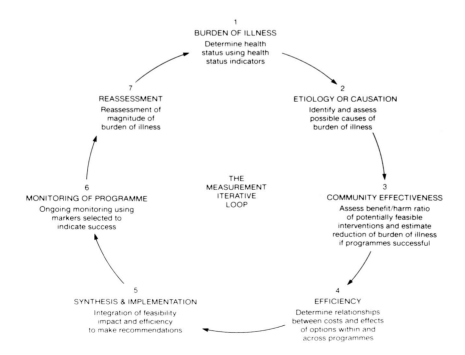

**1**
BURDEN OF ILLNESS
Determine health
status using health
status indicators

**7**
REASSESSMENT
Reassessment of
magnitude of
burden of illness

**2**
ETIOLOGY OR CAUSATION
Identify and assess
possible causes of
burden of illness

THE
MEASUREMENT
ITERATIVE
LOOP

**6**
MONITORING OF PROGRAMME
Ongoing monitoring using
markers selected to
indicate success

**3**
COMMUNITY EFFECTIVENESS
Assess benefit/harm ratio
of potentially feasible
interventions and estimate
reduction of burden of illness
if programmes successful

**5**
SYNTHESIS & IMPLEMENTATION
Integration of feasibility
impact and efficiency
to make recommendations

**4**
EFFICIENCY
Determine relationships
between costs and effects
of options within and
across programmes

**Fig. 21-1.** Measurement iterative loop. A strategy to design, implement, and evaluate health interventions aimed at reducing the burden of illness from hearing loss. This method assists the otologist in appraising critically the needs, benefits, and costs of specific interventions.

## Measuring the Burden of Illness from Hearing Loss

The events of primary interest in clinical epidemiology are the health outcomes of particular concern to patients and those caring for them:

*Death:* A universal health outcome, the timeliness of the event being the issue

*Disease:* A combination of symptoms, physical signs, and laboratory test results

*Disability:* The functional status of patients in terms of ability to live independently and go about their daily lives at home, work, or recreation

*Discomfort:* Uncomfortable symptoms, such as pain, nausea, vertigo, tinnitis, or fatigue

*Dissatisfaction:* Emotional and mental states, such as agitation, sadness, or anger

*Destitution:* Financial consequences of health care to patients

Epidemiologists have devised methods of measuring these key elements to (1) define the burden of illness of a disease in a population; (2) discriminate between individuals along a continuum of health, illness, or disability; (3) predict outcome or prognosis; and (4) evaluate within-person change over time.[12]

The traditional measures of the frequency of health and disease are important to define for considering a problem in a group of patients or population:

*Mortality rate:* Death rate equals the total number of persons dying of a disease (or from all causes) during some period of time (usually a year), divided by the total population (sick and well) alive at the midpoint of the period. (If not subdivided by age, sex, and other factors into age-specific or sex-specific rates, the result is called a crude rate.)

*Case-fatality rate:* The total number of persons dying of a disease during some period of time, divided by the total number of persons who have the disease (Note: Most medical texts get it wrong and use the term mortality rate when they are actually describing the case-fatality rate.)

*Survival rate:* The complement of the case-fatality rate, or 100% (case-fatality rate percentage)

*Incidence (rate):* New cases equals the number of new cases occurring within a specific time period, divided by the number of susceptible persons (the population at risk)

*Prevalence (rate):* All cases equals the total number of cases of a disease at a point in time (point prevalence) or during a period in time (period prevalence), divided by the total population (sick and well) alive at that point or at the midpoint of that period

The interrelationship of these rates is as follows:

$$\text{Prevalence} = \text{incidence} \times \text{duration}$$

$$\text{Mortality} = \text{Case-fatality} \times \text{incidence}$$

Prevalent cases are discovered by surveying a group of people, some of whom are diseased at that point, while others are healthy. The fraction or proportion of the group who are diseased (i.e., cases) constitutes the prevalence of the disease. Such surveys of a population of persons, including cases and noncases, have been termed prevalence or cross-sectional studies.

In contrast to prevalence, incidence is measured by first identifying a population free of the event of interest and then following them through time with periodic examinations for occurrences of the event. In a cohort study, a group of people (a cohort) is assembled, none of whom has experienced the outcome of interest. Upon entry to the study, persons in the cohort are classified according to those characteristics that might be related to outcome. These people are then followed over time to see which of them experience the outcome. It is then possible to see how initial characteristics relate to subsequent outcome events. Other terms for such studies are longitudinal (emphasizing that patients are followed over time), prospective (implying the forward direction in which the patients are pursued), and incidence (calling attention to the basic measure of disease events over time) (Table 21-1).

The prevalence or incidence of hearing disorders in a community depends on the criteria used to define the disorder in terms of impairment, handi-

**Table 21-1. Characteristics of Incidence Rates and Prevalence Rates**

| Rate | Numerator | Denominator | Time of Measurement | Study Design |
|---|---|---|---|---|
| Incidence | New cases occurring during the follow-up period in a group initially free of the disease | All susceptible individuals present at the beginning of the follow-up period (often called the population at risk) | Throughout the follow-up period | Cohort study |
| Prevalence | All cases counted on a single survey or by examination of a group | All individuals examined, including cases and noncases | At a single point in time | Prevalence or cross-sectional study |

cap, and disability. *Hearing loss* is normally used within the context of impairment with many definitions based on averages of specific audiometric frequencies in either or both ears. A number of published studies have examined this question at the national, provincial, and local levels.

A large-scale epidemiologic investigation was carried out under the sponsorship of the Commission for the European Communities[13] in an effort to determine the prevalence of childhood deafness in the nine member countries. The objectives of the survey included a determination of the prevalence of deafness in 8-year-old children who had a hearing loss averaging 50 dB or worse in the better ear at 0.5, 1, and 2 kHz. The prevalence of this degree of deafness was 0.9 per 1,000 live births in 1969, 92 percent of which were of the sensorineural type. When the etiology was known, rubella was the largest single cause. By contrast, a mass survey of 15,890 Navajo schoolchildren was examined between 1978 and 1980[14] by a mobile team of technicians. The prevalence of tympanic membrane perforations was found to be 4.0 percent, 2.3 percent middle ear effusions, 1.9 percent tympanic membrane atalectasis, and 0.4 percent had sensorineural hearing loss. Early detection and follow-up of hearing loss in this age group is crucial, as deafness in infancy and early childhood can have catastrophic consequences for language ability and mental, emotional, and social development.[15] In a U.S. National Census of the Adult Deaf Population, Schein and Delk[16] found wide regional variation of prevalence rates for prevocational deafness ranging from 173/100,000 in the northeast to 242/100,000 in the north central areas.[21] In a National Hearing Study in Great Britain,[17] 6,804 adults were selected from the electoral lists of Southampton, Nottingham, Glasgow, and Cardiff and sent questionnaires regarding hearing loss and tinnitus. About 25 percent of the sample reported some hearing difficulty and about 17 percent reported tinnitus that was more than a transitory experience. Audiometric investigation of a subsample of the study population found that $19.9 \pm 4.4$ percent had hearing impairment greater than 25 dB hearing level in the better ear averaged across 0.5, 1, 2, and 4 kHz. The Canada Health Survey[18] reported overall prevalence rates of approximately 40 hearing-impaired Canadians per 100,000 of the population. The prevalence rates varied with age but are likely to be underestimates due to the nature of self-reporting of hearing disability. A Danish cross-sectional prevalence survey of 5,050 men, aged 45 to 65 years, was done as part of study of heart disease among workers in Copenhagen.[19] A random sample of 206 subjects underwent audiologic examination. The prevalence of hearing impairment, based on the same criteria used in the MRC Study in Great Britain, was $35 \pm 5$ percent, which compared fairly well with the number of $44 \pm 7$ percent complaining of subjective hearing impairment.[20]

## Clinical Measurement, Diagnosis, and Disagreement

In contrast to classic epidemiology, clinicians see patients who are sick and help them most when they recognize that their sickness has three elements: the disease or target disorder, the illness, and the predicament. It is therefore important to define these entities.

> *Disease or target disorder:* Anatomic, biochemical, physiologic, or psychological derangement the etiology (if known), maladaptive mechanisms, presentation, prognosis, and management of which we read about in medical texts (Although this entity is generally called the "disease," the usefulness of that ambiguous term is hampered by the inability of both patients and health scientists to agree on its application to specific situations)
>
> *Illness:* The cluster of symptoms (manifestations of the target disorder perceived by the patient) and signs (manifestations perceived by the clinician) exhibited by the patient as a result of having, and responding to, the target disorder (We shall call this cluster the illness.)
>
> *Predicament:* The social, psychological, and economic fashion in which the patient is situated in the environment

The act of clinical diagnosis focuses on the second element of a sickness (the illness), in order to identify the first (the target disorder), while keeping an eye on the third (the predicament). Put more formally, the act of clinical diagnosis is classification for a purpose: an effort to recognize the class or group to which a patient's illness belongs, so that, based on our prior experience with that class, the subsequent clinical acts we can afford to carry out, and the patient is willing to follow, will maximize that patient's health.

When otologists consider the burden of illness from hearing loss, these traditional measures of frequency often do not yield satisfactory information about the target disorder, illness, and predicament. Standard audiometric methods have been used to define a patient's level of hearing impairment. These diagnostic procedures, however, are not measures of predicament of the patients we seek to help. Measures of handicap and disability from hearing loss across large populations have therefore been limited.

The basic purpose of clinical epidemiology is to foster methods of clinical observations and interpretation that will lead to valid conclusions. Whenever a clinical question is answered by observing human beings, there are three possible explanations for the answer. The observation may be incorrect because of bias or chance (random variation), or it may be correct. There are three main types of bias[22]:

> *Selection bias:* The method by which patients were selected for observation
>
> *Measurement bias:* The method by which the observation or measurement was made
>
> *Confounding bias:* The presence of another variable that accounts for the observation

For example, audiometric threshold determination demonstrates these types of clinical measurement problems (Fig. 21-2).

A clinical observation is valid if it corresponds to the true state of affairs. For the observation to be valid, it must be neither biased nor incorrect due to chance. It is useful to distinguish between two general kinds of validity: internal validity and external validity, or generalizability.

### Internal Validity

Internal validity is the degree to which the results of an observation are correct for the patients being studied. It is internal because it applies to the

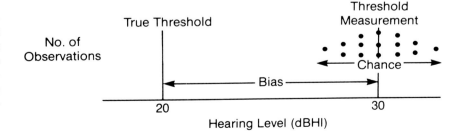

**Fig. 21-2.** Types of measurement errors in audiometric threshold determination. Errors may be random due to chance alone or biased due to introduction of a systematic factor, such as poor calibration of an audiometer.

particular conditions of the particular group of patients being observed, and not necessarily to others. The internal validity of clinical observations is determined by how well they are carried out, and is threatened by all the biases and random variation. For a clinical observation to be useful, internal validity is a necessary but often insufficient condition.

### Generalizability

Generalizability, or external validity, is the degree to which the results of an observation hold true in other settings. For an individual physician, it is an answer to the question: Assuming the results of a study are true, do they apply to my patient as well? Generalizability expresses the validity of assuming that patients in a study are comparable to other patients.

### Reliability

Reliability is the extent to which repeated measurements of a relatively stable phenomenon fall closely to each other. Repeatability, reproducibility, and precision are synonyms for this property.

Validity and reliability are not necessarily related to each other. It is possible to have an instrument (e.g., laboratory machine or questionnaire) that is on the average valid (accurate) but not reliable, because its results are widely scattered about the true value. By contrast, an instrument can be very reliable yet systematically off the mark (inaccurate). The sources of variation in making a diagnosis come from a number of sources (Table 21-2).

The principal scales used for measuring clinical

**Table 21-2. Sources of Variation in Making a Diagnosis**[a]

| Source | Definition |
| --- | --- |
| | **Measurement** |
| Instrument | The means of making the measurement |
| Observer | The person making the measurement |
| | **Biologic** |
| Within individuals | Changes in subjects with time and situation |
| Among individuals | Biologic differences from subject to subject |

[a] See Clinical Disagreement I and II.[23,24]

phenomena are *nominal, ordinal, interval,* and *ratio.* Data that can only be placed into categories, without any inherent order, are called nominal data. Relatively few clinical phenomena can be categorized with such sharp distinction that they might be considered truly nominal or are dramatic, discrete events (death or surgery). Such data can be placed in categories without much concern about misclassification.

Data that are ordered, but for which the size of the intervals cannot be specified, are called ordinal data. Interval data are both ordered and represented by intervals of known size. If there is a clearly understood zero point, such scales have been called ratio rather than interval.

The primary goal of diagnostic tests initiated by clinicians is to establish whether a disease is truly present. The accuracy of a diagnostic test is of prime importance. A simple way of looking at the relationship between test results and the true diagnosis shown in Figure 21-3. This shows the relation between a diagnostic test result and the occurrence of disease. There are two possibilities for the result to be correct (true positive and true negative) and two possibilities for the result to be incorrect (false positive and false negative).

The validity of a particular audiometric outcome and whether it bears any relationship to true impairment of auditory ability is difficult to assess due to a lack of a true "gold standard" for deafness. As in the case of a diagnostic test for cancer, ultimately a tissue diagnosis (either a biopsy or autopsy specimen) will provide the truth; however, with hearing loss, tissue samples of the cochlea are not possible. Thus, we are left only with comparisons of various methods of assessing hearing function. This cannot be merely termed a substitution game, as objective measurement of psychoacoustic events necessitates such methods.

We must rely on agreement among observers or instruments (internal consistency, reliability, or precision) rather than on agreement between the observers with a gold standard (external consistency, validity, or accuracy). Some attempts to use estimates of speech discrimination or communication ability as an external standard have been done, however, these estimates of the "gold standard" are inherently unreliable.

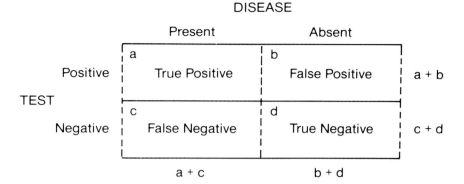

**Fig. 21-3.** Relationship between a diagnostic test result and the occurrence of disease. The goal is to reduce false-positive and false-negative results so as to maximize the accuracy of the test.

## Diagnostic Test Characteristics

The characteristics of a diagnostic test are important to consider: sensitivity, specificity, and accuracy.

*Sensitivity* is defined as the proportion of subjects with the disease who have a positive test for the disease. A sensitive test will rarely miss those who have the disease:

$$\text{Sensitivity} = \frac{a}{a + c}$$

*Specificity* is the proportion of subjects without the disease whose test proves negative. A specific test will rarely misclassify people without the disease as diseased.

$$\text{Specificity} = \frac{d}{b + d}$$

The probability of disease, given the results of a test, is called the *predictive value* of the test. Positive predictive value is the probability of disease in a patient with a positive (abnormal) test result. Negative predictive value is the probability that the patient does not have the disease when the test result is negative (normal). Predictive value is an answer to the question: If my patient's test result is positive (negative), what are the chances that my patient does/does not have the disease?

$$\text{Positive predictive value} = \frac{a}{a + b}$$

$$\text{Negative predictive value} = \frac{d}{c + d}$$

The predictive value of a test is not a property of the test alone. It is determined by the sensitivity and specificity of the test and by the prevalence of disease in the population being tested, where *prevalence* has its customary meaning: the proportion of persons in a defined population at a given point in time with the condition in question:

$$\text{Prevalence} = \frac{a + c}{a + b + c + d}$$

*Accuracy* is the proportion of all test results, both positive and negative, that are correct:

$$\text{Accuracy} = \frac{a + d}{a + b + c + d}$$

(see diagnostic tests I and II).[25]

The definitions in Table 21-3 are commonly used to describe either the central tendency or dispersion of clinical observations.

Ideally, a test result would provide the clinician with an accurate estimate of the diagnosis, prognosis, or therapeutic status of a patient. Unfortunately, most test results are provided with what is termed a "range of normal," and the connection of the result to various aspects of clinical care is left entirely up to the clinician.

The range of normal for many tests is set up by collecting observations from a number of healthy or unhealthy people and calculating the mean and standard deviation of the values obtained from the specimens. The range of normal is then defined as the mean value ±2 SD. The 2 SD is intended to provide a range within which 95 percent of the

**Table 21-3. Expressions of Central Tendency and of Dispersion[a]**

| Expression | Definition | Advantages | Disadvantages |
|---|---|---|---|
| **Central tendency** | | | |
| Mean | Sum of observations; number of observations | Well suited to mathematical manipulation | Easily influenced by extreme values |
| Median | The point where the number of observations above equals the number below | Not easily influenced by extreme values | Not well suited to mathematical manipulation |
| Mode | Most frequently occurring value | Simplicity of meaning | Either no or many most-frequent values |
| **Dispersion** | | | |
| Range | From lowest to highest value in a distribution | Includes all values | Affected by extreme values |
| Standard deviation[a] | The absolute value of the average difference of individual values from the mean | Well suited to mathematical manipulation | non-Gaussian distributions, does not describe a known proportion of observations |
| Percentile decile, quartile, etc. | The proportion of all observations | Describes the "unusualness" of a value without assumptions about the shape of a distribution | Not well suited to statistical manipulation |

[a] Where N = 1; X = each observation; X = mean of all observations; and N = number of observations.

values tested lie. That is, arbitrarily, 5 percent of the values are outside this range of normal and are therefore considered to be abnormal.

This is where the difficulty begins. Consider what would happen if the test were "standardized" for all healthy people. Five percent of them would suddenly become "unhealthy." And what if you do more than one test on a person? On each test there is a 5 percent probability of an abnormal result being found, so that for two tests the probability that the results of one will be abnormal is 10 percent (and for 10 tests there is a 40 percent probability that the results of one will be abnormal on statistical grounds alone).

What is the justification for saying that unusual results (i.e., those that occur less than 5 percent of the time) are *abnormal?* Before it can be said that a result is abnormal, we must know (1) the population from which the result was derived (epidemiologic variation), (2) individual variability (biologic variability), (3) test variability, and (4) tester variability.[26]

### Assessing the Causes of Hearing Loss

Elucidation of causal factors requires a careful review of all biologic and behavioral attributes that might contribute to a problem. By exploring the hypothesis space, the most likely potential causes can be identified. For example, such factors as age, noise exposure, and family history would be important causal factors to consider for hearing loss (Fig. 21-4).

When dealing with multicausal problems, the relative contribution of each factor is often difficult to estimate unless sophisticated multivariate statistical models are used.

Risk generally refers to the probability that some unfortunate event will occur. However, it can be defined more specifically as the likelihood that people who are disease free but exposed to certain risk factors will acquire the disease.

Often there are conditions for which clinical experience is insufficient to confirm exposure–risk relationships:

Long latency period between exposure and disease
Frequent exposure to risk factor
Low incidence of disease
Small risk from exposure
Common disease
Multiple causes of disease

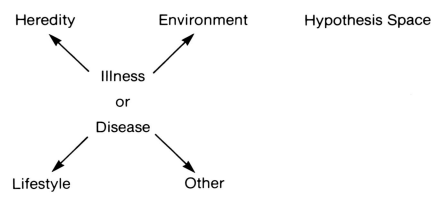

**Fig. 21-4.** Assessing causation of an illness or disease and exploring the hypothesis space. This encourages the otologist to consider the multifactorial nature of chronic disease, such as hearing loss.

A *cause* is something that brings about an effect or a result and is considered by biological scientists in the definition of pathogenesis of basic mechanisms. Information about causation is important to clinicians in guiding their approach to prevention, diagnosis, and treatment. When more than one cause act together, their effects may be complex, resulting in a risk greater than would be expected by simply adding the effects of separate causes. Interactions may occur with the implication than removal of one factor may result in a substantial reduction in risk.

Specific criteria are used for the assessment of cause–effect relationships in the literature. Much weight is placed on the study designs used (Table 21-4). The main types are shown in Figures 21-5 through 21-7.

Figure 21-8 compares how the various designs can be used in establishing a causal relationship. Figure 21-9 summarizes research designs used to establish cause.[27]

### Deciding on the Best Therapy for the Patient

Preventative and therapeutic interventions include actions intended to change the clinical course of disease for the better. Although many seem as though they ought to work, fewer actually do when put to a formal test.

**Table 21-4.    The Nine Diagnostic Tests for Causation**[a]

1. Is there evidence from true experiments in humans?

    Yes: Class 1 evidence: randomized controlled trial

    No: Class 2 evidence: cohort studies; before–after studies
    Class 3 evidence: case-control studies
    Class 4 evidence: descriptive studies

    a. Were the major sources of bias avoided or if present measured?

    b. Were the sampling, assessment of exposure, and analysis at an acceptable level?

2. Is the association strong? Is the association stronger than for alternative explanations?
3. Do other investigators consistently find this same result?
4. Is the temporal relationship in the proper direction?
5. Is there a gradient or dose–response relationship?
6. Does the association make epidemiologic sense?
7. Is the association biologically sensible?
8. Is the association specific?
9. Is the relationship analogous to another, well-accepted relationship?

[a] See under To Determine Etiology or Causation.[27]

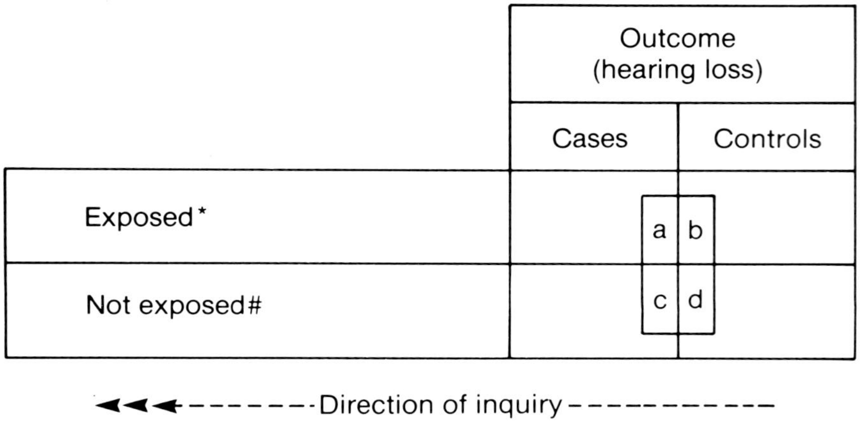

**Fig. 21-5.** Basic structure of a case-control study. Cases are identified and matched to persons who do not have the disease. History of partial exposure to specific agents is sought from both groups and compared in order to calculate relative odds (ad/bc).

The three principal decisions that determine the rational treatment of any patient are as follows:

1. *Identifying the ultimate objective of treatment:* Is the ultimate objective to achieve cure, palliation, symptomatic relief, or some other end?
2. *Selecting the specific treatment:* Does the patient require any treatment at all? What sorts of evidence, from what sources, should determine the choice of the specific treatment to be used to reach this goal?
3. *Specifying the treatment target:* How will you know when to stop treatment, change its intensity, or switch to some other treatment?

The following six objectives, singly or in combination, comprise the ultimate objectives of treatment:

1. Cure the patient (e.g., kill the microbe, cut out the tumor).
2. Prevent a recurrence (e.g., give prophylactic antibiotics following recovery from acute infection).
3. Limit structural or functional deterioration (e.g., reconstruct, rehabilitate).
4. Prevent the later complication (e.g., myringotomy).
5. Relieve the current symptom (e.g., give painkillers, and antiinflamatory drugs).
6. Allow the patient to die with comfort and dignity (e.g., cancel further diagnostic testing and focus on the relief of current symptoms and the preservation of self-esteem).

Treatment is usually considered what physicians prescribe (e.g., drugs, surgery) for patients with

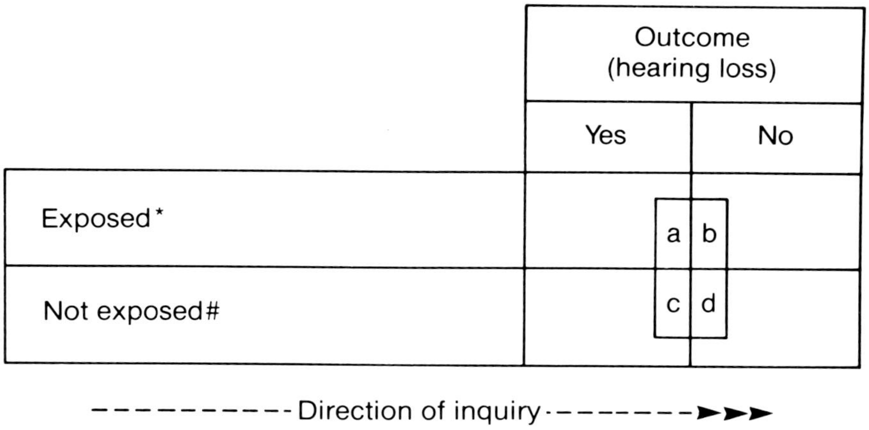

**Fig. 21-6.** Basic structure of a cohort study. A population exposed to an agent(s) is followed forward in time along with an appropriate control group. The incidence of a specific disease or outcome is compared between the groups in order to calculate a relative risk:

$$\frac{a/(a+b)}{c/(c+d)}$$

This population may be selected from a larger population in a number of ways.

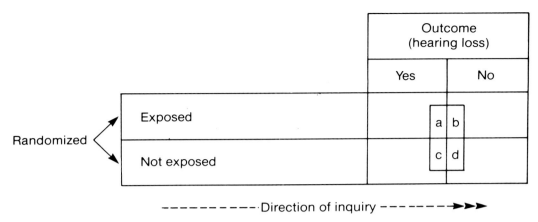

**Fig. 21-7.** Basic structure of a randomized trial. This is a specialized type of cohort study in which the process of randomization may minimize any systematic difference between exposed and nonexposed populations.

established disease. It should be evident, however, that there are a great many other ways of intervening to improve health (Fig. 21-10).

One can prevent disease before it is established, by controlling risk factors (primary prevention). Disease can be detected early and treated when it is more likely to respond (secondary prevention). One can also intervene to change the organization of financing health care and render its delivery more effective.

Clinical trials are a special kind of cohort study in which interventions are specifically introduced by the investigators in ways that improve the possibility of observing treatment effects that are free of bias. The reason for making a distinction between clinical trials and cohort studies is that if investigators can introduce the intervention, they can also control the conditions of the study in other ways in order to give a more accurate assessment of the effects of an intervention. Clearly, clinical trials are more highly structured than are cohort studies. Investigators are in effect conducting an experiment, analogous to those done in the laboratory. Investigators take it upon themselves (with their subject's

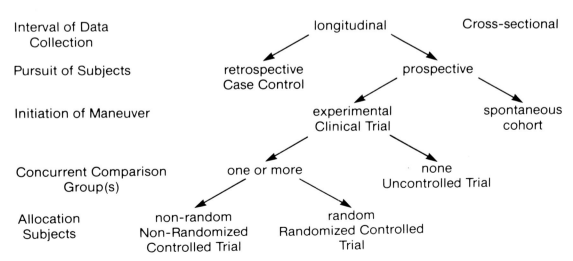

**Fig. 21-8.** Summary of research designs to establish cause. The preferred design is clearly a randomized trial, but often that is neither feasible nor ethical.

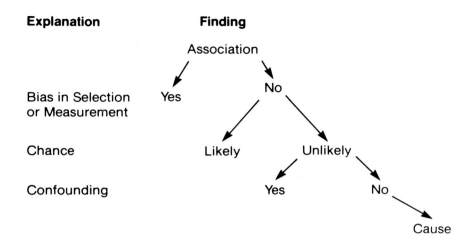

**Explanation**    **Finding**

Association

Bias in Selection    Yes        No
or Measurement

Chance                   Likely        Unlikely

Confounding                          Yes              No

Cause

**Fig. 21-9.** Explanation of an association: bias, chance, confounding, and cause. The otologist needs to appraise critically the evidence before concluding that an observed relationship is causal.

permission) to isolate for study the unique contribution of one factor by holding constant, as much as possible, other determinants of the outcome. Thus, other terms for clinical trials are *intervention* and *experimental studies.*[5]

The structure of a clinical trial, in a simplified form, is shown. The patients to be studied are first selected from a larger number of patients with the condition of interest. They are then divided into two groups of comparable prognosis. One group, the experimental or treated group, is exposed to some intervention that is believed to be helpful. The other group, the *control* or *comparison* group, is treated the same in all ways except that its members are not exposed to the intervention. The clinical course of both groups is then observed and any differences attributed to the intervention (Fig. 21-11).

The main reason for structuring clinical trials in this way is to avoid bias, or systematic error, when comparing the respective value of the two or more approaches to patient management. The validity of clinical trials depends on how well they result in an equal distribution of all determinants of prognosis, other than the one being tested, in treated and control patients.

In general, evaluation of treatment is less likely to be biased if the investigator can establish the conditions of treatment in a clinical trial. A comparison (control) group of patients should be explicitly identified because the clinical course of disease is often not predictable. If treated, and control patients are taken from the same time and place, it is possible to avoid a variety of factors other than treatment that can affect outcome. Patients should be allocated into treated and control groups in such a way that they would have the same outcomes if it were not for the treatment. The surest way to do this is by randomization. It is preferable but not always possible) to arrange that participants in a trial are "blind" (i.e., unaware of individual patients' treatment), so that knowledge of treatment cannot affect their responses. In sum, the soundest approach to a clinical trial is a randomized double-blind controlled trial.

The extent to which the results of a clinical trial can be applied to other patients depends on how patients were sampled for inclusion in the trial. On

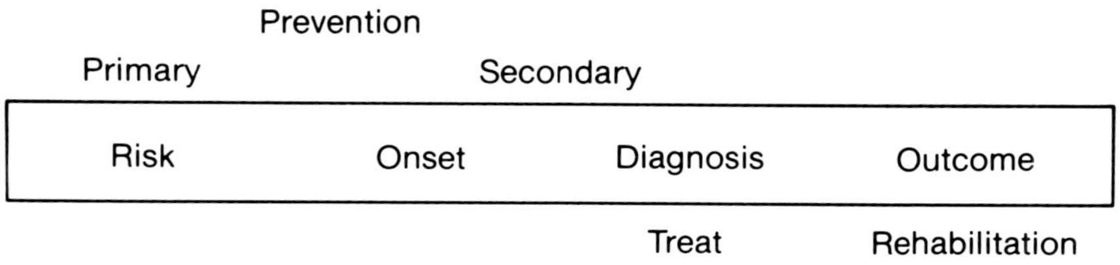

Prevention
Primary                   Secondary

| Risk | Onset | Diagnosis | Outcome |

Treat            Rehabilitation

**Fig. 21-10.** Interventions in the course of disease. The otologist can intervene at a number of points along the natural history of a chronic disease such as hearing loss.

**Fig. 21-11.** The basic structure of a clinical trial. Patients are randomly allocated to receive a treatment or placebo and follow-up and the results of therapy are compared.

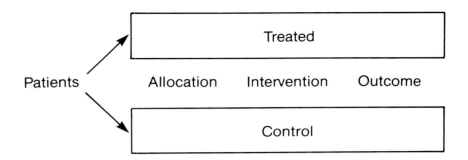

the one hand, efficacy is established in highly cooperative patients and shows whether an intervention can work under specially favorable circumstances, although not necessarily in practice. By contrast, effectiveness is whether treatment (prevention) does more good than harm in those to whom it is offered. The potential sources of bias are illustrated in Figure 21-12.

The results of current treatment are sometimes compared with experience with similar patients in the past—historical or nonconcurrent controls. While this may be done well, there are many pitfalls. Methods of diagnosis and treatment change with time, and with them the average prognosis.

If historical controls are used, the shorter period of time between selection of treated and control groups and the less other aspects of medical care have changed during the interval, the safer an historical control can be. In general, however, choosing concurrent controls (i.e., subjects being treated during the same period of time) eliminates a potential source of bias.

It is preferable to choose both treated and control patients from the same setting because a variety of factors (e.g., referral patterns, organization, and skill of staff) often result in very different prognoses in different settings.

The best way to allocate patients is by means of randomized controlled trials, clinical trials in which patients are randomly allocated to treated and control cohorts. Randomization is done by one of a variety of disciplined procedures—analogous to flipping a coin—whereby each subject has an equal chance of appearing in any of the treatment groups.

Random allocation of subjects is preferred be-

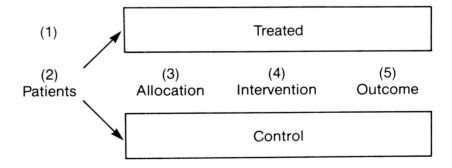

**Fig. 21-12.** Sources of bias in a clinical trial. The otologist must be aware of possible types and source of bias in critically evaluating a study comparing treatments, such as a new drug or surgical procedure.

(1) Comparison group:
(2) Patients from same time and place;
(3) Unbiased allocation of intervention;
(4) Intervention as intended;
(5) Outcome assessed equally.

cause randomization assigns patients to one group or the other(s) without bias. Patients in one group are, on the average, as likely to possess a given characteristic as patients in another. This is so for all factors related to prognosis, whether or not they are known before the study takes place.

However, random allocation does not guarantee that the groups will be similar. While the process of random allocation is unbiased, the results may not be. Dissimilarities between groups can arise, albeit infrequently, by chance alone. The risk of dissimilar groups is particularly great when the number of randomized patients is small.

Before randomization, stratification is often used, so that at least some of the most important characteristics known to be associated with outcome will appear equally in treated and control groups. Patients are first gathered into groups (strata) of similar prognosis and then randomized separately within each stratum. The groups are then bound to be comparable, at least for factors dealt with in this way. After patients are allocated to treatment groups, it is intended that they actually take their treatment and remain in their assigned group.

When analyzing the results of a trial in which patients have not remained in their original (randomized) groups, a dilemma arises. Should patients who changed treatment groups be counted against the treatment they were originally offered or against the one they ultimately received? The answer depends on the clinical question the trial is intended to answer. Trials can ask two different sorts of questions. The first deals with explanations and asks such questions as: "Can drug A reduce tumor size?" The second deals with management and asks such questions as: "Does prescribing drug A to patients with tumors do more good than harm?" These two types of trials have contrasting attributes. The explanatory trial seeks to describe how a treatment produces its effects and to determine whether it can work, often under ideal or restricted circumstances. Conversely, the management trial seeks to describe all the consequences, both good and bad, of treating an illness in a certain way and to determine whether therapy does work, usually under as close to usual clinical circumstances as possible.[28]

Thus, in an explanatory trial, the effects of treatment are analyzed only in those patients who actually receive the treatment, regardless of the group to which they were originally assigned. Conversely, in a management trial, we are interested in the effects of treatment plans, whether they are followed or not, and would compare patient groups according to their original allocation.

The participants in a clinical trial include those who give treatment (clinicians), those who receive it (patients), and those who assess its effects (investigators). Often the clinicians and investigators are the same people. Clinicians in a trial may change their behavior in a systematic way (i.e., become biased) if they are aware of which patients receive which treatment. Therefore, often they are "blinded" in a figurative sense, to knowledge of treatment.

Most patients are anxious to please their physicians and to get well. This leads to difficulty when assessment of outcome is heavily dependent on what patients report. They may exaggerate their improvement if they know they have received a specific treatment.

To avoid bias from this source, an effort is made to conceal from patients the treatment they are actually receiving. Control patients are given a placebo: an intervention that is indistinguishable from the active treatment but that does not possess its specifically active component. For example, a placebo pill would have the same size, shape, color, and taste as the active drug. In one study of a surgical procedure for Menière's disease, investigators even went so far as to perform a sham operation.[29] When placebos are successful, it becomes impossible for patients' responses to be biased by knowledge of their treatment. The placebo effect is therefore a response to a medical intervention that is definitely a result of the intervention, but not because of its specific mechanism of action.

The question of whether a treatment can work is one of efficacy. An efficacious treatment is one that does more good than harm among those who receive it. Efficacy is established by restricting patients in a study to those who will cooperate fully with medical advice.

An effective treatment does more good than harm in those to whom it is offered. Effectiveness is established by offering a treatment or program to patients and allowing them to accept or reject it as they might ordinarily do. Only a small proportion of clinical trials set out to answer questions of effectiveness. If a treatment proves ineffective, it may be due to lack of efficacy, lack of patient acceptance, or both. Compliance is the extent to which patients follow medical advice. Patient compliance intervenes between an efficacious treatment and an effective one.

Having decided that the patient's sickness does warrant treatment and having selected the goal of this treatment, the clinician must now select the specific drug, operation, splint, exercise, or conversation that will best achieve this goal:

1. On the basis of retrospective analyses of uncontrolled clinical experience or the extension of current concepts of mechanisms of disease: The clinician can logically arrive at the therapy that seems to work or ought to work.
2. On the basis of prospective analyses of formal randomized clinical trials designed to expose worthless or dangerous treatments: The clinician can select the therapies that successfully withstand formal attempts to demonstrate their worthlessness;
3. On the basis of recommendations from teachers, consultants, colleagues, advertisements, or pharmaceuticals representatives: The clinician can simply accept a treatment on faith.

For the best information on whether a given treatment does more good than harm to patients with a given disorder, the clinician should rely on the results of a randomized clinical trail in which patients with a given disorder were randomly allocated to receive either the given treatment or a placebo (or conventional therapy) and then followed up for clinically relevant outcomes of their disease and its treatment. Fortunately, randomized clinical trials are becoming very much more common and have demonstrated dramatically the efficacy of many treatments and the uselessness or even harmfulness of several others. However, the proper evaluation of therapy requires more than randomization alone. Other guides for sorting out therapeutic claims are as follows:[3]

1. Was the assignment of patients to treatment truly randomized?
2. Were all clinically relevant outcomes reported?
3. Were the patients participating in the study recognizably similar to your own?
4. Were both clinical and statistical significance considered?
5. Is the therapeutic maneuver feasible in your practice?
6. Were all the patients who entered the study accounted for at its conclusion?

# REFERENCES

1. Sackett DL: Clinical epidemiology. Am J Epidemiol 89:125, 1969
2. Feinstein AR: Why clinical epidemiology? Clin Res 20:821, 1972
3. Department of Clinical Epidemiology and Biostatistics: McMaster University Health Sciences Centre. Clinical Epidemiology Rounds. How to read clinical journals. I–IV. Can Med Assoc J 124:555, 703, 869, 985, 1156, 1981
4. Feinstein AR: Clinical Judgment. Williams & Wilkins, Baltimore, 1967
5. Sackett DL, Haynes, RB, Tugwell P: Clinical Epidemiology: A Basic Science for Clinical Medicine. Little, Brown, Boston, 1985
6. Murphy EA: The Logic of Medicine. Johns Hopkins University Press, Baltimore, 1976
7. Feinstein AR: Clinical Biostatistics. CV Mosby, St. Louis, 1977
8. Cochrane AL: Effectiveness and Efficiency: Random Reflections on Health Services. Nuffield Provincial Hospital Trust, 1977
9. Evans JR: Measurement and Management in Medicine and Health Services. (Mimeo.) Rockefeller Foundation, New York, 1981
10. Tugwell P, Bennett K, Sackett DL, Haynes RB: The measurement iterative loop: A framework for the critical appraisal of need, benefits and costs of health interventions. J Chronic Dis 38:4:339, 1987
11. World Health Organization: Development of indicators for monitoring progress towards health for all by the year 2000. WHO Tech Rep Ser 4, 1981
12. Kirshner B, Guyatt G: A methodological framework for assessing heath indices. J Chronic Dis 38(1):27, 1985
13. Martin JAM, et al: Childhood deafness in the European community. Scand Audiol 10:165, 1981

14. Nelson SM, Berry, RI: Ear disease and hearing loss among Navajo children—A mass survey. Laryngoscope 94:316, 1984

15. Wong D,Shah C: Identification of impaired hearing in early childhood. Can Med Assoc J 121:529, 1979

16. Schein J, Delk M: The Deaf Population in the United States. National Association for the Deaf, Baltimore, 1974

17. Davis AC: Hearing disorders in the population: First phase findings of the MRC National Study of Hearing, p. 35. In (eds): Hearing Science and Hearing Disorders. Lutman ME, Haggard MP Academic Press, London, 1983

18. Canada Health Survey: The Health of Canadians—Report on the Canada Health Survey. Health and Welfare Canada, Statistics Canada, Ministry of Supply and Services, 1981

19. Parving A, Ostri J, Poulsen J,Gyntelberg F: Epidemiology of hearing impairment in male adult subjects at 49–69 years of age. Scand Audiol 12:191, 1983

20. Hinchcliffe R: Prevalence of the commoner ear, nose, and throat conditions in the adult rural population of Great Britain. Br J Prev Soc Med 15:128, 1961

21. NCHS: Basic Data on Hearing Levels of Adults 25–74 Years United States, 1971–75, Vital Health Statistics 11-26. DHEW 80-1663 40 pp., 1980

22. Sackett DL, Vessey MP: Bias in analytic research. J Chron Dis 32:51, 1979

23. Department of Clinical Epidemiology and Biostatistics: McMaster University, Hamilton, Ontario. Clinical Disagreement. I. How often it occurs and why. Can Med Assoc J 123:499, 1980

24. Department of Clinical Epidemiology and Biostatistics: McMaster University, Hamilton, Ontario. Clinical disagreement II: how to avoid it and how to learn from one's mistakes. Can Med Assoc J 123:613, 1980

25. Department of Clinical Epidemiology and Biostatistics: McMaster University, Hamilton, Ontario. How to read clinical journals. II. To learn about a diagnostic test. Can Med Assoc J 124:703, 1981

26. Feinstein AR: The derangements of the "range of normal." Clin Pharmacol Ther 14:528, 1974

27. Department of Clinical Epidemiology and Biostatistics: McMaster University, Hamilton, Ontario. How to read clinical journals. IV. To determine etiology or causation. Can Med Assoc J 124:985, 1981

28. Sackett DL, Gest M: Controversy in counting and attributing events in clinical trial. N Engl J Med 301:1410, 1979

29. Thomsen J, Bretlau P, Tos M, Johnsen NJ: Placebo effect in surgery for Meniére's disease. Arch Otolaryngol 107:271, 1981

# Pathology of the External and Middle Ear

# 22

## Leslie Michaels

## MALFORMATIONS OF THE EXTERNAL AND MIDDLE EAR

Malformations of the external ear include (1) partial or complete absence of the auricle; (2) accessory auricles; (3) preauricular sinus, which frequently shows a squamous epithelial lining, external to which the connective tissue is chronically inflamed, often with elastic cartilage in the deep wall of the sinus (Fig. 22-1); (4) atresia of the external auditory canal, which may present as a blind protrusion or may be completely absent; and (5) abnormalities of the shape and size of the auricle, which may be ascribed to defects of fusion of the knoblike protrusions and flaws in the hollowing out of the first branchial groove.

In the middle ear, the malleus is more often malformed than the stapes and incus. It may be fused with the body of the incus or fixed to the epitympanum by bone. The incus may also be fixed to the medial wall of the epitympanum. Its long process can be short and placed in an abnormal position in the middle ear cleft. The stapes may be congenitally fixed or the crura distorted. The stapes may show a variety of other anomalies, including complete absence. We have found a particular form of stapedial anomaly to be quite common in the temporal bones of fetuses that had died perinatally.[1] In this lesion, the anterior crus of the stapes is markedly bowed, so that the whole of it appears to be curved forward over the promontory. There is also frequently fusion of the crura (Fig. 22-2). Congenital dehiscence of the bony facial canal in the region of the oval window often occurs. Persistence of the stapedial artery and total absence of the round window are rare conditions. The whole middle ear cavity may be incompletely developed, retaining primitive mesenchyme. Anomalies of the internal and external ear are usually present in conjuction with this lesion.

### Syndromes Involving the Middle Ear

A number of congenital syndromes are seen in which middle ear lesions are combined with abnormalities elsewhere.

#### Treacher Collins' Syndrome

Treacher Collins' syndrome (mandibular dysostosis) is a hereditary malformation, predominantly due to abnormal development of the first branchial arch. The ossicles may be small, deformed, or absent, producing mainly conductive deafness. Other anomalies of this syndrome include notching of the lower eyelids, diminished frontonasal angle, flat-

583

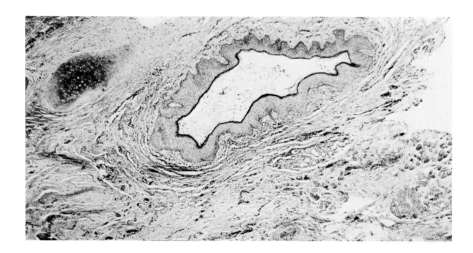

**Fig. 22-1.** Preauricular sinus lined by squamous epithelium. Note cartilage in wall. (H & E, original magnification X 44.)

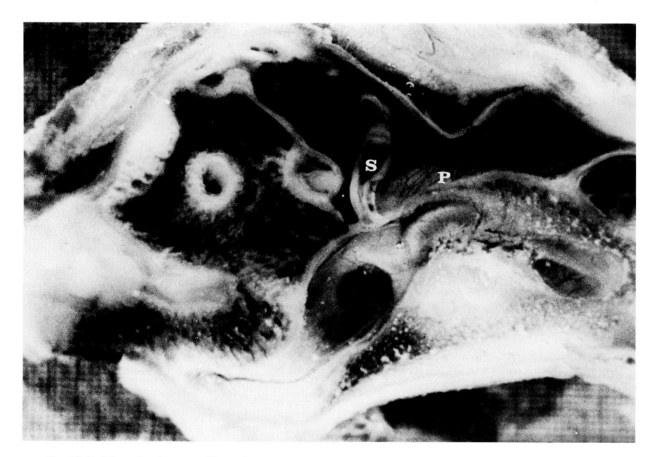

**Fig. 22-2.** Microsliced temporal bone from premature newborn infant showing bowing of stapes with fusion of crura. S, stapes; P, promontory. (Michaels L, Gould SJ, Wells M: The microslicing method in the study of temporal bone changes in the perinatal period. Acta Otolaryngol (Stockh) 423 [suppl]:9, 1985.)

ness of the cheeks, receding mandible, anomalies of the teeth, and deformity of the auricle. The defects are usually bilateral but may be unilateral.

### Crouzon's Syndrome

Crouzon's syndrome (craniofacial dysostosis) is characterized by hypertelorism, exophthalmos, optic atrophy, underdeveloped maxillae, and craniosynostosis. Convulsions and dementia can also occur. Conductive deafness is due to fixation of the stapes footplate and deformed crura. The malleus and incus may also be fixed.

### Hunter-Hurler Syndrome

Hunter-Hurler syndrome (gargoylism) is an inborn metabolic disease characterized by skeletal deformity, blindness, deafness, low-set ears, mental deficiency, and hepatosplenomegaly. The changes are due to the deposition of mucopolysaccharide in many tissues. Deafness is conductive and sensorineural. The middle ear mucosa and vestibular and spiral ganglia of the inner ear may be filled with foamy histiocytes containing one of the abnormally metabolized mucopolysaccharides in their cytoplasm, the so-called gargoyle cells. This material stains positively by the periodic acid-Schiff (PAS) reaction.[2]

### Klippel-Feil Syndrome

Klippel-Feil syndrome consists of congenital fusion of the cervical vertebrae, causing shortening of the neck, low hairline posteriorly, and deafness. The conductive component in the deafness is due to deformed and ankylosed ossicles, and the sensorineural to a rudimentary cochlea and labyrinth.

---

## INFLAMMATORY LESIONS OF THE EXTERNAL EAR

The external ear is subject to a wide variety of inflammatory lesions. Some of these are identical to those that occur elsewhere on the skin. Other lesions are specific to, or most common in, the region of the external ear; only these are considered here.

## Infections

### Diffuse External Otitis

Diffuse external otitis is a common condition affecting the external auditory canal. A variety of organisms, but most commonly *Pseudomonas aeruginosa*, have been recovered from the inflammatory exudate in diffuse external otitis. It is likely that bacterial infection is only one of the causative factors. Equally significant are a hot humid environment and local trauma to the ear canal.[3]

The skin of the ear canal is erythematous and edomatous and gives off a greenish discharge. In the severe form of the condition, histologic examination of the epidermis reveals marked acanthosis, hyperkeratosis, and an acute inflammatory exudate in the dermis, particularly around the apocrine glands.

### Perichondritis

Perichondritis most commonly affects the pinna, where it may follow surgical trauma. As in the diffuse acute inflammation of the ear canal, *Pseudomonas aeruginosa* is the most common infecting organism. Pus accumulates between the perichondrium and cartilage of the pinna, interfering with the blood supply of the cartilage and leading to necrosis.

### Malignant External Otitis

Malignant external otitis was first described by Chandler[4] in 1968, who defined it as a severe infection of the external auditory canal, usually in elderly diabetics, resulting in unremitting pain, purulent discharge and invasion of cartilage, nerve, bone, and adjacent soft tissue. The causative agent in all cases is said to be *Pseudomonas aeruginosa*. The condition frequently goes on to 9th, 10th, 11th, and 12th cranial nerve palsies, as well as meningitis and death.

A study of the histopathologic changes in the temporal bones of three patients diagnosed clinically as having malignant external otitis thought to have died of this condition demonstrated that the changes were those of a severe otitis media with involvement of the jugular foramen by the inflammatory process[5] (Fig. 22-3). The jugular bulb was

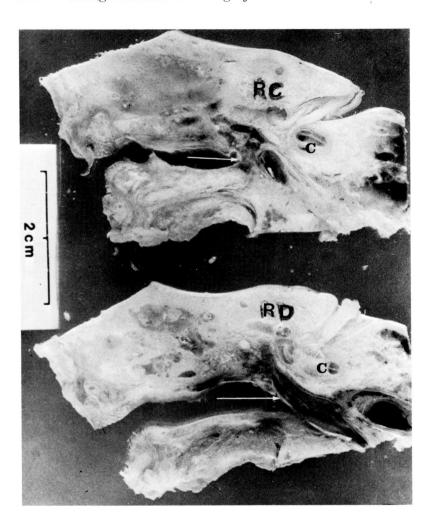

**Fig. 22-3.** Microsliced temporal bone from patient diagnosed clinically as having malignant otitis media. The external auditory canal shows no inflammation. The epithelium of the posterior and anterior wall is well defined in each slice. The middle ear is filled with purulent exudate, which was the source of the inflammation in the jugular foramen region. Arrow points to the tympanic membrane. C, cochlea: RC, upper and RD, lower temporal bone slices.

thrombosed and inflamed in each case. We could find no pathway for the spread of infection to the apex of the temporal bone by injection of toluidine blue solution under pressure, into the wall of the external auditory canal of fresh cadavers.

It seems likely that the manifestations of malignant external otitis are due to the spread of inflammation from the middle ear to the petrous apex via air cells, through the bone marrow spaces by a process of osteomyelitis or by thrombophlebitis of the jugular bulb. The frequency of this condition in elderly patients with diabetes mellitus is probably due to the tendency of diabetics and old people to suffer serious degrees of otitis media. Otitis externa is a common complication of otitis media, the clini-

cal effects of which may overshadow the middle ear inflammation. The role of *Pseudomonas aeruginosa* is poorly understood. It is a frequent cause of infection in diabetics and commonly infects the external ear. It seems unlikely that it is the basis for the deep-seated necrotic lesions described in association with malignant otitis externa. Evidence of infection by anaerobic organisms has been discovered in several cases with such a diagnosis at our hospital.

**Fungus Infections**

Fungi are uncommon causes of external otitis. Superficial pathogenic fungi that occasionally infect the external ear include *Trichophyton rubrum*,

*Microphyton audouini*, and *Candida albicans*, The latter not uncommonly produces a low-grade infection after radical mastoidectomy. *Aspergillus fumigatus* and *A. nigrans* are also cultivated with some frequency from infected ear canals. Deep pathogenic fungus infections are rare and include North American blastomycosis (*Blastomyces dermatidis*), histoplasmosis (*Histoplasma capsulatum*), coccidiodomycosis (*Coccidioides immitis*), and cryptococcosis (*Cryptococcus neoformans*).

### Viral Infections

**Bullous Myringitis.** Presumed to be caused by a virus, bullous myringitis is characterized by the development of vesicular or hemorrhagic bullae on the external aspect of the tympanic membrane. The lesion develops during an acute upper respiratory infection and is associated with severe pain.[3]

**Herpes Simplex.** Both type 1 and type 2 herpes virus (HSV-1 and HSV-2) may cause blisters in the ear canal. Microscopic diagnosis may be made by examination of scrapings from the vesicles. The presence of giant cells with intranuclear inclusions is suggestive of herpes simplex, but identical changes may be found in herpes zoster. The virus may be detected in the epidermal cells by direct immunofluorescence.[6] The histologic appearance is characterized by an intraepidermal vesicle produced by acantholysis of epidermal cells. Ballooning degeneration, in which the swollen cells have a homogeneous eosinophilic cytoplasm, and reticular degeneration, in which the epidermal cells are distended by intracellular edema, are characteristic of the epidermis surrounding the vesicle.[7]

**Herpes Zoster.** This condition is caused by the virus of chicken pox—herpes varicella virus—which travels from the nerve ganglia to the skin along the nerves. When the geniculate ganglion is affected, a vesicular eruption of the pinna, ear canal, postauricular skin, uvula, palate, and anterior tongue is produced. When combined with disturbances of hearing and balance due to involvement of the ganglia of the 8th nerve, the condition is termed Ramsay Hunt syndrome. The skin lesions are histologically similar to those of herpes simplex virus.

### Parasitic Infestation

Parasitic infestations of the external ear are usually part of more general skin infestations. Pediculosis capitis due to the head louse, *Pediculus humanus*, and scabies due to *Sarcoptes scabii* are most likely to affect the external ear.[3]

## Noninfective Inflammatory Lesions

### Starch Granuloma

Granulomatous inflammatory lesions due to contamination by cornstarch glove powder have commonly been encountered in the peritoneum and pleura after surgical operations. Granulomatous inflammatory lesions in reaction to starch granules may also be seen in ear canal and middle ear. The starch in the latter cases is derived not from surgical glove powder but insufflations of antibiotic in which it is used as a vehicle. The antibiotic with its base is insufflated into the external ear in the treatment of external or middle ear otitis. Microscopically, there is an exudate of histiocytes and lymphocytes. Granules of starch are easily recognized as spherical or polyhedral basophilic bodies, 10 to 20 $\mu$m in diameter, often within histiocytes. The granules show a Maltese cross birefringence and a brilliant red coloration after staining with PAS reagent[8] (Figs. 22-4 and 22-5).

### Hair Granuloma

Biopsy sections taken from inflammatory lesions of the ear canal commonly reveal a granulomatous reaction of foreign-body type. Within the granuloma, foreign-body giant cells are seen surrounding and engulfing hair shafts (Figs. 22-6 and 22-7). I have also seen such lesions deep in the ear canal in postmortem temporal bone specimens in which there is no middle ear inflammation and the tympanic membrane is intact.

The hairs in hair granulomas of the ear canal are derived from the patient's own hair, possibly by ingrowth from those near the orifice of the canal, in the same fashion as occurs in cases of pilonidal sinus of the sacroiliac skin. In some instances, the hair may enter the ear canal after hair-cutting. Here one finds very short cuttings of hair, which have been

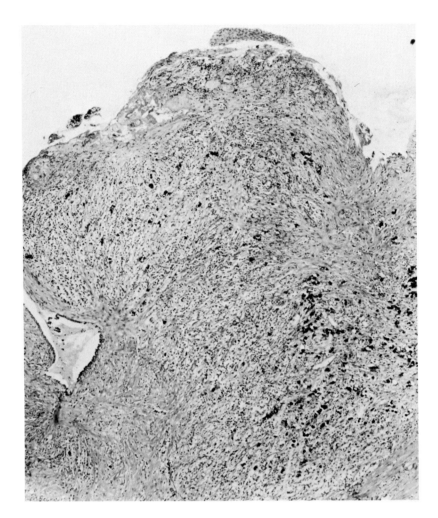

**Fig. 22-4.** Starch granuloma of the mucosa of the middle ear. There is an active chronic inflammation within which are numerous starch granules which appear black in the photograph and red in the original. (Periodic acid–Schiff, original magnification X 75.)

observed to reach as far as the tympanic membrane, where they may cause tinnitus.

## Inflammatory Lesions of Unknown Origin

### Relapsing Polychondritis

Relapsing polychondritis is a disease characterized by recurring bouts of inflammation affecting cartilaginous structures and the eye. Although the cartilage of the external ear is most frequently involved, it is the inflammation with destruction of the cartilage of the respiratory tract, particularly the larynx, which is life-threatening; in most cases

in which death has resulted from this condition, it was caused by respiratory obstruction due to damage to the cartilage.

**Age and Sex Incidence.** Relapsing polychondritis may commence at any age, but 80 percent of patients experience their first symptoms between the ages of 20 and 60. The incidence is equal between the sexes.

**Clinical Features.** Presenting symptoms of relapsing polychondritis are related to inflammation of a wide variety of cartilages, the various tissues of the eye, and the aortic valve. The structures involved in the inflammation are as follows, in descending order of frequency[9]:

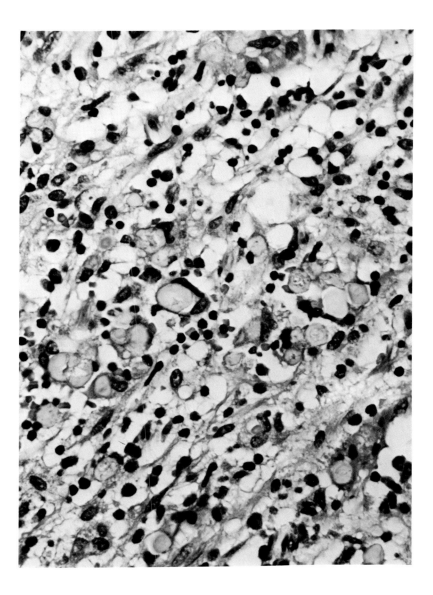

**Fig. 22-5.** Starch granuloma of middle ear. Starch grains are oval, pale gray structures (basophilic in the original), and are often within the cytoplasm of histiocytes. Lymphocytes and plasma cells are also present. (H & E, original magnification X 700.)

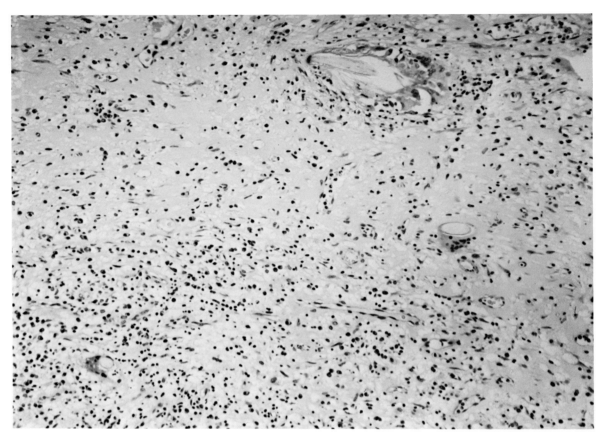

**Fig. 22-6.** Hair shaft granuloma from skin of ear canal. Within the chronic inflammatory tissue, three hair shafts are seen, each engulfed by a foreign-body type giant cell. (H & E, original magnification X 175.)

Ear cartilage
Joint cartilage
Nasal cartilage
Laryngeal and tracheal cartilages
Eye (various tissues)
Costal cartilages
Cardiac valves (usually aortic; occasionally mitral and tricuspid)

The most common site of the disease is the cartilage of the pinna, which becomes inflamed recurrently. A conductive or, more rarely, sensorineural deafness and attacks of vertigo may take occur, but the pathologic bases for these symptoms are unknown. After numerous attacks of inflammation, the pinna shrinks and falls forward. Inflammation of the joints is usually manifested as transient arthralgia, pri-marily involving the large joints of the extremities. The nasal cartilages are often affected, and the in-flammation of the nasal septum causes this struc-ture to sink, producing a saddle-nose appearance. Involvement of laryngeal and tracheal cartilages is associated with tenderness over the larynx. Inflam-mation of the eye usually takes the form of epis-cleritis or scleritis, but iritis, conjunctivitis, or ker-atitis may also be found in relapsing polychondritis. The involvement of the rib cartilages is manifested as tenderness over the ribs anteriorly and the xi-phoid process. Cardiac lesions are characteristi-cally aortic, showing signs of regurgitation. Mitral and tricuspid dilatations are also encountered oc-casionally in some patients. Features of rheumatoid arthritis, systemic lupus erythematosus (SLE), an-kylosing spondylitis, and Reiter's disease have

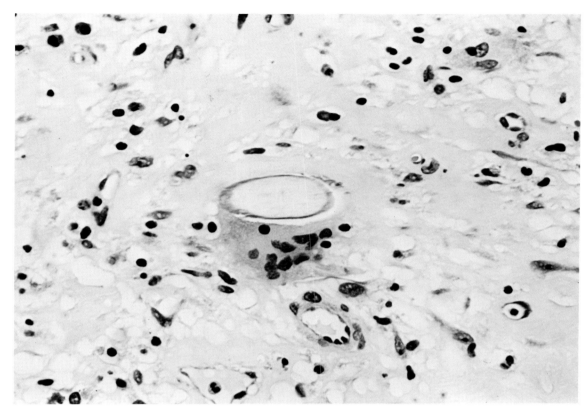

**Fig. 22-7.** Higher-power view of part of Fig. 22-6 showing hair shaft and foreign-body type giant cell. (H & E, original magnification X 700.)

been seen in some cases to coexist with relapsing polychondritis.[9]

**Gross Appearance.** The lobule is usually normal in relapsing polychondritis. In the acute stage, the auricle is erythematous. The anterior surface may have a cobblestone appearance[3] (Fig. 22-8), and it may eventually become atrophic. In the larynx, the epiglottic, thyroid, and cricoid cartilages show loss of cartilage substance and fibrosis. The result may be loss of normal cartilaginous support, particularly in the cricoid region, which may lead to laryngeal obstruction.

**Microscopic Appearance.** The histologic appearance of relapsing polychondritis suggests a primary change of cartilage prior to invasion by inflammatory tissue. The ground substance of the cartilage becomes acidophilic, except for basophilia around some surviving lacunae, and shows deeper staining by the PAS method. In the cartilage near the interface with inflammatory tissue, there is compression of lacunae, which often appear linear. Verity et al.[10] mentioned focal calcification and dystrophic ossification of the degenerate cartilage in their autopsied cases. The early inflammatory exudate is composed of neutrophils. Later, it is formed mainly by plasma cells and lymphocytes, with some areas of histiocytes (Fig. 22-9). Fibroblasts multiply, and eventually a dense, poorly cellular scar results. Hughes et al.[9] described in one of their cases an endstage of cystic spaces containing gelatinous fluid in the degenerated cartilage.

**Immunologic Findings.** Autoantibodies to type II collagen have been found in cases of relapsing polychondritis.[11] It is of interest, in view of the frequent occurrence of ocular inflammation in relapsing polychondritis, that type II collagen is a

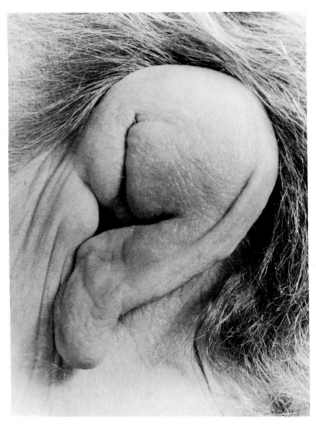

**Fig. 22-8.** Pinna in a case of relapsing polychondritis. Note contractures producing distortion and cobblestone appearance of skin.

constituent of both eye and cartilage. Autoantibodies to cartilage[9] and cell-mediated immunity to cartilage have been described in the lymphocytes of cases of relapsing polychondritis.[12] The significance of these general immunologic findings specifically for relapsing polychondritis is doubtful. Autoantibodies to cartilage, for instance, may be detected in the serum of cases of rheumatoid arthritis and after infectious mononucleosis.[9]

Increasing evidence derived from direct tissue studies indicates that relapsing polychondritis may be related to deposition of immune complexes in the vicinity of chondrocytes. Using fluorescence methods, Valenzuela et al.[13] were able to find immunoglobulins and the C3 component of complement at the chondrofibrous junction in biopsies of inflamed ear cartilage. In unpublished observa-

tions, I have found using the immunoperoxidase method in cartilage biopsies of the cricoid and pinna, each from separate cases of relapsing polychondritis, that IgG and C3 component of complement are present in the lacunae of the cartilage (Fig. 22-10). Chondrocytes from normal auricular cartilage and a variety of inflammatory lesions of the ear and larynx did not show such deposits. The findings lend support to the possibility that immune complexes play a part in the pathogenesis of relapsing polychondritis.

**Keratosis Obturans**

In keratosis obturans, cholesteatoma of the external auditory canal, keratin implantation granuloma, the keratin produced by exfoliation from the skin of the ear canal is retained on the epithelial surface and forms a solid plug. This enlarges and may cause erosion of the bony ear canal. Cholesterol deposition and secondary infection with *Pseudomonas* sp., *Proteus* sp., or *Staphylococcus aureus* may occur within the keratinous mass. The conditions labelled keratosis obturans and cholesteatoma of the external auditory meatus have been considered to be the same process. Piepergerdes et al.,[14] however, suggest that the term keratosis obturans be preferred for the condition described above. It is usually associated with a thickened tympanic membrane and the patients also frequently suffer from chronic sinusitis or bronchiectasis. By contrast, cholesteatoma of the ear canal is a process of localized erosion of the inferior and posterior ear canal wall by a squamous epithelial-lined sac derived from the epidermis of the canal.

The etiologic basis of both conditions is obscure. It is possible that there may be a defect of the normal migratory properties of the squamous epithelium of tympanic membrane and adjacent ear canal that leads to the accumulation of keratinous debris.

Hawke and Jahn[15] describe a granulomatous process that may occur in the external ear canal in reaction to keratin squames, which become implanted into the deeper tissues following traumatic laceration of the ear canal. The granuloma contains foreign-body giant cells, histiocytes, lymphocytes, plasma cells, and flakes of keratin. Aural polyps frequently contain such granulomas, but the keratin is often derived from a middle ear cholesteatoma.

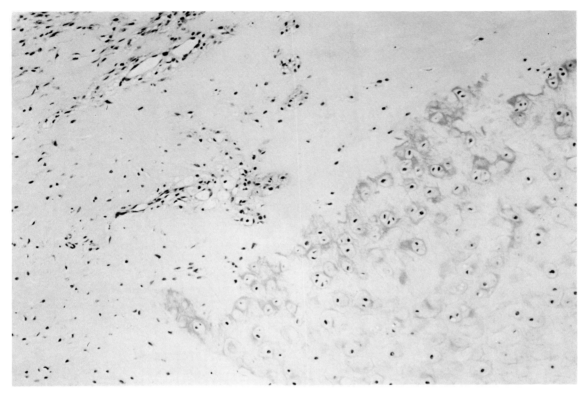

**Fig. 22-9.** Relapsing polychondritis of elastic cartilage of pinna. The cartilage (above) is eroded by histiocytes, lymphocytes and collagen material. (H & E, original magnification X 175.)

## METABOLIC CONDITIONS

A number of metabolic conditions may become manifest in the tissues of the ear.

### Porphyria Cutanea Tarda

The porphyrias are characterized by a disturbance of porphyrin metabolism with resultant increased excretion of porphyrin or its precursors. The defect is the result of an overproduction of intermediates of haem biosynthesis. Porphyria cutanea tarda is a form of porphyria associated with chronic skin disease. Vesicular and ulcerative lesions are common on the external ear. The urine may be brown or pink and contains high levels of uroporphyrin.

The histologic appearance of the affected skin is one of deposits of hyaline material on the basement membrane of the floor of the vesicle and around blood vessels. The hyaline deposits are best seen by the PAS stain, when they appear bright red.[7] PAS positivity of these deposits persists after treatment of the section with diastase.

### Gout

Gout is usually manifested as an acute arthritis. It is related to deposits of urates in the joint capsule —most frequently in the big toe joint—and as tophi containing urates in nonarticular tissues. The external ear is one of the most frequent places for the latter and deposits may occur in the helix and anthelix. They may ulcerate, discharging a creamy white material within which needlelike crystals of sodium urate may be detected on microscopy.

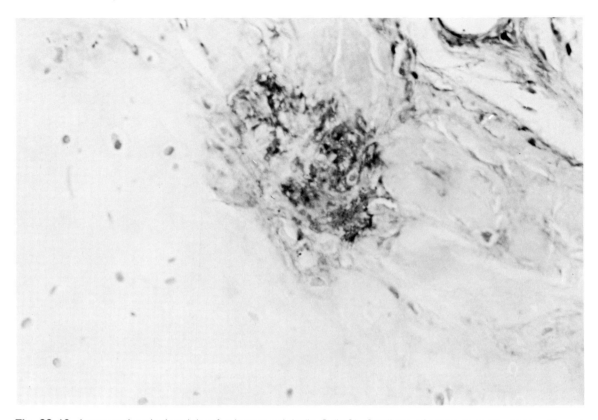

**Fig. 22-10.** Immunochemical staining for immunoglobulin G (IgG). Cartilage of pinna near interface with perichondrium in a case of relapsing polychondritis. Many of the cartilage lacunae are reactive for IgG. (Immunoperoxidase, original magnification X 700.)

Histologically, the gouty tophus is composed of basophilic masses of amorphous material surrounded by foreign-body giant cells and histiocytes. The sodium urate crystals are soluble in water and so are dissolved in the formaldehyde usually used for fixation. For this reason, fixation in alcohol is preferred when a gouty tophus is suspected. A few crystals may then remain and be identified as brownish, closely packed, needlelike structures that are birefringent.

## Ochronosis

Ochronosis (alkaptonuria) is an inherited disease of metabolism in which a step in tyrosine metabolism is disturbed, resulting in accumulation of homogentisic acid in a variety of places, but especially cartilages. The substance is colorless in the urine when first passed but darkens to a black or brown polymer on standing. The disease is inherited as an autosomal-recessive trait.

In the external ear, there may be one or both of two manifestations: (1) dark color of the wax (when seen in a child, this may be the first manifestation of ochronosis); or (2) dark color of the aural cartilage due to the binding of the homogentisic acid to the cartilage ground substance.

## Xanthoma Associated with Hyperlipoproteinemia

Hyperlipoproteinemia is classified into types I through V, depending on which fraction of lipoprotein is prominent on electrophoretic fractionation of the plasma. All the hyperlipoproteinemic conditions are transmitted by inheritance as a dom-

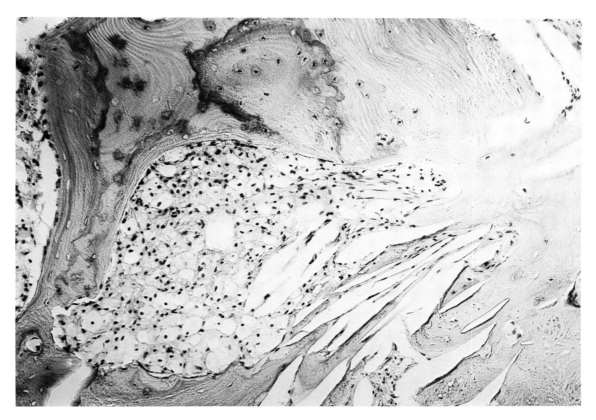

**Fig. 22-11.** Xanthomatous deposit in mastoid associated with type V hyperlipoproteinemia. Marrow spaces and bone trabeculae are infiltrated by foam cells and cholesterol clefts, the latter accompanied by a foreign-body type giant cell reaction. (H & E, original magnification X 175.)

inant or recessive trait. Some of the types are associated with cutaneous and tendinous xanthomas and severe atherosclerotic coronary artery disease. In rare cases, deposits of lipid with an associated histiocytic reaction may be found in the temporal bone.[16]

A 67-year-old man seen at the Royal National Throat, Nose and Ear Hospital, exhibited an extensive destructive and reparative process involving the petromastoid on radiography. The patient was found to have high plasma triglyceride, cholesterol, and very-low-density lipoproteins (VLDLs) indicating a diagnosis of type V hyperlipoproteinemia. Histologic examination of a surgical biopsy of mastoid bone showed infiltration of bone trabeculae and marrow spaces by numerous foam cells and needlelike clefts with foreign-body giant cell reaction. The bone trabeculae showed fraying by the

lipid granuloma and irregular cement lines (Fig. 22-11). The appearances were similar to those of cholesterol granuloma except that there was no trace of hemorrhage or hemosiderin, foam cells were more numerous than usual in cholesterol granuloma, and the lipid deposits and their cellular reaction mainly involved the bone itself and not the mucosa of the mastoid air cells.[17]

## LESIONS SIMULATING NEOPLASMS

A variety of lesions may be found in the external and middle ears that may show some similarity to neoplasms.

## Malacoplakia

Malacoplakia is a chronic inflammatory condition characterized by accumulation of macrophages and presence of characteristic bodies. The lesion may be confused with neoplasm. Only a single case has been described in which this lesion affected the ear.[18] The patient was a 10-year-old boy with a 7th nerve palsy, a mass of vascular tissue in the ear canal, postauricular swelling, and the presence of abnormal tissue in the mastoid. Microscopic examination showed malacoplakia characterized by macrophages with abundant cytoplasm containing diastase-resistant PAS-positive granules (von Hansemann cells). Lamellated, calcified (Michaelis-Guttmann) bodies, often with macrophages were also frequently present (Fig. 22-12).

Malacoplakia is usually associated with a coliform infection and a defective response to phagocytized *Escherichia coli* has been identified in that condition. It is possible that malacoplakia may be commoner in the middle and external ears than would appear by the sole case report, since otologists frequently do not submit for histologic examination material from chronic inflammatory conditions of the ear.

## Chondrodermatitis Nodularis Chronica Helicis

In chondrodermatitis nodularis chronica helicis, sometimes known as Winkler's disease,[19] a small nodule forms on the auricle, usually in the superior portion of the helix. About 70 percent of the pa-

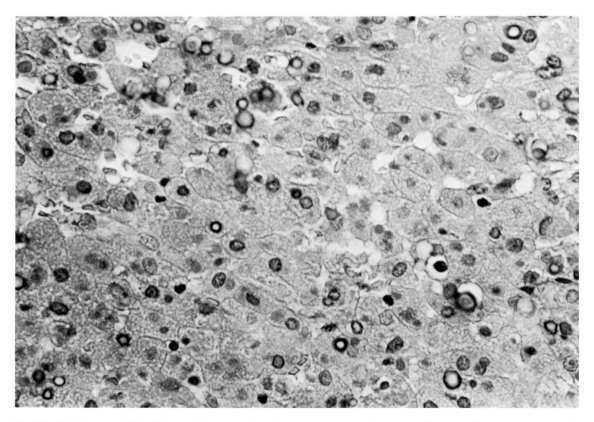

**Fig. 22-12.** Malacoplakia of the middle ear. The tissue is composed of macrophages with abundant granular cytoplasm. Note also numerous calcified Michaelis-Guttmann bodies. (H & E, original magnification X 700.)

tients are males.[20] The lesion is found in middle or older-aged patients. Pain is often a prominent feature. Histologically, the nodule usually shows ulceration with marked irregular acanthosis at its margins. The collagen at the center of the dermis shows increased eosinophilia, is often degenerate, and is surrounded by chronic inflammatory granulation tissue. The perichondrium adjacent to the lesion is usually involved by the inflammatory tissue and the elastic cartilage of the auricle is also often degenerated (Figs. 22-13 and 22-14).

It seems most likely that chondrodermatitis nodularis is related to poor blood supply at the periphery of the auricle and in the opinion of Winkler[19] there was an association with frostbite; this opinion is still commonly held by many, although some published reports do not support this.[20] Injection of corticosteroids into the lesion has been recommended before resorting to surgery for this condition.[20]

## Spectacle Frame Acanthoma

Spectacle frame acanthoma (granuloma fissuratum) occurs behind the ear in the region of the postauricular groove, where it is commonly mistaken for basal cell carcinoma at clinical examination. A similar reaction may occur on the bridge of

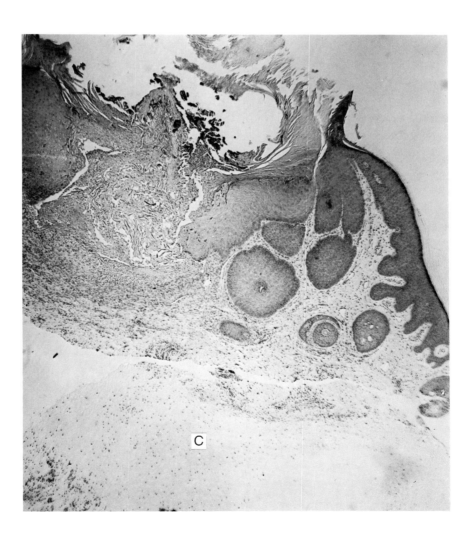

**Fig. 22-13.** Chondrodermatitis nodularis chronica helicis. There is an irregular acanthosis at the margins of an ulcer, the crater of which is occupied by necrotic eosinophilic material. Inflammation extends down into the cartilage of the pinna (C). (H & E, original magnification X 44.)

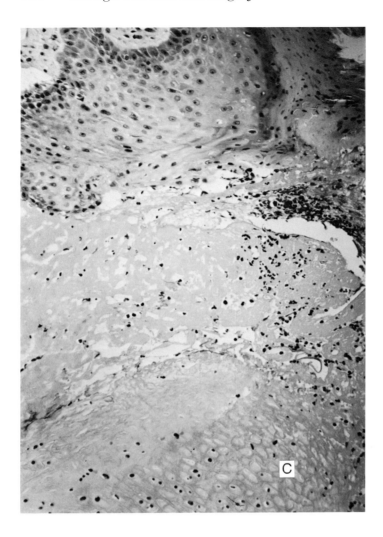

**Fig. 22-14.** Chondrodermatitis nodularis chronica helicis. In this example the cartilage (C) is eroded by the acute inflammation. Note the acanthotic squamous epithelium nearby. (H & E, original magnification X 175.)

the nose or above the malar area. The cause is irritation by the frame of spectacles. Grossly, there is a raised pink nodule with a linear depression running through its center (Fig. 22-15). The spectacle frame usually fits exactly into the depression when in its usual position.[21] Histologically, there is acanthosis and chronic inflammation of the dermis. A shallow sulcus may be seen at the center of the specimen containing keratin and parakeratotic material (Fig. 22-16).

The acanthoma is readily treated by making appropriate alterations in the shape of the spectacle frame, so that it no longer presses into the skin.

## Benign Angiomatous Nodules of Face and Scalp

Benign angiomatous nodules of the face and scalp (atypical pyogenic granuloma and Kimura's disease) may occur anywhere in the skin, particularly on the scalp and face, but there is a particular predilection for the external auricle and external auditory canal.[22] It is a lesion of young and middle aged of both sexes.

Grossly, there are sessile or plaquelike red or reddish-blue lesions from 2 to 10 mm in diameter, which may coalesce to form large plaques that ob-

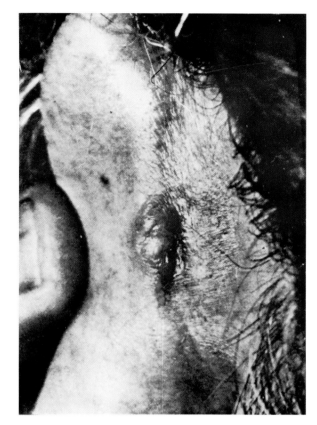

**Fig. 22-15.** Spectacle frame acanthoma producing a nodule in postauricular groove. Note the linear depression running across it. (Barnes HM, Calman CD, Sarkany I: Spectacle frame acanthoma (granuloma fissuratum). Trans St Johns Hosp Dermatol Soc 60:99, 1974.)

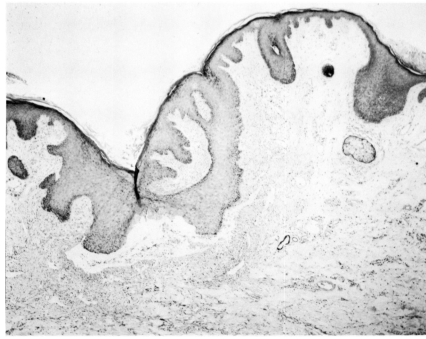

**Fig. 22-16.** Spectacle frame acanthoma. Note moderate acanthosis and inflammation of dermis. The sulcus in the epidermis corresponds to the linear depression seen grossly (see Fig. 22-15) (H & E, original magnification X 44.)

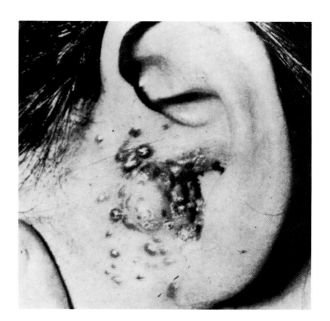

**Fig. 22-17.** Benign angiomatous nodules (Kimura's disease) of external ear. Reddish nodules have formed on and near the tragus and in the ear canal. (Medonca DR: Pseudo (atypical) pyogenic granuloma of the ear. J Laryngol Otol 87:577, 1973.)

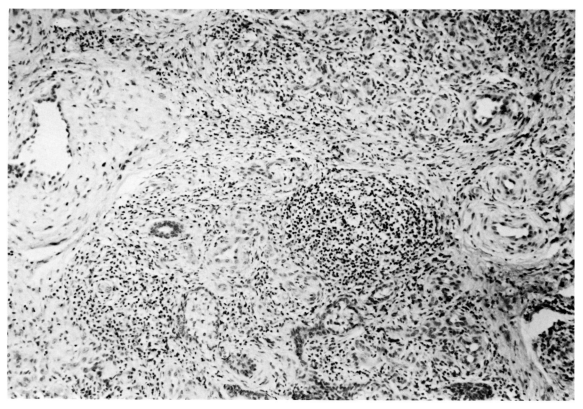

**Fig. 22-18.** Benign angiomatous nodules (Kimura's disease) of external ear. Note abundant capillaries and lymphoid tissue. (H & E, original magnification X 175.)

struct the ear canal (Fig. 22-17). Microscopically, there is a mixture of two proliferated elements in the dermis: blood vessels and lymphoid tissue. The blood vessels are often capillaries lined by plump, sometimes multilayered, endothelial cells. Occasionally, an artery or vein showing intimal fibrous thickening is part of the vascular component. The lymphoid tissue may possess germinal centers. Eosinophils, mast cells, and macrophages may also be prominent (Figs. 22-18 and 22-19). Direct immunofluorescence has shown that deposits of IgA, IgG, and C3 are present around small vessels of the lesion, suggesting that there may be an immunologic basis to the condition.[23]

### Idiopathic Cystic Chondromalacia

Idiopathic cystic chondromalacia (pseudocysts) is an unusual lesion of the cartilage of the auricle that has been the subject of but little investigation.[24,25] It occurs mainly in young and middle-aged adults, usually males but occasionally females. The gross appearance is one of a localized swelling of the auricular cartilage. Cut surface shows a well-defined cyst cavity in the cartilage distended with yellowish watery fluid. Microscopically, the cyst is a simple space with a lining of normal cartilage. There is no inflammation nor any type of lining cellular layer. Simple curettage cures the lesion.

### Keloid

Keloid is a common benign skin lesion that follows injury to the skin on the ear, particularly after incision, even by piercing of the lobule for wearing an earring. It is very frequent in blacks. Grossly, there is a lobulated swelling covered by normal

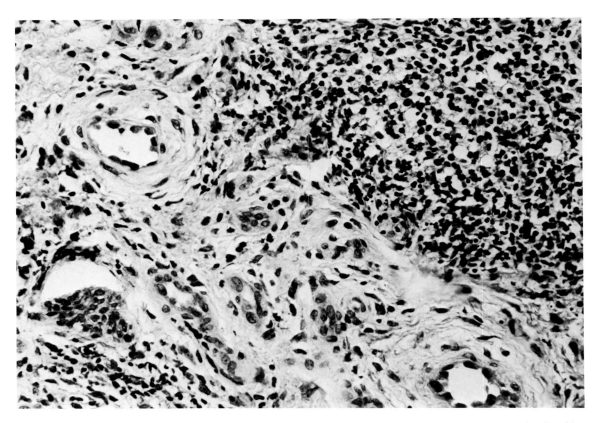

**Fig. 22-19.** Benign angiomatous nodules (Kimura's disease) of external ear. Note abundant capillaries lined by plump endotheilial cells and lymphoid tissue. Capillary in the bottom left-hand corner is lined by multilayered endothelium. (H & E, original magnification X 440.)

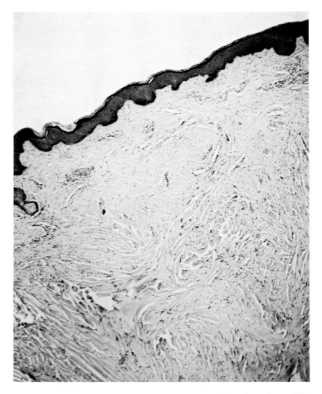

**Fig. 22-20.** Keloid of lobule of ear from a black patient. The dermis is expanded by deposits of eosinophilic hyaline collagen. (H & E, original magnification X 44.)

skin. Microscopically, the dermis is enlarged by deposits of eosinophilic poorly cellular collagen (Fig. 22-20).

## OTITIS MEDIA

Infection of the middle ear causes not only generally known inflammatory changes but also other changes peculiar to the site. Otitis media is one of the most common of all diseases, particularly in young children. The clinical forms of the acute and chronic condition correspond to the pathologic changes, but intermediate or mild states are frequent. The presence or absence of perforation of the tympanic membrane accounts for the two initial subgroups. A third subgroup of otitis media involves an intact membrane but the presence of effusion in the middle ear:

1. Otitis media without effusion or perforation of the tympanic membrane
2. Otitis media with effusion, but without perforation of the tympanic membrane (serous otitis media)
3. Otitis media with perforation of the tympanic membrane

These conditions may be acute, subacute, or chronic.

### Microbiology

In the acute phase, *Streptococcus pneumoniae* and *Hemophilus influenzae* are the most common causative organisms. Epidemiologic studies have indicated certain respiratory viruses as possible agents in the early phases of the illness.[26] In the chronic phase, gram-negative organisms, particularly *Proteus* and *Pseudomonas*, are found, although *Staphylococcus pyogenes* and β-hemolytic streptococci are sometimes isolated from the discharging pus of chronically inflamed ears.

Although much less frequent than the above organisms *Mycobacterium tuberculosis* may be the causative agent of chronic inflammation of the middle ear. In such cases, the inflammatory reaction is quite distinct.

### General Pathologic Changes

The acute phase of otitis media is characterized by a severe congestion of the mucosa of the middle ear and the tympanic membrane (Table 22-1). It is not generally realized that congestion of the mucosa is frequently also a marked feature of chronic otitis media. Congestion of blood vessels (i.e., increased local blood flow) is the means by which phagocytic and other immunologically significant inflammatory cells and substances are brought to the site of the infection. The passage of both the fluid and solid constituents from the blood is called exudation. The fluid portion of blood, plasma, may leave a deposit of fibrin in the tissues. A fluid exudate in the middle ear cavity is frequently a prominent component of the inflammatory reaction—a specific form of the disease known as otitis media with effusion. In these cases, mucus may be secreted by newly formed glands in the middle ear mucosa and contributes to the fluid exudate. In

**Table 22-1. Pathologic Processes in Otitis Media**

| Process | Cell or Tissue | Pathologic Change |
|---|---|---|
| Congestion | | |
| Exudation | Plasma | Serous otitis media |
| | Histiocytes, lymphocytes, plasma cells | Chronic inflammation |
| | Red cells | Hemorrhage Cholesterol granuloma |
| Proliferation | Columnar epithelium | Glandular change |
| | Squamous cell epithelium | Cholesteatoma |
| | Blood vessels, fibroblasts, mononuclear cells | Granulation tissue |
| | Fibroblasts, collagen | Adhesive otitis |
| | Bone | Woven and lamellar bone formation |
| Necrosis | Tympanic membrane | Perforation |
| | Bone | Rarefying osteitis |

acute inflammation, neutrophils are prevalent. In chronic inflammation histiocytes (derived from monocytes of the blood), lymphocytes and plasma cells (derived from lymphocytes) are the characteristic cells. Organisms are seen very rarely in histologic sections of acute or chronic inflammation of the middle ear. In newborn infants, an inflammatory reaction may be the result of contamination of the middle ear by inhaled amniotic squames. In these cases, the histiocytes reacting to the foreign material fuse to form giant cells. Hemorrhage is a common result of the congestion of otitis media. It may lead to cholesterol granuloma.

Local tissue cells frequently react to the inflammatory process by dissolution or proliferation. Necrosis may occur, as is characteristic of perforation of the tympanic membrane or in rarefying osteitis of the ossicles. Several processes may produce the necrosis. It is likely that rupture of the tympanic membrane takes place as a result of ischemic necrosis caused by pressure at a focal point. By contrast, ossicular loss may be caused by substances such as collagenase produced by the inflammatory connective tissue on the surface of the ossicle.[27]

Simultaneous to the process of necrosis, proliferative activity of middle ear tissue occurs and may become an important part of the pathologic picture. The columnar epithelium of the middle ear has in the presence of inflammation the remarkable property of invaginating itself to produce glands that often develop luminal secretion. The glandular transformation of the middle ear mucosa may be seen in any part of the cleft including the mastoid air cells. Fibrous tissue proliferation may also occur in combination with glandular transformation — a process that Schuknecht[28] called fibrocystic sclerosis. Squamous cell epithelium may likewise proliferate in the middle ear — a process known as cholesteatoma. A specific form of reparative reaction following inflammation is the development of granulation tissue. In this process the endothelium of blood vessels and fibroblasts are the newly formed cells. Mononuclear inflammatory cells usually accompany the latter. Fibroblasts and collagen are abundant in the terminal phase of the reparative stage. A normal degree of cellularity in the fibrous reaction is seen in adhesive otitis. A peculiar form of scar tissue production occurs in the middle ear, in which the collagen is poorly cellular and hyalinized. This condition, known as tympanosclerosis, is also characterized by deposition of calcium salts in the hyaline fibrous tissue. The bony walls of the middle ear frequently react to the inflammatory process by a new formation of bone. This is woven during the early stages and lamellar later.

## Acute Otitis Media

### Incidence and Clinical Features

The incidence of acute otitis media as seen in hospital practice in developed countries has declined over the past 25 years because of the ready availability of antibiotics and improved socioeconomic conditions. Children are more often affected than adults.

The clinical features are general signs of infection, pain (particularly in the mastoid area), tenderness and swelling in the postauricular region, and edema of the posterosuperior wall of the external auditory canal. The tympanic membrane is initially hyperemic and then bulges as more pus collects in the middle ear, until eventually it may burst.

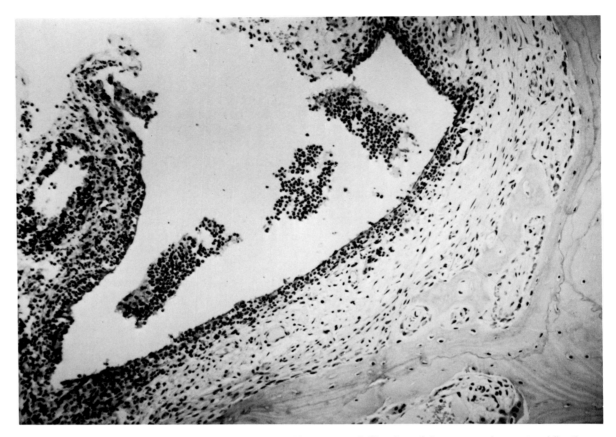

**Fig. 22-21.** Acute inflammation of mastoid air cell. Note severe infiltration of the mucosa by neutrophils; these cells are present in the lumen. Osteoid is deposited on the right and osteoclastic resorption of bone can be identified at the bottom right. (H & E, original magnification X 175.)

### Pathologic Appearance

The appearance of the middle ear mucosa as seen in the bone chips removed at mastoidectomy has been described by Friedmann.[27] The mucosa of the mastoid air cells is congested and edematous. Hemorrhage may be severe and the mucosa and air cells are filled with neutrophils. Loss of bone tissue occurs, the actual dissolution being carried out by osteoclasts. At the same time, new bone formation takes place, commencing as osteoid, later becoming woven and finally lamellar (Fig. 22-21). Fibrosis may also be active, even in the acute stage.

Acute inflammatory changes are also prominent in other parts of the middle ear. The tympanic membrane shows marked congestion, the dilated vessels distending the connective tissue layer. Pus cells fill the middle ear cavity. The acute inflammation may spread deep into the temporal bone as osteomyelitis.

## Chronic Otitis Media

### Clinical Features

The inflammation, while often indolent, may give rise to serious complications and even cause death. The hearing loss that is a constant concomitant also contributes to the immense socioeconomic problem. Chronic otitis media sometimes, but not always, follows an attack of the acute disease.

The major feature is discharge from the middle ear. Sometimes polyps may occlude the external auditory canal. The tympanic membrane is usually perforated in the pars tensa.

## Gross Appearance

There has been little study of the gross appearances of chronic otitis media, except at surgical operation, when the examination of the middle ear cleft is limited to the operation field. With the use of the microslicing method a more complete gross examination of the whole middle ear may be carried out at postmortem. An important feature of chronic otitis media is the variation in the degree and extent of the inflammation. The tubotympanic region is the most frequently involved; mastoid air cells may also be affected, and there is variation in the groups of air cells so inflamed. Mucopurulent material often fills the middle ear in the tubotympanic region and may also be seen in mastoid air cells. In the inflamed regions the mucosa is thickened and congestion may be severe. Granulation tissue formation may be extensive, showing as red thickened areas, particularly on the promontory, in the epitympanum, in the round and oval window niches and in the mastoid. The granulation tissue on the promontory mucosa may be of sufficient thickness to protrude through the perforation in the tympanic membrane. Such a lesion is the common aural polyp presenting clinically in the ear canal.

A variable degree of loss of ossicular bone may be observed. The most frequently affected ossicle is the incus, particularly in the region of its long process, but dissolution of other ossicles may occur as well.

In postmortem temporal bones with chronic otitis media, large surgically produced cavities are sometimes present in the mastoid region. These are the results of operations to remove infected parts of the mastoid to drain the middle ear cleft and they may or may not be accompanied by evidence of other surgical procedures involving the ossicles, depending on the severity of the clearance of the middle ear undertaken by the surgeon.

Yellow localized areas seen anywhere in the middle ear cleft are regions of cholesterol granuloma and pearly white patches, particularly in the attic, are likely to be cholesteatomas which are frequently present in association with chronic otitis media.

## Microscopic Appearance

The most characteristic feature of chronic otitis media is the presence of inflammatory granulation tissue. This cellular reaction has two components. On the one hand there is the presence of leukocytes characteristic of chronic inflammation (i.e., lymphocytes, plasma cells, and histiocytes). The latter are characterized by their phagocytic propensity, continuing the work of polymorphonuclear neutrophils that had taken place early in the infection of enclosing and destroying bacteria and also of clearing up debris produced by the destructive effects of the inflammation. On the other hand, there is granulation tissue constituted by newly formed capillaries and by fibroblasts. Granulation tissue formation takes place in the early stages of healing after the inflammatory destruction of tissue. The chronic inflammatory leukocytes and the granulation tissue may be found in the middle ear in chronic otitis media independently of each other. The two forms of cellular reaction are seen together in aural polyps (Fig. 22-22). This lesion is frequently subjected to biopsy in the investigation of cases of chronic otitis media. The polyp is usually covered by columnar epithelium, which is often ciliated. Sometimes the epithelium is squamous. This may be produced by metaplasia in the middle ear or by irritation of the polyp when it reaches the ear canal. The core of the polyp is made up of chronic inflammatory granulation tissue.

The middle ear cleft is normally lined by a single layer of cubical or columnar epithelium which may bear cilia. Tos and Bak-Pedersen[29,30] studied the normal and pathologic middle ear epithelia by a whole-mount method in which the entire mucosa was removed and stained with PAS-alcian blue. By this method goblet cells appear as oval to round sharply demarcated blue structures on a pale background. A few goblet cells were found in the normal middle ear, but in chronic otitis the numbers were greatly increased, to a level similar to those in other parts of the respiratory tract.

Unlike other parts of the respiratory tract, including the cartilaginous portion of eustachian tube, where tubuloalveolar glands, mucous and

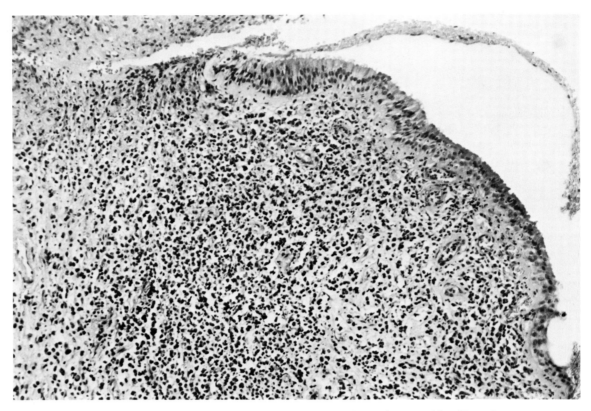

**Fig. 22-22.** Aural polyp, composed of chronic inflammatory granulation tissue and lined by columnar epithelium which is partially ciliated. (H & E, original magnification X 175.)

serous type, are present, the middle ear is normally devoid of such glands. Under conditions of chronic inflammation, however, the middle ear epithelium comes to resemble the rest of the respiratory tract by the formation of glands. They consist usually of a simple tubule of mucus-producing cells. Gland formation is particularly active in children with secretory otitis media.[31] Glandular transformation may take place in the mastoid air cells as well as the main middle ear cavity (Fig. 22-23). The secretion derived from the glands is an important component of the aural discharge in chronic otitis media.

The mastoid air cells show fibrosis and their bony walls are markedly thickened. Cement lines in the lamellar bone are profuse and irregular, often forming a mosaic pattern (Fig. 22-23). This indicates the recent active deposition and resorption of bone as a result of the inflammatory process. The product of these reparative processes in the mastoid is a patchy sclerosis with some cystic cavities representing distended air cells. The obliteration of mastoid air cells as a result of chronic otitis is referred to as secondary sclerosis.

In some ears, the mastoid air cells lack pneumatization from an early age. This has been ascribed to inflammatory change,[32] but such an interpretation has been doubted by others who have regarded the sclerosis as primary, perhaps due to genetic factors.[33] The sclerosis has also been ascribed to local defects in ventilation.[34] The appearance of the mastoid in primary arrest of pneumatization is unlike that following otitis media in that in the former the mastoid air cell system is small and the bone is diffusely sclerotic.

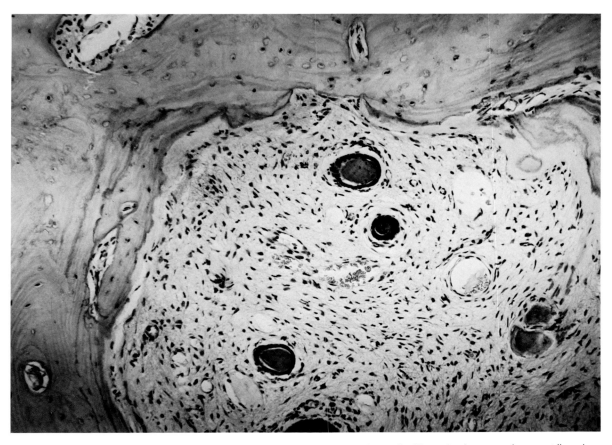

**Fig. 22-23.** Glands and fibrosis of mastoid air cells in the chronic otitis media. Note also increased cement lines in bony wall. (H & E, original magnification X 100.)

Inflammatory tissue, glandular tissue, and fibrosis may be also seen in any part of the middle ear mucosa, including that investing the ossicles. Underlying bone may undergo rarefaction or new formation (Figs. 22-24 and 22-25).

## Cholesterol Granuloma

Yellow nodules are found in the tympanic cavity and mastoid in many cases of chronic otitis media. These are composed microscopically of cholesterol crystals (dissolved away to leave empty clefts in paraffin-embedded histologic sections) surrounded by foreign-body giant cells and other chronic inflammatory cells (Fig. 22-26). Such cho-

lesterol granulomas are almost always found in the midst of hemorrhage in the middle ear mucosa. That hemorrhage is the cause of cholesterol granuloma has been denied by Sadé,[35] who thought the blood seen in the biopsies of such lesions to be the result of surgery. There can be no doubt, however, that hemorrhage is associated with cholesterol granuloma. Red cells are localized to the granuloma and are not usually found elsewhere in the tissues. Hemosiderin is frequently present. Hemorrhage is also a frequent concomitant of cholesterol granuloma in the maxillary antrum and in thyroid adenomas. Cholesterol granuloma in the mastoid air cells must be distinguished from lipid deposits of hypercholesterolemic xanthomatosis.

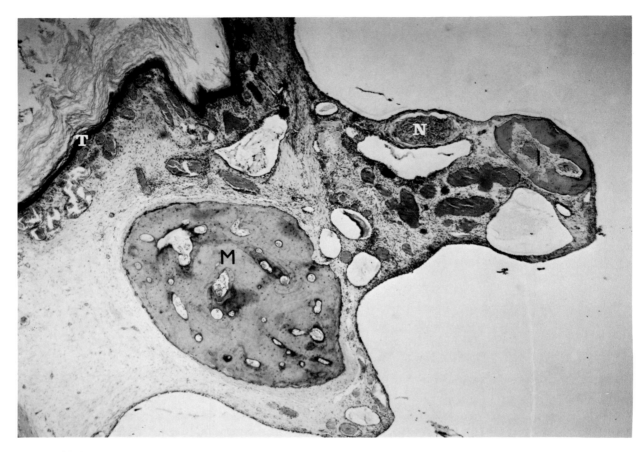

**Fig. 22-24.** Horizontal section of middle ear in chronic otitis media. Fibrous bands between malleus and incus show congestion and glands containing mucus. Note erosion of edge of malleus and incus. T, tympanic membrane; N, chorda tympani nerve; I, incus: M, handle of malleus. (H & E, original magnification X 44.)

## Pathogenesis

Cholesterol granuloma has been produced experimentally by obstructing natural air-filled spaces in bone — the humerus of cockerels[36] — and in the eustachian tube of squirrel monkeys.[37,38] Thomas et al.[37] conducted a study in which hemorrhages were observed to accompany the cholesterol granulomas. While suggesting that lowered air pressure in the middle ear might be associated with cholesterol granuloma, these experiments do not exclude the possibility of hemorrhage resulting from lowered pressure as a precursor.

Sadé and Teitz[39] found the lipid in cholesterol granulomas of the middle ear to be mainly cholesterol with only very small amounts of cholesterol esters. In serum the reverse is the case: a high proportion of cholesterol ester is present, but little cholesterol. These findings are compatible with an origin of the lipid material in cholesterol granuloma from red cell membranes, in which cholesterol exists mainly in the free, not esterified, state.

## Tympanosclerosis

Tympanosclerosis is a special form of fibrosis, often encountered in chronic otitis media. Deposits of dense white tissue are laid down in the middle ear mucosa, not only on the tympanic side

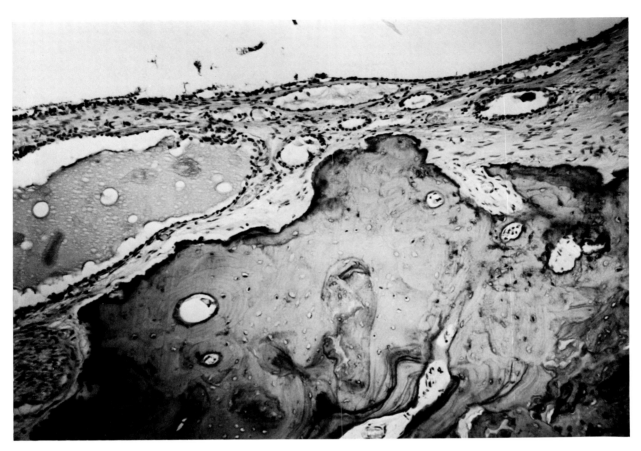

**Fig. 22-25.** Mucosa and middle ear surface of bone of promontory in chronic otitis media. Note irregular edge of bone with multiple cement lines in some areas and glands in mucosa. (H & E, original magnification X 44.)

of the tympanic membrane, which is particularly likely to occur in otitis media with effusion, but also, following chronic suppurative otitis media, on the crura of the stapes, within the tympanic cavity and sometimes in the mastoid. On dissection, the tympanosclerotic deposit may show a lamellated onion skin-like structure.

Microscopically, the material is composed of hyaline collagen deposited in the mucosa. The collagen stains with acid aniline dyes and is birefringent. Deposits of calcium salts, appearing as basophilic dustlike areas, are irregularly distributed through the collagen. A multilayered structure corresponding to the gross appearance of lamellation is frequently observed. Bone is also often

present in the tympanosclerotic plaques (Fig. 22-27).

Ultrastructurally, the tympanosclerotic plaque shows degeneration of collagen and reticulin fibrils with calcified deposits of electron-dense spindle-shaped or spherical material in the areas of degeneration. I have observed the calcium salts to be deposited as crystalline formations. It has been suggested that deposits of calcium salts occur initially in extracellular membrane-bound vesicles[40] in a fashion similar to the postulated mechanism of bone salt deposition during the general process of ossification.[41] Hussl and Lim,[42] however, have been unable to confirm this finding.

Although the result of otitis media, tympanoscle-

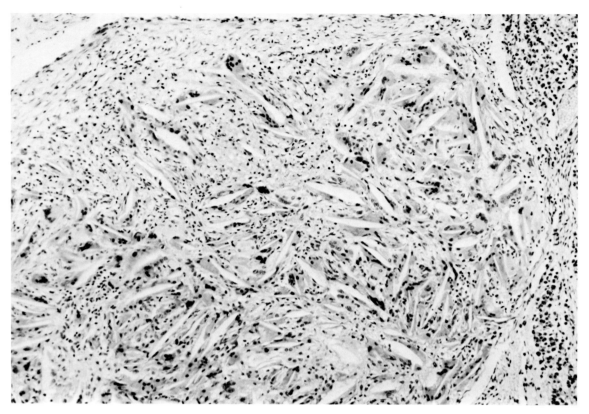

**Fig. 22-26.** Cholesterol granuloma of middle ear. The lesion is composed of cholesterol clefts surrounded by foreign-body giant cells and other chronic inflammatory cells. (H & E, original magnification X 170.)

rosis is not an ordinary form of fibrous tissue reaction, but resembles the type of collagen seen in the silicotic nodules of the lung and leiomyomas of the uterus. There may be an autoimmune factor in its development, which leads to degeneration of collagen. This is possibly enhanced by trauma, as in the use of ventilating tubes, which have been observed to lead to the development of tympanosclerosis of the tympanic membrane.[43]

## Cholesteatoma

Cholesteatoma (keratoma),[28] is an important concomitant in one-third to one-half of cases of chronic otitis media. It is a cyst lined by squamous epithelium within the middle ear cavity. The term *cholesteatoma* is an unfortunate one, because the entity it designates bears no relationship to cholesterol granuloma or to a neoplasm. It is usual to separate a congenital or primary form of cholesteatoma (in which a cyst is present behind an intact tympanic membrane) from an acquired form (in which there is a perforation of the tympanic membrane through which the epidermal squames of the cholesteatoma drain).

### Clinical Features

A small cholesteatoma may be present with normal hearing and no discharge. Typically, however, there is foul-smelling discharge as well as hearing loss. On examination of the tympanic membrane there is, in most cases, a perforation of the superior or posterosuperior margin.

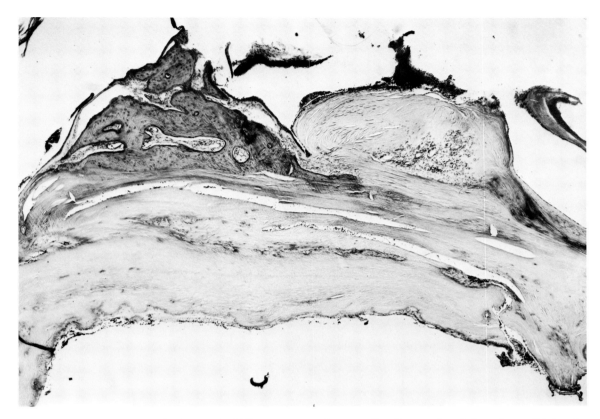

**Fig. 22-27.** Tympanosclerotic plaque of middle ear mucosa. Layers of hyaline poorly cellular collagen thicken the mucosa. Darker areas (basophilic in the original) represent zones of calcification. An area of ossification is seen in the top left. (H & E, original magnification X 170.)

## Gross Appearance

The cholesteatoma appears as a pearly white or yellow cystlike structure in the middle ear cavity (Fig. 22-28). The wall of the cyst may often be seen as a thin membrane.

The congenital (primary) form of cholesteatoma appears as a cyst in the anterior superior part of the middle ear, unrelated to the pars flaccida of the tympanic membrane. It is not typically associated with inflammation of the middle ear mucosa. The term congenital cholesteatoma is also applied to a squamous epithelial cyst arising deep in the temporal bone and elsewhere, causing damage by erosion of the skull. This entity is quite different from the middle ear cholesteatoma; the description epidermoid for the deep lesion is more appropriate.[44]

The sites of involvement of congenital cholesteatoma, a lesion which has recently become more frequently recognized, have been reviewed and indicate that there is a propensity for its occurrence, especially when small, in the anterior superior part of the middle ear.[43a,43b] The same situation is the precise location of an epidermoid cell rest, the epidermoid formation. This is seen in most fetal ears at the junction of the Eustachian tube with the middle ear near the anterior limb of the tympanic ring, until 33 weeks gestation, when it disappears.[43c] Its origin has been traced to early fetal life from the ectoderm of the first branchial groove. In embryonic and early in fetal life it seems to act as an organizer in the development of the tympanic membrane and middle ear.[43d]

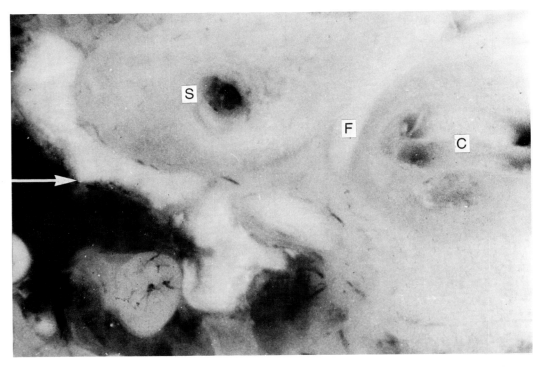

**Fig. 22-28.** Cholesteatoma sac (arrows) in microslice of upper part of middle ear of a 9-year-old child. The middle ear cavity is filled with purulent debris. C, cochlea; F, facial nerve proximal to genu; S, superior semicircular canal.

The much more frequent acquired form of cholesteatoma is usually situated in the upper part of the middle ear cleft and discharges through a perforation of the pars flaccida of the tympanic membrane. The cholesteatoma may extend through the aditus into the mastoid antrum and mastoid air cells. Frequently the outline of the cholesteatomatous sac is adapted to that of normal structures, such as ossicles. Chronic inflammatory changes are always present. At least one ossicle is often seriously damaged, thereby interrupting the continuity of the ossicular chain. The scutum, the upper part of the bony ring of the tympanic opening, is eroded in 42 percent of ears with cholesteatoma.[45]

### Microscopic Appearance

Microscopically the pearly material of the cholesteatoma consists of dead fully differentiated anucleate keratin squames. This is the corneal layer of the squamous cell epithelium. Sometimes biopsy material shows only squames when the so-called capsule has not been excised. The capsule, often called the matrix, is composed of fully differentiated squamous epithelium similar to the epidermis of skin and resting on connective tissue. There is a basal layer of small cuboidal cells, above which is a spinal or malpighian layer composed of five or six rows of cells with intercellular prickles. A thin granular layer in which the cells display prominent cytoplasmic keratohyaline granules separates the malpighian layer from the extensive corneal layer (Fig. 22-29).

The eroded ossicles that are frequently present in cholesteatoma may be invested by the squamous epithelial wall of the sac. Even in these circumstances, there is always a layer of granulation tissue in contact with the bone, and it seems likely that it is the chronic inflammatory covering, not the squamous epithelium, that produces the erosion (Figs. 22-30 and 22-31).

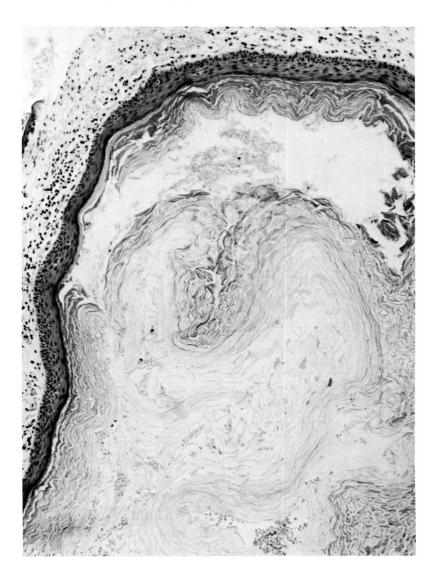

**Fig. 22-29.** Cholesteatoma sac, composed of squamous epithelium enclosing keratinous debris. (H & E, original magnification X 175.)

## Retraction Pocket

A retraction pocket is an invagination of part of the tympanic membrane into the middle ear cavity as a result of chronic otitis media. It is usually the pars flaccida that is so indented. It frequently becomes adherent to the posterior wall of the middle ear in the region of the facial nerve or stapes (Fig. 22-32). Histologic section of the wall of the retraction pocket shows an absence of the normal connective tissue layer of the tympanic membrane. the

latter perhaps having been destroyed by inflammation.[28] We found small keratinizing squamous cell foci in a fibrous band attached to the retraction pocket in two cases[46] (Figs. 22-33 and 22-34).

## Secretory Otitis Media

Secretory otitis media (serous otitis media, otitis media with effusion, catarrhal otitis media, tubotympanitis) has attracted much attention in recent years because of its frequency as a cause of hearing

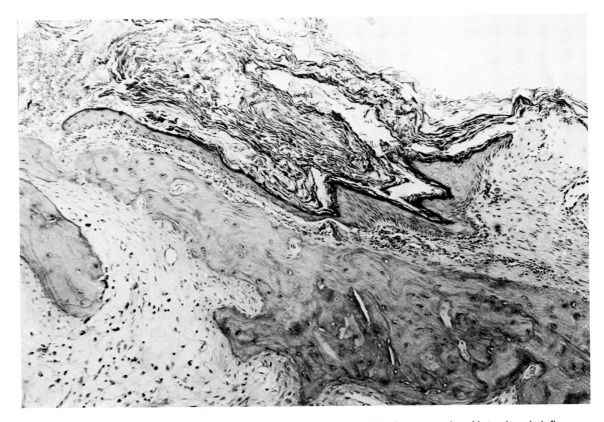

**Fig. 22-30.** Cholesteatoma growing on the surface of the incus, which shows erosion. Note chronic inflammatory infiltrate between the bone and the cholesteatoma and in the marrow space of the bone. (H & E, original magnification X 175.)

loss in children. It is defined by Sadé as a "condition in which an effusion is present behind an intact drum in the absence of frank symptoms of acute infection."[47]

The lesion is said to affect 5 to 10 percent of all children, many of whom have no symptoms. Adults may complain of shifting fluid in the ear. The importance of adenoid enlargement as a cause has been disputed, while the question of eustachian tube obstruction as an important precursor is still open.

The pathologic changes associated with the clinical syndrome of secretory otitis media read like a review of the alterations described earlier in this chapter. Cholesterol granuloma, chronic inflammatory granulation tissue, ossicular destruction, and tympanosclerosis are all important features, and the tympanic membrane itself often changes with the progress of the disease, becoming atelectatic (i.e., adherent to the medial wall of the middle ear) or even forming a retraction pocket. Cholesteatoma may develop behind the intact tympanic membrane or with the formation of a small perforation in the pars flaccida.

Chronic otitis media is an extremely common malady. In a pathologic study of 123 temporal bones with chronic otitis meda, 19.5 percent showed no perforation.[48] Secretory otitis media is one form of chronic otitis media without perforation. Its current epidemiclike frequency may be the result of the treatment of acute otitis with antibiotics in recent years.

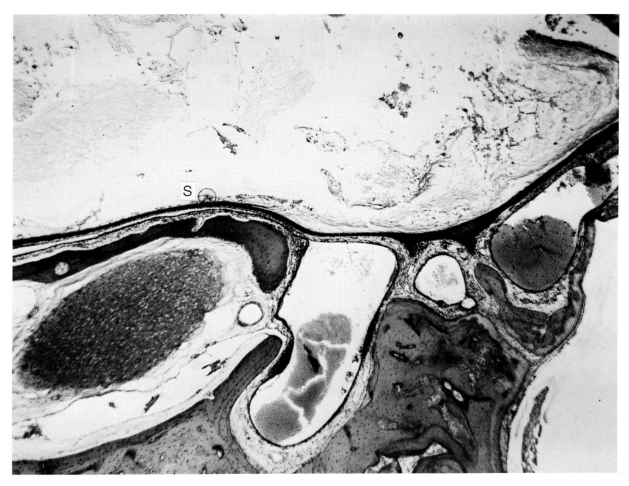

**Fig. 22-31.** Cholesteatoma sac (S) attached to posterior wall of middle ear in the region of the facial nerve (bottom left). The sac is partly separated from the mucosa of the middle ear by a thin space. Note glands in the middle ear mucosa and chronic inflammatory tissue deep to the cholesteatoma. (H & E, original magnification X 44.)

## Complications

The inflammatory process may extend from the middle ear to involve adjacent structures. Inflammation of the labyrinth may occur as a result of extension of the infection through the round or oval windows. The petrous bone may become involved by spread of the inflammation through the bone marrow or air cells. Adjacent intracranial structures may become inflamed by spread of the infection outside of the temporal bone. Meningitis, sinus thrombophlebitis, extradural abscess, or brain abscess are important possible sequelae of otitis media.

## Tuberculous Otitis Media

Tuberculous otitis media is an unusual form of chronic otitis media, generally associated with active pulmonary tuberculosis. In the initial stages, multiple perforations of the tympanic membrane develop. Granulations in the middle ear are pale

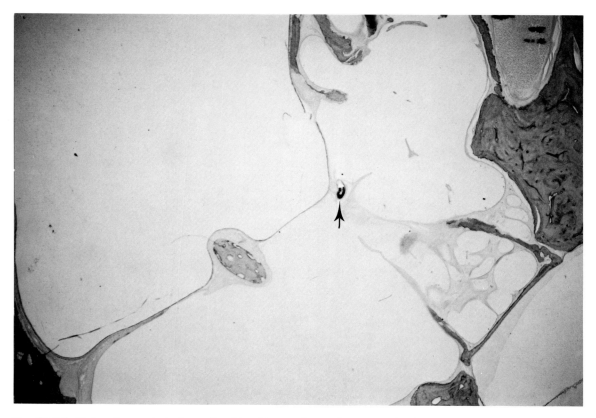

**Fig. 22-32.** Retraction pocket of pars flaccida of tympanic membrane attached to stapes by a fibrous band. Note keratin cyst (arrow) within the band. (H & E, original magnification X 18.)

and profuse; complications, especially involvement of the facial nerve, are more frequent than in the more common form of chronic otitis media.

Culture of the middle ear tissue may produce tubercle bacilli. Histologic examination shows tuberculoid granulation tissue composed of epithelioid cells, Langhans giant cells, and areas of caseation situated in the middle ear mucosa as well as in the bone marrow.[49] There is much bone destruction (Fig. 22-35). Acid-fast bacilli are found with difficulty in the granulomatous material.

Sections from two remarkable cases of tuberculous otitis media were recently observed in my laboratory. Both were otherwise healthy adult men with no evidence of tuberculosis of lung or other internal organ. Each case showed sclerosis of temporal bone on radiography. Vast numbers of acid-fast bacilli were present in the granulomas (Figs.

22-36 and 22-37), confirmed as *Mycobacterium tuberculosis hominis* by culture.

## NEOPLASMS OF THE EXTERNAL EAR

The external ear is a specialized appendage of the skin with a cartilaginous skeleton, attached to a skin-lined tube reinforced by cartilage and bone in its wall. It would therefore be expected that neoplasms of the external ear were mainly those of skin, cartilage, and bone. Indeed, any skin tumor may occur on the external ear. This section deals only with those that have a special predilection for that organ and those that pose special diagnostic histologic and clinical problems. Moreover, the

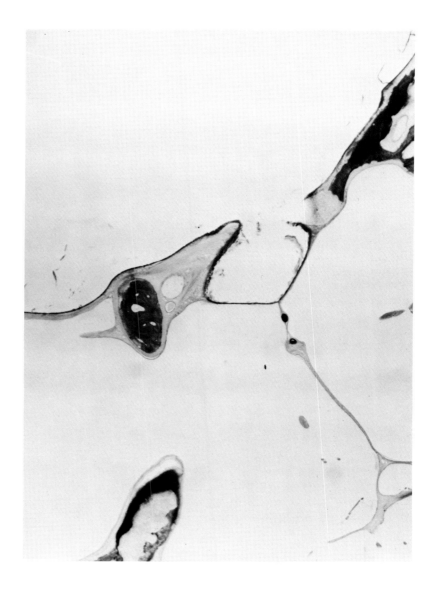

**Fig. 22-33.** Small retraction pocket of tympanic membrane. Note two keratinous cysts within fibrous band attached to pocket. (H & E, original magnification X 44.)

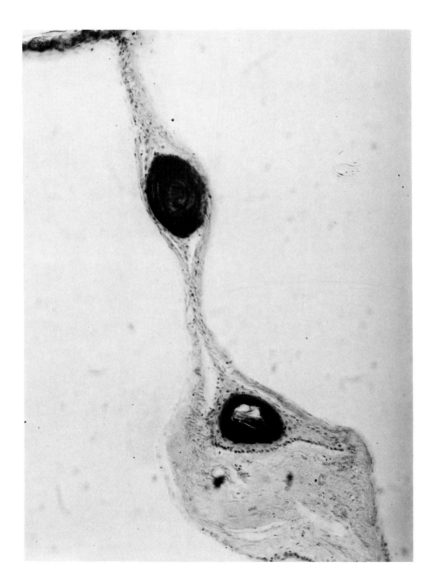

**Fig. 22-34.** Higher-power view of keratinous cysts shown in Fig. 22-33. (H & E, original magnification X 175.)

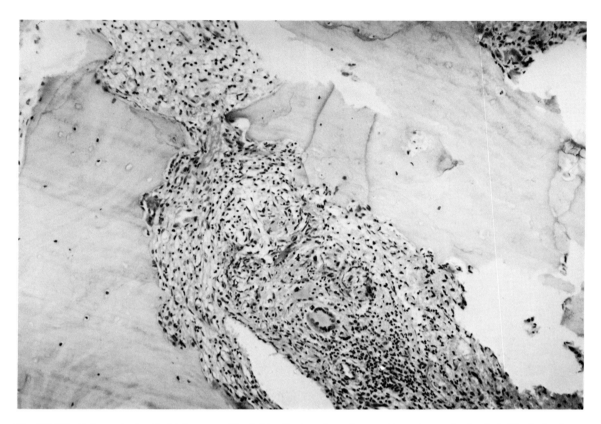

**Fig. 22-35.** Tuberculosis of middle ear. epithelioid cells, lymphocytes, and Langhans giant cells infiltrate the bone surrounding the middle ear. Contrast Langhans giant cells with osteoclast eroding bone on left. (H & E, original magnification X 175.)

presence of ceruminal glands in the ear canal contributes a group of neoplasms unique to that area.

## Epidermoid Neoplasms

### Solar Keratosis

Solar keratosis usually occurs in whites as multiple lesions in areas of the body, such as the face and dorsa of the hands, that are particularly exposed to sunlight over many years with inadequate protection. The pinna of the ear is occasionally involved and, rarely, the commencement of the external auditory canal.

The lesion takes the form of a small erythematous flat plaque. Histologically, hyperkeratosis, epidermal hyperplasia, and dysplasia of the epidermis are exhibited. The upper dermis shows elastic tissue

degeneration and a chronic inflammatory exudate. There is a decided tendency to malignant change. Early squamous carcinomas arising in solar keratosis, however, rarely metastasize.[7]

### Basal Cell Papilloma

Basal cell papilloma (seborrheic keratosis) is very common on the trunk and face. It is sometimes present on the pinna or in the ear canal. This well-demarcated pigmented elevation looks as though it has been stuck onto the skin surface.

Histologically, it is elevated above the surrounding skin such that the lower border with dermis forms a straight line. The proliferated tissue is composed of basal cells with numbers of keratin cysts embedded within them. In the cysts, keratinization occurs by sudden transformation from the basal

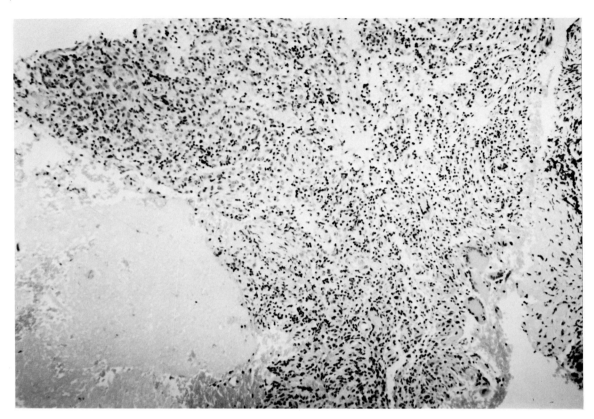

**Fig. 22-36.** Tuberculosis of middle ear. Note caseation on left to the right of which there are epithelioid cells, lymphocytes, and some Langhans giant cells. (H & E, original magnification X 175.)

cells without interposition of a stratum granulosum. Melanocytes are frequently present. The condition is benign.

### Pilomatricoma

Pilomatricoma (pilomatrixoma, calcifying epithelioma of malherbe) is a tumor of the skin of children or young adults with a decided preference for the skin of the external ear, although it is also seen elsewhere on the face, neck, and arms. It often assumes the form of a cyst with a lumen of cheesy material but may show a solid pinkish cut surface. Pilomatricoma is usually situated under the skin.

The peripheral part contains islets and columns of basophilic cells with little cytoplasm and prominent nucleoli. These cells blend with, or are sharply demarcated from ghost cells, which appear to be groups of degenerated epidermal cells stain-

ing only in a faintly eosinophilic fashion. The central part of the lesion contains amorphous debris, keratin, and often calcified and even ossified areas (Fig. 22-38). The neoplasm is almost always benign, although an invasive malignant variant has recently been described.[50]

### Squamous Papillomas

Squamous papillomas are common tumors of the external auditory canal that do not differ significantly from similar tumors growing from the mucous surface of the nasal septum or vocal cord. They show inverted cylinders of squamous epithelium growing on central cores of fibrous tissue. Sometimes the fibrous component is more prominent in an ear canal tumor, meriting the term fibroepithelial polyp. Neither of these lesions is malignant.

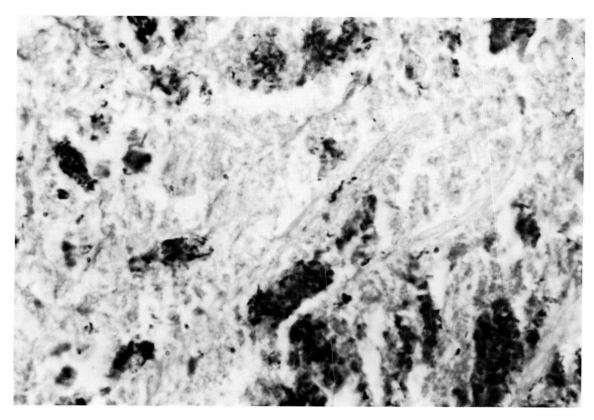

**Fig. 22-37.** Another section from biopsy of middle ear shown in Fig. 22-36, stained by the Ziehl-Nielsen method for acid-fast organisms. Numerous clumps of acid-fast organism are present. These were cultured and confirmed as *Mycobacterium tuberculosis hominis*. (Ziehl-Nielsen, original magnification X 1,000.)

### Keratoacanthoma

Keratoacanthomas may occur on the external ear as well as the skin of the face. The special features of these neoplasms are (1) a resemblance to low-grade squamous carcinoma of the skin, and (2) a tendency to disappear spontaneously after 6 to 8 weeks of growth.

Microscopically, the center of the lesion is composed of a crater of keratin, surrounded by well-differentiated trabeculae of squamous cell epithelium. The outer edge of the lesion is clear cut, with no extension of tongues of growth. In surgical pathology practice, keratoacanthoma is frequently difficult to distinguish from low-grade squamous carcinoma; Lever and Schaumburg-Lever[7] suggest that when in doubt it is safer to diagnose squamous carcinoma.

### Sebaceous Adenoma

Well-defined tumors of sebaceous gland origin may be found in the external auditory canal. The neoplasm is made up of lobules of tumor cells comprising two types of cells. Situated around the periphery of the lobules are undifferentiated germinative cells. More centrally, the cells can be recognized as sebaceous (Fig. 22-39).

### Sebaceous Epithelioma

A malignant variant of sebaceous adenoma, sebaceous epithelioma is sometimes seen. Although locally infiltrative, it does not metastasize and may be a form of basal cell carcinoma (Fig. 22-40).

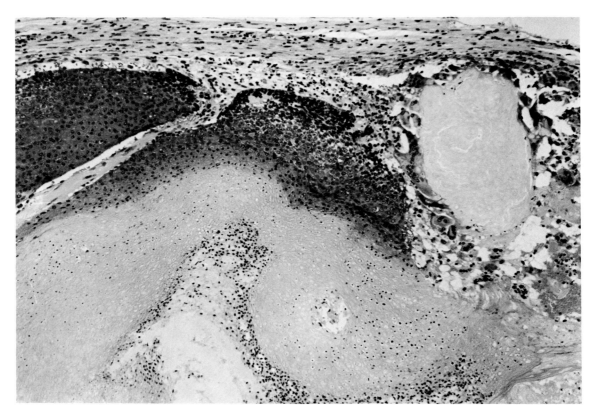

**Fig. 22-38.** Pilomatricoma (pilomatrixoma) of external ear. Note basophilic squamous epithelial cells and ghost cells in which most nuclei have lost their staining property. A keratin cyst surrounded by foreign-body giant cell reaction is present at the top left. (H & E, original magnification X 175.)

## Basal Cell Carcinoma

The great majority of malignant epithelial neoplasms of the pinna are basal cell carcinomas a small number only being squamous cell carcinomas. The few basal cell carcinomas that occur in the ear canal arise near the external opening. Their preference for the exposed part of the external ear is in keeping with the accepted view that sunlight is in most cases a causal factor in skin insufficiently protected by melanin pigment, as it is in solar keratosis. In the series of 71 cases of basal cell carcinoma of the pinna described by Metcalf,[51] 29 were on the posterior surface, 22 on the helix and anthelix, 10 on the concha, and 10 on the anterior pinna (crus, tragus, and antitragus) and lobule.

**Gross Appearance.** The gross appearance of basal cell carcinoma is usually one of a pearly waxlike nodule that eventually ulcerates. Twenty-five percent of basal cell carcinomas of the pinna are of the morphea type. The importance of this variety is that the edge of the tumor tends to infiltrate subcutaneously but that this cannot be recognized clinically or on gross pathologic examination.

**Microscopic Appearance.** The classic and most fequent form of basal cell carcinoma is composed of solid masses of cells seen to be arising from the basal layers of the epidermis or the outer layers of the hair follicles (Fig. 22-41). The cells are uniform with basophilic nuclei and little cytoplasm. At the periphery of the neoplastic lobules, the cells tend to be palisaded (Fig. 22-42). Mitoses are often numerous. Alveolar or cystic spaces are frequently present. Squamous cell differentiation is also common. The splitting up of cell groups by much hyalin

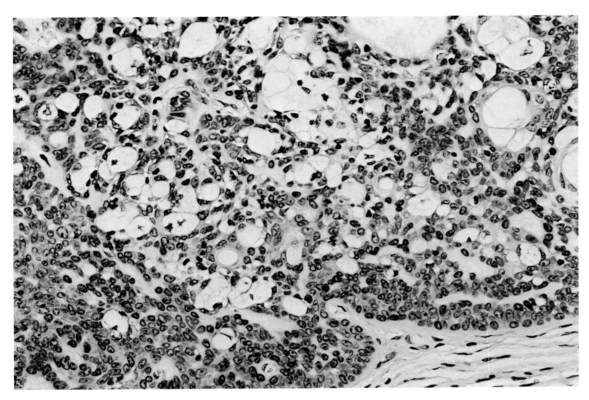

**Fig. 22-39.** Sebaceous adenoma of ear canal. Around the periphery of the tumor lobule are undifferentiated cells. More centrally, the cells are of sebaceous type. (H & E, original magnification X 440.)

fibrous tissue such that the carcinoma appears compressed into thin strands is referred to as the morphea type of basal cell carcinoma. The suggestion that tumors with this histology have a worse outlook is probably related to its tendency of insidious infiltration. There is no convincing evidence of the relationship of any particular histologic appearance to prognosis in basal cell carcinoma.

**Natural History.** Basal cell carcinoma is not an aggressive neoplasm, and in at least 90 percent of cases a 3-year cure can be easily achieved by surgical excision.[51] In a few cases, deep extension to the middle ear, mastoid, and even cranial cavity may recur repeatedly but metastasis is rare.

#### Squamous Cell Carcinoma

**Incidence.** Squamous cell carcinoma is a common form of malignancy, accounting for 7 percent of all squamous carcinomas of the head and neck re-

gion.[51] Squamous carcinomas of the pinna occur predominantly in males; those of the ear canal mainly in females.[53] Ear canal cancers, moreover, grow at a markedly younger age than those of the pinna.[54]

The verrucous form of squamous cell carcinoma has been seen in the external ear.[55] As at other sites where this neoplasm occurs, the diagnosis may be delayed until after several biopsies have been performed.

**Etiology.** Solar exposure has been regarded as a predisposing factor in the etiology of this neoplasm, which may be regarded as an invasive stage following the in situ lesion of solar keratosis. Frostbite has been noted as a cause in some cases.[54]

**Gross Appearance.** The gross appearance of the lesion is similar to that elsewhere in the skin and range from a papular nodule to an ulcerating mass. Its appearance in the ear canal is not diagnostic because of the narrowness of this structure.

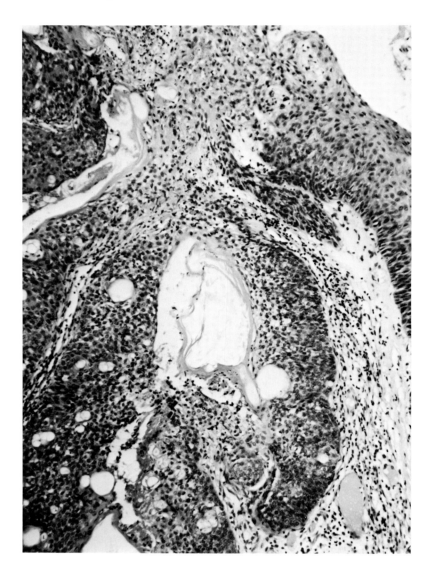

**Fig. 22-40.** Sebaceous epithelioma of external ear. The neoplasm is arising as a downgrowth from the epidermis. Sebaceous cells can be recognized among the invading cells. (H & E, original magnification X 177.)

**Microscopic Appearance.** This form of epidermoid carcinoma usually shows significant degrees of keratinization. Evidence of origin from local epidermis is usually present. In cases arising deeply within the ear canal, there is usually a concomitant origin in the middle ear epithelium and dissolution of the tympanic membrane. An adenoid (pseudoglandular) pattern is not uncommonly seen in this neoplasm. Such tumors are said to have a better prognosis than those with the more usual structure.

**Natural History.** Metastastic spread of squamous carcinoma of the pinna and external auditory canal takes place in 8 to 25 percent of cases.[51,54] Such

spread is an important feature in the prognostic evaluation. Most tumors confined to the external ear have a good outlook after surgical therapy.

**Neoplasms of Ceruminous Glands**

External ear neoplasms derived from ceruminous glands are very uncommon. They can be benign or malignant. Table 22-2 presents a classification of these neoplasms.

**Adenoma.** Adenoma (ceruminoma) usually presents with a blockage of the lateral part of the external auditory canal, often associated with deaf-

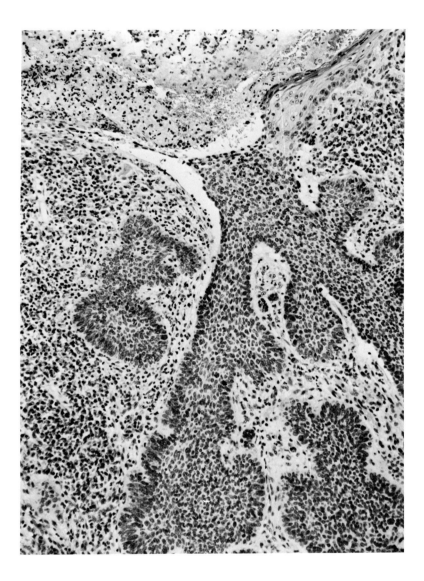

**Fig. 22-41.** Basal cell carcinoma of pinna. Downgrowths of dark-staining undifferentiated cells arise from skin epithelium. (H & E, original magnification X 175.)

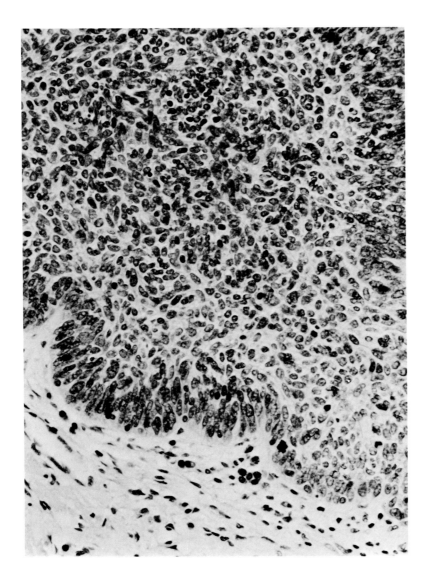

**Fig. 22-42.** Higher-power view of basal cell carcinoma showing palisaded cells at periphery of tumor lobule and occasional mitotic figure. (Original magnification X 440.)

**Table 22-2. Neoplasma of the Ceruminous Glands**

Benign
  Adenoma (ceruminoma)
  Syringocystadenoma papilliferans
  Chondroid syringoma-mixed tumor

Malignant
  Mucoepidermoid carcinoma
  Adenocarcinoma
  Adenoid cystic carcinoma

ness and discharge. An important part of the clinical investigation of all glandular neoplasms of the ear canal is exclusion of origin in the parotid gland.

The gross appearance is that of a superficial gray mass up to 4 cm in diameter, covered by skin. Microscopically, this neoplasm lacks a definite capsule. It is composed of regular glands sometimes with intraluminal projections (Fig. 22-43). The glandular epithelium is bilayered, the outer layer being myoepithelial, but this may not be obvious in all parts of the neoplasm. The cells in some areas show decapitation secretion (Fig. 22-44). The glands are often arranged in groups surrounded by fibrous tissue. In some ceruminomas, acid-fast fluorescent pigment may be found in the tumor cells. This finding is similar to that found in normal ceruminous glands.[56,57] The adenoma of ceruminous glands is a benign neoplasm. Recurrence should not be expected if it is carefully excised.

**Syringocystadenoma Papilliferum.** This benign lesion is usually seen in children or young adults and is usually found on the scalp or face. Occasionally, it occurs in the ear canal. The histologic appearance of the neoplasm is that of an invagination from the surface epithelium forming a cystlike structure. Projecting into the lumen are papillae lined by bi-

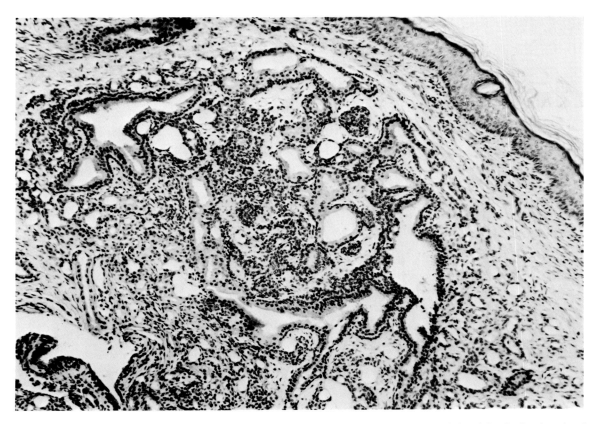

**Fig. 22-43.** Ceruminal adenoma. The neoplasm has a bilayered glandular structure. It is arising in the dermis of the skin of the ear canal. (H & E, original magnification X 175.)

layered glandular epithelium showing decapitation secretion. Apocrine (ceruminous) glands are present in the wall of the cyst.

**Mixed Tumor.** A benign neoplasm of the skin with a structure simiilar to that of pleomorphic adenoma of salivary glands is also occasionally seen in the external auditory canal. Cartilage and myoepithelial and adenomatous structures are features of this neoplasm (Fig. 22-45). The origin is probably from eccrine not apocrine glands[7] so that this tumor should not strictly speaking be grouped with ceruminous gland neoplasms.

**Malignant Salivary Gland Type Neoplasms.** Malignant glandular tumors of salivary gland type are sometimes seen in the ear canal, and an origin in ceruminous glands may then be assumed. Exclusion of a primary site in the parotid gland is crucial

in such cases. The most frequent of such tumors is adenoid cystic carcinoma. This malignant neoplasm has the gross and microscopic features of the corresponding major or minor salivary gland neoplasm (Fig. 22-46), including its tendency to invade along nerve sheaths. A tendency to relentless recurrence and eventual bloodstream metastasis is also a feature of this cancer.

Mucoepidermoid carcinoma arising as primary neoplasm of the ear canal has been described.[58] A malignant glandular neoplasm without adenoid cystic or mucoepidermoid structure may also arise in the ear canal. Its histology bears some similarity to adenoma of ceruminous glands, but the presence of nuclear atypia and mitotic figures enjoins the diagnosis of a malignant glandular neoplasm. A myoepithelial layer and decapitation secretion are not usually recognized in the malignant tumors.

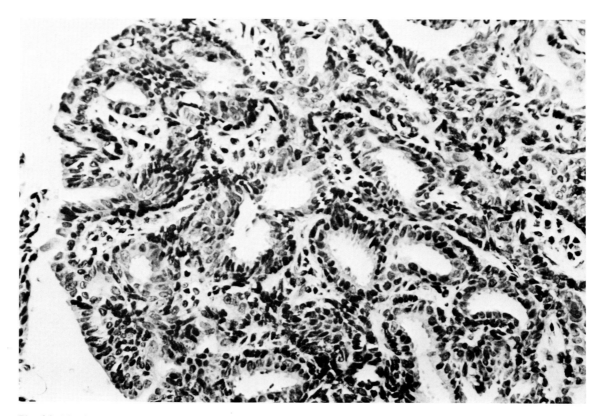

**Fig. 22-44.** Ceruminal gland adenoma. Note epithelial and myoepithelial layers in each gland and the presence of decapitation secretion (pinching off of cytoplasm on luminal side) in some of glandular cells. (H & E, original magnification X 440.)

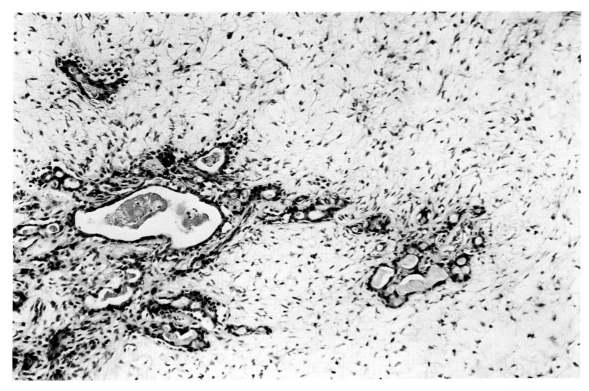

**Fig. 22-45.** Mixed tumor of external auditory canal. Note glandular epithelial elements and loosely lying myoepithelial cells. (H & E, original magnification X 175.)

## Melanotic Neoplasms

Tumors composed of melanin-producing cells are common in the skin. The benign forms are made up of nevus cells, which are modified melanocytes. Nevi are subdivided into junctional, compound, or intradermal depending on the degree of dropping off of nevus cells from the lower epidermis, this being most in the case of junctional nevi and absent in the case of intradermal ones. Malignant melanomas are the malignant counterparts of nevi. In all cases, the melanocytic neoplasm originates in the epidermis. Many malignant melanomas show extensive in situ epidermal change. The current practice for assessment of the prognosis and extent of surgical resection required in a particular case of malignant melanoma is to measure the thickness of the neoplasm.[59]

The occurrence of a melanotic neoplasm in the external ear is unusual. Nevi arise mainly in the ear canal, but are rare on the auricle. Malignant melanomas usually arise on the auricle.[60] The latter authors found a 3 : 1 ratio of males to females and an average of 49.6 percent for malignant melanomas arising on the auricle; 33 percent of patients show metastases to regional lymph nodes at their first visit. The presence of S100 protein on immunocytochemical staining is often of value in histologic diagnosis of malignant melanoma.

## Neoplasms of Bone and Cartilage

### Benign Fibro-osseous Lesion

Ossifying fibroma (fibrous dysplasia) is a solitary intraosseous neoplasm composed of islands of woven bone in a background of fibroblastic cells. Fibrous dysplasia is a bone condition of similar ap-

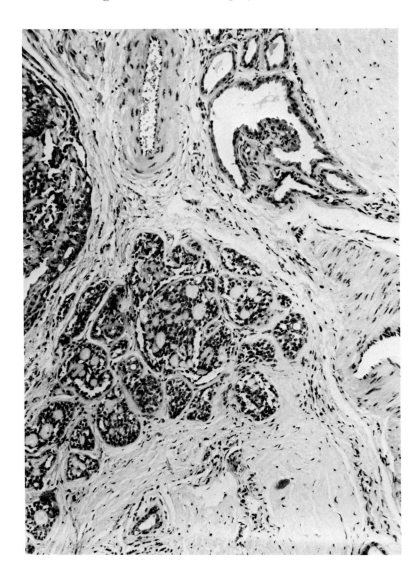

**Fig. 22-46.** Adenoid cystic carcinoma of external auditory canal. Lobules of neoplasm showing a cribriform pattern. Note normal ceruminous glands at top right. (H & E, original magnification X 44.)

pearance, but in which many patients also have multiple lesions of this type together with excessive skin pigmentation and endocrine disturbances. A solitary bone deposit without any accompanying extraosseous changes cannot be fitted into one or other of the two categories with certainty. At our teaching center, there is a tendency to use the term *benign fibro-osseous lesion* for such an entity. Bone tumors both of the latter type and of the generalized type are encountered in the temporal bone.

Nager et al.[61] provided a detailed description of "fibrous dysplasia" and its involvement of the temporal bone. Sixty-nine patients were reviewed, of whom 26 had the monostotic form of fibrous dysplasia. Unless these latter had an endocrine or pigmentary disturbance there would seem to be no essential difference from benign fibro-osseous lesion. Whatever name is given to the lesion, the comprehensive account given by Nager and coworkers is an excellent guide to its pathology in the temporal bone.

**Extraskeletal Manifestations.** Abnormal cutaneous and mucosal melanin pigmentation, usually in the midline of the body, is the most common extraskeletal manifestation of fibrous dysplasia. It occurs in more than 50 percent of polyostotic cases. McCune-Albright syndrome is the association of precocious sexual development with polyostotic fibrous dysplasia. Goiter, hyperthyroidism, acromegaly, Cushing's disease, extrainsular hypothalamic diabetes mellitus, and hyperparathyroidism are other endocrine lesions associated with polyostotic fibrous dysplasia.

**Pathologic Appearance.** The gross appearance of fibrous dysplasia is one of yellowish-white resilient tissue, which occasionally includes small cysts filled with an amber-colored fluid. The transition to normal bone is sharp. Microscopically, irregular trabeculae of woven bone are embedded in a con-

nective tissue stroma (Figs. 22-47 and 22-48). The bony trabeculae are said to lack osteoblasts around their periphery, but this is by no means invariable.

**Malignant Transformation.** Fibrous dysplasia has rarely been associated with malignant disease, such as osteogenic sarcoma, fibrosarcoma, chondrosarcoma, and giant cell tumor. The incidence of such neoplasm has been estimated at less than 0.5 percent. The temporal bone is not one of the sites at which this change has been described.

**Incidence.** Nager et al. reviewed 69 recorded cases of fibrous dysplasia of the temporal bone. These cases showed a male to female relationship of about 2 : 1. Twenty-six of the 69 patients had the monostotic form of fibrous dysplasia, 15 the polyostotic form, and 28 an unspecified type. The age at first consultation ranged from 3 to 80 years, with

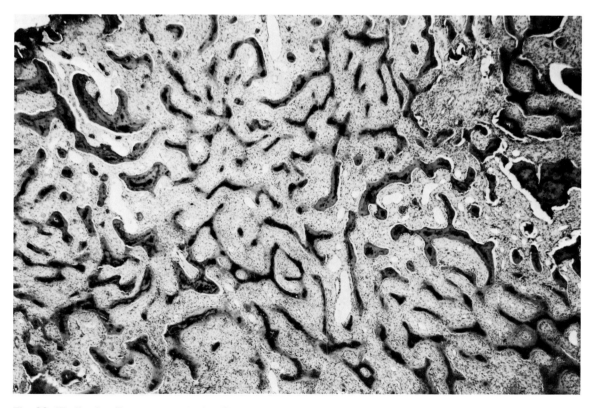

**Fig. 22-47.** Benign fibro-osseous lesion (fibrous dysplasia) of temporal bone. Irregular trabeculae of woven bone forming a Chinese letter pattern. Between the bony trabeculae is a stroma of cellular connective tissue. (H & E, original magnification X 44.)

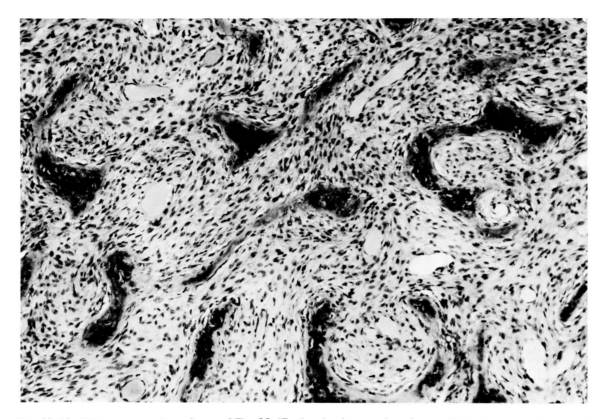

**Fig. 22-48.** Higher-power view of part of Fig. 22-47, showing bony trabeculae partly lined by osteoblasts and cellular fibrous stroma. (H & E, original magnification X 175.)

a mean of 28 years. In the polyostotic form of fibrous dysplasia, the incidence of temporal bone involvement was 50 percent depending upon how generalized the skeletal involvement was. Both temporal bones may be affected.

**Clinical Features.** The most common presenting symptoms of fibrous dysplasia were (1) progressive loss of hearing; (2) enlargement of the temporal bone; and (3) progressive bony occlusion of the external auditory canal. Most had a conductive hearing loss, nine cases a total loss of cochlear function and one a profound sensorineural hearing loss. The constriction of the ear canal had caused an external epidermoid cyst in seven patients. Five had peripheral ipsilateral facial nerve palsy. In one patient the lesion presented as an intracranial space-occupying lesion. Radiographic examination revealed an enlargement of the temporal bone associated with sclerosis or a uniform ground-glass

appearance of the swollen bone. The external auditory canal was confirmed as being constricted by radiography. Two of the patients personally observed by Nager et al. exhibited involvement of the ossicles by the fibrous dysplastic process.

**Treatment.** Forty-one of the 69 patients with fibrous dysplasia of the temporal bone required surgery, 20 of whom underwent two or more operative procedures. At operation, the diseased bone had a soft crumbly and gritty consistency and was uniformly very vascular. In those patients who did not develop a recurrence, the impression was of a decreased activity of the disease rather than that of a surgical cure.

## Osteoma and Exostosis

Two types of benign bony enlargement of the deeper bony portion of the external auditory canal are recognized: osteoma and exostosis.[62,63] Osteoma is a dome-shaped mass arising in the region of the tympanosquamous or tympanomastoid suture line by a distinct bony pedicle. The age range is 12 to 62 years, and 62 percent of patients are under 50 years of age. A few of these lesions occur in females. Symptoms are usually those of ear canal obstruction. Microscopically, the osteoma is composed of lamellar bone and may show outer cortical and inner cancellous trabeculated areas, the latter with marrow spaces. I have seen osteomas of the ear canal that show a thin layer of woven bone on the surfaces of the lamellar bone. The osteoma is covered by the normal squamous epithelium of the meatus.

Exostosis is a broad-based lesion that is often bilateral and symmetric.[62] It is usually situated deeper in the ear canal than are osteomas. Ages range from 18 to 60 years, with 75 percent below 50 years. In Sheehey's series of 64 patients with this lesion, only three were women.[62] A strong clinical impression exists that the exostoses are related to frequent swimming. It seems possible that the repeated contact with cold water during swimming stimulates the development of adjacent bone. Unlike osteoma, the bone formations of exostosis are said not to possess any marrow spaces.

### Chondrosarcoma and Osteosarcoma

Chondrosarcoma and osteosarcoma are rare tumors of the temporal bone. Leedham and Swash[64] described an extensive chondrosarcoma of that structure that invaded extensively downward into the neck and produced multiple metastases by the cerebrospinal fluid (CSF) to the spinal cord.

### Giant Cell Tumor

Involvement of the temporal bone by this neoplasm is rare. In any tumorlike lesion composed of giant cells and fibroblasts, consideration must be given to a nonneoplastic lesion, particularly giant cell reparative granuloma or the brown tumor of hyperparathyroidism. A few cases of genuine giant cell tumor in the temporal bone have been reported.[65]

## Neural Neoplasms

The only common neural neoplasm of the temporal bone is the schwannoma of the 8th cranial nerve. A schwannoma of the facial nerve is occasionally seen. Clinically, the patient may present with facial palsy. I have encountered a patient in whom this did not occur until after the biopsy procedure. Histologically, the features are those of a typical neurilemmoma.

## Neoplasms of Muscle

### Rhabdomyosarcoma

Rhabdomyosarcoma is seen occasionally in the temporal bone; other muscle tumors do not occur in that structure. Jaffee et al.[66] reviewed 40 cases affecting the middle ear and mastoid and reported the usual age incidence to be 1 to 12 years, with an average of 4.4 years. In most cases, the ear canal is involved by the neoplasm, but the middle ear is also invaded, making the precise site of origin difficult to determine. The child usually complains of discharge from the ear, which is often bloody, and a polyp is often present in the external auditory canal.

Grossly, the tumor is lobulated and dark red with a hemorrhagic cut surface. Almost all temporal bone rhabdomyosarcomas are histologically of the embryonal type. The cells of the neoplasm are often concentrated near the surface, forming a cambial layer. The tumor cells are round or elongated primitive cells, often with vacuolated cytoplasm containing much glycogen, imparting a foamy appearance to the cytoplasm. Large cells with eosinophilic granular cytoplasm are always present, although their numbers vary. Cross-striations are usually absent. Immunochemical demonstration of desmin and myoglobin is of most assistance in making the diagnosis. The presence of actin and myosin fibrils and Z-bands within the tumor cells revealed by electron microscopy, may also be of diagnostic assistance.

Rhabdomyosarcoma of the temporal bone is highly malignant and spreads extensively into the cranial cavity, externally, or to the pharyngeal region. Lymph node and bloodstream metastases frequently develop in these patients.

## Histiocytosis X

Histiocytosis X is a proliferative disorder of the reticuloendothelial system, thought by many pathologists to comprise three distinct forms: eosinophilic granuloma of bone, Hand-Schüller-Christian disease, and Letterer-Siwe disease. Only the first two conditions may affect the temporal bone. Eosinophilic granuloma is a solitary bone-destroying lesion of children formed by histiocytes with abundant eosinophilic cytoplasm and nuclei with fine folds together with numerous eosinophils. Hand-Schüller-Christian disease is characterized by multifocal proliferation of histiocytes with many foam cells (Fig. 22-49). Eosinophils are often prominent. Polymorphonuclear leukocytes and plasma cells may also be abundant. A distinct feature on electron microscopy of all three forms of histiocytosis X is the presence of a rod-shaped inclusion in the cytoplasm of the histiocytes. Known as the Birbeck granule, it is identical with the structures seen in the cytoplasm of the Langerhans cell of the epidermis.

In the temporal bone, the disease is usually manifested as a bony lesion of the medial part of the external auditory canal in children often with ear discharge.[67] In patients under 3 years of age, the disease process is more likely to be multifocal in the skull, that is, to be of the Hand-Schüller-Christian disease variety, and therefore to have a much worse outlook.

## NEOPLASMS AND SIMILAR LESIONS OF THE MIDDLE EAR

The middle ear is only occasionally the site of a new growth. Because of its deep-seated position, primary malignant tumors of the middle ear are not

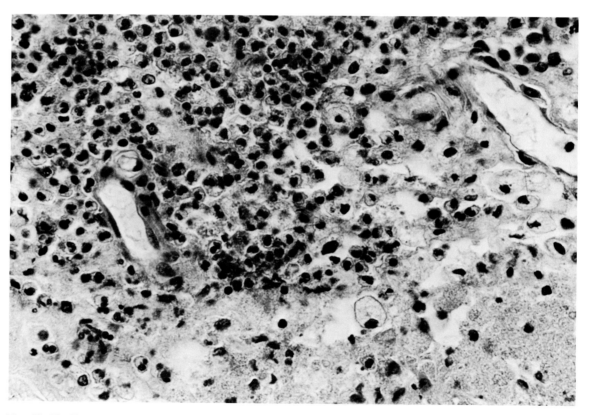

**Fig. 22-49.** Eosinophilic granuloma of temporal bone. The component cells are foamy histiocytes and eosinophils. (H & E, original magnification X 440.)

**Table 22-3. Neoplasms and Similar Lesions of the Middle Ear**

Developmental tumorlike anomalies
  Salivary choristoma
  Glial deposit
  Porencephalic cyst

Neoplasms
  Adenoma
  Inverted papilloma
  Meningioma
  Paraganglioma
  Squamous cell carcinoma
  Papillary adenocarcinoma
  Metastatic neoplasms

generally manifested until at an advanced stage. Table 22-3 presents the neoplastic and tumorlike developmental anomalies located in the middle ear.

## Tumorlike Development Anomalies

A hamartoma is a focal overgrowth in improper proportions of tissues normally present in that part of the body. A choristoma is similar to hamartoma, except that the tissues of which it is composed are not normally present in the part of the body in

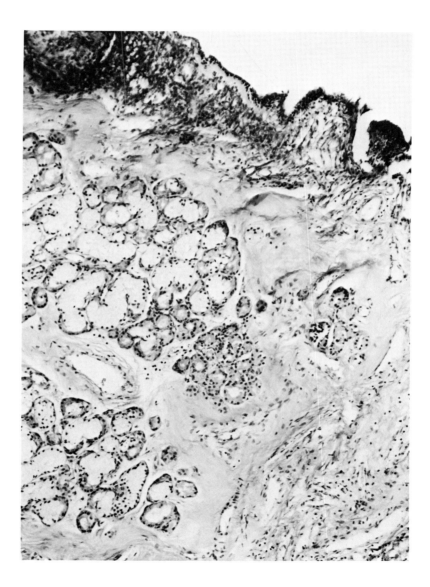

**Fig. 22-50.** Salivary choristoma of middle ear. Lobules of salivary gland tissue are present in the mucosa of the middle ear. The salivary gland acini are composed of both mucous and serous glandular elements. (Original magnification X 175.)

which it is found.[68] Choristomas are occasionally seen in the middle ear. They are usually composed of one or other of two types of tissue: (1) salivary gland, or (2) glial tissue. Salivary gland choristomas in the middle ear are usually composed of mixed mucous and serous elements like the normal submandibular or sublingual gland, but unlike the parotid gland[69] (Fig. 22-50).

Glial masses are composed largely of astrocytic cells (Fig. 22-51), the identity of which may be confirmed by immunochemical staining for glial acidic fibrillary protein. When such masses are identified in biopsy material from the middle ear a

bony deficit with consequent herniation of brain tissue into the middle ear should be ruled out.[70] Porencephalic cysts are leptomeningeal-lined cysts that present in the middle ear canal long after trauma.[71]

## Neoplasms

### Adenoma

A benign glandular neoplasm confined to the middle ear and originating in its epithelium was not recognized until 1976.[72,73] The epithelium of the

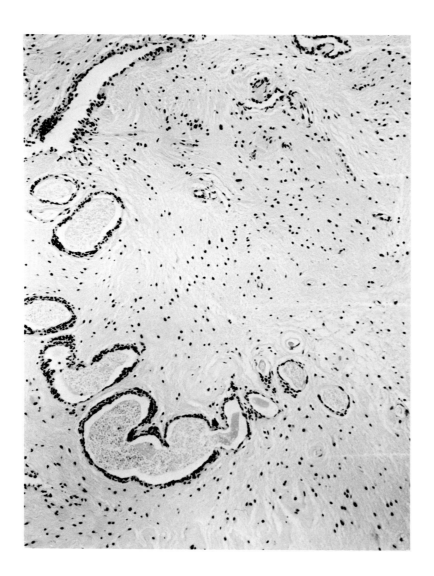

**Fig. 22-51.** "Glioma" of middle ear. The deposit is composed of fibrillary astrocytes. Glands formed by irritated middle ear mucosa are also present. (H & E, original magnification X 175.)

middle ear has a propensity for gland formation in otitis media, and adenoma would seem to represent a benign neoplastic transformation of this epithelium along the same lines.

**Incidence.** In the series described by Hyams and Michaels,[74] patients with this lesion ranged in ages from 14 to 80 years, three in the second to the fourth decades. There was an equal sex distribution. Most patients complained of hearing loss of conductive type. Pain, facial palsy, and ear discharge were usually absent. The tympanic membrane was intact in most cases and the neoplasm was confined to the middle ear, sometimes extending to the mastoid spaces, although in a few cases it did extend through a perforation into the ear canal. A rare example of penetration through the intact tympanic membrane has been described.[74]

**Gross Appearance.** The neoplasm appears white, gray, or reddish brown at operation and, unlike paraganglioma, is not vascular. It seems to peel away from the walls of the surrounding middle ear with ease, although ossicles may sometimes be entrapped in the tumor mass and may even show destruction.

**Microscopic Appearance.** Adenoma is composed of small glands closely apposed with a back-to-back appearance (Fig. 22-52). In some places, a solid or trabecular arrangement is present. Sheetlike disorganized areas are seen in which the glandular pattern appears to be lost (Fig. 22-53). This finding may be artifactual and related to the effects of the trauma of the biopsy on the delicate structure of this neoplasm, but the appearance can cause anxiety as regards the possibility of a more malignant

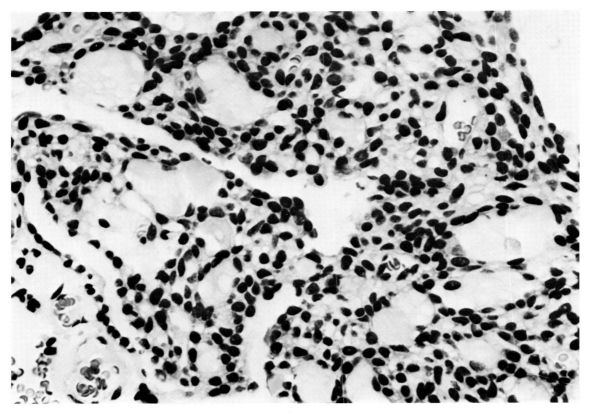

**Fig. 22-52.** Adenoma of middle ear. The tumor is composed of glands composed of a single layer of cells. There is secretion in many gland lumina. (H & E, original magnification X 700.)

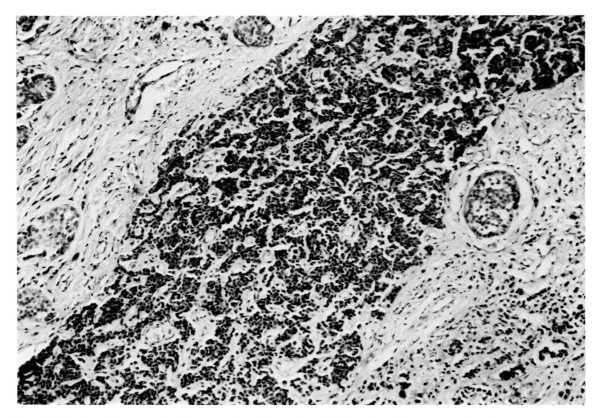

**Fig. 22-53.** Sheetlike area of adenoma of middle ear in which the glandular structure has been lost. (H & E, original magnification X 175.)

lesion. The cells are regular, cuboidal, or columnar. The glands may enclose a luminal secretion. No myoepithelial layer is seen. Sometimes a papillary pattern is present. Mills and Fechner[75] found lysozyme in each of five adenomas stained for this enzyme by an immunochemical method. We have examined four adenomas for lysozyme using the same antiserum as that reported by Mills and Fechner, but we used a sandwich technique for the further stages of the test. We found no lysozyme present in the cells of the adenomas. Electron microscopic examination shows microvilli projecting from the luminal surfaces of the cells. Desmosomes are present at points of contact with other cells at the base. Large electron-dense granules, probably secretory in character, are present in many cells.

**"Carcinoid Tumor".** There has been a report of "carcinoid tumors" arising in the middle ear on the basis of neuroendocrine granules found within the tumor cells on electron microscopy.[76] Apart from this ultrastructural feature, this neoplasm is otherwise typical of adenomas as described above; there seems little justification for invoking the term *carcinoid* with its suggestion of an endocrine aspect and a more aggressive behavior of the neoplasm, which this tumor did not possess.

**Differential Diagnosis.** The important differential diagnosis of adenoma of the middle ear is from adenocarcinoma. In the great majority of cases, the latter neoplasm is metastatic to the middle ear. The distinction can usually be made easily on the basis of the benign cellular pattern of the adenoma and the lack of destructive features clinically and on radiography. Ceruminoma grows in the ear canal and shows a myoepithelial layer and decapitation secretion.

**Treatment.** The treatment by simple excision of all growth in the cases described by Hyams and Michaels[72] resulted in recurrence in only one case. There was no recurrence on follow-up of this latter case 10 years after further resection of the growth.

### Inverted Papilloma

Three cases of a benign tumor with appearances resembling the inverted papilloma of the nose were seen at the Armed Forces Institute of Pathology in Washington, D.C. These neoplasms had a benign course (VJ Hyams, personal communication).

### Meningioma

Most meningiomas are intracranial. Extracranial meningiomas are sometimes seen, particularly in the nose and ear. Like the intracranial variety, they are thought to arise in the arachnoid villi. These structures may be formed at a number of sites in the temporal bone, including the internal auditory canal, the jugular foramen, the geniculate ganglion region, and the roof of the eustachian tube. Thus, meningiomas may arise from a wide area within the temporal bone itself.[77] The commonest temporal bone site for primary meningioma is in the middle ear cleft. Symptoms are usually those of otitis media; involvement of the chorda tympani and facial nerve may also occur.

The gross appearance is that of a granular or even gritty mass. Microscopically, the neoplasm takes the same forms as any of the well-described intracranial types of meningioma (Fig. 22-54). The most common variety seen in the middle ear is the meningothelial type, in which the tumor cells form reg-

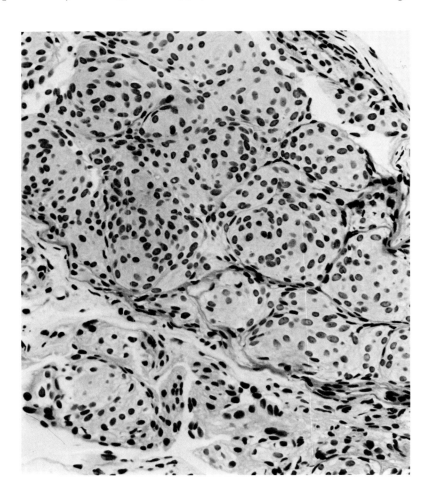

**Fig. 22-54.** Meningioma of middle ear. The tumor cells form regular epithelioid groups with a tendency to a whorled arrangement. (H & E, original magnification X 440.)

ular epithelioid masses with a whorled structure. Fibroblastic and psammomatous varieties are also sometimes seen in the middle ear.

Nager's review of temporal bone meningioma indicated that only two of 30 cases survived the 5-year period. More recent experience of middle ear meningiomas indicates a more favorable outlook after careful local excision. Nevertheless, I have seen three meningiomas presenting in the middle ear at the Royal National Throat, Nose and Ear Hospital, London, in which there were repeated recurrences, until it became clear that the tumor was arising from outside the petrous bone, probably on its external surface, and was actually invading the middle ear. Such tumors need not reveal symptoms related to space-occupying lesions of the intracranial cavity.

### Jugulotympanic Paraganglioma

Jugulotympanic paraganglioma (chemodectoma) presents in the middle ear in most cases; it is slightly less frequent than squamous cell carcinoma in this situation.

**Site of Origin.**   Most jugulotympanic paragangliomas arise from the paraganglion which is situated in the wall of the jugular bulb; a few of the tumors arise from the paraganglion situated near the middle ear surface of the promontory. The distinction between jugular and tympanic paragangliomas is easily made radiologically. The jugular neoplasm shows evidence of invasion of the petrous bone. The tympanic neoplasm is confined to the middle ear.

**Sex and Age Incidence.**   These neoplasms arise predominantly in females. Alford and Guilford[78] give the proportion of female patients as 75 percent. The neoplasm has been seen at ages between 13 and 85 years with a mean age of 50 years.

**Clinical Features.**   Most patients present with conductive hearing loss. Pain in the ears, as well as facial palsy, hemorrhage, and tinnitus, are also described as symptoms of this lesion. On examination, a red vascular mass is seen either behind the intact tympanic membrane or sprouting through the lat-

ter into the external auditory canal. Surgical approach to the mass, as at biopsy, results in severe bleeding.

**Gross Appearance.**   The neoplasm is a reddish sprouting mass at its external surface. In the jugular variety, the petrous temporal bone is largely replaced by red, firm material, the middle ear space is occupied by soft reddish neoplasm as far as the tympanic membrane. The bony labyrinth is rarely invaded by paraganglioma. In a case of jugular paraganglioma that I was able to examine grossly by the microslicing method, the shape of the jugular bulb was still outlined, but it was completely replaced by neoplasm (Figs. 22-55 and 22-56).

**Microscopic Appearance.**   The neoplasm in a typical section shows some resemblance to carotid body tumor. Epithelioid, rather uniform, cells are separated by numerous blood vessels. The tumor cells often form clusters, or *Zellballen* (Fig. 22-57). Nuclei are usually uniform and small, but a diagnosis is sometimes made difficult by the presence of bizarre or multinucleate cells. These appearances do not denote a malignant origin. I have not encountered an alveolar pattern in paragangliomas, such as that reported by Chen and Dehner,[79] to resemble adenoma of the middle ear. A fibrous stroma is sometimes encountered in these tumors. Reticulin stain usually shows groups of tumor cells outlined by reticulin, without reticulin fibers between the cells. Neuron-specific enolase, as demonstrated by the immunoperoxidase method, is positive in the cells of this neoplasm. Formalin fluorescence has been detected in paragangliomas of the middle ear by a similar touch preparation technique to that which I have used for the demonstration of olfactory neuroblastomas.[80] Electron microscopic examination shows membrane-bound electron-dense granules in the cytoplasm of these cells. Such granules may even be found in the cells of this neoplasm at autopsy (Fig. 22-58).

**Spread and Natural History.**   Jugulotympanic paraganglioma is a neoplasm of slow growth. The jugular variety infiltrates the petrous bone, but distant metastasis is rare, reportedly occurring in only 2 percent of cases.[78] Recurrence is stated to occur in

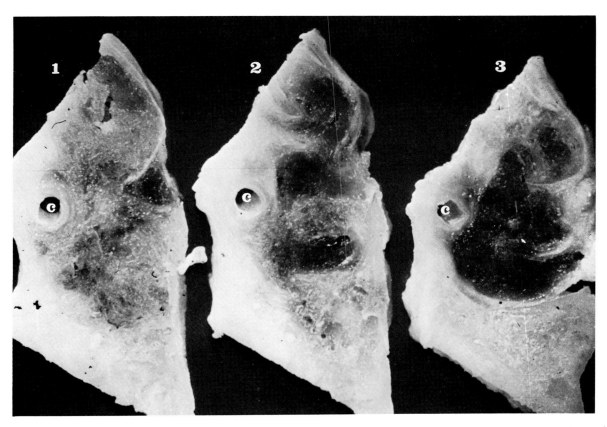

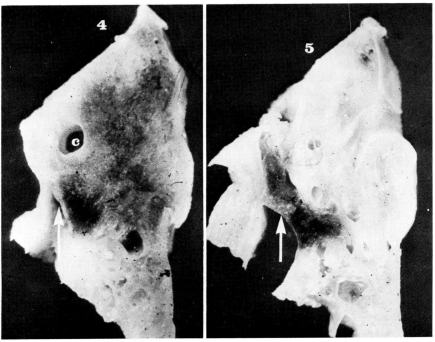

**Fig. 22-55.** Microslices of temporal bone in a case of jugular paraganglioma. The tumor appears as dark areas, bright red in the original. It is seen in slice 1 on the posterior wall and by slice 3, higher in the temporal bone it has expanded to the shape and position of the jugular bulb. c, internal carotid artery.

**Fig. 22-56.** Higher-level microslices of temporal bone in the case of jugular paraganglioma shown in Fig. 22-54. In slices 4 and 5, tumor occupies the middle ear cavity. Arrow points to tympanic membrane. c, internal carotid artery.

from one-third to one-half of treated cases, and the mortality is about 17 percent.[81] Death usually results from spread of the tumor to the intracranial cavity.

### Squamous Carcinoma

Squamous carcinoma, although the most frequent of the neoplasms of the neoplasms of the middle ear, is nevertheless very uncommon. Approximately 40,000 cases of chronic otitis media were seen at the Royal National Throat, Nose and Ear Hospital, London, between 1962 and 1978. Yet, during the same period, only 28 cases of squamous cell carcinoma of the middle ear were seen at this hospital.[82] The following description is taken from the report of this hospital's experience of this disease.

**Age and Sex Incidence.** Incidence is equal in the two sexes. The age range is 34 to 85 years, with an average of 60 years.

**Clinical Features.** Aural discharge and conductive hearing loss are present in all patients. Pain in the ear as well as bleeding and facial palsy are common. None of the patients seen at our hospital had cholesteatoma.

**Site of Origin and Microscopic Appearance.** In microscopic sections of squamous carcinoma of the middle ear, tumor may be seen arising from the surface squamous epithelium (Fig. 22-59). In some

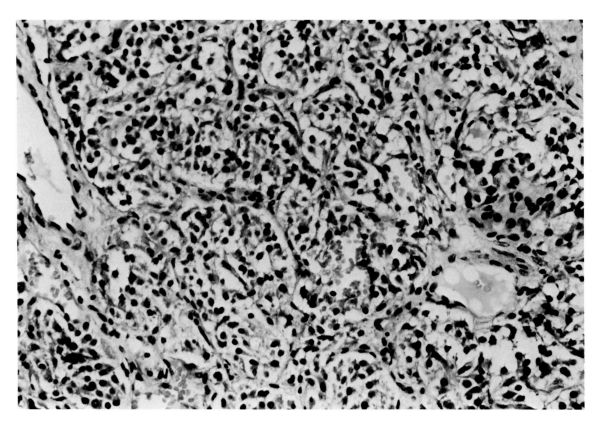

**Fig. 22-57.** Jugular paraganglioma. The tumor cells form small clusters with numerous intervening blood vessels. (H & E, original magnification X 440.)

areas an origin from the basal layers of cubical or columnar epithelium may be seen. This feature is also present in some cases of squamous carcinoma of the larynx. In some, the tumor appears to arise from external ear as well as middle ear and the squamous epithelium of the ear canal with its sebaceous and apocrine adnexa is confirmed histologically as the source of part of the tumor. There is no doubt that such cases arise concomitantly from both external and middle ear epithelia, rather than by subepithelial spread of tumor from one to the other.

The neoplasm is an epidermoid carcinoma similar in range of keratinization and epithelial differentiation to similar neoplasms elsewhere in the upper respiratory tract. Carcinoma in situ may be seen in some parts of the middle ear epithelium adjacent to the growth.

**Spread.** The mode of spread of the neoplasm from the middle ear epithelium was worked out in temporal bone autopsy sections by Michaels and Wells[82] and subsequently confirmed radiologically in living patients with squamous carcinoma of the middle ear.[83] The carcinoma tends to grow into and erode the thin bony plate which separates the medial wall of the middle ear at its junction with the eustachian tube, from the carotid canal (Figs. 22-60 and 22-61). This bony wall is normally up to 1 mm in thickness and may be recognized radiologically. Having reached the carotid canal, the growth will extend rapidly along the sympathetic nerves and the tumor is now impossible to eradicate surgically. Another important method of spread is through the bony walls of the posterior mastoid air cells to the dura of the posterior surface of the temporal bone. From there it travels me-

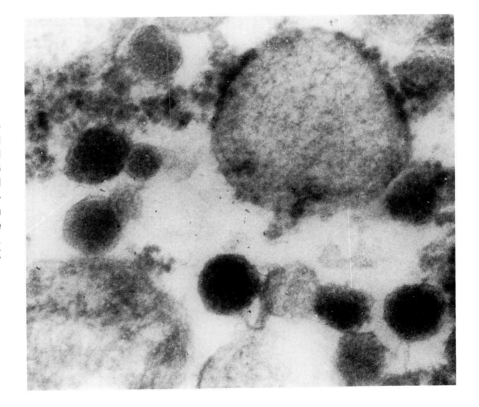

**Fig. 22-58.** Postmortem electron micrograph of formalin fixed paraganglioma from temporal bone tumor shown in Fig. 22-56 and 22-57. Membrane-bound granules of about 120 nm diameter are present in the cytoplasm of the tumor, confirming the diagnosis of paraganglioma. (Original magnification X 140,000.)

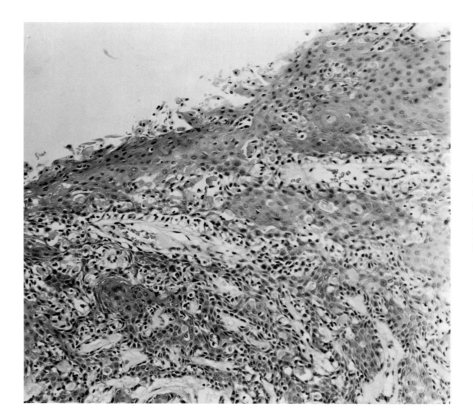

**Fig. 22-59.** Squamous carcinoma of middle ear. Note origin of malignant downgrowths from metaplastic malignant epithelium. (H & E, original magnification X 175.)

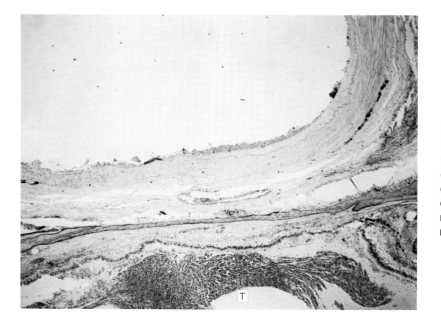

**Fig. 22-60.** Eustachian tube (T) and carotid canal with internal carotid artery in a case of squamous carcinoma of the middle ear. At this level, a thin bar of bone separates the tube from the carotid canal. The tube contains a large number of neutrophils. (H & E, original magnification X 44.)

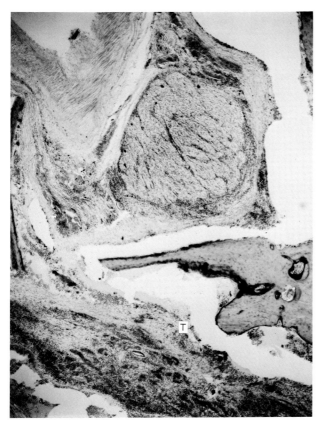

**Fig. 22-61.** Squamous carcinoma of middle ear at a lower level than shown in Fig. 22-60. Squamous carcinoma growing from the epithelium of the eustachian tube (T) has penetrated the thin bar of bone separating it from the carotid canal and is growing in the nerve plexus around the internal carotid artery. (H & E, original magnification X 44.)

When invasion does occur, it takes place after entry of the tumor into the internal auditory canal and penetration of the bone by way of the filaments of the vestibular and cochlear divisions of the 8th nerve. In the later stages, tumor grows extensively in the middle cranial fossa and may invade the condyle of the mandible. Death is usually due to direct intracranial extension. Lymph node metastasis is unusual and spread by the bloodstream even more so.

### Papillary Adenocarcinoma

Many glandular neoplasms in which a diagnosis of primary adenocarcinoma of the middle ear is initially suspected shows features that permit their eventual classification as adenomas of the middle ear. Some, however, show too many atypical cellular features for a benign tumor and adenocarcinoma must be considered. In such cases, every effort must be made to exclude the possibility of the middle ear neoplasm representing a secondary metastatic deposit. A group of eight cases showing a distinctive primary glandular neoplasm of the middle ear has been seen in the Otolaryngic Division of the Armed Forces Institute of Pathology (VJ Hyams, personal communication). These neoplasms display a papillary adenocarcinomatous pattern with a close resemblance to papillary adenocarcinoma of the thyroid. The behavior is that of a slow-growing but invasive neoplasm that responds well to surgical therapy. Similar tumors have been mentioned in recent publications.[84,85]

### Metastatic Neoplasms

Metastasis of malignant neoplasms to the temporal bone is not uncommon. Hill and Kohut[86] listed breast, lung, kidney, stomach, and larynx as primary sources of metastatic tumors in that order of frequency. Jahn et al.[87] drew attention to malignant melanoma as a common source of metastasis and noted two distinct modes of spread of all metastatic neoplasms within the temporal bone. These correspond to the two modes of spread described in primary squamous carcinoma above: (1) along vascular channels in the petrous bone, and (2)

dially, enters the internal auditory canal, and may invade the cochlea and vestibule from the internal canal. Spread into the lamellar bone in both situations is along vascular channels between bone trabeculae. A similar type of bone invasion may also occur from other parts of the middle ear surface such as in the region of the facial nerve. By contrast the special bone of the bony labyrinth is peculiarly resistant to direct spread of growth from tumor within the middle ear (Fig. 22-62); even the round window membrane is not invaded (Fig. 22-63).

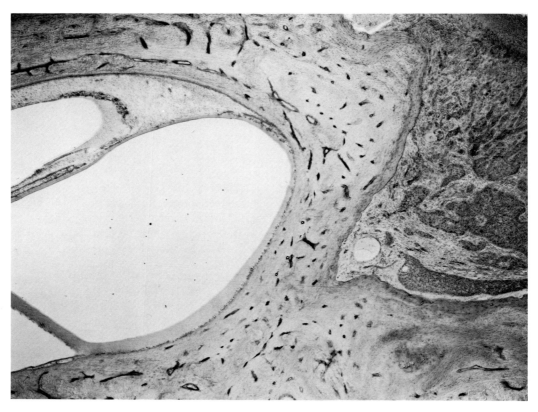

**Fig. 22-62.** Squamous carcinoma of the middle ear. Tumor has eroded the periosteal layer of the bony cochlea but has not entered the endochondral layer. (H & E, original magnification x 44.)

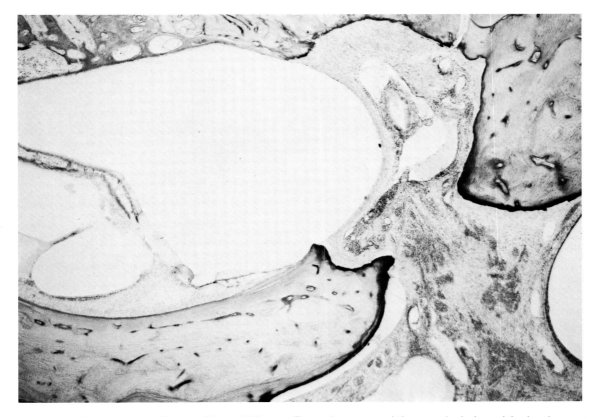

**Fig. 22-63.** Squamous carcinoma of the middle ear. Tumor has entered the round window niche but has not invaded the round window membrane. (Original magnification X 44.)

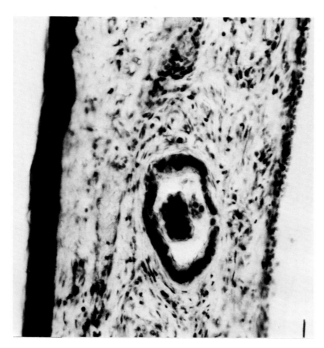

**Fig. 22-64.** Metastatic adenocarcinoma of temporal bone. Section of tympanic membrane. Adenocarcinoma has grown from the bony tympanic ring into the connective tissue layer of the membrane. (H & E, original magnification X 440.)

along nerves emanating from the internal auditory meatus into the labyrinthine structures and bone. I have seen a case of metastatic adenocarcinoma in which the neoplasm grew along the connective tissue of the tympanic membrane between the squamous and cuboidal epithelia (Fig. 22-64).

## REFERENCES

1. Michaels L, Gould SJ, Wells M: The microslicing method in the study of temporal bone changes in the perinatal period. Acta Otolaryngol (Stockh) 423[Suppl]:9, 1985
2. Zechner G, Altmann F: The temporal bone in Hunter's syndrome (gargoylism). Arch Klin Exp Ohren Nasen Kehlkopfheilkd 192:137, 1968
3. Senturia BH, Marcus MD, Lucente FE: Diseases of the External Ear. An Otologic–Dermatologic Manual. Grune & Stratton, Orlando, FL, 1980
4. Chandler JR: Malignant external otitis. Laryngoscope 78:1257, 1968
5. Wells M, Michaels L: "Malignant otitis externa" — A form of chronic otitis media with complications? Clin Otolaryngol 9:131, 1984 (abst)
6. Liu C, Llanis-Rodas R: Application of the immunofluorescent technic to the study of pathogenesis and rapid diagnosis of virus infections. Am J Clin Pathol 57:829, 1972
7. Lever WF, Schaumberg-Lever G: Histopathology of the Skin. 6th Ed. JB Lippincott, Philadelphia, 1983
8. Michaels L, Shah N: Dangers of corn starch powder. (Letter.) Br Med J 2:714, 1973
9. Hughes RA, Berry CL, Seifert M, et al: Relapsing polychondritis. Three cases with a clinico-pathological study and literature review. J Med 41:363, 1972
10. Verity MA, Larson WM, Madden SC: Relapsing polychondritis. Report of two necropsied cases with histochemical investigation of the cartilage lesion. Am J Pathol 42:251, 1963
11. Foidart JM, Abe S, Martin GR, et al: Antibodies to type 11 collagen in relapsing polychondritis. N Engl J Med 299:1203, 1978
12. Rajapakse DA, Bywaters EG: Cell mediated immunity to cartilage proteoglycan in relapsing polychondritis. Clin Exp Immunol 16:497, 1974
13. Valenzuela R, Cooperrider PA, Gogate P, et al: Relapsing polychondritis. Immunomicroscopic findings in cartilage of ear biopsy specimens. Hum Pathol 11:19, 1980
14. Piepergerdes JC, Kramer BM, Behnke EE: Keratosis obturans and external auditory canal cholesteatoma. Laryngoscope 90:383, 1980
15. Hawke M, Jahn AF: Keratin implantation granuloma in external ear canal. Arch Otolaryngol 100:317, 1974
16. Koch HJ, Lewis JJ: Hyperlipemic xanthomatosis with associated osseous granulomas. A clinical report. N Engl J Med 255:387, 1956
17. Emery PS, Gore M: An extensive solitary xanthoma of the temporal bone associated with hyperlipoproteinaemia. J Laryngol Otol 96:451, 1982
18. Azadeh B, Ardehali S: Malakoplakia of middle ear: A case report. Histopathology 7:129, 1983
19. Winkler M: Knötchenformige Erkrankung am Helix (Chondermatitis Nodularis Chronica Helicis). Arch Dermatol 12:278, 1915
20. Metzger SA, Goodman ML: Chondermatitis helicis. A clinical re-evaluation and pathological review. Laryngoscope 86:1402, 1976

21. Barnes HM, Calman CD, Sarkany I: Spectacle frame acanthoma (granuloma fissuratum). Trans St John's Hosp Dermatol Soc 60:99, 1974

22. Mendonca D: Pseudo (atypical) pyogenic granuloma of the ear. J Laryngol Otol 87:577, 1973

23. Grimwood R, Swinehart SM, Aeling JL: Angiolymphoid hyperplasia with eosinophilia. Arch Dermatol 115:205, 1979

24. Hansen JE: Pseudocysts of the auricle in Caucasians. Arch Otolaryngol 85:13, 1967

25. Santos VB, Polisar IA, Ruffy ML: Bilateral pseudocysts in a female. Ann Otol 83:9, 1974

26. Henderson FW, Collier AM, Sanyal MA, et al: A longitudinal study of respiratory viruses and bacteria in the etiology of acute otitis media with effusion. N Engl J Med 306:1377, 1982

27. Friedmann I: The pathology of otitis media. J Clin Pathol 9:229, 1956

28. Schuknecht HF: Pathology of the Ear. Harvard University Press, Cambridge, MA, 1974

29. Tos M, Bak-Pedersen K: Goblet cell population in the normal middle ear and Eustachian tube of children and adults. Ann Otol 85(Suppl 25):44, 1976

30. Tos M, Bak-Pedersen K: Goblet cell population in the pathological middle ear and Eustachian tube of children and adults. Ann Otol 86:209, 1977

31. Tos M: Production of mucus in the middle ear and Eustachian tube. Ann Otol 83:44, 1974

32. Wittmaak K: Über die normale und die pathologische Pneumatisation des Schlafbeins. G Fischer, Jena, 1918

33. Albrecht W: Pneumatisation und Konstitution. Z Hals-Nasen Ohrenheilkd 10:51, 1954

34. Brock W: Trommelfelbild und Pneumatisation der Warzenteile: eine rontgenologische Studie. Z Hals-Nasen Ohrenheilkd 15:241, 1926

35. Sadé J: The blue drum (idiopathic hemotympanum) and cholesterol granulomas. p. 12. In Sadé J (ed): Secretory Otitis Media and Its Sequelae. Churchill Livinstone, New York, 1979

36. Beaumont GD: The effect of exclusion of air from pneumatised bones. J Laryngol Otol 80:236, 1966

37. Thomas SM, Shimada T, Lim DJ: Experimental cholesterol granuloma. Arch Otolaryngol 91:356, 1970

38. Kuipers W, van der Beek JMH, Willart ECT: The effect of experimental tubal obstruction on the middle ear. Preliminary report. Acta Otolaryngol (Stockh) 87:345, 1979

39. Sadé J, Teitz A: Cholesterol in cholesteatoma and in the otitis media syndrome. p. 125 In Sadé J (ed): Cholesteatoma and Mastoid Surgery. Proceedings

of the Second International Conference. Kugler, Amsterdam, 1982

40. Friedmann I, Galey FR: Initiation and stages of mineralization in tympanosclerosis. J Laryngol Otol 94:1215, 1980

41. Katchburian E: Membrane bound bodies as initiators of mineralization of dentine. J Anat 116:285, 1973

42. Hussl B, Lim DJ: Fine morphology of tympanosclerosis. pp. 348–353. In Lim DJ, Bluestone CD, Klein JO, Nelson JD (eds): Recent Advances in Otitis Media with Effusion. BC Decker, Philadelphia, 1984

43. Poliquin JF, Catanzaro A, Robb J, Schiff M. Adaptive immunity of the tympanic membrane. Am J Otolaryngol 2:94, 1981

43a. Cohen D: Locations of primary cholesteatoma. Am J Otology 8:61, 1987

43b. Levenson MJ, Parisier SC, Chute P, Wenig S, Juarbe C: A review of twenty congenital cholesteatomas of the middle ear in children. Otolaryngol Head Neck Surg 94:560, 1986

43c. Michaels L: An epidermoid formation in the developing middle ear; possible source of cholesteatoma. J Otolaryngol 15:169, 1986

43d. Michaels L: Evolution of the epidermoid formation and its role in the development of the middle ear and tympanic membrane during the first trimester. J Otolaryngol 1987, in press

44. Nager GT: Epidermoids involving the temporal bone. p. 41. In Sadé J (ed): Cholesteatoma and Mastoid Surgery. Proceedings of the Second International Conference. Kugler, Amsterdam, 1982

45. Sadé J, Berco E, Buyanover D, Brown M: Ossicular damage in chronic middle ear inflammation. p. 347. In Sadé J (ed): Cholesteatoma and Mastoid Surgery. Proceedings of the Second International Conference. Kugler, Amsterdam, 1982

46. Wells MD, Michaels L: Role of retraction pockets in cholesteatoma formation. Clin Otolaryngol 8:39, 1983

47. Sadé J: The clinical picture. pp. 1–11. In Sadé J (ed): Secretory Otitis Media and Its Sequelae. Churchill Livingstone, New York, 1979

48. Meyerhoff WL, Kim CS, Paparella MM: Pathology of chronic otitis media. Ann Otol Rhinol Laryngol 87:749, 1978

49. Proctor B, Lindsay JR: Tuberculosis of the ear. Arch Otolaryngol 35:221, 1942

50. Lopansri S, Mihm MC Jr: Pilomatrix carcinoma or calcifying epitheliocarcinoma of Malherbe. A case report and review of the literature. Cancer 45:2368, 1980

51. Metcalfe PB Jr: Carcinoma of the pinna. N Engl J Med 251:91, 1954

52. Goodwin WC, Jesse RH: Malignant neoplasms of the external auditory canal and temporal bone. Arch Otolaryngol 106:675, 1980

53. Lewis JS: Squamous carcinoma of the ear. Arch Otolaryngol 97:41, 1973

54. Johns ME, Headington JT: Squamous cell carcinoma of the external auditory canal. Arch Otolaryngol 100:45, 1974

55. Woodson GE, Jurco S III, Alford BR, McGavran MH: Verrucous carcinoma of the middle ear. Arch Otolaryngol 107:63, 1981

56. Wetli CV, Pardo V, Millard M, Gersdon K: Tumors of ceruminous glands. Cancer 29:1169, 1972

57. Cankar V, Crowley H: Tumors of ceruminous glands: A clinicopathological study of 7 cases. Cancer 17:67, 1964

58. Pulec JL: Glandular tumors of the external auditory canal. Laryngoscope 87:1601, 1977

59. Bagley FH, Cady B, Lee A, Legg MA: Changes in clinical presentation and management of malignant melanoma. Cancer 47:2126, 1981

60. Pack GT, Conley J, Oropega R: Melanoma of the external ear. Arch Otolaryngol 92:106, 1970

61. Nager GT, Kennedy DW, Kopstein E: Fibrous dysplasia: A review of the disease and its manifestations in the temporal bone. Ann Otol Rhinol Laryngol 91[suppl 92]: pp. 1–52, 1982

62. Sheehy JL: Diffuse exostoses and osteomata of the external auditory canal: A report of 100 operations. Otolaryngol Head Neck Surg 90:337, 1982

63. Graham MD: Osteomas and exostoses of the external auditory canal. A clinical, histopathologic and scanning electron microscopic study. Ann Otol 88:566, 1979

64. Leedham PW, Swash M: Chondrosarcoma with subarachnoid dissemination. J Pathol 107:59, 1972

65. Moyes PD, Bratty PJA, Dolman CJ: Osteoclastoma of the jugular foramen. J Neurosurg 32:255, 1970

66. Jaffee BF, Fox JE, Batsakis JG: Rhabdomyosarcoma of the middle ear and mastoid. Cancer 27:29, 1971

67. Tors M: A survey of Hand-Schüller-Christian disease in otolaryngology. Acta Otolaryngol (Stockh) 62:217, 1966

68. Diamandopolous GTh, Meissner WA: Neoplasia. p. 515. In Kissane JH (ed): Anderson's Pathology. 8th Ed. CV Mosby, St Louis, 1984

69. Quaranta A, Mininni F, Resta L: Salivary gland choristoma of the middle ear. A case report. J Laryngol Otol 95:953, 1981

70. Kamerer DB, Caparosa RJ: Temporal bone encephalocele — Diagnosis and treatment. Laryngoscope 92:878, 1982

71. Konrad HR, Pearson DH, VanWinkle R, Hopla D: Traumatic porencephalic cysts of the ear canal: Diagnosis and therapy. Otolaryngol Head Neck Surg 89:477, 1981

72. Hyams VJ, Michaels L: Benign adenomatous neoplasms (adenoma) of the middle ear. Clin Otolaryngol 1:17, 1976

73. Derlacki EL, Barney PL: Adenomatous tumors of the middle ear and mastoid. Laryngoscope 86:1123, 1976

74. Jahrsdoerfer RA, Fechner RE, Selman JW, et al: Adenoma of the middle ear. Laryngoscope 93:1041, 1983

75. Mills SE, Fechner RE: Middle ear adenoma. A cytologically uniform neoplasm displaying a variety of architectural patterns. Am J Surg Pathol 8:677, 1984

76. Murphy GE, Pilch BZ, Dickersin GR, et al: Carcinoid tumour of the middle ear. Am J Clin Pathol 73:816, 1980

77. Nager GT: Meningiomas Involving the Temporal Bone. Charles C Thomas, Springfield, IL, 1963

78. Alford BR, Guilford FR: A comprehensive study of tumors of the glomus jugulare. Laryngoscope 72:765, 1962

79. Chen KTK, Dehner LP: Primary tumors of the external and middle ear. 11. A clinicopathologic study of 14 paragangliomas and three meningiomas. Arch Otolaryngol 104:253, 1978

80. DeLillis RA, Roth JA: Norepinephrine in a glomus jugulare tumor. Arch Pathol Lab Med 92:73, 1971

81. Rosenwasser H: Long-term results of therapy of glomus jugulare tumors. Arch Otolaryngol 97:49, 1973

82. Michaels L, Wells M: Squamous cell carcinoma of the middle ear. Clin Otolaryngol 5:235, 1980

83. Phelps PD, Lloyd GAS: The radiology of carcinoma of the ear. Br J Radiol 54:103, 1981

84. Pallanch JF, McDonald TJ, Weiland LH, et al: Adenocarcinoma and adenoma of the middle ear. Laryngoscope 92:47, 1982

85. Stone HE, Lipa M, Bell RD: Primary adenocarcinoma of the middle ear. Arch Otolaryngol 101:702, 1975

86. Hill BA, Kohut RI: Metastatic adenocarcinoma of the temporal bone. Arch Otolaryngol 102:568, 1976

87. Jahn AF, Farkashidy J, Berman JM: Metastatic tumors in the temporal bone — A pathophysiologic study. J Otolaryngol 8:85, 1979

# Pathology of the Inner Ear

# 23

## Leslie Michaels

This chapter presents a review of the pathologic changes in the human inner ear and some of the clinical correlations. The lesions of this anatomic region include some of the common disorders of humankind. Nevertheless, the postmortem study of these conditions has received less attention than that given to any other part of the body. A large part of the field of temporal bone pathology, in consequence, remains a terra incognita. Much of the material presented is based on small numbers of case reports and is offered rather cautiously. Until a much greater contribution of original observations has been made in this difficult field, a more confident statement will not be possible.

## MALFORMATIONS

### Pathogenesis of Malformations in Relation to Development

The development of the inner ear does not depend on branchial arch structures, but rather on an ectodermal invagination, the otocyst, which becomes separated from the surface ectoderm, and,

by a system of branching and coiling, gives rise to the whole endolymphatic system. The sensory epithelium, cochlear duct, and vestibular and endolymphatic duct areas are differentiated from the inner lining surface cells. The bony labyrinth is formed from the surrounding mesoderm, with the prior development of a cartilaginous framework as in the long bones. Thus, malformations may relate to (1) deficiencies in the degree of branching and coiling of the otocyst-derived tubular structures, (2) absence or poor development ("dysplasia") of the sensory epithelium, and (3) deficiencies in the cartilaginous and bony framework. The first two etiologies may exist separately or together, but if the third is present, the underlying membranous structures are always defective or, more often, absent. Neural elements of the inner ear are derived from the neuroectoderm and its coverings. Malformations of these structures will thus tend to be associated with other brain and skull deformities.

### Problems in Classification

Malformations of the inner ear form a large group of entities, the classification of which is particularly difficult. Attempts have been made to allocate genetic bases for many of these conditions,[1] but the decision is derived frequently from exami-

651

nation of only a single or small number of patients. In many cases, the pathologic basis is unknown. Frequently, the anomaly is classified on the basis of changes elsewhere in the body, if such exist.

The structure and function of the inner ear of patients with developmental malformations are singularly difficult to investigate. The standard clinical tests of hearing are inappropriate in many of these patients, and only recently have modern electrophysiological methods such as electrocochleography shown promise of some improvement in the clinical recognition of these lesions. Surgical exploration is usually not indicated and, even when it is, little can be learned of pathologic changes in the inner ear at middle ear surgery. Radiologic studies have recently provided dramatic advances,[2] but this form of study of the living patient cannot be expected to reveal the finer anomalies of the inner ear tissues. Postmortem investigation of inner ear pathology is difficult and is carried out at only a few centers. Patients with inner ear malformations do not usually die of their ear disturbances, and the need for removal and pathologic examination of the temporal bones will often not be pressing for the pathologist or the medical attendants at the autopsy. Finally, even when the temporal bone has been removed and pathologic changes meticulously analyzed, the findings may appear to be more trivial than suggested by the severe hearing disability suffered by the patient.

Although clear-cut morphologic anomalies have been established in numbers of malformed ears, such information has not yet led to the discovery of many similar anomalies in living patients. This is in strong contrast with the situation in other organs, such as the heart, the seat of a wide range of congenital anomalies. The pathologic bases of cardiac anomalies were worked out in the early twentieth century, leading to the development of physiologic and hemodynamic methods by means of which such anomalies could be recognized in living patients and in some cases, on the basis of clear cut morphologic diagnoses, successfully treated surgically. In the inner ear, in spite of advances in radiology and electrophysiology, similar precise morphologic diagnosis cannot be made nearly so often in the living patient.

It is likely that a whole range of developmental disturbances exists in the human comparable to those in animals. Grüneberg[3] described a mutant form of mice in which the inner ear appears to develop normally until about 8 to 12 days after birth, when "degeneration" occurs in the organ of Corti and the animals do not hear. Since vestibular sensory epithelium is also sometimes affected and there is some recent evidence that in fact there may be an earlier developmental defect, the term *neuroepithelial abnormality* is perhaps more appropriate than *degeneration* for this condition.[4] If it affected humans, a disturbance of this sort might be suspected, but would be difficult to confirm as a distinct entity on the basis of the sequence of morphologic abnormalities. It is conceivable that genetically determined inner ear disease with a similar natural history may occur not only in the early years of life, corresponding to the newborn mouse, but also later in life and even in old age. Even the broad group of patients labeled as having presbycusis may include some patients with that kind of deafness.

Another difficulty is the autolytic changes suffered by the structures of the membranous labyrinth when postmortem examination is delayed. This may lead not only to apparent loss of hair cells in the organ of Corti, the most frequent appearance, but also to collapse and adhesion of Reissner's membrane and degeneration of strial and vestibular cells. These are, however, the very changes that characterize the Scheibe or cochleosaccular type of anomaly. This anomaly undoubtedly exists as a true human developmental defect and has its counterparts in animals,[4] but some cases have been wrongly placed into this and similar categories on account of autolysis.

## Structural Forms of Malformation

Among the attempts made to classify malformations of the inner ear, that of Ormerod has, perhaps, aroused the most interest.[5] He delineated four broad types of lesion:

1. Michel type: complete lack of development
2. Mondini-Alexander, more usually known as the Mondini, type: development of only a single curved tube representing the cochlea and the

presence of similar immaturity of the vestibule and canals (Fig. 23-1)

3. Bing-Siebenmann type: underdevelopment of the membranous labyrinth, particularly its sense organ, with a well-formed otic capsule
4. Scheibe type: malformation restricted to organ of Corti and saccular neuroepithelium (Fig. 23-2)

Reference to this developmental schema above suggests that (1) corresponds to (a), (b), and (c) combined; (2) corresponds to (a) above; and both (3) and (4) correspond to (b).

Many defects within this classification are not described. Suehiro and Sando[6] listed a large number of congenital lesions and proposed a new and more detailed system based on the presence of structural anomalies of parts of the bony or membranous labyrinth or both. This classification is outlined in Table 23-1.

### Etiology of Malformations

Many of the malformations of the inner ear represent part of a disease or syndrome usually associated with other defects. These diseases may be classified on an etiologic basis and a summary of these and some notes on important examples are given in Table 23-2. Further details on the pathology of these conditions will be found in the works of Konigsmark,[7] Konigsmark and Gorlin,[1] and Suehiro and Sando.[6]

An index of those malformations of the inner ear that have been studied in temporal bone specimens, with notes on the changes found, is presented alphabetically in Table 23-3.

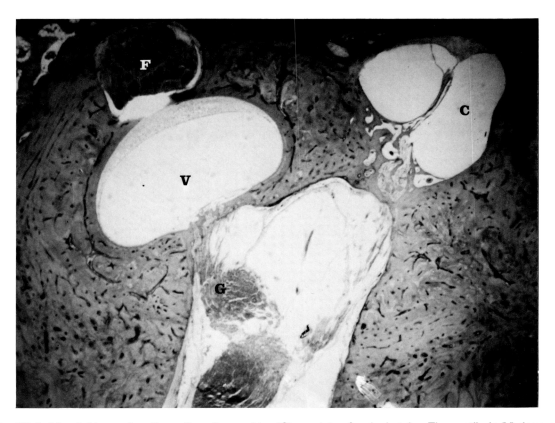

**Fig. 23-1.** Mondini type of malformation. The cochlea (C) consists of a single tube. The vestibule (V) does not contain endolymphatic sacs. Note the anomalous position of the facial nerve (F). G, vestibular ganglion. (H & E, original magnification × 18.)

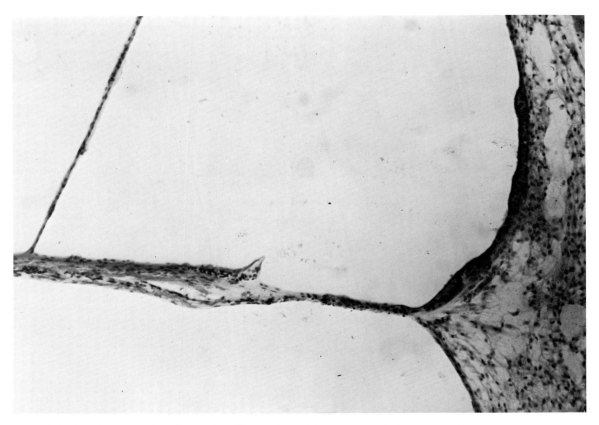

**Fig. 23-2.** Scheibe type of malformation. The outline of the scala media is present, but the organ of Corti is absent. (H & E, original magnification × 175.)

## HEMORRHAGE INTO THE INNER EAR IN VERY-LOW-BIRTHWEIGHT INFANTS

Very-low-birthweight infants are known to be at increased risk of sensorineural hearing loss. This has been found in 4 to 18 percent of such babies.[69] There has been little postmortem study on those infants who do not survive to ascertain the possible pathologic basis for the hearing loss. In cases of hyperbilirubinemia, it is well known that the cochlear nucleus may be damaged by the toxic effect of unconjugated bilirubin. The use of anti-D prophylaxis has greatly reduced the incidence of this complication.

Attention has recently been focused on the possibility of hemorrhage into the hearing portion of the inner ear as a cause of this deafness. Spector et al.[70] studied the temporal bones of 52 neonatal infants of whom 28 had respiratory distress. Hemorrhage had extended from the subarachnoid space into perilymphatic spaces of the inner ear in 23 of these cases by a variety of pathways, including the internal auditory canal and cochlear aqueduct. A study is under way in my department in which the temporal bones of neonatal deaths, many of which are of low birthweight, are examined by the microslicing method and subsequent histology. In an interim report,[71] 49 cases had been so examined, in 12 which hemorrhage was observed within the 8th nerve. This was always composed of bright red blood that had exuded at the apex of the fundus within the cochlear division of the nerve. In three

## Table 23-1. Anatomic Classification of Malformations of Inner Ear

**Inner ear as a whole**
  Absence and underdevelopment of labyrinth

**Cochlea**
  Cochlea in general
    Absent, underdeveloped, or anteriorly displaced
  Osseous cochlea
    Osseous cochlea in general, such as deformity
    Round window absent, displaced, or partitioned by bony bar
    Scala tympani underdeveloped
    Scala vestibuli absent or underdeveloped
    Modiolus absent, underdeveloped, or focally thickened
    Cochlear aqueduct absent, underdeveloped, or widened
  Membranous cochlea
    Cochlear duct in general absent or underdeveloped
    Organ of Corti absent or underdeveloped
    Tectorial membrane underdeveloped or rolled and covered by single epithelial layer
    Spiral limbus partially absent
    Stria vascularis absent, deformed, underdeveloped or displaced
    Spiral ligament absent, deformed, or calcified
    Reissner's membrane absent or displaced
    Basilar membrane elongated, absent, or displaced
    Ductus reuniens absent or enlarged

**Vestibule**
  Vestibule in general underdeveloped
  Osseous vestibule
    Osseous vestibule in general underdeveloped or malformed
    Oval window absent, thin, malformed, calcified annular ligament
    Vestibular aqueduct underdeveloped or displaced
  Membranous vestibule
    Utricle absent, underdeveloped, large, or malformed; anomalies of macule
    Saccule absent, undeveloped, or malformed; anomalies of macule
    Endolymphatic duct and sac, including underdevelopment, shortening and widening, and anomalies of utriculoendolymphatic valve

**Semicircular canal**
  Semicircular canal in general
    Absent, underdeveloped, or enlarged
  Superior semicircular canal
    In general, absence of canal or parts of it
    Osseous superior semicircular canal; underdeveloped or widened
    Membranous superior semicircular canal; absence of part or widening of part of it; absence or underdeveloped crista
  Posterior semicircular canal
    Posterior semicircular canal generally absent, underdeveloped, displaced superiorly, or deformed
    Osseous posterior semicircular canal narrow or enlarged
    Membranous posterior semicircular canal absent, widened, narrowed, or crista malformed
  Lateral semicircular canal
    Lateral semicircular canal in general absent, underdeveloped, or malformed
    Osseous lateral semicircular canal absent or underdeveloped and widened
    Membranous lateral semicircular canal absent, underdeveloped, or flat; crista undeveloped or flat and maculalike

**Internal auditory canal**
  Absent, underdeveloped, displaced, or deformed

**Nerves**
  Facial nerve
    Absent, underdeveloped, displaced
  Eighth nerve
    In general, absent or underdeveloped
    Cochlear nerve absent or displaced
    Vestibular nerve absent or displaced

**Vessels**
  Displaced (e.g., crossing perilymphatic space of cochlea)

**Subarcuate fossa**
  Absent, underdeveloped, displaced, or enlarged

(After Suehiro S, Sando I: Congenital anomalies of the inner ear. Introducing a new class of labyrinthine anomalies. Ann Otol Rhinol Laryngol 88(suppl 59):1, 1979.)

655

**Table 23-2.   Etiology of Diseases with Inner Ear Anolamies**

Unknown Etiology
 Without associated anomalies (e.g., congenital absence of round window)
 With other associated anomalies (e.g., chromosomal anomalies, anomalies of cochlea, vestibule and semicircular canals, congenital heart disease)

Hereditary Characteristics
 Associated with heart disease (e.g., cardioauditory syndrome—Jervell-Lange-Nielsen syndrome)
 Associated with integumentary system disease (e.g., interoculoiridodermato auditive dysplasia—Waardenburg syndrome)
 Associated with eye disease (e.g., retinitis pigmentosa—Usher's syndrome)
 Associated with nervous system disease (e.g., acoustic neuroma)
 Associated with skeletal disease (e.g., Paget's disease of bone)
 Associated with renal disease (e.g., nephritis and sensorineural hearing loss—Alport's disease)
 Associated with goiter (e.g., goiter and profound sensorineural deafness—Pendred's syndrome

Prenatal infections (e.g. rubella, syphilis)

Iatrogenic ototoxicity (e.g., chloroquine, thalidomide)

**Table 23-3.   Index of Malformations of Inner Ear That Have Been Studied in Temporal Bone Section[a]**

Acrocephalosyndactyly (Apert's syndrome)
 Large, open subarcuate fossa[8]
Alport's syndrome
 *See* Nephritis and sensorineural hearing loss
Anencephaly
 Defects of cochlea, vestibule, semicircular canals, and internal auditory canal[9]
Apert's syndrome
 *See* Acrocephalosyndactyly
Arachnodactyly (Marfan's syndrome)
 Bony lip projecting into vestibular aqueduct[10]
Arnold-Chiari malformation
 Defects of cochlea, vestibule, and semicircular canals[11]
Atresia auris congenita
 Hypoplasia of cochlea, semicircular canals, and internal auditory canal[12]
Bing-Siebenmann defect
 Underdevelopment of membranous labyrinth; well-formed bony labyrinth[13]
Bony vestibule
 *See* Osseous vestibule
Brevicollis (Klippel-Feil syndrome)
 Defects of cochlea, vestibule, semicircular canals, and internal auditory canal[14]
Cardioauditory syndrome (Lange-Nielsen Jervell syndrome)
 Atrophy of organ of Corti and stria vascularis[15]
Cervico-oculoacoustic dysplasia (Wildervanck's syndrome)
 Defects of cochlea, vestibule, and semicircular canals[16]
Cholesteatoma, congenital
 Defects of cochlea, vestibule, and semicircular canals[17]
Cleft palate, micrognathia, and glossoptosis (Pierre-Robin syndrome)
 Defects of cochlea, vestibule, semicircular canals, and internal auditory canal[18]
Cochlea
 Absent[19]
 Absent apical turn[20,21]
 Absent hook portion[22] Anterior displacement[9,23]
 Deformity[9,16,24]
 Underdevelopment[16,25]
Cochlear aqueduct
 Absent[11]
 Hypoplasia[23]
 Wide[6]
Cochlear duct
 Absent[26]
Conjoined twin
 Absense of inner ear and oval window[33]

*(Table continues)*

**Table 23-3** *(continued)*

Craniofacial dysostosis (Crouzon's disease)
    Underdeveloped periosteal layer of labyrinth[31]
Craniometaphyseal dysplasia (Pyle's disease)
    Narrow internal auditory canal[32]
Crouzon's disease
    *See* Craniofacial dysostosis
Deafness, congenital, spiny hyperkeratosis, and universal alopecia
    Defects of tectorial membrane and otolithic membrane[61]
Deleted chromosome D syndrome
    Hypoplastic cochlear aqueduct[23]
DiGeorge syndrome
    *See* Third and fourth pharyngeal pouch syndrome
Dominant progressive early-onset sensorineural hearing loss
    Hydrops[42]
Edward's syndrome
    *See* Trisomy 18 syndrome
Endolymphatic duct
    Shortened[11,16]
    Underdeveloped[11]
    Wide[26,30,36]
Gargoylism (Hurler's syndrome)
    Resorption of perichondrial and periosteal layers[37]
Generalized spiny hyperkeratosis, universal alopecia, and congenital sensorineural deafness
    Cochleosaccular abnormality of Scheibe type[61]
Goiter and profound sensorineural hearing loss (Pendred's syndrome)
    Defects of cochlea, vestibule, and semicircular canals[20]
Goldenhar's syndrome
    *See* Oculoauriculovertebral dysplasia
Gonadal dysgenesis (Turner's syndrome)
    Mondini defect in[38]
Heart disease, congenital
    Defects of cochlea, vestibule, and semicircular canals[39]
Hemifacial microsomia
    *See* Oculoauriculovertebral syndrome
Hereditary hemorrhagic telangiectasia (Rendu-Osler-Weber disease)
    Hypoplasia of vestibular aqueduct and endolymphatic sac[40]
Heredopathia atactica polyneuritiformis (Refsum's syndrome)
    Degeneration of stria vascularis, atrophy of organ of Corti and loss of spiral ganglion cells[41]
Hurler's syndrome
    *See* Gargoylism
Hydrops
    In dominant progressive early-onset sensorineural hearing loss[42]
Hypophosphatasia
    Calcified spiral ligament[43]
Internal auditory canal
    Absent[45]
Interoculoiridodermato auditive dysplasia (Waardenburg's syndrome)
    Absence of organ of Corti and most neurons in spiral ganglion[44]
Interscalar septum
    Absent between apical and middle coils[9,16]
    Absent between middle and basal coils[9,25]
Jervell and Lange-Nielsen syndrome
    *See* Cardioauditory syndrome
Klippel-Feil syndrome
    *See* Brevicollis
Labyrinth
    Absent[33,45]
    Underdeveloped, thalidomide induced[45]
Lateral semicircular canal
    Absent[11,14]
    Dilated[11]
    Flat crista[22,30]
    Undeveloped crista[16,46]
    Wide[9,47]

*(Table continues)*

**Table 23-3** *(continued)*

Macula of utricle
    Small[16]
Mandibulofacial dysostosis (Treacher-Collins syndrome)
    Short cochlea, wide aqueduct, large utricle, absent lateral canal[48,49]
Marfan's syndrome
    *See* Arachnodactyly
Michel's defect
    Complete absence of labyrinth[50] Microstomia, aglossia, agnathia, and synotia
    Wide cochlear aqueduct and bony lateral canal[51]
Mid-frequency sensorineural hearing loss
    Loss of organ of Corti, atrophic stria vascularis, and loss of spiral ganglion cells in basal coil[52]
Modiolus
    Absent in apical turn[54]
    Absent in apical and middle coils[25,53]
    Absence of whole[14,16,24]
    Broad base[16,36]
Mondini's defect
    In Turner's syndrome[38]
    One and a half turns of cochlea[55]
Mondini-Alexander defect
    *See* Mondini's defect
Muckle-Wells syndrome
    *See* Nephritis, urticaria, amyloidosis, and sensorineural hearing loss
Nephritis, urticaria, amyloidosis, and sensorineural deafness (Muckle-Wells syndrome)
    Absent organ of Corti and vestibular sensory epithelium; ossification of basilar membrane[56]
Nephritis and sensorineural hearing loss
    Minor defects of cochlea and vestibule[9]
Oculoauriculovertebral dysplasia (Goldenhar's syndrome)[57]
Organ of Corti
    Absent[9]
Osseous spiral lamina
    Absent[9,14]
Osseous vestibule
    Large[14,16]
    Small[46]
Oval window
    Absent[33,57,62]
    Malformed[34]
Patau's syndrome
    *See* Trisomy 13-15 syndrome
Pendred's syndrome
    *See* Goiter and profound sensorineural deafness
Pierre-Robin's syndrome
    *See* Cleft palate, micrognathia, and glossoptosis
Posterior semicircular canal
    Absent[58]
Preauricular pit, branchial fistula, and hearing loss
    Defects of cochlea, vestibule and semicircular canal[36]
Pyle's disease
    *See* Craniometaphyseal dysplasia
Refsum syndrome
    *See* Heredopathia atactica polyneuritiformis
Reissner's membrane
    Absent[67]
Rendu-Osler-Weber disease
    *See* Hereditary hemorrhagic telangiectasia
Retinitis pigmentosa and congenital sensorineural hearing loss
    Hypoplasia of organ of Corti and stria vascularis[13]
Round window
    Congenital absence of[59]
Saccule
    Absent[14,60]

*(Table continues)*

**Table 23-3** *(continued)*

Adhesion of wall to macula[9]
    Large[16,53]
    Undeveloped[16]
Saccular macula
    Otolithic membrane in fibrous envelope[61]
Scala tympani
    Undeveloped[16]
Scala vestibuli
    Malformed[22]
    Underdeveloped (wide)[46]
Scheibe's defect
    Abnormality of organ of Corti and saccule[69]
Semicircular canals
    Absent[2,60]
    Underdeveloped[16,25]
Sensory radicular neuropathy and progressive sensorineural deafness
    Atrophy of stria vascularis and loss of hair cells in organ of Corti[41]
Sickle cell disease and sensorineural hearing loss
    Degeneration of organ of Corti and stria vascularis (ischemia)[63]
Spiral ligament
    Absent in apical and middle coils[58]
    Calcified[43]
Spiral limbus
    Absent[58]
Stria vascularis
    Absent[16,19]
    Atrophic[21]
Superior semicircular canal
    Absent[14]
    Absent crista[23]
    Absent crus commune[11,36]
Tectorial membrane
    Rolled and covered by epithelium[27,61,65,65]
    Underdevelopment[53]
Third and fourth pharyngeal pouch syndrome
    Defects of cochlea and lateral semicircular canal and internal auditory canal; absent oval window[66]
Treacher Collins' syndrome
    *See* Mandibulofacial dysostosis
Trisomy 13-15 syndrome, Patau's syndrome
    Defects of cochlea, vestibule, semicircular canals, internal auditory canal[22]
Trisomy 18 syndrome
    Defects of cochlea, vestibule, semicircular canals, and singular nerve
Trisomy 21 syndrome
    Shortened cochlea, vestibular defects, superiorly displaced internal auditory meatus[47]
Turner's syndrome
    *See* Gonadal dysgenesis

Usher's syndrome
    *See* Retinitis pigmentosa and congenital sensorineural hearing loss
Utricle
    Absent[14,19]
    Large[11,16]
Vestibular aqueduct
    Bony lip[10]
    Hypoplastic[16,28]
    Large[16,36]
Waardenburg's syndrome
    *See* Interoculoiridodermato auditive dysplasia
Wildervanck's syndrome
    *See* Cervico-oculoacoustic syndrome

---

[a] For each malformation, the second line summarizes morphologic changes. Sources cited appear in the Reference list. This index was drawn up with he aid of Suehiro and Sando,[6] Konigsmark and Gorlin,[1] and Konigsmark.[7]

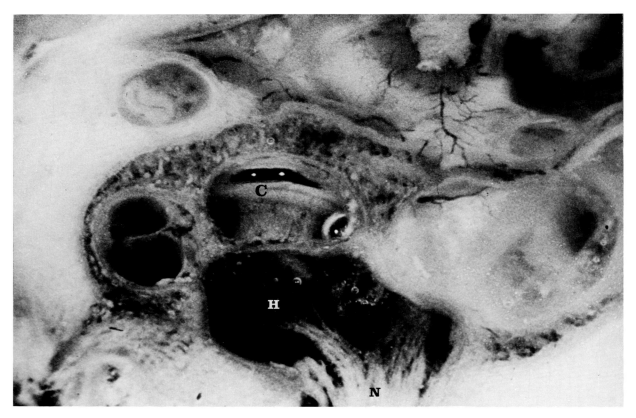

**Fig. 23-3.** Microsliced specimen of temporal bone showing hemorrhage (H) into fundus of internal auditory canal of premature infant. C, cochlea; N, 8th cranial nerve.

cases, the vestibular division of the eighth cranial nerve was also affected by hemorrhage (Fig. 23-3). Histologic examination showed the hemorrhage to be of fresh blood only, with no hemosiderin. The hemorrhage in these cases is probably the result of anoxia, like the intracranial hemorrhage in this age group, which is a frequent concomitant.

## TRAUMA

### Fractures

In most patients with fractures of the base of the skull, the rigid and more brittle wedge of bone occupying about one-third of the skull base, the temporal bone, is the seat of a fracture. Although such material at autopsy provides a large potential source for research into the mechanism of cochlear damage by trauma, this had been hardly used, and what knowledge there is has been largely derived from clinical and radiologic observations.

Fractures of the petrous portion of the temporal bone fall within two anatomic groups: longitudinal and transverse. The effects on the cochlea of these two types of lesion are quite different. Longitudinal fractures arise as a result of direct blows to the temporal and parietal areas of the head. The fracture line starts in the squamous portion of the temporal bone and usually involves the external auditory canal, the tympanic membrane and one or more of the ossicles of the middle ear, and ends up in the region of the foramen lacerum near the apex of the petrous temporal bone. The cochlea is not involved. The transverse fractures are caused by blows to the front or back of the skull, producing a sideways tearing effect. The fracture line in these cases passes from the dural membrane on the posteromedial aspect of the petrous temporal bone, often through the internal auditory canal to involve the 7th and 8th cranial nerves and then into the cochlea in the region of the basal turn at its posterolateral side. The adjacent vestibule and round and oval windows are also frequently involved. Thus, in the case of the longitudinal fracture, the hearing loss is usually mild or moderate, of the conductive type, which may be helped by surgery. The hearing loss caused by a transverse fracture, involving as it does both the sensory organ and the afferent nerve derived from it, produces a severe sensorineural deafness from which little improvement is to be expected. A further serious effect of transverse fractures is the production of a communication between the meninges and the middle ear. Thus, there is a leak of cerebrospinal fluid (CSF), which invariably leads to infection spreading to the meninges, causing death if not controlled by antibiotic therapy. Another form of fluid disturbance in transverse fractures, that involving endolymph, may be associated with the symptoms of Meniere's disease. The pathologic changes in these cases probably arise from the inflammation of perilymph with secondary endolymphatic hydrops. Reissner's membrane is seen to be grossly distended throughout the cochlear duct, and the saccule may be dilated.

In the temporal bone, callus does not seem to form; the union of the two fractured portions is by fibrous tissue, not bone. This type of fracture healing seems to be general in skull fractures and may be related to the immobility of the affected bones.

Small fractures that may or may not be united by fibrous tissue are often found in sections of temporal bone at postmortem examination in cases demonstrating no history of trauma and no symptoms related to the bone damage which is usually insignificant. These healed fractures are found most frequently between the vestibule or cochlea and the middle ear. Their pathogenesis is unknown.

## Microscopic Cochlear Damage in Head Injury

After a head injury, a sensorineural type of deafness may develop without any detectable macro-scopic damage to the cochlea. The hearing loss is in the higher frequency, ranging from 3,000 to 8,000 Hz. Experimental studies have revealed microscopic cochlear damage following direct head injury.[72] Anesthetized animals were given a blow to the exposed skull in the midline, via a 2-lb metal rod 1 inch in diameter, by a 1-lb mallet. The animals were allowed to recover and then tested audiometrically until they were killed some weeks after trauma had been inflicted. All animals had hearing losses at least between 3,000 to 8,000 Hz, and some had an even more widespread damage. The cochleae of all the animals were examined histologically by serial section. A constant change was found to be a loss of external hair cells in the upper basal coil region. In some animals, damage was more marked and in a few there was a complete disappearance of internal and external hair cells in some areas. Nerve fibers and ganglion cells were correspondingly reduced in these areas.

## Blast and Gunshot Injury

Peripheral damage to the ear, particularly rupture of the tympanic membrane, is the most striking result of explosive blast and gunshot injury and vestibular damage frequently takes place; however, permanent damage to the internal ear and its hearing mechanism is also a likely sequela. In the experimental study of injury from this source and other types of injury to the hair cells of the cochlea, a particularly useful technique has been the examination of surface preparations of the spiral organ. By this method, the precise distribution of hair cell damage can be mapped out easily and correlated with functional studies of sound reception. The effects of blast and gunshot injury are initially on the external hair cells of the basal coil. When this type of trauma is particularly severe, outer hair cells in long stretches of the cochlea may be destroyed and the supporting cells in these areas may become disrupted.[73]

## Sound Wave Injury

Sound waves of high intensity damage the cochlea. Again, the pathologic changes are destruction of hair cells. The earliest changes affect isolated outer hair cells. As the intensity of the sound is increased, large groups of outer hair cells die and their supporting cells are lost with them. The basal coil is once more the main center for external hair cell loss. These findings have been obtained mainly by animal experiments, but there is some material from human pathology indicating the same pattern of injury.

### Stimulation Deafness

The changes in the inner ear following the trauma of direct blows to the head, of explosive blasts, and of high-intensity sound waves, which together produce a condition that may be categorized as stimulation deafness,[74] all seem to be directed particularly to the external hair cells of the basal coil. Internal hair cells and higher cochlear coils may be affected by greater degrees of these insults to the inner ear. Although there have been a number of studies of stimulation deafness to determine its pathogenesis, the mechanism of hair cell damage is not understood.

# OTOTOXIC DAMAGE

Ototoxic injury to the inner ear has been observed with a variety of drugs. There are five classes of substances, the ototoxicity of which has been carefully investigated clinically and experimentally because they are so frequently used in medical practice: (1) aminoglycoside antibiotics; (2) loop diuretics; (3) salicylates; (4) quinine and its derivatives; and (5) cytotoxic drugs used in the treatment of malignant disease.

## Pathogenesis of Ototoxic Damage

### Aminoglycoside Antibiotics

The aninoglycosides are in common clinical use in the treatment of a variety of infections. The following members of this group have all been found to be associated with ototoxic effects on the inner ear: streptomycin, kanamycin, gentamicin, tobramycin, viomycin, and amikacin.

The aminoglycosides produce toxic effects on the renal tubules as well as the inner ear. Excretion is mainly by glomerular filtration. Disturbance of renal function may lead to impaired excretion of the drug. The raised blood levels so produced will increase the tendency for ototoxicity of the drug. It would seem from numerous animal studies that the ototoxicity of aminoglycosides is the result of a direct effect of the drug on the sensory cells of the cochlea and vestibule. To reach these cells, the substance must usually pass from the bloodstream into the endolymph probably via the stria vascularis or spiral lamina. High levels of streptomycin in the subarachnoid space were found during the early days of therapy for tuberculous meningitis to be particularly dangerous for the development of ototoxicity. This finding suggests that there was transport of the substance to the perilymph via the cochlear aqueduct. No such ototoxic effects were observed, however, more recently, when gentamycin was given intrathecally in the treatment of gram negative meningitis.[75]

Experimentally in a wide variety of mammalian species, including guinea pigs, cats, chinchillas, and monkeys, the ototoxic effects of aminoglycoside antibiotics have been shown to occur in the hair cells of the organ of Corti and in the ampulla of the semicircular canals. In the hair cells of the organ of Corti, the lesion produced in the early stages is one of degeneration and death of the outer hair cells principally in the basal coil. In the later stages, internal hair cells, supporting cells, and nerve elements may be involved. A sequence of hair cell destruction has been observed in many experiments in the following order of decreasing susceptibility: first-row outer hair cells, second-row outer hair cells, third-row outer hair cells, and finally inner hair cells.[76] At a later stage, the spiral ganglion cells degenerate.[77]

### Human Aminoglycoside Ototoxicity

Table 23-4 records the histopathologic findings in the few human cases of ototoxicity due to aminoglycosides studied at postmortem. Clinical investigations would suggest that aminoglycosides damage the hair cells, particularly of the basal coil of the cochlea, as well as some vestibular structures.

**Table 23-4. Histopathologic Changes in Human Aminoglycoside Ototoxicity**

| Investigators | Patient's Age | Aminoglycoside Antibiotic | Destruction of Hair Cells | Loss of Spiral Ganglion Cells | Vestibular Structures |
|---|---|---|---|---|---|
| Lindsay et al.[79] | 50 | Neomycin | Most IHC | — | Normal |
| Matz et al.[85] | 73 | Kanamycin | Occ. IHC; most OHC | Basal coil | Normal |
| Michaels (unpublished observations)[1] | 68 | Gentamicin | Most IHC; Most OHC | Left side | Atrophy, cristae, and maculae |
| Michaels (unpublished observations)[2] | 54 | Gentamicin | Most IHC; most OHC | — | Atrophy, cristae, and maculae |
| Keene et al.[80] | 48 | Gentamicin | Most OHC | Basal coil | Vacuolization; hair cells in cristae |
| Tange and Huizing[78] | 24 | Gentamicin[a] | Most IHC; most OHC | Middle and basal coils | Not observed |

IHC, inner hair cells; OHC, outer hair cells.

[a] Surface preparation used to observe hair cells.

In all postmortem studies, the outer hair cells throughout the cochlea are destroyed. In most studies it is stated that the inner hair cells also are almost completely lost. Histologic observations of unperfused human hair cells are of doubtful validity because of their autolytic degeneration. However, the report by Tange and Huizing[78] is based on surface preparation studies of the hair cells of the cochlea in a patient with gentamycin ototoxity. In this patient, most inner and outer hair cells were lost. There is a need for further surface preparation study of human cases with aminoglycoside ototoxicity, particularly during the early stages of cochlear damage.

The four cases indicated in Table 23-4 demonstrated loss of spiral ganglion nerve cells. In two of these, the patients were aged 73 and 68 years; thus, the ganglion cell loss may have been a manifestation of presbycusis. In the other two cases, the patients were 48 and 24 years of age and it is possible that the ganglion cell loss was a late manifestation of ototoxic change, particularly since the basal coils were involved. Metz and Lerner[76] cite the case of a 29-year-old patient who had a moderate hearing deficit due to ototoxic damage by gentamicin; the spiral ganglion cells were reduced on both sides, but the cochlear hair cells were normal in all areas on histologic examination. The possibility that ototoxic drugs might produce direct nerve and ganglion cell damage leaving hair cells intact can only be settled by further studies of human temporal bones using both surface and histologic sectioning techniques.

In some temporal bone studies in cases of aminoglycoside ototoxicity, there were changes in the sensory epithelium of the maculae and/or cristae. This again is in accordance with clinical findings of vestibular disturbances and with findings in experimental studies of damage to vestibular structures, but much more information is required in human cases of the nature of the change and the particular anatomic sites affected. The sensory epithelia of maculae and cristae are subject to similar autolytic changes to those described in Chapter 2 in the cochlear hair cells; surface preparations studies will perhaps be required also for postmortem analysis in these regions.

## Loop Diuretics

Ethacrynic acid, a loop diuretic, has been associated with ototoxicity. In laboratory animals, the first sign of cochlear damage is in the stria vascularis. The earliest changes are seen only by the electron microscope,[81] but later changes become visible by light microscopy. At a further stage of ethacrynic acid-induced ototoxicity, the hair cells of cochlea and vestibular structures are affected.[82] In humans the clinical effects of ototoxicity of ethacrynic acid, like the aminoglycosides, are those of both hearing loss and vestibular disturbance.

Studies of histopathologic changes in the human temporal bone are even fewer than with aminoglycoside ototoxicity and they are listed in Table 23-5. Two of the three cases showed outer hair cell dam-

**Table 23-5.** **Histopathologic Changes in Human Ethacrynic Acid Ototoxicity**

| Investigators | Patient's Age | Destruction of Hair Cells | Loss of Spiral Ganglion Cells | Vestibular Structures |
|---|---|---|---|---|
| Matz et al.[83] | 53 | OHC in both basal turns | Normal | Normal |
| Meriwether et al.[84] | 65 | Normal | Normal | Normal |
| Matz[82] | 49 | OHC in basal turn[a] | Normal | Cystic change cupula, post. semi-circular canal and saccule |

OCH, outer hair cells. N, normal.
[a] Also showed edema of stria vascularis.

age in the basal cochlear turn. In the case of Matz,[82] there were edematous changes in the cells of the stria vascularis in addition to damage to outer hair cells. Vestibular changes were also observed in the case of Matz, but not in the other two case reports. These vestibular changes took the form of cyst formation in the sensory epithelium of the posterior semicircular canal and the saccular macula. This very small number of observations would indicate that ethacrynic acid ototoxicity in the human shows similar cellular changes to ototoxicity due to aminoglycoside antibiotics, as far as evidence for hair cell damage by histologic study can be accepted. In addition, there is some evidence in human material that, as in experimental studies, the stria vascularis may be damaged.

## Salicylate Ototoxicity

The ototoxic effect of salicylates is well known in clinical practice, but no morphologic changes have been noted in experimental animals in cochlear or vestibular structures after salicylate overdose.[86] No human autopsy temporal bone studies have been conducted.

## Quinine Ototoxity

Sensorineural hearing loss of temporary duration with smaller doses, but permanent with heavier doses, is an important complication of treatment with quinine, the first and oldest drug known to cause deafness. In experimental animals, severe degeneration of the organ of Corti, particularly in the basal coil, cochlear nerves, and stria vascularis, has been observed.[87] There have been no human autopsy temporal bone studies.

## Ototoxicity Due to Cytotoxic Drugs

Nitrogen mustard, an alkylating agent, has been observed to have ototoxic properties when administered by total body perfusion. Experimental studies with cats given carotid perfusion with nitrogen mustard showed loss of both inner and outer hair cells in basal and middle turns of the cochlea.[88] Examination of the cochlea in case of ototoxicity in a patient who had been perfused with nitrogen mustard showed shrinkage of the organ of Corti without actual loss of hair cells.[89]

Cisplatin (cis-platinum) is a cytotoxic drug that has been recently used in the treatment of advanced malignant disease. Ototoxic effects have been noted clinically. In guinea pigs outer hair cell damage at first and later inner hair cell damage was found over the whole length of the cochlea.[90] Definite degenerative changes were seen in the stria vascularis of the animals. I have had the opportunity to examine the temporal bones of a 7-year-old boy who died of multiple metastases of neuroblastoma. The hair cells, inner and outer, of all cochlear coils appeared to be absent (but this was a histologic preparation). The cells of the stria vascularis showed degeneration and cystic change (Fig. 23-4 through 23-6). The spiral ganglion cells and vestibular structures were normal. These changes are similar to those described in experimental animals.

## INFECTIONS

Infection of the inner ear may be produced by viruses, by bacteria and treponemes, and by fungi.

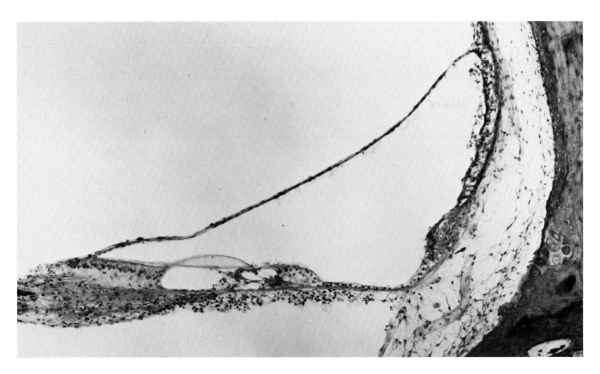

**Fig. 23-4.** Cochlea of 7-year-old boy who died of multiple metastases of neuroblastoma, treated by cis-platinum. Note changes in the organ of Corti and stria vascularis. (H & E, original magnification × 175.)

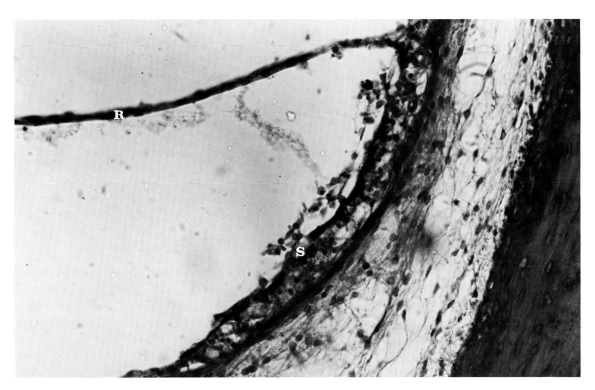

**Fig. 23-5.** Higher-power view of part of Fig. 23-4, showing cystic degeneration of stria vascularis (S). R, Reissner's membrane. (H & E, original magnification × 380.)

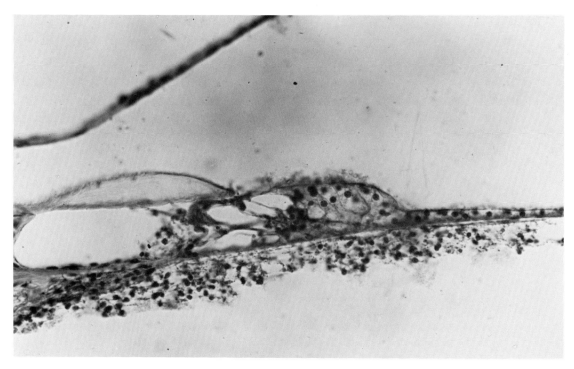

**Fig. 23-6.** Higher-power view of part of Fig. 23-4 showing apparent absence of inner and outer hair cells in organ of Corti. (H & E, original magnification × 380.)

### Viral Infections

Infecting viruses may reach the inner ear via the bloodstream, along the nerves, from the middle ear, or along the meninges. In fact, it is likely that only the first two of these routes are valid. The direct application of a culture of mumps virus through the opened oval window of rhesus monkeys did not produce any evidence of labyrinthine infection.[91] Four viral infections are known to affect the labyrinth by the bloodstream route: cytomegalovirus (CMV) infection, measles, mumps, and rubella. The histopathologic changes in the labyrinth in known cases of infection are listed in Table 23-6. The virus of herpes zoster oticus, varicella virus, enters the inner ear along the 7th and 8th cranial nerves.

Cytomegaloviruses are DNA-containing members of the herpesvirus group. CMV infection is very common and, since primary infection of pregnant women is particularly frequent (30 to 50 per 1,000 pregnancies[92]), intrauterine infection is a strong possibility. In a study of 551 congenitally deaf children, 40 (7.3 percent) were found to be excreting CMV in the urine.[93] A few case reports have described the characteristic lesions of cytomegalic inclusion disease — large basophilic inclusions in nuclei — in the stria vascularis and Reissner's membrane of infants who have died of generalized cytomegalic inclusion disease[94] (Fig. 23-7).

Measles is caused by an RNA myxovirus in which the main lesions are in the upper respiratory tract and lymphoid tissue. Involvement of the inner ear is rare. In two of the very few reported cases with pathological study, the cochlea was involved.[95] In one of these there was severe loss of nerve fibers and spiral ganglion cells associated with atrophy of the organ of Corti. The cases both showed adhesions of Reissner's membrane. A case of labyrinthitis due to measles has been described in which there were two projecting nodules of inflammatory cells in the wall of the utricle.[96]

Mumps is caused by an RNA virus that usually attacks the salivary glands and sometimes the testes, ovaries, or pancreas. Sensorineural hearing

Table 23-6. Histopathology of the Inner Ear in Four Viral Infections

| Infection | Reissner's Membrane | Organ of Corti | Spiral Ganglion | Tectorial Membrane | Stria Vascularis | Vestibular Structures |
|---|---|---|---|---|---|---|
| Cytomegalovirus[93,94] | Viral inclusions | Normal | Normal | Normal | Viral inclusions | Normal |
| Measles[95,96] | Adherent | Atrophic | Loss | Normal | Atrophic | Collapsed granulomas in utricle |
| Mumps[97] | Collapsed | Mainly atrophi | Loss | Normal | Atrophic | Normal |
| Rubella[98,99] | Partially collapsed | Probably normal | Normal | Rolled up | Atrophic, cystic areas | Saccule collapsed |

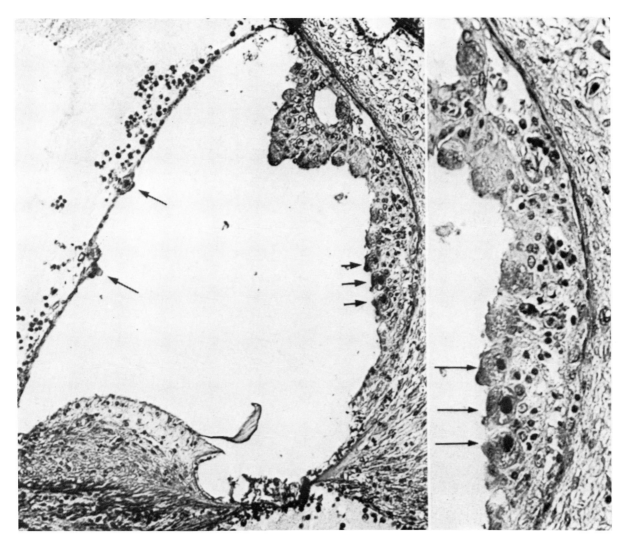

**Fig. 23-7.** Cytomegalovirus infection in the cochlea of an infant. Note characteristic basophilic distention of nuclei and swelling of cytoplasm (arrows). The smaller photograph on the right is a higher power view of the stria vascularis. (Davis G: Cytomegalovirus in the inner ear. Case report and electron microscopic study. Ann Otol Rhinol Laryngol 78:1179, 1969.)

loss is a well-known complication. In a temporal bone of such a case[97] there was atrophy of most of the basal coil of the cochlea, with corresponding nerve fiber and spiral ganglion cell loss.

Maternal rubella occurs in 1 to 22 per 1,000 pregnancies, so, like CMV infection, congenital hearing loss is a risk. It is caused by an RNA virus. A number of temporal bone reports is available, mainly from premature or young infants. A fairly uniform finding was partial collapse of Reissner's membrane with adherence to the stria vascularis and organ of Corti. The tectorial membrane was rolled up. The stria vascularis was usually atrophic, often with cystic areas. In two cases, there were inflammatory collections at the upper and near the junction with Reissner's membrane and adherent to it[98] (Fig. 23-8). The organ of Corti was mainly normal. Collapse of the saccule has been observed in some cases.[99]

The herpes zoster auris (Ramsay Hunt syndrome), the virus (the DNA herpes varicella virus) enters the inner ear along the 7th and 8th cranial nerves, presumably from nerve ganglia, where it has been dormant until a change in the immunologic status of the patient. In the five histopathologic studies previously described there were extensive pathologic changes mainly in those two nerves in accordance with the mode of transmission of the virus. In the case described by Blackley et al.,[100] there were extensive lymphocytic infiltrates in the nerves, modiolus, and skin of the external auditory canal.

## Conditions of Possible Viral Origin

There are reports in the literature of temporal bone pathology in patients who developed sudden

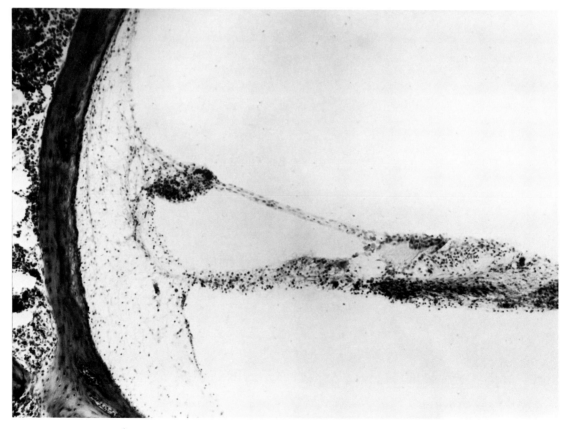

**Fig. 23-8.** Cochlea of newborn with rubella showing inflammatory focus at junction of stria vascularis with Reissner's membrane. Case reported by Friedman and Wright.[98] (H & E, original magnification × 175.)

hearing loss of sensorineural type in the course of a head cold, pharyngitis, or other symptoms suggestive of viral infection. Some of the patients had had no previous symptoms whatsoever. Temporal bone findings have been similar to those of measles, mumps, or rubella, and it has been thought that these inner ear lesions were of viral origin.[101,102]

Another condition that may be due to an, as yet unidentified, viral infection in the inner ear is that of Bell's palsy, which is manifest clinically as a peripheral facial paralysis. There has been a very small number of reports of temporal bone studies from patients with Bell's palsy. In Fowler's report[103] of a patient who died 14 days after the onset of facial paralysis, there was evidence of degeneration of the myelin sheaths and axis cylinders throughout the course of the nerve in the temporal bone. There were fresh hemorrhages in and around the facial nerve, but no evidence of inflammation. I have seen two, as yet unpublished, serially sectioned temporal bones from cases of Bell's palsy in which the histologic findings were similar. In the genu region there was constriction of the nerve by granulation tissue, which formed a sheath around it and encroached on its interior. The adjacent bone showed foci of resorption with abundant osteoclasts. The tissue of the geniculate ganglion was infiltrated by large numbers of lymphocytes (Figs. 23-9 and 23-10). In some areas, the nerve tissue appeared severely edematous, and nerve cells were shrunken and showed eosinophilic cytoplasm. The descending part of the affected facial nerve showed swelling and vacuolation of myelin sheaths and some loss of axis cylinders when compared with sections of the contralateral facial nerve taken in the same region. These findings are compatible with a geniculate ganglionitis, possibly of viral origin, with secondary periostitis of the adjacent bony canal and edema and degeneration of the nerve.

## Bacterial Infections

### Petrositis

Bacterial infections of the inner ear may involve both the petrous bone itself or the labyrinthine structures within it. Bacterial infection of the petrous bone is always derived by extension from middle ear infection. There are four possible routes by which infection may extend from the middle ear into the petrous bone:

1. Via air cells (In recent gross observations of 50 adult temporal bones by the microslicing method I found that eight (16 percent) showed air cells in the apical region. It is therefore possible that infection to the petrous apex mostly travels by air cells.)
2. By direct extension of the inflammatory process through a process of bone necrosis (osteitis)
3. By extension through the bone marrow of the petrous bone (osteomyelitis)
4. Along vessels and nerves

In addition to inflammatory infiltration, the pathologic changes of petrositis comprise three main processes in relationship to the bone tissue, all of which may be seen simultaneously: (1) bone necrosis, (2) bone erosion, and (3) new bone formation (Fig. 23-11). It should be noted that these three processes are frequently seen in the bony wall of the middle ear in many cases of otitis media in which extensive petrositis has not taken place. The inflammatory changes that accompany the bony changes may be acute (i.e., showing largely neutrophils), or they may be chronic (i.e., with lymphocytes, plasma cells, histiocytes, and fibroblasts forming fibrous tissue). These two forms of inflammatory infiltrate are frequently found in the same ear in the very variegated pathologic picture of otitis media when the whole temporal bone is examined in section.

Petrositis is of great importance because of the large numbers of vital structures embedded in and surrounding the petrous bone that may be involved, causing serious symptoms and perhaps death:

1. Extension to the labyrinth may lead to labyrinthitis with destruction of the organs of hearing and balance.
2. Important nerves may be damaged. The facial nerve is early at risk. Involvement of the trigeminal ganglion and the 6th cranial nerve lead to Gradenigo's syndrome. Involvement of the jugular foramen region by the inflammatory process leads to palsy of the 9th, 10th, and 11th

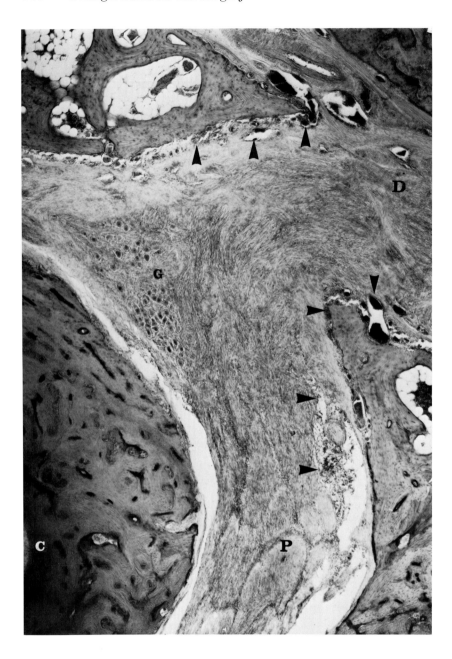

**Fig. 23-9.** Horizontal section of temporal bone in genu region of facial nerve from a patient with Bell's palsy who died of unrelated causes 1 week after onset. C, upper part of cochlea; G, geniculate ganglion; P, proximal end of facial nerve in photograph; D, distal end of facial nerve. Arrowheads indicate sites of inflammation and osteoclastic bone resorption. (H & E, original magnification × 38.)

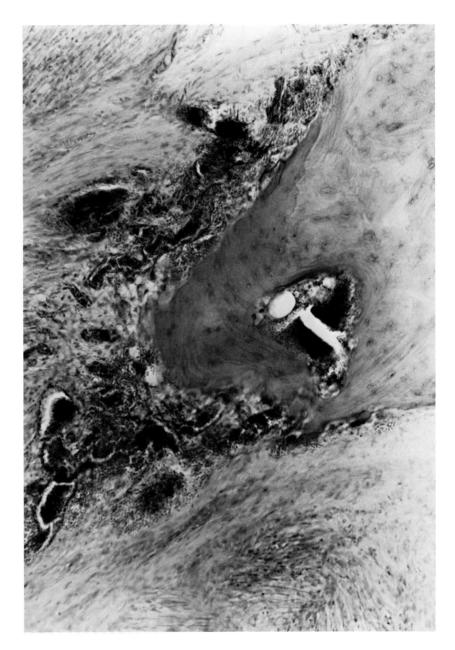

**Fig. 23-10.** Interface between facial nerve and bone in region of genu from the patient with Bell's palsy shown in Fig. 23-9. Note inflammation and osteoclasts with evidence of bone resorption. (H & E, original magnification × 380.)

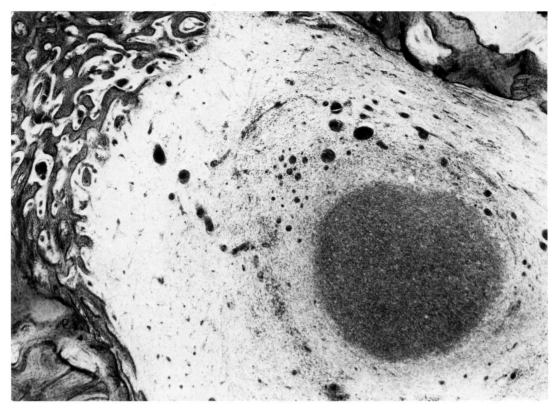

**Fig. 23-11.** Abscess in bone at apex of petrous bone. Note new bone formation at periphery. From patient with jugular foramen syndrome with otitis media. (H & E, original magnification × 38.)

cranial nerves (jugular foramen syndrome) (Fig. 23-12).

3. The wall of the internal carotid artery may become inflamed, which may lead to thrombosis of the blood flow in the lumen.

4. Similarly, the lateral sinus may become thrombosed; this complication or extension of the thrombus to the superior sagittal sinus, or both, may be associated with the somewhat arcane syndrome of otitic hydrocephalus.

5. Extension of the infection to the immediately adjacent cranial structures will lead to meningitis and cerebral abscess.

It should be pointed out that patients with diabetes mellitus are especially susceptible to the development and extension of otitis media. An erroneous concept of malignant otitis externa has grown up in regard to diabetics: because of the presence of external otitis that frequently coexists with otitis otitis media, it is postulated that the infection (usually by *Pseudomonas aeruginosa*) spreads from the ear canal to the petrous apex beneath the temporal bone. No such pathway exists, however, and it is likely that spread of infection in these cases is from otitis media and thrombophlebitis of jugular bulb.

### Labyrinthitis

Most instances of labyrinthitis owe their source to otitis media, as does petrositis. Infection may enter the labyrinth by penetrating the oval or the round window. An infected air cell may rupture into the labyrinthine system at some point of its complex periphery. Occasionally, damage to bone by the inflammation may produce a fistula between the middle ear and the labyrinth, usually in the lateral semicircular canal, the nearest vulnerable point to the middle ear. The latter complication

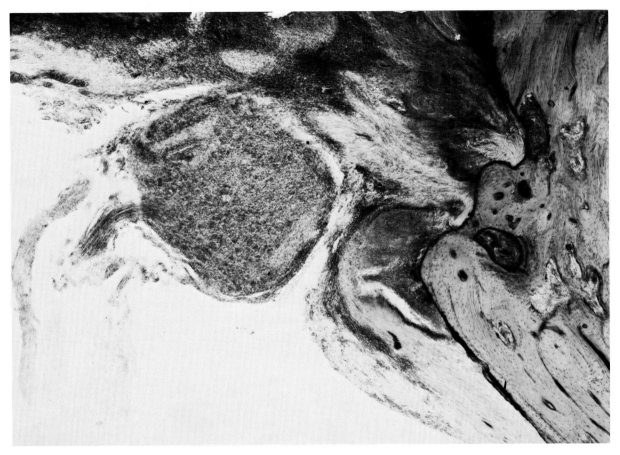

**Fig. 23-12.** Jugular ganglion and vagus nerve from case depicted in Fig. 23-11. The ganglion and surrounding tissue are inflamed. (H & E, original magnification × 25.)

takes place in most cases when a cholesteatoma is present that has the effect of stimulating the inflammatory process. Another possible source of infection of the labyrinth is the meninges and the two tracts that link them, the cochlear aqueduct and internal auditory canal, which may convey infection from meningitic lesions into the labyrinth.

A toxic form of labyrinthitis is recognized in which bacteria and inflammatory products have not actually entered the labyrinth, but some toxin derived from one or other of them produces exudation of serous fluid into the labyrinthine spaces. Hydrops, particularly in the cochlea, is a common accompaniment of toxic labyrinthitis.

In suppurative labyrinthitis, the perilymph spaces display usually a massive outpouring of neutrophils (Fig. 23-13). If the process extends to the endolymphatic spaces, there is concomitant destruction of membranous structures and irreparable damage to sensory epithelia.

Healing is at first by fibrosis, but later osseous repair is frequent, leading to a condition of labyrinthitis ossificans. In this condition, the spaces of the bony labyrinth are filled in by a newer bone, which appears in striking contrast to the normal bone surrounding the bony labyrinth (Fig. 23-14).

### Mycotic Infection

Fungal infections of the inner ear are rare; only a few cases have been described in temporal bone pathology studies. Mycotic infections are increasing due to the widespread use of immunosuppressive therapy in the treatment of malignant and

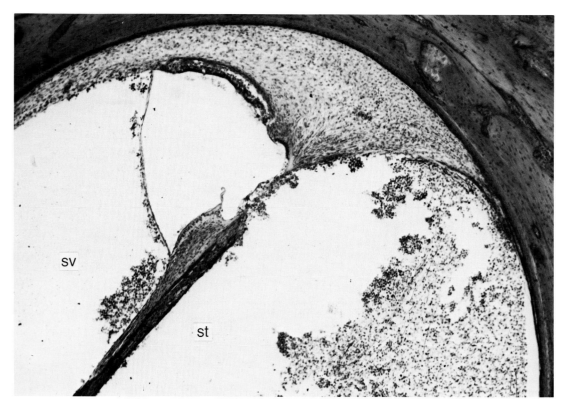

**Fig. 23-13.** Suppurative labyrinthitis. The scala vestibuli (sv) and scala tympani (st) contain numerous pus cells. (H & E, original magnification × 175.)

renal disease. Mucor infection is frequently seen in the head and neck and Meyerhoff et al.[104] described a case in which such an infection reached the inner ear, probably by the bloodstream. Three other cases of inner ear infection by *Candida* are also described in the same work. The route of infection in these cases was from the middle ear and meninges. Cryptococcosis is a fungal infection that is not generally related to immunologic deficiency. It usually infects the meninges. Igarashi et al.[105] described a case involving extension of infection by the organism *Cryptococcus neoformans*, from the meninges along the internal auditory canal and then into the cochlea via the modiolus.

## Syphilis

Syphilis has not been fully eradicated by penicillin treatment; the incidence is, in fact, rising. Sensorineural hearing loss is common in all forms of acquired syphilis. In secondary syphilis, the pathologic changes of the labyrinth are described as part of a lymphocytic meningitis.[106] In tertiary syphilis, the pathologic changes are similar to those of late congenital syphilis. Hearing loss is also an important feature of late congenital syphilis, forming one of the constituents of Hutchinson's triad (interstitial keratitis, deformed incisor teeth, and deafness). More than one-third of patients with congenital syphilis develop this symptom.[107] In infantile congenital syphilis the labyrinthine features are an insignificant aspect of a widespread and often fatal illness.

### Late Congenital Syphilis

"Late congenital syphilis is essentially a bone disease of the ear." This quotation from Mayer and Fraser[108] gives the key to the most important aspect of the complex pathologic processes that account for the lesions of congenital syphilis. The

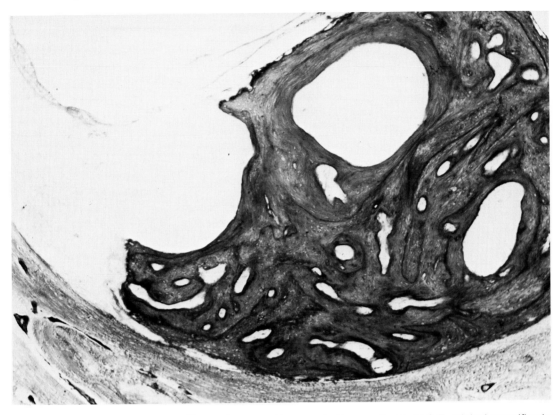

**Fig. 23-14.** Labyrinthitis ossificans. The scala tympani is occupied by new bone. (H & E, original magnification ×110.)

osseous nature of the disease process is emphasized by the finding of treponemes *(Treponema pallidum)* in the temporal bone at autopsy in 48-year-old man with syphilis.[109] The spirochetes were usually found within the bone surrounding the cochlear duct and semicircular canals. In most places, there was no inflammatory reaction to the organisms. Syphilis of the temporal bone is unrelated to inflammation of the middle ear mucosa, unlike septic petrositis or the rare cases of tuberculous involvement of the bony labyrinth, in which the source of the infection is usually in the middle ear.

The bony lesions of congenital syphilis have two forms: (1) gummatous involvement of bone marrow and periosteum, and (2) diffuse periostitis. Gummatous involvement is seen most frequently external to the bony cochlea. Gummata are foci of epithelioid cells, occasional giant cells of Langhans type, lymphocytes, and plasma cells, frequently arranged around blood vessels. They widen the bone marrow spaces by bone destruction in the region around the bony cochlea and vestibule and occur also in relationship to the outer periosteum of the petrous bone. These inflammatory foci vary in size; in some cases, they spread centrally to erode the bony labyrinth. Tongues of inflammatory tissue even reach the endosteum in some places. Inflammation may also involve the vestibular aqueduct and lead to replacement of the endolymphatic duct.[110] Areas of necrotic bone may be seen in the inflammatory tissue. Fibrosis is a prominent component of the lesion. Also new bone formation, both lamellar and woven types, contribute to the complex appearance of the pathology of syphilitic osteitis.

In the second form of bony labyrinthine involvement in congenital syphilis, a diffuse periostitis is present. This lesion is seen most often in the semicircular canals. It is characterized by a formation of bony and fibrous tissue continuous with the bony capsule of the semicircular canals that may completely obliterate their canal lumen.

Although the main emphasis in the pathology of congenital syphilis is on bony lesions, the membranous cochlea always undergoes changes that are clinically more apparent than those of bone. There is frequently a process of hydrops identical in appearance to that seen in Meniere's disease. This affects endolymphatic channels in both cochlea and vestibule and may be severe.[110] The organ of Corti is always atrophic, and the spiral ganglion cells are greatly depleted.

## PRESBYCUSIS

In only a few pathologic studies of presbycusis has there been a correlation with hearing losses in patients measured during life; these have been with subjective audiometric tests only, which are often difficult to carry out and interpret in the older patients.

### Inner Ear Structures

Particular attention has been paid in pathologic analyses to several inner ear structures: spiral ganglion cells, nerves of the basilar membrane, the organ of Corti; cells of the basilar membrane, stria vascularis, otic capsule, and cochlear nuclei of the brain stem.

### Spiral Ganglion Cells

Most authorities have found loss of spiral ganglion cells to be the most definite feature in the pathology of presbycusis (Figs. 23-15 and 23-16). Clear-cut findings of loss of spiral ganglion cells were obtained by Guild et al.,[111] Suga and Lindsay,[112] and others. Guild et al. used a painstaking method in which careful counts of ganglion cells and measurements of positions in the cochlea were made of histologic sections, the results of which were plotted on charts. They correlated the loss of

acuity of hearing for high tones with diminution by atrophy of the numbers of spiral ganglion cells in the lower part of the basal turn of the cochlea. In all subsequent studies, the numbers of ganglion cells have been assessed approximately and their numbers recorded at different measured levels of the cochlear coil.

In a study of 17 aged patients who had spontaneous and progressive bilateral sensorineural hearing loss, Suga and Lindsay[112] also found the most prominent histologic change to be a decrease in the population of the spiral ganglion cells. This loss was never complete in spite of apparently total hair cell loss in the organ of Corti.

### Nerves of the Basilar Membrane

The fine nerve fibers in the osseous spiral lamina have also been studied. The nerve bundles are easily located in histologic section in the osseous spiral lamina, where their thickness may be assessed at different levels of the cochlear spiral. Degeneration of nerve fibers is usually seen with loss of spiral ganglion nerve cells but at a more advanced age than the latter.[113]

Nerve fiber patterns are seen particularly well in a surface view (see Ch. 2). Johnsson and Hawkins[114] indicated that loss of nerve fibers may take place as a feature of presbycusis in both the major radial and the minor spiral nerve network. In the radial nerve network, nerve fiber losses have a clear-cut outline. Johnsson and Hawkins stated that in presbycusis, lesions are found mainly in the lower half of the basal coil symmetrically in the two ears, and apparently following hair cell loss in the corresponding part of the organ of Corti. Degeneration of spiral fibers is much more unusual and occurs with severe hair cell and radial fiber loss involving most of the length of the cochlea.

### Organ of Corti

There has been much emphasis on changes in the organ of Corti as a manifestation of presbycusis. The hair cells are quite susceptible to autolytic changes and to the damaging effects of the acid used in decalcification, facts that have not been adequately considered in pathologic interpretations. Confident statements about hair cell damage

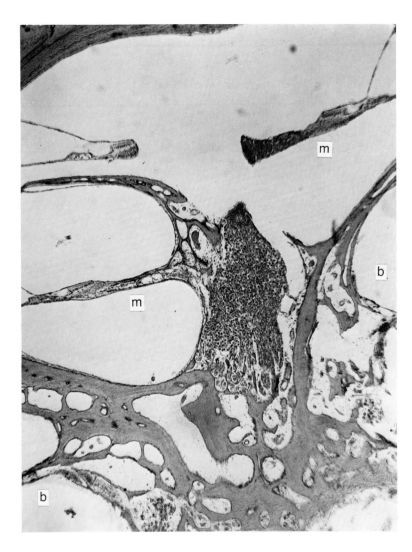

**Fig. 23-15.** Temporal bone from patient with presbycusis. Numerous ganglion cells are present in relation to the middle coil (m) but are lacking in the modiolus in relation to the basal coil (b). (H & E, original magnification, × 38.)

based only on histologic study of decalcified material are put forward in the literature.[115-117] These views indicate that damage to hair cells and often to supporting cells in the basal coil of the cochlea are characteristic of presbycusis. Such views have not gone uncontested.[113] Surface preparations in which fixation has been carried out by perilymph perfusion carry more validity (Figs. 23-17 and 23-18). Such studies were undertaken by Johnsson and Hawkins,[114] using the surface specimen technique after osmic acid fixation. Hair cell loss was indeed found in some cases in the basal coil, in association with degeneration of radial nerve fibers. The process was symmetric in the two ears

and seldom extended above the lower half of the basal turn. When this did occur, it involved the whole cochlea. A surprising finding in all cases of presbycusis studied by Johnsson and Hawkins was complete loss of outer hair cells at the upper end of the apical turn accompanied by only mild nerve degeneration. The pillar cells and Dieter cells were found to degenerate at a much later stage and in fact their presence contributed locally to the development of a scar soon after the loss of the hair cell.

In an electron microscopic examination of the organ of Corti by in three temporal bones of patients with presbycusis, only one showed hair cell damage in the basal turn.[119] The other two cases

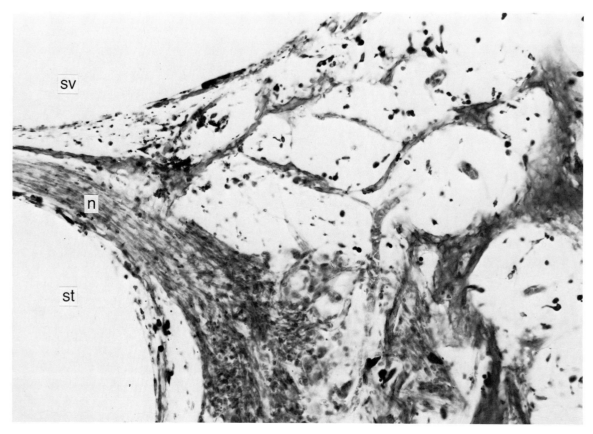

**Fig. 23-16.** Modiolus in region of basal coil. A radial nerve bundle (n) enters a group of ganglion cells, but adjacent spaces in the modiolus, normally occupied by ganglion cells, contain loose connective tissue only. sv, scala vestibuli; st, scala tympani. (H & E, original magnification × 380.)

showed normal hair cells but marked degenerative changes in spiral bundles and spiral ganglion cells. Thus, it would appear that hair cell loss is quite common in the basal coil, but it is by no means a necessary accompaniment of presbycusis.

### Cells of the Basilar Membrane

Little attention has been paid to pathologic changes in this structure, apart from the organ of Corti. Schuknecht[120] suggested that a descending type of curve of sensorineural hearing loss may be associated with such changes, but this has not been confirmed. Calcification, fluorescent pigment, and vascular sclerosis have been described in the basilar membrane of older people, but the significance of such findings in the pathogenesis of presbycusis has not been adequately assessed.

### Stria Vascularis

Atrophic changes of the stria vascularis have been observed and correlated with a flat type of hearing curve.[120] There is atrophy of strial cells, particularly those of marginal ones, small cysts or basophilic deposits also may be found (Figs. 23-19 and 23-20).

### Otic Capsule

Spicules of bone in the spiral tract[121] have been suggested as a possible source of pathologic interference with hearing in old age. The concept put forward is that the nerves of the spiral tract are compressed by these new bodies, causing hearing loss. There has been no rush of supporters, however, for this challenging suggestion, and the matter requires careful scrutiny by further observers.

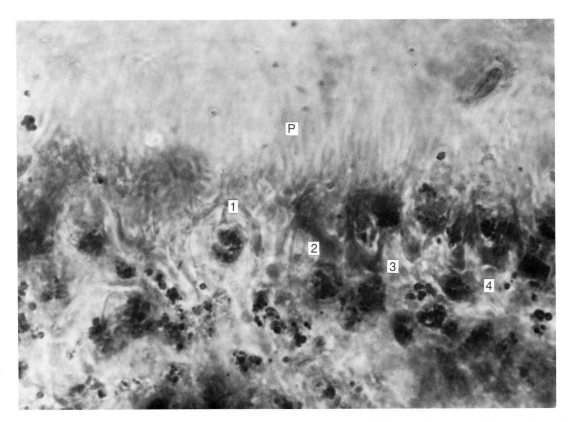

**Fig. 23-17.** Surface preparation of organ of Corti from basal coil region of 86-year-old woman with sensorineural deafness. P, pillar cells. Outer hair cells in focus are designated 1, 2, 3, and 4. Most of the other outer hair cells are absent. From perilymph perfused, microsliced specimen exposed to osmic acid solution after removal. (Original magnification × 1,700.)

## Cochlear Nuclei of the Brain Stem

Studies of the most central parts of the auditory pathway are few in presbycusis. Arnesen[122] counted the nerve cells in the ventral and dorsal cochlear nuclei of the brain stem in patients in whom he had found audiometric evidence of presbycusis. He compared the total counts with those of the normal patients established earlier by Hall.[123] The latter counted the cells in cases of neonatal asphyxia, finding that the average number for both nuclei was 96,400 (87,700 to 112,500). Arnesen found that in his 12 cases the total was on average only one-half that of Hall's normal cases.

## Changes in Blood Vessels

Thickening of the arteries, arterioles, and capillaries supplying the internal ear has been noted at several anatomic levels. There appears to be little correlation between vascular alterations and the presence of other abnormalities. Hyaline and fibrous thickening of walls of small blood vessels is often seen, particularly in the internal auditory canal, and atherosclerotic changes in the blood vessels surrounding the facial nerve are sometimes severe. It must be admitted that the qualitative and quantitative assessment of blood vessels in any organ is notoriously difficult. Attempts also to correlate local vascular changes with generalized thickening have proved well-nigh impossible in other organs and the problem does not seem to be any more soluble in the inner ear.

There would seem to be a variety of pathologic changes in the hearing pathways which, although characteristic, are by no means constantly present in presbycusis. The significance of these changes

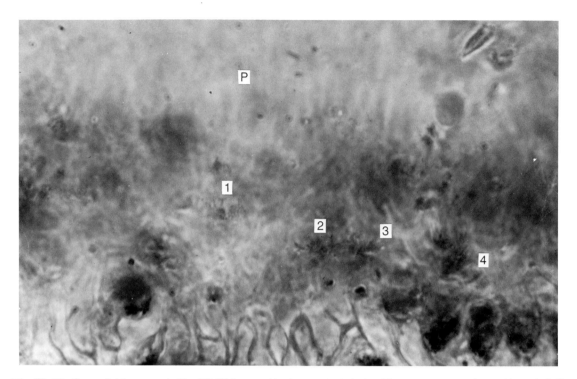

**Fig. 23-18.** Same field as seen in Fig. 23-17 focused to demonstrate hairs. These are present in positions 1, 2, 3, and 4, identical to the cell bodies. P, pillar cells. (Original magnification × 1,700.)

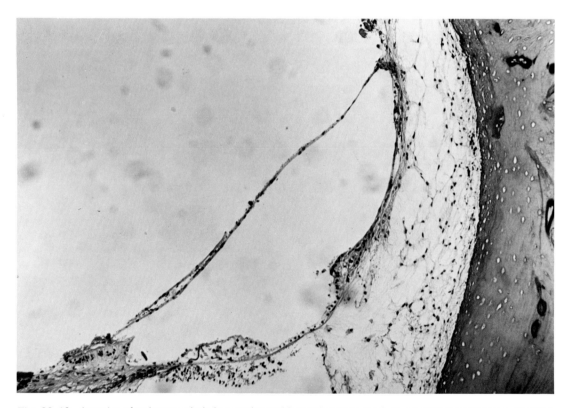

**Fig. 23-19.** Atrophy of stria vascularis in a patient with presbycusis. (H & E, original magnification × 175.)

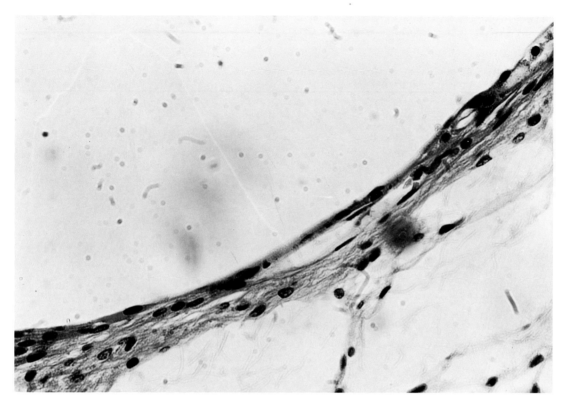

**Fig. 20.** Higher-power view of atrophic stria in presbycusis. (H & E, original magnification × 700.)

cannot be estimated; indeed, the definition of the term presbycusis is debated. The possibility of correlation of patterns of audiometric hearing loss with different pathologic changes[120] is open to serious doubt. Patients with presbycusis are frequently uncooperative or even demented, and reliance should not be placed on tests requiring their active cooperation. A study of presbycutic patients by hearing tests based on objective criteria would be more accurate. The correlation of such findings with pathologic alterations in the inner ear and brain stem would be more acceptable than those hitherto proffered. The vestibular structures are also subject to aging changes and are discussed later in this chapter.

Work has been carried out in my department on the electrophysiologic and pathologic features of presbycusis. The following is a summary of these studies.

In an investigation of the brain stem evoked responses of 111 ears from 90 subjects the pattern of the waveforms suggested a peripheral origin for the hearing loss. A technique for extratympanic electrocochleography was developed and used in 42 elderly subjects and 22 controls. Analysis of the findings of action potentials, cochlear microphonics and summating potentials gave strong evidence of disturbed cochlear function, probably emanating from the hair cells.[123a,123b]

A technique was devised for sampling, locating and staining the hair cells from the organ of Corti of elderly subjects in whom perilymphatic perfusion had been carried out soon after death. In 57 cochleas examined by those means the following changes were detected and analyzed quantitatively: atrophy of the terminal part of the basal coil of the cochlea, including all hair cells and radial nerve fibers and severe loss of outer hair cells and mild loss of inner hair cells throughout the whole cochlea. In all specimens of elderly cochleas severe elongation and fusion of some of the stereocilia of outer and inner hair cells were present, indicating a specific ageing aberration of the hair cells prior to their death.[123a,123c]

This work has suggested that hearing loss in the aged is an endogenous condition affecting all subjects and it is primarily a process of degeneration of the outer hair cells of the cochlea, with complete loss of structure at the basal end. It is the latter pathologic change that leads to the emphasis on higher tone loss, which characterizes the clinical disorder of presbyacusis.

## MENIERE'S DISEASE

### Hydrops and Its Causes

Meniere's disease is an affection of both the hearing and balance organs of the inner ear, characterized by episodes of vertigo, hearing loss, and tinnitus. Its pathologic basis is now firmly estab-

lished as hydrops, that is, fluid distention of the endolymphatic spaces of the labyrinth. The cause of the hydrops in Meniere's disease is unknown. There are, however, a number of disease entities of known etiology in which hydrops may be present as a complication. The common feature of these conditions is presence of inflammatory or neoplastic involvement of the perilymphatic spaces. Thus otitis media complicated by perilymph labyrinthitis (Fig. 21–21) syphilitic involvement of the labyrinth or leukemic deposits in the perilymphatic spaces may be associated with hydrops.[124]

### Location of Hydrops in Meniere's Disease

The hydrops of Meniere's disease may affect one or both inner ears. In most cases, the cochlear duct and saccule are involved. Utricular and semicircu-

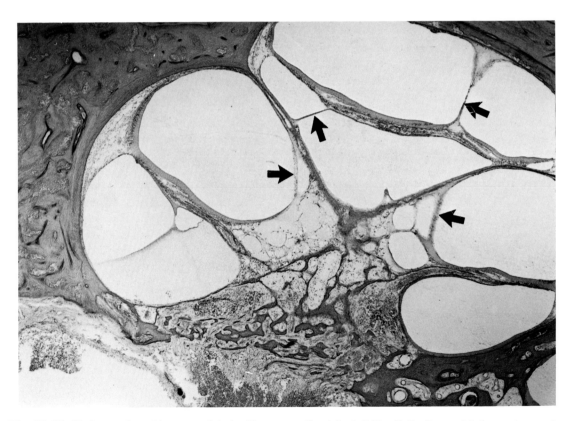

**Fig. 23-21.** Hydrops of cochlea associated with suppurative labyrinthitis. Collections of inflammatory cells (neutrophils) are present in the fundus of the internal auditory canal. Positions of distended Reissner's membranes are shown by arrows. (H & E, original magnification × 38.)

lar duct hydrops are unusual. In some cases, the cochlear duct alone is hydropic. A rare and debatable form of Meniere's is thought to affect the vestibule but not the cochlea. Symptoms are those of vertigo, but not hearing loss. I have recently studied such a case observing a questionable saccular, but no evidence of cochlear, hydrops.

In the hydropic cochlear duct, the elastic Reissner's membrane shows bulging of various degree. In the most severe cases, Reissner's membrane reaches the top of the scala vestibuli and may be in contact with a wide area of cochlear wall (Fig. 21-22). In the apical region it may bulge to such an extent that it fills the helicotrema, while the distended scala media may even enter the scala tympani. The saccule swells up from its position on the medial wall of the vestibule and frequently touches the vestibular surface of the footplate of the stapes (Fig. 21-23). The utricle may be compressed in the process. In some cases, the swollen saccule may herniate into the semicircular canals from the vestibule. Less frequently, the utricle may be distended, sometimes with small infoldings producing a scalloped appearance.[125]

## Changes in the Walls of Membranous Labyrinth in Hydrops

Changes may be seen in the thin distended membranes of the hydropic endolymphatic spaces. Ruptures may be present, particularly in Reissner's membrane, and the terminal end of the ruptured membrane may be curled up. Such ruptures have been incriminated as possible pathologic bases of the fluctuations in pure-tone thresholds which patients with Meniere's disease may suffer. It has been suggested that the flooding of the perilymph with endolymph with its high potassium level, may inhibit the bioelectric activity of the cochlea.[120] It

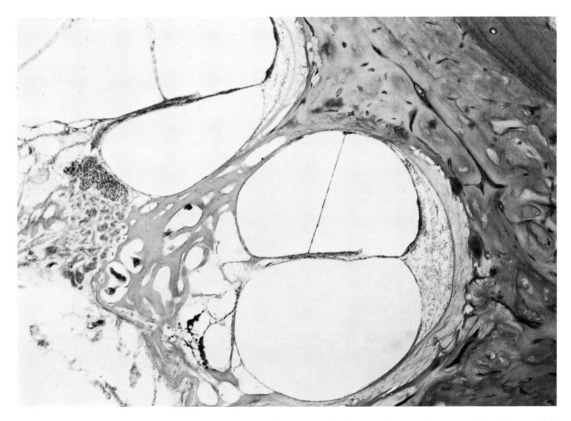

**Fig. 23-22.** Cochlear hydrops in Meniere's disease. The distended Reissner's membrane reaches the top of the scala vestibuli. (H & E, original magnification × 38.)

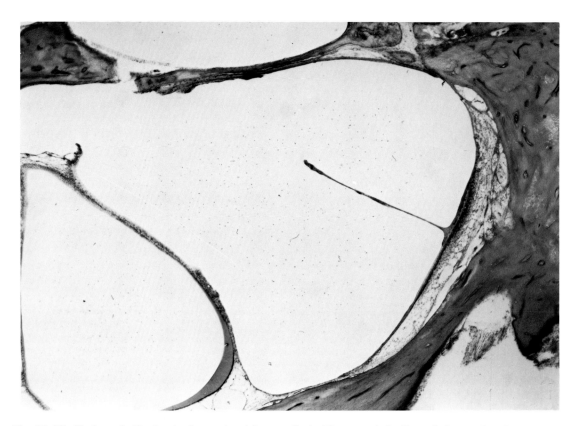

**Fig. 23-23.** Hydrops in Meniere's disease involving vestibule. The saccule is distended to such a degree that it lines the base of the footplate of the stapes (artifactually fractured). A thin membrane, possibly the result of rupture, projects into the vestibule. (H & E, original magnification × 38.)

is likely, however, that most of these ruptures are artifactual. They may be found in nonhydropic labyrinths. They are often multiple in the same membranous labyrinth; it is conceivable that one of them only could be nonartifactual.[126] Outpouchings are often seen in which dilatation of part of the wall of the membranous labyrinth takes place and a lining is present here that is thinner than elsewhere. These outpouchings have been explained as healed ruptures but, because of their regular features, it is more likely that they simply represent increased distention of parts of the labyrinthine wall, which are normally thinner. The presence of fibrous tissue in cases of Meniere's hydrops external to the endolymphatic space has been described in the scala vestibuli by Hallpike and Cairns,[127] and by Schuknecht[120] in the vestibule deep to the footplate of the stapes. It is possible that these foci of connective tissue represent reactions to irritation produced by repeated distention and subsidence of the adjacent cochlear duct and saccule, respectively.

## Changes in Vestibular Aqueduct and Endolymphatic Duct

While hydrops involving the thinner-walled structures of the membranous labyrinth is accepted by all as a basic feature of the pathology of Meniere's disease, there is no such unanimity with regard to the alterations in the endolymphatic duct and its surrounding vestibular aqueduct. There have been many descriptions of obstructive or potentially obstructive lesions of these structures in Meniere's disease, and it has been suggested that the obstruction to endolymphatic flow may cause the hydrops in these cases. The following list gives a brief indication of the lesions to which considerable attention is devoted in the literature:

Fibrosis[128,129]
Metastatic breast carcinoma[130]
Decreased vascularity[131]
Partial atresia of the intermediate portion of the vestibular aqueduct with decreased amounts of endolymphatic duct tissue[132]
Irregularity of the osseous wall of vestibular aqueduct, sometimes with blockage of the orifice of vestibule[133]
Blockage of the vestibular aqueduct by syphilitic microgummata (perivascular round cell infiltrations[134])

Finally, I have seen a tumorlike papillary lesion resembling choroid plexus that was removed surgically from the endolymphatic sac. No Meniere's symptoms were present in this case. Similar lesions were described in cases of Meniere's disease by Schuknecht within the ductus reuniens region of the hydropic cochlear duct[120] and by Gussen[132] in the hydropic crus commune. It is possible that such structures may secrete an excess of endolymph and so produce lesions and symptoms of hydrops. In contrast to these observations, it must be pointed out that in many careful studies of Meniere's hydropiic temporal bones no changes whatever have been noted in the endolymphatic duct or vestibular aqueduct.[135]

Ultrastructural alterations of a degenerative nature have been observed in the epithelial cells of the endolymphatic sac in cases of Meniere's disease,[136] but similar changes were also seen in cases of acoustic neuroma suggesting that the changes are the result of the disease process, and not its cause.

## Changes in the Sensory Epithelia of the Labyrinth

Alterations of the sensory cells of the organ of Corti are cited by Hallpike and Cairns,[127] but these workers warn that such changes may be the result of postmortem autolysis. The effect of acid used in decalcification of the temporal bone is another possible source of damage to these cells after death. Such possibilities of artefacts have been ignored in some reports. Changes, particularly in the apical region have been described and associated with low frequency hearing loss.[120] In a recent study of 23 temporal bones from 17 patients with Meniere's, however, no direct correlation was found between endolymphatic hydrops and hair cell loss.[134] Atrophy of the macula of the saccule may also be found (Fig. 23-24) which does not appear to be artifactual.

The significance of electron microscopic findings of utricular sensory epithelial changes supposedly related to Meniere's disease[137] has been reduced by the observation of similar alterations in cells at the same situation in cases of acoustic neuroma.[138]

## Relationship of Symptoms to Pathologic Changes

Image analysis of the areas in histologic section of the cochlear duct (corresponding to volume in the whole structure) has been carried out in two studies and related to the hearing loss. In Antoli-Candela's[139] study, the area of the cochlear duct was significantly related to the degree of hearing loss. Losses of more than 70 dB showed a particularly high degree of hydropic expansion. Fraysse et al.[134] found a similar relationship between cochlear duct size and the total average hearing loss. Their study also found a correlation between those dimensions with the duration of the disease: the longer the history of symptoms, the more pronounced the cochlear duct dilatation. A relationship was also found between the amount of dilatation of vestibular contents and response to caloric tests and the presence of positional nystagmus, but this was less definite than the cochlear duct/hearing loss association.

## Pathogenesis

Ablation of the endolymphatic sac in guinea pigs results in endolymphatic hydrops within 3 months.[140] In cats the same result can only be attained by survival times of 6 months to 3 years.[141] In humans, operations for drainage of endolymph into the subarachnoid space are sometimes of value in the treatment of Meniere's disease. These facts

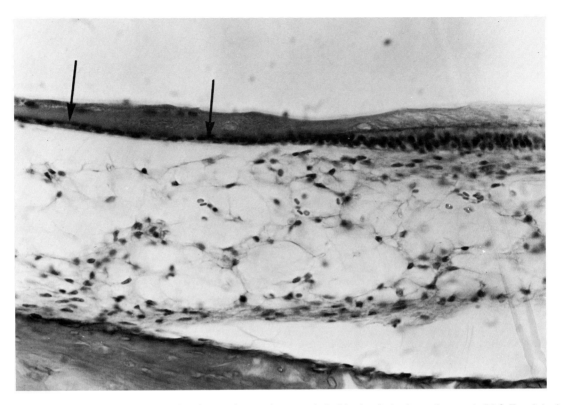

**Fig. 23-24.** Atrophy of sensory cells of part of saccular macula in Meniere's hydrops (arrows). (H & E, original magnification × 380.)

suggest than obstruction of the endolymphatic duct may play a part in the pathogenesis of Meniere's disease. Endolymphatic duct obstruction is sometimes, but not consistently, present on histopathologic examination of serial sections of temporal bones in cases of hydrops. It is possible that studies of further cases at autopsy using modern techniques such as radiography of microsliced bones (see Ch. 2), histochemistry, and electron microscopy may yet establish a definite lesion of the endolymphatic duct as the cause of the hydrops.

## NEOPLASMS

Neoplasms arising primarily in the inner ear are rare. More usually neoplasms reach the inner ear by growth from outside, either by direct invasion from adjacent structures or as metastasis by the bloodstream.

### Primary Neoplasms in Inner Ear

The cellular constituents of the inner ear, apart from bone are, for the most part, fully differentiated nonmitotic structures, such as nerve cells and sensory epithelia, so that neoplasms would not be expected to arise in them. Indeed, primary neoplasms are rare except for acoustic neuroma (schwannoma), which, in most cases probably arises from Schwann cells at the neurilemmal-glial junction of the 8th nerve within the internal auditory canal. Acoustic neuroma is dealt with in Chapters 24 and 25. On rare occasions, a schwannoma arises within the cochlea. I have seen one case of this condition in a patient with concomitant Paget's disease of the temporal bone (Fig. 23-25). A similar combination of pathologic conditions is described by Nager.[142]

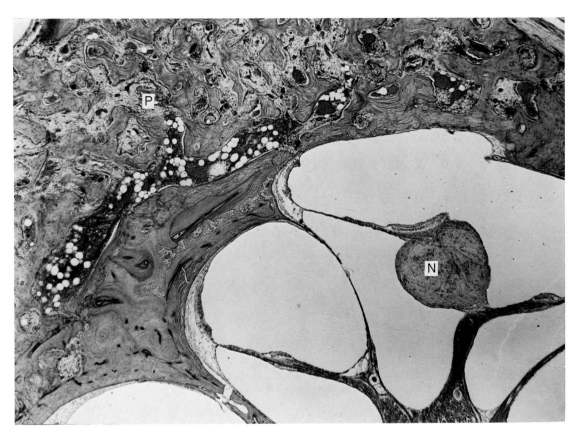

**Fig. 23-25.** Neuroma (schwannoma) of apical portion of cochlea (N). The surrounding bone shows a severe degree of involvement by the changes of Paget's disease (P). (H & E, original magnification × 38.)

Meningiomas are tumors that generally form intracranial masses. They arise from arachnoid villi which are small protrusions of the arachnoid membranes into the venous sinuses. Arachnoid villi may be found in parts of the temporal bone, including the inner ear, and on occasion meningiomas may arise from these structures as primary neoplasms of the inner ear region, although the commonest site of origin of temporal bone meningioma is the middle ear. The histologic appearance of a meningioma is that of a tumor with a whorled arrangement of cells: meningotheliomatous if the tumor cells appear epithelioid, psammomatous if calcification of the whorled masses is prominent (Fig. 23-26), and fibroblastic if the tumor cells resemble fibroblasts. Meningiomas as well as acoustic neuromas may appear in the vicinity of the inner ear in von Recklinghausen's syndrome. The meningioma is a slow-growing tumor of the temporal bone which has had a reputation for complete benignity. My recent experiences with this neoplasm, however, have indicated its propensity for local recurrence and invasion.

## Neoplasms Directly Invading Inner Ear

There are two routes by which tumors invading from outside may reach the inner ear. The first route is directly through the petrous bone. It is rare for tumors invading by this route to reach the membranous labyrinth. The otic capsule seems to provide a particularly strong barrier against invasion.[143] Neoplasms that may enter the inner ear by the bony route are jugular paraganglioma and squamous carcinoma. Jugular paraganglioma arises from paraganglia situated in the wall of the jugular

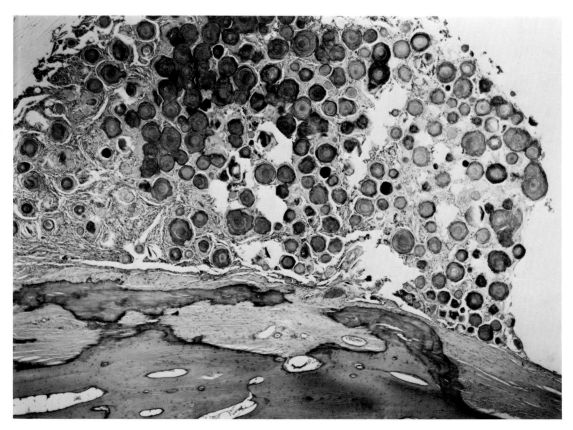

**Fig. 23-26.** Psammomatous meningioma arising from the posterior surface of the temporal bone in a case of von Recklinghausen's disease. (H & E, original magnification × 38.)

bulb (see Ch. 2) and then invades the temporal bone. The pathway of invasion of this tumor usually bypasses the cochlea and vestibule traversing rapidly the floor of the middle ear (Fig. 23-27). Squamous carcinoma originating in the middle ear soon erodes the thin bony plate on the anterior wall separating the eustachian tube from the carotid canal. Superficial invasion of the bone around the middle ear takes place, but the otic capsule is not invaded directly until very late in the disease process[143]

Tumors entering the inner ear by the other route arrive from the meninges and enter the internal auditory canal, proceeding to its lateral end and then passing through the foramina in the anteroinferior part of the cribriform plate alongside the filaments of the cochlear nerves. Tumor cells thus infiltrate the modiolus and even the osseous spiral lamina of the basal coil. The vestibule appears to be more resistant to invasion by a similar mechanism,

perhaps because there are fewer foramina communicating with the internal auditory canal. Squamous carcinoma originating from the middle ear is more likely to invade the inner ear in this fashion than by the mode described above. After penetrating the thin bony walls of the posterior mastoid air cells, squamous carcinoma reaches the dura of the posterior surface of the temporal bone. From there it spreads medially along the posterior surface of the temporal bone and enters the internal auditory canal between bone and dura and then penetrates the cochlea by way of the foramina of the cochlear nerves.[143] This route provides, in fact, a mode of entry into the inner ear for any solid neoplasm which may be infiltrating widely along the meninges. I have seen a secondary signet ring adenocarcinoma (primary origin unknown) infiltrate into the deepest parts of the cochlea in this fashion (Figs. 23-28 through 23-30).

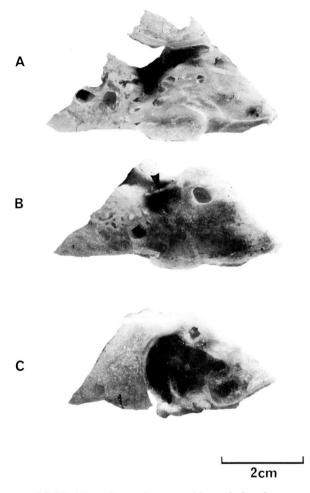

A

B

C

2cm

**Fig. 23-27.** Microslices of temporal bone in jugular paraganglioma. **(A)** The neoplasm fills the middle ear in the region of the cochlea but does not invade the otic capsule. **(B)** At a lower level, the tumor fills the hypotympanum but has not eroded the tympanic membrane (arrowhead). **(C)** The tumor, bright red in the original, is seen with a rounded edge, corresponding to the jugular fossa.

### Neoplasms Metastatic to Inner Ear

The temporal bone is frequently the site of blood-borne metastasis for carcinomas originating in the breast, kidney, lung, stomach, larynx, prostate, and thyroid. The internal auditory canal is a common location for such growth. Once the metastasis is deposited, further spread into the cochlea may take place by the route outlined above.

### Leukemia

Leukemia may involve the inner ear in several ways. The most important is by hemorrhage into the membranous spaces, to which leukemic patients are particularly prone. The hemorrhage may be into the perilymph space alone or into both perilymphatic and endolymphatic spaces. If the patient survives a massive intracochlear leukemic hemorrhage for several months, the organ of Corti and spiral ganglion will appear severely degenerated. There is also fibrous tissue and new bone growth in the scalae.[144] I have seen severe leukemic infiltration of the perilymph spaces of the cochlea in chronic lymphocytic leukemia, which is probably due to leukemic cells being conveyed to that location from the cerebrospinal fluid via the cochlear aqueduct (Figs. 23-31 and 23-32).

### Malignant Lymphoma, Lymphoplasmacytic Type

Malignant lymphoma of the lymphoplasmacytoid/lymphoplasmacytic type (Waldenström's macroglobulinemia)[145] is a primary dyscrasia of B-type lymphoid cells producing an excess of monoclonal macroglobulin of the IgM variety. Hearing loss and vertigo are present in some patients with this disorder. These symptoms are probably related to increased blood viscosity. One such case showed complete disruption of the labyrinth by hemorrhage.[146]

## PATHOLOGY OF THE VESTIBULAR SYSTEM

The pathology of the vestibular system in humans has been even less adequately investigated than the auditory system. Table 23-7 lists conditions the pathologic basis of which have been established by direct observation at autopsy or surgery; affections such as vestibular neuronitis in which the possible structural changes have been only guessed from the clinical symptoms are not

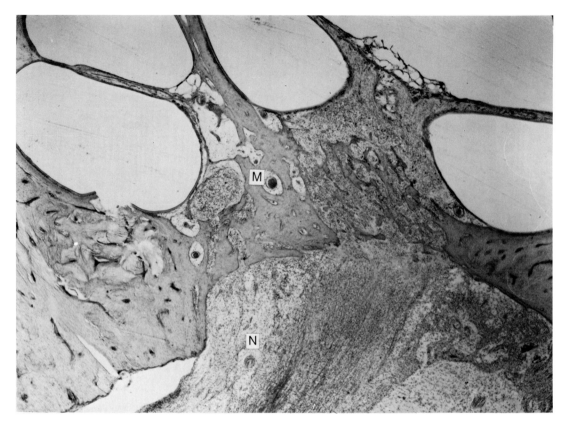

**Fig. 23-28.** Invasion of 8th cranial nerve (N) and modiolus (M) by signet ring neoplasm. (H & E, original magnification × 38.)

considered. Further details of many of the conditions are given elsewhere in this chapter.

## Malformations

A wide variety of malformations may affect the vestibular structures and semicircular canals (Tables 23-1 and 23-3).

**Table 23-7.    Pathology of the Vestibular System**

Malformations
Aging changes
Trauma
Ototoxicity
Infections (viral, bacterial, syphilis)
Osseous lesions (Paget's disease, otosclerosis)
Hydrops (Meniere's disease, syphilis, bacterial infection)
Positional vertigo (atrophy of superior division of vestibular nerve, atrophy of utricle, cupulolithiasis)
Neoplasms (acoustic neuroma, metastatic carcinoma)

## Aging Changes

Changes comparable to the cochlea in presbycusis have been described for the vestibular structures. With advancing age there is degeneration of the saccular macula and, to a lesser degree, of the utricular macula. These changes are accompanied by a loss of otoconia.[114] Epithelial cysts have been seen in the sensory epithelium of the posterior and superior cristae in advanced old age.[147] There does not appear to be a reduction of vestibular ganglion cell numbers in old age comparable to that seen in the spiral ganglion.[148]

## Trauma

Fractures may involve the vestibular system. Surgical operations may be complicated by accidental penetration of vestibule or semicircular

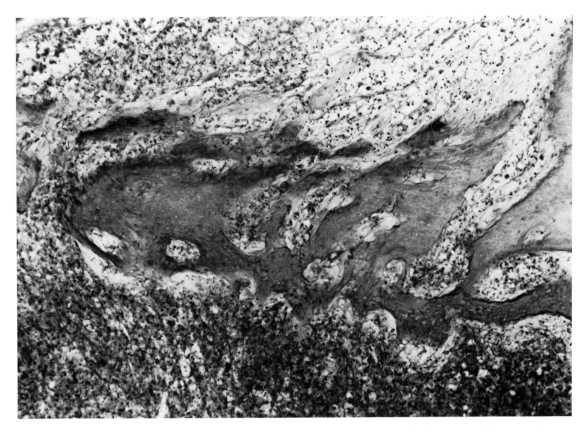

**Fig. 23-29.** Higher-power view of modiolus region of specimen shown in Fig. 23-28 showing infiltration of tumor cells between trabeculae of modiolus. (H & E, original magnification × 100.)

canals. The production of a fistula from the lateral semicircular canals, by design, into the middle ear was part of the now-abandoned operation of fenestration for otosclerosis. A temporary fistula may occur as the result of the still-practiced operation of stapedectomy.

### Ototoxicity

Part of the damage produced by aminoglycoside antibiotics, such as gentamicin, implicates the sensory epithelium of the cristae and maculae (Tables 23-4 and 23-5).

### Viral Infection

In measles and rubella, changes have been observed in the utricle and saccule (Table 23-6).

### Bacterial Infection

Bacterial infection may involve the vestibular system as part of labyrinthitis. In most bacterial infections, spread occurs from the middle ear via the oval window. A direct fistula resulting from the bone erosion of otitis media may occur in the lateral semicircular canal, particularly in the presence of cholesteatoma.

### Syphilis

The diffuse periostitic form of syphilis has a special tendency to involve semicircular canals. The lumina of the canals may be completely obliterated by bone and fibrous tissue.

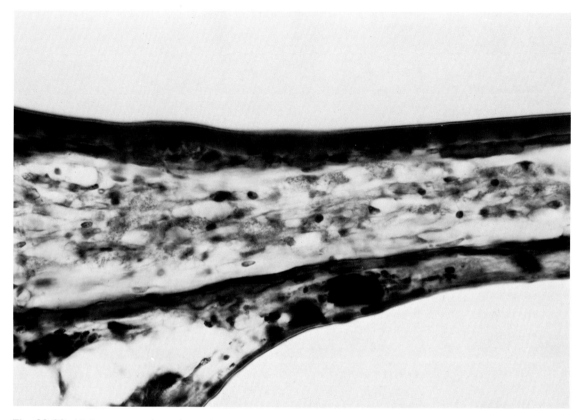

**Fig. 23-30.** Higher-power view of specimen shown in Figs. 23-28 and 23-29 showing infiltration of signet ring tumor cells in connective tissue of osseous spiral lamina. (H & E, original magnification × 700.)

### Bone Diseases

Paget's disease frequently involves the bony vestibule and semicircular canals to a severe degree and as a result clinical symptoms referable to this system are well known. Otosclerosis, although frequently present in relationship to the bony wall of the vestibule, rarely involves the membranous structures of the vestibular system, hence the rarity of vestibular symptoms in this condition.

### Hydrops

Hydrops of the saccule and sometimes the utricle represents the major pathologic feature of Meniere's disease. Saccular hydrops may also be a manifestation of syphilitic and bacterial inflammation involving the labyrinth.

### Positional Vertigo

Positional vertigo is a condition in which vertigo is induced in the patient by alteration in the position of the head. Since nystagmus is used clinically as an objective test of this condition, the term positional nystagmus is often preferred.[149]

A temporal bone study of a patient who suffered a bout of severe vertigo without deafness, followed by the features of positional vertigo, was carried out by Lindsay and Hemenway[105] in 1956. The findings were those of atrophy of the superior division of the vestibular nerve, utricle, and crista of

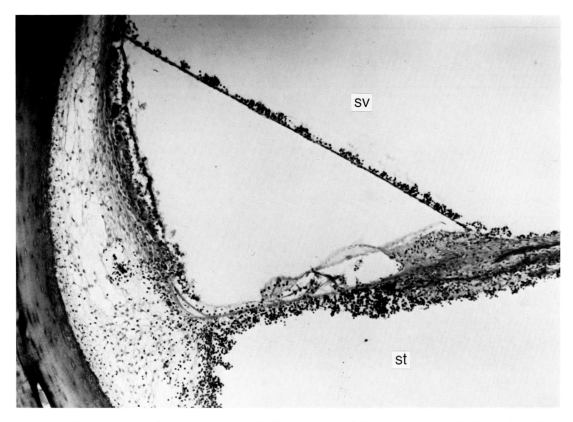

**Fig. 23-31.** Cochlea in chronic lymphatic leukemia. Numerous lymphoid cells are present in the scala vestibule adjacent to Reissner's membrane, in the scala tympani (st) adjacent to the basilar membrane, and in the spiral ligament. sv, scala vestibuli (H & E, original magnification × 175.)

the lateral semicircular canal. Lindsay and Hemenway attributed these changes to occlusion of a vessel supplying the vestibular labyrinth, but pathologic change in such a vessel was not actually observed.

A temporal bone study of two cases of positional vertigo at the National Hospital, Queen's Square, London, conducted in 1952 and 1957, revealed degeneration of the macula of the utricle and of the cristae of the horizontal and superior semicircular canals and of the superior vestibular nerve.[151,152] In these two cases, the changes were also attributed to atherosclerosis of supplying arteries, although such changes were not actually seen in the temporal bone sections.

Schuknecht[153] in 1969 described the temporal bone findings in two cases of postional vertigo. Attached to the posterior surface of the cupula of the left posterior semicircular canal in each of the cases

was a basophilic staining homogeneous deposit measuring 300 μm in one case and 350 μm in the other, in their greatest diameter. On the basis of these cases, Schuknecht built up an explanation of the symptomatology of positional vertigo. He postulated that the calcific material derived from otoconia in a degenerated utricular macula will descend by gravity along the endolymph and form on the crista of the posterior semicircular canal, the lowest part of the labyrinth. Schuknecht suggested that such a mechanism was responsible for the positional vertigo in the three other cases described, even though cupulolithiasis was not observed in the serial sections.

This ingenious theory has attracted much interest, and the term cupulolithiasis is frequently used as a synonym for positional vertigo. A surgical operation to denervate the posterior semicircular canal in cases of positional vertigo has been devised

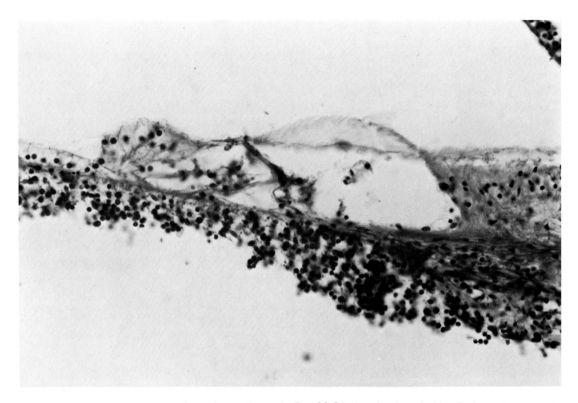

**Fig. 23-32.** Higher-power view of specimen shown in Fig. 23-31 showing lymphoid cells in scala tympani in relation to basilar membrane and organ of Corti. (H & E, original magnification × 250.)

and is claimed to be successful.[154] It is disturbing, however, that no further autopsy studies of positional vertigo have been described since Schuknecht's 1969 paper. Indeed, in a study of 391 temporal bones, 125 small cupular calcific deposits, 21 medium-size deposits, and four large ones were found by Schuknecht and Ruby.[155] Positional vertigo (nystagmus) is not a pathologic entity but a clinical symptom (and sign). Pathologic lesions outside the vestibular system are known to give rise to this condition, particularly those in the cerebellum.[149] I would urge that further study of human posterior canal cupulas in cases of postural vertigo should be carried out before Schuknecht's theory becomes embedded in established dogma.

### Neoplasms

The most important neoplasm of the vestibular system is schwannoma of the vestibular division of the 8th cranial nerve (acoustic neuroma). This does not usually invade the vestibule. The saccule and utricle usually show an exudate of proteinaceous fluid in the presence of a neuroma in the internal auditory canal. Acoustic neuroma is discussed in Chapters 24 and 25. Other primary neoplasms of the vestibular system are extremely rare and metastatic deposits are unusual.

## BONY ABNORMALITIES

### Paget's Disease

Paget's disease (osteitis deformans) is a common condition affecting particularly the skull, pelvis, spine, and femur in people over 40 years of age. The cause is unknown, but the presence in many cases of viruslike structures in osteoclasts has given rise to the suggestion that Paget's disease may be of viral etiology. The pathologic change is one of active bone formation simultaneous to active bone destruction. The affected bones are enlarged, porous, and deformed. Microscopically, bone formation is seen as trabeculae of bone with a lining of numerous osteoblasts. A mosaic appearance is formed by the frequent successive deposition of bone, cessation of deposition resulting in thin, blue cement lines, followed by resumption of deposition and cessation, and so production of further cement lines. Bone destruction is shown by the presence of numerous, large osteoclastic giant cells with Howship's lacunae. Areas of chronic inflammatory tissue intermixed with the bone are common.

The pathology of involvement of the temporal bone by Paget's disease was well described by Davies[156] and by Nager.[142] The petrous apex, the mastoid, and the bony part of the eustachian tube are most frequently affected. The periosteal part of the bony labyrinth is its first part to undergo pagetoid changes. The endochondral layer is also affected in many cases and the endosteal layer and modiolus least frequently (Figs. 23-33 and 23-34). The internal auditory canal may show protuberances into its lumen of pagetoid tissue. In a few cases cited by Davies and by Nager, the stapes may be tethered by involvement of its footplate by pagetoid tissue. Calcification of the annulus fibrosis was cited as another cause of such fixation. Involvement of other ossicles is unusual. Davies drew attention to the possibility of an alternative means of ossicular fixation by involvement of the malleus by pagetoid tissue in the epitympanum. Both Davies and Nager believed that fissure fractures occurring during life are more frequent in the temporal bone of patients with Paget's disease. The round window niche may be narrowed by the bony overgrowth.

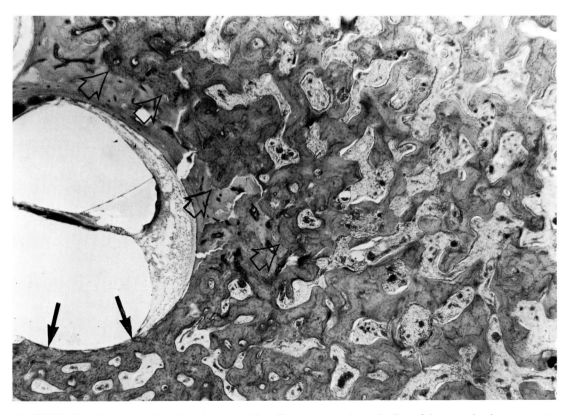

**Fig. 23-33.** Paget's disease involving bony cochlea. Open arrows show the line of demarcation between pagetoid tissue and endochondral bone. The black arrows indicate where pagetoid tissue has reached the endosteum. (H & E, original magnification × 38.)

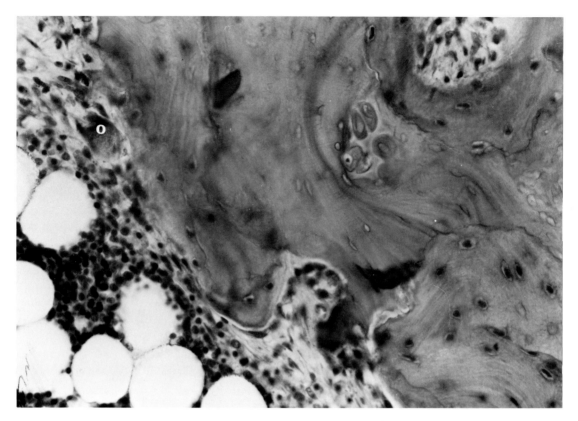

**Fig. 23-34.** Paget's disease of bony cochlea, showing mosaic pattern of cement lines, osteoclastic giant cell (O) with Howship's lacunae, and chronic inflammatory tissue in marrow space. (H & E, original magnification × 250.)

Involvement of the membranous labyrinth by the changes of Paget's disease was cited by both investigators. It is likely that the changes described are in fact associated with concomitant presbycusis.

Patients with Paget's disease are predisposed to neoplasms of bone, particularly osteosarcoma and fibrosarcoma. Nager described a spindle cell sarcoma of the temporal bone in one of his Paget's disease patients. He also described a benign neuromatous lesion of the cochlea associated with Paget's disease of the temporal bone and a similar case is also present in the files of my department (Fig. 23-25).

## Osteogenesis Imperfecta

Osteogenesis imperfecta is a general bone disease with a triad of clinical features: multiple fractures, blue sclerae, and conductive hearing loss.

There is a congenital recessive form, which is often rapidly fatal, and a tardive form in adults, which is inherited in a dominant fashion and is more benign.

The pathology is well seen in long bones in which resoption of cartilage in the development of bone is normal, but the bony trabeculae themselves are poorly formed although often abundant in the cortical part of the bone. It seems that there is a general disturbance in the development of collagen, hence the thin (blue) sclerae as well as poorly formed bone tissue.

In the temporal bone, the bony labyrinth is said to sometimes be affected by deficient bone formation,[157] but the membranous structures of the inner ear are normal, except for basophilic deposits in the stria vascularis in some cases,[158] a feature I have seen in a variety of pathologic conditions and regard as being of little or no pathologic significance. The major pathologic change is in the ossicles, which are very thin and subject to fracture. There is also very frequently fixation of the footplate of the stapes. The nature of the bony tissue causing fixation is problematic. Claims have been put forward that it is conventional otosclerotic bone. On the other hand, it has been maintained that it is a specific type of bone formed as part of the process of osteogenesis imperfecta. In favor of the latter view is that the histologic appearance has been described as being less organized than in otosclerosis.[159] It should be said in this connection that the histologic appearance of otosclerosis is by no means specific and shows a range of changes. Little is known of etiologic factors in otosclerosis; in fact, it has been suggested that otosclerosis may also be part of a general connective tissue disturbance.[160]

### Osteopetrosis

Osteopetrosis (often called marble bone disease) is a rare disease of bone in which there is a failure to absorb calcified cartilage and primitive bone. Recent evidence suggests that there is a deficient activity of osteoclasts. A relatively benign dominantly inherited form occurs in adults and a malignant recessively inherited one in infants and young children. Patients with the benign form often survive to old age and present prominent otologic symptoms.

The intermediate, endochondral portion of the otic capsule is swollen and appears as an exaggerated thickened form of the normal state. Globuli ossei composed of groups of calcified cartilage cells are normally present in this region, and in osteopetrosis they are present in greatly increased numbers and form a zone of increased thickness (Fig. 23-35). The periosteal bone is normal. The organ of Corti may be normal but in some cases has been described as atrophied. The ossicles are of fetal shape and are filled with unabsorbed, calcified cartilage. The canals for the 7th and 8th cranial nerves

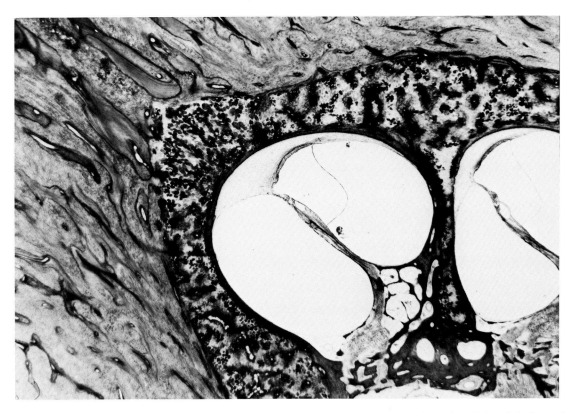

**Fig. 23-35.** Osteopetrosis involving bony cochlea. The endochondral layer is enlarged, and the globuli ossei (calcified cartilage cells) are excessively basophilic. (H & E, original magnification × 38.)

are severely narrowed by the expanded cartilaginous and bony tissue.[161,162]

## Achondroplasia

In this condition, which is an inherited and congenital disorder, there is a deficiency of growth of cartilage, so that the patient is a dwarf with stunted growth of the long bones, but there is normal growth of bones formed in membrane. Hearing loss of the conductive and sensorineural type is frequent. The temporal bone in such a case was described as showing a normal endochondral layer but thickened middle and periosteal layers composed of dense thick trabeculae without globuli ossei.[163]

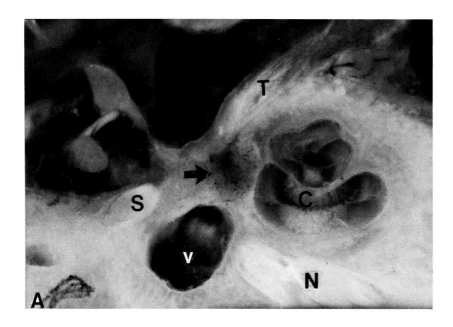

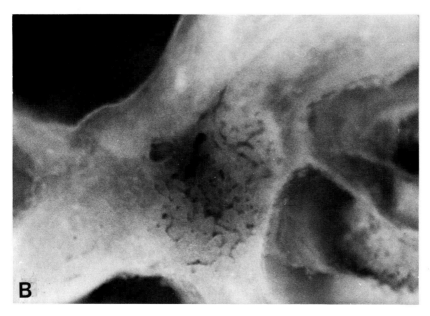

**Fig. 23-36. (A)** Microsliced temporal bone showing focus of otosclerosis (arrow). T, tensor tympani muscle; C, cochlea; N, 8th cranial nerve; V, vestibule, stapedius muscle. **(B)** Higher-power view of area of otosclerotic focus. Note marked vascularity.

# OTOSCLEROSIS

Otosclerosis is a common focal lesion of the otic capsule of unknown etiology found principally in relationship to the cochlea and footplate of the stapes. Otosclerotic deposits, not associated with hearing loss, are found in about 10 percent of all adult temporal bones in white people, on histological examination at autopsy.[164] Otosclerosis usually affects both ears symmetrically. The lesion mainly attacks whites and is said to be unusual in blacks and Mongolian peoples. The disease process is probably confined to the temporal bone; a similar bony change often appears, however, in a position similar to that of otosclerosis in the generalized bone disease, osteogenesis imperfecta.

## Gross Appearance

In cases with prominent otosclerotic involvement of the otic capsule region, the lesion may be observed, through the middle ear, as a smooth prominence of the promontory area. The stapes is sometimes fixed on handling. The pink swelling of the otosclerotic focus may sometimes be seen through a particularly translucent tympanic membrane.

In microsliced temporal bones showing otosclerosis, the focus appears well demarcated and pink. Blood vessels are prominent and evenly distributed. Radiographs show the well-defined lesion as a patch of mottled translucency in the temporal bone (Figs. 23-36 through 23-38).

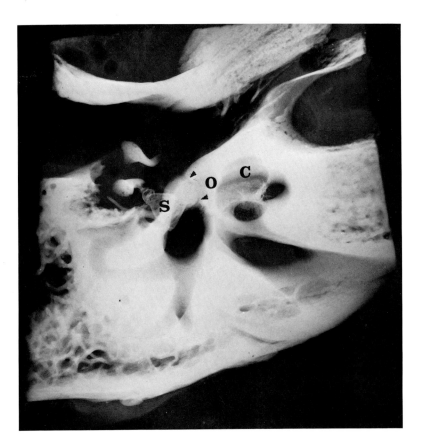

**Fig. 23-37.** Radiograph of microslice shown in Fig. 23-36. The otosclerotic focus (O) appears as a mottled, translucent area. S, stapes; C, cochlea. Arrowheads indicate fissula ante fenestram.

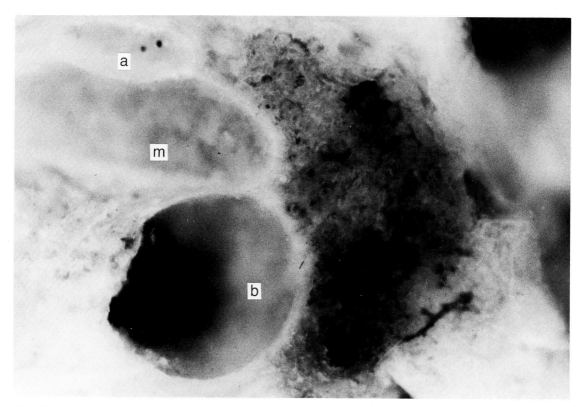

**Fig. 23-38.** Microslice of temporal bone showing large focus of otosclerosis closely associated with the apical (a), middle (m), and basal (b) coils of the cochlea.

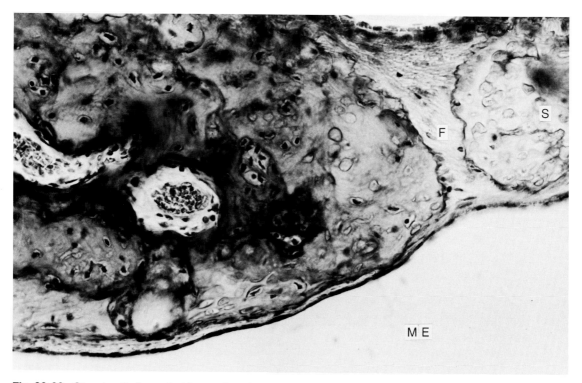

**Fig. 23-39.** Otosclerotic focus that has replaced the normal bone to the epithelial surface of the middle ear (ME) but has not involved the annulus fibrosis (F), its cartilaginous borders or the footplate of the stapes (S). (H & E, original magnification × 380.)

## Microscopic Appearance

The histologic characteristic of otosclerosis is the presence of trabeculae of new bone, which is for the most part of woven type. This appearance contrasts with the well-developed bone of the outer periosteum, the endochondral middle layer, and the endosteal layer of the otic capsule (see Ch. 2), a sharply demarcated edge being a prominent feature. The pathologic bony tissue has a variable appearance with areas of differing bony cellularity. In most areas, osteoblasts are very abundant within the woven bone. Osteoclasts may be present, and there is evidence of bony resorption. Marrow spaces in the focus contain prominent blood vessels and connective tissue. In a few areas, the bone within the otosclerotic focus may be more mature and less cellular, and even lamellar bone may be found. In these latter areas, marrow spaces are small. Thus active (more cellular and more vascular) and inactive (less cellular and less vascular) otosclerotic foci, may be recognized[165] (Figs. 23-39 and 23-40).

The most common site for the formation of otosclerotic foci is the bone anterior to the oval window. This region normally bears the fissula ante fenestram (Fig. 23-37), but this anatomic relationship does not necessarily denote any developmental connection. Cartilaginous rests are also found normally in this area and may be seen in relationship to the otosclerotic focus (Figs. 23-41 and 23-42). Otosclerosis may also be seen in the bone near the round window membrane (Fig. 23-43), in the inferior part of the cochlear capsule or in the bone around the semicircular canals.

Otosclerotic involvement of the stapes footplate leading to functional fixation of the stapes may occur in two ways. First, there may be actual partic-

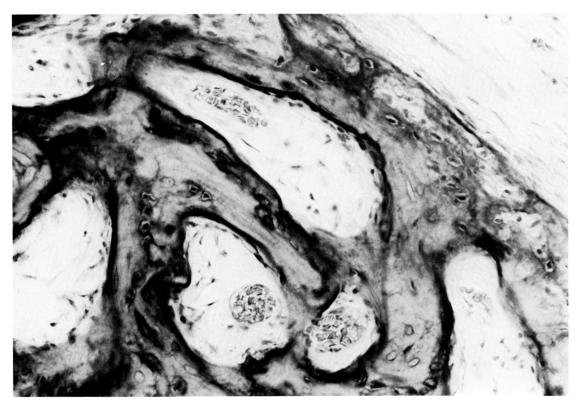

**Fig. 23-40.** Otosclerotic focus. Note numerous osteocytes and prominent blood vessels and fibrous tissue in marrow spaces. (H & E, original magnification × 380.)

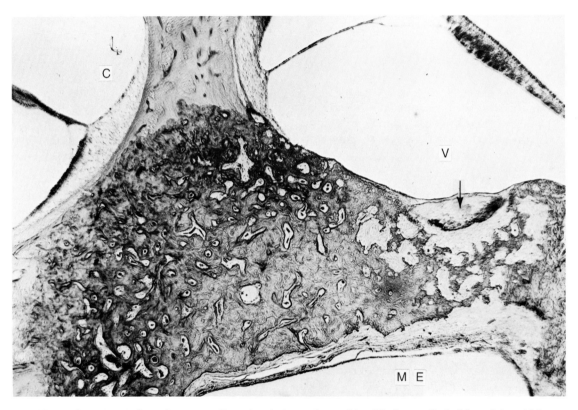

**Fig. 23-41.** Otosclerotic focus in temporal bone in relation to the cochlea (C), the vestibule (V), and the middle ear cavity (ME). Note cartilaginous rest (arrow) adjacent to focus. (H & E, original magnification × 380.)

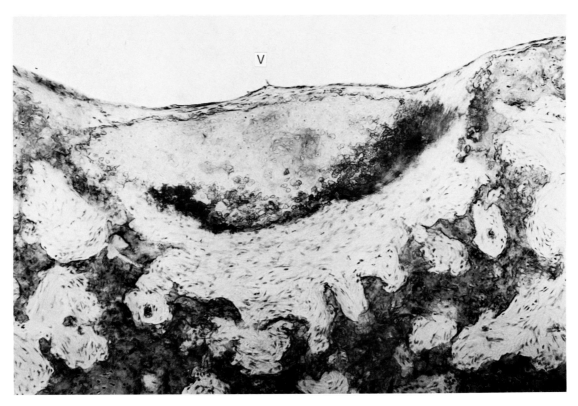

**Fig. 23-42.** Cartilaginous rest and otosclerosis from Fig. 23-41. V, vestibule. (H & E, original magnification × 175.)

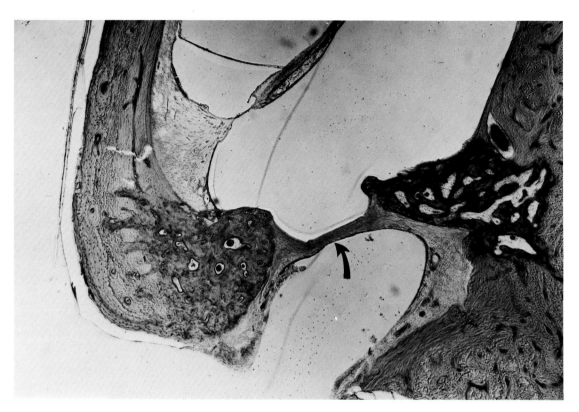

**Fig. 23-43.** Otosclerotic bone surrounding round window membrane (arrow). (H & E, original magnification × 38.)

ipation by the stapes footplate in the formation of otosclerotic bone so that the otic capsular focus of pathologic bone is continuous with the former. This is often described as an invasion of otosclerotic bone from otic capsule to footplate, but it is unlikely that extension takes place in such a tumorlike manner. It is more likely that a field change of new bone formation affects footplate as well as otic capsule. Involvement of the oval window takes place at any point of its circumference, or indeed around most of it. The process may also be associated with similar alterations in the lower parts of the stapedial crura.

Second, the footplate is frequently not party to the otosclerotic process, but the bone surrounding the footplate proliferates to such an extent that the oval window is distorted and narrowed. Fibrous thickening of the annulus fibrosis may be prominent. The otosclerotic focus may also encroach on the round window, narrowing it in the same fashion as the oval window.

Otosclerotic bone frequently reaches the endosteum of the cochlear capsule. In some cases it may lead to a fibrous reaction deep to the spiral ligament (Fig. 23-44). Overgrowth of otosclerotic bone may, rarely, cause distortion of the cochlear contours and may even affect the modiolus and lead to spontaneous fractures of the modiolar septa.[166]

Much emphasis has been placed on the presence of lesions known as blue mantles in otosclerosis. At

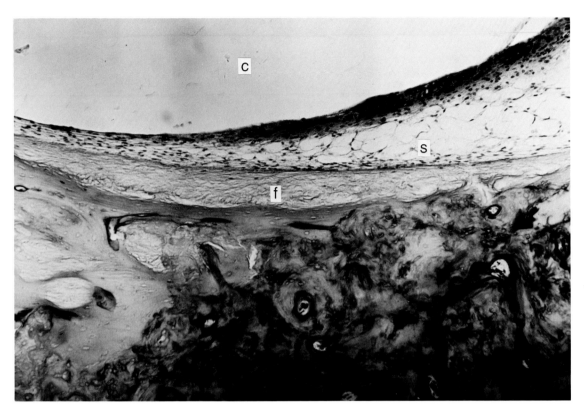

**Fig. 23-44.** Fibrous area (f) between otosclerotic focus and spiral ligament (s) of cochlea (c). (H & E, original magnification × 175.)

the center of each such lesion is a small blood vessel, and the mantle is represented by a blue-staining (i.e., hematoxyphil) deposit around the blood vessel (Fig. 23-45). Schuknecht[120] warned against confusing blue mantles, which are actually formations of bone, with the thin blue-staining membranes found on the inner surfaces of lacunae in cartilage and canaliculi in bone and in the walls of bony vascular channels. Schuknecht called these membranes *Grenzscheiden* (boundary partitions). Lindsay[167] observed blue mantles in almost all cases of localized otosclerosis and in a few cases without the usual type of otosclerosis. They are present usually in the bony capsule around the semicircular canals.[167] The pathologic process rep-

resented by the designation "blue mantle" would seem to be similar to the conventional form of otosclerosis and, indeed, areas of blue mantle formation may be present within the otosclerotic focus at the classic sites. There is very little evidence that blue mantles represent a distinct pathologic entity.

### Hearing Loss in Relationship to Otosclerotic Foci

By far the most common form of hearing loss in otosclerosis is related to oval window disturbance and is of the conductive type. Depression of air

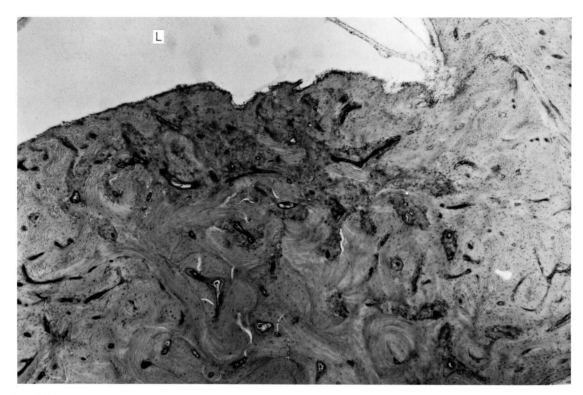

**Fig. 23-45.** Blue mantles (darker areas) in bone of lateral semicircular canal (L), which shows a frayed edge. (H & E, original magnification × 175.)

conduction of sound waves is also the result of obstruction of the round window by otosclerosis. The possibility of sensorineural hearing loss by otosclerotic involvement of the cochlea has been much discussed. It seems possible that a biochemical change may occur in the labyrinth from the proximity of the otosclerotic focus, which could damage the hearing mechanisms.

## REFERENCES

1. Konigsmark BW, Gorlin RJ: Genetic and Metabolic Deafness. WB Saunders, Philadelphia, 1976
2. Phelps PD, Lloyd GAS: Radiology of the ear. Blackwell Scientific Publications, Oxford, 1983
3. Grüneberg H: Hereditary lesions of the labyrinth in the mouse. Br Med Bull 12:153, 1956
4. Steel KP, Bock GR: Hereditary inner ear abnormalities in animals. Relationships with human abnormalities. Arch Otolaryngol 109:22, 1983
5. Ormerod F: The pathology of congenital deafness. J Laryngol Otol 74:919, 1960
6. Suehiro S, Sando I: Congenital anomalies of the inner ear. Introducing a new classification of labyrinthine anomalies. Ann Otol Rhinol Laryngol 88[suppl 59]:1, 1979
7. Konigsmark BW: Pathology of hereditary deafness. N Engl J Med 281:713, 1969
8. Lindsay JR, Black FO, Donnelly WH Jr: Acrocephalosyndactly (Apert's syndrome): Temporal bone findings. Ann Otol Rhinol Laryngol 84:174, 1975
9. Lindsay JR: Profound childhood deafness. Inner ear pathology. Ann Otol Rhinol Laryngol 82[suppl 5]:1, 1973
10. Kelemen G: Marfan's syndrome and hearing organ. Acta Otolaryngol (Stockh) 59:23, 1965
11. Altmann F: The inner ear in genetically determined deafness. Report and analysis of 2 new cases. Acta Otolaryngol (Stockh) [Suppl] 187:1, 1964

12. Altmann F: Congenital atresia of ear in man and animals. Ann Otol Rhinol Laryngol 64:824, 1955

13. Siebermann F, Bing R: Über den Labyrinth und Hirnbefund bei einem an Retinitis Pigmentosa erblindeten Angeboren Taubstummen. Z Hals Nasen Ohrenheilkd 54:265, 1907

14. Zeitzer LD, Lindeman RC: Multiple branchial arch anomalies. Case report and temporal bone study. Arch Otolaryngol 93:562, 1971

15. Friedmann I, Froggatt P, Fraser GR: Pathology of the ear in the cardio-auditory syndrome of Lange-Nielsen and Jervell. J Laryngol Otol 82:883, 1968

16. Lindsay JR: Inner ear pathology in congenital deafness. Otolaryngol Clin North Am 4:249, 1971

17. Peron DL, Schuknecht HF: Congenital cholesteatomata with older anomalies. Arch Otolaryngol 101:498, 1975

18. Igarashi M, Filippone MV, Alford BR: Temporal bone findings in Pierre-Robin syndrome. Laryngoscope 86:1679, 1976

19. Paparella MM, el-Fiky FM: Mondini's deafness. Arch Otolaryngol 95:134, 1972

20. Hvidberg-Hansen J, Jorgensen MB: The inner ear in Pendred's syndrome. Acta Otolaryngol (Stockh) 66:129, 1968

21. Wells M, Michaels L: Congenital abnormalities of the ear in perinatal deaths. Clin Otolaryngol 7:107, 1982

22. Sando I, Lieberman A, Bergstrom L: Temporal bone histopathological findings in trisomy 13 syndrome. Ann Otol Rhinol Laryngol 84[suppl 21]:1, 1975

23. Bergstrom L, Hemenway WG, Sando I: Pathological changes in congenital deafness. Laryngoscope 82:1777, 1972

24. Maniglia AJ, Wolff D, Herques AJ: Congenital deafness in 13-15 trisomy syndrome. Arch Otolaryngol 92:181, 1970

25. Valvassori GE, Naunton RF, Lindsay JR: Inner ear anomalies, clinical and histopathological considerations. Ann Otol 78:929, 1969

26. Miglets AW, Schuller D, Ruppert E, et al: Trisomy 18: A temporal bone report. Arch Otolaryngol 101:433, 1975

27. Kos AO, Schuknecht HF, Singer JD: Temporal bone studies in 13-15 and 18 trisomy syndromes. Arch Otolaryngol 83:439, 1966

28. Egami T, Sando I, Black FO: Hypoplasia of the vestibular aqueduct and endolymphatic sac in endolymphatic hydrops. ORL 86:327, 1978

29. Davies DG: Paget's disease of the temporal bone. Acta Otolaryngol (Stockh) [Suppl] 242:1, 1968

30. Sando I, Bergstrom L, Wood RP: Temporal bone findings in trisomy 18 syndrome. Arch Otolaryngol 91:552, 1970

31. Baldwin J: Dysostosis craniofacialis of Crouzon. (A summary of recent literature and case reports with emphasis on involvement of the ear.) Laryngoscope 78:1660, 1968

32. Kietzer G, Paparella MM: Otolaryngologic disorders in craniometaphyseal dysplasia. Laryngoscope 79:921, 1969

33. Igarashi M, Singer DB, Alford BR, Cook TA: Middle and inner ear anomalies in a conjoined twin. Laryngoscope 84:1188, 1974

34. Altmann F: The ear in severe malformations of the head. Arch Otolaryngol 66:7, 1957

35. Myers EN, Stool S: The temporal bone in osteopetrosis. Arch Otolaryngol 89:460, 1969

36. Fitch, N, Lindsay JR, Srolovitz H: The temporal bone in the preauricular pit, cervical fistula, hearing loss syndrome. Ann Otol 85:268, 1976

37. Kelemen G: Hurler's syndrome and the hearing organ. J Laryngol Otol 80:791, 1966

38. Windle-Taylor PC, Buchanan G, Michaels L. The Mondini defect in Turner's syndrome. A temporal bone report. Clin Otolaryngol 7:75, 1982

39. Egami T, Sando I, Myers EN: Temporal bone anomalies associated with congenital heart disease. Ann Otol Rhinol Laryngol 88:72, 1979

40. Sando I, Holinger LD, Balkany TJ, Wood RP: Unilateral endolymphatic hydrops and associated abnormalities. Ann Otol 85:368, 1976

41. Hallpike CS. Observations on the structural basis of two rare varieties of hereditary deafness. p. 285 In de Reuch AVS, Knight J (eds): Myotatic, Kinesthetic and Vestibular Mechanisms. CIBA Foundation Symposium. Little, Brown, Boston, 1967

42. Gussen R. Delayed hereditary deafness with cochlear aqueduct obstruction. Arch Otolaryngol 90:429, 1969

43. Nomura Y, Mori W: Hypophosphatasia. Histopathology of human temporal bones. J Laryngol Otol 82:1129, 1968

44. Fisch L: Deafness as part of an hereditary syndrome. J Laryngol Otol 73:355, 1959

45. Jorgensen MB, Kristensen HK, Buch TH: Thalidomide-induced aplasia of the inner ear. J Laryngol Otol 78:1095, 1964

46. A case of congenital deafness showing malformation of the bony and membranous labyrinths on both sides. J Laryngol Otol 42:315, 1927

47. Igarashi M, Takahashi M, Alford B: Inner ear morphology in Down's syndrome. Acta Otolaryngol (Stockh) 83:175, 1977

48. Ruben RJ, Toriyama M, Dische MR, et al: External

and middle ear malformations associated with mandibulo-facia dysostosis and renal abnormalities. A case report. Ann Otol Rhinol Laryngol 78:605, 1969

49. Sando I, Hemenway WG, Morgan WR: Histopathology of the temporal bones in mandibulofacial dysostosis (Treacher-Collins syndrome). Trans Am Acad Ophthalmol Otolaryngol 72:913, 1968

50. Michel EM: Gas Med Strasbourg 3:55, 1963. Arch Ohrenheilkd 1:353, 1864 (abst)

51. Black FO, Myers EN, Rorke LB: Aplasia of the first and second branchial arches. Arch Otolaryngol 98:124, 1973

52. Paparella MM, Saguira S, Hoshino T: Familial progressive sensorineural deafness. Arch Otolaryngol 90:44, 1969

53. Beal DD, Davey FR, Lindsay JR: Inner ear pathology of congenital deafness. Arch Otolaryngol 85:134, 1967

54. Karmody CS, Schuknecht HF: Deafness in congenital syphilis. Arch Otolaryngol 83:18, 1966

55. Mondini C: Anatomico surdi nati sectio: Die Bononiensi Scientiarum et articum instituto atque academii commentarii. Bononiae 7:429, 1791

56. Muckle TJ, Wells M: Urticaria, deafness and amyloidosis: A new heredofamilial syndrome. Q J Med 31:235, 1962

57. Wells M, Phelps PD, Michaels L: Oculo-auriculovertebral dysplasia. A temporal bone study of a case of Goldenhar's syndrome. J Laryngol Otol 97:689, 1983

58. Murakami Y, Schuknecht HF: Unusual congenital anomalies in the inner ear. Arch Otolaryngol 87:335, 1968

59. Hough JVD: Malformations and anatomical variations seen in the middle ear during the operation for mobilization of the stapes. Laryngoscope 68:1337, 1968

60. Wolff D: Malformations of the ear. Arch Otolaryngol 79:288, 1964

61. Myers EN, Stool SE, Koblenzer PJ: Congenital deafness, spiny hyperkeratosis and universal alopecia. Arch Otolaryngol 93:68, 1971

62. Adkins WY, Gussen R: Oval window absence, bony closure of round window and inner ear anomaly. Laryngoscope 84:1210, 1974

63. Morgenstein KM, Manace EO: Temporal bone histopathology in sickle cell disease. Laryngoscope 79:2172, 1969

64. Saito H, Okano Y, Furuta M, et al: Temporal bone findings in trisomy D. Arch Otolaryngol 100:386, 1974

65. Ward PH, Kinney CE, Lindsay JR: Inner ear pathology and congenital deafness. Laryngoscope 72:435, 1962

66. Adkins WY Jr, Gussen R: Temporal bone findings in the third and fourth pharyngeal pouch (DiGeorge) syndrome. Arch Otolaryngol 100:206, 1974

67. Kelemen G: Malformation involving external, middle and internal ear, with otosclerotic focus. Arch Otolaryngol 37:183, 1943

68. Scheibe A: Ein Fall von Taubstummheit mit Acusticusatrophie und Bildungsanomalien in hautigen Labyrinth beiderseits. Z Hals Nasen Ohrenheilkd 22:11, 1892

69. Abramovitch SJ, Gregory S, Slemick M, Stewart AL: Hearing loss in very low birthweight infants treated with neonatal care. Arch Dis Child 54:421, 1979

70. Spector GJ, Pettit WJ, Davis G, et al: Fetal respiratory distress causing CNS and inner ear hemorrhage. Laryngoscope 88:764, 1978

71. Michaels L, Gould SJ, Wells M: The microslicing method in the study of temporal bone changes in the perinatal period: An interim report. Acta Otolaryngol. (Stockh) 423:9, 1985.

72. Schuknecht HF, Neff WO, Perlman HB: An experimental study of auditory damage following blows to the head. Ann Otol 60:273, 1951

73. Engstrom H, Ades HW, Bredberg G: Normal structure of the organ of Corti and the effect of noise induced cochlear damage. p. 127. In Wolstenholme GEW, Knight J (eds): Sensorineural Hearing Loss. J and A Churchill, London, 1970

74. Paparella MM, Melnick W: Stimulation deafness. p. 427. In Graham AB (ed): Sensorineural Hearing Processes and Disorders. Little, Brown, Boston, 1967

75. Rahal JJ, Hyams PJ, Simberkoff MS, Rubinstein E: Combined intrathecal and intramuscular gentamicin for gram negative meningitis. N Engl J Med 29:1394, 1974

76. Matz GJ, Lerner SA: Drug ototoxicity. p. 573. In Beagley HA (ed): Audiology and Audiological Medicine. Vol. 1. Oxford University Press, Oxford, 1981

77. Wicke W, Welleschik B, Firbus W, Sinzinger H: Zur Streptomycinschadigung des Ganglion spirale. Acta Otolaryngol (Stockh) 85:360, 1978

78. Tange RA, Huizing EH: Hearing loss and inner ear changes in a patient suffering from severe gentamycin ototoxicity. Arch Otorhinolaryngol 228:113, 1980

79. Lindsay JR, Proctor LR, Work WP: Histopathologic inner ear changes in deafness due to neomycin in a human. Laryngoscope 70:382, 1960
80. Keene M, Hawke M, Barber HO, Farkashidy J: Histopathological findings in clinical gentamycin ototoxicity. Arch Otolaryngol 108:65, 1982
81. Forge A: The endolymphatic surface of the stria vascularis in the guinea pig and the effects of ethacrynic acid as shown by scanning electron microscopy. Clin Otolaryngol 5:87, 1980
82. Matz GJ: The ototoxic effects of ethacrynic acid in man and animals. Laryngoscope 86:1065, 1976
83. Matz GJ, Beal DD, Krames L: Ototoxicity of ethacrynic acid—demonstrated in a human temporal bone. Arch Otol 90:152, 1969
84. Meriwether WD, Manji RJ, Serpick AA: Deafness following standard intravenous dose of ethacrynic acid. JAMA 216:795, 1971
85. Matz GJ, Wallace TH, Ward PH: The ototoxicity of kanamycin. A comparative histopathologic study. Laryngoscope 75:1690, 1965
86. Myers E, Bernstein J, Fostiropolous G: Salicylate ototoxicity. A clinical study. N Engl J Med 273:587, 1965
87. Ruedi L, Furrer W, Luthy F, et al: Further observations concerning the toxic effects of streptomycin and quinine on the auditory organ of guinea pigs. Laryngoscope 62:333, 1952
88. Cummings C: Experimental observations on the ototoxicity of nitrogen mustard. Laryngoscope 78:530, 1968
89. Schuknecht H: The pathology of several disorders of the inner ear which cause vertigo. South Med J 57:1161, 1964
90. Tange RA, Conijin EAJG, van Zeyl LEPM: Differences in the cochlear degeneration pattern in the guinea pig as result of gentamicin and cis-platinum intoxication. Clin Otolaryngol 8:138, 1983 (abst)
91. Karmody CS: Viral labyrinthitis—An experimental study. Ann Otol 84:179, 1975
92. Glascow LA: Virus infections of the fetus and newborn infant. J Pediatr 77:315, 1970
93. Institute of Laryngology and Otology Clinicopathological Meeting: Cytomegalovirus and congenital hearing loss. Clin Otolaryngol 6:219, 1981
94. Davis G: Cytomegalovirus in the inner ear. Case report and electron microscopic study. Ann Otol Rhinol Laryngol 78:1179, 1969
95. Bordley JE, Kapur YP: Histopathologic changes in the temporal bone resulting from measles infection. Arch Otolaryngol 103:162, 1977
96. Lindsay JR, Hemenway W: Inner ear pathology due to measles. Ann Otol Rhinol Laryngol 63:754, 1954
97. Smith GA, Gussen R: Inner ear pathologic features following mumps infection. Report of a case in an adult. Arch Otolaryngol 102:108, 1976
98. Friedmann I, Wright MI: Histopathological changes in the foetal and infantile inner ear caused by maternal rubella. Br Med J 2:20, 1966
99. Brookhouser PE, Bordley JE: Congenital rubella deafness. Pathology and pathogenesis. Arch Otolaryngol 98:252, 1973
100. Blackley B, Friedmann I, Wright I: Herpes zoster auris associated with facial nerve palsy and auditory nerve symptoms. A case report with histopathological findings. Acta Otolaryngol (Stockh) 6:533, 1967
101. Sando I, Harada T, Loehr, Sobel JH: Sudden deafness. Histopathologic correlation in temporal bone. Ann Otol 86:269, 1977
102. Lindsay JR: Histopathology of deafness due to postnatal viral disease. Arch Otolaryngol 98:258, 1973
103. Fowler EP: The pathologic findings in a case of facial paralysis. Trans Am Acad Ophthalmol Otol 67:187, 1963
104. Meyerhoff WL, Paparella MM, Oda M, Shea D: Mycotic infections of the inner ear. Laryngoscope 89:1725, 1979
105. Igarashi M, Weber SC, Alford BR et al: Temporal bone findings in cryptococcal meningitis. Arch Otolaryngol 101:577, 1975
106. Goodhill V: Syphilis of the ear. A histopathological study. Ann Otol Rhinol Laryngol 48:676, 1939
107. Karmody C, Schuknecht H: Deafness in congenital syphilis. Arch Otolaryngol 83:18, 1966
108. Mayer O, Fraser JS: Pathological changes in late congenital syphilis. J Laryngol Otol 51:683 and 755, 1936
109. Mack LW, Smith JL, Walter EK, et al: Temporal bone treponemes. Arch Otolaryngol 90:37, 1969
110. Belal A, Linthicum FH: Pathology of congenital syphilitic labyrinthitis. Am J Otolaryngol 1:109, 1980
111. Guild SR, Crowe SJ, Bunch CC, Polvogt LM: Correlations of differences in the density of innervation of the organ of Corti with differences in the acuity of hearing, including evidence as to the location in the human cochlea of the receptors for certain tones. Acta Otolaryngol (Stockh) 15:269, 1939
112. Suga F, Lindsay J: Histopathological observations of presbycusis. Ann Otol 85:169, 1976

113. Jorgensen MB: Changes of aging in the inner ear. Histological studies. Arch Otolaryngol 74:164, 1961

114. Johnsson L, Hawkins JE: Sensory and neural degeneration with aging, as seen in microdissection of the human inner ear. Ann Otol Rhinol Laryngol 81:179, 1972

115. Schuknecht HF: Presbycusis. Laryngoscope 65:402, 1955

116. Belal A: Presbycusis: Physiological or pathological. J Laryngol Otol 89:1011, 1975

117. Hansen CC, Reske-Nielsen E: Pathological studies in presbycusis. Cochlear and central findings in 12 aged patients. Arch Otolaryngol 82:115, 1965

118. Bredberg G: Cellular patterns and nerve supply of the human organ of Corti. Acta Otolaryngol (Stockh) [Suppl] 236:6, 1968

119. Nadol JB: Electron microscopic findings in presbycusic degeneration of the basal turn of the human cochlea. Otolaryngol Head Neck Surg 6:818, 1979

120. Schuknecht HF: Pathology of the Ear. Harvard University Press, Cambridge, MA, 1974

121. Stern-Padovan R, Vukicevic S: Histologic changes in the ageing spiral tract. J Laryngol Otol 94:255, 1980

122. Arnesen AR: Presbycusis—Loss of neurons in the human cochlear nuclei. J Laryngol Otol 96:503, 1982

123. Hall JG: The cochlea and the cochlear nuclei in neonatal asphyxia. A histological study. Acta Otolaryngol (Stockh) [Suppl] 194:1, 1964

123a. Soucek S, Michaels L, Frohlich A: Evidence for hair cell degeneration as the primary lesion in hearing loss of the elderly. J Otolaryngol 15:175, 1986

123b. Soucek S, Mason SM: A study of hearing in the elderly using non-invasive electrocochleography and auditory brainstem responses. J. Otolaryngol, 1987, In press

123c. Soucek S, Michaels L, Frohlich A: Pathological changes in the organ of Corti as revealed by microslicing and staining. Acta Otolaryngol (Stockh) [Suppl] 436:93, 1987

124 Lindsay JR, Kohut RI, Sciarra PA: Ménière's disease: Pathology and manifestations. Ann Otol Rhinol Laryngol 76:5, 1967.

125. Kohut RI, Lindsay JR: Pathologic changes in idiopathic labyrinthine hydrops. Acta Otolaryngol (Stockh) 73:402, 1972

126. Altmann F, Kornfeld M: Histologic studies of Ménière's disease. Ann Otol 74:915, 1965

127. Hallpike KS, Cairns H: Observations on the pathology of Ménière's disease. J Laryngol Otol 53:625, 1938

128. Hallpike CS, Wright AJ: On the histological changes in the temporal bones of a case of Méniére's disease. J Laryngol Otol 55:58, 1940

129. Gussen R: Ménière's syndrome. Compensatory collateral venous drainage with endolymphatic sac fibrosis. Arch Otolaryngol 99:414, 1974

130. Rollin H: Zur Kenntis des Labyrinthhydrops und des durch ihn bedingten Ménière. Hals Nasen Ohren 31:73, 1940

131. Shambaugh GE Jr: Surgery of the endolymphatic sac. Arch Otolaryngol 83:305, 1966

132. Gussen R: Ménière's disease. New temporal bone findings in two cases. Laryngoscope 81:1695, 1971

133. Keleman G: Anatomical observations on the distal extremity of the vestibular aqueduct. J Laryngol Otol 90:1071, 1976

134. Frayse BG, Alonso A, House WF: Ménière's disease and endolymphatic hydrops. Clinical–histopathological correlations. Ann Otol Rhinol Laryngol 8[suppl 76]:2, 1980

135. Arenberg IK: Marovitz W, Shambaugh G Jr: The role of the endolymphatic sac in the pathogenesis of endolymphatic hydrops in man. Acta Otolaryngol (Stockh) [Suppl] 275:7, 1970

136. Schindler RA: The ultrastructure of the endolymphatic sac in man. Laryngoscope 90[Suppl 21]:1, 1980

137. Friedmann I, Cawthorne K, McLay K, Bird ES: Electron microscopic observations on the human membranous labyrinth with particular reference to Ménière's disease. J Ultrastruct Res 9:123, 1963

138. Hilding DA, House WF: An evaluation of the ultrastructural findings in the utricle in Ménière's disease. Laryngoscope 74:1135, 1964

139. Antoli-Candela F: The histopathology of Ménière's disease. Acta Otolaryngol (Stockh) suppl 340:5, 1976

140. Kimura RS, Schuknecht HF: Membranous hydrops in the inner ear of the guinea pig after obliteration of the endolymphatic sac. Pract Otorhinolaryngol (Basel) 27:343, 1956

141. Schuknecht HF, Northrop C, Igarashi M: Cochlear pathology after destruction of the endolymphatic sac in the cat. Acta Otolaryngol (Stockh) 65:479, 1968

142. Nager GT: Paget's disease of the temporal bone. A clinical and histopathological survey. Acta Otolaryngol (Stockh) [Suppl] 242:1, 1968

143. Michaels L, Wells M: Squamous carcinoma of the middle ear. Clin Otolaryngol 5:235, 1980

144. Druss JG: Aural manifestations of leukemia. Arch Otolaryngol 42:267, 1945

145. Wright DH, Isaacson PG: Biopsy Pathology of the

Lymphoreticular System. Chapman and Hall, London, 1983

146. Wells M, Michaels L, Wells DG: Otolaryngeal disturbances in Waldenström's macroglobulinaemia. Clin Otolaryngol 2:327, 1977

147. Rosenhall U: Epithelial cysts in the human vestibular apparatus. J Laryngol Otol 88:105, 1974

148. Fleischer K: Morphological aspects of the ageing ear. HNO 20:103, 1972

149. Rudge P: Clinical Neuro-otology. Churchill Livingstone, Edinburgh, 1984

150. Lindsay JR, Hemenway WG: Postural vertigo due to unilateral sudden partial loss of vestibular function. Ann Otol 65:692, 1956

151. Dix R, Hallpike CS: The pathology, symptomatology and diagnosis of certain common disorders of the vestibular system. Ann Otol 61:987, 1952

152. Cawthorne TE, Hallpike CS: A study of the clinical features and pathological changes within the temporal bones, brain stem and cerebellum of an early case of positional nystagmus of the so-called benign paroxysmal type. Acta Otolaryngol (Stockh) 48:89, 1957

153. Schuknecht HF: Cupulolithiasis. Arch Otolaryngol 90:113, 1969

154. Gacek RR: Transection of the posterior ampullary nerve for relief of benign paroxysmal positional vertigo. Ann Otol Rhinol Laryngol 83:596, 1974

155. Schuknecht H, Ruby R: Cupulolithiasis. Adv Otorhinolaryngol 20:434, 1973

156. Davies DG. Paget's disease of the temporal bone. A clinical and histopathological survey. Acta Otolaryngol (Stockh) [Suppl] 242:1, 1968

157. Igarashi M, King AI, Schwenzfeier CW, et al: Inner ear pathology in osteogenesis imperfecta congenita. J Laryngol Otol 94:697, 1980

158. Zajtchuk JT, Lindsay JR: Osteogenesis imperfecta congenita et tarda: A temporal bone report. Ann Otol Rhinol Laryngol 84:350, 1975

159. Brosnan M, Burns H, Jahn AF, Hapke M: Surgery and histopathology of the stapes in osteogenesis imperfecta tarda. Arch Otolaryngol 103:294, 1977

160. Arslan M, Ricci V: Histochemical investigations of otosclerosis with special regard to collagen disease. J Laryngol Otol 77:365, 1963

161. Myers EN, Stool S: The temporal bone in osteopetrosis. Arch Otolaryngol 89:44, 1969

162. Hamersma H: Ostopetrosis (marble bone disease) of the temporal bone. Laryngoscope 80:1518, 1970

163. Schuknecht HF: Pathology of sensorineural deafness of genetic origin. p. 79. In McDonnell F, Ward PH (eds): Deafness in Childhood. Vanderbilt University Press, Nashville, TN, 1967

164. Guild SR: Histologic otosclerosis. Ann Otol 53:246, 1944

165. Nager GT: Histopathology of otosclerosis. Arch Otolaryngol 89:157, 1969

166. Nager GT: Sensorineural deafness and otosclerosis. Ann Otol 75:481, 1966

167. Lindsay JR: Blue mantles in otosclerosis. Ann Otol 83:33, 1974

# Pathology of the Central Auditory Pathways and Cochlear Nerve

# 24

## Dikran Horoupian

The pathology of the two divisions of the eighth nerve are discussed in two separate chapters; therefore, some degree of repetition is unavoidable. To minimize this and because of space limitations, certain subjects are presented at some length in one chapter and briefly covered in the other. In essence, this and the following chapter complement each other. In this chapter, pathologic alterations encountered in sensorineural hearing loss are presented with special emphasis on the central portion of the auditory pathway. The developmental and hereditary disorders of the cochleovestibular system are stressed particularly as this subject is not covered in Chapter 25. Infectious diseases that affect the auditory system more than the vestibular are reviewed. The pathology of demyelinating diseases and vascular disorders, aging, and dementia is covered in some detail. Neoplasia is mentioned only briefly, and the pathology is reviewed in depth in Chapter 25.

## DEVELOPMENTAL AND HEREDITARY DISORDERS

### Chromosomal Aberrations

Structural abnormalities of the central nervous system (CNS) are well established in all three major autosomal trisomies. In *Downs syndrome*, these include reduction in total brain weight, simplified convolutional pattern, bilateral narrow superior temporal gyrus in 50 percent of patients, and disproportionately small brain stem and cerebellum[1] (Fig. 24-1). Reports of pathologic studies pertaining the central auditory pathway are scarce. Using the computer image analyzer, Gandolfi et al.[2] reported a reduction in the number of neurons in the ventral cochlear nucleus, a small nuclear volume, low cell-packing density, and abnormally large mean neuronal diameter.

*Trisomy E (17-18)* (Edwards syndrome) resembles Downs syndrome in that it has a bimodal distribution of maternal ages, but unlike Downs it has a $3:1$ preference for females, and the life expectancy is much reduced.[3] Anomalous lobar and gyral patterns, heterotopias, and disorganization of the lateral geniculate nuclei are a few of the neuropathologic findings encountered in this condition.[4,5] Although structural disorders of the peripheral auditory system are well documented, little is known about the central pathways.[6,7] Morphometric and Golgi studies in two cases of trisomy E showed maturational retardation of both the ventral cochlear nucleus and the dendritic arbors of the pyramidal cells of the auditory cortex. The small size of the ventral cochlear nucleus was also consistent with the overall smallness of the brain.[2]

*Trisomy D, 13-15* (Patau syndrome) is less common than the previous two types. Most infants are

713

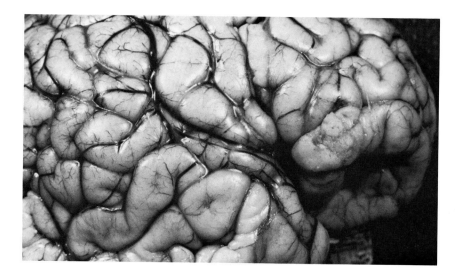

**Fig. 24-1.** Lateral view of a brain of a patient with Downs syndrome. The superior temporal gyrus is very thin, and the orbital surface of the frontal lobe is slanted upward.

females with a very low life expectancy.[8] Holoprosencephaly is the characteristic developmental anomaly of the CNS.[9] These infants fail to respond to sound and are presumed deaf. Exceptionally large nests of matrix cells have been described.[10] Maturational retardation of neurons in the auditory cortex[2] was similar to Marin-Padilla's observations in the motor cortex.[11]

## Skeletal and CNS Deformities

### Arnold-Chiari Malformation

Arnold-Chiari malformation is characterized by a disproportionately small posterior cranial cavity with tightly packed brain stem and cerebellum extending to a variable degree into an enlarged funnel-shaped foramen magnum and upper cervical canal[10] (Fig. 24-2). Hydrocephalus and various dysraphic conditions of the spine, particularly lumbosacral meningomyelocele, are common. The caudal shifting and elongation of the medulla oblongata stretch the acoustic nerves, kinking them over the margin of the internal acoustic meatus.[12] Compression of the seventh and eighth nerves at the cerebellopontine angle by the ventral edge of the foramen magnum has also been described.[13] These nerves, along with other cranial nerves, may become compressed from crowding in the posterior fossa. Dislocated blood vessels could also lead

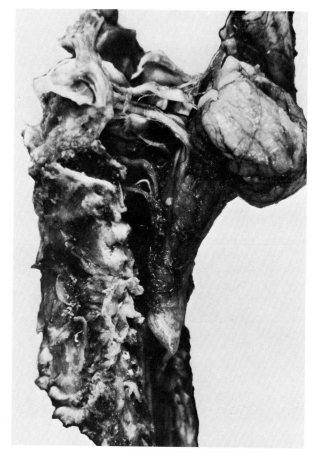

**Fig. 24-2.** Arnold-Chiari malformation. The cerebellum is displaced into the upper cervical cord; the cranial nerves are stretched and kinked.

to ischemic changes in the brain stem.[14] Auditory symptoms may appear in about 20 percent of cases.[15] Saez et al.[12] reported that in their series, 7 of 60 patients with Arnold-Chiari malformation had hearing loss.

### Bony Abnormalities in the Floor of the Posterior Fossa

Deformities of the floor of the posterior fossa and upper cervical vertebra, such as in Klippel-Feil syndrome, may cause serious neurologic complications, including dizziness and deafness.[16] Basilar impression or invagination is the most serious abnormality and may be associated with platybasia and sometimes with fusion of two or more cervical vertebrae. In basilar impression, the medulla and lower cranial nerves may become kinked and compressed.[7]

### Hereditary Deafness

Hereditary sensorineural deafness comprises a large number of disorders, some congenital and others having their onset in childhood and early adult life. It is estimated that about one-third of all hereditary deafness represents recognizable syndromes.[18] Konigsmark[19] classified them on the basis of associated neurodegenerative diseases, oc-

ular abnormalities, or cutaneous disorders. Only conditions that have pathologic documentation pertaining to the auditory pathways are presented.

### Cockayne's Syndrome

Cockayne's syndrome is one of the four syndromes of deafness with retinitis pigmentosa that Konigsmark has distinguished from other neurodegenerative disorders. This autosomal-recessive condition is characterized by dwarfism, microcephaly, mental retardation, peculiar facies, premature senility, photosensitive dermatitis, pigmentary retinal degeneration, and deafness.[20] Hearing impairment usually becomes apparent during the course of the disease, along with the gradual failure of cognitive functions. Gandolfi et al.[21] reported atrophy of the spiral ganglion (Fig. 24-3) and changes in the first three auditory relay nuclei probably due to anterograde transsynaptic degeneration (Fig. 24-4). In addition, areas of demyelination and gliosis were present in the auditory radiation.

### Sylvester's Disease

Sylvester's disease (dominant optic atrophy, ataxia, and progressive hearing loss) is one of the four syndromes characterized by hereditary deaf-

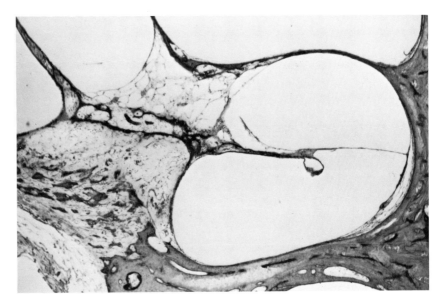

**Fig. 24-3.** Modiolus of a deaf patient with Cockayne's syndrome. The spiral ganglion is severely depleted of neurons. (H & E, original magnification × 4.)

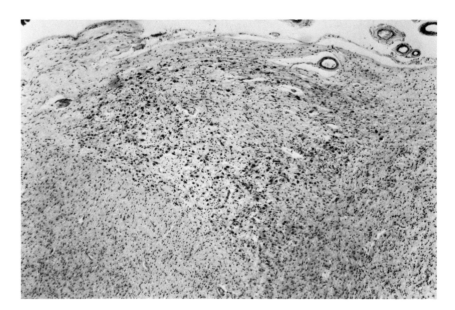

**Fig. 24-4.** Ventral cochlear nucleus of the same patient as in Fig. 24-3, showing reduction in the size of the nucleus and marked neuronal loss. (Nissl stain, original magnification × 10.)

ness and optic atrophy in Konigsmark's classification. It is an autosomal-dominant syndrome in which auditory and visual deficits are associated with variable degrees of mental retardation, peripheral extremity weakness, and ataxia. Skeletal abnormalities such as kyphosis, pes cavus, and claw hands, have been described. Limited neuropathologic study of a 2.5-year-old girl with this syndrome demonstrated atrophy of the dorsal and ventral spinocerebellar tracts, the corticospinal tracts, posterior funiculi, and optic nerves.[19]

### Norrie's Disease

In Norrie's disease (oculo-acoustico-cerebral degeneration), blindness is present at birth. It is due to gliovascular proliferation in the pigmentary layer of the retina and is associated with optic atrophy. Cataracts occur later. Mental retardation is present in about one-half of patients, making evaluation of hearing impairment difficult to assess. Hearing loss usually develops in the second or third decade of life. The brain changes in two reports consisted of abnormal arrangement of the cortical neurons and atrophy of the optic nerves and lateral geniculate bodies.[22,23]

### Waardenburg's Syndrome

In this autosomal-dominant syndrome, the congenital deafness is associated with a white forelock,

heterochromia iridis, and lateral displacement of the medial canthi. Fisch[24] found a Mondini-type malformation with secondary atrophy of the acoustic division, the vestibular division was normal.

### Alport's Syndrome

This form of hereditary congenital deafness is associated with renal disease. The condition is more common in males, and its prognosis is worse than in female siblings with the disease. There are conflicting pathologic reports about the locus of hearing impairment. Johnson and Arenburg[25] reported atrophy of the stria with minimal neuronal atrophy.

### Hereditary Deafness of Later Onset

*Friedrich's ataxia* is one of the few heredofamilial spinocerebellar disorders in which some morphologic documentation of the auditory pathways are available. Friedrich's ataxia is usually an autosomal-recessive disorder with average age of onset at 11.75 years. In the dominant form, the age of onset is at 20.4 years.[26] It is characterized by progressive ataxia, dysarthia, absence of vibration and position senses, skeletal deformities, and extensor plantar responses. Hearing impairment is common. If it is not clinically overt, Friedrich's ataxia can often be detected by electrophysiologic studies such as brain stem auditory evoked responses (BAER).[27]

Urich et al.[28] described degeneration in the auditory pathways in one patient. Van Bogaert and Martin[29] observed definite degeneration of the superior olive in one patient and degeneration of the ventral cochlear nucleus, striae medullaris, and superior olives in that patient's sister. The lower quadrigeminal body and medial geniculate nuclei were normal. In a series of 13 patients, four of whom had deafness, Oppenheimer[30] found variable degrees of cell loss and gliosis in more than one of the auditory relay nuclei in the brain stem. On the other hand, Boudin et al.[31] reported normal cochlear nuclear complex in a 36-year-old woman with the disease.

### Hick's Disease

Hick's disease (Denny-Brown syndrome, dominant sensory radicular neuropathy) is usually a dominant familial disorder characterized by progressive sensory neuropathy, trophic ulcers of the extremities, neuropathic joints, and sensorineural deafness. Although progressive hearing impairment was noted in all affected members of some families,[32] it was not regularly observed in others.[33] Hallpike[34] found degeneration of the organ of Corti in one patient; in another case, Hallpike and associates[35] found the degeneration to affect the cochlear nerves and spiral ganglion and not the organ of Corti. In a patient with audiometrically verified sensorineural deafness and peripheral neuropathy of the Hick's type, cell count and cell size determinations of the ventral cochlear nucleus were normal. In Golgi preparations, however, the dendritic arbor and the dendritic spines of the pyramidal cells of Heschl's gyrus were abnormal.[35a]

### Progressive Bulbar Palsy with Neural Deafness

Progressive bulbar palsy with neural deafness (Vialetto-van Laere syndrome) is an autosomal-recessive disorder characterized by progressive sensorineural hearing loss, usually beginning in the second and third decade, followed shortly after by gradual weakness of the facial and bulbar muscles. Peripheral muscle weakness, ataxia, vestibular manifestations, and pyramidal signs, to a variable extent, have also been described in some patients. This condition should be distinguished from Fazio-Londe disease and juvenile forms of amyotrophic lateral sclerosis. Autopsy findings showed neuronal atrophy and gliosis of the eighth nerve nuclei, motor nuclei of brain stem, and anterior horns.[36] There was also degeneration of the pyramidal, spinocerebellar, and fasciculus gracilis fibers.[37]

## INFECTIONS

### Intrauterine

#### Congenital Rubella Syndrome

Gregg[38] was first to recognize the embryopathy associated with maternal rubella infection. The first 4 weeks of gestation are the period of risk. The embryopathy is characterized by microcephaly, cataracts, dental anomalies, and congenital heart disease. Neurologically, affected children have microcephaly, intracranial calcification, mental retardation, focal neurologic deficits, seizures, and deafness. Hearing loss is common, 52 percent according to Cooper and Krugman,[39] and may be the only defect caused by this intrauterine infection. Deafness is largely due to destruction of the cochlea, and sometimes to middle ear abnormalities. The chronic meningitis, the small foci of necrosis, and the vasculopathy of the intracerebral vessels[40] may also contribute to the hearing impairment in these children, but a definite clinical pathologic study is lacking.[41]

#### Cytomegalovirus Infection

Generalized intrauterine infection with cytomegalovirus is characterized by hepatosplenomegaly, jaundice, anemia, thrombocytopenia, petechiae, and diarrhea.[42] The CNS is at risk in about 50 percent of cases; these children may display microcephaly, cerebral calcifications, seizures, chorioretinitis, mental retardation, and deafness.[43,44] The inflammatory lesions are mainly periventricular, where large cells probably astrocytes, show enlarged nuclei with a voluminous round or oval Cowdry type A inclusion, and an abundant cytoplasm containing basophilic stipplings (Fig. 24-5). Inner ear involvement, particularly of the labyrinth, has been described.[45] Hearing impairment,

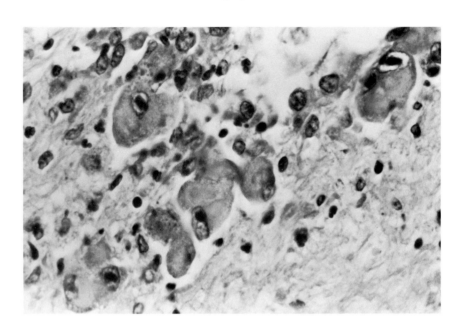

**Fig. 24-5.** Ventriculitis due to cytomegalovirus infection. The large cells are probably reactive astrocytes displaying the characteristic owl-eye intranuclear inclusion. (H & E, original magnification × 100.)

either alone or in conjunction with other stigmata of the disease, is said to be a common complication of congenital cytomegalovirus disease.[46,47] Possible CNS lesions that may be responsible for hearing loss in such patients have not been investigated.

## Meningitides

### Acute Bacterial Meningitis

The organisms responsible for hematogenous purulent meningitis are often age dependent. Group B streptococcus or *Escherichia coli* meningitis commonly occurs in the perinatal period and *Hemophilus influenzae* is encountered almost exclusively in children between 2 months and 7 years of age. Meningitis due to *Neisseria meningitidis* (meningococcus) occurs most often in children and young adults. Pneumococcal meningitis predominates in the very young and in adults over 40 years of age. Macroscopically, a creamy exudate is frequently confined to the fissures and spares the crowns of the gyri over the convexities of the brain (Fig. 24-6). The exudate is also present in the basal cisternae.Microscopically, the exudate consists mainly of polymorphonuclear leukocytes, variable numbers of lymphocytes, plasma cells, and macrophages, depending on the stage of the disease and the type of organism. Bacteria may be seen in and among the pus cells. Purulent meningitis accounts for about 20 percent of unilateral and bilateral acquired deafness and is usually the direct result of labyrinthine destruction.[48] Inflammation spreads from the subarachnoid space via the base of the modiolus or the cochlear duct.[49] The eighth nerve itself may also be affected by the pyogenic exudate which is largely contained in the subarachnoid space. Occasionally, thrombophlebitis or actual arteritis may complicate bacterial meningitis, causing focal neurologic symptoms.[50] Lechevalier et al.[51] reported cortical deafness in a patient with pneumococcal meningitis who had developed bilateral temporal lobe lesions demonstrated on CT scan. In meningitis due to *Listeria monocytogenes*, abscesses may develop in the rhombencephalon, which in turn may destroy the cochlear nucleus. Infections of the CNS with *Listeria* usually occurs in terminally ill patients especially with lymphoproliferative disorders.

### Viral Meningitides

Deafness due to mumps is one of the causes of acquired unilateral sensorineural deafness in children.[54] It is usually due to destruction of the cochlea and rarely, if ever, secondary to the meningoencephalitis.

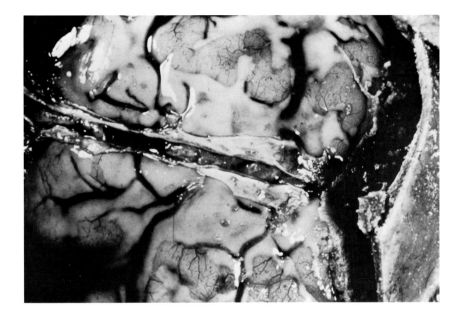

**Fig. 24-6.** Creamy exudate covers the sulci and obscures the blood vessels in a patient with purulent meningitis. The superior sagittal sinus is incised to demonstrate the complicating thrombophlebitis.

## Chronic Granulomatous Meningitides

**Tuberculosis.** Tuberculous meningitis or meningoencephalitis is invariably secondary to primary tuberculous infection elsewhere in the body. In children, it is a complication of miliary tuberculosis but in adults, especially in the elderly, it is due to reactivation or reinfection. The meningitis results from rupture of a superficial cortical tuberculoma, discharging bacteria into the subarachnoid space. Small discrete gray white tubercles are sometimes visible over the surface of the brain. A thick exudate, mainly at the base, often obliterates the cisterna ambiens and interpeduncularis and leads to hydrocephalus (Fig. 24-7). Microscopically, the tubercles display central caseation surrounded by epithelioid cells with rare Langhan giant cells and rimmed peripherally by lymphocytes and plasma cells. Depending on the stage of the disease, there is connective tissue proliferation. Tuberculous endarteritis is a frequent complication that accounts for focal areas of cerebral infarctions. Because of the basal distribution of the inflammation, cranial nerve palsies, usually ocular and less frequently acoustic, may occur.[55] If untreated, tuberculous meningitis is invariably fatal, death occurring within 4 to 8 weeks of onset. *Tuberculomas* are still the most common intracranial space-occupying lesions in areas of the world in which milk is not

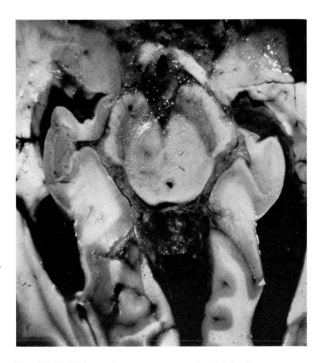

**Fig. 24-7.** Tuberculous meningitis. A thick feltlike organizing exudate surrounds the midbrain section.

pasteurized and bacille Calmette-Guérin (BCG) vaccination is not enforced.[56] They have special predilection to the posterior fossa and may involve the pontocerebellar region.

**Syphilis.** Before the advent of penicillin, a large percentage of children with congenital syphilis complained of hearing impairment.[57] Deafness was usually bilateral and of sudden onset. In addition to destruction of the cochlea, the acoustic nerves were sometimes entrapped in the leptomeningeal fibrosis or destroyed by endarteritis or gummata. In acquired syphilis, involvement of the central afferent auditory pathways by any one of the several forms of meningovascular syphilis or parenchymatous degeneration may account for deafness in syphilitic patients.[55,58]

### Fungal Infections

Fungal infections may occur in healthy persons but often complicate diseases and therapies that impair the immune system of patients. In recent years, fungal infections have been reported in large numbers in patients with acquired immune deficiency syndrome (AIDS).[59,60] Patients at risk are male homosexuals, drug addicts, hemophiliacs, and Haitians. A fungal infection that may affect the mastoid bone or cerebellopontine angle is mucor-

mycosis.[61] Mucormycosis is also known to complicate diabetic ketoacidosis. Mucormycosis-causing fungi have nonseptate hyphae and have the propensity to invade and grow in blood vessels causing thromboses and infarctions. Similarly, Aspergillosis may affect the middle cranial fossa or cerebellopontine angle.[62] It may form granulomatous masses that display dichotomically branching septate hyphae.[63] *Cryptococcus neoformans*[64] *(Torula histolytica)* infection and coccidioidomycosis[65] are sometimes responsible for indolent basal meningitis, which can entrap the lower cranial nerves including the eighth nerve. For more details, refer to Chapter 26.

---

# METABOLIC DISORDERS

## Anoxia/Ischemia

The phenomena of selective vulnerability of the CNS are particularly striking in anoxia/ischemia. The cerebral cortex at the depth of the sulci, especially its third laminar layer, is most susceptible. The pyramidal cells within Ammon's horn and the

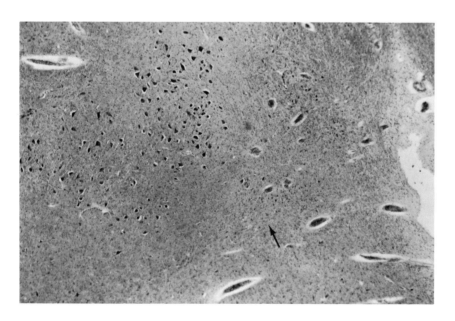

**Fig. 24-8.** Kernicterus in Crigler-Najjar syndrome. The superior olivary nucleus (arrow) is depleted of neurons; those surviving are shrunken and atrophic. Compare these neurons with those of the adjacent facial nucleus, which was not affected by the disorder. (H & E, original magnification × 40.)

Purkinje cells are also vulnerable.[66] The brain stem nuclei in adults are relatively resistant to anoxia, but in infants and young children destruction of the ventral cochlear nucleus[67] and inferior colliculi may take place and similar changes have been reproduced in term monkey fetuses.[68] In *double athetoid syndrome*, which complicates in utero hypoxia, hearing impairment is well recognized.[69] According to Dublin, there is a gradient of involvement of the ventral cochlear nucleus similar to kernicterus. Topistic susceptibility of octopoid cells is said to account for some cases of central loudness recruitment.

## Kernicterus

This complication of erythroblastosis fetalis due to Rh or ABO blood incompatibilities is now rare because of the vigorous policy of exchange transfusion and phototherapy in neonatal centers.[71] Anoxia in conjunction with the toxic action of unconjugated bilirubin causes topistic destruction of certain regions of the brain, notably, the subthalamic nuclei, the pallida, and Ammon's horn. In the auditory pathway, the inferior colliculi and less frequently the cochlear nuclei are affected. The deafness commonly present in the surviving children has been attributed to degeneration of the cochlear nucleus. In two deaf patients, however, Haymaker[72] found no such lesions. Dublin[73] reported cell loss mostly in the superior ventral segment of the nucleus and the spheroid cells appeared to be chiefly affected.

In *hereditary hyperbilirubinemia*, gross pigmentation and microscopic lesions consistent with kernicterus may take place.[74] In a 5-year-old patient with Crigler-Najjar, the ventral cochlear nucleus was replaced by a dense gliotic patch with a few surviving shrunken neurons. The trapezoid body and the superior olivary nuclear complex were markedly attenuated (personal communication) (Fig. 24-8).

## Refsum's Disease

This rare autosomal-recessive condition is due to a defect in the utilization of dietary phytol. Failure of oxidation of phytanic acid results in its accumulation in tissues and may constitute 5 to 30 percent of the total fatty acids of the serum lipids. It may

have its onset in late childhood, adolescence, or early adulthood. The syndrome consists of retinitis pigmentosa, cerebellar ataxia, chronic polyneuropathy, and sensorineural deafness. Other manifestations, such as cardiomyopathy, cataracts, and ichthyosis, may be present as well.[75] The cerebrospinal fluid (CSF) protein is almost constantly raised. The changes in the peripheral nerves are those of Schwann cell proliferation with onion-bulb formation.[76,77] Hallpike[34] described degeneration of the sense organs in the cochlea and saccule, but there was no mention of hypertrophic changes in the nerves. In a more recent study, demyelination and gliosis of the auditory nerves were reported, but it was not possible to establish whether they were primary changes or secondary to end-organ degeneration.[78]

## Hypothyroidism

Auditory dysfunction has been described in congenital hypothyroidism and myxedema. The consensus is that the cochlea is the locus of sensorineural hearing loss in children with endemic goiter or with Pendred's syndrome, which results from genetic defects in thyroxine synthesis.[48,79,80] No detailed studies of the afferent auditory pathways are available. There are experimental studies, however, to indicate that thyroxine deficiency delays both synaptogenesis[81] and myelination.[82] It is possible that similar structural changes in the CNS may be partially responsible for the auditory dysfunction in cretins.

## Diabetes Mellitus

Diabetes mellitus per se does not seem to be associated with higher incidence of hearing loss.[83] It is most likely that the complicating arteriosclerosis and hypertension account for loss of hearing in some diabetics.

## Avitaminosis B

Denny-Brown[84] found that 10 percent of prisoners of war who had neuropathy had also deafness. There was demyelination of the cochlear nerves and end-organ changes. It is possible that the changes in the eighth nerve described by Ylikoski[85] in a chronic alcoholic with peripheral neuropathy is due to vitamin deficiency rather than due to the direct toxic effect of alcohol. It should be emphasized that cranial neuropathies in general are very rare in alcoholics.

### Mitochondrial Cytopathies

Mitochondrial cytopathies are heterogeneous conditions putatively attributed to mitochondrial dysfunction.[86] A few of these disorders, such as *Kearn-Sayre's syndrome*, are often associated with deafness. Kearn-Sayre's syndrome is characterized by progressive external ophthalmoplegia, pigmentary degeneration of the retina, and heart block, usually beginning before age 20 years. Neurosensory hearing loss and vestibular dysfunction were present in 54 percent and 33 percent of cases reviewed, respectively, and in 85 percent of patients tested.[87] Muscle biopsy regularly shows ragged-red fibers in Engel's modified trichrome stain and aberrant mitochondria on electron microscopy (Fig. 24-9). Lindsay and Hirojosa[88] have reported secondary cochlear nerve degeneration. *Usher's syndrome*, a recessively inherited condition of congenital deafness and retinal degeneration that has been classified by Konigsmark as one of the hereditary deafness with retinitis pigmentosa, may in some ways be related to this heterogeneous group of disorders.

---

## DEMYELINATING DISEASES

Demyelinating diseases have in common destruction specifically of the myelin sheath with relative preservation of the other elements of the nervous system such as axons and neurons. Diseases included in this category are (1) multiple sclerosis and its variants, (2) acute disseminated encephalomyelitis either postvaccinal or postexanthematous, and (3) acute hemorrhagic leukoencephalopathy.

*Multiple sclerosis* is by far the most common of the demyelinating diseases.[89] It is more common in temperate climates, and its onset is usually in the third or fourth decades of life. The etiology and pathogenesis remain obscure. Infection, possibly

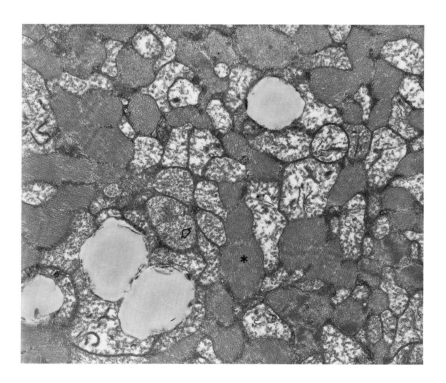

**Fig. 24-9.** Electron micrograph of a cross section of a muscle biopsy from a patient with Kearn-Sayre's syndrome. Aberrant enlarged mitochondria (arrow) displace the myofibers (asterisk) and are associated with globules of neutral lipid. (Original magnification × 14,000.)

viral, has been postulated mostly on circumstantial evidence, such as migration studies. Attempts to demonstrate such an agent by morphologic or immunologic means have failed. Delayed hypersensitivity is another prevailing hypothesis; it may occur in acute disseminated encephalomyelitis, but no target autoantigen that reacts with immune cells from patients with multiple sclerosis has yet been identified.[90] It is possible that infection by a specific virus or several unrelated viruses[91] may trigger in susceptible individuals (say, with certain HLA-linked determinants) an aberrant immune response aimed at central myelin[92,93] (myelin produced by oligodendrocytes). Peripheral myelin derived from Schwann cells is generally spared. The pathologic hallmark of multiple sclerosis are the plaques, which are often discrete in early stages and may become confluent as the disease progresses or remits.[94] Plaques occur in large concentration around the lateral ventricles (Fig. 24-10) and on the pial surface of the brain stem, optic nerves, and spinal cord. Microscopically, the typical plaque is sharply demarcated and displays complete loss of myelin and oligodendroglia, the axons being relatively well preserved. Early plaques are hypercellular due to proliferation of astrocytes and mononuclear cells. Perivascular lymphocytic cuffs are present in and around the lesions.[95] Plaques

occur frequently in the brain stem (Fig. 24-11) and can account for hearing impairment in some patients.[96,97] They have been described at the root entry zone of the eighth nerve.[98] Deafness in multiple sclerosis is rare, but in approximately 10 percent of patients some detectable hearing loss will become apparent in late stages of the disease.[99] Deafness is rarely an initial manifestation of the disease; however, two recent studies have shown otherwise.[100,101] Deafness may be incapacitating during the acute exacerbations.[101] Auditory hallucinations, possibly attributable to involvement of cochlear connections, have been described. Hearing problems in multiple sclerosis are largely caused by the cumulative effects of the plaques which can be seen all along the auditory pathways interfering thus with integrative processes.[102] Although plaques have generally been incriminated in loss or impaired functions, the symptoms are sometimes difficult to correlate with the autopsy findings.

*Acute disseminated encephalomyeloneuropathy* is considered an immune-mediated complication of infection (usually viral) or inoculation of foreign protein, such as vaccines.[103] The pathologic findings in the CNS are very similar to those of a laboratory model of the disease, experimental allergic encephalomyelitis, which can be induced by ino-

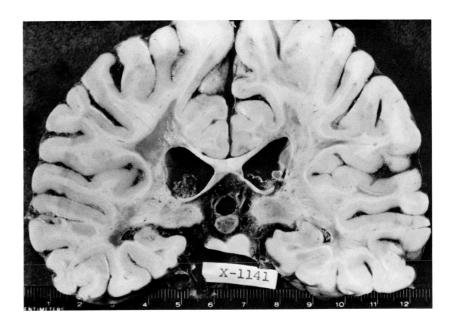

**Fig. 24-10.** Coronal section of the brain of a patient with multiple sclerosis. Large, confluent plaques of demyelination are present in the white matter and are most accentuated around the ventricles.

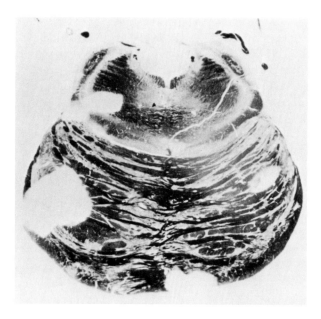

**Fig. 24-11.** Cross section of the pons in a patient with multiple sclerosis, stained for myelin. The plaques are represented by punched-out clear areas. They have a predilection to the subpial zone.

culating the animal with brain tissue of another species mixed with Freund's complete adjuvant.[104] The demyelinated lesions are characteristically perivenular and associated with inflammatory infiltrates. They are about 0.1 to 1 mm in diameter, with a preferential distribution in the subpial surface of the spinal cord and brain stem.[105] Acute disseminated encephalomyeloneuropathy has been incriminated in hearing loss, but a detailed pathologic verification is lacking. This mechanism may explain the sudden deafness that complicates tetanus immunization[106] or some of the more obscure encephalomyeloradiculoneuropathies.[107]

# TRAUMA

The eighth nerve may be injured in fractures of the temporal bone, which are classified into transverse and longitudinal types.[108] Both cochlear and vestibular divisions are often lacerated in the transverse type.[109] The facial nerve is also involved in approximately 50 percent of these cases.[110] Longitudinal fractures, which are more common than transverse fractures, do not generally result in eighth nerve injury.[111] Local infection or the meningitis complicating some of these compound fractures may further aggravate the symptoms. In closed head injuries due to rapid angular acceleration or deceleration of the head, shearing forces generated within the brain can cause diffuse axonal injuries[112,113] or tears of blood vessels. The axonal injury is only apparent shortly after the accident and may disappear when the reparative process is completed. The injured axons take the form of "retraction bulbs." Many affected patients sustain severe damage to the brain stem, and the retraction bulbs are seen in large concentration in the lateral tegmental areas and periaqueductal gray matter of the midbrain and upper pons. Such lesions were shown to cause "midbrain deafness."[114]

# VASCULAR DISORDERS

By and large, vascular disorders are due to hypertensive/arteriosclerotic cerebrovascular disease or embolism.

## Cerebral Hemorrhages and Infarctions

Deafness is rarely a manifestation of cerebral hemispheric lesion because of the bilateral representation of hearing functions. There are autopsy verified examples, however, of bilateral infarctions of the middle third of the superior temporal gyrus and rare instances of unilateral lesion of the auditory cortex of the dominant hemisphere associated with "pure" word deafness[5,11,51] (Fig. 24-12). Patients with this uncommon disorder, which is also referred to as auditory verbal agnosia, are unable to hear, yet audiometric testing shows no hearing defects.

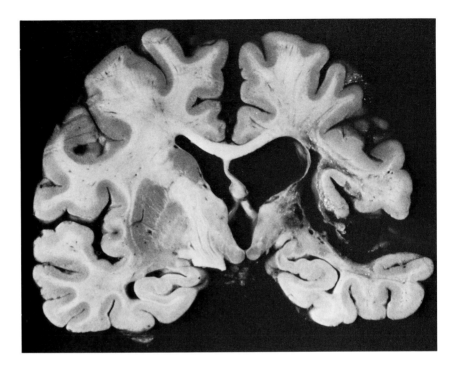

**Fig. 24-12.** Old cystic infarction of the temporal lobe extensively involving the superior temporal gyrus.

## Brain Stem Lesions

Occlusion of either the superior cerebellar artery or the anterior inferior cerebellar artery (AICA) can lead to deafness. In the former condition it is usually partial, whereas in the latter it is more severe. The extent of infarction is unpredictable because of the great variation in the areas supplied by each vessel and the considerable overlapping of adjacent fields of blood supply.[6,11] The cochlear nuclear complex or the cochlear nerve itself is invariably involved in *AICA syndrome*[117] (lateral pontomedullary syndrome). In this syndrome, the patient complains not only of ipsilateral deafness but of facial weakness, tinnitus, vertigo, nausea, vomiting, nystagmus, and cerebellar ataxia. Depending on the extent of the infarction, there may also be ipsilateral Horner's syndrome, paresis of conjugate gaze, and contralateral loss of pain and temperature sense. The internal auditory artery, which is often a branch of the AICA, may also become occluded by emboli or in hyperviscosity syndromes.[118] Deafness in such cases is usually due to infarction of either the cochlea or the eighth nerve, or both. The role of such vascular occlusion accounting for sudden deafness in adults with no other signs of vertebrobasilar insufficiency is disputed, however.[119]

## Aneurysms

Fusiform aneurysms are caused by severe arteriosclerotic disease, resulting in marked ectasia and tortuosity of the affected vessels. Fusiform aneurysms of the basilar artery acting as a mass lesion can compress the brain stem or cause cranial neuropathies[120] (Fig. 24-13). They rarely rupture and bleed in the subarachnoid space. Saccular (berry) aneurysms, presumed to be due to developmental defects of the media at sites of branchings, may occur, albeit infrequently, at the origin of AICA and may compress the acoustic nerve[121] (Fig. 24-14). In addition to causing subarachnoid hemorrhages, ruptured berry aneurysms can dissect cranial nerves, including the acoustic. Mycotic and dissecting aneurysms[122] of the cerebellar arteries are rare.

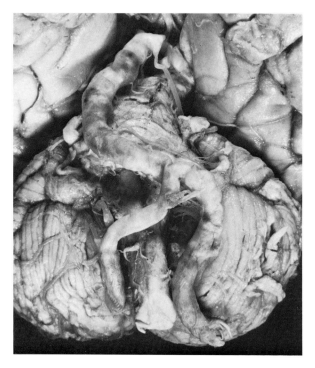

**Fig. 24-13.** Ectatic arteriosclerotic vertebrobasilar arteries. The tortuous vertebral artery is impinging on the nerves emanating from the left cerebellopontine angle.

## Arteriovenous Malformations

Arteriovenous malformations are developmental anomalies of blood vessels representing persistence of embryonic sinusoids. Due to abnormal hemodynamics with shunting of blood from arterial to venous system, these channels enlarge and form tortuous tangles of dilated vessels in the subarachnoid space and underlying brain parenchyma (Fig. 24-15). The respective arteries and veins which feed and drain these AVMs also enlarge. The abnormal vessels consist of variable-sized arteries and arterialized veins.[123] They are more frequent in males, and rare familial cases have been described.[124] In the large majority of patients, the first clinical manifestation is hemorrhage, either subarachnoid and/or intracerebral, which usually takes place in the first two decades of life. Infratentorial arteriovenous malformations,[125] like any other arteriovenous malformation, may also undergo thrombosis or gradual enlargement[126]; they can also cause focal symptoms, such as deafness, vertigo, ataxia, and hemiplegia and sometimes have simulated multiple sclerosis.[127]

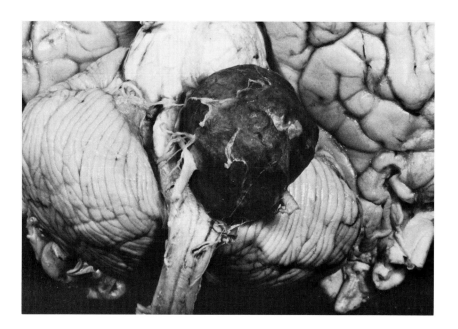

**Fig. 24-14.** Giant berry aneurysm of the left vertebral artery near its junction with the basilar artery. The aneurysm is compressing and indenting the pontomedullary junction.

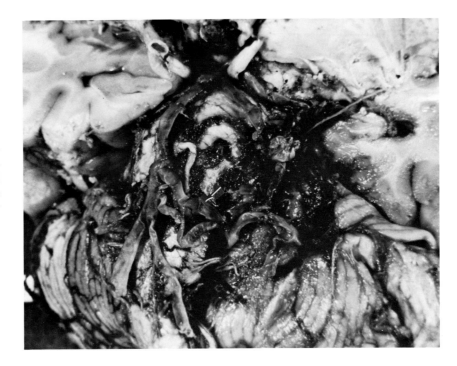

**Fig. 24-15.** Arteriovenous malformation of the left cerebellopontine angle. Note the enlarged feeding vessels, particularly the anterior inferior cerebellar artery (arrow).

## STORAGE DISEASES

Deafness has been reported in a few of the storage diseases, particularly those dominated by white matter degeneration (leukodystrophies).[128,129] These disorders are usually due to enzymatic defects in the catabolic pathway of sphingolipids and, depending on the site of the enzymatic block, various forms of glycolipids accumulate in the tissues.[130] The lysosomes become gradually distended with the storage material and appear as cytoplasmic inclusions. Ultrastructurally, these inclusions have been variously designated, based on the arrangement of the dense lines representing layers of polar lipid separated from each other by an aqueous phase, as multilamellar cytoplasmic bodies in gangliosidoses, zebra bodies in mucopolysaccharidoses, tuffstone bodies, and prismatic inclusions in metachromatic leukodystrophies.[131] Deafness and abnormal brain auditory evoked responses (BAER) have been reported in metachromatic leukodystrophy due to multiple ar-

ylsulfatase deficiency,[132] adrenoleukodystrophy, Gaucher's disease,[133] and cherry red spot myoclonus syndrome, especially those with type II sialidosis.[134] In infantile Gaucher's disease, histologic examination of the brain stem auditory relay nuclei and connecting pathways did not demonstrate any obvious pathologic changes despite the abnormal BAER obtained when the infant was alive.[135]

## AUTOIMMUNE DISORDERS

There are a number of ill-defined syndromes, largely believed to be *auto*immune in nature, in which deafness may be a feature. They include Vogt-Kyanagi-Harada syndrome, Behçet's disease, and Logan's syndrome. In Vogt-Kyanagi-Harada syndrome,[136–138] there is bilateral uveitis, depigmentation of the skin and hair, meningitis, and auditory impairment. The condition is common in the Japanese[139] and rare in whites. Auditory and less frequently vestibular symptoms appear when the uveitis is well established. CSF pleocytosis with up to 500 cells/mm³, mostly lymphocytes, has been reported. There is an intense inflamatory change about melanocytes of the uveal tract, but no pathologic studies of the ear are available.

In Behçet's disease, the uveitis is associated with mucocutaneous ulceration of the oral and genital tract.[140] Neurologic complications are not uncommon.[141,142] Neuropathologic findings include diffuse meningoencephalitis with perivascular infiltration by lymphocytes and plasma cells; microinfarcts, particularly adjoining blood vessels; and phlebothrombosis of cerebral blood vessels.[143,144] The degree of auditory dysfunction varies from one report to another.[145,146] The condition is more common in the Middle East and Japan.

Cogan's syndrome[147] is characterized by interstitial keratitis, episodic vertigo, tinnitus, and deafness. The onset is usually abrupt, with vertigo, vomiting, and hearing loss. Within a few weeks to months, bilateral deafness is often well established. This condition is commonly associated with polyarteritis nodosa or other forms of collagen vascular diseases.[148] The inner ears have displayed degeneration of all neural elements, but no vasculitis has been demonstrated.[149]

---

## AGING AND DEMENTIA

Hearing impairment is a frequent manifestation of aging and often referred to as *presbycusis*. Inner ear changes in aging are well documented, but pathologic studies of the central auditory pathway are scant and sometimes controversial. Kirikae et al.[150] described atrophy and degeneration of nerve cells in the various relay nuclei throughout the auditory pathway, a view endorsed by Dublin.[70] By contrast, Konigsmark[151] showed no loss of neurons in the ventral cochlear nucleus in the aged but a definite reduction in the mean volume of the nucleus after 50 years of age. He attributed this gradual shrinkage to loss of neuropil.[152] This was also the conclusion reached by Gandolfi et al.[153] on a limited number of cases studied by the computer image analyzer. Similar controversy exists concerning cell loss in the superior temporal gyrus in elderly patients. Brody,[154] for instance, reported marked neuronal loss, but Terry and De Teresa[155] found no change in neuron density per unit area in the course of normal aging. There was, however, a substantial decrease in the number of neurons in the large cell category (greater than 90 $\mu$m²). These workers assumed that the large neurons have shrunken into the smaller size classes. Their findings in normal aging were significantly different from those of senile dementia of Alzheimer type, in which a total loss of neurons expressed particularly in the large neuron category was found.

In both aged and senile patients, the neurons in the ventral cochlear nucleus, as in many brain stem nuclei, often display large accumulation of lipofuscin. This increase in senile dementia of Alzheimer type is no different than in the normal aged.[156] Studies have shown that as the lipofuscin increases, cytoplasmic RNA declines.[157] Nevertheless, there is no direct evidence to indicate that lipofuscin is cytotoxic to neurons. In senile dementia of Alzheimer type, certain structural changes are seen in the cortex that are most severe in the hippocampus. Of particular interest are the neurofibrillary degeneration and senile (neuritic) plaques. Although these lesions are seen in small numbers in the hippocampus of the aged, a large concentration of plaques and tangles (Fig. 24-16) in the neocortex show a high correlation with dementia.[158] Neurofibrillary degeneration appears as masses of coarse tangled fibers within the cytoplasm of affected neurons. They are best demonstrated with silver impregnation techniques, such as that of Bodian and Bielschowsky. Each coarse fiber is composed of a pair of twisted filaments, hence the term paired helical filaments. Each filament measures 10 nm in width and usually crosses each other at regular 80-nm intervals. The nature of the protein making up these tangles is the object of considerable current research. The senile or neuritic plaques have a central core of amyloid surrounded by abnormal neurites distended with lamellar lysosomes and often paired helical filaments. Most of the abnormal neurites are preterminal axons.[159]

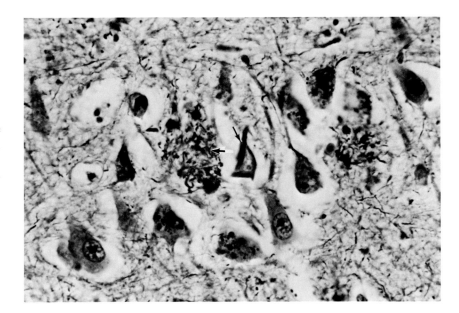

**Fig. 24-16.** The hallmarks of Alzheimer's disease are neurofibrillary degeneration (arrow) and senile "neuritic" tangles (white arrow).

## TUMORS

The various types of gliogenous and nongliogenous tumors can compress, irritate, invade, or destroy the temporal lobe cortex, including Heschl's gyrus and the auditory radiation. Detailed histologic account of some of these tumors is considered beyond the scope of the present review. Tumors frequently involving the auditory cortex are meningiomas, metastases, astrocytomas, and glioblastoma multiforme.

Unilateral destruction of the auditory receptive zone does not cause deafness because of the bilateral central auditory representations. Recent studies have shown, however, that variable degrees of the integrative aspect of hearing is altered.[18] Auditory illusions and hallucinations may occur if the tumor distorts the auditory cortex without completely destroying it. The effect of generalized increased intracranial pressure on hearing is controversial. Saxena et al.[160] found variable degrees of hearing impairment that resolved in some patients following reduction of the intracranial pressure. Deafness results if both inferior colliculi and lateral lemnisci are destroyed by tumor, as was reported by Sloane et al.[161] Mid-brain tumors, however, are rare compared with those arising in the pons.[162] It is therefore more common to encounter hearing dysfunction with pontine tumors, especially the astrocytomas, which form the predominant neoplasm affecting the brain stem. The main tumors that frequently cause deafness are those that occur in the cerebellopontine angle, especially the acoustic schwannomas and meningiomas. All these tumors are reviewed in some detail in Chapter 25.

## REFERENCES

1. Crome L, Cowie V, Slayer E: A statistical note on cerebellar and brain stem weight in mongolism. J Ment Defic Res 10:69, 1966
2. Gandolfi A, Horoupian D, DeTeresa R: Pathology of the auditory system in autosomal trisomies with morphometric and quantitative study of the ventral cochlear nucleus. J Neurol Sci 50:443, 1981
3. Weber WW, Mamunes P, Day R, Miller P: Tisomy 17-18 (E): Studies in long term survival with report of two autopsied cases. Pediatrics 34:533, 1964
4. Sumi SM: Brain malformations in the trisomy 18 syndrome. Brain 93:821, 1970
5. Michaelson PS, Gilles FH: Central nervous system

abnormalities in trisomy E (17-18) syndrome. J Neurol Sci 15:193, 1972

6. Passarge E, True CW, Sueoka WT, et al: Malformations of the central nervous system in trisomy 18 syndrome. J Pediatr 69:771, 1966

7. Gacek R: The pathology of hereditary sensorineural hearing loss. Ann Otol Rhinol Laryngol 80:289, 1971

8. Taylor AI: Patau's, Edward and cri du chat syndromes: A tabulated summary of current findings. Dev Med Child Neurol 9:78, 1967

9. Warkany J, Passarge E, Smith LB: Congenital malformations in autosomal trisomy syndromes. Am J Dis Child 112:502, 1966

10. Friede RL: Developmental Neuropathology. Springer-Verlag, New York, 1975

11. Marin-Padilla M: Structural organization of the cerebral cortex (motor area) in human chromosomal aberrations. A Golgi study. Part 1 (D,(13-15) trisomy, Patau syndrome). Brain Res 66:375, 1974

12. Saez RJ, Onofrio BM, Yanagihara T: Experience with Arnold-Chiari malformation, 1960 to 1970. J Neurosurg 45:416, 1976

13. Penfield W, Coburn DF: Arnold-Chiari malformation and its operative treatment. Arch Neurol Psychiatry 40:328, 1938

14. Sieben RL, Ben Hamida M, Shulman K: Multiple cranial nerve deficits associated with the Arnold-Chiari malformation. Neurology (NY) 21:673, 1971

15. Rydell RE, Pulec JL: Arnold-Chiari malformation. Neuro-otologic symptoms. Arch Otolaryngol 94:8, 1971

16. McLay K, Maran AGD: Deafness and the Klippel-Feil syndrome. J Laryngol 83:175, 1969

17. Hughes JT: Diseases of the spine and spinal cord. p. 652. In Blackwood W, Corsellis JAN (eds): Greenfield's Neuropathology. Edward Arnold, London, 1976

18. Adams RD, Victor M: Principles of Neurology. McGraw-Hill, New York, 1977

19. Konigsmark BW: System disorders and atrophies. Part II. p. 499. In Vinken PJ, Bruyn GW, DeJong JMBV (eds): Handbook of Clinical Neurology. Vol. 22. North-Holland, Amsterdam, 1975

20. Soffer D, Grotsky HW, Rapin I, Suzuki K: Cockayne syndrome: Unusual neuropathological findings and a review of the literature. Ann Neurol 6:340, 1979

21. Gandolfi A, Horoupian D, Rapin I, et al: Deafness in Cockayne's syndrome, morphological, morphometric and quantitative study of the auditory pathway. Ann Neurol 15:135, 1984

22. Whitnall SE, Norman RM: Microphthalmia and the visual pathways. A case associated with blindness and imbecility and sex-linked. Br J Ophthalmol 24:229, 1940

23. Warburg M: Norrie's disease: A congenital progressive oculo-acoustico-cerebral degeneration. Acta Ophthalmol (Copenh) 89 (suppl):1, 1966

24. Fisch L: Deafness as a part of a hereditary syndrome. J Laryngol 73:355, 1959

25. Johnson LG, Arenburg IK: Cochlear abnormalities in Alport syndrome. Arch Otolaryngol 107:340, 1981

26. Bell JM, Carmichael EA: On hereditary ataxia and spastic paraplegia. p. 141. In Treasury of Human Inheritance. Vol. 4. Cambridge University Press, London, 1939

27. Satya-Murti S, Cacace A, Hanson P: Auditory dysfunction in Friedreich ataxia: Result of spiral ganglion degeneration. Neurology (NY) 30:1047, 1980

28. Urich H, Norman RM, Lloyd OC: suprasegmental lesions in Friedreich's ataxia. Conf Neurol 6:360, 1957

29. Van Bogaert L, Martin L: Optic and cochleovestibular degeneration in the hereditary ataxias. I. Clinicopathological and genetic aspects. Brain 97:15, 1974

30. Oppenheimer DR: Quebec cooperative study of Friedreich's ataxia. Brain lesions in Freidreich's ataxia. Can J Neurol Sci 6:173, 1979

31. Boudin G, Grossiord A, Guillard A, et al: Maladie de Friedreich avec atteintes systématisées sus-médullaires. Rev Neurol 127:441, 1972

32. Hicks EP: Hereditary sensory neuropathy. Neurology (NY) 5:15, 1955

33. Spillane JD, Wells CEC: Acrodystrophic neuropathy: A critical review of the syndrome of trophic ulcers, sensory neuropathy, and bony erosion together with an account of 16 cases in South Wales. Oxford University Press, London, 1969

34. Hallpike CS: Observations on the structural basis of two rare varieties of hereditary deafness. p. 285. In DeReuck AVS, Knight J (eds): Ciba Foundation Symposium on Myotatic, Kinesthetic and Vestibular Mechanisms. Churchill, London, 1967

35. Hallpike CS, Harriman DGF, Wells CEC: A case of afferent neuropathy and deafness. J Laryngol Otol 94:945, 1980

35a. Horoupian DS: Pathology of the auditory pathway in hereditary sensory neuropathy and deafness (HSANI). J Neuropath Exp Neurol 46:386, 1987 (abstr.)

36. Gallai V, Hockaday JM, Hughes JT, et al: Pontobul-

bar palsy with deafness (Brown-Vialetto-van Laere syndrome). A report on 3 cases. J Neurol Sci 50:250, 1981

37. Alberca R, Montero C, Ibanez A, et al: Progressive bulbar paralysis associated with neural deafness. A nosologic entity. Arch Neurol 37:214, 1980

38. Gregg NM: Congenital cataract following German measles in the mother. Trans Ophthalmol Soc Aust 3:35, 1942

39. Cooper LZ, Krugman S: Clinical manifestations of postnatal and congenital rubella. Arch Ophthalmol 77:434, 1967

40. Rorke L, Spiro A: Cerebral lesions in congenital rubella syndrome. J Pediatr 70:243, 1967

41. Peckham CS, Martin JAM, Marshall WC, Dudgeon JA: Congenital rubella deafness: A preventable disease. Lancet 1:258, 1979

42. Medearis DN Jr: Cytomegalic inclusion disease: Analysis of clinical features based on literature and six additional cases. Pediatrics 19:467, 1957

43. Weller TH, Hanshaw JB: Virologic and clinical observations on cytomegalic inclusions disease. N Engl J Med 266:1233, 1962

44. McCracken GH Jr, Shinefield HR, Cobb R, et al: Congenital cytomegalic inclusion disease. Am J Dis Child 117:522, 1969

45. Davis LE, Johnsson L-G, Kornfeld M: Cytomegalovirus labyrinthitis in an infant. Morphological, virological and immunofluorescent studies. J Neuropathol Exp Neurol 40:9, 1981

46. Hanshaw JB, Scheiner AP, Moxley AW, et al: School failure and deafness after "silent" congenital cytomegalovirus infection. N Engl J Med 295:468, 1976

47. Saigal S, Lunyk O, Larke RPB, Chernesky MA: The outcome in children with congenital cytomegalovirus infection. Am J Dis Child 136:896, 1982

48. Paparella MM, Capps MJ: Sensorineural deafness in children—Non-genetic. p. 309. In Paparella MM, Shumrick DA (eds): Otolaryngology, vol. 2. WB Saunders, Philadelphia, 1973

49. Igarashi M, Saito R, Alford BR, et al: Temporal bone findings in pneumococcal meningitis. Arch Otolaryngol 99:79, 1974

50. Igarashi M, Gilmartin RC, Gerald B, et al: Cerebral arteritis and bacterial meningitis. Arch Neurol 41:531, 1984

51. Lechevalier B, Rossa Y, Eustache F, et al: Un cas de surdité corticale épargnant en partié la musique. Rev Neurol 140:190, 1984

52. Duffy PE, Sassin JF, Summers DS, Lourie H: Rhombencephalitis due to Listeria monocytogenes. Neurology (NY) 14:1067, 1964

53. Weinstein AJ, Schiavone WA, Furlan AJ: Listeria rhombencephalitis. Report of a case. Arch Neurol 39:514, 1982

54. Lindsay JR, Davey PR, Ward PH: Inner ear pathology in deafness due to mumps. Ann Otol 69:918, 1960

55. Morrison AW: Management of Sensorineural Deafness. Butterworth, London, 1975

56. Dastur HM, Desai AD: A comparative study of brain tuberculomas and gliomas based on 107 case records of each. Brain 88:375, 1965

57. Rodger TR: Syphilis as seen by the aural surgeon. J Laryngol Otol 55:168, 1940

58. Vercoe GS: The effect of early syphilis on the inner ear and auditory nerves. J Laryngol Otol 90:853, 1976

59. Reichert CM, O'Leary TJ, Levens DL, et al: Autopsy pathology in the acquired immune deficiency syndrome. Am J Pathol 112:357, 1983

60. Snider WD, Simpson DM, Nielsen S, et al: Neurological complications of acquired immune deficiency syndrome: Analysis of 50 patients. Ann Neurol 14:403, 1983

61. Smith BH: Infections of the cranial dura and the dural sinuses. p. 149. In Vinken PJ, Bruhn GW (eds): Handbook of Clinical Neurology. Vol. 33: Infections of the Nervous System. North-Holland, Amsterdam, 1978

62. Beal MF, O'Carroll CP, Kleinman GM, Grossman RI: Aspergillosis of the nervous system. Neurology (NY) 32:473, 1982

63. Schwarz J: The diagnosis of deep mycoses by morphologic methods. Hum Pathol 13:519, 1982

64. Felter BF, Klintworth GK, Hendry WS: Mycoses of the Central Nervous System. Williams & Wilkins, Baltimore, 1967

65. Winn WA: Coccidioidal meningitis. A follow-up report. p. 55. In Ajello L (ed): Coccidioidomycosis. University of Arizona Press, Tucson, 1965

66. Brierley JB: Cerebral hypoxia. p. 43. In Blackwood W, Coresellis JAN (eds): Greenfield's Neuropathology. Edward Arnold, London, 1976

67. Hall JG: The cochlea and the cochlear nuclei in neonatal asphyxia. Acta Otolaryngol (suppl)194, 1964

68. Myers RE: Two patterns of perinatal brain damage and their conditions of occurrence. Am J Obstet Gynecol 112:246, 1972

69. Flottorp G, Morley DE, Skatvedt M: The localization of hearing impairment in athetoids. Acta Otolaryngol 48:404, 1957

70. Dublin WB: Fundamentals of Sensorineural Audi-

tory Pathology. Charles C Thomas, Springfield, IL, 1976

71. Pearlman MA, Gartner LM, Lee K, et al: Absence of kernicterus in low-birth-weight infants from 1971 through 1976: Comparison with findings in 1966 and 1967. Pediatrics 62:460, 1978

72. Haymaker W, Margoles C, Pentschew A, et al: Pathology of kernicterus and posticteric encephalopathy. Presentation of 87 cases, with a consideration of pathogenesis and etiology. p. 21. In Kernicterus in Cerebral Palsy. Charles C Thomas, Springfield, IL, 1961

73. Dublin WB: Cytoarchitecture of the cochlear nuclei. Report of an illustrative case of erythroblastosis. Arch Otolaryngol 100:355, 1974

74. Gardner WA, Konigsmark B: Familial nonhemolytic jaundice: Bilirubinosis and encephalopathy. Pediatrics 43:365, 1969

75. Djupesland G, Flottorp G, Refsum S: Phytanic acid storage disease: Hearing maintained after 15 years of dietary treatment. Neurology (NY) 33:237, 1983

76. Fardeau M, Engel WK: Ultrastructural study of a peripheral nerve biopsy in Refsum disease. J Neuropathol Exp Neurol 28:278, 1969

77. Flament-Durand J, Noel P, Rutsaert J, et al: A case of Refsum disease: Clinical, pathological, ultrastructural and biochemical study. Pathol Eur 6:172, 1971

78. Allen IV, Swallow M, Nevin NC, McCormick D: Clinicopathological study of Refsum's disease with particular reference to fatal complication. J Neurol Neurosurg Psychiatry 41:323, 1978

79. Illum P, Kiaer HW, Hvidberg-Hansen J, Sondergaard T: Fifteen cases of Pendred's syndrome. Congenital deafness and sporadic goiter. Arch Otolaryngol 96:297, 1972

80. Milutinovic PS, Stanbury JB, Wicken JV, Jones EW: Thyroid function in a family with the Pendred Syndrome. J Clin Endocrinol 29:962, 1969

81. Rebière A, Dainat J: Répercussions de l'hypothyroïdie sur la synaptogenèse dans le cortex cerebelleux du rat. Acta Neuropathol (Berl) 35:117, 1976

82. Rosman NP, Malone MJ, Helfenstein M, Kraft E: The effect of thyroid deficiency on myelination of brain. A morphological and biochemical study. Neurology (NY) 22:99, 1972

83. Harner SG: Hearing in adult onset diabetes mellitus. Otolaryngol Head Neck Surg 89:322, 1981

84. Denny-Brown D: Neurological conditions resulting from prolonged and severe dietary restrictions. Medicine (Baltimore) 26:41, 1947

85. Ylikoski JS, House JW, Hernandez I: Eighth nerve alcoholic neuropathy. A case report with light and electron microscopic findings. J Laryngol Otol 95:613, 1981

86. Egger J, Lake BD, Wilson J: Mitochondrial cytopathy: A disorder with ragged red fibers on muscle biopsy. Arch Dis Child 56:741, 1981

87. Berenberg RA, Pellock JM, DiMauro S, et al: Lumping or splitting? "Ophthalmoplegia-plus" or Kearns-Sayre Syndrome? Ann Neurol 1:37, 1977

88. Lindsay JR, Hinojosa R: Histopathologic features of the inner ear associated with Kearns-Sayre syndrome. Arch Otolaryngol 102:747, 1976

89. McFarlin DE, McFarland HF: Multiple sclerosis. N Engl J Med 307:1246, 1982

90. Paterson PY: The demyelinating diseases: Clinical and experimental studies in animals and man. p. 1400. In Samter M, Talmadge DW, Rose B, Austen KF, Vaughan JH (eds): Immunological Diseases. Little, Brown, Boston, 1978

91. Johnson RT: The possible viral etiology of multiple sclerosis. Adv Neurol 13:1, 1975

92. Stewart GJ, McLeod JG, Basten A, Bashir HV: HLA family studies and susceptibility to multiple sclerosis: A common gene, dominantly expressed. Hum Immunol 3:13, 1981

93. Waksman BH: Viruses and immune events in the pathogenesis of multiple sclerosis. p. 155. In Mims C (ed): Viruses and Demyelinating Diseases. Academic Press, London, 1983

94. Adams CWM: The onset and progression of the lesion in multiple sclerosis. J Neurol Sci 25:165, 1975

95. Prineas J: Pathology of the early lesion in multiple sclerosis. Hum Pathol 6:531, 1975

96. Colletti V: Stapedius reflex abnormalities in multiple sclerosis. Audiology 14:63, 1975

97. Luxon LM: Hearing loss in brainstem disorders. J Neurol Neurosurg Psychiatry 43:510, 1980

98. Dix MR: Observations upon the nerve fiber deafness of multiple sclerosis with particular reference to the phenomenon of loudness recruitment. J Laryngol Otol 69:608, 1965

99. Noffsinger D, Olsen WO, Carhart R, et al: Auditory and vestibular aberrations in multiple sclerosis. Acta Otolaryngol 303(suppl 1):1, 1972

100. Daugherty WT, Lederman RJ, Nodar RH, Conomy JP: Hearing loss in multiple sclerosis. Arch Neurol 40:33, 1983

101. Fischer C, Joyeux O, Haguenauer JP: Surdité et acouphènes lors de poussées dans 10 cas de sclérose en plaques. Rev Neurol 140:117, 1984

102. Dix MR, Hood JD: Symmetrical hearing loss in brainstem lesions. Acta Otolaryngol (Copenh) 75:165, 1973

103. Poser Ch M: Neurological complications of swine

influenza vaccination. Acta Neurol Scand 66:413, 1982

104. Raine CS: Multiple sclerosis and chronic relapsing EAE: comparative ultrastructural neuropathology. p. 413. In Hallpike JF, Adams CWM, Tourtelotte WW (eds): Multiple Sclerosis. Williams & Wilkins, Baltimore, 1983

105. Raine CS: Biology of disease. Analysis of autoimmune demyelination: Its impact upon multiple sclerosis. Lab Invest 50:608, 1984

106. Wirth G: Reversible Kochlear isschadigung nach Tetanol-injektion. MMW 107:379, 1965

107. Wendt JS, Burks JS: An unusual case of encephalomyeloradiculoneuropathy in a young woman. Arch Neurol 38:726, 1981

108. Schuknecht HF: Pathology of the Ear. Harvard University Press, Cambridge, 1974

109. Fischer J, Wolfsen L: The Inner Ear. Grune & Stratton, Orlando, FL, 1943

110. Grove WE: Skull fractures involving the ear: A clinical study of 211 cases. Laryngoscope 49:678, 1939

111. Kelemen G: Fractures of the temporal bone. Arch Otolaryngol 40:333, 1944

112. Adams JH, Graham DI, Murray LS, Scott G: Diffuse axonal injury due to nonmissile head injury in humans: An analysis of 45 cases. Ann Neurol 12:557, 1982

113. Gennarelli TA, Thibault LE, Adams JH, et al: Diffuse axonal injury and traumatic coma in the primate. Ann Neurol 12:564, 1982

114. Howe JR, Miller CA: Midbrain deafness following head injury. Neurology (NY) 25:286, 1975

115. Coslett HB, Brashear HR, Heilman KM: Pure word deafness after bilateral primary auditory cortex infarcts. Neurology (NY) 12:564, 1982

116. Atkinson WJ: The anterior inferior cerebellar artery. Its variations pontine distribution and significance in the surgery of the cerebellopontine angle tumors. J Neurol Neurosurg Psychiatry 12:137, 1949

117. Adams RD: Occlusion of the anterior inferior cerebellar artery. Arch Neurol Psychiatry 49:765, 1943

118. Jaffe B: Sudden deafness—A local manifestation of systemic disorders: Fat emboli, hypercoagulation and infections. Laryngoscope 80:788, 1970

119. Polus K: The problem of vascular deafness. Laryngoscope 82:24, 1972

120. Deek ZL, Jannetta PJ, Rosenbaum AE, et al: Tortuous vertebrobasilar arteries causing cranial nerve syndromes. Screening by computed tomography. J Comput Assist Tomog 3:774, 1979

121. Nishimoto A, Fujimoto S, Tsuchimoto S, et al: Anterior inferior cerebellar artery aneurysm: Report of three cases. J Neurosurg 59:697, 1983

122. Kalyan-Raman UP, Kowalski RV, Lee RH, Fierer JA: Dissecting aneurysm of superior cerebellar artery. Its association with fibromuscular dysplasia. Arch Neurol 40:120, 1983

123. Pool JL: Arteriovenous malformations of the brain. p. 227. In Vinken P, Bruyn G (eds): Handbook of Clinical Neurology. Vol. 12. North-Holland, Amsterdam, 1972

124. Snead OC, Acker JD, Morawetz R: Familial arteriovenous malformation. Ann Neurol 5:585, 1979

125. Matsumura H, Makita Y, Someda K, Kondo A: Arteriovenous malformations in the posterior fossa. J Neurosurg 47:50, 1977

126. Delitala A, Delfini R, Vagnozzi R, Esposito S: Increase in size of cerebral angiomas. J Neurosurg 57:556, 1982

127. Stahl SM, Johnson KP, Malamud N: The clinical and pathological spectrum of brain stem vascular malformations: Long-term course simulates multiple sclerosis. Arch Neurol 37:25, 1980

128. Schaumburg HH, Powers JM, Raine CS, et al: Adrenoleukodystrophy. A clinical and pathological study of 17 cases. Arch Neurol 32:577, 1975

129. Dunn HG, Dolman CL, Farrell DF, et al: Krabbe's leukodystrophy without globoid cells. Neurology (NY) 26:1035, 1976

130. Stanbury JB, Wyngaarden JB, Fredrickson DS, et al: Metabolic Basis of Inherited Diseases. McGraw-Hill, New York, 1983

131. Suzuki K: Electron microscopy in human medicine. p. 3. In Johannessen JV (ed): Nervous System, Sensory Organs and Respiratory Tract. Vol. 6. McGraw-Hill, New York, 1979

132. Thomas PK: Other inherited neuropathies. p. 1745. In Dyck PJ, Thomas PK, Lambert EH, Bunge R (eds): Peripheral Neuropathy. Vol 2. WB Saunders, Philadelphia, 1984

133. Ochs R, Markand ON, De Myer WE: Brainstem auditory evoked responses in leukodystrophies.

134. Lowden JA, O'Brien JS: Sialidosis: A review of human neuraminidase deficiency. Am J Hum Genet 31:1, 1979

135. Kaga M, Azuma Ch, Imamura T, Murahami T: Auditory brainstem responses (ABR) in infantile Gaucher's disease. Neuropediatrics 13:207, 1982

136. Vogt A: Fruhzeitiges Ergrauen der Zilien und Bemerkungen über den sogenanten plötzlichen Eintritt dieser Veranderung. Klin Mbl Augenheilkd 44:228, 1906

137. Harada E: Clinical study of non suppurative choroiditis: A report of acute diffuse choroiditis. Acta Soc Ophthalmol (Jpn) 30:351, 1926

138. Kyanagi Y: Dyscousia, Alopecia and Poliosis bei Schwerer Uveitis nich traumatischen Ursprunges. Klin Mbl Augenheilkd 82:194, 1929

139. Sugiura S: Vogt Kyanagi Horada disease: J Jpn Ophthalmol 22:9, 1978

140. Behçet H: Some observations on the clinical picture of so-called triple symptom complex. Dermatologica 81:73, 1949

141. Pallis CA, Fudge BJ: The neurological complications of Behçet's syndrome. Arch Neurol Psychiatry 75:1, 1956

142. Rougemont D, Bousser MG, Wechsler B, et al: Manifestations neurologiques de la maladie de Behçet. Vingt-quatre observations. Rev Neurol 138:493, 1982

143. McMenemey W, Lawrence BJ: Encephalomyelopathy in Behçet's disease. Lancet 2:353, 1957

144. Kawakita H, Nishimura M, Satoh Y et al: Neurological aspects of Behçet's disease. J Neurol Sci 5:417, 1967

145. Dinning WJ: Behçet's disease and the eye: Epidemiological considerations. In Lehner T, Barnes CG (eds): Behçet's Syndrome. Academic Press, London, 1979

146. Brama I, Fairnaru: Inner ear involvement in Behçet's disease. Arch Otol Laryngol 106:215, 1980

147. Cogan DG: Syndrome of non symphilitic interstitial keratitis and vestibuloauditory symptoms. Arch Ophthalmol 33:144, 1945

148. Fisher E, Hellstrom H: Cogan's syndrome and systemic vascular disease: Analysis of pathologic features with reference to its relationship to thromboangiitis obliterans (Buerger). Arch Pathol Lab Med 75:572, 1961

149. Wolff D, Bernhard WG, Tsutsumi S, et al: The pathology of Cogan's syndrome causing profound deafness. Trans Am Otol Soc 53:94, 1965

150. Kirikae I, Soto T, Shitara T: Study of hearing in advanced age. Laryngoscope 74:205, 1964

151. Konigsmark B, Murphy E: Neuronal populations in the human brain. Nature (Lond) 228:1335, 1970

152. Konigsmark B, Murphy E: Volume of the ventral cochlear nucleus in man and its relationship to neuronal population and age. J Neuropath Exp Neurol 31:304, 1972

153. Gandolfi A, Horoupian DS, DeTeresa R: Quantitative and cytometric analysis of the ventral cochlear nucleus in man. J Neurol Sci 50:443, 1981

154. Brody H: Organization of the cerebral cortex. Study of aging in human cerebral cortex. J Comp Neurol 102:511, 1955

155. Terry R, DeTeresa R: Neocortical cell counts in normal human aging. J Neuropathol Exp Neurol 43:331, 1984 (abst)

156. Mann DMA, Yates PO: Lipoprotein pigments— Their relationship to aging in the human nervous system. I. The lipofuscin content of nerve cells. Brain 97:481, 1974

157. Mann DMA, Sinclair KGA: The quantitative assessment of lipofuscin pigment, cytoplasmic RNA and nucleolar volume in senile dementia. Neuropathol Appl Neurobiol 4:129, 1978

158. Blessed G, Tomlinson BE, Roth M: The association between quantitative measurements of dementia and of senile changes in the cerebral gray matter of elderly subjects. Br J Psychiatry 114:797, 1968

159. Terry RD, Katzman R: Senile dementia of the Alzheimer type: defining a disease. p. 51. In Katzman R, Terry RD (eds): The Neurology of Aging. FA Davis, Philadelphia, 1983

160. Saxena RK, Tandon PN, Sinha A, et al: Auditory functions in raised intracranial pressure. Acta Otolaryngol (Copenh) 68:402, 1969

161. Sloane P, Persky A, Saltzman M: Midbrain deafness: Tumor of the midbrain producing sudden and complete deafness. Arch Neurol Psychiatry 49:237, 1943

162. Zülch KJ: Biologic and Pathologic der Hirngeschwülste. Der Vorzugssitz der Hirngeschwülste. In Handbuch der Neurochirurgie. Vol. 3. Springer-Verlag, Berlin, 1956

# Pathology of the Vestibular Nerve and Its Central Nervous System Pathways

# 25

## Dikran Horoupian

This chapter discusses pathologic alterations involving the vestibular nerve and its central connections. To avoid repetition, the pathology of certain disorders that affect both the cochlear and vestibular divisions of the 8th nerve is not covered, and the reader is referred to Chapter 24. Subjects not mentioned in this chapter include the developmental and hereditary disorders, the storage diseases, the pathology of aging and dementia, and some of the obscure collagen diseases that may affect the eighth nerve. The pathology of certain infectious, metabolic, and vascular disorders that preferentially involve the vestibular system is reviewed. The section on neoplasia provides extensive coverage of the various tumors that occur in the cerebellopontine angle and adjoining structures, with the exception of the paragangliomas, epidermoid cysts (cholesteatomas), and arachnoid (leptomeningeal) cysts, which are presented in Chapter 26.

## INFECTIONS

### Herpes Simplex Virus Encephalitis

Herpes simplex virus (HSV), which has a propensity to affect the temporal lobes, frequently causes dizziness, but rarely vertigo. The portal of entry of the virus, whether by bloodstream or by way of the olfactory nerves or the branches of the trigeminal nerve supplying the dura of the middle cranial fossa that may serve to explain this unique localization of HSV to the temporal lobes, remains unsettled.[1-3] HSV encephalitis occurs at any age but has its highest incidence in young adults. Grossly, the acute lesion consists of swollen hemorrhagic necrotic brain tissue selectively involving one or both temporal lobes, insular cortices, inferior frontal lobes, and the cingulate gyri[4] (Fig. 25-1). Microscopically, the lesion may resemble a hemorrhagic infarct, but more peripherally, where necrosis is less severe, perivascular cuffing with inflammatory cells, rare glial nodules, and occasional neuronophagia may be present. The pathologic hallmark is the finding of the typical Cowdry type A inclusions, usually within neurons but occasionally in glial cells as well (Fig. 25-2). Immunocytochemical techniques, especially Sternberger's peroxidase–antiperoxidase method using anti-HSV sera, have proved helpful in establishing a precise diagnosis, since ultrastructurally HSV cannot be distinguished morphologically from the other members of the herpes group.[5]

### Brain Stem Viral Encephalitis

Brain stem viral encephalitis may cause vertigo. In several epidemics of viral illnesses in Denmark,

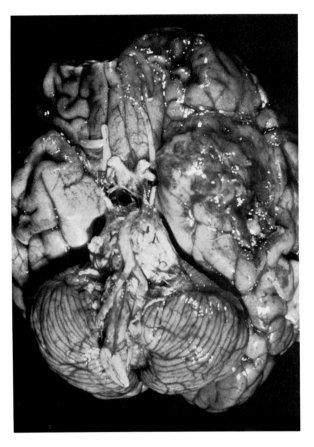

**Fig. 25-1.** Herpes simplex encephalitis. The left temporal lobe is swollen and hemorrhagic.

Pedersen[6] noted the occurrence of vertigo either as an isolated symptom or in association with other brain stem findings. He suggested that the vestibular nuclei and/or vestibular nerve roots might be focally affected by the viral infection, and he concluded that focal brain stem viral encephalitis is a common cause of epidemic vertigo. Brain stem encephalitis has also been described as complicating carcinoma, either as an isolated manifestation[7] or as part of a diffuse paraneoplastic encephalomyelitis. In the latter, destruction of the vestibular nuclei with gliosis has been documented histologically by Halperin et al.[8]

## Vestibular Neuronitis

*Vestibular neuronitis* is the term introduced by Dix and Hallpike[9] to describe patients with paroxysmal vertigo and impaired vestibular function on caloric testing. These workers inferred that an infective process plays a role in this disorder, since many patients with this condition had experienced prior ear, nose, and throat infection. The fact that none of the patients had deafness despite abnormal galvanic responses led these investigators to conclude that the lesion is proximal to Scarpa's ganglion. Pathologic verification to support their hypothesis has been inconclusive,[10] and most authors

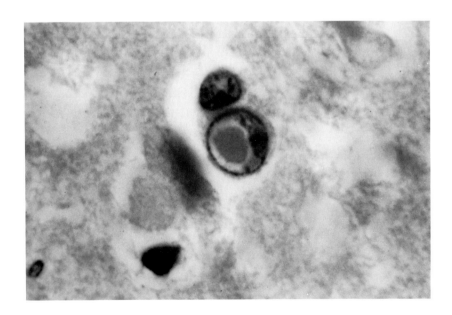

**Fig. 25-2.** Cowdry type A inclusion. (H & E; original magnification × 400.)

now believe that this type of vestibular dysfunction can be produced by a variety of disorders, such as vascular, demyelinating, toxic and many other conditions. Other noncommittal terms such as *vestibulopathy*[11] and *acute vestibular failure*[12] have been suggested to describe this syndrome. It is not clear, however, how this condition can be distinguished from the so-called isolated viral mononeuritis of the vestibular nerve, since in both conditions episodic vertigo with impaired caloric tests and normal hearing are found and an antecedent upper respiratory tract infection is frequently elicited. This syndrome, however, occurs more often in epidemics (epidemic vertigo), and several members of the same family may be affected by this disorder.[13] It has been suggested that the condition is due to a viral infection, but attempts to isolate an infectious agent have proved unsuccessful.[14] *Cerebritis*, a term used to indicate inflammation of brain tissue by pyogenic organisms, is uncommon in the brain stem. In *Listeria monocytogenes* infections, however, which frequently occur in immunosuppressed patients, the brain stem is especially vulnerable. Focal or confluent areas of necrosis with microcytic changes and large numbers of phagocytes are found. The inflammatory cellular response include polymorphonuclear leukocytes and mononuclear cells.[15] Fungal infections, such as candidiasis and mucormycosis, can affect the brain

stem as part of a more diffuse central nervous system (CNS) involvement or as the result of extension of aural mycotic infection into the cerebellopontine angle. (See also Chapter 26.)

## CIRCULATORY DISORDERS

### Mechanical Distortion of Brain Stem

The mechanical distortion of the brain stem from transtentorial herniations secondary to a rapidly expanding supratentorial mass leads to stretching of the perforating vessels of the mid-brain and pons.[16,17] The resulting vascular compromise causes ischemic changes and multiple hemorrhages (Duret hemorrhages) in the tegmentum of the mid-brain and upper pons, particularly in the midline (Fig. 25-3). These lesions interrupt the pathways connecting the vestibular nuclear complex to the extraocular motor nuclei and account for the loss of oculocephalic (doll's head maneuver) and oculovestibular reflexes.[18] Microscopically, no significant cellular reaction is detected in and around these hemorrhages, attesting to the terminal character of these hemorrhages.

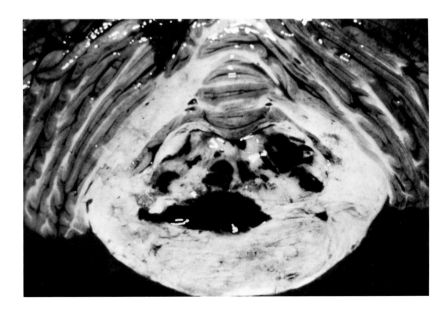

**Fig. 25-3.** Secondary brain stem hemorrhages (Duret hemorrhages) in tentorial herniation. The hemorrhages are multiple, mostly midline and in the tegmentum.

## Vascular Diseases

*Vertebrobasilar Insufficiency* is a frequent cause of vertigo in elderly patients. Transient ischemic attacks (TIAs) are frequent manifestations of vertebrobasilar insufficiency. TIAs are defined as periods of temporary loss of function due to inadequate circulation of the corresponding regions of the brain. They tend to repeat, and each episode may last a few seconds to 24 hours with total functional recovery. They are usually harbingers of strokes. The symptomatology of TIAs of the vertebrobasilar system is complex, but dizziness is an almost constant feature.[19]

TIAs are thought to be due to platelet emboli originating from atherosclerotic intimal ulcers, but altered hemodynamics from atherosclerotic narrowing of the vertebrobasilar system has been suggested as an alternate explanation. Vertebrobasilar insufficiency due to hypoperfusion frequently occurs in Stokes-Adams attacks. In about 4 percent of patients with occlusion of the first segment of the subclavian artery (i.e., proximal to the origin of the vertebral artery), vertebrobasilar insufficiency may be precipitated with strenuous exercise of the upper extremity on the affected side. This phenomenon which is referred to as subclavian steal phenomenon is due to siphoning of blood down the vertebrobasilar system to the brachial artery.[20]

Infarction of the medulla dorsolateral to the inferior olivary nucleus[21] causes lateral medullary syndrome (Wallenberg's syndrome). The infarction roughly corresponds to the territorial supply of the posterior inferior cerebellar artery (PICA) (Fig. 25-4). Fisher et al.,[22] however, demonstrated that the infarction is usually due to occlusion of the vertebral artery and not of PICA.[22] In addition to destruction of the vestibular nuclei, which accounts for the vertigo, nystagmus, and oscillopsia, interruption of the spinothalamic tract leads to loss of pain and temperature sensation over the opposite half of the body. Involvement of the descending sympathetic tract causes Horner's syndrome and the nucleus ambiguus and the fibers of ninth and tenth nerves results in dysphagia and dysphonia. Ipsilateral cerebellar manifestations and facial hypoesthesia are due to involvement of the inferior cerebellar peduncle and the descending tract and nucleus of the fifth nerve, respectively. Deafness is not a feature of this syndrome because the infarction is caudal to the cochlear nuclei and cochlear nerve entry zone.

An infarction in the distribution of the anterior inferior cerebellar artery (AICA) occupies the dor-

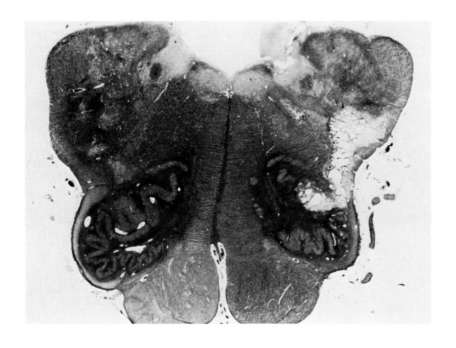

**Fig. 25-4.** Incomplete infarction of the dorsolateral medulla (Wallenberg's syndrome). (Heidenhain; original magnification × 4.)

solateral pontomedullary region and variable portions of the inferolateral cerebellum.[23] Damage to this artery is a serious complication following removal of an acoustic schwannoma, and proven cases of arteriosclerotic occlusion of AICA are rare.[24] The severity of brain stem and cerebellar dysfunctions depends on the extent of infarction, which is quite variable. The severe vertigo that frequently accompanies this syndrome (lateral pontomedullary or AICA syndrome) is largely caused by the infarction of the membranous labyrinth, which is supplied by the labyrinthine artery, a branch of AICA. (See also Chapter 24.) Intraparenchymal bleeding involving the vestibular nuclei is rare; most reports have attributed it to anticoagulant therapy,[25] vascular malformations,[26] or caudal extension of a pontine hemorrhage.[27] Hypertensive hemorrhage of the medulla is extremely rare.[28]

usually subpial, and the vestibular nuclei are sometimes involved (Fig. 25-5). There is a remarkable disparity in the susceptibility of the auditory and vestibular components of the eighth nerve system. Vertigo is a common complaint of patients with multiple sclerosis, whereas only a few present with deafness. McAlpine et al.[29] found 5 percent to have vertigo as an initial symptom. A similar figure was reported by Shibasaki et al.[30] The vestibular signs may remit or exacerbate, depending on the activity of the disease. It is said that as many as 50 percent of patients will experience vertigo at some time during the course of illness. Pathologic nystagmus is found in 90 percent of patients with longstanding disease and is due not only to brain stem lesions but also to involvement of the cerebellum and its connections as well.

## DEMYELINATING DISEASES

Multiple sclerosis is the most common of the demyelinating diseases (See Chapter 24). The vestibular pathways are maximally affected in the brain stem. The plaques in this region of the brain are

## METABOLIC DISORDERS

### Thiamine Deficiency

Thiamine (vitamin $B_1$) deficiency is secondary to malnutrition, particularly in chronic alcoholics, and may present as Wernicke's encephalopathy.

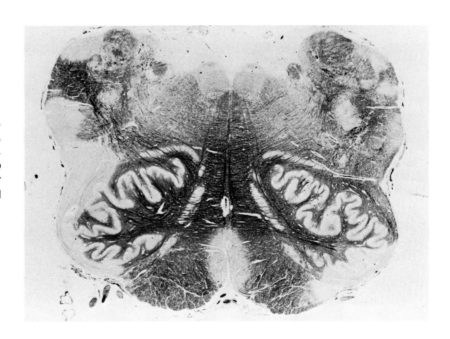

**Fig. 25-5.** Multiple sclerosis. Multiple demyelinating plaques, mostly subpial in distribution. Some of the plaques are also seen in the vestibular nuclear complexes. (Heidenhain; original magnification × 4.)

The incidence of Wernicke's encephalopathy seems to be increasing, but only 20 percent are diagnosed clinically.[31] It is characterized by a triad of mental confusion, ataxia, and ophthalmoplegia. The clinical manifestations correlate satisfactorily with the neuropathologic findings.[32] In the acute stages of the encephalopathy, symmetric lesions are consistently found in the mamillary bodies and walls of the third ventricles. The anteroventral thalamic nuclei, fornices, periaqueductal gray matter, and floor of the fourth ventricle are also frequently involved.[33] Microscopically, the neuropil appears spongy because of many tiny optically empty spaces. In experimentally induced Wernicke's encephalopathy, Blank et al.[34] found that this microvacuolar change in the monkey was due to intramyelinic blebs, whereas Watanabe and Kanabe[35] attributed the spongy changes in mice to hydropic swelling of the glial cells and their processes. Contrary to common perception, macroscopic petechial hemorrhages in the mamillary bodies occur in only 12 percent of patients; massive hemorrhages are rare and presumably secondary to associated bleeding diathesis.[36,37] In the experimental model using pyrithiomine-induced acute thiamine-deficient encephalopathy of the mouse, however, red cell diapedesis occurred at a higher rate.[38] Capillary proliferation with plump endothelial lining is another histologic feature of Wernicke's encephalopathy. The neurons in the mammillary bodies show variable degeneration, but they are sometimes relatively spared. The affected regions show a high nuclear density due to proliferation of astrocytes, microglia, and occasional macrophages. In chronic Wernicke's encephalopathy, the mamillary bodies are shrunken and brownish (Fig. 25-6) due to marked loss of neuropil and atrophy of neurons. The pathogenesis of the lesions remains obscure. Some workers have suggested increased requirements of the vitamin by the areas affected, and others have attributed the changes to the toxic effects of pyruvates, which are consistently elevated in untreated cases of Wernicke's disease.[39] Although vertigo and hearing loss are uncommon complaints in these patients, the vestibular nuclei are frequently involved. The medial vestibular nucleus is affected in 71 percent of cases, with the lateral, superior, and spinal vestibular nuclei involved in 50 percent, 36 percent, and 30 percent of cases, respectively. Experimentally, the lateral vestibular nucleus is also shown to be vulnerable to thiamine deficiency.[40] This may explain the constant impairment of vestibular function as measured by the response to ice-water caloric test in acute Wernicke's disease. Injection of thiamine improves the clinical signs and often restores the vestibular function, as measured by serial caloric testing, to normal.

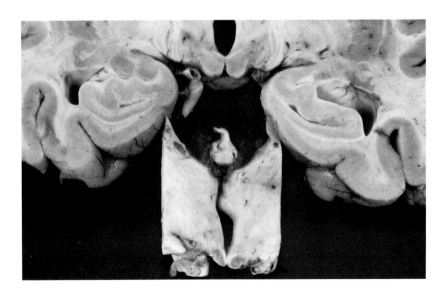

**Fig. 25-6.** Wernicke's encephalopathy, old. The mammillary bodies (bottom) are smaller and darker than in a normal brain (top).

## Diabetes Mellitus

Brain stem findings accounting for vestibular dysfunction in diabetics are largely due to the complicating atherosclerotic cerebrovascular disease, with ischemic lesions that interrupt the central vestibular pathways.[41]

---

## TRAUMA

In severe cases of closed head injuries, the brain stem may be involved. The contusions characteristically occur at the periphery of the mid-brain and pons and around the aqueduct of Sylvius.[42] Often, the corpus callosum in its center shows petechial hemorrhages and focal area of necrosis. Some of these patients do not manifest signs of increased intracranial pressure, but their level of consciousness remains markedly decreased.[43] These patients were assumed to suffer from primary brain stem injury. Recent studies, however, have shown the so-called primary brain stem contusion to be only part of a more diffuse process that disrupts axons throughout the brain—diffuse axonal injury.[44] This was also confirmed experimentally in mon-

keys.[45] Caloric stimulations in such patients are invariably abnormal, and their absence is regarded as an ominous sign.[46]

---

## TUMORS

Vertiginous seizures, albeit rare, may occur with tumors invading the region of the intraparietal sulcus and posterior segment of the superior temporal gyrus.[47] Primary CNS neoplasms common to this area are convexity meningiomas, astrocytomas, and glioblastoma multiforme.

### Brain Stem Gliomas

Brain stem gliomas may destroy the vestibular nuclei or invade their pathways. Fibrillary (pilocytic) astrocytoma is the predominant glioma involving the brain stem. The pons is by far the most frequent site of origin.[48] Grossly, the pons is enlarged—"pontine hypertrophy"—and with further growth of the tumor, the basilar artery becomes gradually encased and the surface of the pons acquires a bosselated appearance (Fig. 25-7). As the tumor spreads along the neuraxis, lobulated

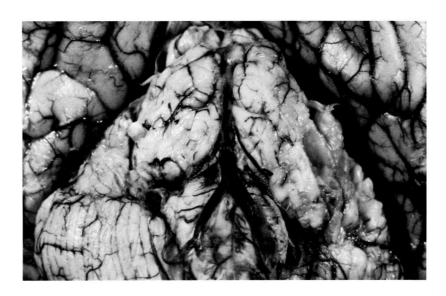

**Fig. 25-7.** Pontine glioma. The surface of the pons is irregular and focally bosselated. The middle segment of the basilar artery is almost totally encased by the growth.

masses of tumor gradually fill the cerebellopontine angle and interpeduncular fossa. The cut surface sometimes fails to display a discrete mass but sometimes gelatinous areas of cystic degeneration with or without hemorrhages may be present. In later stages, the medulla, mid-brain, and often the cerebellum are replaced by a diffuse gray tumor tissue. Microscopically, the tumor is made up of neoplastic fibrillar astrocytes. The cells grow along the pre-existing fiber tracts often sparing the nerve fibers and the neurons. The better differentiated tumors have slender long processes and mildly pleomorphic nuclei. They are generally classified as grade I or II astrocytomas. Pontine gliomas frequently occur during the first two decades of life, and 80 percent become symptomatic before 20 years of age.[49] Cranial nerve palsies and long tract signs are the usual manifestations. Vestibular and cochlear complaints occur in approximately 50 percent of cases.[50] Although the typical history is that of a relentless, gradual neurologic deterioration, rapid or sudden changes may be due to either malignant transformation of the tumor into a glioblastoma multiforme[51] (Fig. 25-8) or hemorrhage within the tumor. Glioblastoma multiforme is distinguished by the marked anaplasia of the cells, endothelial proliferation resulting in tufted ag-

glomerations, and pseudo-palisading of the tumor cells around necrotic foci. Life expectancy in pontine gliomas has been extended by radiation and ventricular shunting.[52,53]

## Cerebellar Astrocytomas

Unlike astrocytomas of the cerebral hemispheres, cerebellar astrocytomas occur predominantly during the first two decades of life and tend to be discrete and cystic.[54] The large cystic tumors sometimes display a mural nodule in which most of the neoplastic tissue is found (Fig. 25-9). If these tumors occur in the vermis, they grow in the cavity of the fourth ventricle and may involve its floor. More laterally placed tumors may extend along the inferior cerebellar peduncle and invade the vestibular nuclear complex or its projections. The tumor often displays spongy areas alternating with areas in which the cells are more compactly arranged. In the loosely reticulated foci, the cells are stellate-shaped reminiscent of protoplasmic astrocytes, whereas in the densely cellular areas, the tumor cells are elongated and bipolar with glial processes arranged in parallel bundles as in pilocytic astrocy-

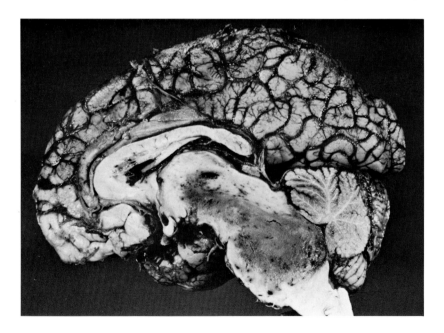

**Fig. 25-8.** Glioblastoma multiforme developing in a pontine glioma that has extended up to the diencephalon.

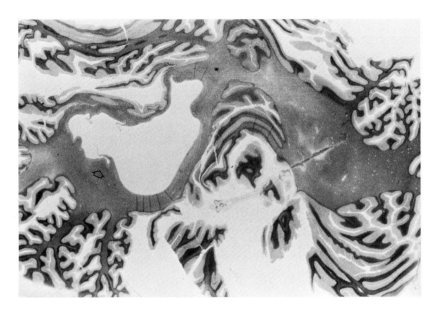

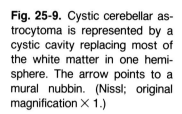

**Fig. 25-9.** Cystic cerebellar astrocytoma is represented by a cystic cavity replacing most of the white matter in one hemisphere. The arrow points to a mural nubbin. (Nissl; original magnification × 1.)

tomas. Rosenthal fibers, eosinophilic homogeneous formations in astocytic processes, are sometimes seen in the compact areas. In the spongy areas, microcysts coalescing to form larger cavities are common[55] (Fig. 25-10). Diffuse fibrillary astrocytomas may also occur in the cerebellum, usually in the older age group; according to some workers, the prognosis is less favorable than with the cystic variant.[56] Gilles et al.[57] attempted to delineate histologically the few patients who had a less favorable outcome; however, the prognostic value of such predictive discriminants has yet to be determined.[58,59] Cystic cerebellar astrocytomas, if completely removed, have an excellent prognosis, with total cure in some cases.[60] Malignant transformation to glioblastoma multiforme of childhood cerebellar astrocytomas or de novo anaplastic astrocytomas of cerebellum are exceedingly rare.[61,62]

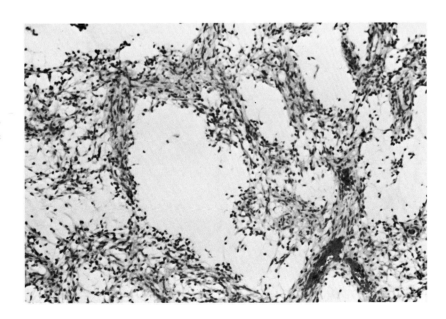

**Fig. 25-10.** Cystic cerebellar astrocytoma. Spongy microcystic areas alternate with more densely arranged tumor cells. The microcysts fuse to form larger cysts. (H & E; original magnification × 40.)

## Miscellaneous Tumors Originating in the Fourth Ventricle or Cerebellum

Other tumors originating in the fourth ventricle or cerebellum may also invade or compress the vestibular nuclear complex and its connections. These include medulloblastomas, ependymomas, choroid plexus papillomas and carcinomas, dermoid and epidermoid cysts, and capillary hemangioblastomas.

### Medulloblastomas

Medulloblastoma is a primitive tumor that originates either in cell rests in the posterior medullary velum or in the fetal remnants of the external granular layer of the cerebellum.[63,64] It usually appears in the posterior part of the cerebellar vermis, grows into the cavity of the fourth ventricle, and infiltrates its floor (Fig. 25-11). These tumors are gray and moderately demarcated from the adjacent brain tissue. Microscopically, they are formed of tightly packed sheets of anaplastic cells. In about 20 percent of cases, the tumor cells may display

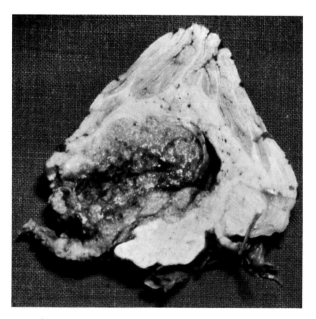

**Fig. 25-11.** A medulloblastoma fills the cavity of the fourth ventricle. It extends into one of the lateral recesses of the ventricle and infiltrates the floor.

concentric arrangements known as rosettes of the Homer-Wright type, especially if the tumor exhibits attempts of neuroblastic differentiation (Fig. 25-12). Medulloblastoma rosettes are distinguished from the ependymal rosettes by their central fibrillated core rather than a central lumen. The tumor cells have scant cytoplasm and hyperchromatic nuclei, either round or oval, depending on the plane of section. Mitotic figures are always present but variable in numbers. Electron microscopic studies have shown that in most cases the tumor cells lack any features suggesting differentiation[65]; however, occasionally glial, ganglionic or rhabdomyoblastic differentiation may be found.[66] Rarely, the tumor may consist almost exclusively of neuroblasts.[67] The tumor has the propensity to seed along the CSF pathways, and tumor implants may be seen in the ventricular lining and in the meninges of terminal or untreated patients. Extracranial spread has been reported, but it is rare.[68,69] Medulloblastomas occur primarily in children during the second part of the first decade of life; another peak of incidence is seen in young adults 20 to 24 years old. These tumors are more common in males. Positional vertigo and nystagmus are frequent. The tumor is radiosensitive; in recent years, combined surgical extirpation and radiation therapy have improved the survival figures.[70] Adjuvant chemotherapy is promising in prolonging life.[71,72] The concept of period of risk for recurrence formulated by Collins et al. often holds true in medulloblastomas.[73]

### Ependymomas

*Ependymomas* comprise about 6 percent of all gliomas and occur predominantly during the first three decades of life. About 70 percent occur infratentorially,[74] and as they grow they fill up the cavity of the fourth ventricle and protrude into the cisterna magna as tonguelike processes (Fig. 25-13). Gritty foci of calcification may be found. In classic cases, the tumor cells are arranged along tubular channels which seemingly recapitulate the central canal ependymal rosettes (Fig. 25-14). These cells often display cilia and basal bodies along their free borders. More often, however, the tapering processes of the tumor cells converge

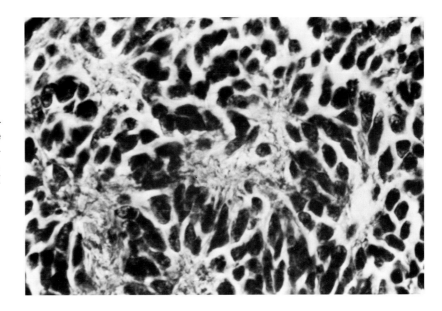

**Fig. 25-12.** Homer-Wright rosettes of medulloblastoma. The anaplastic tumor cells are arranged around fibrillated cores. (H & E; original magnification × 100.)

toward centrally placed blood vessels with the nucleated cell bodies equidistantly arranged around these vessels—perivascular pseudo-rosettes. In the more differentiated examples, the nuclei except for slight pleomorphism, have the same chromatin distribution as in normal ependymal cells. In the less differentiated forms the round or oval nuclei contain abundant dense chromatin which help in distinguishing ependymomas from astrocytomas. Glial fibrillary acidic protein, which is believed to be a specific marker for fibrillary astrocytes, has occasionally been demonstrated in small amounts in ependymomas.[75] Ultrastructural studies of ependymomas demonstrated several features common to the normal ependyma, namely, variable presence of cilia, basal bodies, junctional complexes, and intermediate cytoplasmic filaments.[76] There are several histologic variants of ependymomas based largely on cell density and patterns of arrangement of the tumor cells. The histology of these tumors is of limited value in assessing prognosis, since both benign and the less differentiated types have the propensity to disseminate along the CSF pathways introducing thus an unpredictable factor.[77] It is a general rule, however, that infratentorial ependymomas are well differentiated; their prognosis is better than those situated in the supratentorial space.[78]

Ependymoblastomas are considered to be more anaplastic than ependymomas. Rubinstein[79] reserves the term *ependymoblastoma* for a more specific type of tumor of ependymal origin that occurs in childhood.

Nystagmus and vertigo often occur with ependymomas. In one series of intracranial ependymomas in children, 8 of 43 had vestibular dysfunction.[80]

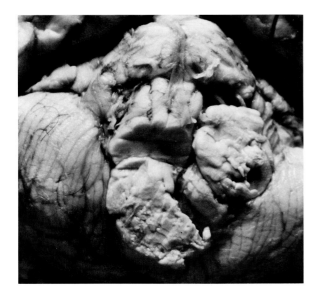

**Fig. 25-13.** Ependymoma protruding from the left lateral recess and roof of the fourth ventricle.

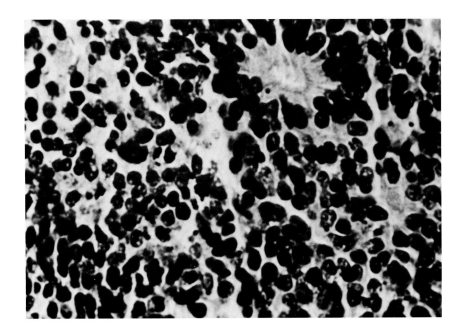

**Fig. 25-14.** Ependymoma showing a typical ependymal rosette(top). (H & E; original magnification × 100.).

## Choroid Plexus Papilloma and Carcinoma

Tumors originating in the choroid plexus are rare—usually less than 1 percent of all verified intracranial tumors.[81] In adults they occur predominantly in the fourth ventricle, whereas in children they are by and large situated in the lateral ventricles. Choroid tumors of the fourth ventricle sometimes extend into the cerebellopontine angle[82] and may cause hearing loss and/or vestibular dysfunction in addition to ataxia and manifestations of obstructive hydrocephalus. These tumors sometimes secrete large amounts of CSF and account for the rapid development of hydrocephalus in such cases. Grossly, choroid plexus tumors are pink-gray with an irregular granular or tufted surface. Microscopically, they recapitulate the features of normal choroid plexus. The frondlike projections are made up of vascular connective tissue lined externally by a single layer of cuboidal epithelium. Ultrastructurally, the cells display microvilli and basement lamina.[83] They are to be distinguished from fronds of papillary ependymomas, which have a gliovascular core, and the lining cells exhibit blepharoplasts and cilia.[84] The more anaplastic forms, also called choroid plexus carcinomas, may be misinterpreted as a metastatic carcinoma or vice-versa.[85] Both benign and malignant choroid plexus tumors may seed along the CSF pathways.

## Capillary Hemangioblastomas

Capillary hemangioblastomas constitute about 7.3 percent of all adult primary tumors of the posterior fossa.[86] They usually occur in the paravermal region, from which they may extend into the cavity of the fourth ventricle. Those originating in the medulla arise from the area postrema. They can be single or multiple and, if multiple, a genetic background of Lindau's syndrome is suggested.[87] Other stigmata of the syndrome include pancreatic cysts, renal and suprarenal tumors, and angiomatosis retinae (von Hippel's disease).

The tumor is discrete and often undergoes cystic degeneration. In the cyst, the neoplastic cells may only be demonstrable in an eccentric nubbin called the mural nodule (Fig. 25-15). The fluid in the cyst is often clear yellow, but sometimes it may be hemorrhagic. Two cellular components are identified in hemangioblastomas, the stromal cells, usually rich in neutral lipids, and the endothelial cells (Fig. 25-16). Reticulin stain readily outlines the sinusoidal spaces and discloses the highly vascular nature of the tumor. Ultrastructural studies have at-

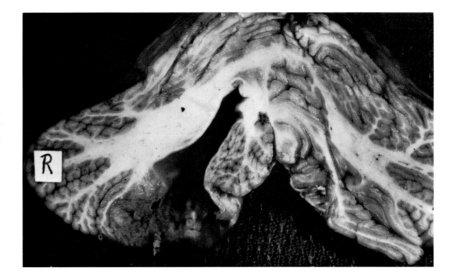

**Fig. 25-15.** Capillary hemangioblastoma. Most of the tumor is replaced by a cystic cavity, but tumor tissue can be appreciated near the surface.

tempted to determine the histogenesis of the stromal cells, but the results have been somewhat conflicting.[88] Recent immunocytochemical studies suggest that the stromal cells are of endothelial origin.[89] The prognosis after surgical extirpation is favorable; however, recurrences if incompletely removed or development of new primaries are to be anticipated. In such cases, radiotherapy is recommended.[90] Rarely, hemangioblastoma may seed along the CSF pathways.[91] Ten percent of patients may show erythropoiesis or actual polycythemia that resolves after total resection of the tumor.[92]

## Extraaxial Tumors

Extraaxial tumors, which frequently occur in the cerebellopontine angle, are the acoustic schwannomas, meningiomas and epidermoid cysts.

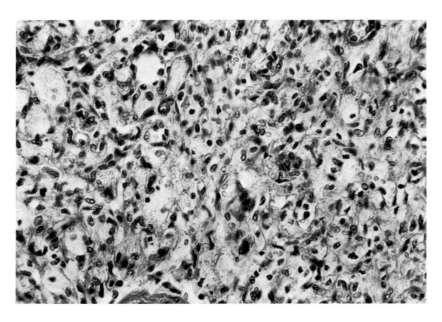

**Fig. 25-16.** Capillary hemangioblastoma. The stromal cells are vacuolated and the tumor is rich in capillaries that have a prominent endothelial lining. (H & E; original magnification × 40.)

## Acoustic Schwannoma

The cytogenesis of acoustic schwannoma (neuroma, neurilemmoma, neurofibroma) has been clarified by the advent of electron microscopy[93] and by advances in tissue culture.[94] There is ample reason to believe that it originates from Schwann cells and should therefore be appropriately designated as schwannoma. These tumors form about 8 percent of all primary intracranial tumors, and their favorite site is the cerebellopontine angle (Fig. 25-17). In Revilla's[95] series, they accounted for 78 percent of all tumors in this region, but figures reported by otologists are much higher, well over 90 percent in one series.[96] The term *acoustic* is a misnomer, as in about 90 percent of cases, these tumors originate in the vestibular nerve.[97,98] They are twice as common in females than in males,[81] and the mean age of presentation is usually between 40 and 45 years. Small schwannomas are occasionally seen in older patients as an incidental finding at necropsy. They are often situated in the internal auditory canal. When they enlarge, they gradually protrude through a widened funnel-shaped canal. They stretch adjacent nerve roots over their surface and eventually compress and deform the brain stem and cerebellum. Schwannomas are encapsulated and firm tumors with smooth surface, but as they grow they acquire an irregularly lobulated appearance. Hemorrhages and cystic degeneration are not infrequent in the larger schwannomas. Deafness and tinnitus are the initial symptoms in more than 90 percent of patients.[99]

Deafness is usually progressive, but occasionally it may have an acute onset, suggesting a vascular complication and possibly an interference with the blood supply of the cochlea or the nerve itself. Vestibular dysfunction is less common than auditory impairment. Vertigo is present in only 20 percent of patients,[100] but some degree of imbalance or dizziness develops in 50 percent of patients as the illness progresses.[101] Compression of the fifth or seventh nerves may be an initial symptom in a small number of patients. When the tumor reaches massive proportions, the lower cranial nerves may be compromised, and deformation of the brain stem may lead to obstructive hydrocephalus with manifestations of increased intracranial pressure. Bilateral acoustic neuromas are sometimes seen in von Recklinghausen's disease either in the presence of peripheral nerve and dermal lesions or in association with multiple intracranial and intraspinal tumors with no apparent peripheral lesions — so-called central neurofibromatosis. It is estimated that 5 percent of patients with von Recklinghausen's disease have bilateral acoustic schwannomas; often they are the sole manifestation of the disease.[102] In such instances, the acoustic tumor may become symptomatic as early as the first decade of life. Microscopically, two distinct architectural patterns are often identified, namely, Antoni types A and B[103] (Fig. 25-18). In Antoni A, the cells are arranged in compact interwoven bundles with the nuclei often focally aligned in linear configuration referred to as palisading. One or more consecutive

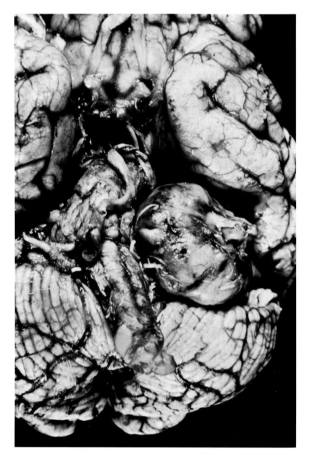

**Fig. 25-17.** Schwannoma of the left accoustic nerve indenting and displacing the brain stem and cerebellum.

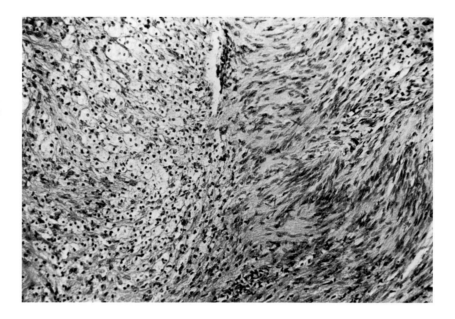

**Fig. 25-18.** The two patterns of a schwannoma are clearly distinguished. On the right the cells are densely packed and are spindle shaped (Antoni A), and on the left they are loosely arranged, round, and foamy (Antoni B).

rows of similarly aligned nuclei may be separated by anucleated zones made up of elongated cytoplasmic processes. These formations are known as Verocay bodies (Fig. 25-19). Palisading and Verocay bodies are more common in spinal schwannomas than in acoustic tumors. The cells have spindle-shaped cytoplasm with long bipolar processes giving these tumors a fibrillated appearance. The

nuclei are ovoid or rod shaped, often with one or more shallow indentations. They contain variable amounts of chromatin and inconspicuous nucleoli. The tumor is very rich in reticulin, which ultrastructurally may correspond to the abundant undulating basement membrane material that invests the cell processes[104] (Fig. 25-20).

Antoni B tissue consists of spongy meshwork of

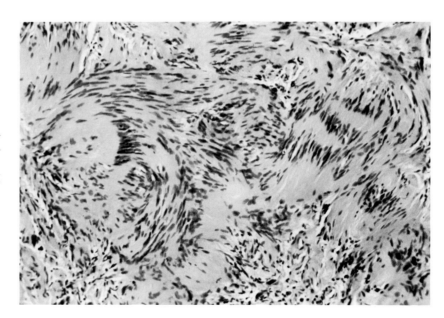

**Fig. 25-19.** Schwannoma displaying striking nuclear palisading and several Verocay bodies. (H & E; original magnifications ✕ 40.)

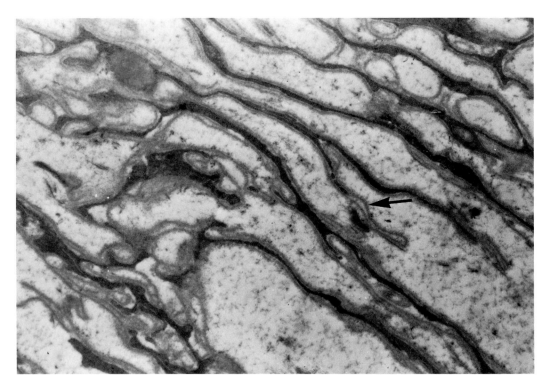

**Fig. 25-20.** Schwannoma with interdigitating cell processes invested with basal lamina (arrow). (Original magnification × 14,000.) (Courtesy of Dr. A. Hirano.)

vacuolated cells with round often hyperchromatic nuclei. Foam cells may be present. Although the appearance suggests degeneration of Antoni A tissue, tissue culture studies have proved otherwise.[105] Xanthomatous degeneration accounts for the yellowish areas often seen in the tumor. The blood vessels are usually sinusoidal and thin walled. Occasional vessels may have hyalinized adventitia. Ultrastructurally, the endothelium has numerous pores in contrast to the nonfenestrated endothelium of the blood vessels in normal nerves.[106] Another feature observed in electron microscopic studies of schwannomas is the presence of long-spacing collagen.[107] It consists of fibrils with cross-banding of periodicity between 120 and 150 nm. It was originally thought to be highly characteristic of schwannomas but was later found in other lesions.[108] Axons are usually not present in schwannomas; however, occasional randomly arranged unmyelinated axons may be seen. Malignant acoustic nerve tumors are exceptionally rare.[109]

## Meningiomas

Meningiomas are next in frequency after schwannomas in occupying the cerebellopontine angle. They comprise approximately 6 to 8 percent of all tumors occurring in this region and represent well over 50 percent of all posterior fossa meningiomas. Several reports of meningiomas of the cerebellopontine angle were recently analyzed by Sekhar and Jannetta.[110] Meningiomas occur more frequently in women. In the series by Grand and Bakay,[111] 25 of 30 patients with posterior fossa meningiomas were women. These tumors are seen mostly in the fifth and sixth decades. If found in children, they have some special predilection to the posterior fossa and are frequently associated with neurofibromatosis.[112]

The most common complaints are headache, ataxia, and hearing loss. Facial pain or spasm may also be a presenting symptom. Meningiomas originate in the arachnoid cap cells that abound in the arachnoid villi, hence the propensity of these tumors to be located along major sinuses. Those occurring in the cerebellopontine angle frequently arise in the margin of the sigmoid or petrosal sinuses over the posterior aspect of the petrous bone.[113] As these tumors grow, they displace cranial nerves and compress the brain stem and cerebellum. They are tenaciously adherent to the dura and never invade the brain tissue unless they undergo sarcomatous degeneration. On the other hand, they do invade venous sinuses and bone. In the case of the petrous pyramid, this may produce hyperostosis with labyrinthine involvement[114] in addition to compressing the eighth nerve at the cerebellopontine angle. Meningiomas in this location are often flat or en plaque, but occasionally are globoid with a bosselated surface. They are firm and may be gritty on sectioning. Focal areas of yellowish discoloration may be seen. Microscopically, several patterns have been identified; these bear little prognostic significance except for the angioblastic variant.

A simple classification distinguishes four types: syncytial, fibroblastic, transitional, and angioblastic. The syncytial (meningothelial) variant is formed of meningothelial cells with indistinct cellular borders arranged in whorls (Fig. 25-21). The nuclei are relatively large and spheroidal. They display a pale nucleoplasm with delicate chromatin meshwork and inconspicuous nucleoli. A gray inclusion body that represents cytoplasmic invagination imparts an empty appearance to some of the nuclei. These nuclear inclusions may help in the interpretation of frozen sections. Reticulin is confined to the vascularized trabeculae that intersect the tumor lobules or whorls. Xanthomatous cells in small clusters are frequently present.

In the fibroblastic variant, the neoplastic cells have long processes which are aligned in parallel intersecting bundles. Whorls and psammomas are absent, but careful sampling may disclose these features in a few foci. The nuclei are elongated and usually compressed, accounting for the slightly higher chromatin density than in the syncytial variant. Reticulin is seen between individual cells and is not confined to the blood vessels.

The transitional meningioma has features intermediate between the previous two types. Characteristic whorls are seen, but the cell processes are longer and the cell borders are better outlined than in the syncytial type. In some meningiomas, particularly in the posterior fossa and spinal cord, psammoma bodies are seen in great numbers (Fig. 25-22). Psammomas represent dystrophic calcifi-

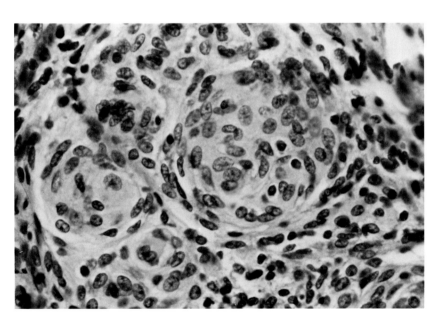

**Fig. 25-21.** Meningothelial meningioma. The cells with indefinite cell borders are arranged in whorls. (H & E; original magnification × 40.)

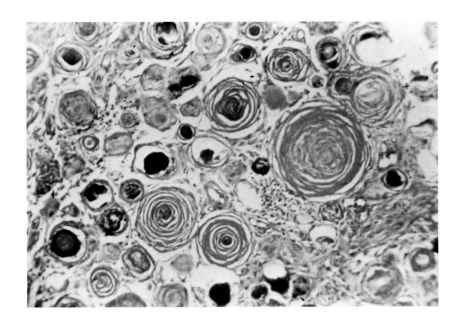

**Fig. 25-22.** Psammomatous meningioma. The tumor is largely formed of psammomas with few islets of residual tumor cells. (H & E; original magnification × 40.).

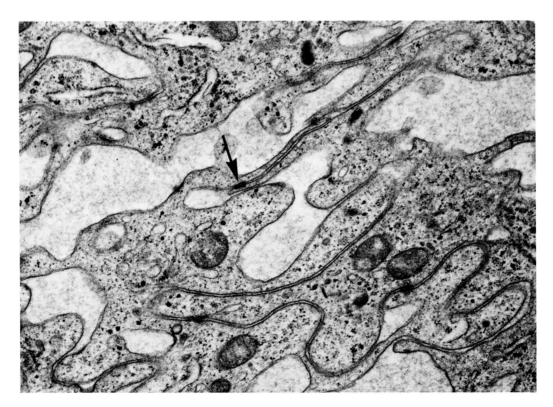

**Fig. 25-23.** Meningioma with intertwining cell processes displaying junctional complexes (arrow). (Original magnification × 30,000.) (Courtesy of Dr. A. Hirano.)

cation in the center of the whorls. Several theories have been proposed to explain their genesis. Recent studies suggest that matrix vesicles serve as the initial mineralization focus for these psammomas.[115,116] Ultrastructurally, meningiomas are characterized by interdigitating cell processes linked by various types of junctional complexes, particularly desmosomes[117] (Fig. 25-23). The cytoplasm and its processes contain abundant intermediate filaments.

In the angioblastic variant, whorl formation is absent and the tumor cells are supported by a rich network of reticulin permeated by sinusoidal vascular spaces. The nuclei are hyperchromatic and the chromatin is coarser than in the previous types. Moderate degree of nuclear pleomorphism and variable number of mitotic figures are present. Sometimes, they resemble hemangiopericytomas (Fig. 25-24) or capillary hemangioblastomas, hence the controversy concerning the nomenclature of these lesions.[118] Angioblastic meningiomas are aggressive tumors, especially if they display papillarylike projections, focal areas of necrosis, and more than a few mitoses. They tend to recur after incomplete excision or infiltrate the brain parenchyma (Fig. 25-25). Frank sarcomatous change, often indistinguishable from fibrosarcoma, can take place.[119] Radiation therapy to the head

might be involved in the induction of intracranial meningioma.[120,121]

## Dermoid and Epidermoid Cysts

*Dermoid cysts*[122] usually occur in the midline between the cerebellar hemispheres or in the fourth ventricle. A dermal sinus in the occipital region overlying the cerebellar dermoid cyst may act as a route for pyogenic infection. The wall of the cyst contains sebaceous cysts and hairs. The content is made up of laminated desquamated epithelium. Focal calcifications are common, and teeth are rare. (For a detailed description of the epidermoid cysts of the cerebellopontine angle, see Chapter 26.)

## Metastatic Tumors

In theory, vertigo can be produced by metastases that irritate the cortex of the posterior superior gyrus of the temporal lobe, since Penfield et al.[123,124] were able to produce a sense of rotation by stimulating this region in patients undergoing surgery. Clinically, however, this association has been difficult to prove. Metastases may involve the brain stem, including the cerebellopontine angle. The

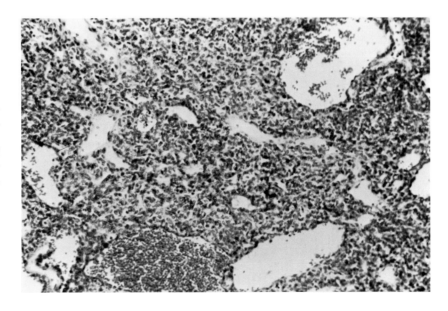

**Fig. 25-24.** Angioblastic meningioma resembling a hemangiopericytoma. No whorls are seen. The tumor is very cellular and heavily permeated by vascular spaces. (H & E; original magnification × 10.)

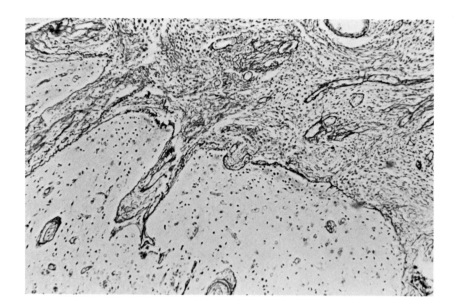

**Fig. 25-25.** Invasive meningioma. Prongs of tumor cells from the meninges are extending along the Virchow-Robin spaces into the brain parenchyma. (reticulin; original magnification × 40.)

most common sites of origin of carcinomas that metastasize to the brain, in order of decreasing frequency, are the bronchus, breast, and kidney.[125] Malignant melanomas and choriocarcinomas deserve special mention, since both have a special predilection to affect the brain.[126,127] It appears that the incidence of cerebral metastases in patients with sarcomas has increased due to improved survival.[128,129] Leukemic or lymphomatous deposits may also affect the brain stem nuclei, including the vestibular complex.

# REFERENCES

1. Baringer JR, Swoveland P: Recovery of herpes simplex virus from human trigeminal ganglions. N Engl J Med 288:648, 1973

2. Davis LE, Johnson RT: An explanation for the localization of herpes simplex encephalitis. Ann Neurol 5:2, 1979

3. Lach B, Gilbert J, Monpetit VA, et al: Significance of tissue distribution of viral antigen in pathogenesis of human herpes simplex virus (HSV) encephalitis. J Neuropathol Exp Neurol 43:333, 1984

4. Haymaker W: Herpes simplex encephalitis in man.

With a report of three cases. J Neuropathol Exp Neurol 8:132, 1949

5. Swanson JL, Craigherd JE, Reynolds ES: Electron microscopic observation on herpes virus hominis (herpes simplex virus) encephalitis in man. Lab Invest 15:1966, 1966

6. Pedersen E: Epidemic vertigo. Clinical picture and relation to encephalitis. Brain 83:566, 1959

7. Henson A, Urich H: Cancer and the Nervous System. The Neurological Manifestations of Systemic Malignant Disease. Blackwell Scientific Publications, Oxford, 1982

8. Halperin JJ, Richardson Jr EP, Ellis J, et al: Paraneoplastic encephalomyelitis and neuropathy. Report of a case. Arch Neurol 38:773, 1981

9. Dix M, Hallpike C: The pathology, symptomatology and diagnosis of certain common disorders of the vestibular systems. Ann Otol Rhinol Laryngol 61:987, 1952

10. Morgenstein K, Seung H: Vestibular neuronitis. Laryngoscope 81:131, 1971

11. Drachman DA, Hart CW: An approach to the dizzy patient. Neurology (NY) 22:323, 1972

12. Rudge P: Clinical Neuro-otology. Clinical Neurology and Neurosurgery. Vol. 4. Churchill Livingstone, New York, 1983

13. Williams S: Epidemic vertigo in children. Med J Aust 2:660, 1963

14. Merifield D: Self-limited idiopathic vertigo (epidemic vertigo). Arch Otolaryngol 81:355, 1965

15. Duffy PE, Sassin JF, Summers DS, Lourie H:

Rhombencephalitis due to Listeria monocyto-genes. Neurology (NY) 14:1067, 1964

16. Lindenberg R: Compression of brain arteries as a pathogenetic factor for tissue necrosis and their areas of predilection. J Neuropathol Exp Neurol 14:223, 1955

17. Johnson RT, Yates PO: Brain stem hemorrhages in expanding supratentorial conditions. Acta Radiol (Stockh) 46:250, 1956

18. Plum F, Posner JB: The Diagnosis of Stupor and Coma. FA Davis, Philadelphia, 1980

19. Hutchinson EC, Acheson EJ: Major Problems in Neurology. Vol. 4: Strokes. Natural History, Pathology, and Surgical Treatment. WB Saunders, London, 1975

20. Contorni L: The vertebrobasilar circulation in obliteration of the subclavian artery at its origin. Minerva Chir 15:268, 1960

21. Foix C, Hillemand P, Schalit I: Sur le syndrome latéral du bulbe et l'irrigation du bulbe supérieur. Rev Neurol 1:160, 1925

22. Fisher CM, Karnes WE, Kubik CS: Lateral medullary infarction—The pattern of vascular occlusion. J Neuropathol Exp Neurol 20:323, 1961

23. Atkinson WJ: Anterior inferior cerebellar artery, its variations, pontine distribution and significance of cerebellopontine angle tumors. J Neurol Neurosurg Psychiatry 12:137, 1949

24. Adams RD: Occlusion of anterior inferior cerebellar artery. Arch Neurol Psychiatry (Chicago) 49:765, 1943

25. Mastaglia FL, Edis B, Kakulas BA: Medullary hemorrhage: A report of two cases. J Neurol Neurosurg Psychiatry 32:221, 1969

26. Kempe LG: Surgical removal of an intramedullary hematoma simulating Wallenberg's syndrome. J Neurol Neurosurg Psychiatry 27:78, 1964

27. Martin P, Noterman J: L'hematome bulboprotu-berantiel operable. Acta Neurol (Belg) 71:261, 1971

28. Neumann PE, Mehler MF, Horoupian DS: Primary medullary hypertensive hemorrhage. Neurology (NY) 34[Suppl 1]:90, 1984 (abst)

29. McAlpine D, Lumsden CE, Acheson ED: Multiple Sclerosis. A Reappraisal. Churchill Livingstone, Edinburgh, 1972

30. Shibasaki K, Okihiro M, Kuroiwa Y: Multiple sclerosis among orientals and caucasians in Hawaii: A reappraisal. Neurology (NY) 28:113, 1978

31. Harper C: The incidence of Wernicke's encephalopathy in Australia—A neuropathological study of 131 cases. J Neurol Neurosurg Psychiatry 46:593, 1983

32. Riggs HE, Boles RS: Wernicke's disease: A clinical and pathological study of 42 cases. Q J Stud Alcohol 5:361, 1944

33. Victor M, Adams RD, Collins EH: The Wernicke-Korsakoff Syndrome. FA Davis, Philadelphia, 1971

34. Blank NK, Vick NA, Schulman S: Wernicke's encephalopathy. An experimental study in the rhesus monkey. Acta Neuropathol (Berl) 31:137, 1975

35. Watanabe I, Kanabe S: Early edematous lesion of pyrithiamine induced acute thiamine deficient encephalopathy in the mouse. J Neuropathol Exp Neurol 37:401, 1978

36. Grunnett ML: Changing incidence distribution and histopathology of Wernicke's polioencephalopathy. Neurology (NY) 19:1135, 1969

37. Rosenblum WI, Feigin I: The hemorrhagic component of Wernicke's encephalopathy. Arch Neurol 13:627, 1965

38. Watanabe I, Iwasaki Y, Aikawa H, et al: Hemorrhage of thiamine deficient encephalopathy. J Neuropathol Exp Neurol 40:566, 1981

39. Thompson RH, Johnson RE: Blood pyruvate in vitamin $B_1$ deficiency. Biochem J 29:694, 1935

40. Tellez I, Terry RD: Fine structure of the early changes in the vestibular nuclei of the thiamine-deficient rat. Am J Pathol 52:777, 1968

41. Makishima K, Tanaka K: Pathological changes of the inner ear and antral auditory pathways in diabetics. Ann Otol Rhinol Laryngol 80:218, 1971

42. Tomlinson BE: Brain-stem lesions after head injury. J Clin Pathol 23[Suppl]4:154, 1970

43. Mitchell DE, Adams JH: Primary focal impact damage to the brain stem in blunt head injuries. Does it exist? Lancet 2:215, 1973

44. Adams JH, Graham DI, Murray LS, Scott G: Diffuse axonal injury due to non-missile head injury in humans. An analysis of 45 cases. Ann Neurol 12:557, 1982

45. Gennarelli TA, Thibault LE, Adams JH, et al: Diffuse axonal injury and traumatic coma in the primate. Ann Neurol 12:564, 1982

46. Poulen J, Zilstrorff K: Prognostic value of the caloric vestibular test in the unconscious patients with cranial trauma. Acta Neurol Scand 48:282, 1972

47. Spiegel EA, Alexander A: Vertigo in brain tumors with special reference to results of labyrinth examination. Ann Otol Rhinol Laryngol 45:979, 1936

48. Mantravadi RV, Phatak R, Bellur S, et al: Brain stem gliomas: An autopsy study of 25 cases. Cancer 49:1294, 1982

49. Panitch HS, Berg BO: Brain stem tumors of childhood and adolescence. Am J Dis Child 119:465, 1970

50. Barnett HJ, Hyland HH: Tumors involving the brain stem. Q J Med 21:265, 1952

51. Golden GS, Ghatak NR, Hiram A, French JH: Malignant glioma of the brain stem. J Neurol Neurosurg Psychiatry 35:732, 1972

52. Lassman LP, Arjona VE: Pontine gliomas of childhood. Lancet 1:913, 1967

53. Albright AL, Price RA, Guthkelch N: Brain stem gliomas of children. A clinicopathological study. Cancer 52:2313, 1983

54. Bucy PC, Gustafson WA: Structure, nature and classification of cerebellar astrocytomas. Am J Cancer 35:327, 1939

55. Russell DS, Rubinstein LJ: Pathology of Tumors of the Nervous System. Williams & Wilkins, Baltimore, 1977

56. Gjerris F, Klinken L: Long term prognosis in children with benign cerebellar astrocytoma. J Neurosurg 49:179, 1978

57. Gilles FH, Winston K, Fulchiero A, et al: Histological features and observational variation in cerebellar gliomas in children. J Natl Cancer Inst 58:175, 1977

58. Leviton A, Fulchiero A, Gilles FH et al: Survival status of children with cerebellar gliomas. J Neurosurg 48:29, 1978

59. Auer RN, Rice GP, Hinton GG, et al: Cerebellar astrocytoma with benign histology and malignant clinical course. J Neurosurg 54:128, 1981

60. Griffin TW, Beaufort D, Blasko JC: Cystic cerebellar astrocytomas in childhood. Cancer 44:276, 1979

61. Alpers CE, Davis RL, Wilson CB: Persistence and late malignant transformation of childhood cerebellar astrocytoma. Case report. J Neurosurg 57:548, 1982

62. Kopelson G: Cerebellar glioblastoma. Cancer 50:308, 1982

63. Stevenson L, Echlin F: Nature and origin of some tumors of the cerebellum. Medulloblastoma. Arch Neurol Psychiatry 31:93, 1934

64. Kadin ME, Rubinstein LJ, Nelson JS: Neonatal cerebellar medulloblastoma originating from the fetal external granular layer J Neuropathol Exp Neurol 29:583, 1970

65. Matakas F, Cervós-Navarro J, Gullota F: The structure of medulloblastomas. Acta Neuropathol (Berl) 16:271, 1970

66. Dickson DW, Hart MN, Menezes A, Cancilla PA: Medulloblastoma with glial and rhabdomyoblastic differentiation. J Neuropath Exp Neurol 42:639, 1983

67. Shin W-Y, Laufer H, Lee Y-C, et al: Fine structure of a cerebellar neuroblastoma. Acta Neuropathol (Berl) 42:11, 1978

68. Kleinman GM, Hochberg FH, Richardson Jr EP: Systemic metastases from medulloblastoma, report of two cases and review of the literature. Cancer 48:2296, 1981

69. McComb JG, Davis RL, Isaacs H Jr, Landing PH: Medulloblastoma presenting as neck tumors in 2 infants. Ann Neurol 7:113, 1980

70. Park TS, Hoffman HJ, Hendrick EB, et al: Medulloblastoma: Clinical presentation and management. Experience at the Hospital for Sick Children, Toronto 1950–1980. J Neurosurg 58:543, 1983

71. Mealey J Jr, Hall PV: Medulloblastoma in children. Survival and treatment. J Neurosurg 46:56, 1977

72. Thomas PRM, Duffner PK, Cohen ME, et al: Multimodality therapy for medulloblastoma. Cancer 45:666, 1980

73. Quest DO, Brisman R, Antunes JL, Housepian EM: Period of risk for recurrence in medulloblastoma. J Neurosurg 48:159, 1978

74. Mørk S, Løken AC: Ependymoma. A follow-up study of 101 cases. Cancer 40:907, 1977

75. Duffy PE, Graf L, Huang Y-Y, Rapport MM: Glial fibrillary acidic protein in ependymomas and other brain tumors. J Neurol Sci 40:133, 1979

76. Goebel HH, Cravioto H: Ultrastructure of human and experimental ependymomas. J Neuropathol Exp Neurol 31:54, 1972

77. Svien HJ, Mabon RF, Kernohan JW, Craig W McK: Ependymoma of brain (pathological aspects). Neurology (NY) 3:1, 1953

78. Liu HM, Boggs J, Kidd J: Ependymomas of childhood. I. Histological survey and clinicopathological correlation. Childs Brain 2:92, 1976

79. Rubinstein LJ: The definition of the ependymoblastoma. Arch Pathol Lab Med 90:35, 1970

80. Coulon RA, Till K: Intracranial ependymomas in children. A review of 43 cases. Childs Brain 3:154, 1977

81. Zülch KJ: Biologie und Pathologie der Hirngeschwültse. In Olivecrona H, Tönnis W (eds): Handbuch der Neurochirurgie. Vol 3. Springer-Verlag, Berlin, 1956

82. Naguib MG, Chou SN, Mastri A: Radiation therapy of a choroid plexus papilloma of the cerebellopontine angle with bone involvement. J Neurosurg 54:245, 1981

83. Matsushima T: Choroid plexus papilloma and

human choroid plexus. A light and electron microscopic study. J Neurosurg 59:1054, 1983

84. Rubinstein LJ, Brucher J-M: Focal ependymal differentiation in choroid plexus papillomas. Acta Neuropathol (Berl) 53:29, 1981

85. Nakashima N, Goto K, Takeuchi J: Papillary carcinoma of choroid plexus. Light and electron microscopic study. Virchows Arch [A] 395:303, 1982

86. Olivecrona H: Cerebellar angioreticulomas. J Neurosurg 9:317, 1952

87. Palmer JJ: Hemangioblastomas. A review of 81 cases. Acta Neurochir (Wien) 27:125, 1972

88. Kawamura J, Garcia JH, Kamijyo Y: Cerebellar hemangioblastoma: Histogenesis of stromal cells. Cancer 31:1528, 1973

89. Jurco S, Nadji M, Harvey DG: Hemangioblastomas: Histogenesis of the stromal cell studied by immunocytochemistry. Hum Pathol 13:13, 1982

90. Sung DI, Chang CH, Harisiadis L: Cerebellar hemangioblastomas. Cancer 49:553, 1982

91. Mohan J, Brownell B, Oppenheimer DR: Malignant spread of hemangioblastoma: Report on two cases. J Neurol Neurosurg Psychiatry 39:515, 1976

92. Waldmann TA, Levin EH, Baldwin M: The association of polycythemia with a cerebellar hemangioblastoma. The production of an erythropoiesis stimulating factor by the tumor. Am J Pathol 31:318, 1961

93. Waggener JD: Ultrastructure of benign peripheral nerve sheath tumors. Cancer 19:699, 1966

94. Cravioto H, Lockwood R: The behavior of acoustic neuroma in tissue culture. Acta Neuropathol (Berl) 12:141, 1969

95. Revilla GA: Differential diagnosis of tumors at the cerebellopontine recess. Bull Johns Hopkins Hosp 83:187, 1948

96. Selters WA, Brookman DE: Acoustic tumor detection with brainstem electric response audiometry. Arch Otolaryngol 103:181, 1977

97. Schuknecht HJ: Pathology of the Ear. Harvard University Press, Cambridge, 1974

98. Morrison AW, Gibson WPR, Beagley HA: Transtympanic electrocochleography in the diagnosis of retrocochlear tumors. Clin Otolaryngol 1:153, 1976

99. Erickson L, Sorenson G, McGavran M: A review of 140 consecutive neurinomas (neurolemmomas). Laryngoscope 75:601, 1965

100. Edwards CH, Paterson JH: A review of the symptoms and signs of acoustic neurofibromata. Brain 74:144, 1951

101. Ozsahinoglu C, Harrison MS: The symptoms of

neurofibroma of the 8th nerve. J Laryngol Otol 88:493, 1974

102. Young D, Eldridge R, Gardner W: Bilateral acoustic neuroma in a large kindred. JAMA 214:347, 1970

103. Antoni N: Ueber Rückenmarkstumoren und Neurofibrome. Bergmann, Münich, 1920

104. Thomas PK: Changes in the endoneurial sheaths of peripheral myelinated nerve fibers during Wallerian degeneration. J Anat 98:175, 1964

105. Murray MR, Stout AP: Schwann cell versus fibroblasts as origin of specific nerve sheath tumor; observations upon normal nerve sheaths and neurilemmomas in vitro. Am J Pathol 16:41, 1940

106. Hirano A, Dembitzer HM, Zimmerman HM: Fenestrated blood vessels in neurilemmoma. Lab Invest 27:305, 1972

107. Luse SA: Electron microscope studies of brain tumors. Neurology (NY) 10:881, 1960

108. Ramsey HJ: Fibrous long-spacing collagen in tumors of the nervous system. J Neuropathol Exp Neurol 24:40, 1965

109. Kudo M, Matsumoto M, Terao H: Malignant nerve sheath tumor of acoustic nerve. Arch Pathol Lab Med 107:293, 1983

110. Sekhar LN, Jannetta PJ: Cerebellopontine angle meningiomas. Microsurgical excision and follow-up results. J Neurosurg 60:500, 1984

111. Grand W, Bakay L: Posterior fossa meningiomas, a report of 30 cases. Acta Neurochir (Wien) 32:219, 1975

112. Merten DF, Gooding CA, Newton TH, Malamud N: Meningiomas of childhood and adolescence. J Pediatr 84:696, 1974

113. Igarashi M, Alford BR, Herndon JW, Saito R: Cerebellopontine meningiomas and the temporal bone. Arch Otolaryngol 94:224, 1971

114. Nager GT: Meningiomas Involving the Temporal Bone, Clinical and Pathological Aspects. Charles C Thomas, Springfield, IL, 1964

115. Lipper S, Dalzell JC, Watkins PJ: Ultrastructure of psammoma bodies of meningioma in tissue culture. Arch Pathol Lab Med 103:670, 1979

116. Kubota T, Hirano A, Yamamoto S, Kajikawa K: The fine structure of psammoma bodies in meningocytic whorls. J Neuropathol Exp Neurol 43:37, 1984

117. Copeland DD, Bell SW, Shelburne JD: Hemidesmosome-like intercellular specializations in human meningiomas. Cancer 41:2242, 1978

118. Horten BC, Urich H, Rubinstein LJ, Montague SR: The angioblastic meningioma: A reappraisal of a nosological problem. J Neurol Sci 31:387, 1977

119. Jellinger K, Slowik F: Histologic subtypes and

prognostic problems in meningiomas. J Neurol 208:279, 1975

120. Soffer D, Pittaluga S, Feiner M, Beller AJ: Intracranial meningiomas following low-dose irradiation to the head. J Neurosurg 59:1048, 1983

121. Iacono R, Apuzzo M, Davis R, Tsai F: Multiple meningiomas following radiation therapy for medulloblastoma. J Neurosurg 55:282, 1981

122. Tytus JS, Pennybacker I: Pearly tumors in relation to the central nervous system. J Neurol Neurosurg Psychiatry 19:241, 1956

123. Penfield W, Kristiansen K: Epileptic Seizure Patterns: A Study of the Localizing Value of Initial Phenomena in Focal Cortical Seizures. Charles C Thomas Springfield, IL, 1951

124. Penfield W, Jasper H: Epilepsy and the Functional Anatomy of the Human Brain. Little, Brown, Boston, 1954

125. Willis RA: The Spread of Tumors in the Human Body. Butterworths, London, 1973

126. Gupta TD, Brasfield R: Metastatic melanoma. A clinico-pathologic study. Cancer 17:1323, 1964

127. Shuangshoti S, Panythanya R, Wichienkur P: Intracranial metastases from unsuspected choriocarcinoma. Onset suggesting of cerebrovascular disease. Neurology (NY) 24:649, 1974

128. Gercovich FG, Luna MA, Gottlieb JA: Increased incidence of cerebral metastases in sarcoma patients with prolonged survival from chemotherapy. Report of cases of leiomyosarcoma and chondrosarcoma. Cancer 36:1843, 1975

129. Zuker DK, Katz R, Koto A, Horoupian DS: Sarcomas metastatic to the brain: Case report of a metastatic fibrosarcoma and review of literature. Surg Neurol 9:177, 1978

# Pathology of the Facial Nerve and Its Central Nervous System Pathways

# 26

## Dikran Horoupian

Lesions that affect the facial nerve and its central nervous system (CNS) pathways have been broken down into three anatomic sites: supranuclear, nuclear, and peripheral. The pathology of the supranuclear lesions is only briefly stated. In the brain stem, the pathology of some of the developmental, vascular, and infectious disorders is discussed at some length, but the demyelinating conditions receive only brief mention, since these are covered in Chapter 24. The section on the peripheral segment of the nerve includes many disorders specific to the facial nerves or in which the facial nerves are frequently affected along with other peripheral nerves. Of the neoplasias, only the schwannomas of the facial nerve, the paragangliomas, and the epidermoid/arachnoid cysts are discussed in this chapter; the rest are covered in Chapter 25.

nervations from both hemispheres. There is also a dissociation of emotional and voluntary facial movements. Strokes due to infarctions or hypertensive hemorrhages are the most frequent causes of supranuclear palsies. They destroy either the facial center in the motor strip or its projection fibers as they course through the centrum semiovale or internal capsule (Fig. 26-1). Other causes of supranuclear facial palsies include inflammatory processes (such as pyogenic or tuberculous abscesses) and tumors (either primary CNS neoplasms, notably gliomas, or metastases).

## BRAIN STEM (NUCLEAR) LESIONS

### Congenital or Developmental Disorders

Lower facial palsy possibly due to aplasia of facial nucleus has sometimes been associated with cardiac anomalies.[2,3] By contrast, Pape and Pickering[4] found that facial palsy is an index of other congenital anomalies not exclusively restricted to the heart.

## CEREBRAL HEMISPHERIC (SUPRANUCLEAR) LESIONS

Facial palsy caused by a supranuclear lesion is characterized by relative preservation of the functions of the frontalis and orbicularis oculi muscles because the facial nuclei receive upper motor in-

759

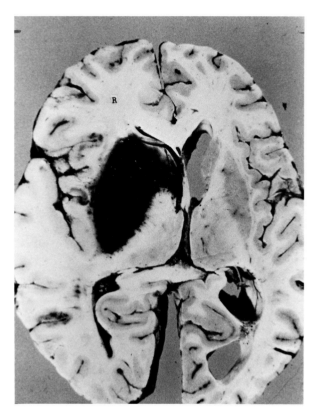

**Fig. 26-1.** Hypertensive intracerebral hemorrhage disrupting the internal capsule.

### Möbius syndrome

Möbius syndrome, or congenital facial diplegia, is a congenital nonprogressive condition of bilateral facial palsies frequently associated with abducens nerve paralysis.[5] The definition has been broadened to include unilateral facial palsy as well.[6] Möbius syndrome is usually sporadic, but it has been reported in twins[7] and occasionally in families.[8] It has been likened to arthrogryposis multiplex congenita,[9] with which it has occasionally been reported.[10] Both myopathic and neuropathic forms of the syndrome are assumed to exist. In recent years, however, several well-documented neuropathologic studies have shown that most patients with this syndrome had foci of necrosis in the brain stem[11] (Fig. 26-2). Dystrophic calcifications were frequently present in these lesions, suggesting an encephaloclastic process.[12] Hypoxia or hypoperfusion of the fetus during a crit-

ical period of its development is believed to result in selective necrosis of the tegmental nuclei, including the facial nuclei.[13,14] This explains the frequent bilaterality of the palsies and the presence of other cranial nerve deficits.

### Vascular Accident

Hypertensive brain stem hemorrhages involving the pons account for about 10 percent of all primary CNS hemorrhages.[15] In massive pontine hemorrhage, more often seen in accelerated malignant hypertension,[16] death usually occurs within a few hours, and facial palsy is obscured by the more life-threatening condition.[17] There are exceptions, however, in which a small hemorrhage is not associated with coma and cranial nerve palsies, including facial paresis with crossed sensory or motor signs, may prevail.[18,19] Charcot-Bouchard microaneurysms may be found in the pons of severely hypertensive patients.[20] These outpouchings of arterioles 250 to 450 $\mu$m in diameter are the result of fibrinoid necrosis, which in turn causes weakening of the vessel walls (Fig. 26-3). They are frequently surrounded by hemorrhages, recent or old, but their role in initiating a massive intracerebral hemorrhage is less certain.[21] Lacunae in the basis pontis are also frequently encountered in the brains of hypertensive patients. These cavitary lesions, about 5 to 15 mm in diameter, represent remnants of small infarcts, according to Fischer[22] (Fig. 26-4). Lacunes may interrupt the intraaxial course of the facial nerve and can account for facial palsy of the lower motor neuron type. Facial palsy is often part of the lateral pontomedullary syndrome, which results from ischemic infarction in the distribution of the anterior inferior cerebellar artery[23] (see also Chapter 24). Rarely, a pontine infarction may manifest as isolated cranial nerve palsies, including the 7th cranial nerve.[24]

### Infections

#### Viral Infections

In bulbar forms of anterior poliomyelitis,[25] the facial nucleus was involved in more than 50 percent of patients and was frequently associated with

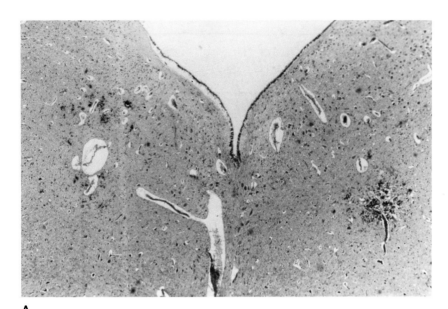

A

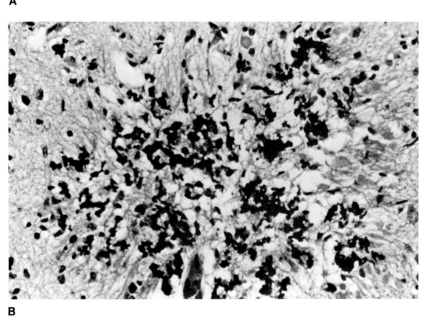

B

**Fig. 26-2. (A)** Pontine tegmentum in Möbius syndrome at the level of the facial nuclei shows multifocal areas of necrosis with dystrophic calcifications interrupting the course of the facial nerves. (H & E; original magnification × 40.) **(B)** Higher magnification of one of the calcific foci in Möbius syndrome displaying in addition axonal swellings and reactive astrocytes. (H & E; original magnification × 100.)

other cranial nerve palsies, particularly of the glossopharyngeal and vagal nerves. The facial nerve along with other lower cranial nerves may be affected in subacute brain stem encephalitis[26] either of putative viral origin[27] or as a remote effect of carcinoma.[28,29] The lesions in this condition are like those in most viral encephalitides and consist of collections of mononuclear cells (glial nodules), neuronophagia, microglial proliferation, and perivascular lymphocytic cuffings. The pathology is largely restricted to the brain stem and cerebellum. Isolated 7th nerve palsy, possibly due to viral infection, has also been described in the recently recognized condition of acquired immune deficiency syndrome (AIDS).[30] Cerebritis, which refers to inflammation of brain tissue by pyogenic organisms, rarely affects the brain stem. In *Listeria monocytogenes* infection, however, the brain stem may be-

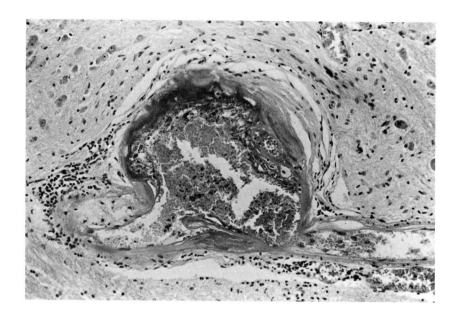

**Fig.    26-3.** Charcot-Bouchard microaneurysm in the pons of a hypertensive patient. The wall of the aneurysm displays fibrinoid changes and adventitial fibrosis. (H & E; original magnification × 100.)

come specially vulnerable—*Listeria* rhombencephalitis.[31,32] In such cases, the facial nucleus or nerve may be destroyed. Although *Listeria monocytogenes* occurs mostly in immunosuppressed persons, it has also been described in healthy subjects. Tuberculomas can occur in the brain stem

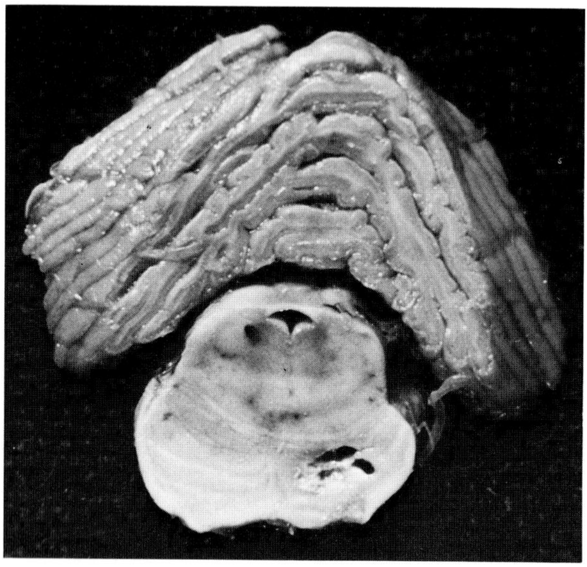

**Fig. 26-4.** Lacunar infarct in the basis pontis of a hypertensive patient.

and cause facial palsy. *Syphilis* has also been implicated in causing facial nerve palsy.[33]

## Fungal Infections

Fungal infections may involve the brain stem. Candidiasis or monilial infection due to *Candida* is one of the most common cerebral mycosis encountered at postmortem and is often not recognized clinically.[34] Predisposing factors include major surgery, steroid therapy, and deep venous lines—intravenous alimentation. Gram-negative sepsis complicating cancer and prolonged antibiotic therapy are also frequent underlying causes. Prematurity and prior treatment with antibiotics have also accounted for the increased incidence of systemic candidiasis during the perinatal period.[35,36] The portal of entry appears to be either the gastrointestinal (GI) tract or deep venous lines, or both.

It usually causes intracerebral microabscesses (Fig. 26-5) and noncaseating granulomas.[37] *Candida* leptomeningitis per se is uncommon, and *Candida* pachymeningitis is rare.[36,38] The most common species in cases CNS moniliasis for which the infecting strains were reliably identified was *C. albicans.* Facial paresis may result from either destruction of the facial nucleus by a microabscess or entrapment of the nerve by the inflammatory process in its subarachnoid course.[39]

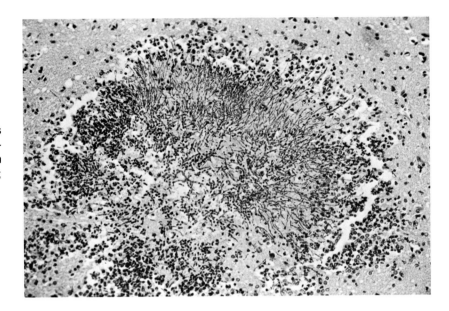

**Fig. 26-5.** Monilial abscess shows abundant polymorphonuclear leukocytes enmeshed in yeast pseudo-hyphae. (H & E; original magnification × 40.)

Aspergillosis is second only to candidiasis in frequency of mycoses among patients with cancer in general and leukemia in particular. Patients with collagen diseases and those on immunosuppression and chemotherapy are also susceptible to aspergillosis.[40] Intravenous narcotic abuse is another significant factor.[41,42] Most patients with CNS aspergillosis have infections elsewhere in the body, especially the lungs, but aspergillosis limited to the CNS has also been described. In such cases, cerebral involvement is sometimes secondary to an orbital,[43] paranasal,[44] or otic infection.Pathologically, vascular thrombosis, hemorrhages, and infarctions are common findings and are due to invasion of the walls of blood vessels by the fungus. Other tissue responses include meningitis, abscesses, and granulomas. Granulomatous masses may occur in the cerebellopontine angle and cause facial nerve dysfunction.[45] Brain stem and/or cerebellar findings were presenting features in three patients and were eventually seen in five others in a series of 12 patients with cerebral aspergillosis analyzed by Beal et al.[44] Although there are 350 species of *Aspergillus*, the vast majority of clinically significant infections are caused by *A. fumigatus*, which is known to produce an endotoxin. *Aspergillus niger* and *A. flavus* are less frequent pathogens.[46] The organisms appear as branched septate hyphae in affected tissue (Fig. 26-6).

*Cryptococcus neoformans* is a yeast measuring 5 to 15 $\mu$m; it has a thick mucoid capsule that stains positively with mucicarmine and periodic acid–Schiff (PAS). CNS infection with the *Cryptococcus* is usually hematogenous, and the portal of entry is believed to be the lungs. Factors predisposing to this opportunistic infection are Hodgkin's disease[47] and immunosuppression. Recently, cryptococcal CNS involvement was described in a few patients with AIDS.[30,48] Pigeon breeders are also at special risk, since the fungus has been isolated in bird nests and excrement[49] in many parts of United States. Cryptococcal meningitis has been reported, however, from many parts of the world.[50] The leptomeninges appear thickened, opacified, and gelatinous. The process is often more severe over the base of the brain and the cerebellum. The leptomeningitis may also be diffuse or patchy. The chronic inflammatory response elicited is usually scanty. Most of the organisms are extracellular, but some may be present in multinucleate giant cells[51] (Fig. 26-7). Long survivals in untreated longstanding cryptococcal meningitis have been reported.[52] Solid or cystic nodules may also occur deep in the brain parenchyma, particularly the basal ganglia. These cysts are flask shaped and contain large collections of organisms floating in gelatinous material with very little reaction visible in the surrounding tissues. Granulomatous meningitis or small, single

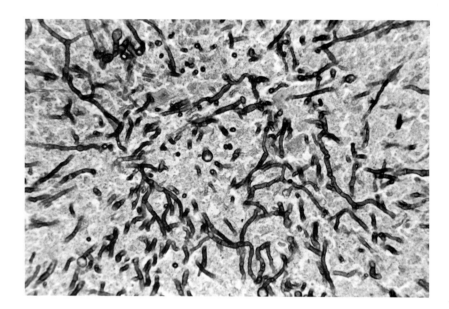

**Fig. 26-6.** Aspergillus hyphae growing in necrotic brain tissue. (Methenamine silver; original magnification × 40.)

or multiple, parenchymal granulomas can occur in some patients, who very often do not have recognized factors predisposing to opportunistic infections.[53] Cranial nerve disturbances, including disturbances of the facial and eighth nerves, occur, though irregularly.[54]

Phycomycosis (mucormycosis) is another saprophytic fungus infection that may attack debilitated hosts. Patients with diabetes mellitus account for up to 80 percent of all reported cases.[55] This infection has also been described in narcotic addicts.[56] Most patients suffer from rhino-orbitocerebral involvement,[57] but mastoid bone infection has been recognized as well.[58] Three genera of Phycomycetes have been isolated: *Rhizopus*, *Mucor*, and *Absidia*. In tissues the fungi appear as nonseptate

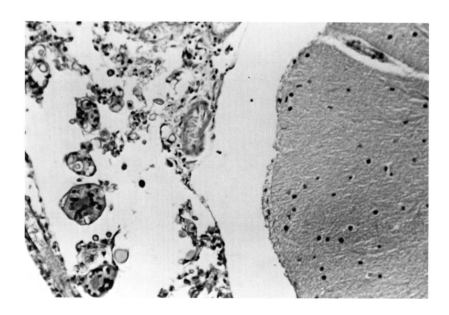

**Fig. 26-7.** Cryptococcosis of the leptomeningitis. Note paucity of inflamatory reaction and presence of the yeast in multinucleated giant cells. (PAS; original magnification × 40.)

coarse hyphae tangled in masses that fill the lumina of vessels (Fig. 26-8), causing thrombosis and ischemic infarctions.

### Demyelinating Diseases

Facial paralysis due to interruption of the intraaxial course of the facial nerve by a multiple sclerosis plaque or lesions of perivenous leukoencephalopathy has been documented. In multiple sclerosis, facial palsy appears usually when the disease is well established; rarely, it is a presenting symptom. Facial palsy was present in 15 percent of patients in Müller's series.[59] If it is an isolated early manifestation of the disease, it may be readily confused with idiopathic Bell's palsy.[60] (The pathogenesis and pathology of demyelinating diseases are covered in Chapter 24.)

### Tumors

The facial nucleus or the intraaxial segment of the facial nerve may be invaded by primary tumors of the CNS or destroyed by metastases. Pontine gliomas are by far the most common primary tumors (see discussion in Chapter 25).

## PERIPHERAL LESIONS

Tschissny's scheme[61] or one of its modifications is helpful in localizing with some accuracy the site of facial nerve lesions. If the lesion of the facial nerve is at the stylomastoid foramen, there is paralysis of all facial muscles, including the orbicularis oculi and frontalis muscles, but taste is preserved. Interruption of the nerve between its junction with the chorda tympani and geniculate ganglion leads to facial paralysis and ipsilateral loss of taste over the anterior two-thirds of the tongue and hyperacusis. Lacrimation is affected if the lesion is situated at the geniculate ganglion.

### Trauma

Facial paresis, usually transient, has been observed in newborn infants, especially after forceps delivery.[62] Injury to the nerve is usually in the peripheral segment as it emerges from the skull. Hemorrhage and edema in the nerve ordinarily resolve, and the functions are totally restored. More serious and often permanent facial nerve palsy has been reported following otologic or parotid sur-

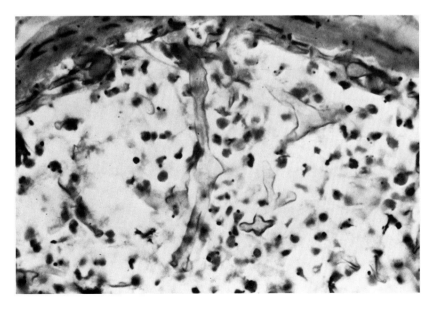

**Fig. 26-8.** Mucormycosis. Nonseptate coarse hyphae filling the lumen of an artery. (PAS; original magnification × 100.)

gery.[63] The facial nerve may also be severed in head injuries, particularly injuries involving fractures of the middle cranial fossa. Facial palsy is more frequent when fractures of the petrous bone are transverse than longitudinal and is frequently associated with deafness and vertigo because of the 8th nerve involvement[64] (see also Chapter 24).

## Idiopathic Polyneuropathy

Cranial nerve dysfunctions have been reported in about one-third of patients with idiopathic polyneuropathy (Landry-Guillain-Barré syndrome). Facial nerve is most frequently involved, and some degree of facial weakness occurs in approximately 50 percent of cases. In one series, more than one-half had bilateral facial palsies.[65] Asbury[66] suggests that if only the facial nerves are involved, certain criteria should be fulfilled to consider such cases as Landry-Guillain-Barré syndrome. Landry-Guillain-Barré syndrome is considered a cell-mediated immunologic disorder. Viral infection has been implicated as a trigger for the reaction, since two-thirds of Landry-Guillain-Barré syndrome patients in most series had experienced an upper respiratory tract infection or a GI ailment 1 to 3 weeks earlier. Serologic studies strongly point to cytomegalovirus (CMV) or Epstein-Barr virus (EBV) infection at least in some reports.[67] Other predisposing conditions include inoculation of foreign proteins such as anti-rabies vaccination, viral exanthemata, and surgical procedures.[68] It has also been reported in patients with neoplasia, particularly Hodgkin's disease.[69]

The lesions are notably seen in the spinal roots, dorsal root ganglia, and major nerve plexuses, largely because these are more accessible for pathologic examination. They consist of focal areas of demyelination with relative preservation of axons and perivascular lymphocytic infiltrates. Myelin damage is carried out largely by macrophages assumed to be sensitized to peripheral myelin.[70] Landry-Guillain-Barré syndrome is usually an acute monophasic disease, but in 3 to 5 percent of patients it has a chronic relapsing or slowly progressive course.[71] The pathologic findings in the peripheral nerves during the exacerbations are essentially the same as in the acute phase. In addition, "onion-bulbs" consisting of supernumerary Schwann cell processes surrounding a segment of an axon usually reflect recurrent demyelination and remyelination.

## Bell's Palsy

The etiology of Bell's palsy, or idiopathic facial paralysis, is unknown. In the acute phase of this common ailment, the nerve is said to be swollen and constricted at the stylomastoid foramen[72,73] and to bulge upon incision of its sheath.[74] However, other investigators have questioned these findings.[75] It has been suggested that viral infection may be responsible,[76,77] and herpes simplex virus (HSV) is strongly suspected.[78,79] Experimental inoculation of different viruses by various routes has shown that several human viruses can infect the facial nerve and geniculate ganglion.[80] Such studies, however, do not quite clarify the cause of Bell's palsy in humans, since facial palsy can also be induced in animals by a variety of methods other than infection, such as application of ice over the mastoid region of rabbits sensitized to horse serum.[81] Furthermore, attempts to culture viruses from geniculate ganglia of patients with Bell's palsy have been unsuccessful.[82] The notion that Bell's palsy is due to inflammation is derived from a very limited number of autopsy and surgical studies. Maximal pathologic changes were present in the geniculate ganglion and adjoining segments of the facial nerve.[83,84] It is possible, however, that the changes described as inflammatory may well represent Wallerian-like degeneration. Whichever factor triggers the inflammation, the congestion and edema that follow cause the nerve to swell and, since it is confined to a rigid canal, entrapment or ischemic neuropathy sets in. A possible correlation of Bell's palsy with diabetes mellitus,[85] hypertension,[86] and pregnancy[87] has been recognized.

## Ramsay Hunt Syndrome

Ramsay Hunt syndrome (geniculate or cephalic herpes zoster), is characterized by herpetic eruptions of the external auditory meatus with or without facial paralysis, vertigo, and deafness. Hunt[88] proposed that the condition is due to inflammation of the geniculate ganglion by varicella zoster virus (VZV) analogous to the dorsal root ganglionitis in spinal zoster. Pathologic studies, however, have shown either completely normal ganglia or variable degenerative or inflammatory changes. The pathology of geniculate ganglionitis was reviewed by Aleksic et al.[89]

## Infections

Acute inflammation of the facial nerve may either occur in acute pyogenic meningitis, the result of extension of the meningeal infection along its roots, or it may be secondary to acute otitis media.[90] In chronic otitis media complicated with a cholesteatoma, the prognosis for recovery of the facial palsy is less favorable.[91] Frequently deafness coexists with the facial palsy. The nerve displays fragmentation of myelin, axonal degeneration, and infiltration with neutrophils. Bilateral facial palsies may also occur in lymphocytic meningoradiculitis, also known as Bannwarth's syndrome.[92] The condition is characterized by pain and sensorimotor disturbances in the distribution of the peripheral nerves, especially the facial nerve. Erythematous skin lesions, sometimes related to a tick bite, often precede the symptoms.

In basal meningitis due to tuberculosis or syphilis, the facial nerves are sometimes affected (see Chapter 24). Sarcoidosis, a granulomatous disease of unknown etiology, also frequently involves the basal meninges, particularly the floor of the third ventricle and the posterior fossa.[93] The facial nerves are therefore frequently implicated; facial palsy is considered the most common neurologic manifestation of sarcoidosis. Colover[94] found facial palsies in 50 percent of his patients. In Delaney's[95] series, however, the frequency was 22 percent. Facial palsy may either be unilateral or bilateral. The onset may be sudden, and the palsy often resolves spontaneously. The frequent occurrence of parotitis in sarcoidosis has led to the belief that the facial nerve was involved during its course in the parotid gland. More recently, however, CNS sarcoidosis was shown to occur with no evidence of disease outside the cranial cavity.[96,97] It is possible that in such instances the facial palsy is due to entrapment of the nerve by the basal leptomeningitis (Fig. 26-9) or concomitant osseous sarcoidosis of the skull bones.[98] It has also been shown that the perivascular (Virchow-Robin) spaces of the brain stem may be distended with granulomas. Such lesions may affect the intraparenchymal course of the facial nerve or its nucleus.

The presence of sarcoid granulomas in the peripheral segment of the facial nerve has not so far been documented histologically. The sarcoid granulomas of peripheral nerves are closely related to

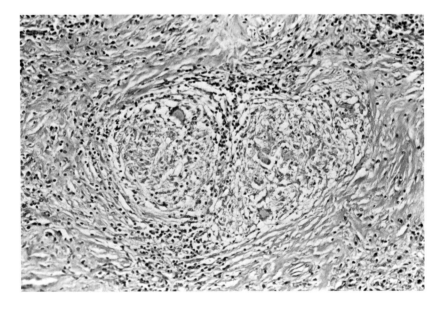

**Fig. 26-9.** Sarcoid granulomas associated with thickened leptomeninges of the brain stem. Granulomas characteristically lack central necrosis. (H & E; original magnification × 40.)

blood vessels and formed of epithelioid cells with occasional multinucleated giant cells. Unlike tuberculous granulomas, caseous necrosis is absent in the center.[99]

### Leprosy

In addition to the cutaneous and superficial mucous membrane manifestations, the peripheral nerves are frequently involved by *Mycobacterium leprae.*[100] Of the cranial nerves, the facial and trigeminal are most susceptible to damage by the disease. Leprosy is a common cause of facial paralysis in endemic regions and may even be a presenting symptom.[101-103] The Madrid classification[104] distinguishes at least four clinical types that largely depend on the host immune reaction to the *Mycobacterium.* In the lepromatous form, which is associated with low immunity, nerve involvement is often symmetric. The nerves are uniformly thickened in the early stages,[105] but later in the course of the disease they become thin and fibrotic. Characteristically there are no inflammatory cells, but rather a marked proliferation of Schwann cells and foamy macrophages. Large numbers of acid-fast bacilli are present within the cytoplasm of these cells, and loss of axons is severe.[106] When the facial nerves are involved, the small superficial branches are affected first. As the leprous neuropathy progresses, lagophthalmos and ectropion of the lid develop.[107] The tuberculoid form occurs in patients with high immunity. Peripheral nerve involvement is focal and usually asymmetric leading to irregular focal enlargement of the affected nerves. Superficially situated nerves, such as the ulnar and lateral popliteal, become palpable. This form of leprous neuropathy is characterized by the formation of epithelioid cell granulomas with central caseation and prominent lymphocytic infiltration. In classic cases, acid-fast bacilli are absent; however, in ultrastructural studies on nerve biopsies from eight early cases, Dastur et al.[108] found acid-fast bacilli in only one case. The granulomas cause only focal destruction of the nerve tissue and Wallerian degeneration distal to the lesions. In dimorphous (or borderline) leprosy,[109] and in the indeterminate[110] group, the cellular reaction and bacterial content of the nerves depend on the immunologic status of the patient.

### Vascular Lesions

Redundant arterial loops[111] or vascular abnormalities[112] in the cerebellopontine angle compressing or stretching the facial nerve have been implicated as one of the causes of hemifacial spasm. In such cases, surgical intervention seems to relieve this distressing condition.[113]

The facial nerve, like the 8th nerve, may be compressed or destroyed by aneurysms (either fusiform or saccular) and by arteriovenous malformations. (See also Chapter 24.)

### Metabolic

Facial palsies occur in metabolic disorders as part of the polyneuropathy.

#### Porphyric Neuropathy

The porphyrias are complex metabolic disorders, usually genetically determined and characterized by increased production of porphyrins and porphyrin precursors in the liver or bone marrow.[114] The peripheral nervous system is principally affected,[115] but the precise mechanism of porphyric neuropathy remains controversial. Earlier researchers were impressed by the segmental demyelination and suggested that the process is essentially a demyelinating neuropathy.[116,117] In recent years, however, the prevailing opinion is that the basic lesion is a dying-back degeneration of the peripheral nerves,[118,119] and is most likely due to neurotoxic effects of porphyrin precursors.[120] In patients with fully developed porphyric neuropathy, cranial nerve involvement may be present. The seventh and tenth cranial nerves are most frequently involved.

#### Diabetic Mononeuropathy

The facial nerves rank fourth after the oculomotor, trochlear, and abducens nerves (in order of decreasing frequency) in likelihood to be affected in diabetes mellitus. It may take the form of a cranial mononeuropathy or may present with multiple cranial nerve involvement.[121,122] In general, diabetic cranial neuropathies occur more often in older patients. Although no pathologic studies are available to determine the nature of the lesion of facial palsy in these cases, it can be assumed that the pathogenesis is similar to the oculomotor palsy in diabetes mellitus and is therefore most likely vascular ischemic in nature.[123] The role of diabetes in predisposing to, or causing, Bell's palsy, however, has been controversial. On the basis of his findings of a higher incidence of abnormal glucose tolerance in patients with Bell's palsy, Korczyn[124] considered diabetes an important factor; however, Takahashi and Sobue[125] disagree with this contention.

### Amyloidotic Cranial Neuropathy

In certain hereditary forms of amyloidosis, cranial nerve palsies may occur. The facial nerves are particularly involved in some Finnish kindred with familial amyloidosis who present with latice corneal dystrophy in their third decade and paresis of the upper branch of the facial nerves in the fifth decade.[126] Autopsy studies showed marked amyloid deposition in the cranial nerves, especially the facial nerves, with only moderate amyloid infiltration of the peripheral nervous system, meninges, and meningeal vessels.[127] Visceral amyloidosis, primarily in the blood vessels, was also present. Facial nerve involvement is also seen in familial oculoleptomeningeal amyloidosis,[128] in which extensive amyloid deposition is found in the adventitia of leptomeningeal vessels as well as in leptomeninges.

### Degenerative

Facial weakness has been described in several disorders characterized by degeneration of the lower motor neurons.[129] These conditions are collectively referred to as *hereditary motor neuropathies*.[130-132] Facial paresis is particularly prominent in type II hereditary motor neuropathies (Kugelberg-Welander disease or chronic proximal spinal muscular atrophy), in facioscapulohumeral hereditary motor neuropathies, in bulbar hereditary motor neuropathies (Vialetto-van Laere syndrome and Fazio-Londe disease), and in X-linked recessive bulbospinal neuropathy. Autopsy reports concerning CNS changes are relatively few, but all stress neuronal loss and gliosis of the bulbar nuclei and anterior horns.[133,134]

## Tumors

### Schwannomas

The facial nerve may be compressed by a schwannoma arising from the 8th nerve as it grows out of the internal auditory canal and extends into the cerebellopontine angle. Sometimes the schwannoma originates in the facial nerve itself.[135] About 2 percent of all schwannomas in the petrous bone arise from the facial nerve.[136] If the growth is too advanced, however, it is difficult to determine with certainty the nerve from which it has originated. In such cases, it fills up the tympanic cavity; if it spreads into the attic of the middle ear it may erode the tegmen tympani and appears as an extradural mass in the middle cranial fossa. Tumors in the vertical portion may destroy the posterior wall of the external auditory canal and the tympanic membrane, thus predisposing to secondary infection. The growth may rarely spread below the base of the skull.[137] If the tumor is in the first or third part of the facial canal, facial palsy occurs with or without loss of taste in the anterior two-thirds of the tongue. If the tumor is in the second part, deafness may be the first presenting symptom.[138] Schwannomas of the facial nerve have been reported in the parotid gland and are usually mistaken for mixed parotid tumors.

### Paragangliomas

Paragangliomas (or chemodectomas) arise from the glomus jugulare (which consists of small clusters of chemoreceptor cells in the adventitia of the jugular bulb[139]) or from the paraganglion tympanicum[140] and vagale.[141,142] Glomus vagale and jugulare tumors cause 9th, 10th, and 11th nerve palsies (jugular foramen syndrome) and sometimes may invade the labyrinth. Glomus tympanicum tumors occur in the middle ear and usually produce conductive hearing loss, pulsatile tinnitus, and facial weakness. Chemodectomas are vascular tumors that cause erosion and destruction of the bony structures of the middle ear. The more aggressive forms may extend into the posterior fossa and compress the brain stem, especially the region of the cerebellopontine angle.[143,144] If they appear in the external auditory canal, they may be mistaken for polyps. Microscopically, they are made up of nests of large monomorphic round or cuboidal cells supported by a reticulin framework. These nests, or *Zellballen*, are separated by richly vascularized fibrous septae (Fig. 26-10). The tumor cells have a granular cytoplasm and, despite their designation as "nonchromaffin tumors," faint chromaffin reaction may be obtained by the Del Rio Hortego technique[145] if the material is optimally fixed. Dense-core secretory granules can be demonstrated ultrastructurally.[146] The nuclei are round and usually regular in shape; however, as in many other endocrine tumors, bizarre nuclei may be seen that should not be interpreted as indicative of malignancy. Two or more chemodectomas may occur simultaneously,[147] and familial incidence has been reported.[148] There are no definite criteria that predict the more aggressive behavior of some 10 percent of all paragangliomas.[149]

### Epidermoid Cysts and Cholesteatomas

Intracranial epidermoid cysts frequently occur in the petrous bone[150,151] and in the cerebellopontine angle.[152] In the latter location, they are only superseded by schwannomas and meningiomas in decreasing order of frequency. There is some controversy as to whether the so-called cholestea-tomas of the middle ear are actually epidermoid cysts derived from squamous epithelial rests in the attic of the petrous bone or are the result of metaplastic changes secondary to chronic ear infection.[153,154] Epidermoid cysts of the cerebellopontine angle vary greatly in size; in extreme cases; they may extend from the perichiasmatic region down to the foramen magnum (Fig. 26-11). The capsule is smooth or focally bosselated and has a characteristic mother-of-pearl sheen. The content is variably described as cheesy or flaky. Focal calcifications may be found in the capsule. The capsule is composed of stretched and compressed stratified squamous epithelium supported externally by a thin layer of connective tissue. The content of the cyst consists of lamellar desquamated keratin. Rupture of epidermoid cysts in the subarachnoid space or in the ventricles may cause foreign-body-type inflammation of the leptomeninges or ependymal lining, respectively[155,156] (Fig. 26-12). Epidermoid cysts in the cerebellopontine angle may occur at any age, but they usually become symptomatic in the fifth decade. Hemifacial spasm may be an early symptom, and erosion of the petrous apex is frequently found on plain radiographs of the skull. In cholesteatomas (keratomas) of the petrous bone, the accompanying chronic ear infection may cause facial nerve dysfunction.

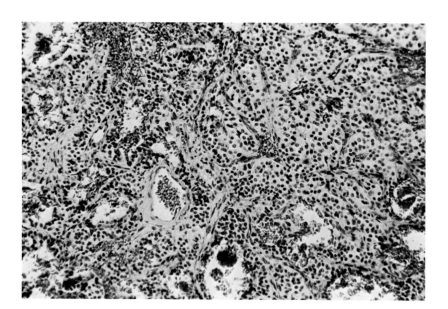

**Fig. 26-10.** Paraganglioma from a patient with jugular foramen syndrome. Tumor cells are arranged in small nests separated by relatively thin vascular septae. (H & E; original magnification × 40.)

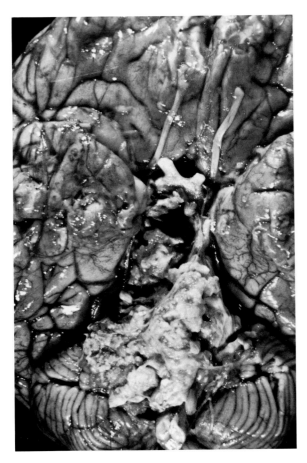

**Fig. 26-11.** Epidermoid cyst of the right cerebellopontine angle. This patient had refused surgery. At autopsy the cyst was found to have extended from the optic chiasm to the foramen magnum.

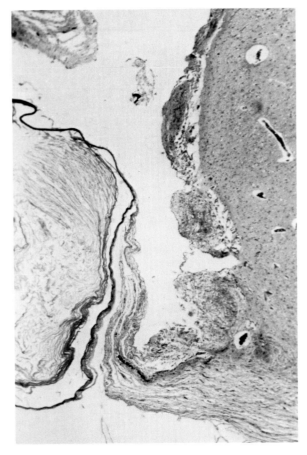

**Fig. 26-12.** Epidermoid cyst (right) had ruptured into the ventricle. The ventricular lining shows several excrescences representing chronic ventriculitis caused by keratin. (H & E; original magnification × 10.)

## Arachnoid or Leptomeningeal Cysts

Arachnoid cysts are loculated collections of fluid in the subarachnoid space. They are usually translucent and filled with clear fluid. Some are acquired but most are congenital.[157,158] Electron microscopic studies have shown that in the congenital type, the cyst lining varies from flattened cells to ependymal-like epithelium (Fig. 26-13). Occasionally, the cells resemble choroidal cells[159]; tufts similar to fronds of a choroid plexus have also been described.[160] The acquired cysts develop as a result of circumscribed pial-arachnoid adhesions usually secondary to meningitis or head trauma. In the posterior fossa, arachnoid cysts have some predilection to the cerebellopontine angle.[157,161]

## Primary Epidermoid Carcinomas of the Cerebellopontine Angle

Primary epidermoid carcinomas of the cerebellopontine angle arise either de novo or from a preexisting epidermoid cyst.[162,163] They are extremely rare and usually occur in the fourth or fifth decade of life. They are more common in males. Other rare primary carcinomas occurring in this region include ceruminous gland adenocarcinomas,[164] adenoid cystic carcinoma, basal cell carcinoma, and

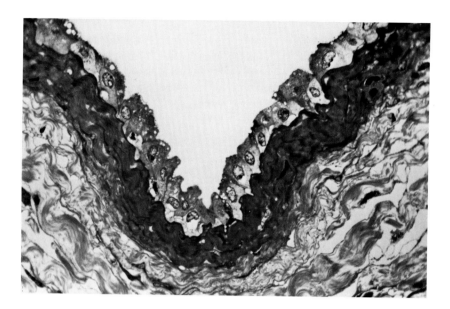

**Fig. 26-13.** Arachnoid cyst of the cerebellopontine angle. The cyst is lined by columnar epithelium; some of the cells are ciliated. (H & E; original magnification × 40.)

mucoepidermoid carcinoma.[165] The facial nerve may be destroyed by primary or secondary neoplasms of the petrous bone.[166]

## Miscellaneous

### Melkersson-Rosenthal Syndrome

Melkersson-Rosenthal syndrome is a rare disorder characterized by a triad of recurrent attacks of facial paralysis indistinguishable from Bell's palsy, usually beginning before 16 years of age, consisting of episodes of facial edema affecting particularly the upper lip, leading to permanent facial enlargement and, less consistently, plication of the tongue (lingua plicata).[167] The facial nerve is swollen and displays lymphocytic infiltration and interstitial edema.[168] Although granulomas are observed in the oral mucosa (cheilitis granulomatosa),[169] no such granulomatous reaction has been described in the facial nerve. The cause of the syndrome is unknown, but occasionally its association with other neurologic dysfunctions (i.e., congenital megacolon and deafness) suggests a congenital defect in the autonomic nervous system.[170]

### Facial Hemiatrophy of Romberg

Facial hemiatrophy of Romberg is a rare and curious condition that affects mainly females and that usually begins during adolescence.[171] It is characterized by a loss of cutaneous fat characteristically on one side of the face. The facial muscles and bones on the affected side may also be involved but to a lesser extent.[172] Autonomic disturbances such as Horner's syndrome have been described in abortive forms of the disease.

## REFERENCES

1. Adams RD, Victor M: Principles of Neurology. McGraw-Hill, New York, 1977
2. Hoefnagel D, Penry JK: Partial facial paralysis in young children. N Engl J Med 262:1126, 1960
3. Cayler GC: An "epidemic" of congenital facial paresis and heart disease. Pediatrics 40:666, 1967
4. Pape KE, Pickering D: Asymmetric crying facies: An index of other congenital anomalies. J Pediatr 81:21, 1972
5. Möbius PJ: Uber angeborene doppelseitige Abducens-Facialis-Lähmung. MMW 35:91, 1888

6. Henderson JL: The congenital facial diplegia syndrome: Clinical features, pathology and etiology. Brain 62:381, 1939

7. Hanissian A, Fuste F, Hayes WT, Duncan JM: Möbius syndrome in twins. Am J Dis Child 120:472, 1970

8. Zitter FA, Wiser WC, Robinson A: Three-generation pedigree of a Möbius syndrome variant with chromosome dislocation. Arch Neurol 34:437, 1977

9. Pitner SE, Edwards JE, McCormick WF: Observations on the pathology of Möbius syndrome. J Neurol Neurosurg Psychiatry 28:362, 1965

10. Sprofkin BE, Hillman JW: Möbius's syndrome — Congenital oculofacial paralysis. Neurology (NY) 6:50, 1956

11. Thakkar N, O'Neil W, DuVally J, et al: Möbius syndrome due to brain stem tegmental necrosis. Arch Neurol 34:124, 1977

12. Towfighi J, Marko K, Palmer E, Vanwucci R: Möbius syndrome. Neuropathologic observations. Acta Neuropathol (Berl) 48:11, 1979

13. Gilles FH: Hypotensive brain stem necrosis. Arch Pathol Lab Med 88:32, 1969

14. Leech R, Alvord EC Jr: Anoxic-ischemic encephalopathy in the human neonatal period: The significance of brain stem involvement. Arch Neurol 34:109, 1977

15. Stehbens WE: Pathology of the Cerebral Blood Vessels. CV Mosby, St. Louis, 1972

16. Russell DS: The pathology of spontaneous intracranial hemorrhage. Proc R Soc Med 47:689, 1954

17. Dinsdale HB: Spontaneous hemorrhage with observations on the pathogenesis. Arch Neurol 10:200, 1964

18. Aleksic S, Budzilovich G: Lateral inferior pontine syndrome. J Neurol Sci 18:317, 1973

19. Kase CS, Maulsby GO, Mohr JP: Partial pontine hematomas. Neurology (NY) 30:652, 1980

20. Charcot JM, Bouchard C: Nouvelles recherches sur la pathogénie de l'hémorrhagie cérébrale. Arch Physiol (Norm) Pathol 1:110, 1868

21. Hutchinson EC, Acheson EJ: p. 86. In Walton JW (ed): Major problems in Neurology. Vol. 4: Pathology and Surgical Treatment. WB Saunders, London, 1975

22. Fischer CM: The arterial lesions underlying lacunes. Acta Neuropathol (Berl) 12:1, 1969

23. Adams R: Occlusion of the anterior inferior cerebellar artery. Arch Neurol Psychiatry 49:765, 1943

24. Bergeron C, Rewcastle NB, Richardson JC: Pontine infarction manifesting as isolated cranial nerve palsies. Neurology (NY) 29:377, 1979

25. Engler CW, Missal SC: Involvement of the cranial nerves in poliomyelitis. Trans Am Acad Ophthalmol Otolaryngol 59:732, 1955

26. Waxman SG, Sabin TD, Embree LJ: Subacute brain-stem encephalitis. J Neurol Neurosurg Psychiatry 37:811, 1974

27. Horoupian DS, Kim Y: Encephalomyeloneuropathy with ganglionitis of the myenteric plexuses in the absence of cancer. Ann Neurol 11:628, 1982

28. Brain L, Adams RD. Epilogue: A guide to the classification and investigation of neurological disorders associated with neoplasms. p. 216. In Brain L, Norris FH (eds): Contemporary Neurology Symposia. Vol. 1: The Remote Effects of Cancer on the Nervous System. Grune & Stratton, Orlando, FL, 1965

29. Henson RA, Hoffman HL, Urich H: Encephalomyelitis with carcinoma. Brain 88:449, 1965

30. Snider WD, Simpson DM, Nielsen S, et al: Neurological complications of acquired immune deficiency syndrome: Analysis of 50 patients. Ann Neurol 14:403, 1983

31. Duffy PE, Sassin JF, Summers DS, Lourie H: Rhombencephalitis due to Listeria monocytogenes. Neurology (NY) 14:1067, 1964

32. Weinstein AJ, Schiavone WA, Furlan AJ: Listeria rhombencephalitis. Report of a case. Arch Neurol 39:514, 1982

33. Goodhill V: Syphilis of the ear: A histopathologic study. Ann Otol Rhinol Laryngol 48:676, 1939

34. Parker JC Jr, McCloskey JJ, Lee RS: Human cerebral candidosis — A postmortem evaluation of 19 patients. Hum Pathol 12:23, 1981

35. Seelig MS: The role of antiobiotics in the pathogenesis of candida infections. Am J Med 40:887, 1966

36. Lilien LD, Ramamurthy RS, Pildes RS: Candida albicans meningitis in a premature neonate successfully treated with 5-fluorocytosine and amphotericin B: A case report and review of the literature. Pediatrics 61:57, 1978

37. Block JT: Cerebral candidiasis: Case report and review of literature. J Neurol Neurosurg Psychiatry 33:864, 1970

38. Bayer AS, Edwards JE, Seidel LB, et al: Candida meningitis. Medicine (Baltimore) 55:477, 1976

39. Gorell JM, Palutke WA, Chason JL: Candida pachymeningitis with multiple cranial nerve paresis. Arch Neurol 36:719, 1979

40. Young RC, Bennet JE, Vogel CL, et al: Aspergil-

losis: The spectrum of the disease in 98 patients. Medicine (Baltimore) 49:147, 1970

41. Burston J, Blackwood W: A case of aspergillosis infection of the brain. J Pathol 86:225, 1963

42. Kaufman DM, Thal LJ, Farmer PM: Central Nervous system. Aspergillosis in two young adults. Neurology (NY) 26:484, 1976

43. Hedges TR, Leung L-SE: Parasellar and orbital apex syndrome caused by aspergillosis. Neurology (NY) 26:117, 1976

44. Beal MF, O'Carroll CP, Kleinman GM, Grossman RI: Aspergillosis of the nervous system. Neurology (NY) 32:473, 1982

45. Iyer S, Dodge PR, Adams RD: Two cases of aspergillus infection of the central nervous system. J Neurol Neurosurg Psychiatry 15:152, 1952

46. Mukoyama M, Gimple K, Poser CM: Aspergillosis of the central nervous system. Report of a brain abscess due to A. fumigatus and review of the literature. Neurology (NY) 19:967, 1969

47. Collins VP, Gellhorn A, Tremble JR: Coincidence of cryptococcosis and diseases of the reticuloendothelial and lymphatic systems. Cancer 4:883, 1951

48. Reichert CM, O'Leary TJ, Levens DL, et al: Autopsy pathology in the acquired immune deficiency syndrome. Am J Pathol 112:357, 1983

49. Halde C, Fraher MA: Cryptococcus neoformans in pigeon feces in San Francisco. Cal Med 104:188, 1966

50. Tay CH, Chew WLS, Lim LCY: Cryptococcal meningitis: Its apparent increased incidence in the Far East. Brain 95:825, 1972

51. Mosberg WH Jr, Arnold JG Jr: Torulosis of the central nervous system: Review of literature and report of five cases. Ann Intern Med 32:1153, 1950

52. Marshall M, Teed RW: Torula histolytica meningoencephalitis: Recovery following bilateral mastoidectomy and sulfonamide therapy. (Preliminary report.) JAMA 120:527, 1942

53. Markham JW, Alcott DL, Manson RM: Cerebral granuloma caused by cryptococcus neoformans. Report of a case. J Neurosurg 15:562, 1958

54. Roberts M, Rinaudo PA, Tilton RC, Vilinskas J: Treatment of multiple intracerebral cryptococcal granulomas with 5-fluorocytosine. (Case report.) J Neurosurg 37:229, 1972

55. Kasper LH, Bernat JL, Nordgren RE, Reeves AG: Bilateral rhinocerebral phycomycosis. Ann Neurol 6:131, 1979

56. Masucci EF, Fabaro JA, Saini N, Kurtzke JF: Cerebral mucormycosis (phycomycosis) in a heroin addict. Arch Neurol 39:304, 1982

57. Pillsbury HC, Fischer ND: Rhinocerebral mucormycosis. Arch Otolaryngol 103:600, 1977

58. Gregory J, Golden A, Haymaker W: Mucormycosis of central nervous system: Report of three cases. Bull Johns Hopkins Hosp 73:405, 1943

59. Müller R: Studies on disseminated sclerosis with special reference to symptomatology, course and prognosis. Acta Med Scand 133[suppl]:222, 1949

60. Hallpike JF: Clinical aspects of multiple sclerosis. p. 129. In Hallpike JK, Adams CWM, Tourtellotte WW (eds): Multiple Sclerosis. Williams & Wilkins, Baltimore, 1983

61. Tschiassny K: Eight syndromes of facial paralysis and their significance in locating the lesions. Ann Otol Rhinol Laryngol 62:677, 1953

62. Hepner WR Jr: Some observations on facial paresis in the newborn infant: Etiology and incidence. Pediatrics 8:494, 1951

63. Miehlke A: Typical sites of facial nerve lesions. Arch Otolaryngol 89:122, 1969

64. Grove WE: Skull fractures involving the ear: A clinical study of 211 cases. Laryngoscope 49:678, 1939

65. Soffer D, Feldman S, Alter M: Clinical features of the Guillain-Barré syndrome. J Neurol Sci 37:135, 1978

66. Asbury A: Diagnostic considerations in Guillain-Barré syndrome. Ann Neurol 9[suppl]:1, 1981

67. Dowling PC, Cook SD: Role of infection in Guillain-Barré Syndrome: Laboratory confirmation of herpes viruses in 41 cases. Ann Neurol 9[suppl]:44, 1981

68. Arnason BGW: Acute inflammatory demyelinating polyradiculoneuropathies. p. 2050. In Dyck PJ, Thomas PK, Lambert EH, Bunge R (eds): Peripheral Neuropathy. Vol. II. WB Saunders, Philadelphia, 1984

69. Lisak RP, Mitchell M, Zweiman B, et al: Guillain-Barré syndrome and Hodgkin's disease: Three cases with immunologic studies. Ann Neurol 1:72, 1977

70. Prineas JW: Pathology of the Guillain-Barré syndrome. Ann Neurol 9[suppl]:6, 1981

71. Dyck PJ, Lais AC, Ohta M, et al: Chronic inflammatory polyradiculoneuropathy. May Clin Proc 50:621, 1975

72. Cawthorne T: Peripheral facial paralysis: Some aspect of its pathology. Laryngoscope 56:653, 1946

73. Jongkees LBW: On peripheral facial nerve paralysis. Arch Otolaryngol 95:317, 1972

74. Pulec J: Discussion. Arch Otolaryngol 95:414, 1972

75. Sadé J, Levy E, Chaco J: Surgery and pathology of Bell's palsy. Arch Otolaryngol 82:594, 1965

76. Adour KK, Byl FM, Hilsinger RL, et al: The true nature of Bell's palsy. Analysis of 1000 consecutive patients. Laryngoscope 88:787, 1978

77. Djupesland G, Berdal P, Johannessen TA et al: Viral infection as a cause of acute peripheral facial palsy. Arch Otolaryngol 102:403, 1976

78. Adour KK, Bell DN, Hilsinger RL: Herpes simplex virus in idiopathic facial paralysis (Bell's palsy). JAMA 233:527, 1975.

79. Sapiro SM: Bell's palsy associated with acute herpetic gingivostomatitis. Oral Surg 39:403, 1975

80. Davis LE: Experimental viral infections of the facial nerve and geniculate ganglion. Ann Neurol 9:120, 1981

81. Karnes WE: Diseases of the seventh cranial nerve. p. 1266. In Dyck PJ, Thomas PK, Lambert EH, Bunge R (eds): Peripheral Neuropathy. Vol. II. WB Saunders, Philadelphia, 1984

82. Palva T, Hortling L, Ylikoski J, et al: Viral culture and electron microscopy of ganglion cells in Ménière's disease and Bell's palsy. Acta Otolaryngol (Stockh) 86:269, 1978

83. Antoli-Candela F, Stewart TJ: The pathophysiology of otologic facial paralysis. Otolaryngol Clin North Am 7:309, 1974

84. Brackman DE: Bell's palsy. Incidence, etiology and results of medical treatment. Otolaryngol Clin North Am 7:357, 1974

85. Korczyn AD: Bell's palsy and diabetes mellitus. Lancet 1:108, 1971

86. Vassalo L, Galea-Debono A: An etiology of Bell's palsy. (Letter to the editor.) Lancet 2:383, 1972

87. Korczyn AD: Bell's palsy and pregnancy. Acta Neurol Scand 47:603, 1971

88. Hunt JR: On herpetic inflammation of the geniculate ganglion: A new syndrome and its complications. J Nerve Ment Dis 34:73, 1907

89. Aleksic SN, Budzilovich GN, Lieberman AN: Herpes zoster oticus and facial paralysis (Ramsey Hunt syndrome). Clinicopathologic study and review of literature. J Neurol Sci 20:149, 1973

90. McGovern FH, Fitz-Hugh GS: Diseases of the facial nerve. Laryngoscope 66:187, 1956

91. Riskaer N: The course of the otitic facial palsy under adequate treatment of the disease of the ear. Acta Otolaryngol (Stockh) 34:280, 1946

92. Wulff CH, Hansen K, Strange P, Trojaburg W: Multiple mononeuritis and radiculitis with erythema, pain, elevated CSF protein and pleocytosis (Bannwarth's syndrome) J Neurol Neurosurg Psychiatry 46:485, 1983

93. Widerholt WC, Siekert RG: Neurological manifestations of sarcoidosis. Neurology (NY) 15:1147, 1965

94. Colover J: Sarcoidosis with involvement of the nervous systems. Brain 71:451, 1948

95. Delaney P: Neurologic manifestations in sarcoidosis: Review of the literature, with a report of 23 cases. Ann Intern Med 87:336, 1977

96. Griggs RC, Markesbery WR, Condemi JJ: Cerebral mass due to sarcoidosis; regression during corticosteroid therapy. Neurology (NY) 23:981, 1973

97. Lax, F, Tabaddor K: Extraparenchymal sarcoid mass: A case report. Neurosurgery 5:604, 1979

98. Case records of the Massachusetts General Hospital: N Engl J Med 307:1257, 1982

99. Oh SJ: Sarcoid polyneuropathy: A histologically proven case. Ann Neurol 7:178, 1980

100. Sabin TD, Sweift TR: Leprosy. p. 1955. In Dyck PJ, Thomas PK, Lambert EH, Bunge R (eds): Peripheral Neuropathy. Vol. II. WB Saunders, Philadelphia, 1984

101. Bosher SK: Leprosy presenting as facial palsy. J Laryngol Otol 76:827, 1962

102. Dastur DK, Antia NH, Diverkar SC: The facial nerve in leprosy. II. Pathology, pathogenesis, electromyography, and clinical correlations. Int J Lepr 34:118, 1968

103. Van Droogenbroeck JBA: The surgical treatment of lower facial palsy in leprosy. Ann Soc Belg Med Trop 50:653, 1970

104. Madrid classification. Technical resolutions. Int J Lepr 21:504, 1953

105. Job CK, Desikan KV: Pathologic changes and their distribution in peripheral nerves in lepromatous leprosy. Int J Lepr 36:257, 1968

106. Job CK: Mycobacterium Leprae in nerve lesions in lepromatous leprosy. An electron microscopic study. Arch Pathol Lab Med 89:195, 1970

107. Sabin TD: Neurologic features of lepromatous leprosy. Am Fam Physician 4:84, 1971

108. Dastur DK, Ramamohan Y, Shah JS: Ultrastructure of nerves in tuberculoid leprosy. Neurology (India) 20[suppl 1]:89, 1972

109. Finlayson MH, Bilbao JM, Lough JO: The pathogenesis of the neuropathy in dimorphous leprosy: Electron microscopic and cytochemical studies. J Neuropath Exp Neurol 33:446, 1974

110. Boddingius J: Ultrastructureal changes in blood vessels of peripheral nerves in leprosy neuropathy. I. Tuberculoid and borderline tuberculoid leprosy patients. Acta Neuropathol (Berl) 35:159, 1976

111. Jannetta PJ: Microsurgical exploration and decom-

pression of the facial nerve in hemifacial spasm. Curr Top Surg Res 2:217, 1970

112. Maroon JC: Hemifacial spasm, a vascular cause. Arch Neurol 35:481, 1978

113. Jannetta PJ: Observations on the etiology of trigeminal neuroalgia, hemifacial spasm, and acoustic nerve dysfunction and glossopharyngeal neuralgia. Definite microsurgical treatments and results in 117 patients. Neurochirurgia (Stuttg) 20:145, 1977

114. Schmidt R, Schwartz S, Watson CT: Porphyrin content of bone marrow and liver in the various forms of porphyria. Arch Intern Med 93:167, 1954

115. Wochnik-Dyjas D, Niewiadamska M, Kostrzewska E: Porphyric polyneuropathy and its pathogenesis in the light of electrophysiological investigations. J Neurol Sci 35:243, 1978

116. Denny-Brown D, Sciarra D: Changes in the nervous system in acute porphyria. Brain 68:1, 1945

117. Campbell JAH: The pathology of South African genetic porphyria. S Afr J Lab Clin Med 9:197, 1963

118. Cavanagh JB, Mellick RS: On the nature of the peripheral nerve lesions associated with acute intermittent porphyria. J Neurol Neurosurg Psychiatry 28:320, 1965

119. Thorner PS, Bilbao JM, Sima AAF, Briggs S: Porphyric neuropathy: An ultrastructural and quantitative case study. Can J Neurol Sci 8:281, 1981

120. Goldberg A, Paton WDM, Thompson JW: Pharmacology of the porphyrins and porphobilinogen. Br J Pharmacol 9:91, 1954

121. Garcin R, Lapresle J: Complications nerveuses péripheriqnes et centrales du diabète sucré. Assises Med 14:346, 1956

122. Justin-Besancon L, Cornet A, Contamin F et al: Attente aiguë bilatérale et partiellement reversible de plusieurs paires craniennes (7-8-9-10) chez une diabétique ayant presenté sept ans auparavant une atteinte encéphalique aiguë reversible. Bull Soc Med Hop (Paris) 114:985, 1963

123. Asbury AK, Aldredge H, Hershberg R, Fisher CM: Oculomotor palsy in diabetes mellitus: A clinicopathological study. Brain 93:55, 1970

124. Korcyzn AD: Bell's palsy and diabetes mellitus. Lancet 1:108, 1971

125. Takahashi A, Sobue I: Concurrence of facial paralysis and diabetes mellitus: Prevalence, clinical features and prednisone treatment. p. 173. In Goto Y, Horiuchi A, Kogure K (eds): Diabetic Neuropathy Excerpta Medica, Amsterdam, 1982

126. Meretoja J: Familial systemic paramyloidosis with lattic dystrophy of the cornea, progressive cranial neuropathy, skin changes and various internal symptoms. Ann Clin Res 1:314, 1969

127. Meretoja J, Teppo L: Histopathological findings of familial amyloidosis with cranial neuropathy as principal manifestation. Acta Pathol Microbiol Immunol Scand [A] 79:432, 1971

128. Goren H, Steinberg MC, Farboody GH: Familial oculoleptomeningeal amyloidosis. Brain 103:473, 1980

129. Emery AEH: Review: The neurology of the spinal muscular atrophies. J Med Genet 8:481, 1971

130. Pearn JH: Classification of the spinal muscular atrophies. Lancet 1:919, 1980

131. Harding AE: Inherited neuronal atrophy and degeneration predominantly of lower motor neurons. p. 1537. In Dyck PJ, Thomas PK, Lambert EH, Bunge R (eds): Peripheral Neuropathy. Vol II. WB Saunders, Philadelphia, 1984

132. Kennedy WR, Alter M, Sung JH: Progressive proximal spinal and bulbar muscular atrophy of late onset. A sex linked recessive trait. Neurology (NY) 18:671, 1968

133. Alberca R, Montero C, Ibanez A, et al: Progressive bulbar paresis associated with neural deafness. A nosologic entity. Arch Neurol 37:214, 1980

134. Gallai V, Hockaday JM, Hughes JT, et al: pontobulbar palsy with deafness (Brown-Vialetto-Van Laere syndrome). A report on 3 cases. J Neurol Sci 50:250, 1981

135. Pulec JL: Facial nerve tumors. Ann Otol 78:962, 1969

136. House WF, Luetje CM: Evaluation and preservation of facial function. Post operative results. In House WF, Luetje CM (eds): Acoustic Tumors. Vol. 2. University Park Press, Baltimore, 1979

137. Shambaugh GE, Arenberg IK, Burney PL: Facial neurilemmomas. A study of four diverse cases. Arch Otolaryngol 90:742, 1969

138. Bogdasarian RM: Neurinoma of the facial nerve. Arch Otolaryngol 40:291, 1944

139. Guild S: The glomus jugulare, a nonchromaffin paraganglion in man. Ann Otol Rhinol Laryngol 62:1045, 1953

140. Lattes R, Waltner JG: Nonchromaffin paraganglioma of the middle ear (carotid-body-like tumor; glomus jugulare tumor) Cancer 2:447, 1949

141. Rosenwasser H: Glomus jugulare tumors. Arch Otolaryngol 88:1, 1968

142. Shermer KL, Pantino EE, Dziabis MD, McQuistan RJ: Tumors of the glomus jugulare and glomus tympanicum. Cancer 19:1273, 1966

143. Bickerstaff ER, Howell JS: The neurological importance of tumors of the glomus jugulare. Brain 76:576, 1953

144. Hawk WA, McCormack LJ: Nonchromaffin paraganglioma of the glomus jugulare. Review of the

literature and report of six cases. Cleve Clin Q 26:62, 1959

145. Barroso-Moguel R, Costero I: Argentaffin cells of the carotid body tumor. Am J Pathol 41:389, 1962

146. Grimley PM, Glenner GG: Histology and ultrastructure of carotid body paragangliomas; comparison with the normal gland. Cancer 20:1473, 1967

147. Kipkie GF: Simultaneous chromaffin tumors of the carotid body and glomus jugulare. Arch Pathol Lab Med 44:113, 1947

148. Zacks SI: Chemodectomas occurring concurrently in the neck (carotid body), temporal bone (glomus jugulare) and retroperitoneum; report of a case with histochemical observations. Am J Pathol 34:293, 1958

149. Whimster WF, Masson AF: Malignant carotid body tumor with extradural metastases. Cancer 26:239, 1970

150. Jefferson G, Smalley AA: Progressive facial palsy produced by intratemporal epidermoids. J Laryngol 53:417, 1938

151. Pennybacker J: Cholesteatoma of the petrous bone. Br J Surg 32:75, 1944

152. Mahoney W: Die epidermoide des Zentral nerven systems. Z Gesamte Neurol Psychiat 155:416, 1936

153. Tytus JS, Pennybacker J: Pearly tumors in relation to the central nervous system. J Neurol Neurosurg Psychiatry 19:24, 1956

154. Sadé J: Pathogenesis of attic cholesteatomas. J R Soc Med 71:716, 1978

155. Schwartz JF, Benlentine DJ: Recurrent meningitis due to an intracranial epidermoid. Neurol 28:124, 1978

156. Horoupian DS, Wisniewski HM, Gamble R, Liebskind AL: Aqueductal gliosis caused by keratin and cholesterol in a case of craniopharyngioma. Can J Neurol Sci 1:185, 1974

157. Rengachary SS, Watanabe I: Ultrastructure and pathogenesis of intracranial arachnoid cysts. J Neuropathol Exp Neurol 40:61, 1981

158. Patrick BS: ependymal cyst of the Sylvian fissue. Case report. J Neurosurg 35:751, 1971

159. Koto A, Horoupian DS, Shulman K: Choroidal epithelial cyst. Case report. J Neurosurg 47:955, 1977

160. Lewis AJ: Infantile hydrocephalus caused by arachnoidal cyst. Case report. J Neurosurg 19:431, 1962

161. Gomez MR, Yanagihara T, McCarty CS: Arachnoid cysts of the cerebellopontine angle and infantile spastic hemiplegia. J Neurosurg 29:87, 1968

162. Wong SW, Ducker TB, Powers JM: Fulminating parapontine epidermoid carcinoma in 4 year old. Cancer 37:1525, 1976

163. Garcia CA, McGarry PA, Rodriguez F: Primary intracranial carcinoma of the right cerebellopontine angle. J Neurosurg 54:824, 1981

164. Cilluffo JM, Harner SG, Miller RH: Intracranial ceruminous gland adenocarcinoma. J Neurosurg 55:952, 1981

165. Heffelfinger MJ, Dahlin DC, MacCarty CS, Beabont JW: Chordomas and cartilaginous tumors at the skull base. Cancer 32:410, 1973

166. Proctor B, Lindsay J: Tumors involving the petrous pyramid of the temporal bone. Arch Otolaryngol 46:180, 1974

167. Melkersson E: Ett fall ar recidiverande facialispares i samband med angioneurotiskt ödem. Hygie 90:737, 1928

168. Hornstein OP: Melkersson-Rosenthal syndrome. p. 205. In Vinken PJ, Bruyn GW (eds): Handbook of Clinical Neurology. Vol. 8: Disease of Nerves. Part II. North-Holland, Amsterdam 1970

169. Meischer G: Über essentielle granulomatose Makrocheilie (cheilitis granulomatosa). Dermatologica (Basel) 91:57, 1945

170. Klaus SN, Brunsting LA: Melkerson's syndrome (persistent swelling of the face, recurrent facial paralysis, and lingua plicata): Report of a case. Mayo Clin Proc 34:365, 1959

171. Romberg MH: Klinische Ergebnisse. A Förstner, Berlin, 1846

172. Wartenberg R: Progressive facial hemiatrophy. Arch Neurol 54:75, 1945

# Pathogenesis and Pathology of Otitis Media

# 27

David J. Lim
Thomas F. DeMaria

## HISTORICAL BACKGROUND

Otitis media was well recognized as one of the major causes of death during the late 1800s[1]: one in every 158 postmortems in London's Guy's Hospital, one in every 232 in Vienna General Hospital, and one in every 303 in Communal Hospital in Copenhagen. Of those treated, the fatality rate ranged from 0.2 to 2.5 percent. Bezold and Siebenmann[1] believed these figures to be lower than the true incidence of mortality due to otitis media. Because routine postmortems did not include temporal bone examination, many cases of otogenic cause of death could have been missed, particularly in young children. This supposition was borne out by the later observation by von Troeltsch that inflammatory changes with gathering of secretion in the middle ear was found in nearly every postmortem examination in infants during the first few years.[1] Presyng found pathologic changes in the middle ear in 81 of 100 postmortem examinations of children under 3 years of age.[1]

The bacteriology of otitis media was already well established in the latter part of the nineteenth century. Bezold and Siebenmann[1] stated:

The presence of organized germs of infection has been established with such regularity that we can not doubt of their causative importance as to the pathogenesis of all inflammations of the middle ear. The numerous bacteriological examinations made since *Zaufal's* initiative showed that germs were never absent in the slight cases which do not perforate, as well as in the serious perforating forms of inflammations.

*Zaufal* and later investigators only exceptionally succeeded in raising cultures of some few germs from the normal drum-cavity. We are justified in the supposition that so small a quantity of germs are powerless against the living cells of the normal lining of the middle ear. We also found the transudations formed ex vacuo in the middle ear after prolonged occlusion of the tubes, to be free of the germs. The exudations which form while symptoms of inflammation are present and which always contain more or less cells, on the contrary are regularly impregnated with one or more forms of pathogenic micro-organisms.

Diplococcus pneumoniae [currently *Streptococcus pneumoniae*] and streptococcus pyogenes are found the most frequently. The different forms of staphylococcus pyogenes [currently *Staphylogoccus aureus*] usually appear secondarily after a suppuration has lasted for a while, although some-

779

times they seemed to be the primary infection. . . . Even the germs which usually cause some general acute infectious disease like influenza, typhoid, diphtheria bacillus and meningococcus intracellularis were found in the purulent secretions of the middle ear.

An early account of the detailed bacteriology was also given by Barr,[2] who listed the following bacteria as important:

(1) The streptococcus pyogenes . . . , which seems to be most frequently associated with chronic purulent disease and with cranial suppurations attending it. This is one of the most virulent microorganisms found in the ear. (2) Frankel's pneumococcus or diplococcus . . . (3) The pneumo-bacillus of Friedlander [currently *Hemophilus influenzae*]. These two latter organisms seem to be most frequently associated with the acute forms of purulent middle ear disease, and are both encapsuled when found in the body. (4) The staphylococcus . . . , albus and aureus, are also frequently found in connection with purulent processes in the middle ear, . . .

Other bacteria mentioned include tubercle bacillus, Löffler's bacillus (diphtheria), and *Micrococcus* of ozena.

The investigators at the turn of the century had already demonstrated that certain bacteria are intimately involved in the pathogenesis of otitis media. They remain so today, with the exception of the generalized infectious disease that plagued the general population at that time, but it is no longer a major public health problem. It is astonishing to note that the bacterial flora involved in acute otitis have not changed much since that time.

## DEFINITION AND CLASSIFICATION

With interest in otitis media growing worldwide, it is necessary to have common definitions and classifications to improve communication among the clinicians and researchers throughout the world. These definitions and classifications should be based on a sound clinical and scientific rationale. For the most part, there is consensus on the terms, with the exception of secretory otitis media, or chronic otitis media with effusion. The disagreement is largely due to differences of opinion as to its pathogenesis and pathologies, but also to linguistic differences.

The classification of otitis media was already advanced in the times of Politzer, Bezold, and Toynbee; however, there is evidence that no consensus was reached. In the fifteenth lecture of his *Text-Book of Otology*,[1] Bezold stated, "There is no agreement amongst authors as to the classification and nomenclature of diseases of the middle ear. All inflammations of the middle ear were called catarrhal in former years." Then he argued that because in postmortem examinations of the ear he found different pathologic anatomic changes in the cartilaginous part of the tube from those in the bony part the use of the generalized term *catarrh* (inflammation of mucous membrane) to denote different diseases of the spaces of the middle ear complicated matters rather than cleared them up. He further stated:

In classifying the diseases of the middle ear, we must therefore first set apart pure *uncomplicated occlusion of the tube*, as an independent disease. . . .

There are other *inflammatory processes* in the middle ear of extremely varying intensity, partly in connection with long lasting occlusion of the tubes, partly independent from it, which are all caused by immigration of germs of infection either from the outside or with the blood.

A classification of the diseases of the middle ear based on the different species of bacilli and cocci which cause them, can not be carried out, because, with the exception of the tubercle bacillus, they all may provoke symptoms of inflammation which are quite similar in quality and may vary in the same species from the mildest to the most severe.

The only remaining principle of a classification is the different clinical and pathologic anatomical appearance. We differentiate two main groups, *otitis media simplex or non perforative*, and *otitis media purulenta* or *suppurative*, or *perforative*.

He then devised the following classification based on consideration of the course of the disease:

1. Occlusion of the tubes and its physiologic consequence
2. Otitis media simplex, acute and subacute

3. Otitis media simplex chronica
4. Otitis media purulenta acuta
5. Otitis media purulenta chronica
6. Residues of otitis media purulenta with permanent perforation
7. Residues of otitis media purulenta with closed perforation[1]

The classification recently proposed by Bluestone and Klein[3] used perforation as a criterion similar to that already proposed by Bezold and Siebenmann[1] at the turn of the century.

In 1983, the panel of clinicians and scientists at the Research Conference on Recent Advances in Otitis Media with Effusion[4] recommended the following classification:

1. Myringitis (with or without external otitis or otitis media)
2. Acute suppurative otitis media (acute purulent otitis media, acute otitis media)
3. Secretory otitis media (chronic otitis media with effusion, nonsuppurative otitis media, catarrh), serous otitis media (serotympanum), mucoid otitis media (mucotympanum)
4. Chronic suppurative otitis media (chronic otitis media)

---

# INCIDENCE, EPIDEMIOLOGY, AND NATURAL HISTORY

## Incidence

Health statistics available from the Department of Health, Education and Welfare (now the Department of Health and Human Services) indicated there were 9.9 million visits to physicians' offices due to otitis media in 1955 and that it ranked second of most common diseases in children, following upper respiratory infection.[5] Kessner et al.[6] estimated the incidence of otitis media to be 30 percent in the 6-month-old to 3-year-old group in the United States, similar to recent data obtained in Finland.[7] Howie et al.[8] observed a higher incidence in Huntsville; 76 percent of the children had at least one bout of ear infection by 6 years of age,

which is similar to findings in Boston[9] and in Denmark.[10] In their cohort study in Denmark, in which 729 children were followed from birth to 9 years of age, Stangerup and Tos[10] showed the incidence of acute otitis media to be about 22 percent in the first year, 15 percent in the second year, 10 percent in the third and fourth years, and 2 percent in the eighth year. By the end of the third year of life, 50 percent of all children had had at least one episode of acute otitis media; by the age of 9, 75 percent had had one. Prevalence was about 25 percent during the first 5 years, dropping to 7 percent during the eighth and ninth years. Most of the attacks (80 percent) during the first 2 years were bilateral, whereas after the sixth year, 86 percent of the children had experienced unilateral disease. Reliable data on the incidence of otitis media with effusion are not available because of its often asymptomatic nature.[11,12]

## Epidemiology

A number of studies in recent years have addressed the epidemiology and natural history of otitis media,[12–23] and an excellent review was recently done by Giebink.[24] Several important factors appear to be closely related to the occurrence of otitis media.

### Age

Otitis media is predominantly a disease of infants and young children. Forty-five percent of children have their first episode of otitis media by age 1 and 61 percent by age 2.[8] Similar results were reported by Teele et al.[14] in Boston, showing 47 percent had their first otitis media at 1 year and 71 percent by 3 years of age.

### Sex

Most studies show a greater frequency of acute otitis media among males (61 to 70 percent),[24] although a few studies have shown no gender-based differences.[25] Similar results have been obtained in patients with otitis media with effusion (59 to 72 percent).[24]

### Race

American Indians, Eskimos, and Hispanic children have a higher incidence of otitis media than do

American whites, while American blacks have a lower rate.[13,14,16,26] The reasons for these differences are not fully known, but one could be differences in tubal anatomy among the races.[27]

### Season

There is ample evidence documenting seasonal patterns in the incidence of acute otitis media and chronic otitis media with effusion.[28-30] The peak season is between October and April, and the low season is during the summer months. There is a slight lag in the incidence of chronic otitis media with effusion (Fig. 27-1). This seasonal incidence coincides with that of upper respiratory infection.

### Family History

Children with a positive sibling or parent history of otitis media had a higher incidence of the disease than did children from families with no histories of otitis media.[4,23] The risk of chronic otitis media with effusion was reported to be two times higher for children with a positive family history than for those with a negative family history.[20] These reports support the notion of a genetic background that may be more susceptible to otitis media.

### Allergy

Although allergy has been considered a risk factor, no definitive evidence has been forthcoming that it is a major risk factor for chronic otitis media with effusion.[15,31-33] However, recent studies suggest that the allergic or atopic child is at increased risk of otitis media.[20,23]

### Other High-Risk Factors

Childen with cleft palate,[34] Downs syndrome,[35] and Kartagener's (or immotile cilia) syndrome[3] are universally considered a high-risk group. For cleft palate and Down's syndrome, the cause of the high incidence is the anatomic defects of the craniofacial structures, which affect tubal function.[36] In Kartagener's syndrome, the defective motility of the cilia in the tubotympanum deprives the ear of mucociliary protection, resulting in easy bacterial invasion.

## Natural History

Accurate information concerning the natural history of otitis media is not readily available, because once diagnosed the treatment cannot be withheld. Thus, most of the studies have involved intervention. A few studies have addressed the disappearance of the effusions after an acute episode of otitis media. After the first episode, 70 percent of children still had otitis media with effusion at 2 weeks, 40 percent at 4 weeks, 20 percent at 8 weeks, and 10 percent at 12 weeks, according to Teele et al.[14]; similar results were reported by Schwartz et al.[17] Thus, 10 percent of acute otitis media is expected to develop into chronic otitis media with effusion, if one defines chronicity as a duration of 12 weeks or longer.[37]

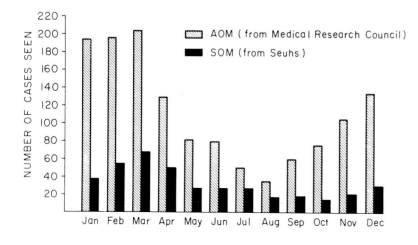

**Fig. 27-1.** Comparison between the monthly pattern of acute otitis media (AOM)[29] and that of serous otitis media (SOM).[28] (Lim DJ, DeMaria TF: Pathogenesis of otitis media. Bacteriology and Immunology. Laryngoscope 92:278, 1982.)

A number of studies have indicated that the incidence of chronic (persistent) middle ear effusion is closely related to a prior history of acute otitis media.[18,20] The chance of persistent middle ear effusion is correlated with the number of episodes. The risk of persistent effusion increases 6.9 times in children with one or two episodes, but it increases 165.7 times in children with more than six episodes.[20] Furthermore, if the acute episodes occurred in children under 2 years of age, the chance of having persistent effusion was four times higher.[38]

Only a few studies have been done on the natural history of chronic otitis media with effusion (or secretory otitis media). A recent study by Tos et al.[22] of three cohorts of children followed by tympanometry for 6 to 8 years after birth showed that (1) 15 percent of the ears had single episodes of 1 to 6 months duration, (2) about 25 percent of the ears developed short but recurring episodes of 1 to 6 months duration, (3) about 15 percent of the ears developed protracted episodes of 6 to 12 months duration, (4) about 15 percent of the ears developed protracted cases that improved but deteriorated again, and (5) about 10 percent of the ears developed very protracted cases of 1 to 4 years duration. These results indicate that about 25 percent of ears that suffer from chronic otitis media with effusion (secretory otitis media) will have rather significant sequelae.

# PATHOGENESIS OF OTITIS MEDIA

There is abundant epidemiologic and clinical evidence supporting the notion that tubal dysfunction, upper respiratory viral infection, and a high incidence of nasopharyngeal bacterial colonization are important predisposing factors in the pathogenesis of otitis media.[3,24]

The tubotympanum is protected by the mucosal defense system common to all mucous membranes exposed to the external environment. The mucosal defense system comprises (1) mechanical defense (e.g., mucociliary transportation system containing the mucous blanket, ciliated cells, and mucous cells); (2) biologic defense (e.g., antibacterial enzyme secretion); (3) immunodefense (e.g., humoral and cellular immune system); (4) phagocytosis (polymorphonuclear neutrophils, macrophages) (Fig. 27-2). The entire length of the eustachian tube and the middle ear mucosa near the tubal opening are provided with a mucociliary as well as a secretory defense system. It is important to understand that when any one of these systems is compromised, the person becomes predisposed to otitis media.

Although it is not fully documented, there is good reason to believe that chronic otitis media with effusion is related to the acute condition.[20] Of those who suffered from chronic otitis media with effusion, 97 percent had histories of acute otitis media.[39] Because the predisposing factors involved in both acute otitis media and chronic otitis media with effusion are similar if not identical, they are dealt with together here.

## Role of Tubal Dysfunction

There is good epidemiologic evidence that persons with high negative middle ear pressure are a high-risk group.[40] Susceptibility to chronic otitis media with effusion parallels the anatomic maturation of the tubal muscles and cartilage.[41] Patients with increased tubal compliance (lack of stiffness) are susceptible to the development of chronic otitis media with effusion,[42] and in one study tubal dysfunction was found in all 38 otitis media patients studied.[43] Obviously children with high negative pressure due to poor tubal function represent a high-risk group.[12]

Bluestone and Beery[42] demonstrated that patients with an increase of compliance of the tube (floppy tube) are prone to develop serous otitis media, and the younger the children the floppier the tube. A maturing process of the tube takes place in the young age group, and proper stiffness and adequate muscle strength will be attained by age 10 or so.[41]

Casselbrant et al.[12] further documented that a larger number of children develop high negative middle ear pressure during the winter months, supporting an earlier epidemiologic observation that the prevalence of acute otitis media as well as

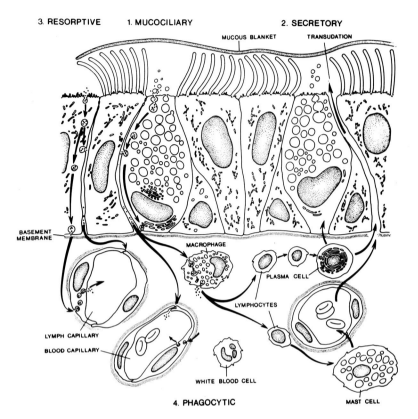

3. RESORPTIVE    1. MUCOCILIARY    2. SECRETORY

MUCOUS BLANKET    TRANSUDATION

BASEMENT
MEMBRANE

MACROPHAGE

PLASMA CELL

LYMPHOCYTES

LYMPH CAPILLARY

BLOOD CAPILLARY

WHITE BLOOD CELL

4. PHAGOCYTIC

MAST CELL

**Fig. 27-2.** Mucosal defense systems illustrated graphically. (Drawing by Nancy Sally.)

chronic otitis media with effusion has seasonal fluctuations that correlate with high negative pressure.[44-46] A study conducted by Bylander and colleagues[40] indicated that children who develop otitis media with effusion show a greater incidence of hypomuscular tubal function, but these workers suggested that these children may become a high-risk group when additional risk factors are superimposed.

Poor tubal function has been suggested to cause transudation in the tympanum because of negative pressure after the absorption of air by the mucosa,[47] and absorption of gas in the tympanic cavity has been documented.[48] Tubal occlusion in animal experiments resulted in middle ear transudation.[49] Besides its contribution to middle ear transudation, such negative pressure may also increase the chance of a bolus of mucus containing bacteria being sucked in from the pharynx, causing ear infection.[50,51]

## Role of Mucosal Secretion

Whether the middle ear effusion is secreta or transudate has been hotly debated. Because of their different biologic activities, determination of the origin of middle ear effusion is important. The presence of numerous secretory cells in the middle ear mucosa of cases of chronic otitis media with effusion[52-55] and the high concentration of hexosamine (mucopolysaccharides)[56] and secretory immunoglobulins (SIgA) and bactericidal substances (e.g., lysozyme and lactoferrin)[57-60] in the effusions strongly suggest a secretory origin, at least in part, for middle ear effusion, particularly of the mucoid type (Fig. 27-3). Furthermore, when these secretory products were compared with the bacterial recovery rate in the middle ear effusion they were inversely related.[61] This finding supports the hypothesis that the middle ear secretory defense (mucociliary and immune) systems may mature

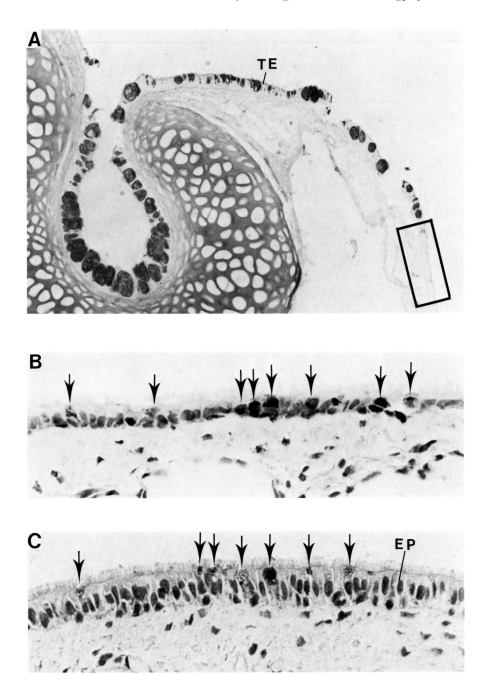

**Fig. 27-3.** **(A)** Cross-sectional view of the eustachian tube near the tympanal orifice showing transitional epithelium (TE) following Alcian blue-PAS staining. **(B)** Enlarged view of the boxed area in **A**, stained for lactoferrin, showing of the cuboidal area of the transitional zone with cells strongly positive for lactoferrin (arrows), which are AB-PAS negative. CA, capillary, **(C)** Epithelium (Ep) of the transitional zone (near eustachian tube) of chinchilla middle ear mucosa showing lysozyme-positive secretory cells (arrows). (Original magnifications: B × 480, C × 400.) (Hanamure Y, Lim DJ: Normal distribution of lysozyme- and lactoferrin-secreting cells in the chinchilla tubotympanum. Am J Otolaryngol 7:410, 1986. Reprinted with permission from WB Saunders Co.)

with age.[62,63] This concept is compatible with the current understanding of mucosal immunity.[64,65] It can also be postulated that these immunoglobulins and their amplification factors (e.g., lysozyme, lactoferrin) may modify the behavior of the infection, resulting in chronic otitis media with effusion.

## Role of Transudation

Serous effusions have been postulated to be transudates and mucoid effusion to be serous fluid condensed by the middle ear mucosa. Albumin is a serum protein marker often used as a measure for transudation. The ratio of effusion albumin to serum albumin concentrations was about equal in both mucoid and serous effusions.[62] When effusion immunoglobulin profiles were examined, the highest concentration of immunoglobulin was IgG, followed by IgA and IgM, a similar pattern to that of internal fluids such as cerebrospinal fluid (CSF), synovial fluid, and peritoneal fluid (Fig. 27-4). However, the fact that effusion IgG and IgA are significantly greater than those of sera suggests the local production of immunoglobulins that are exudated. Thus, it appears that middle ear effusion is a mixture of secreta, exudates, and transudates (sera), but the proportions may vary. However, mucoid effusions tend to contain more secreta and, conversely, serous effusions tend to contain more transudate.

## Role of Bacteria

### Nasopharyngeal Flora

The normal tubotympanal mucosa is protected by the mucociliary transportation system and by surface mucosal immunoglobulins (SIgA), that inhibit bacterial adhesion to the mucosal surfaces. Therefore, for otitis media to occur, three conditions must be met: (1) bacterial adherence to the nasopharynx, (2) bacterial entry to the tubotympanum, and (3) bacterial replication in the tympanum (Fig. 27-1). There is ample evidence suggesting that there is a higher incidence of bacterial colonization (pathogens) in the nasopharynx among patients with histories of acute otitis media

(90 percent), as well as chronic otitis media with effusion (80 percent), compared with the low incidence (2 percent) of nasopharyngeal colonization of normal patients.[50,66,67]

### Bacterial Adhesion

A fundamental understanding of bacterial adhesion is important in understanding the pathogenesis of all mucosal infections. A considerable body of knowledge has accumulated in recent years concerning the mechanism by which bacteria adhere to host cells. The bacteria mediate adherence to the host cells by adhesive appendages (adhesins or ligands), which interact with host cell receptors.[68-74] Adhesins are defined as molecular adhesive structures on the surface of a microorganism and have been shown to be generally composed of protein, lipid, or carbohydrates. Adhesins are often associated with bacterial appendages that project outward from the cell, such as fibrillae, which are short, hairy, irregular filamentous structures of some gram-positive organisms, or fimbriae, which are large structures of uniform size and shape often associated with gram-negative bacteria. In addition to fimbrial or fibrillar adhesins, however, bacteria may adhere to host cells via interactions of their glycocalyx, a polysaccharide-rich external network of fibers.[75] This structure is capable of interacting with the host cell through a variety of specific and nonspecific associations.

The host receptors are usually sugar residues (e.g., mannose, fucose, sialic acid) and most likely exist as either glycolipids or glycoproteins in the cell membrane. Host receptors for the bacterial pathogens involved in otitis media have not been fully characterized, with the exception of *Streptococcus pneumoniae*, which is reported to bind to GlcNAc$\beta$1 $\rightarrow$ 3Gal sugar residue of the host cell surfaces.[76]

Because the bacterial appendages (fibrillae and fimbriae) are often intimately involved in bacterial adhesion to the mucosal surfaces, including the nasopharyngeal epithelium, it should be possible to develop monoclonal antibodies against the specific bacterial appendages. Attempts have made to purify the bacterial appendage (pilus) of *Hemophilus influenzae* type b, and it is reported to be a protein with a molecular weight of 24,000.[77] Theoreti-

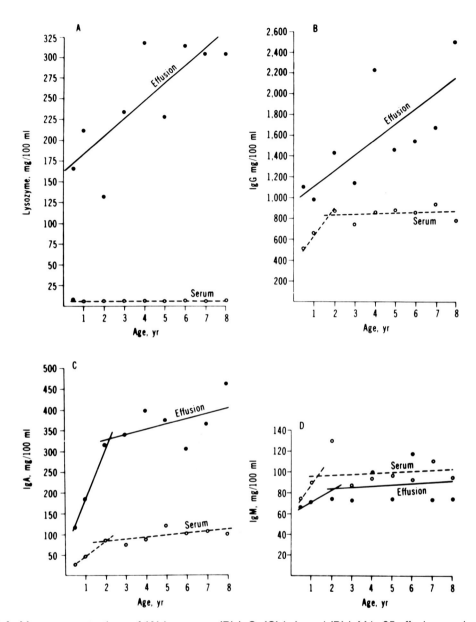

**Fig. 27-4.** Mean concentrations of **(A)** lysozyme, **(B)** IgG, **(C)** IgA, and **(D)** IgM in 95 effusions and sera from patients suffering from chronic otitis media with effusion (serous otitis media), grouped by age. (Liu YS, Lim DJ, Lang RW, Birck HG: Chronic middle ear effusions: Immunochemical and bacteriological investigation. Arch Otolaryngol 101:278, 1975. Copyright 1975, American Medical Association.)

cally, antibodies against bacterial appendages can block adherence, thereby preventing bacterial infection. Such a strategy would be worthwhile because elicitation of host antibody using capsular polysaccharide as an antigen has serious limitations due to the poor immune response obtained in human subjects in the age group under 2 years.[78,79]

### Specific Bacteria Pathogens

**Acute Otitis Media.** Studies of the etiology of acute otitis media have not indicated any major changes in the relative frequency of the major bacterial species for over 40 years.[80] *Strep. pneumoniae* and *H. influenzae* remain the major pathogens of acute otitis media in all age groups. Group A β-hemolytic streptococci, *Staphylococcus aureus*, and gram-negative enteric bacilli are infrequent causes of otitis media. The incidence of *Branhamella catarrhalis°*-induced otitis media is on the rise in certain regions of the United States. Recent data indicate that approximately 10 percent of effusions from cases of acute otitis media are sterile, and an additional 21 percent contain a bacterium, whose pathogenic role in otitis media has not been conclusively established, such as *Staphylococcus epidermidis* or various diphtheroid species.[81] Whether these organisms are contaminants is currently the subject of much debate.[82] Recent epidemiologic data indicate that upper respiratory tract virus, *Mycoplasma*, anaerobes, and *Chlamydia* may also be etiologic agents, in varying degrees, of acute otitis media.

*Streptococcus pneumoniae* is the most important cause of acute otitis media and the subject of numerous investigations. The number of serotypes responsible for approximately 85 percent of infections of the middle ear is limited to 11 of the 86 known serotypes. The six most common types, in order of decreasing frequency, are 19, 23, 6, 14, 3, and 8. The reason only a limited number of serotypes are responsible for most cases of otitis media is not known. Recent data suggest that a differential ability for each serotype to attach and colonize the upper respiratory tract may be responsible for this

association of a limited number of serotypes. Perhaps the most important development in recent years has been the emergence of strains of *Pneumococcus* that are relatively resistant to amoxicillin and other antimicrobial agents. Although resistant *Strep. pneumococci* account for fewer than 1 percent of all cases of acute otitis media, there is reason to suspect that these resistant strains will become more prevalent in the future.

*Hemophilus influenzae* rank as the second most frequently isolated pathogen from cases of acute otitis media and accounts for approximately 20 percent of the bacteria isolated.[81] Although six serotypes of *H. influenzae* (types a–f) are recognized, approximately 90 percent of all cases of *H. influenzae* acute otitis media are due to nontypable strains. Type b *H. influenzae*, a major pathogen in other pediatric infectious diseases, accounts for slightly less than 10 percent of the acute otitis media associated with this pathogen. This pathogen was previously thought to have limited importance; it was designated a significant cause of otitis media primarily in preschool-age children. However, recent studies indicate that this is not the case and that nontypable *H. influenzae* is a significant pathogen in all age groups. Recent epidemiologic evidence indicates that approximately 15 to 30 percent of the *H. influenzae* middle ear isolates produce β-lactamase.[3]

Group A streptococci have been recognized as pathogens. *Strep. pyogenes* has been reported as a significant pathogen in epidemiologic studies from Japan and Scandanavia but not in the United States.[80] The reason for this geographic difference is unknown. In the United States, group A streptococcus accounts for only 2 percent of the bacterial species isolated from cases of otitis media. A similar discrepancy exists in the reported incidence of *Staph. aureus* isolation from middle ear effusions due to acute otitis media. Several reports from Japan stated an incidence of 19 percent from *Staph. aureus*,[83,84] whereas in numerous other studies over the past 10 years *Staph. aureus* isolates approximate the same low incidence as that for *Strep. pyogenes*. *Branhamella catarrhalis* isolation from cases of acute otitis media has been the focus of much debate in recent years. Evidence has been accumulating that this bacteria is a true pathogen in the middle ear, and its incidence is increasing in

---

° Genus *Branhamella* has recently been changed to *Moraxella*.

certain geographic areas in the United States. Reports indicate an incidence ranging from 8 percent in Dallas to 22 percent and 27 percent in Cleveland[85] and Pittsburgh,[86] respectively. Perhaps the most convincing evidence is a study from Finland by Leinonen et al.[87] that demonstrated IgA antibody to *B. catarrhalis* in 42 percent of middle ear effusion specimens and found a significant rise in serum IgG antibodies in 53 percent of children whose middle ear specimens contained *B. catarrhalis*. In more than half of the case reports, *B. catarrhalis* is isolated in pure culture. Together, the culture and serologic evidence lend credence to the argument that this bacteria is indeed capable of initiating acute otitis media. In addition, approximately 80 percent of *B. catarrhalis* strains produce β-lactamase,[85] which may account for the increasing number of therapeutic failures with amoxicillin.

Coagulase-negative staphylococci is a generic term that includes 11 different species as defined by the identification scheme proposed by Kloos and Schleifer.[88] Although they represent 21 percent of the bacteria isolated from cases of acute otitis media, the role of coagulase-negative staphylococci in the pathogenesis of this disease remains uncertain. These organisms are usually considered commensals and are part of the skin flora of the external ear canal. However, as with *B. catarrhalis*, specific antibody has been found bound to *Staph. epidermidis* in middle ear effusions from cases of acute otitis media. The precise contribution of contamination of middle ear effusions with coagulase-negative staphylococci to the overall incidence of these bacteria isolated from acute middle ear effusion is yet to be determined. One possibility is that they are bona fide pathogens capable of invading and causing disease in the middle ear, as proposed by Feigen et al.[89] Another is that they are opportunistic pathogens that invade the middle ear only under certain circumstances, such as persistent effusion.

Gram-negative enteric bacilli are responsible for approximately 2 percent of all cases of acute otitis media but for 21 percent of cases in infants under 6 weeks of age. This predilection for neonates has been attributed to colonization of the infant during birth, together with overall immature or inadequate immune system. In all cases, acute otitis media caused by this group of organisms is associated with a high rate of complications, including bacteremia, mastoiditis, and osteomyelitis.[90]

Anaerobic bacteria have rarely been identified as pathogens of acute otitis media. The initial report of a significant number of anaerobic isolates was subsequently refuted by the original authors.[91,92] Disinfection of the auditory canal prior to tympanocentesis drastically reduced the incidence of positive anaerobe cultures, suggesting that the initial high incidence of positive anaerobic cultures can be attributed to contamination of middle ear effusions with anaerobes from the external auditory canal.

**Chronic Otitis Media with Effusion (Secretory Otitis Media).** Although middle ear effusions of chronic otitis media with effusion are presumably sterile bacteriologically,[93] recent data have demonstrated that 22 to 40 percent of cases show culturable bacteria,[18,28,29,39,57,61,86,94–101] and 80 percent of the samples had bacteria present in Gram-stained smears.[61] This wide range of bacterial recovery rates in otitis media with effusion may result in part from differences in culture technique, in patient population, and/or in the definition of pathogens.

A large number (20 to 50 percent) of young children with acute otitis media may be left with chronic otitis media with effusion.[8,102] Giebink et al.[39] found 97 percent of cases of chronic otitis media with effusion to have histories of prior acute otitis media, strongly suggesting the relatedness of chronic otitis media with effusion to acute otitis media and thus a bacterial pathogenesis of chronic otitis media with effusion. The striking similarity between the monthly incidence of acute otitis media and chronic otitis media with effusion[28,29] further supports this relatedness. The high incidence of pathogenic flora in the nasopharynx among acute otitis media (98 percent) and chronic otitis media with effusion (84 percent) patients, compared with the low incidence in healthy persons (18 percent), further suggests a bacterial pathogenesis for chronic otitis media with effusion.[103] Additional supportive evidence is that effusions with positive bacterial culture were associated with a significantly high number of polymorphonuclear neutrophils in the effusions,[18,104] and the presence of specific antibodies to bacteria in the effusions from patients with chronic otitis media with effusion.[105]

Data from Lim and DeMaria[106] based on a study of 957 middle ear effusions collected over a 5-year period from patients aged 3 months to 11 years suffering from chronic otitis media with effusion show that 54 percent of middle ear effusions were culture negative and 46 percent culture positive. Among the positive cultures, *H. influenzae* represented the single most common organism recovered (24.6 percent). *B. catarrhalis* represented 14 percent, *Strep. pneumoniae* represented 9.4 percent, and *Staph. aureus* was cultured in 0.7 percent of middle ear effusions. These four organisms are commonly considered pathogens and represent 34.7 percent of the total bacteria recovered. However, diphtheroids were cultured in 14.2 percent and *Staph. epidermidis* in 20.5 percent of middle ear effusions, and these organisms are often considered nonpathogens for otitis media. If one considers them nonpathogens, the bacterial recovery rate is drastically reduced. However, recent studies have suggested that both diphtheroids and *Staph. epidermidis* are not contaminants. Specific IgA antibody to diphtheroids was found in some effusions but not in the matching sera.[105] On the basis of various biologic characteristics, Bernstein et al.[82] concluded that coagulase-negative staphylococci *(Staph. epidermidis)* found in middle ear effusions are different from those found in the external canal skin or behind the ear. In another study, Bernstein and Ogra,[107] also observed specific antibodies against *Staph. epidermidis* in the effusions in certain cases of chronic otitis media with effusion, also suggesting that this organism may be a pathogen.

Information concerning anaerobes in chronic otitis media with effusion is contradictory, and no conclusion can be drawn as to their role. Fulghum et al.[108] reported that four of 10 (40 percent) effusions obtained from patients with chronic otitis media with effusion yielded anaerobes (*Propionibacterium acnes* being the most prominent organism), often found as mixed flora with aerobes, particularly *Staph. epidermidis.* Others have failed to duplicate these results.[14,39,80,98] Recently, experimental otitis media with anaerobes was successfully produced in guinea pigs.[109] Further study is clearly needed.

Although there are many similarities in the species of bacteria isolated from cases of chronic otitis media with effusion and acute otitis media, there are also several striking differences, as pointed out by Giebink et al.[39] *H. influenzae* is the predominant pathogen isolated from cases of chronic otitis media with effusion, and this organism is associated primarily with serous effusions. *Staph. epidermidis* is the second most frequently isolated pathogen and is clearly most prevalent in mucoid effusions.

**Chronic Suppurative Otitis Media.** Chronic suppurative otitis media is most often a recurrent rather than a constant infection associated with a tympanic membrane perforation and/or cholesteatoma. The bacterial pathogens associated with this condition by and large represent contaminants that invade the middle ear via the external canal through the tympanic membrane perforation. More than 50 percent of cases of chronic suppurative otitis media represent mixed infections, with two to five organisms typically present.[110] Mixed aerobic and anaerobic infections and aerobic infection alone are common.

*Pseudomonas aeruginosa* is the most frequent aerobic bacteria associated with cases of chronic suppurative otitis media, followed by *Staph. aureus.* The balance of aerobic isolates is a mixed flora of *Escherichia coli, Proteus,* and other enteric organisms. The most frequently isolated anaerobic pathogens are various species of the genus *Bacteroides,* in 13 percent of cases, followed by various anaerobic species of *Staphylococcus* and *Streptococcus.*[111] It should be noted that unlike the case in acute otitis media or chronic otitis media with effusion, anaerobes are important pathogens in chronic suppurative otitis media.

### Role of Mycoplasma

Originally it was reported that *Mycoplasma* is the causative agent of bullous myringitis when Rifkind et al.[112] induced this condition in nonimmune volunteers inoculated with *Mycoplasma pneumoniae.* Subsequent studies by Sobeslavsky et al.[113] indicated that *Mycoplasma* was not present in more than 700 middle ear effusions examined, and Roberts[114] indicated in a thoroughly documented review that mycoplasmas play no role in bullous myringitis and no significant role in acute otitis media.

## Role of Chlamydia

*Chlamydia trachomatis* is the etiologic agent of a mild but prolonged pneumonitis in infants. The first indication *C. trachomatis* could induce acute otitis media was reported by Dawson et al. in 1967.[115] Eleven of 17 adult volunteers, during experiments designed to induce experimental eye infections, developed otitis media. Subsequently, it was shown by Schachter et al.[116] and Tipple et al.[117] that children with chlamydial pneumonia also have otitis media. In studies of children over 1 year of age with chlamydial pneumonitis, the organism is rarely recovered from middle ear fluid. No systematic study of infants under 6 months of age — the peak period for chlamydial infection — has been reported. However, it is assumed that *Chlamydia* are important etiologic agents of acute otitis media in this age group.

## Role of Viral Infection

Even though viruses are not frequently recovered from middle ear effusions, there is epidemiologic evidence to suggest that upper respiratory infection predisposes the ear to infection.[118] Although upper respiratory viral infection has been suspected of being associated with the pathogenesis of otitis media, only recently has evidence been found of the close association between respiratory viruses (e.g., respiratory syncytial virus, influenza A, and adenovirus) and acute otitis media.[19] Using a sensitive radioimmunoassay, Meurman et al.[118] demonstrated local IgA class antibodies against respiratory virus in middle ear effusions. Adenovirus and respiratory syncytial virus antibodies were detected in 50 percent and parainfluenza 3 antibodies in about 20 percent of the 52 patients studied. Using the enzyme-linked immunosorbent assay (ELISA) method, similar results were observed in 52 children with acute otitis media in the United States (R.H. Yolken, personal communication). Furthermore, Yamaguchi et al.[119] demonstrated positive secretory viral antibodies (SIgA) to respiratory viruses in 24 percent of the chronic middle ear effusions studied, indicating that these respiratory viruses may have an immediate as well as a long-term effect on the pathogenesis of otitis media.

Experimental evidence supporting the role of influenza A virus in the pathogenesis of acute otitis media was presented by Giebink et al.[120] When the nasopharynges of chinchillas were instilled with *Strep. pneumoniae*, only 13 percent developed acute otitis media, whereas the incidence of acute otitis media was more than 62 percent when the middle ear was also deflated. When the nasopharynges were instilled with *Strep. pneumoniae* together with influenza A virus, the incidence of otitis media was 67 percent. The follow-up investigation documented that the influenza A virus caused immediate destruction of the tubal mucosal lining,[121] and even 2 weeks after viral inoculation of the middle ear the mucosal epithelium of the tube had not established normal morphology on the ultrastructural level (D.J. Lim and T.F. DeMaria, unpublished data) (Fig. 27-5). Therefore, it appears that an individual whose tubotympanum suffers from influenza A infection becomes highly vulnerable to a secondary bacterial infection from the nasopharynx. Although we are not certain whether all respiratory viruses have similar pathologic effects, it is conceivable that the pathogenic respiratory viruses may damage the integrity of the ciliated epithelium. Further critical study is needed in this area.

There is some supporting evidence that respiratory viral infection may also enhance bacterial adherence to the host epithelia cell surfaces,[122,123] thereby increasing the chance of bacterial infection. This enhancement is presumbly mediated by the presence of the virus-induced glycoproteins on the host cell surface. The possible immunosuppressive effects of the respiratory viruses by various alterations of immunocompetent cell function[124] could also have an influence on the pathogenesis of acute otitis media. Although such an influence has not been well documented in otitis media, poor functional states of the middle ear macrophages in chronic middle ear effusions have been described.[125]

## Role of Immunology

Available evidence strongly suggests the existence of a distinct age-related systemic and local immune system (humoral and cell mediated) in the tubotympanum, consisting of B cells and antibody,

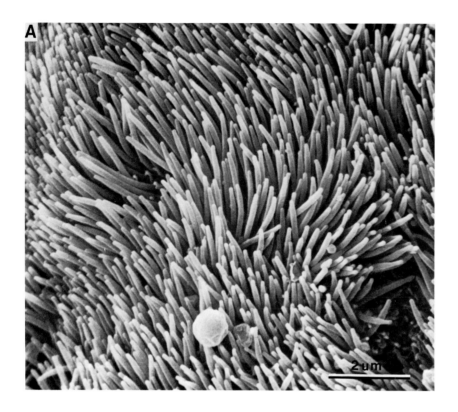

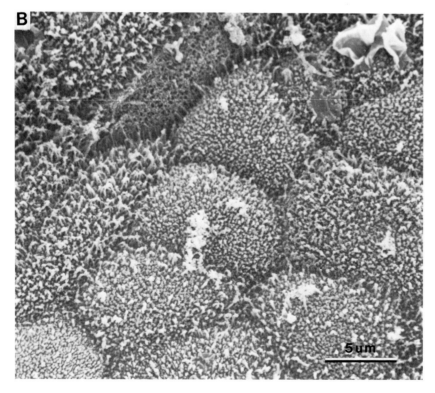

**Fig. 27-5. (A)** Scanning electron micrograph showing normal chinchilla ciliated eustachian tube mucosa. **(B)** Regeneration of ciliated cells of the tubal mucosa following experimental influenza A infection that destroyed the ciliated epithelium (2 weeks after infection).

T lymphocytes and cell-mediated immunity, and components of the complement system.[106,126,127] In addition, chemotactic factor and macrophage migration inhibitory factor are found in the effusions.[128] There is ample evidence to suggest that the middle ear can produce antibacterial (and antiviral) antibodies,[65,96,119,129-132] and clearance of the bacteria is related to the presence of the antibody in the effusion[133,134] and in serum[135,136] or complement.[137] However, while antibodies do provide some immune protection, there is ample evidence that some bacteria persist, even in the presence of specific antibody, in many cases of chronic otitis media with effusion. The reason for this persistence is not clear, but it could be due either to immune suppression[138] or to phagocytic cell dysfunction. A lack of information regarding the antigens of the key pathogens that confer protection to the host has hampered progress in this area.

It has become increasingly clear over the past 5 years that all the major effector cells and proteins of the classic inflammatory and immune response have been found in the middle ear but are not totally effective in eliminating the invading pathogen. A logical conclusion from this observation is that some sort of suppressive activity, in the generic sense, is taking place in the middle ear. A recent report by Bernstein and Park[139] indicates that a defective immunoregulatory mechanism may contribute to the pathogenesis of otitis media, in particular in those patients with persistent middle ear effusions. These investigators noted an imbalance of T-cell subsets and decreased interleukin-2 (IL-2) production, suggesting defects in humoral immunity.

Additional reports of other humoral defects indicate that IgG$_2$ is significantly depressed in otitis-prone children,[140,141] that complement abnormalities may be present in children with recurrent otitis media,[142] and that certain forms of chronic otitis media there is a relative predominance of mononuclear cells that are actively immunosuppressive for B lymphocytes.[125]

A separate but related issue is the defects noted in various phagocytic cells in patients with otitis media. Defects in polymorphonuclear neutrophil function, including chemotaxis and phagocytosis, have been reported in children with recurrent episodes of otitis media.[18,143] Diminished phagocyto-

sis would also result in possible ineffective stimulation of the host's immune system, since phagocytosis and transport of antigens by polymorphonuclear neutrophils and macrophages to the regional lymph nodes is a pivotal component of the afferent limb of the humoral antibody response.

Evidence has accumulated over the past 10 years that immune injury may contribute to the pathogenesis of otitis media, especially chronic otitis media with effusion. Four basic mechanisms of immune injury that may be involved are outlined below.

Allergy (type I response) has been suggested to be involved in chronic otitis media with effusion, based on clinical observations[144] and on the finding of elevated IgE in middle ear effusions,[145] but other workers have failed to substantiate these observations.[31-33] However, the finding of low IgE levels in middle ear effusions does not rule out the possibility that specific IgE antibodies may occur in middle ear effusions and may be of significance in the development of chronic otitis media with effusion. Sloyer et al.[146] reported the presence of IgE antibodies to pneumococcal antigens in middle ear effusion. Mogi[129] also reported a few cases of IgE antibodies to mites in middle ear effusions. Berger et al.[147] reported significantly higher histamine levels in chronic effusions than in sera but failed to correlate with respiratory allergy status. They concluded that a type I response is the least likely mechanism involved. Our morphologic findings show that the middle ear contains a large number of mast cells and they become degranulated during the course of chronic otitis media with effusion. The mechanism by which this degranulation occurs in chronic otitis media with effusion is unknown.

In a guinea pig model, Poliquin et al.[148] found that trauma to the tympanic membrane evoked an immune response of the type II (or type III) variety in the membranes of animals that had been passively immunized with antitympanic membrane antibody. This immune response was suggested to be the underlying mechanism for the pathogenesis of tympanosclerosis in chronic otitis media with effusion. Ultrastructural study of human tympanosclerosis revealed two types, one involved with cell degeneration and the other with collagen fibers (D.J. Lim, unpublished data), consistent with the concept of type II immune injury.

The role of complement as a pathogenetic factor has not been clearly established. However, a number of investigators have shown the presence of abnormal C1 complement complexes in the sera of children with acute otitis media[149] and recurrent otitis media.[150] The possibility that the complement system, through the immune complex, might play a role in the pathogenesis of chronic otitis media with effusion has been proposed.[8,11,151,152] We found inflammatory response in chinchilla middle ear mucosa when immune complexes were introduced.[153] Similar results were obtained using sensitized animals challenged with antigen.[154] Prellner and Nilsson[150] observed the presence of C1q-binding substances in the serum samples of patients with chronic otitis media with effusion[155] and associated this activity with components of pneumococci.[156-158] The high concentration of rheumatoid factor found in the effusions[159] may also support this possibility. However, Bernstein et al.[82] currently doubt the role of immune complexes in chronic otitis media with effusion because only 6 percent (4 of 70) of middle ear effusions in their study contained soluble immune complex, and

they failed to demonstrate immune complex deposition in the biopsied tissue. A recent study of Meri et al.[160] on components of complement in middle ear effusions demonstrated evidence of activation of both classic and alternate pathways. These investigators suggested that the bacterial components rather than immune complexes are responsible. Another possible mechanism of complement activation is suggested by the finding that C-reactive protein can react with C-polysaccharide of *Strep. pneumoniae*,[161] and endotoxin derived from gram-negative organisms, as demonstrated in this laboratory.[162] These data together suggest that the complement system may play an important role in chronic otitis media with effusion.

The contribution of cellular immune mechanisms to the defense of the middle ear or their possible role in the pathogenesis of otitis media with effusion has also been suggested because of the recent evidence indicating the presence of a local (mucosal) cell-mediated immune system[163] and the fact that lymphocytes are cells commonly found in middle ear effusions and submucosal connective tissue (Fig. 27-6).[164,165] While it is possible that

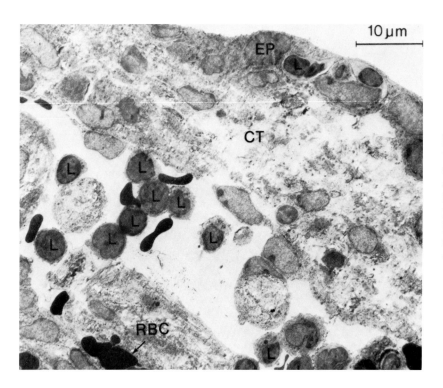

**Fig. 27-6.** Heavy lymphocyte (L) infiltration in a mucosal biopsy specimen obtained from a patient with chronic otitis media with effusion. Ep, epithelium; CT, connective tissue; RBC, red blood cell. (Lim DJ: Normal and pathological mucosa of the middle ear and eustachian tube. Clin Otolaryngol 4:213, 1979.)

culture-negative and lymphocyte-rich fluid represents the resolution stage of the middle ear infection,[166] it is also possible that the suppressed cell-mediated immune response could have contributed to the sustained inflammation, leading to chronic otitis media with effusion.[138] Bernstein et al.[164] demonstrated that mucoid effusions contain more T cells and serous effusions are dominated by B cells. The results from our laboratory show that there are about twice the number of T cells as B cells, regardless of effusion type.[50] Palva et al.[167] showed that the lymphocytes in effusions are predominantly T lymphocytes, which could be viewed as positive evidence of a possible delayed hypersensitivity, as suggested by Bryan and Bryan.[168] An analysis of subsets of T lymphocytes from chronic middle ear effusions and mucosal biopsies showed the dominance of helper cells over suppressor cells in most cases, with a small amount of natural killer cells, suggesting that the normal immune response is operative in the middle ears of these patients.[169] By contrast, Bernstein et al.[138] recently reported that the helper/suppressor cell ratio in the effusions is indictive of an imbalanced immunoregulatory function. These reports are superficially contradictory and no conclusion can be drawn; more detailed studies of the cell-mediated immune system are obviously required.

## SUMMARY

Despite the fact that otitis media has been studied for more than a century and a number of risk factors have been identified as contributing to its pathogenesis, many research questions remain unanswered. Numerous studies have dealt with each facet of otitis media, testifying to the complexity of the disease involved. Currently available research tools enable us to probe deeply into the fundamental molecular mechanisms involved in the pathogenesis. Once we understand these mechanisms, we should be able to devise better approaches to treatment and prevention.

## ACKNOWLEDGMENT

This work was supported in part by a grant from NINCDS/NIH (NS08854). Dr. Lauren O. Bakaletz critically reviewed a portion of the manuscript. We gratefully acknowledge the invaluable help of Shakuntala Lamgaday, Smokey Lynn Bare, and Katherine Adamson in preparing the manuscript.

## REFERENCES

1. Bezold F, Siebenmann F: Text-Book of Otology for Physicians and Students (Holinger J, trans). EH Colegrove, Chicago, 1908
2. Barr T: Pathogenic organism in the middle ear (1901). p. 187. In García-Ballester L, Olagüe G, Ciges M (eds): Classics in Modern Otology. University Press, Granada, 1978
3. Bluestone CD, Klein JO: Otitis media with effusion, atelectasis, and eustachian tube dysfunction. p. 356. In Bluestone CD, Stool SE (eds): Pediatric Otolaryngology. WB Saunders, Philadelphia, 1983
4. Paparella MM, Bluestone CD, Arnold W, et al: Definition and classification. Ann Otol Rhinol Laryngol 94(suppl 116):8, 1985
5. DHEW: Advance Data from Vital and Health Statistics. No. 12. U.S. Department of Health and Human Services, Washington DC, 1977
6. Kessner DM, et al: Assessment of Medical Care in Children, Contrasts in Health Status. Vol. 3. National Academy of Science. Washington, DC, 1973
7. Pukander J, Sipilä M, Karma P: Occurrence of and risk factors in acute otitis media. p. 9. In Lim DJ, Bluestone CD, Klein JO, Nelson JD (eds): Recent Advances in Otitis Media with Effusion. BC Decker, Philadelphia, 1984
8. Howie VM, Ploussard JH, Sloyer J: The otitis prone condition. Am J Dis Child 129:676, 1975
9. Klein JO: Epidemiology of otitis media. p. 18. In Wiet RJ, Coulthard SW (eds): Proceedings of the Second National Conference on Otitis Media. Ross Laboratories, Columbus, OH, 1979
10. Stangerup S-E, Tos M: Epidemiology of acute suppurative otitis media, Am J Otolaryngol 7:47, 1986

11. Fiellau-Nikolajsen M: Tympanometry and secretory otitis media: Observations on diagnosis, epidemiology, treatment, and prevention in prospective cohort studies of three-year-old children. Acta Otolaryngol (Stockh) [suppl 394], 1983

12. Casselbrant ML, Okeowo PA, Flaherty MR, et al. Prevalence and incidence of otitis media in a group of preschool children in the United States. p. 16. In Lim DJ, Bluestone CD, Klein JO, Nelson JD (eds): Recent Advances in Otitis Media with Effusion. BC Decker, Philadelphia, 1984

13. Griffith T: Epidemiology of otitis media: An interracial study. Laryngoscope 89:22, 1979

14. Teele DW, Rosner BA, Klein JO: Epidemiology of otitis media in children. Ann Otol Rhinol Laryngol 89[suppl 68]:5, 1980

15. Virolainen E, Puhakka H, Aantaa E, et al: Prevalence of secretory otitis media in seven to eight-year-old school children. Ann Otol Rhinol Laryngol 89[suppl 68]:7, 1980

16. Wiet RJ, DeBlanc GB, Stewart J, Weider DJ: Natural history of otitis media in the American native. Ann Otol Rhinol Laryngol 89[suppl 68]:14, 1980

17. Schwartz RH, Schwartz DM, Rodriguez WJ: Otitis media with effusion (OME): Natural course in untreated children. Pediatr Res 15:556, 1981

18. Giebink GS, Le CT, Paparella MM: Epidemiology of otitis media with effusion in children. Arch Otolaryngol 108:563, 1982

19. Henderson FW, Collier AM, Sanyal MA, et al: A longitudinal study of respiratory viruses and bacteria in the etiology of acute otitis media with effusion. N Engl J Med 306:1377, 1982

20. Kraemer MJ, Richardson MA, Weiss NS, et al: Risk factors for persistent middle ear effusions: Otitis media, catarrh, cigarette smoke exposure, and atopy. JAMA 249:1022, 1983

21. Ingvarsson L, Lundgren K, Olofsson B: Epidemiology of acute otitis media in children—A cohort study in an urban population. p. 19. In Lim DJ, Bluestone CD, Klein JO, Nelson JD (eds): Recent Advances in Otitis Media with Effusion. BC Decker, Philadelphia, 1984

22. Tos M, Stangerup S-E, Andreassen UK, et al: Natural history of secretory otitis media. p. 36. In Lim DJ, Bluestone CD, Klein JO, Nelson JD (eds): Recent Advances in Otitis Media with Effusion. BC Decker, Philadelphia, 1984

23. Visscher V, Mandel JS, Batalden PB, et al: A case-control study exploring possible risk factors for childhood otitis media. p. 13. In Lim DJ, Bluestone CD, Klein JO, Nelson JD (eds): Recent Advances in

Otitis Media with Effusion. BC Decker, Philadelphia, 1984

24. Giebink GS: Epidemiology and natural history of otitis media. p. 5. In Lim DJ, Bluestone CD, Klein, JO, Nelson JD (eds): Recent Advances in Otitis Media with Effusion. BC Decker, Philadelphia, 1984

25. Paradise JL: Otitis media in infants and children. Pediatrics 65:917, 1980

26. Bush PJ, Rabin DL: Racial differences in encounter rates for otitis media. Pediatr Res 14:1115, 1980

27. Doyle WJ: A functiono-anatomic description of eustachian tube vector relations in four ethnic populations: An osteologic study. Doctoral dissertation, University of Pittsburgh, 1977

28. Suehs OW: Secretory otitis media. Laryngoscope 62:998, 1952

29. Medical Research Council: Acute otitis media in general practice. Lancet 2:510, 1957

30. Lemon AN: Serous otitis media in children. Laryngoscope 72:32, 1962

31. Lewis DM, Schram JL, Lim DJ, et al: Immunoglobulin E in chronic middle ear effusions: Comparison of results obtained by RIST, PRIST, and RIA techniques. Ann Otol Rhinol Laryngol 87:197, 1978

32. Mogi G, Maeda S, Yoshida T, Watanabe N: Immunochemistry of otitis media with effusion. J Infect Dis 133:125, 1976

33. Reisman RE, Bernstein JM: Allergy and secretory otitis media. Pediatr Clin North Am 22:251, 1975

34. Paradise JL, Bluestone CD, Felder H: The universality of otitis media in 50 infants with cleft palate. Pediatrics 44:35, 1969

35. Schwartz DM, Schwartz RH: Acoustic impedance and otoscopic findings in young children with Down's syndrome. Arch Otolaryngol 104:652, 1978

36. Sando I, Harada T: Temporal bone histopathologic findings in Down syndrome. Arch Otolaryngol 107:96, 1981

37. Senturia BH et al: Panel I-A: Definition and classification. Ann Otol Rhinol Laryngol 89[suppl 69]:4, 1980

38. Shurin PA, Pelton SI, Donner A: Persistence of middle ear effusion after acute otitis media in children. N Engl J Med 300:1121, 1979

39. Giebink GS, Mills EL, Huff JS, et al: The microbiology of serous and mucoid otitis media. Pediatr Pediau 63:915, 1979

40. Bylander A, Tjernström Ö, Ivarsson A, Ingvarsson L: Eustachian tube function in children with and

without otologic history. p. 56. In Lim DJ, Blue-stone CD, Klein JO, Nelson JD (eds): Recent Advances in Otitis Media with Effusion. BC Decker, Philadelphia, 1984

41. Holborow C: Eustachian tubal function: Change throughout childhood and neuromuscular control. J Laryngol Otol 89:47, 1975

42. Bluestone CD, Beery QC:Concepts on the pathogenesis of middle ear effusions. Ann Otol Rhinol Laryngol 85[suppl 25]:182, 1976

43. Holmquist J, Renwall U: Eustachian tube function in secretory otitis media. Arch Otolaryngol 99:59, 1974

44. Fiellau-Nikolajsen M, Lous J: Prospective tympanometry in 3-year-old children: A study of the spontaneous course of tympanometry types in a nonselected population. Arch Otolaryngol 105:461, 1979

45. Lous J, Fiellau-Nikolajsen M: Epidemiology of middle ear effusion and tubal dysfunction. A one-year prospective study comprising monthly tympanometry in 387 non-selected 7-year-old children. Int J Pediatr Otol Rhinol Laryngol 3:303, 1981

46. Tos M, Holm-Jensen S, Sørensen CH: Changes in prevalence of secretory otitis from summer to winter in four-year-old children. Am J Otol 2:324, 1981

47. Holmgren L: Experimental tubal occlusion. Acta Otolaryngol 28:587, 1940

48. Cantekin EI, Doyle WJ, Phillips DC, Bluestone CD: Gas absorption in the middle ear. Ann Otol Rhinol Laryngol 89[suppl 68]:71, 1980

49. Paparella MM, Hiraide F, Juhn SK, Kaneko Y: Cellular events involved in middle ear fluid production. Ann Otol Rhinol Laryngol 79:766, 1970

50. Lim DJ, DeMaria TF: Pathogenesis of otitis media. Bacteriology and immunology. Laryngoscope 92:278, 1982

51. Kuijpers W, van der Beek JMH: Experimental occlusion of the eustachian tube: The role of short- and long-term infection and its sequelae. p. 204. In Lim DJ, Bluestone CD, Klein JO, Nelson JD (eds): Recent Advances in Otitis Media with Effusion. BC Decker, Philadelphia, 1984

52. Lim DJ, Birck H: Ultrastructural pathology of the middle ear mucosa in serous otitis media. Ann Otol Rhinol Laryngol 80:838, 1971

53. Lim DJ, Viall J, Birck H, St Pierre R: The morphological basis for understanding middle ear effusions. Laryngoscope 82:1625, 1972

54. Tos M, Bak-Pedersen K: Goblet cell population in the normal middle ear and eustachian tube of children and adults. Ann Otol Rhinol Laryngol 85[suppl 25]:44, 1976

55. Sadé J: The middle ear mucosa—Its biology and pathology. p. 23. In Sadé J (ed): Secretory Otitis Media and Its Sequelae. Churchill Livingstone, New York, 1979

56. Senturia BH, Gessert DF, Carr CD, Baumann ES: Studies concerned with tubotympanitis. Ann Otol Rhinol Laryngol 67:440, 1958

57. Juhn SK: Huff JS, Paparella MM: Lactate dehydrogenase activity and isoenzyme patterns in serous middle ear effusions. Ann Otol Rhinol Laryngol 82:192, 1973

58. Mogi G, Yoshida T, Honjo S, et al: Middle ear effusions—quantitative analysis of immunoglobulins. Ann Otol Rhinol Laryngol 82:196, 1973

59. Bernstein JM, Tomasi TB Jr, Ogra P: The immunochemistry of middle ear effusions. Arch Otolaryngol 99:320, 1974

60. Lim DJ: Functional morphology of the mucosa of the middle ear and eustachian tube. Ann Otol Rhinol Laryngol 85[suppl 25]:36, 1976

61. Liu YS, Lim DJ, Lang RW, Birck HG: Chronic middle ear effusions: Immunochemical and bacteriological investigation. Arch Otolaryngol 101:278, 1975

62. Lim DJ: Normal and pathological mucosa of the middle ear and eustachian tube. Clin Otolaryngol 4:213, 1979

63. Mogi G, Maeda S, Watanabe N: The development of mucosal immunity in guinea pig middle ear. Int J Pediatr Otorhinolaryngol 1:331, 1980

64. Tomasi TB Jr: The Immune System of Secretions. Prentice-Hall, Englewood Cliffs, NJ, 1976

65. Ogra PL, Fishaut M, Welliver RC: Mucosal immunity and immune response to respiratory viruses. p. 225. In Weinstein, BN Fields (eds): Seminars in Infectious Disease. Vol III. Thieme, New York, 1980

66. Howie VM, Ploussard J: Bacterial etiology and antimicrobial treatment of exudative otitis media. South Med J 64:233, 1971

67. Nylén O: Otitis media acuta. Thesis, University of Göteborg, Göteborg, Sweden, 1975

68. Beachey EH, Ofek I: Epithelial cell binding of group A streptococci by lipoteichoic acid on fimbriae denuded of M-protein. J Exp Med 143:759, 1976

69. Weed WP, Williams RC: Bacterial adherence: First step in pathogenesis of certain infections. J Chronic Dis 31:67, 1978

70. Beachey EH: Bacterial Adherence. Chapman and Hall, London, 1980

71. Beachey EH: Bacterial adherence: Adhesin-receptor interactions mediating the attachment of bacteria to mucosal surfaces. J Infect Dis 143:325, 1981

72. Andersson B, Eriksson B, Falsen E, et al: Adhesion of *Streptococcus pneumoniae* to human pharyngeal epithelial cells in vitro: Differences in adhesive capacity among strains isolated from subjects with otitis media, septicemia, or meningitis or from healthy carriers. Infect Immun 32:311, 1981

73. Lampe RM, Mason EO Jr, Kaplan SL, et al: Adherence of *Haemophilus influenzae* to buccal epithelial cells. Infect Immun 35:166, 1982

74. Anderson PW, Pichichero ME, Connor EM: Enhanced nasopharyngeal colonization of rats by piliated *Haemophilus influenzae* type b. Infect Immun 48:565, 1985

75. Costerton JW, Geesey GG, Cheng KJ: How bacteria stick. Sci Am 238:86, 1978

76. Andersson B, Leffler H, Jørgensen F, et al: Molecular mechanisms of adhesion of *Streptococcus pneumoniae* to human oropharyngeal epithelial cells. p. 132. In Lim DJ, Bluestone CD, Klein JO, Nelson JD (eds): Recent Advances in Otitis Media with Effusion. BC Decker, Philadelphia, 1984

77. Stull TL, Mendelman PM, Haas JE, et al: Characterization of *Haemophilus influenzae* type b fimbriae. Infect Immun 46:787, 1984

78. Austrian, R: Pneumococcal infections. p. 257. In Germanier R (ed): Bacterial Vaccines. Academic Press, Orlando, FL, 1984

79. Robbins JB, Schneerson R, Pittman M: *Haemophilus influenzae* type b infections. p. 289. In Germanier R (ed): Bacterial Vaccines. Academic Press, Orlando, FL, 1984

80. Klein JO: Microbiology of otitis media. Ann Otol Rhinol Laryngol 89[suppl 68]:98, 1980

81. Nelson JD: Microbiology of otitis media: The American experience. p. 25. In Presymposium on Management of Otitis Media, Kyoto, Japan, January 12, 1985

82. Bernstein JM, Dryja D, Neter E: The role of coagulase-negative staphylococci in chronic otitis media with effusion. Otolaryngol Head Neck Surg 90:837, 1982

83. Sugita R: Bacteriological study of suppurative otitis media and chemotherapy. p. 30. In Presymposium on Management of Otitis Media, Kyoto, Japan, January 12, 1985

84. Yamamoto E: Bacteriology of otitis media from surgical stand point. p. 21. Presymposium on Management of Otitis Media, Kyoto, Japan, January 12, 1984

85. Shurin PA, Marchant CD, Kim CH, et al: Emergence of beta-lactamase-producing strains of *Branhamella catarrhalis* as important agents of acute otitis media. Pediatr Infect Dis 2:34, 1983

86. Rohn DD, Vatman F, Cantekin EI: Incidence of organisms in otitis media. Ann Otol Rhinol Laryngol 92[suppl 107]:17, 1983

87. Leinonen M, Luotonen J, Herva E, et al: Preliminary serologic evidence for a pathogenic role of *Branhamella catarrhalis.* J Infect Dis 144:570, 1981

88. Kloos WE, Schleifer KH: Simplified scheme for routine identification of human staphylococcus species. J Clin Microbiol 1:82, 1975

89. Feigin RD, Shackelford PG, Campbell TO, et al: Assessment of the role of *Staphylococcus epidermidis* as a cause of otitis media. Pediatrics 52:569, 1973

90. Ostfeld E, Rubinstein E: Acute gram-negative bacillary infections of middle ear and mastoid. Ann Otol Rhinol Laryngol 89:33, 1980

91. Brook I: Bacteriology and treatment of chronic otitis media. Laryngoscope 89:1129, 1979

92. Brook I, Schwartz R: Anaerobic bacteria in acute otitis media. Acta Otolaryngol (Stockh) 91:111, 1981

93. Siirala U: The problem of sterile otitis media. Pract Otorhinolaryngol 19:159, 1957

94. Bernstein JM, Hayes ER: The middle ear mucosa in health and disease. Arch Otolaryngol 94:30, 1971

95. Kokko E: Chronic secretory otitis media in children: A clinical study. Acta Otolaryngol (Stockh) [suppl 327]:1, 1974

96. Liu YS, Lang RW, Lim DJ, Birck HG: Microorganisms in chronic otitis media with effusion. Ann Otol Rhinol Laryngol 85[suppl 25]:245, 1976

97. Palva T, Holopainen E, Karma P: Protein and cellular pattern of glue ear secretions. Ann Otol Rhinol Laryngol 85[suppl 25]:103, 1976

98. Healy BG, Teele DW: The microbiology of chronic middle ear effusions in children. Laryngoscope 87:1472, 1977

99. Riding KH, Bluestone CD, Michaels RH, et al: Microbiology of recurrent and chronic otitis media with effusion. J Pediatr 93:739, 1978

100. Sundberg L, Cederberg A, Edén T, Ernstson S: Bacteriology in secretory otitis media. Acta Otolaryngol (Stockh) [suppl 384]:18, 1981

101. Sipilä P: Inflammatory cells and bacteria in mucoid middle ear effusion of patients with secretory otitis

media. Doctoral dissertation, University of Oulu, Finland, 1982

102. Pelton SI, Shurin PA, Klein JO: Persistence of middle ear effusion after otitis media. Pediatr Res 11:504, 1977

103. Lundgren K, Rundcrantz H: Microbiology in serous otitis media. Ann Otol Rhinol Laryngol 85[suppl 25]:152, 1976

104. Lim DJ, Lewis DM, Schram JL, Birck HG: Otitis media with effusion: Cytological and microbiological correlates. Arch Otolaryngol 105:404, 1979

105. Lewis DM, Schram JL, Birck HG, Lim DJ: Antibody activity in otitis media with effusion. Ann Otol Rhinol Laryngol 88:392, 1979

106. Lim DJ, DeMaria TF: Pathogenesis and pathology of chronic otitis media with effusion. p. 275. In Myers E (ed): New Dimensions in Otorhinolaryngology—Head and Neck Surgery. Elsevier Science Publishing, New York, 1985

107. Bernstein JM, Ogra PL: Mucosal immune system: Implications in otitis media with effusion. Ann Otol Rhinol Laryngol 89[suppl 68]:326, 1980

108. Fulghum RS, Daniel JH, Yarborough JG: Anaerobic bacteria in otitis media. Ann Otol Rhinol Laryngol 86:196, 1977

109. Thore M: Studies on experimental anaerobic infections of the middle ear and on the polymorphonuclear leukocyte function under anaerobic conditions. Doctoral dissertation. Umeå University, Sweden, 1984

110. Harker LA, Koontz FP: The bacteriology of cholesteatoma. p. 264. In McCabe BF, Sade J, Abramson M (eds): Cholesteatoma: First International Conference. Aesculapius, Birmingham, Alabama, 1977

111. Fairbanks DNF: Antimicrobial therapy for chronic suppurative otitis media. Ann Otol Rhinol Laryngol 90[suppl 84]:58, 1981

112. Rifkind DR, Chanock RM, Kravetz H, et al: Ear involvement (myringitis) and primary atypical pneumonia following inoculation of volunteers with Eaton agent. Am Rev Respir Dis 85:479, 1962

113. Sobeslavsky O, Syrucek L, Bruckoya M, Abrahamovic M: The etiological role of *Mycoplasma pneumoniae* in otitis media in children. Pediatrics 35:652, 1965

114. Roberts DB: The etiology of bullous myringitis and the role of mycoplasmas in ear disease: A review. Pediatrics 65:761, 1980

115. Dawson D, Wood TR, Rose L, et al: Experimental inclusion conjunctivitis in man. III. Keratitis and other complications. Arch Ophthalmol 78:341, 1967

116. Schachter J, Grossman M, Holt J, et al: Prospective study of chlamydial infection in neonates. Lancet 2:377, 1979

117. Tipple MA, Beem MO, Saxon EM: Clinical characteristics of the afebrile pneumonia associated with *Chlamydia trachomatis* infection in infants less than 6 months of age. Pediatrics 63:192, 1979

118. Meurman OH, Sarkkinen HK, Puhakka HJ, et al: Local IgA-class antibodies against respiratory viruses in middle ear and nasopharyngeal secretions of children with secretory otitis media. Laryngoscope 90:304, 1980

119. Yamaguchi T, Urasawa T, Kataura A: Secretory immunoglobulin A antibodies to respiratory viruses in middle ear effusion of chronic otitis media with effusion. Ann Otol Rhinol Laryngol 93:73, 1984

120. Giebink GS, Berzins IK, Marker SC, Schiffman G: Experimental otitis media after nasal inoculation of *Streptococcus pneumoniae* and influenza A virus in chinchillas. Infect Immun 30:445, 1980

121. Giebink GS, Ripley ML, Wright PF: Eustachian tube histopathology during experimental influenza A virus infection in the chinchilla. Ann Otol Rhinol Laryngol 96:199, 1987

122. Fainstein V, Musher DM, Cate TR: Bacterial adherence to pharyngeal cells during viral infection. J Infect Dis 141:172, 1980

123. Ramphal R, Small PM, Shands JW Jr, et al: Adherence of *Pseudomonas aeruginosa* to tracheal cells injured by influenzae infection or by endotracheal intubation. Infect Immun 27:614, 1980

124. Friedman H, Specter S, Bendinelli M: Viruses and the immune response. p. 119. In Falcone G, Campa A, Smith H, Scott GM (eds): Bacterial and Viral Inhibition and Modulation of Host Defenses. Academic Press, London, 1984

125. Yamanaka T, Bernstein JM, Cumella J, Ogra PL: Lymphocyte-macrophage interaction in otitis media with effusion. p. 173. In Lim DJ, Bluestone CD, Klein JO, Nelson JD (eds): Recent Advances in Otitis Media with Effusion. BC Decker, Philadelphia, 1984

126. Branefors-Helander P, Nylén O, Jeppsson J-H: Acute otitis media: Assay of complement-fixing antibody against *Haemophilus influenzae* as a diagnostic tool in acute otitis media. Acta Pathol Microbiol Scand [B] 81:508, 1973

127. Johnston RB, Stroud RM: Complement and host defense against infection. J Pediatr 90:169, 1977

128. Bernstein JM: Biological mediators of inflamma-

tion in middle ear effusions. Ann Otol Rhinol Laryngol 25[suppl 85]:90, 1976

129. Mogi G: Secretory IgA and antibody activities in middle ear effusions. Ann Otol Rhinol Laryngol 85[suppl 25]:97, 1976

130. Lewis DM, Schram JL, Meadema SJ, Lim DJ: Experimental otitis media in chinchillas. Ann Otol Rhinol Laryngol 89[suppl 68]:344, 1980

131. Watanabe N, DeMaria TF, Lewis DM, et al: Experimental otitis media in chinchillas. II. Comparison of the middle ear immune responses to *S pneumoniae* types 3 and 23. Ann Otol Rhinol Laryngol 91[suppl 93]:9, 1982

132. Bernstein JM, Moore LL, Ogra P: Defective phagocytic and antibacterial activity of middle ear neutrophils. p. 129. In Lim DJ, Bluestone CD, Klein JO, Nelson JD (eds): Recent Advances in Otitis Media with Effusion. BC Decker, Philadelphia, 1984

133. Sloyer JL Jr, Cate CC, Howie VM, et al: The immune response to acute otitis media in children. II. Serum and middle ear fluid antibody in otitis media due to *Hemophilus influenzae.* J Infect Dis 132:685, 1975

134. Sloyer JL Jr, Ploussard JH, Howie VM: Immunology and microbiology in acute otitis media. Ann Otol Rhinol Laryngol 85[suppl 25]:130, 1976

135. Giebink GS, Quie PG: Comparison of otitis media due to types 3 and 23 *Streptococcus pneumoniae* in the chinchilla model. J Infect Dis 136:S191, 1977

136. Shurin PA, Marchant CD, Howie VM: Bactericidal antibody to antigenically distinct nontypable strains of *Hemophilus influenzae* isolated from acute otitis media. p. 155. In Lim DJ, Bluestone CD, Klein JO, Nelson JD (eds): Recent Advances in Otitis Media with Effusion. BC Decker, Philadelphia, 1984

137. Crosson FJ, Winkelstein JA, Moxon ER: Participation of complement in the non-immune host defense against experimental *Haemophilus influenzae* type b septicemia and meningitis. Infect Immun 14:882, 1976

138. Bernstein JM, Yamanaka T, Cumella J, et al: Some observations on lymphocyte and macrophage function in middle ear effusions. p. 51. In Veldman JE, McCabe BF, Huizing EH, Mygind N (eds): Immunobiology, Autoimmunity and Transplantation in Otorhinolaryngology. Kugler, Amsterdam, 1985

139. Bernstein JM, Park BH: Defective immunoregulation in children with chronic otitis media with effusion. Otolaryngol Head Neck Surg 94:334, 1986

140. Oxelius V: Chronic infections in a family with hereditary deficiency of IgG$_2$ and IgG$_4$. Clin Exp Immunol 17:19, 1974

141. Freijd A, Oxelius V, Rynnel-Dagöö B: IgG subclass levels in otitis-prone children. p. 153. In Lim DJ, Bluestone CD, Klein JO, Nelson JD (eds): Recent Advances in Otitis Media with Effusion. BC Decker, Philadelphia, 1984

142. Prellner K, Kalm O, Pedersen FK: Complement and pneumococcal antibodies during and after recurrent otitis media. p. 162. In Lim DJ, Bluestone CD, Klein JO, Nelson JD (eds): Recent Advances in Otitis Media with Effusion. BC Decker, Philadelphia, 1984

143. Hill HR, Book LS, Hemming VG, Herbst JJ: Defective neutrophil chemotactic response in patients with recurrent episodes of otitis media and chronic diarrhea. Am J Dis Child 131:433, 1977

144. Clemis JD: Identification of allergic factors in middle ear effusions. Ann Otol Rhinol Laryngol 85[suppl 25]:234, 1976

145. Phillips MH, Knight NJ, Manning H, Abbott AL: IgE and secretory otitis media. Lancet 2:1176, 1975

146. Sloyer JL, Ploussard JH, Karr LJ: Otitis media in the young infant: An IgE-mediated disease? Ann Otol Rhinol Laryngol 89[suppl 68]:133, 1980

147. Berger G, Hawke M, Proops DW, et al: Histamine levels in middle ear effusions. p. 195. In Lim DJ, Bluestone CD, Klein JO, Nelson JD (eds): Recent Advances in Otitis Media with Effusion. BC Decker, Philadelphia, 1984

148. Poliquin JF, Catanzaro A, Robb J, et al: Adaptive immunity of the tympanic membrane. Am J Otolaryngol 2:94, 1981

149. Johnson U, Kamme C, Laurell AB, et al: C1 subcomponents in acute pneumococcal otitis media in children. Acta Pathol Microbiol Scand [C] 85:10, 1982

150. Prellner K, Nilsson NI: Complement aberrations in serum from children with otitis due to *S. pneumoniae* or *H. influenzae.* Acta Otolaryngol (Stockh) 94:275, 1982

151. Veltri RW, Sprinkle PM: Secretory otitis media: An immune complex disease. Ann Otol Rhinol Laryngol 85[suppl 25]:135, 1976

152. Palva T, Lehtinen T, Rinne J: Immune complexes in the middle ear fluid in chronic secretory otitis media. Ann Otol Rhinol Laryngol 92:42, 1983

153. Mravec J, Lewis DM, Lim DJ: Experimental otitis media with effusion: An immune complex-mediated response. Trans Am Acad Ophthalmol Otolaryngol 86:ORL-258, 1978

154. Takasaka T, Kaku Y, Shibahara Y, et al: Experimental otitis media with effusion: An immunoelectron microscopic study. p. 88. In Lim DJ, Bluestone CD, Klein JO, Nelson JD (eds): Recent Advances in Otitis Media with Effusion. BC Decker, Philadelphia, 1984

155. Prellner K, Johnson U, Nilsson NI, et al: Complement and Clq binding substances in otitis media. Ann Otol Rhinol Laryngol 89[suppl 68]:129, 1980

156. Prellner K: Complement activation by pneumococci associated with acute otitis media. Acta Pathol Microbiol Scand [C] 87:213, 1979

157. Prellner K: Bacteria associated with acute otitis media have high Clq binding capacity. Acta Pathol Microbiol Scand [C] 88:178, 1980

158. Prellner K: Clq binding and complement activation by capsular and cell wall components of *S. pneumoniae* type XIX. Acta Pathol Microbiol Scand [C] 89:359, 1981

159. DeMaria TF, McGhee RB Jr, Lim DJ: Rheumatoid factor in otitis media with effusion. Arch Otolaryngol 110:279, 1984

160. Meri S, Lehtinen T, Palva T: Complement in chronic secretory otitis media: C3 breakdown and C3 splitting activity. Arch Otolaryngol 110:774, 1984

161. Kaplan MH, Volanakis JE: Interaction of C-reactive protein complexes with the complement system. J Immunol 112:2135, 1974

162. DeMaria TF, Prior RC, Briggs BR, et al: Endotoxin in middle-ear effusions from patients with chronic otitis media with effusion. J Clin Microbiol 20:15, 1984

163. Brandtzaeg P: Immune functions of human nasal mucosa and tonsils in health and disease. p. 28. In J Bienenstock (ed): Immunology of the Lung and Upper Respiratory Tract. McGraw-Hill, New York, 1984

164. Bernstein JM, Szymanski C, Albini B, et al: Lymphocyte subpopulations in otitis media with effusion. Pediatr Res 12:786, 1978

165. Palva T, Häyry P, Ylikoski J: Lymphocyte morphology in middle ear effusions. Ann Otol Rhinol Laryngol 89[suppl 68]:143, 1980

166. Lim DJ: Microbiology and cytology of otitis media with effusion: A review. p. 125. In Sadé J (ed): Secretory Otitis Media and Its Sequelae. Churchill Livingstone, New York, 1979

167. Palva T, Häyry P, Ylikoski J: Lymphocyte morphology in mucoid middle-ear effusions. Ann Otol Rhinol Laryngol 87:421, 1978

168. Bryan MP, WTK: Cytologic and immunologic response revealed by middle ear effusions. Ann Otol Rhinol Laryngol 85[suppl 25]:238, 1976

169. Palva T, Taskinen E, Häyry P: T lymphocytes in secretory otitis media. p. 45. In Veldman JE, McCabe BF, Huizing EH, Mygind N (eds): Immunobiology, Autoimmunity and Transplantation in Otorhinolaryngology. Kugler, Amsterdam, 1985

# The Natural History of Cholesteatoma

# 28

Maxwell Abramson
Takafumi Sugita
Cheng C. Huang

Middle ear cholesteatoma is a saclike structure composed of keratinizing squamous epithelium known as the matrix, a variable amount of epithelial debris, and a subepithelial connective tissue layer or perimatrix. This structure, which is usually in the form of a diverticulum, extends medially from the canal wall into the middle ear, attic, and mastoid cavity. Cholesteatoma, misnamed as a cholesterol-associated tumor in 1836 by Müller,[1] is not a tumor histologically, and yet the name cholesteatoma is still used. The tumor derivation of the name is not entirely inappropriate since, in a biologic sense, cholesteatoma behaves very much like a benign tumor. Cholesteatoma exhibits three characteristics that are decidedly tumorlike: (1) the structure grows progressively, exhibiting loss of growth control; (2) it grows at the expense of the underlying bone and is therefore characterized by bone resorption; and (3) it is a tenacious process that tends to persist and recur in spite of attempts at total removal. Although skin forms a junction with other forms of epithelium at all the body openings, the most frequent derangement of the epithelial junction occurs in the ear.[2] The incidence of cholesteatoma ranges from 6 per 100,000 per year in

Iowa to 0.92 percent per year in cleft palate patients[3] followed from birth to age 10. The external and middle ear have certain unique characteristics that predispose to this disease. The ear canal is the only skin-lined bony cul-de-sac in the body. The middle ear is the source of frequent inflammation, contains numerous bony crevices, and is subject to variable pressures.

## ORIGIN OF CHOLESTEATOMA

### Congenital Cholesteatoma

Cholesteatoma behind an intact tympanic membrane with absent history of suppuration is considered to be of congenital origin. Congenital cholesteatomas, usually quite large when diagnosed, are uncommon, comprising fewer than 5 percent of cholesteatomas.[4,5] Recently, small cholesteatomas have been reported within or just medial to the tympanic membrane, usually anterior to the malleus.[6,7] They occur in children with little or no history of otitis media. The 53 cases reported in two recent series appear to represent an increase in incidence. Whether these are truly congenital or primary cholesteatomas is not entirely clear, since acquired cholesteatomas could occur within the tympanic membrane without perforation from rupture of the basement membrane of the epithelium, in response to middle ear pressure changes, or from inflammation without perforation.

## Metaplasia

The metaplasia theory of the pathogenesis of cholesteatoma was described as early as 1873 by Wendt,[8] modified by Tumarkin,[9] and recently revised by Sade.[10] This theory is based on the fact that pluripotent or undifferentiated epithelial cells of the mucous membrane can in fact produce keratin and stratified squamous epithelium. Biopsy of the middle ear mucosa in patients with chronic otitis media has demonstrated islands of squamous epithelium.[11] The possibility exists that metaplastic epithelium could differentiate into keratinizing squamous epithelium and grow laterally through the tympanic membrane. Although squamous epithelium can occur from metaplasia of the mucosa of the middle ear, there is no good histologic or clinical evidence that islands of keratinizing epithelium grow into a three-dimensional structure and take the form of a cholesteatoma. The metaplastic theory for cholesteatoma pathogenesis is not widely held today. Further evidence against the metaplastic theory is that certain specialized cells found only in skin, such as Merkel cells and Langerhans cells,[12] are found in cholesteatomas. Merkel cells are sensory cells related to the touch receptor of the skin. Langerhans cells present in the skin function in the immune system by processing antigens. These cells would not normally be found in the mucosa of the middle ear.

## Immigration

Most of the clinical and histologic evidence support the concept that acquired cholesteatomas originate from immigration of canal wall skin. This etiology was first described by Habermann[13] and then by Bezold,[14] Wittmaack,[15] and others.[16,17] Immigration is what skin attempts to do when it is disrupted or injured. Histologic reconstruction of cholesteatoma from temporal bone sections and operative findings shows their origin as diverticula of ear canal skin.[18] Studies using animal models of cholesteatoma[19] have shown that isolated explants of skin do not grow into a sac or cyst but remain circumscribed. The exception is with immunodeficient nude mice in which human cholesteatoma can grow if transplanted into the middle ear of these animals.[20] Cholesteatoma in other animal models showing progressive growth and bone resorption[21,22] are characterized by some form of compression as well as connection to canal wall skin.[19]

Cholesteatomas are commonly divided into primary acquired and secondary acquired. The primary acquired cholesteatoma is the extension of an attic retraction pocket that grows medially, while the secondary acquired cholesteatoma originates in the pars tensa following otitis media that destroys the margin of the tympanic membrane and fibrous annulus. The distinction as to primary versus secondary serves no useful purpose, since all forms of acquired cholesteatoma follow certain events and are therefore secondary. However, we do not precisely know what the primary events are. Cholesteatomas are best described anatomically in terms of the site of perforation and the extent of the sac within the middle ear and mastoid. Cholesteatomas are therefore pars flaccida or pars tensa in origin, occupying the middle ear, attic, antrum, or mastoid and any combination thereof.

Most cholesteatomas seen today develop in the pars flaccida. They often occur in patients who are under medical observation during the early stages of the disease. These patients exhibit certain features that permit us to make conclusion on the early pathogenic features of the disease. By contrast, pars tensa cholesteatomas are fully developed when first appreciated and are more often associated with active suppuration. The description that follows is based on observations of pars flaccida cholesteatomas. The three principal features of cholesteatoma pathogenesis are eustachian tube dysfunction, middle ear inflammation, and destruction of the connective tissue in the tympanic membrane. Pressure changes in the middle ear are an early pathogenic feature of the disease process.

Cholesteatoma begins or has its origin in childhood and occurs in patients with malfunction of the eustachian tube. In testing eustachian tube function, requiring an active opening in response to positive and negative pressures in the middle ear (e.g., the inflation–deflation test used by Cantekin et al.[23]), all patients with cholesteatomas and retraction pocket show abnormalities. In a recent study of children, Bluestone et al.[24] discovered that upon swallowing, patients with cholesteatoma manifest functional impairment of the eustachian tube characterized by abnormal closing of the eustachian tube, rather than the normal opening. These patients do not manifest mechanical blockage of the eustachian tube. This type of functional abnormality leads to wide swings in middle ear pressure. Wide variations in middle ear pressure are likely to change the position of the tympanic membrane. Stretching and other physical changes result in atrophy and loss of a connective tissue structure. Although certain patients with eustachian tube abnormalities develop flaccidity of the entire pars tensa, leading to generalized atelectasis, patients with cholesteatoma and retraction pocket tend to produce localized areas of connective tissue loss. Eustachian tube function has not yet been adequately characterized in patients with various forms of middle ear disease; hence the difficulty in determining which patient is likely to develop localized retraction, generalized atelectasis, or chronic otitis media without cholesteatoma.

The localized atrophy of the pars flaccida as well as the posterior margin of pars tensa that occurs in cholesteatoma requires more than simple changes in physical pressure. Inflammation is the second feature of cholesteatoma pathogenesis. Under certain conditions, both the suppurative and secretory otitis media can induce chronic inflammatory connective tissue in the attic. Inadequate drainage of inflammatory materials in a confined space, such as Prussak's space, leads to increased local concentration of bacteria and inflammatory cell products, providing further chemotactic stimulation to monocytes and macrophages. Proteolytic enzymes released by these cells result in destruction of collagen and elastic fibers of the tympanic membrane. As the structure in the membrane changes, repeated bouts of negative pressure will draw the membrane medially into contact with the attic mu-

cosa, which is the simple cuboidal type and easily injured. The adhesion occurs between the pars flaccida epithelium, containing a thin atrophic connective tissue layer and inflammatory connective tissue or mesenchyme. This leads to a process described as epithelial–mesenchymal interaction. This interaction occurs in wound healing, in development, and in many disease states. The exact biochemical signal that induces epithelial growth and proliferation in response to inflamed connective tissue is unknown. These initial events in cholesteatoma pathogenesis — eustachian tube dysfunction, negative pressure, and inflammation — are extremely common, yet cholesteatoma is relatively uncommon. When atrophy, eustachian tube dysfunction with wide pressure changes, and inflammation coexist, and especially repeatedly, the seeds of cholesteatoma pathogenesis begin to take root.

## EPITHELIAL GROWTH AND MIGRATION

The ear canal skin must provide for epithelial differentiation growth and outward migration, so that the meatus does not become blocked with epithelial debris. Ear canal skin undergoes both vertical differentiation and a horizontal epithelial migration pattern in a centrifugal direction. The process by which the normal centrifugal direction of skin migration becomes perverted to a medially migrating pattern is a crucial subject in the pathogenesis of cholesteatoma. Under normal circumstances, ink dots placed at the umbo will migrate out in an orderly fashion toward the outer meatus.[25] The precise mechanism of this outward migration is not entirely clear.

Epithelial migration is governed to a great extent by the dermis. All types of epithelium require a substratum of connective tissue for nutrition. The fibers of the subepithelial connective tissue give both physical support and contact guidance to the orderly pathway of epithelial migration. The radial arrangement of collagen fibers of the pars tensa directs epidermal products outwardly. The concept of contact guidance of epithelium by connective tissue[26] forms the physical basis of both normal and abnormal epithelial migration patterns.

The early events in cholesteatoma pathogenesis produce atrophy of localized areas in the pars flaccida and pars tensa. Negative pressure in the middle ear draws in the connective tissue of the tympanic membrane, forming what turns out to be traction diverticulum due to adhesions to the ossicles and medial wall of the attic. Fibroblasts within connective tissue of the adhesions contract, drawing the collagen fibers medially. The medial orientation of the connective tissue fibers provides contact guidance to the epithelium inward. This medial perversion of the epithelial direction results in piling up of epidermal cells and their products, compressing skin in the retraction pocket. Skin likes to be on the outside and not in the inside and, when subjected to compressive forces, responds with an increase in epithelial growth. This fact has become the basis of recent successful animal models of middle ear cholesteatomas by covering skin with middle ear mucosa[19] and with suture ligatures compressing the canal wall skin.[21,23]

Anything that increases the rate of keratinization and the rate of cell division will influence the development of cholesteatoma. Certainly inflammation and infection are important factors, especially chronic inflammation. We recently studied the effect of endotoxin on epidermal cells in vitro.[27] When endotoxin was added to cultured epidermal cells, both the extent of protein synthesis and the amount of protein synthesis diverted into keratin production increased markedly. This process is likely to happen in the attic, especially in an ear in which the barrier between the skin and the middle ear has broken down or become markedly thin through atrophy.

Epithelium will not tolerate a free edge. Epidermis at the edge of a wound will migrate until the epidermis contacts similar cells, thereby sealing the defect. The epithelium of the wound becomes thin rather than piling up as it does in middle ear cholesteatoma. What is there in the middle ear that interferes with contact inhibition, preventing further epithelial growth and migration? One probable source of the persistent growth stimulus is the nature of mesenchymal interaction with the epidermis in the ear. The presence of a nondraining area in Prussak's space maintains connective tissue in a chronic inflammatory state, providing continuous stimulation for epithelial growth.

## Bone Resorption

Bone resorption is a characteristic feature of chronic otitis media with or without cholesteatoma. Ruedi[28] believed that direct pressure on the bone from cholesteatoma was the major cause of bone resorption; but there is no direct evidence to support this theory.

Walsh et al.[29] postulated that bone-dissolving enzymes are involved in bone resorption. Because collagen constitutes more than 90 percent of bone protein, collagenase appears to be a major factor in degradation of the organic matrix of bone. Abramson[30] demonstrated high collagenase activity in cultures of human cholesteatoma tissue.

Demineralization must be the first step in bone resorption, since hydroxyapatite, the calcium phosphate–hydroxide crystal of bone, normally protects collagen from denaturation and enzymatic degradation.[31] Thomsen et al.[32] proposed that bone resorption is carried out by the activity of lysosomal enzymes, such as acid phosphatase, and through the local accumulation of metabolic acids, such as lactic and citric acids. Parathyroid hormone, osteoclast-activating factor from stimulated lymphocytes,[33] endotoxin from gram-negative microorganisms,[34] and prostaglandins[35] have all been shown to increase bone decalcification.

Clinical evidence[36–38] as well as studies with animal models[19] have shown that chronic otitis media with cholesteatoma causes greater bone resorption than does chronic otitis media without cholesteatoma. This finding suggests that keratinized epithelium in the cholesteatoma sac or products of the epithelium play a role in enhancing bone destruction. Epithelial debris (keratin) seems to play two roles: (1) exerting physical force (pressure) within cholesteatoma sac, and (2) as an inflammatory stimulus to form granulation tissue.

Kaneko et al.[39] noted that epithelial debris and keratin in human cholesteatoma can induce foreign-body granulation tissue in the middle ear. In an animal model, we placed keratin into the rat tympanic cavity, producing a large granulation tissue containing numerous macrophages and foreign-body giant cells.[40] Bone resorption was observed in the cochlear wall. Macrophages, fibroblasts, and osteoclasts were seen in the area of bone resorption, and these cells produced collagenase (Fig. 28-1).

Macrophages play an important role in bone resorption in chronic inflammation because of their phagocytic activity, secretory function, and participation in immunologic events. In culturing macrophages in the presence of endotoxin,[41] we found that macrophages alone, even when stimulated by endotoxin, produce very little collagenase. Macrophages may require other agents to stimulate colla-

genase production, such as a lymphokine, which is a soluble protein factor released by stimulated lymphocytes.[42] By contrast, macrophages may function as effector cells to stimulate collagenase production in fibroblasts. Our studies showed that conditioned medium obtained from endotoxin-activated macrophages considerably enhances production of fibroblast collagenase. Since macrophages and fibroblasts are always seen to be associated with bone resorption in the middle ear cholesteatoma, it is possible that cellular interaction between macrophages and fibroblasts is necessary to produce collagenase, which in turn appears to cause bone resorption.

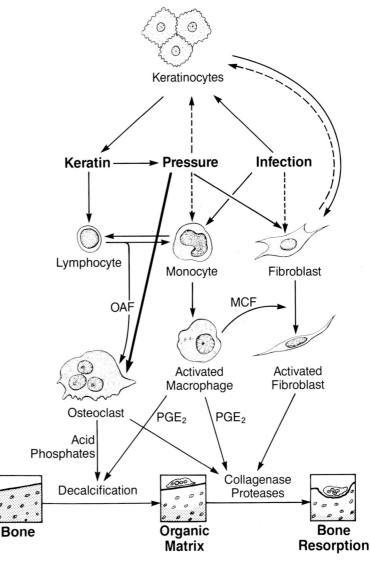

**Fig. 28-1.** Bone resorption in cholesteatoma. OAF, osteoclast activating factor; MCF, monocytic cell factor; PGE, prostaglandin E.

Although pressure does not directly cause bone resorption, it stimulates cells within bone as well as adjacent cells, causing resorption. We have demonstrated the effect of pressure in the rat middle ear by inserting an expandable seaweed (*Laminaria*).[43] Pressure created by seaweed was found to cause extensive bone resorption of cochlea and bulla, with formation of a layer of granulation tissue. Collagenase appears to be produced by osteoclasts, fibroblasts, and macrophages,[43] as demonstrated immunocytochemically. As pointed out previously by Sade and Halvey,[37] the most important cause of bone resorption in chronic otitis media is the inflammatory process, which gives rise to granulation tissue. Cholesteatoma membrane and pressure are not directly responsible for the resorption. This finding is supported by our studies in which indomethacin, an antiinflammatory agent and an inhibitor or prostaglandin synthesis, was given to animals after insertion of *Laminaria*.[43] Indomethacin given to rats subcutaneously (5 mg/kg body weight) on a daily basis after implantation of *Laminaria*, was found to inhibit the formation of granulation tissue as well as bone resorption.

What is the relative role of osteoclasts compared with macrophages in bone resorption associated with cholesteatoma? In a recent histologic study of human and gerbelline cholesteatoma, Chole[44] showed bone resorption only adjacent to osteoclasts and osteoblasts and not at other sites adjacent to the cholesteatoma. Other histologic studies have failed to demonstrate osteoclasts at bone-resorption sites. For example, Bretlau et al.,[20] using immunodeficient nude mice, and Thomsen et al.,[32] with human cholesteatoma, failed to show osteoclasts at bone-resorption sites. In our recent study of pressure-induced bone resorption using an expanding seaweed (*Laminaria*),[43] active resorbing bone appeared to be lined by osteoclast under the inflamed granulation tissue. The presence or absence of osteoclast on histologic sections have much to do with sampling and with timing, since osteoclasts are present for 48 hours or less and then die, leaving a defect. Are osteoclasts derived from bone cells or from the circulation? Osteoclasts are similar to macrophages in both function and form and are most likely derived from circulating monocytes transformed into macrophages. Multinucleation of macrophages has previously been demon-

strated using anti-macrophage serum.[45] In a recent in vitro experiment, we induced fusion of macrophages into multinucleated giant cells with an inflammatory stimulus using anti-type II collagen antiserum.[46] Fusion of macrophages into osteoclasts probably occurs in cholesteatomas in response to inflammation.

## CHOLESTEATOMA IN CHILDREN

Cholesteatomas in children are considered a different and more virulent disease than cholesteatomas in adults.[47] The pathogenic features of cholesteatoma are particularly prominent in children, including abnormalities of the eustachian tube as well as a higher incidence of otitis media. In addition, cholesteatomas in young children tend to occur within pneumatized mastoids. The increased number of air cells provides more places for cholesteatomas to grow, more areas for compression of epithelium, and a readily available blood supply, making total extirpation of disease more difficult. Since surgery treats the results of the disease but not the causes of cholesteatoma, postoperative cholesteatoma is more common in children. Canal-down surgery, which generally provides greater exposure and eliminates some of the original sites for epidermal migration, is the preferred treatment for cholesteatomas in children.

## TREATMENT OF RETRACTION POCKETS

Retraction pockets that are dry, shallow, and do not contain epithelial debris are generally considered harmless. However, the potential for this benign structure to become transformed into a growing cholesteatoma remains. The crucial ingredient is inflammation. We tend to think of inflammation as being middle ear in origin. The reason cholesteatomas occur in all ages is based on the presence of retraction pockets from childhood lying in the attic or sinus tympane that can become infected at any time. This infection can occur from without and result from a external otitis, producing moisture, swelling, increased keratin debris, compression, and stimulation of skin growth. Patients with retraction pockets should be observed throughout life and should be advised to keep water out of their ears.

When retraction pockets are adherent to the incudostapedial joint or extend beyond view, especially in children, early surgery should be considered to prevent widespread disease as well as resorption of the incudostapedial joint. A simple exploration with insertion of perichondrium and cartilage under the retraction pocket and placement of a pressure-equalizing tube can prevent a serious problem at the cost of a relatively minor operation.

## TREATMENT OF CHOLESTEATOMAS

The choice between canal-up versus canal-down surgery as treatment for cholesteatoma continues to be a controversial question. Canal-up surgery appears to have a better functional results, but with a higher incidence of postoperative disease. Canal-down surgery is less likely to need revision operations but requires more care and is somewhat less successful in restoring hearing.

We recommend canal-down surgery (1) for children under 8 years of age, (2) whenever exposure is difficult, (3) whenever there is a strong likelihood of incomplete removal of disease, or (4) when for any reason the operation is difficult to perform with the canal-up procedure. We tend to reserve the canal-up approach for (1) patients with hearing loss in the other ear, in which we are trying to get the best possible functional result; (2) patients who are physically active and like to swim; and (3) patients who are willing to accept the increase risk in recurrence. Since aditus and attic retraction pockets can occur only when the canal wall is left intact, we have prevented this particular complication with the use of cartilage blocks placed from the mastoid cavity into the attic and aditus acting as a barrier to retraction of epithelium. We have not had postoperative retraction pocket cholesteatomas, since this change was instituted approximately 7 years ago.

## INNER EAR FISTULAS

The treatment of fistulas of the semicircular canals remains controversial. Should one remove the matrix over the fistula or leave it in place? It is very important to maintain a high index of suspicion in all cases of cholesteatoma and to approach the bottom of the antrum at the end of the operation when all other disease is removed. We remove the matrix as long as we are sure that the cholesteatoma is not attached to the endosteal membrane and that no perilymph leak will occur. The matrix is left in patients who have only one hearing ear or when there may be some adherence of the cholesteatoma to the endostium. The patient should then have a revision after 6 to 9 months. In some of these cases, the cholesteatoma had disappeared at the time of revision.

## FUTURE DIRECTIONS IN TREATMENT OF CHOLESTEATOMAS

Clinicians are usually in the position of treating the disease after it has already been established, as opposed to preventing the disease. In the case of cholesteatoma, the future requires us to understand eustachian tube function and dysfunction; to recognize those forms of dysfunction that are most likely to result in severe disease, such as cholesteatoma, and to attempt to treat the middle ear prophylactically. It is hoped that improved permanent indwelling tympanostomy tubes will become available. It may soon be possible to reverse the differentiation of keratin in an already established cholesteatoma, using vitamin A derivatives in the form of retinoic acid and various keratolytic agents (e.g., 5-fluorouracil) and in some cases prevent the destruction caused by the disease. In any case, cholesteatoma will remain a difficult problem, both biologically and therapeutically. It will always be necessary to have a high degree of technical skill to eliminate the disease while preserving function.

# REFERENCES

1. Müller J: Von der geschicteten perlmutterglanzenden Fettgeschwulst. Cholesteatoma in uber den feineren bau und die formen der krankhaften geschwulste. G. Reimer, Berlin, 1838
2. Harker LA: Cholesteatoma: An incidence study. p. 308. In McCabe B, Sade J, Abramson M (eds): Cholesteatoma. First International Conference. Aesculapius, Alabama, 1977
3. Harker LA, Severeid LR: Cholesteatoma in the cleft palate patient. p. 37. In Sade J (ed): Proceedings of the Second International Conference on Cholesteatoma and Mastoid Surgery. Kugler, Amsterdam, 1982
4. Derlacki EL: Congenital cholesteatoma of the middle ear and mastoid: A third report. Arch Otol 97:177, 1973
5. Sanna M, Zini C: Congenital cholesteatoma of the middle ear. p. 29. In Sade J (ed): Proceedings of the Second International Conference on Cholesteatoma and Mastoid Surgery. Kugler, Amsterdam, 1982
6. Levenson MJ, Parisier SC, Chute P: A review of twenty congenital cholesteatomas of the middle ear in children. Otolaryngol Head Neck Surg. 94:560, 1986
7. Schwartz RH, Grundfast KM, Feldman B, et al: Cholesteatoma medial to an intact tympanic membrane on 34 young children. Pediatrics 74:236, 1984
8. Wendt H: Desquamative entundung des mittelhors. Arch Heilkd 14:428, 1873
9. Tumarkin A: Attic cholesteatosis. J Laryngol 72:593, 1958
10. Sade J: Pathogenesis of attic cholesteatoma. p. 212. In McCabe B, Sade J, Abramson M (eds): Cholesteatoma. First International Conference. Aesculapius, Alabama, 1977
11. Sade J: Cellular differentiation of the middle ear lining. Ann Otol Rhinol Laryngol 80:376, 1971
12. Bremond G, Magnan J: Evidence for the migration theory: Ultrastructural cell types in the epithelial layer of cholesteatoma. p. 187. In McCabe B, Sade J, Abramson M (eds): Cholesteatoma. First International Conference. Aesculapius, Alabama, 1977
13. Habermann J: Zur entschung des cholesteatoms des mittelhors. Arch Ohren Nasen Kehlkopfheilkd 27:42, 1888
14. Bezold F: Cholesteatoma, perforation of shrapnell's membrane, and occlusion of the tubes—An etiological study. Arch Otolaryngol 21:232, 1892
15. Whittmaack K: Wie entsteht ein genuines Cholesteatoma? Arch Ohren Nasen Kehlkopfheilkd 137:306, 1933
16. Ruedi L: Cholesteatoma formation in the middle ear in animal experiments. Acta Otolaryngol (Stockh) 50:233, 1959
17. Fernandez C, Lindsay JR: Aural cholesteatoma. Experimental observations. Laryngoscope 70:1119, 1960
18. Abramson M, Gantz BJ, Asarch RG, Litton WB: Cholesteatoma pathogenesis: Evidence for the migration theory. p. 176. In McCabe B, Sade J, Abramson M (eds): Cholesteatoma. First International Conference. Aesculapius, Alabama, 1977
19. Abramson M, Asarch RG, Litton WB: Experimental aural cholesteatoma causing bone resorption. Ann Otol Rhinol Laryngol 84:425, 1975
20. Bretlan P, Jorgensen MB, Sorensen C, Dabelsteen E: Bone resorption in human cholesteatoma. Ann Otol 91:131, 1982
21. McGinn MD, Chole RA, Henry KR: Cholesteatoma: experimental induction in the mongolian gerbil meriones unguiculatus. Acta Otolaryngol (Stockh) 93:61, 1982
22. Ragheb S, Gantz BJ: Experimental model of an acquired cholesteatoma (unpublished data).
23. Cantekin EI, Bluestone CD, Saez C, et al: Normal and abnormal middle ear ventilation. Ann Otol Rhinol Laryngol 86[Suppl 41]:1, 1977
24. Bluestone CD, Casselbrant ML, Cantekin EI: Functional obstruction of the eustachian tube in the pathogenesis of aural cholesteatoma in children. p. 211. In Sade J (ed): Proceedings of the Second International Conference on Cholesteatoma and Mastoid Surgery. Kugler, Amsterdam, 1982
25. Litton WB: Epidermal migration in the ear: The location and characteristics of the generation center revealed by utilizing a radioactive desoxyribose nucleic acid precursor. Acta Otolaryngol (Stockh) [Suppl]:240, 1968
26. Weiss P: The biologic foundations of wound repair. Harvey Lect 55:13, 1959–1960
27. Sugita T, Huang CC, Abramson M: Effect of endotoxin on keratin production of keratinocytes in vitro. Am J Otolaryngol 7:42, 1986

28. Ruedi L: Cholesteatosis of the attic. J Laryngol Otol 72:593, 1958

29. Walsh TE, Covel WP, Ogura JH: The effect of cholesteatosis on bone. Ann Otol Rhinol Laryngol 60:1100, 1951

30. Abramson M: Collagenase activity in middle ear cholesteatoma. Ann Otol Rhinol Laryngol 78:112, 1969

31. Glimcher MJ, Hodge AJ, Schmitt FD: Macromolecular aggregation states in relation to mineralization: The collagen hydroxyapatite system as studied in vitro. Proc Natl Acad Sci USA 43:860, 1857

32. Thomsen J, Bretlau P, Jorgensen MB, Kristensen HK: Bone resorption in chronic otitis media. p. 136. In McCabe B, Sade J, Abramson M (eds): Cholesteatoma. First International Conference. Aesculapius, Alabama, 1977

33. Raisz LG: Bone resorption in tissue culture: Factors influencing the response to parathyroid hormone. J Clin Invest 44:103, 1965

34. Hausmann E, Weinfeld N, Miller WA: Effect of Lipopolysaccharides on bone resorption in tissue culture. Calcif Tissue Res 9:272, 1972

35. Robinson DR, McGuire MB: Prostaglandins in the rheumatoid disease. Ann NY Acad Sci 256:318, 1975

36. Tos M: Pathology of the ossicular chain in various chronic middle ear disease. J Otolaryngol 93:769, 1979

37. Sade J, Halevy A: The aetiology of bone destruction in chronic otitis media. J Laryngol Otol 88:139, 1974

38. Thomsen J, Tos M, Nielsen M, Jorgensen MB: Bone destruction in inflammatory diseases of the ear. In Sade J (ed): Proceedings of the Second International Conference on Cholesteatoma and Mastoid Surgery. Kugler, Amsterdam, 1982

39. Kaneko Y, Yuasa R, Jse Y, et al: Bone Destruction due to rupture of a cholesteoma sac: A pathogenesis of bone destruction in aura; cholesteatoma. Laryngoscope 90:1865, 1980

40. Moriyama H, Huang CC, Shirahata Y, Abramson M: Effects of keratin on bone destruction in experimental otitis media. Arch Otorhinolaryngol 230:61, 1984

41. Moriyama H, Huang CC, Abramson M: Cell cooperation in bone resorption in chronic otitis media. Arch Otorhinolaryngol 240:89, 1984

42. Wahl LM, Wahl SM, Mergenhagen S: Collegenase production by lymphokine-activated macrophages. Science 187:261, 1975

43. Moriyama H, Huang CC, Kato M, Abramson M: Effects of pressure on bone resorption in the middle ear of rats. Ann Otol Rhinol Laryngol 94:60, 1985

44. Chole RA: Cellular and subcellular events of bone resorption in human and experimental cholesteatoma: The role of osteoclasts. Laryngoscope 94:76, 1984

45. Ptak W, Cichocki T: The mechanism of antimacrophage serum-induced fusion of hamster macrophages. Acta Histochem (Jena) 121:116, 1972

46. Huang CC, Hsu S, Saporta D, Abramson M: Effects of anti-type II collagen antibody on macrophages in vitro. Trans Am Otol Soc. 74:119, 1986

47. Glasscock ME, Dickins JER, Wiet R: Cholesteatoma in children. Laryngoscope 91:1743, 1981

# Immunology of the Ear

# 29

## Jacques F. Poliquin

The application of immunology to otolaryngology is a recent phenomenon, and new immune theories have been advanced to define the pathogenesis of such common disorders as secretory otitis media, autoimmune sensorineural loss, and tympanosclerosis. Immunology has now developed into a mother discipline that encompasses all aspects of medicine and awaits more practical and immediate applications in otolaryngology. Otolaryngologists will then have to familiarize themselves with the immune properties of the various organs of the respiratory tract in order to keep abreast of these recent developments.

The normal immune response has been subdivided into many phases; this subdivision follows a sequence of events that is variable in both time and intensity and may vary from one individual to another and from one organ to the other. Recent developments in research during the past 10 years have defined the immune capacity of each compartment of the ear and now shed light on various syndromes of so-called unknown origin.

This chapter describes the normal and abnormal immune responses, followed by an illustration of how the ear participates in the immune system.

## THE NORMAL IMMUNE RESPONSE

The human body is an abundant reservoir of lymphoid organs in which effector cells originate. These various organs are the thymus gland, the spleen, and the lymph nodes, which represent an internal secretory system, as opposed to an external secretory system of lymphoreticular tissue, located in the salivary glands, the respiratory tract, the mammary glands, and the gastrointestinal (GI) and genitourinary tracts.

These different cells circulate through and between these organs and, upon antigenic stimulation, may give rise to an immune response which, for the sake of clarity, has been divided into two classes. The first class is the nonspecific response mediated by mononuclear phagocytes, granulocytes, and platelets, and the second class is the specific response, which is mediated by T and B cells.

### The Nonspecific Response

In the nonspecific response, the agents responsible for the mobilization of cells (chemotactic factors) produce numerous cell elements, including kallikreins, SRS-A, basic peptides, histaminase, arylsulfatase, phospholipase D, eosinophil-derived inhibitors, and vasoactive amines.[1-4] All elements have one common denominator in the sense that they destroy, partially or completely, the antigen membrane and initiate the specific response.

## The Specific Response

The effector mechanisms of the specific response are the different classes of immunoglobulins and the various lymphokines. In humans, the bone marrow gives rise to T and B cells. Upon antigenic stimulation, the stem cell differentiates into B cells or plasma cells, producing the different immunoglobulins, the effector cells of the humoral response. T cells also originate from the stem cells; when stimulated they produce soluble factors called lymphokines, which are responsible for the cell-mediated response. Antigenic stimulation of T and B precursor cells also produces memory T and B cells that will be active in subsequent antigenic exposure. There is a well-defined interaction between T cells and B cells. B cells are responsible for the humoral immunity and T cells for the delayed cell-mediated immunity.

### Humoral Immunity

Antibodies belong to a group of structurally related protein molecules, known as immunoglobulins. Five classes of immunoglobulins have been identified: IgG, IgA, IgM, IgD, and IgE. These five classes have common antigenic determinants; thus, an antiserum produced by immunization of an animal with one class of immunoglobulin reacts with all other classes. Each immunoglobulin also contains antigenic determinants unique to that same class, which elicit the production of specific antibodies that react only with this class of immunoglobulin.

The basic structural unity of each immunoglobulin class consists of two pairs of polypeptide chains joined by disulfide bonds. Reduction of these disulfide bonds results in the liberation of four polypeptide chains; two light (L) and two heavy (H) chains. The intact molecules may be digested by papain to produce other fragments (Fc and Fab fragments). One fragment that can be crystallized contains most of the IgG specific antigenic determinants of the molecule and is designated the Fc fragment; the other two fragments retain the ability to combine with antigen and are designated Fab fragments. Very slight changes in the Fc region govern the biologic behavior of each immunoglobulin class in a general way. The variation in the constant region has been systematized into a formal classification of immunoglobulin.

IgG (molecular weight 150,000) has the ability to cross the placenta and to provide passive immunity to the newborn infant. IgG is widely distributed within tissue fluids and is equally distributed in the intravascular and extravascular spaces.

IgM (molecular weight 900,000) may be the first immunoglobulin class to appear in primary response following immunization. It is found mainly in the intravascular fluids. It is very efficient in fixing complement.

IgA (molecular weight 170,000) is found in relatively low concentrations in serum and tissue fluid but is present in a high concentration in external secretions, such as colostrum, saliva, tears, and in intestinal and bronchial secretions. In these fluids, the IgA molecules exist in dimer (two four-chain units) joined by an extra fragment (transport piece) that facilitates the secretion of IgA into the external fluids. IgA antibodies are part of the first line of defense against infectious agents and, because they are prominent in external secretions, such antibodies play a major role in the mucosa of the respiratory tract.

IgE (molecular weight 196,000) is present in a very low concentration in serum and tissue fluids but has a particular affinity to fix to tissue. This explains its ability to sensitize certain cells, such as, mast cells leading to degranulation upon contact with antigens.

IgD (molecular weight 150,000) is present in a very low concentration in the serum and is distributed mainly in the intravascular space. Antibody activity in the IgD class has rarely been demonstrated. IgD may serve as a cellular receptor for antigen.

In addition to the five aforementioned classes, subclasses of IgA, IgG, and IgM have been recognized.

## Cell-Mediated Immunity

The term cell-mediated immunity has come to be applied to the destruction of target cells by lymphocytes in vitro. T cells react to the antigen presented by the macrophage membrane. T cell clone multiplies by cell division and maturation and effector T cells appear. Effector cells have different subsets, such as, helper, suppressor, and killer cells. T cells can destroy the antigenic membrane directly by cytotoxic effect or through lymphokines. Lymphokines are mediators released or extracted from sensitized T lymphocytes after exposure to the specific antigen to which they are sensitized. They include migratory inhibitory factor of macrophages, skin-reactive factor, transfer factor, cytotoxic factor, chemotactic factor, lymphocyte-stimulating factor, lymphocyte permeability factor, aggregation factor, proliferation-inhibitory factor, macrophage-activating factor, interferon, and cytophilic antibody.

Delayed hypersensitivity mediated by T cells has numerous applications. Rejection of grafts, defense against viral infections, contact allergy and various autoallergic diseases represent a few of the examples of delayed cell-mediated response.

## Complement System

The complement system consists of immune separate components (C1 through C9) that, when activated, interact sequentially with one another in a waterfall fashion which reminds us of the coagulation sequence. The numbering does not follow their order of activation. The complement can be activated in the classic fashion, going from C1 through C9 in interaction with immunoglobulins, or in the alternate pathway, where C3 activation occurs without the early C components and without immunoglobulins. When the different complement components are activated, they release highly active mediators. The activation of complement leads to the lysis of microorganisms. Interaction of the complement system with the antigen–antibody complex results in swifter and greatly enhanced degradation and elimination of the antigen. Congenital abnormalities of the complement find their application in otolaryngology, such as, in hereditary angioneurotic edema (C1s inhibitor deficiency) and recurrent infections (defect in C3b

inactivator). The role of the complement cascade in middle ear inflammation has not yet been determined and may only represent a phenomenon of elimination of a pathologic process.

## Mucosal Defense System

Local immunity of the mucosa of the respiratory and GI tracts is now regarded as a separate entity from systemic immunity. Mucosal or secretory antibodies have been shown to be predominantly found in lymphoid-plasma cells that lie in an intimate anatomical relationship with the mucous membrane epithelium. The secretory immune system has unique properties and is located in or about the mucous membranes; in certain circumstances, it may function quite independently of the systemic response. Moreover, mucosal delayed hypersensitivity reaction has been described so that the concept of the "secretory system" applies to many types of antibodies, as well as to cellular immune reactions.

Tomasi[5] described the mucosal, secretory, immune system as the first line of defense. As we shall see in more detail (in the section on the humoral response of the ear), all classes of immunoglobulins have been shown to be produced by the middle ear mucosa and IgA in the upper respiratory and digestive systems is the dominant element of defense. The mucosa may therefore be the first effective element in the defense of the organism against antigens. The second line of defense is provided by systemic responses, which may be specific or nonspecific.

## Classification of the Immune Response

The immune response has been classified according to various parameters. There can exist a hyperimmune response, as seen in allergy, a hypoimmune reaction, as seen in congenital immunoglobulin deficiency syndrome and, lastly, autoimmune disorders, in which defense lines against the self are broken down, as in certain forms of glomerulonephritis. This classification, which is based on the degree of response, is not very specific. Most authorities have adopted the Gell and Coombs classification.[6] In this classification, abnormal immune responses have been divided into four categories.

## Type I Reactions

Type 1 is IgE mediated. IgE antibodies are fixed passively on mast cells and basophils. The antigen–antibody reaction liberates powerful pharmacologic mediators, such as histamine. The best examples of this type 1 reaction are anaphylactic shock and atopic asthma.

Allergy may be a cause of intrinsic mechanical obstruction of the eustachian tube.[7] As suggested by Bluestone, allergy may have a role to play in the etiology and pathogenesis of otitis media in four different ways. First, the middle ear could function as a "shock organ" like the lower respiratory tract in asthma. Second, the allergic swelling around the eustachian tube opening could be a cause of obstruction. Third, the eustachian tube could become obstructed in response to an inflammatory obstruction of the nose. Finally, ascending aspiration phenomena of allergic secretions in the tympanum could be a fourth factor.

In a double-blind crossover study, Friedman et al.[8] were able to demonstrate that with antigen challenge, symptoms of allergic rhinitis, including rhinorrhea and nasal obstruction, could be produced in all patients tested, leading to temporary obstruction of the eustachian tube in most patients, but to changes persisting for more than 3 days in a smaller group. No subject developed a middle ear effusion, but the dose and method of administration of the antigen in their study could be responsible for the negative findings.

IgE has been demonstrated in chronic middle ear effusion,[9,10] but there is a lack of fundamental evidence to support the fact that allergy is a major causative factor of middle ear effusion.[11–15] Allergic patients probably develop an obstruction of the eustachian tube, by way of tubal swelling, resulting, in some cases, in middle ear effusions. In some allergic patients, the middle ear mucosa probably reacts as the rest of the respiratory mucosa and becomes the site of local IgE production. IgE levels are usually elevated in the blood when middle ear fluid IgE is elevated.

## Type II Reactions

Immune reactions of type II are characterized by cytotoxicity and neutralization. The antibody binds to antigen found in certain molecules or on cell membranes. In the latter case, the antigen–antibody reaction may activate the complement and attract killer cells, leading to cytolysis. With or without complement, antibodies may neutralize certain molecules found in the membranes. The best example of this type II reaction is the hemolytic reaction caused by anti-red blood cell antibodies (hemolytic reaction of the newborn).

The presence of complement, inflammatory mediators, and lysosomal enzymes in serous otitis media has been well documented, but the likelihood that their source is the result of a cytotoxic type II immune mechanism lacks sufficient evidence in the way of detecting autoantibodies to middle ear tissues. Heterophilic antibodies have been shown in the middle ear fluid of patients with otitis media with effusion.[16] These heterophil antibodies of Forssman specificity may well have been engendered by bacterial infectious agents. An autoantibody to a target antigen in the middle ear has not been identified as yet.

## Type III Reactions

Type III reactions are secondary to the action of immune complexes. These antigen–antibody aggregates may be found in tissues or organs or may be circulating in the blood. In certain instances, particularly when there is an excess of antigen, the immune complex leads to a local inflammatory response. Serum sickness remains the perfect example of a type III reaction.

The type III immune complex reaction necessitates antigen, antibody, complement system, and polymorphonuclear neutrophils. All classes of immunoglobulins have been identified in middle ear effusions. Several studies have demonstrated depressed total complement and normal to increased C3 in middle ear effusions, as well as C3 proactivator and activator. Activation of the complement, both in the classic and external pathways, could result in the formation of immune complexes. Polymorphonuclear neutrophils and monocytes would in turn be attracted and release their intracellular contents, including lysosomal enzymes.

Using the Raji cell test, Maxim et al.[17] were able to demonstrate the presence of soluble immune complexes in middle ear effusions. Immune complexes and C1q reactive substances were also identified by Laurell et al.[18] in middle ear effusions. Similar findings were also reported earlier by Palva et al.[19,20] and Wilson[21] and by Mravec et al.[22]

In a more recent report, Bernstein[23] forwarded contradictory evidence. Using the anti-antibody inhibition assay, immune complexes were found in only 6 percent of cases of middle ear effusion. The techniques employed by Bernstein detect only immune complexes of IgG class. The possibility of immune complexes formed by other immunoglobulins cannot be excluded. It is also possible that the presence of immune complexes in middle ear effusions may only represent a normal immune reaction as a method of antigen elimination.

## Type IV Reactions

The last type of immunologic reaction (type IV of Gell and Coombs) is called cellular or delayed hypersensitivity. In this type of reaction, sensitized T cells act on the antigen without the aid of antibodies, by direct cytotoxicity, or through the liberation of soluble factors called the lymphokines, which in turn activate some effector cells, such as macrophages.

Macrophages play a dominant role in this type of reaction. Macrophages have been identified in middle ear effusions,[24,25] leading to the assumption that local immune mechanisms mediated by the T cells may exist in the middle ear. B and T lymphocytes have also been identified[26,27] in different types of effusions. Histologic, cytologic, and biochemical evidence seems to exist that type IV reactions may play a major role in the maintenance of middle ear effusions. The relationship between the local immunization of lymphocytes and the systemic cell-mediated immunity certainly needs to be explored further. Our own experiment on the cell-mediated response of guinea pig middle ear lead us to believe that the middle ear is capable of a T-cell-mediated response.

# THE IMMUNE FUNCTION OF THE EAR

The interface between the immune response of the ear and other organs of the respiratory tract is not yet fully understood. Much more is known about the immune response of other respiratory organs and the role of the mucosal defense system in general. Attempts to study the immune capacity of the ear have only been initiated during the past 10 years. Here, we shall review the nonspecific and specific responses of the ear, with special emphasis on the recent advances in the immune aspects of serous otitis media, homografts, tympanosclerosis, and autoimmune inner ear disorders.

## Serous Otitis Media

Most of the work in otologic immunology has focused on serous otitis media. The obstruction of the eustachian tube is still regarded as the first mechanism of middle ear effusion, but the chronicity and recurrence of the disease could be due to altered immune phenomena.[28] We shall review the different aspects of the immune response of the middle ear as they became evident in research on serous otitis media.

### Nonspecific Response of Middle Ear Mucosa

Nonspecific immune factors have been extensively studied. In a comparative study of 631 cases of serous otitis media and 361 cases of cholesteatoma, Mortensen et al.[29] were able to demonstrate a preponderance of blood type A and a shortage of phenotype O, suggesting hereditary trends in serous otitis media.

In effusions from patients suffering from otitis media with effusion, Bernstein[30] identified various biologic mediators of inflammation, such as the chemotactic factor(s), macrophage inhibition factor(s), activated complement, and prostaglandins. These factors may be responsible for the formation of new antigenic determinants on the cell surface.

These new antigenic determinants appear in the acute phase of the inflammation and could account for the chronicity of effusions.

In a further study on mediators of inflammation, Bernstein[31] identified an enzyme system, $\beta$-D-N-acetylhexosaminidase, in seromucinous cells of the middle ear mucosa, suggesting the role of lysozomal enzymes in permanent and irreversible damage found in serous otitis media.

The findings of Yamanaka et al.[32] from a study of 95 cases of serous otitis media, suggested that macrophages were the predominating cells in all types of effusion, as compared with the broad range of T cells (11 to 66 percent). It was also shown that the middle ear mucosa has a diminished response to phytohemagglutinin (PHA) and other mitogens, when compared with serum and adenoid cells. This suppressive activity may be attributable to macrophages and monocytes, which may have a marked influence on the regulation of the immune response in the ear of patients with otitis media with effusion.

### Humoral Response

Various studies have demonstrated the production of immunoglobulins by the middle ear mucosa upon antigenic stimulation. Tomasi[5] and Bryan and Bryan[33] exhibited the capacity of the middle ear mucosa to produce immunoglobulins of types A, G, E, and M. In 100 cases of serous otitis media, Liu and Lim[34] established a direct correlation between the rapid course of clinical recovery and the levels of IgA, IgG, and lysozymes.

IgA seems to be the predominant immunoglobulin in the mucosa of the middle ear and the local synthesis of the secretory component is evident in the epithelium. IgA and IgG seem to predominate in mucoid forms of effusion.[35] It has also been shown by Liu that immunoglobulins were present in effusions at a higher level (one to five times) than in serum.

Maturation of the defense system could also play a role in defense of the organism. In Liu's series, 75 percent of effusions reported were in children under 2 years of age and, of these children, 50 percent had not reached their first birthday.

It is a well-known fact that the defense system is immature before the age of 2 years. Liu showed that the production of immunglobulins is low below the age of 6 months but that it increases steadily up to 2 years, reaching a slowly ascending curve from ages 2 through 8. The data are in accordance with the epidemiologic findings and the natural history of serous otitis media.[36]

For some time, the presence of fluid or the type of secretions in middle ear effusions were thought to represent an abnormal immune response. The elevated expression of IgA, the absence of IgE, the participation of various biologic mediators, and the lack of evidence regarding the role of immune complexes all concur to suggest that middle ear effusions could be a normal physiologic response to inflammation. Epidemiologic studies have shown that a certain proportion of middle ear effusions will become chronic and will have a morbid evolution (hearing impairment, chronic purulent otitis, cholesteatoma); the challenge today in immunology is to identify this at-risk population, which could be immunodeficient in some way.

### The Cell-Mediated Response of the Ear

Research on the cell-mediated response of the middle ear mucosa is very scanty. Macrophages were found to be the dominant element in nineteen cases of serous otitis media, as reported by Sipila et al.[25] Activation of macrophages could be lymphokine dependent and a correlation must exist between the inflammatory response and the presence of T cells. In a separate report, Drexhage et al.[37] studied the delayed skin-test reactivity to a somatic antigen of *Hemophilus influenzae* in 21 patients with relapsing chronic purulent otitis media; their results showed that at least 50 percent of patients exhibited other immunologic disorders and that only 9 percent of these patients showed a positive delayed hypersensitivity pattern of skin-test reactivity. Such a study indicated that abnormalities in cell-mediated immunity to *H. influenzae* and also to streptococci form a basis for at least some chronically relapsing upper respiratory tract infections.

The astonishingly high rate of success with middle ear transplants has led some investigators to conclude that the middle ear is a privileged site. Tolerogenesis has been suggested as the mechanism for success in tympano-ossicular homografts.[38–42] The middle ear has a diminished immune response in transplantation, probably due to external factors, such as the preservatives and the poor cellularity of the grafts, but also because of local factors. Besides Kastenbauer's report,[43] very few studies exist on the cell-mediated response of the middle ear: which limb response of the immune response (afferent or efferent) is affected in the middle ear remains the important question.

In an experiment on the cell-mediated response of guinea pig middle ear, Poliquin et al.[44] studied the afferent and efferent responses to skin grafts. The response obtained from stimulating the ear with isografts and allografts was compared with the classic model of skin grafts, in which first- and second-set reactions are best illustrated. Their results showed that the middle ear has a rather low capacity to elicit a second-set rejection of the skin graft. This lack of sensitization in the ear was explained by the concept of tolerance.

In a more recent study, using the mixed lymphocyte response (MLR) to monitor the cell-mediated immunity of the guinea pig's middle ear, Poliquin et al.[45] studied the afferent and efferent limbs of the immune response (Table 29-1). Animals sensitized with an allograft in the ear showed an elevated MLR upon a second antigenic stimulation, contradicting the preliminary data of 1979. In the second part of the experiment (efferent limb), isografts and allografts inserted in the middle ear were studied following a second antigenic exposure (allograft on the back of the animal one month earlier). The results of this second experiment are unavailable at this time, but we hope both to characterize the systemic cell-mediated response by way of the MLR and to define the role of T cells and B cells on the middle ear grafts by the use of monoclonal antibodies and immunoperoxidase staining techniques.

This study clearly establishes the capacity of the middle ear to mount a cell-mediated response. The rejection of allografts in some patients could represent an abnormal immune phenomenon, and a research project is currently under way to help us detect the population of patients who would reject these allografts. Various factors could be at play, such as blocking antibodies and HLA.

## Homografts

Many factors were thought to be responsible for the exceptionally high take of grafts in the middle ear. At first, the middle ear was believed to be an immunologically privileged site, like the anterior chamber of the eye or the hamster cheek pouch. But the eardrum and the middle ear do contain all the necessary elements with which to mount an immune response, as has been shown by various studies on serous otitis media.

Local factors has also been extensively studied to explain this tolerance. These factors were the antigenicity of the graft, the reduced surface of the grafted area, the preservatives, and the positioning of the graft (overlay versus underlay techniques). Finally, studies by Veldman and Kuijpers have[40,41] shown that tolerogenesis is probably responsible for the high rate of success in reconstructive surgery of the ear.

Apart from Kastenbauer's report,[42] very few studies exist on the cell-mediated response of the middle ear. Which limb of the immune response (afferent or efferent) is at play in transplantation in the middle ear remains the important question.[43]

Acquired tolerance could prove an important concept in the field of homografts. Tolerance is an antigen-mediated defense that is based on multiple

**Table 29-1. The Cell-mediated Response of Guinea Pig Middle Ear[a]**

| Day | Series 100 #15 | Series 200 #18 | Series 300 #20 | Series 400 #30 | Series 500 #30 |
|---|---|---|---|---|---|
| 1 | Allograft in middle ear | Isograft in middle ear | Allograft on back | Allograft on back | Allograft on back |
| 28 | Allograft on back | Allograft on back | Allograft on back | Isograft in middle ear | Allograft in middle ear |
| 1, 7, 14, 25, 35, 48 | MLR | MLR | MLR | MLR immune staining | MLR immune staining |

[a] Strain 2 guinea pigs: donors; strain 13 guinea pigs: recipients.
MLR, mixed lymphocyte response.

factors, such as the dose of the antigen or changes in its structure. The so-called afferent inhibition model of transplantation leads us to postulate that the antigen–antibody complexes may cover antigenic sites and thus prevent sensitization of host lymphocytes. Antigen–antibody complexes could bind to the immunocompetent cells and prevent the recognition of an immune reaction against the graft.[44,45]

## Tympanosclerosis

The question of an abnormal immune response in tympanosclerosis became evident to us because tympanosclerosis, in humans, was shown to develop after repeated infections or surgical trauma. Since the incidence of trauma is random, an abnormal immune response may be suspected as the causative factor. It was possible that the infectious agent (as seen in autoimmune glomerulonephritis) or trauma alone (as seen in sympathetic ophthalmia) was responsible for an abnormal antigen–antibody reaction in the tympanic membrane.

Von Troltsch coined the term tympanosclerosis in 1873, but it was not until 1956 that the state of the art was exposed by Zollner.[46] Repeated infections represent a causative factor. Characteristically, changes occur in the submucosa of the tympanic membrane or in the tympanum. The connective tissue undergoes a hyaline degeneration and the hyaline fibers form small islands that tend to calcify. Large numbers of matrix vesicles may be scattered among the intact collagen fibers and bundles. Conductive deafness may be associated with tympanosclerosis. The disease process may extend to the ossicular chain and the ligaments. A close association with cholesteatoma has been reported by Friedmann.[47,48] Again, both basic and clinical research in serous otitis media has led to interesting discoveries about tympanosclerosis.

Haugeto et al.,[49] in 1979, reported a prospective study with a 5-year follow-up of 242 patients who had undergone myringotomy with a ventilation tube for serous otitis media. Of these patients, 42.9 percent showed tympanic scars with retraction and sclerosis. The same type of longitudinal study was performed by Tos[50] on 527 ears evaluated 3 to 8 years following the insertion of ventilation tubes. The incidence of complications was quite high: tympanosclerosis was found in 18.8 percent and a combination of atrophy and tympanosclerosis was found in 9.1 percent of cases. In a further study, Tos confirmed his initial findings, which concurred with those of MacKinnon's[51] study in which 33 percent of eardrums with a ventilation tube showed some degree of tympanosclerosis.

In a study of 54 patients with bilateral otitis media with effusion, Kilby et al.[52] performed a myringotomy with ventilation tube on one side and a myringotomy without ventilation tube on the other. Patients were followed for a 24-month period and, at that time, atrophic scars were already more frequent on the ventilation tube side (32 percent as compared with 11 percent), and hypertrophic scars were present in 30 percent of ventilation tube patients compared with 21 percent in nonventilation tube patients. Tos's study is similar and involves 224 consecutive cases of bilateral serous otitis media[53]; 193 patients were followed for up to 3 years. Tympanosclerosis was found in 48 percent of ventilation tube cases, as compared with 10 percent in nonventilation tube patients ($P < 0.001$). These studies clearly demonstrate the direct correlation between the site of the insertion of the tube and the formation of tympanosclerosis. In a more recent study, Lildholdt[54] revealed similar findings among a population of patients suffering from tympanosclerosis who were followed for up to 5 years. The incidence of tympanosclerosis and atrophy of the pars tensa was 77 percent.

In an effort to identify an antigen–antibody reaction at the site of trauma on the eardrum of sensitized animals, we raised an antiserum to the Hartley guinea pig tympanic membrane. This antiserum was raised in the rabbit (heterologous antiserum) and in the guinea pig (autologous antiserum) and was shown to contain IgG. We then passively immunized 181 Hartley guinea pigs with one of three types of solution (normal saline, heterologous or autologous antisera). Within 1 hour of passive immunization by intracardiac injection, trauma was created on three right-sided organs (tympanic membrane, nasal mucosa, and muscle of the leg). Figure 29-1 describes the sequence of the protocol, and Table 29-2 provides a summary of the techniques performed on day 1 or day 7.

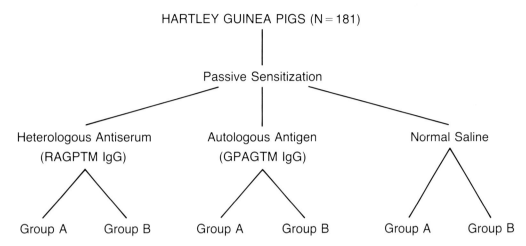

**Fig. 29-1.** Sequence of methods. **(A)** Myringotomy performed on (R) tympanic membrane. **(B)** Infection in (R) middle ear with *Streptococcus pneumoniae*. RAGPTM IgG, rabbit anti-guinea pig tympanic membrane IgG; GPAGTM IgG, guinea pig anti-guinea pig tympanic membrane IgG.

In this experiment, all the rhodamine staining was negative, suggesting the nonconsumption of the complement. Immunoperoxidase staining was mostly positive in all groups and seemed to predominate on the right eardrum, but these results were not statistically significant. Positive immunofluorescence, on the other hand, was obtained on the right tympanic membrane (Fig. 29-2) and was more evident on day 7 with the heterologous antiserum. The muscles and the nasal mucosa failed to demonstrate any immune response and no cross-reactivity between the tympanic membrane and the other organs could be evidenced. The left-sided control organs remained negative throughout the experiment and nonsignificant results were obtained in the normal saline-treated group. Essentially, the purpose of this study was to measure the immune reaction in the traumatized eardrum of a sensitized guinea pig and to identify the factors influencing the degree of this reaction.

Our results also show that passive immunization, preferably with heterologous immunization, yields a positive immune response as measured by immunofluorescence on traumatized tympanic membranes on days 1 and 7. Further studies comparing the heterologous sensitization with Freund's complete adjuvant are in progress to establish the reason for these discrepancies. Our heterologous antiserum was more concentrated than the autologous antiserum, the ratio being 2.6 : 1 and this could explain the difference between the results obtained with the two antisera.[55]

Our antiserum was obtained from the lamina propria of guinea pig tympanic membrane. Fine fibrils and homogenous interfibrillar ground substances constitute the middle layer of the eardrum. In separate reports, Lim[56] and Johnson et al.[57] showed that these fibrils are neither true collagen nor elastin, differing in both size and chemical content. The finer fibrils of the tympanic membrane contain amino acids that are present both in collagen and elastin.

The antigenicity of the connective tissue elements of the guinea pig tympanic membrane has already been established. The antigenic element resides in the fibrous portion or in the ground substance or in both. A microfibrillar protein, widely distributed in connective tissue and associated with both elastin and collagen fibers, could be responsi-

**Table 29-2.    Techniques Performed on Animals Sacrificed at 24 Hours and at 7 Days**

| Tissue[a] | Staining Method |
| --- | --- |
| Tympanic membrane | Immunofluorescence (double direct) |
| Nasal mucosa | Immunoperoxidase |
| Striated muscle of leg | Rhodamine (C3) |

[a] R, side traumatized; L, side intact.

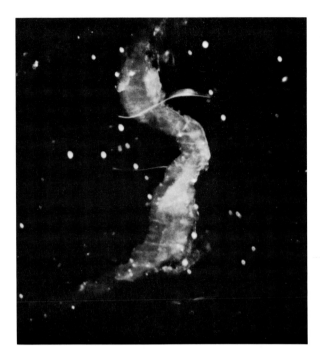

**Fig. 29-2.** Positive immunofluorescence staining (FITC). On the right can be seen traumatized tympanic membrane of the guinea pig passively sensitized with rabbit anti-guinea pig tympanic membrane IgG.

ble for the antigenicity observed in the lamina propria.

After trauma or infection, the lamina propria could become the source of hidden antigen and an antigen–antibody reaction could be precipitated in certain persons. Such an immunopathologic event, as seen in Hashimoto's thyroiditis, could explain the hyaline degeneration seen in tympanosclerosis after multiple myringotomies. In order to apply Witebsy's criteria, more work is needed to pinpoint an autoimmune reaction at the site of the tympanic membrane.

Our study has shown that after a few days, trauma and/or infection favor the homing of antibodies at the site of the trauma. Damage to the lamina propria could increase vascular permeability and favor the leaking of plasma proteins. Circulating antibodies could then enter the tympanic membrane during infection or inflammation.

Tympanosclerosis usually develops following repeated infections or chronic trauma to the drum.

The tympanic membrane could then become antigenic to the organism and produce local changes in the lamina propria and the ground substance by different mechanisms that need to be examined more precisely. Such mechanisms could be complement dependent and specific to certain bacteria or viruses. A genetic predisposition could always play a part. The presence or absence of immune complexes is also important, as seen in serous otitis media.

In the final analysis, the antigen–antibody reaction elicited by the trauma in immunized animals could be autoimmune in origin. More sophisticated methods are needed in order to identify these autoantibodies.

As noted by Schiff et al.[58] the Koch postulate does not always apply in autoimmune disorders. Autoantibodies can be identified, but it becomes difficult to establish scientifically whether these antibodies are the sole cause of the clinical manifestations or whether they are associated with other mechanisms. Autoantibodies could also be the consequence of the disease process itself.

In conclusion, tympanosclerosis has been shown to develop in the eardrum as a sequela of myringotomy and ventilatory tubes and is also known to appear after repeated infections. Our acute experimental model suggests that abnormal antigen–antibody reaction and phenomena of autoimmunity can occur on the traumatized eardrum of sensitized guinea pigs, which is not in itself sufficient to make tympanosclerosis an autoimmune disorder, but strongly suggests it. Further chronic experimental models are now being developed to explore these results.

## Immunology of the Inner Ear

Like the middle ear, the inner ear was thought to lack the anatomic basis necessary to mount an immune response. Recent studies of the immune functions of the inner ear have clearly established the presence of immunocompetent cells around the endolymphatic sac and the role of the perilymph. Indeed, the endolymphatic sac is the site of a lymphocyte–macrophage interaction and IgG seems to be the predominant class of immunoglobulin.[59]

Using keyhole limpet hemocyanin (KLH), immunization in the perilymphatic compartment of the guinea pig inner ear, Harris and Ryan[60] showed that the inner ear is capable of generating primary and secondary local antibody responses. By comparing the humoral and cellular immune responses using KLH immunization in the inner ear, middle ear, and the peritoneum, the same investigators[61] were able to show that the inner ear is as good a route of sensitization (afferent limb) as the peritoneal cavity, when measuring the humoral response. It thus appears that the inner ear has an immune system that functions quite independently. There is still some controversy as to the mechanisms of local production of antibodies in the inner ear. As shown by Mogi et al.[62] in the chinchilla, the main source of immunoglobulin in the perilymph is the filtrate from blood vessels surrounding the perilymphatic space. There seem to be functional and mechanical differences between the blood–labyrinth barrier and the blood–brain barrier. Such experiments will lead to a better understanding of the immune function of the inner ear. For example, animals presensitized with cytomegalovirus (CMV) could preserve their inner ear function when subsequently challenged with CMV in the perilymphatic space.[63] The host and the inner ear seem capable of developing immunity when the antigen is presented to the inner ear.

## Autoimmunity

Autoimmune disorders of the inner ear have been the subject of many recent reports.[64,65] Most of the immune phenomena observed in the inner ear were related to phenomena of autoimmunity; we shall discuss these phenomena in more detail.

The immune system is usually prevented from responding to self-antigen. Autoimmune disease could develop when the regulatory mechanisms are no longer active. Three possible mechanisms may exist. The first, as in sympathetic ophthalmia, occurs when an antigen, usually sequestered during embryogenesis, is later exposed and elicits an immune response as a foreign antigen. A second mechanism could be due to the close similarity that may exist between a self and a non-self-antigen, leading to cross-reactivity of antibodies. A third possible mechanism is the modification of a self-antigen by an external cause, such as a viral infection, leading the immune system to perceive the self-antigen as foreign.

Lindsay and Hinojosa[66] in 1978 reported a case of multiple ear anomalies associated with a poor cell-mediated response. The immunologic parameters used in that study were quite rudimentary. The low lymphoblastic response to PHA stimulation was the only immune parameter used in that one case, although other factors could explain many of the so-called abnormal immune responses.

In a further report, by McCabe,[67] in 1979, the concept of autoimmune sensorineural hearing loss was put forward. Eighteen cases of a bilateral, asymmetric, gradual sensorineural loss associated with manifestations of vestibular and organ dysfunction were reported. The criteria of autoimmunity used in McCabe's report were quite scanty: one case showed signs of vasculitis in the temporal bone, and some patients showed moderate elevation of IgM. The main criterion of autoimmunity was the dramatic improvement in hearing attributable to cortisone and cyclophosphamide. A new test was also advocated in McCabe's report: lymphocyte inhibition assay (LIA) using ear antigen. In this test, the patient's mononuclear leukocytes were placed in contact with the inner ear antigen, and the response was considered positive if migration areas in the presence of antigens were significantly different from those of controls containing medium alone. Only a few patients had a positive LIA test in McCabe's series, and the favorable response to steroid therapy remained the main criterion of autoimmunity.

Caution should be exercised when using the term *autoimmunity*. A response to long-term therapy of steroids is insufficient to warrant such an appellation, and animal studies are needed. Animal models are being developed in order to study the pathophysiology of Menière's syndrome. The failure of the mechanisms regulating the production and disposal of endolymph in these syndromes is thought to be the main pathophysiologic event. In an effort to reproduce an immune animal model of Menière's syndrome, Yoo et al.[68] sensitized Hartley guinea pigs to bovine type II collagen emulsified with Freund's incomplete adjuvant. Antibody titers were assayed by the ELISA method and permanent sections of the temporal bones were ob-

**Table 29-3. Lymphocyte Blastogenesis Assay: Stimulation Index**

| Group | N | PHA | IE Ag 4 μg | IE Ag 500 μg | Skin 4 μg | Skin 500 μg |
|---|---|---|---|---|---|---|
| Menière's syndrome | 14 | 52.8 | 0.95 | 0.98 | 1.17 | 1.05 |
| Control | 11 | 43.9 | 0.90 | 0.95 | 1.19 | 1.12 |

(Harris JP: An immunological profile of Menière's syndrome. In Third World Congress of Otorhinolaryngology, Miami Beach, FL, May 26–31, 1985.)

tained. Histologic changes, compatible with Menière's syndrome and endolymphatic hydrops were found in the spiral ganglion, the organ of Corti, the stria vascularis, the scala media, the endolymphatic duct. Abundant macrophages along with immunofluorescent deposits, complement positive, were identified in the endolymphatic duct. There was increased antibody activity against type II collagen, a component of inner ear tissue. These preliminary reports need to be reproduced with a larger group of animals and in other laboratories before drawing conclusions. They are, however, quite promising.

In a further study, Yoo et al.[69] attempted to demonstrate the sensorineural loss and the cochleovestibular dysfunctions in sensitized rats. The methodology used for determining the auditory threshold had its limitations (auditory brain stem potentials) and further studies will be needed.

### Menière's Syndrome

In a 1983 report by Hughes et al.[70] on 11 cases of Menière's syndrome, two patients were shown to have tests compatible with autoimmune disease. The migration inhibition test and the lymphocyte transformation test were used in this study. This constituted very meager evidence; larger series are needed before recommending steroids and cytotoxic drug therapy for Menière's syndrome. At the Thirteenth World Congress of Otorhinolaryngology, Harris[71] presented 14 cases of Menière's syndrome in which a battery of immune tests had been performed prospectively and evaluated against controls.

As shown in Table 29-3, there was no significant lymphocyte blastogenesis upon exposure to inner ear antigen (two different Ag concentrations) in patients with Menière's syndrome vs. normal control population. As a negative control, their cells were also cultured in the presence of skin antigen obtained from the inner ear antigen donors. Thus there does not appear to be specific recognition of inner ear antigenic determinants by T cells from Menière's patients. This report is contrary to the 1983 report by Hughes and also mitigates against Hughes latest report in which six patients were shown to have Menière's syndrome of autoimmune origin.[72]

## AUTOIMMUNE DISORDERS

Autoimmune disorders that may affect the inner ear vary from connective tissue disorders, hematologic diseases, to endocrine diseases.[73] The double common denominator is the presence of isoantibodies against antigens of a specific organ and vasculitis. The participation of complement may also be pathogenic in the phenomena of vasculitis. When confronted with the possibility of an autoimmune disorder, the clinician could err with a multitude of laboratory data and should consult a fellow immunologist (see Table 29-4). The in vitro response of an individual to an allogenic inner ear antigen, as first suggested by McCabe, has no diagnostic value and has been the source of erring in many cases. The treatment of suspected autoimmune disorders with steroids and other immunosuppressive agents aims at altering favorably the humoral and cell-mediated response but, because the inner ear does not lend itself to biopsies, the clinical response has to be measured in a very indirect manner by way of audiograms, vestibular tests, and immune response in other organs. Logically, most immunologic syndromes that may affect the inner ear are within the province of the clinical

**Table 29-4. Investigation of Autoimmune Disorders**

Hematology
  Total leukocyte count
  Differential
  Sedimentation rate
Biochemistry and immunology
  Immunoglobulins
  Immunoelectrophoresis
  Liver-function tests
  Autoantibodies to various organs
  Complement system
  Circulating immune complexes
  Rheumatoid factors
Virology
  Viral antibodies
Pathology
  Phenomena of vasculitis (skin and heart muscle)
  Antigen markers, T subsets, Ig (immunoglobulins), Complement

immunologist. The otolaryngologist should be aware that the ear may be the site of initial symptoms in immune disorders and that new immunopathologic techniques are being developed to help diagnose and monitor these entities. A good illustration of the recent developments in immunobiology of the ear is the immune profile of Cogan's syndrome. In 1976, Edstrom and Vahlne[74] put forward an autoimmune theory regarding this syndrome, stressing the phenomena of vasculitis, the consumption of complement, and the transient depression of the cell-mediated response, elements that, by themselves, are of suggestive, but not diagnostic, value. In 1984, Arnold and Gebbers[75] added substantial evidence by reporting elevated IgG antibodies against inner ear tissues, IgG and IgA antibodies against human cornea. The role of immune complexes in Cogan's syndrome could be nonspecific and could represent the end point of the disease, but their presence does not necessarily preclude the role of specific antibodies against inner ear antigens. The audiovestibular symptomatology of Cogan's syndrome could be the local manifestation of generalized polyarteritis nodosa.

More and more information is being collected on the immune parameters of otologic syndromes of so-called undetermined nature. The otologic manifestations of Wegener's granulomatosis were well described by Illum and Thorling,[76] and phenomena of vasculitis, granulomata, circulating or deposited immune complexes substantiate the possible immune origin. Otologic changes are often nonspecific on biopsy, but most often the synchronous nasal/sinus involvement permits an appropriate histopathologic examination and may allow the clinician to start treatment early in order to avoid the auditory deficit.

Other forms of vasculitis, such as polyarteritis, may affect the ear, but the otologic manifestations may be clinically discrete. Sudden hearing loss has not yet been shown to be of immune origin, but studies are being conducted in randomized clinical trials, and reports should soon become available.

Table 29-4 illustrates the various tests available for the detection of autoimmune disorders. The cost/benefit of such studies leads us to believe that not all undetermined otologic syndromes warrant such costly investigation.

Clearly, some progress has been made in inner ear biology during the past decade, but clinical applications remain few and sometimes anecdotal. Phenomena of autoimmunity remain to be better defined in otology.

## CONCLUSION

The difficulty for the otolaryngologist confronted with a suspected case of abnormal immune response in otologic practice is still the lack of common definitive laboratory studies. A careful history remains paramount. It will always reveal family tendencies to recurrent infections and angioedema. Symptoms such as dryness of the mouth or conjunctivitis may indicate phenomena of autoimmunity, as seen in Sjögren's syndrome. Sneezing and vasomotor phenomena may be due to an allergic reaction. Recurrent upper respiratory infections and growth disturbances may suggest a defect in the humoral response.

Some laboratory studies may evaluate the circulatory cells but are often found to be nonspecific. Total and differential white blood cell counts and the dinitrochlorobenzene test (DNCB) are perfect examples. On the other hand, it is only by using the different tests available that one will become famil-

**Table 29-5. Otologic Disorders with Abnormal Immune Response**

| | Type I | Type II | Type III | Type IV | Autoimmunity | Complement Deficiency | Other Immune Anomalies |
|---|---|---|---|---|---|---|---|
| Serous otitis media with effusion | ? | X | X | X | | | T cells |
| Merière's syndrome | | | | | ? | | ? |
| Progressive sensorineural loss | | | | | ? | | X |
| Purulent chronic otitis media | | X | X | X | | | T cells |
| Homografts | | | | X | | | |
| Tympanosclerosis | | | | | ? | ? | |
| Allergic otitis media | X | | | | | | ? |
| Recurrent respiratory infection | | | | | | C3B | |
| Cogan's syndrome | | | | | X | X | Immune complexes |
| Wegener's granulomatosis | | | | | ? | | Immune complexes |

iar with the information that they contain. Consultation with the clinical immunologist will become more frequent, and the interaction between immunology and otolaryngology is bound to flourish.

As always, laboratory data have to be interpreted in light of the clinical facts. Electrophoresis, secretions of lymphokines, circulating autoantibodies, identification of immune complexes, consumption of the complement factors, to cite only a few tests, are now readily available in our clinical facilities but, for the time being, should be used judiciously in otology. As seen in McCabe and Hughes's series, the so-called immune disorders of the inner ear may be reflected in abnormal lymphocyte transformation tests or migration inhibition tests, but so far these data are not conclusive, and the inner ear antigen is hard to obtain and the test may vary from one center to another. We are still far from the day when a standard immunology work-up will exist in otology practice. More clinical and research studies are needed to adapt recent discoveries to the daily practice of otolaryngology.

We have reviewed the most recent developments in immunology as they apply to otology. It appears that the external, the middle, and the inner ear have all the necessary elements to mount a normal immune response. Abnormal immune responses and isolated immune phenomena have been shown to exist in the ear and help elucidate certain clinical mysteries in which the pathology and the pharmacopeia remain ill defined and give rise to therapeutic failures. Table 29-5 represents a list of otologic disorders in which abnormal reactions (according to the classification of Gell and Coombs) or isolated immune phenomena have been identified. This list will certainly expand in the years to come, when clinical and basic research will have bridged the gap that has existed for so long between immunology and otolaryngology.

## ACKNOWLEDGMENT

This work was supported in part by MRC grant MA-6961 and PSI grant 84-43.

## REFERENCES

1. Bach JF, Lesavre P: Immunologie. Flamarion, Paris, 1981
2. Richter MA: Clinical Immunology. 2nd Ed. Williams & Wilkins, Baltimore, 1983

3. Bellanti JA: Immunology. Vol II. WB Saunders, Toronto, 1978

4. Guttmann RD: Immunology. Upjohn, Kalamazoo, MI, 1981

5. Tomasi TB: Mucosal immune system. Ann Otol Rhinol Laryngol 85[suppl. 25, pt. 2]:87, 1976

6. Coombs RRA, Gell PGH: Classification of allergic reactions responsible for clinical hypersensitivity and disease. p. 575. In Gell PGH, Coombs RRA (eds): Clinical Aspects of Immunology. 2nd Ed. Blackwell Scientific Publications, Oxford, 1968

7. Bluestone C: Eustachian tube function: Physiology, pathophysiology and the role of allergy in pathogenesis of otitis media. J Allergy Clin Immunol 72:242, 1983

8. Friedman RA, Doyle WJ, Casselbrant ML, et al: Immunologic-mediated eustachian tube obstruction: a double-blind cross-over study. J Allergy Clin Immunol 71:442, 1983

9. Lim DJ, Liu YS, Schram J, Birck HG: Immunoglobulin E in chronic middle ear effusions. Ann Otol Rhinol Laryngol 85[suppl 25, pt 2]:117, 1976

10. Lewis DM, Schram JL, Lim DJ, et al: Immunoglobulin E in chronic middle ear effusions. Ann Otol Rhinol Laryngol 87:197, 1978

11. Bernstein JM, Ellis E, Li P: The role of IgE-mediated hypersensitivity in otitis media with effusion. Otolaryngol Head Neck Surg 89:874, 1981

12. Sloyer JL, Ploussard JH, Karr LH: Otitis media in the young infant: An IgE-mediated disease? (Proceedings of the Second International Symposium, Recent Advances in Otitis Media with Effusion. Ann Otol Rhinol Laryngol 89[suppl 68, pt 2]:133, 1980

13. Sergent JS, Christian CL: Necrotizing vasculitis after acute serous otitis media. Ann Inter Med 81:195, 1974

14. Mogi G, Maeda S, Yoshida T, Watanabe N: Radioimmunoassay of IgE in middle ear effusions. Acta Otolaryngol (Stockh) 82:26, 1976

15. McMahan JT, Calenoff E, Croft J, et al: Chronic otitis media with effusion and allergy: Modified Rast analysis of 119 cases. Otolaryngol Head Neck Surg 89:427, 1981

16. Van Cauwenberge P: Otitis media with effusion. Functional morphology and physiopathology of the structures involved. Acta Otorhinolaryngol Belg 36:1, 1982

17. Maxim PE, Veltri RW, Sprinkle PM, Pusateri RJ: Chronic serous otitis media: An immune complex disease. Trans Am Acad Ophthalmol Otolaryngol 84:234, 1976

18. Laurell AB, Nilsson NI, Prellner K: Immune complexes in serous and mucoid otitis media. Acta Otolaryngol (Stockh) 90:290, 1980

19. Palva T, Lehtinen T, Rinne J: Immune complexes in middle ear fluid in chronic secretory otitis media. Ann Otol Rhinol Laryngol 92:42, 1983

20. Palva T, Lehtinen T, Virtanen H: Immune complexes in the middle ear fluid and adenoid tissue in chronic secretory otitis media. Acta Otolaryngol (Stockh) 95:539, 1983

21. Wilson W: Recurrent acute otitis media in infants — Role of immune complexes acquired in utero. Laryngoscope 93:418, 1983

22. Mravec J, Lewis DM, Lim DJ: Experimental otitis media with media with effusion: An immune-complex-mediated-response. Otol Rhinol Laryngol 86:258, 1978

23. Bernstein JM, Brentjens J, Vladutiu A: Are immune complexes a factor in the pathogenesis of otitis media with effusion? Am J Otolaryngol 3:20, 1982

24. Yamanaka T, Bernstein J, Cumella J, et al: Immunologic aspects of otitis media and effusion: Characteristics of lymphocyte and macrophage reactivity. J Infect Dis 145:804, 1982

25. Sipila P, Sutinen S, Sutinen SH, Karma P: Ultrastructural morphology of mucoid effusion in secretory otitis media. Acta Otolaryngol (Stockh) 90:342, 1980

26. Bernstein JM, Szymanski B, Albini B, et al: Lymphocyte subpopulations in otitis media with effusion. Pediatr Res 12:786, 1978

27. Palva T, Hayry P, Ylikoski J: Lymphocyte morphology in middle ear effusions. Ann Otol Rhinol Laryngol 89[suppl 68]:143, 1980

28. Karma P, Palva A, Kokko E: Immunological defects in children with chronic otitis media. Acta Otolaryngol (Stockh) 82:193, 1976

29. Mortensen EH, Lildholdt T, Gammelgard NP, Christensen PH: Distribution of ABO blood groups in secretory otitis media and cholesteatoma. Clin Otolaryngol 8:263, 1983

30. Bernstein JM: Biological mediators in inflammation in middle ear effusions. Ann Otol Rhinol Laryngol 85[suppl 25, pt 3]:90, 1976

31. Bernstein JM, Villari EM, Rattazzi MC: The significance of lysosomal enzymes in middle ear effusions. Otolaryngol Head Neck Surg 87:845, 1979

32. Yamanaka T, Cumella J, Parker C, et al: Immunologic aspects of otitis media with effusion. II. Nature of cell-mediated immunosuppressive activity in middle ear fluid. J Infect Dis 147:794, 1983

33. Bryan MP, Bryan WTK: Cytologic and immunologic response revealed in middle ear effusions. Ann Otol Rhinol Laryngol 85[suppl 25, pt 2]:238, 1976

34. Liu Y, Lim D, Lang RW, et al: Chronic middle ear effusions. Arch Otolaryngol, 101:278, 1975

35. Watanabe N, Briggs BR, Lim DJ: Experimental otitis

media in chinchillas. I. Baseline immunological investigation. Watanabe N, DeMaria TF, Lewis DM, Mogi G, Lim DJ: II. Comparison of the Middle Ear Immune Responses to S. Pneumoniae Type 3 and 23. Ann Otol Rhinol Laryngol 91:[suppl 93, No. 3, pt 3], 3, 1982

36. Lamothe A, Boudreault V, Blanchette M, et al: Serous otitis media: A six week prospective study. J Otolaryngol 10:371, 1981
37. Drexhage HA, Van de Plassche EM, Kokje M, Leezenberg HA: Abnormalities in cell-mediated immune functions to Haemophilus influenzae in chronic purulent infections of the upper respiratory tract. Clin Immunol Immunopathol 28:218, 1983
38. Marquet JFE: Historical notes on homografts. Otolaryngol Clin North Am 10:479, 1977
39. Plester D, Steinbach E: Histologic fate of tympanic membrane and ossicle homografts. Otolaryngol Clin North Am 10:487, 1977
40. Veldman JE, Kuijpers W, Overbosch HC: Middle ear implantation: Its place in the immunohistophysiology of lymphoid tissue. Clin Otolaryngol 3:93, 1978
41. Veldman JE, Kuijpers W: The middle ear: An immunologically privileged site for tolerance induction in otologic tissue grafting. In Proceedings of the Third Congress of Immunology. Elsevier, Amsterdam, 1977
42. Kastenbauer E, Hochstrasser K: Der einfluss des konservierungsmittel Cialit auf die proteinlos lichkeit und die antigenitat von allogenen und xenogenen gettorknochlchen und trommelfell transplanten. Arch Otorhinolaryngol 203:225, 1973
43. Munster AM: Surgical Immunology. Grune & Stratton, New York, 1976
44. Poliquin J, Ryan A, Bone R, Catanzaro A: Immunocompetence of the guinea pig's middle ear. J Otolaryngol 8:385, 1979
45. Cormier R, Poliquin JF,: The cell-mediated response of the guinea pig's middle ear. J Otol 15:31, 1968
46. Zollner F: Tympanosclerosis. J Laryngol Otol 70:77, 1956
47. Friedmann I, Galey FR: Initiation and stages of mineralization in tympanosclerosis. J Laryngol Otol 64:1215, 1980
48. Friedmann I: Pathology of the Ear. Blackwell Scientific Publications, Oxford, 1974
49. Haugeto OK, Elverland HH, Schroder KE, Mair IWS: Chronic secretory otitis media. Acta Otolaryngol (Stockh) 360:192, 1979
50. Tos M: Upon the relationship between secretory otitis in childhood and chronic otitis and its sequelae in adults. J Laryngol Otol 95:1011, 1981

51. MacKinnon DM: The sequel to myringotomy for exudative otitis media. J Laryngol Otol 85:773, 1971
52. Kilby D, Richards SH, Hart G: Grommets and glue-ears: Two year results. J Laryngol Otol 86:881, 1972
53. Tos M, Bonding P, Poulsen G: Tympanosclerosis of the drum in secretory otitis after insertion of grommets. A prospective comparative study. J Laryngol Otol 97:489, 1983
54. Lildholdt T: Ventilatory tubes in secretory otitis media. Acta Otolaryngol (Stockh) [Suppl 398], 1983
55. Poliquin J: An acute experimental model of autoimmunity in tympanosclerosis. American Laryngological, Rhinological and Otological Society, Inc., thesis, 1985.
56. Lim DJ: Tympanic membrane: Electron microscopic observation. 1. Pars tensa. Acta Otolaryngol (Stockh) 66:181, 1968
57. Johnson FR, McMinn RHM, Atfield GN: Ultrastructural and biochemical observations on the tympanic membrane. J Anat 103:297, 1968
58. Schiff M, Poliquin JF, Catanzaro A, Ryan AF: Tympanosclerosis. A theory of pathogenesis. Ann Otol Rhinol Laryngol 89[suppl 70, pt 2]:1, 1980
59. Rask-Andersen H, Stahle J: Immunodefence of the inner ear? Lymphocyte–macrophage interaction in the endolymphatic sac. Acta Otolaryngol (Stockh) 89:283, 1980
60. Harris JP, Ryan AF: Immunobiology of the inner ear. Am J Otolaryngol 5:418, 1984
61. Harris JP, Woolf NK, Ryan AF: Elaboration of systemic immunity following inner ear immunization. Am J Otolaryngol 6(3):148, 1985
62. Mogi G, Kawauchi H, Suzuki M, Sato N: Inner ear immunology. Am J Otolaryngol 6(3):142, 1985
63. Harris JP, Woolf NK, Ryan AF, et al: Immunologic and electrophysiologic response to cytomegalovirus inner ear infection in the guinea pig. J Infect Dis 150:523, 1984
64. Talal N: Disordered immunologic regulation and autoimmunity. Transplant Rev 31:240, 1976
65. Krakauer RS, Clough JD, Ilfed D: Recent advances in autoimmunity. Cleve Clin Q 47(2):73, 1980
66. Lindsay JR, Hinojosa R: Ear anomalies associated with renal dysplasia and immunodeficiency disease. A histopathological study. Ann Otol Rhinol Laryngol 87:10, 1978
67. McCabe BF: Autoimmune sensorineural hearing loss. Ann Otol Rhinol Laryngol 88:585, 1979
68. Yoo TM, Yazawa Y, Tomoda K, Floyd R: Type II collagen-induced autoimmune endolymphatic hydrops in guinea pigs. Science 222:65, 1983
69. Yoo TM, Tomoda K, Stuart JM, et al: Type II Collagen-induced autoimmune sensorineural hearing

loss and vestibular dysfunction in rats. Ann Otol Rhinol Laryngol 92:267, 1983

70. Hughes GB, Kinney SE, Barna BP, Calabrese LH: Auto-immune reactivity in Menière's disease: A preliminary report. Laryngoscope 93:410, 1983

71. Harris JP: An immunological profile of Menière's disease. In Thirteenth World Congress of Otorhinolaryngology, Miami Beach, FL, May 26–31, 1985

72. Hughes GB, Kinney SE, Barna BP, Calabrese LH: Autoimmune Menière's syndrome. p. 119. In Immunobiology, Autoimmunity, Transplantation in Otorhinolaryngology. Kugler, Amsterdam, 1985

73. Veldman JE, Roord JJ, O'Connor AF, Shea JJ: Au-toimmunity and inner ear disorders: An immune complex mediated sensorineural hearing loss. Laryngoscope 94:501, 1984

74. Edstrom S, Vahlne A: Immunological findings in a case of Cogan's syndrome. Acta Otolaryngol (Stockh) 82:212, 1976

75. Arnold W, Gebbers JO: Serum-antikorper gegen Kornea-und Innenohrgewebe beim Cogan-Syndrom. Laryngol Rhinol Otol (Stuttg) 63:428, 1984

76. Illum P, Thorling K: Otological manifestations of Wegener's granulomatosis. Laryngoscope 92:801, 1982

# Genetics of Hearing Loss $30$

Joann Bodurtha
Walter E. Nance

During the past 30 years, there has been a growing awareness of the importance of genetic factors in the etiology of deafness. With the progressive identification and control of environmental causes, hereditary deafness is likely to assume an even greater relative importance in the future. One of the most important insights to emerge from recent research is the realization that genetic deafness is not a single condition but rather a collection of many fundamentally different diseases that have one symptom in common. In retrospect, this heterogeneity should have come as no surprise. It is currently estimated that the human genome contains 50,000 to 500,000 active genes. Each gene may be thought of as an instruction that contains the information required to direct or regulate the formation of a specific polypeptide or enzyme whose programmed synthesis is required for normal development and function. The precise interaction of literally hundreds, perhaps thousands, of different genes must be required during the embryologic development of a normal ear, so that a defect in any one of many genes or gene pairs can lead to deafness.

Contemporary research on the molecular basis of other genetic diseases has also made it clear that a remarkable variety of different alterations in the structure of a gene can lead to changes in function. Although knowledge about the chromosomal locations, primary products, and mutational alterations involved in the genes that give rise to deafness is virtually nonexistent, it is clear from the progress that has been made with more tractable systems what the future directions of research on genetic deafness will be. Specialists responsible for the care of patients with deafness should not only be sufficiently familiar with the recognized hereditary deafness syndromes to formulate an accurate differential diagnosis but should also be sensitive to unusual opportunities for clinical or genetic research when they present themselves.

Thus, a major goal of this chapter is to present a selective review of the current status of knowledge about hereditary deafness and to emphasize major areas in which information is lacking. As more is learned during the coming decades about the biochemical and underlying genetic abnormalities that can lead to deafness, new possibilities for presymptomatic or antenatal diagnosis and more effective treatment will undoubtedly emerge. This chapter makes no attempt to present a comprehensive description of all recognized genetic entities in

831

which hearing loss can be seen. For authoritative surveys of this type, several reviews are available.[1-4]

---

## MOLECULAR BASIS OF INHERITANCE

In 1973, James D. Watson and Francis H.C. Crick proposed a model for the structure of DNA that elegantly showed how the chemical properties of this macromolecule allow it to encode, evolve, express, and faithfully transmit genetic information from one generation to the next.[5] In nature, DNA is found as a double-stranded coil or helix in which each chain is composed of just four nucleotide subunits: adenine, thymine, guanine, and cytosine. Wherever adenine occurs on one strand, it specifically binds to a thymine residue on the other and vice versa, similarly guanine and cytosine pair in a complementary manner. The strands have polarity and run in opposite directions; they may be thought of as complementary mirror images of each other. Genetic information is encoded in the sequence of the nucelotides of the DNA molecules. When the two strands uncoil and expose previously paired bases, each strand can serve as a template for the assembly of a new strand, explaining how the precise replication of a molecule can occur. When the stored information or instructions are to be used by the cell, a second type of nucleic acid, RNA, is assembled by complementary pairing with a segment of the uncoiled DNA molecule. This process is called transcription. RNA differs from DNA in its component sugar (ribose in place of desoxyribose) and in the substitution of the base uracil for thymine.

Once transcribed, the messenger RNA (mRNA) moves from the nucleus to the cytoplasm, where it is processed and becomes associated with ribosomes. Here the RNA directs the assembly of proteins from amino acids in a process called translation. The 20 amino acids that make up proteins are brought to the ribosomes by small specific RNA molecules called transfer RNA (tRNA) to which they have been enzymatically attached. Each of the amino acids has one or more specific RNA. A sequence of three nucleotides on a tRNA, the *anticodon*, pair up with three complementary nucleotides, a *codon*, of the RNA. In this way, the sequence of triplet codons on the RNA determines the sequence of amino acids in the protein whose synthesis it directs. In humans and other eukaryotic organisms, the segments of a DNA molecule that code for protein may be interrupted by intervening sequences, *introns*, that do not code for amino acid sequences in the resulting protein. The introns must be removed or excised from the RNA by special processing enzymes before the remaining exons can function normally in translation.

The precise function of introns is unknown, but it has already become clear that mutations that interfere with the normal processing of the noncoding regions can lead to grossly abnormal functioning of the gene. Genetic regions known as pseudogenes may well represent evolutionary relics of such events. These nonfunctional genes share sequence homology with adjacent functional genetic loci. They may well arise by gene duplication followed by the accumulation of deleterious mutations, which render them nonfunctional.

Proteins synthesized according to the instructions of the RNA may undergo additional posttranslational modification. For example, polypeptides may be cleaved, have sugar molecules added to them, or be assembled into larger macromolecules. The genes themselves are also subject to regulation and differential expression, which must, in the final analysis, underlie all the numerous steps involved in the development of adult structures from a fertilized egg. To achieve this remarkable result, genes need to be turned on and off at the proper times during development to ensure the production of appropriate proteins.

The ability of DNA to change or mutate and for those changes to be replicated just as faithfully as the original sequence is another essential property of the genetic material upon which all biologic evolution is based. If an error occurs in base pairing at the time of DNA replication in the germ cells, exactly the same mistake will be precisely transmitted to subsequent generation. Were it not for this property, there could be no permanent changes in the genetic material, no selection of the fittest, and no biologic evolution. Although some mutations must obviously have been beneficial for evolution to have occurred, most changes in the genetic material are likely to either be harmful or to have no detectable effect. When mutations occur in somatic or body cells, malignant degeneration is one possible consequence and, during the course of evolution, elaborate mechanisms have arisen to protect and repair the DNA when it becomes damaged. For example, two recognized DNA repair processes include the enzymatic excision of certain error sequences and photoreactivation of sequences that have been damaged by ultraviolet (UV) light.[6]

Remarkable advances in our understanding of the molecular basis of inheritance have taken place during the past 30 years. In the coming years, it seems likely that this knowledge will be increasingly applied to clarify and therapeutically modify the molecular, chromosomal, and genetic causes of deafness.

## PATTERNS OF HUMAN INHERITANCE

### Chromosomal Inheritance

Human DNA is packaged into 46 chromosomes, 22 pairs of autosomes, and the two sex chromosomes. Normal females have two X chromosomes, while males have only a single X and a very much smaller Y chromosome. Each cell contains its own copy of this 46-volume set of genetic instructions. To perform a chromosomal analysis, peripheral lymphocytes are cultured for approximately 72 hours to yield adequate numbers of dividing cells. Cell division is then arrested chemically at metaphase, the stage of mitosis in which the chromosomes are compact and aligned at the equatorial plane in preparation for cell division. The chromosomes are stained, photographed, and arranged in pairs by size according to a standard classification to obtain a karyotype. Several important new techniques have greatly enhanced the resolution and sensitivity of chromosomal analysis. These include the use of special histologic procedures, such as quinacrine staining and pretreatment with trypsin, which reveal highly complex and distinctive banding patterns for each chromosome pair. The use of these procedures on extended or prometaphase preparations now permits the detection of very subtle abnormalities of chromosomal structure that could not have been found with earlier techniques.

Abnormalities in the structure or number of the chromosomes often lead to recognizable clinical phenotypes or syndromes. Trisomy refers to the presence of three copies of a chromosome or chromosomal region instead of the usual pair and may arise from an error (nondisjunction) in meiosis during the formation of the egg or sperm cell such that they receive both members of a chromosome pair instead of one. Another important class of chromosomal abnormalities are those arising from the repair of chromosomal breaks. If multiple breaks occur in different chromosomes, several possible consequences can occur. Translocation refers to the reunion of two different broken chromosomes. If the total amount of genetic material is preserved, the translocation is said to be balanced. Persons who appear normal but who carry a balanced chromosomal rearrangement on karyotyping are said to be balanced translocation carriers. During meiosis, the cell divisions that precede formation of the germ cells, the normal pairing of the chromosomes may be disturbed, such that there is an increased risk of producing eggs or sperm with abnormal amounts of chromosomal material. On the other hand, if chromosomal breaks in a single chromosome are not repaired in a normal manner, the loss (deletion) or inversion of chromosomal material can result. Other more complicated rearrangements that can be seen include the formation of ring chromosomes and complex translocations involving more than two chromosomes.

Ordinarily, chromosomal rearrangements that involve the presence in excess or deficiency of a large amount of chromosomal material (i.e., aneuploidy) result in severe developmental abnormalities and may well be incompatible with extrauterine survival. Thus, it is estimated that at least 40 to 60 percent of first-trimester miscarriages are the consequence of recognizable chromosomal abnormalities. With the application of modern cytogenetic techniques, a growing number of children with a wide variety of malformations are also being iden-

## Table 30-1. More Common Chromosomal Abnormalities Associated with Ear Anomalies

| Chromosomal Disorder Other Features[a] | Hearing/Learning Defect | Ear Anomalies | | | | |
|---|---|---|---|---|---|---|
| | | Size | Folding | Placement | Appendages | Other |
| 4p<br>Monosomy<br>Severe growth retardation, and mental deficiency, microcephaly, "Greek warrior helmet" | ?; indifferent to environment | Normal | Adherent lobe | Normal | Preauricular | — |
| 5p<br>Monosomy<br>Cri-du-chat syndrome Cat cry, microcephaly moonlike face, hypertelerism | May have a few words | Small | Normal | Somewhat lowset | ± pretragal tag | Narrow auditory canals |
| 8<br>Trisomy<br>Long face, thick everted lower lip, osteoarticular anomalies | Language difficulties | Large | Well-defined upper; poorly defined lower | Normal to lowset | — | — |
| 9p<br>Trisomy<br>Brachycephaly, bulbous nose, unilateral grin, worried look | Delayed language to deaf mutism | Large | — | Normal detached | — | — |
| 13<br>Trisomy<br>Cleft lip, microphthalmia, polydactyly, early death | Defects in organ of Corti have been reported | Normal | Flat, poorly defined helix | Low set | — | — |
| 15q<br>Oval face, high cheekbones, deep orbits, seizures | — | Normal to large | Normal | Normal to low set | — | — |
| 18<br>Trisomy | — | Normal | Flat pinnae, | Low set | — | Atresia of |

| | | | | | |
|---|---|---|---|---|---|
| Micrognathia, prominent occiput, overlapping fingers, rockerbottom feet, premature death | | | pointed helix, faunlike | | external auditory canal |
| 18p Monosomy Small size, round face, wide mouth, dental anomalies | Deafness has been reported | Large | Soft, floppy, aplastic, anthelix | Low set, posteriorly, rotated, detached | — |
| 18q Monosomy Depressed mid-face carp-shaped mouth | Language difficulties, hearing loss | Normal | Deep sulcus between helix and anthelix, deep concha, protuberant anti-tragus | Normal | Atresia of external auditory canal |
| 21 Trisomy (Downs' syndrome) Hypotonia, round flat face, eyes with mongoloid, slant flat occiput | Usually normal | Small round | Small adherent lobule, over-folded and straight upper helix | Normal to low set | Small auditory canal |
| 22p Trisomy (cat-eye syndrome) Metacentric supernumerary chromosome, ocular coloboma, anal atresia | — | Normal to large | May protrude | Normal to low set | Preauricular tags and/or pits |
| X0 Turner syndrome Short stature, lack of pubertal development, ovarian agenesis, webbed neck, aortic coarctation | Congenital deafness or hearing difficulties | Normal | — | Normal to low set | — |

[a] All patients, with the exception of Turner's syndrome, have mental retardation.

tified in whom minor deviations from the normal karyotype can be found. Many of these new chromosomal syndromes are associated with malformations of the external ears, and some even appear to be more or less specifically associated with hearing impairment. Two examples are trisomy 13, and 18q− (deletion involving the long (q) as opposed to the short (p) arm of chromosome 18). The major features of trisomy 13 include cleft lip, microphthalmia, and hexadactyly. The ears are low set with abnormal, flat, and poorly defined helices. Mental retardation is severe, and mean life expectancy is 130 days. Structural defects in the organ of Corti and associated deafness have been reported.[7] Partial deletion of the long arm of chromosomes 18 is associated with hypotonia and froglike positioning of the lower extremities in infancy. There is depression of the mid-face, a carp-shaped mouth, and strongly folded ears, with a deep sulcus between the helix and anthelix and a protuberant antitragus. Mental retardation is variable, and psychotic behavior is frequently observed. A husky voice has been described as well as absent speech. Deafness has been associated with this syndrome, but to our knowledge the histologic findings in the cochlea have never been reported.

Structural inner or outer ear defects or hearing abnormalities have been reported to be a component of one or more clinical syndromes arising from partial duplications or deficiencies involving every one of the chromosomes, with the exception of the Y chromosome.[8] These syndromes often include hearing impairment and related language deficits. When autopsies of these patients have been performed, they usually do not include detailed studies of the temporal bone and inner ear. An extraordinary opportunity to learn about the morphologic correlates of these rare chromosomal abnormalities is thus being lost. Unexpected insights into the genetic regulation of cochlear development could arise from systematic study of these patients.

In children with dysmorphic features who are being evaluated for a possible chromosomal abnormality, it can be very helpful for the cytogenetic laboratory to know which chromosome(s) are thought to be involved in the defect. The auricular abnormalities reported in some of the more common complete and partial aneuploidy syndromes are given in Table 30-1 as an aid in the diagnosis of infants in whom these anomalies are a conspicuous part of the malformation complex.

## Mendelian Inheritance

The rules of inheritance first described in plants by Gregor Mendel are applicable to many human disorders associated with deafness. The various gene pairs on homologous chromosomes are responsible for individual traits. The alternative forms that genes at a given locus may take are called alleles. The clinical characteristics of individuals within several generations of a family can be examined in order to characterize the patterns of inheritance for many disorders. The classic patterns are autosomal dominant, autosomal recessive, X-linked, and multifactorial inheritance.

### Autosomal Dominant Transmission

Autosomal dominant inheritance refers to the pattern of transmission that occurs when the possession of only a single abnormal gene is sufficient for full manifestation of the trait (Fig. 30-1). Dominant inheritance is characterized by three properties: (1) all affected individuals have at least one affected parent, unless they are the result of a new mutation; (2) about one-half of the children of an affected individual are also affected; and (3) both sexes are affected with equal frequency. Certain dominant disorders exhibit great variability in the degree to which they are expressed, such that a person with the abnormal gene or allele may fail to exhibit certain, or any, features of the disorder. These differences in the phenotype produced by a gene are termed variable expressivity, and when the gene has no detectable effect at all, it is said to be nonpenetrant. Familiar otologic examples of autosomal dominant inheritance include Waardenburg syndrome, Treacher-Collins syndrome, and otosclerosis. It is important to recognize these entities because affected individuals have a 50 percent chance of passing on the dominant gene to each of their children.

Waardenburg syndrome is characterized by lateral displacement of the inner canthi, a broad, high nasal bridge, partial albinism, and deafness.[9] The partial albinism is most commonly apparent as a white forelock and/or pale blue eyes with hypo-

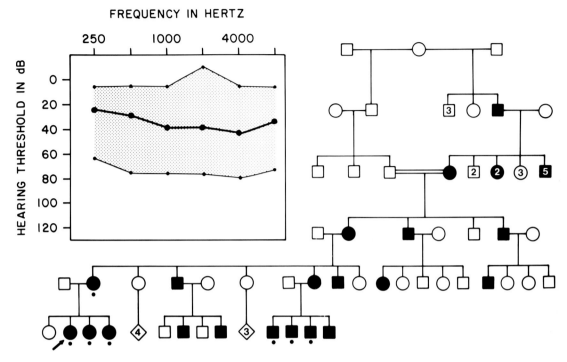

**Fig. 30-1.** Pedigree illustrating dominant transmission of mild to moderate sensorineural hearing loss through five generations. Affected individuals who were examined had mild facial asymmetry and scoliosis with fused cervical vertebrae. The family appears to represent an example of dominant Klippel-Feil syndrome with hearing loss.

plastic irises or eyes of different colors (heterochromia iridum). Approximately 20 percent of affected persons exhibit moderate to severe unilateral or bilateral sensorineural hearing loss. Histologically, the organ of Corti shows atrophic changes in the spiral ganglion and nerve.[10] Vestibular abnormalities are present in nearly all affected persons, even when hearing is normal. It has been suggested that there may be two subtypes of Waardenburg syndrome.[12] In type I, the canthal abnormality is almost invariably present and visceral, and cranial malformations may be found. In type II, the frequency of deafness is higher, but the canthal defect is often absent. On the basis of family studies, some evidence has been reported suggesting that type I Waardenburg syndrome may be determined by a gene located close to the ABO blood group locus on chromosome 9.[13]

Treacher-Collins syndrome, also referred to as mandibulofacial dysostosis, is a craniofacial anom-aly involving the derivatives of the first and second branchial arches. Features of this anomaly include downward-sloping palpebral fissures, depressed cheek-bones, hypoplastic mandible, and lower lid coloboma.[14] Deformities of the external ear occur in more than 75 percent of patients and are frequently associated with malformations of the auditory ossicles that can lead to a conductive or mixed hearing loss. Despite the fact that the disorder is considered an autosomal dominant trait, more than one-half of affected persons have two normal parents, and there is no other history of the disease in the family.[15] These cases are thought to mark the first incidence of new mutations in a given family. If this interpretation is correct, the recurrence risk for the parents, in such a case, would be negligible, while the affected individual would have the expected 50 percent risk of transmitting the trait. Before concluding that an affected child represents a new mutation, careful clinical and possibly audiologic examination of the parents and siblings would be required to exclude minimal signs of the trait in other family members.

Another example of dominant inheritance is otosclerosis. This disorder is initially a spongifying disease beginning in the endochondral layer of the capsular bone. When the lesion is near the foot-plate of the stapes, impaired stapedial mobility produces the characteristic gradually progressive conductive hearing loss.[16] The pathogenesis of the disorder is obscure. The occurrence of a positive family history, frequently in several generations, lends support to the assumption that the disease is transmitted as a dominant trait with incomplete penetrance and variable expressivity. Even identical twins are not invariably concordant in their expression of this trait.[17] Females appear to be more commonly affected, but the frequent occurrence of male to male transmission excludes X-linked transmission.[16]

### Autosomal Recessive Transmission

Autosomal recessive inheritance refers to the pattern of transmission observed when homozygosity or the possession of a double dose of an abnormal gene is required for full expression of the trait. The expected pedigree findings include the following: (1) the parents of affected individuals are usually unaffected carriers or heterozygotes, each of whom carries only a single abnormal allele; (2) the recurrence risk for affected children in marriages between carriers is 25 percent (3) both sexes are equally affected; and (4) if the trait is rare, an increased incidence of consanguinity is observed among the parents of affected children. Recessive disorders are often associated with enzymatic defects.

Although the enzymatic basis for only a few forms of recessive deafness is known, the frequent occurrence of complementation in marriages among the deaf suggests the involvement of many different loci that determine genetically distinct forms of recessive deafness. Complementation refers to the mutual correction in the offspring of recessive phenotypes in both parents when those defects result from mutations involving two distinct gene pairs. It is observed whenever a child with normal hearing is born to parents who both have recessive deafness. In this situation, we may conclude that the parents are homozygous for two fundamentally distinct forms of recessive deafness caused by genes at different loci regardless of whether is is possible to distinguish the two types in the parents by any known clinical criteria. Because of the great frequency of assortative mating that exists among the deaf, marriages of this type are by no means rare and they provide an incisive, though largely unexploited, approach to genetic nosology that is very seldom applicable to other genetic diseases. Approximately 80 percent of genetic deafness is estimated to be autosomal recessive in nature.[18] Familiar examples of recessive deafness include Usher syndrome, Jervell and Lange-Nielson syndrome, and Pendred syndrome.

Usher syndrome refers to the association of congenital sensorineural hearing loss with retinitis pigmentosa.[19] Visual symptoms include night blindness and progressive constriction of the visual field. However, because these symptoms may not develop until late in the first decade of life, periodic examinations of the hearing impaired children are important. An electroretinogram may help confirm the diagnosis long before the onset of overt visual symptoms. Although the term Usher syndrome is usually restricted to patients with profound congenital sensorineural hearing loss, it has become clear from studies of patients with a primary complaint of retinitis pigmentosa that a broader association exists between these two symptoms. Thus, in a survey of 670 patients with retinitis pigmentosa, Boughman[20] found that hearing loss was the most commonly reported extraocular symptom, noted by 71 or 10.6 percent of the patients. In most cases, the losses were of mild to moderate severity and had not interfered with the acquisition of normal speech. Other recognized syndromes in which hearing loss and retinitis pigmentosa may be found include Refsum syndrome, Alstrom syndrome, Laurence-Moon-Biedl syndrome, and Cockyne syndrome.[20]

It is estimated that Jervell and Lange-Nielson syndrome accounts for approximately 1 to 2 percent of the congenitally deaf. In this recessive trait, hearing loss is associated with a cardiac conduction defect manifested by a prolonged QT interval on the electrocardiogram (ECG).[21] Cardiac symptoms may appear as early as 3 to 5 years of age with the onset of fainting spells. The occurrence of sudden arrhythmic death in 50 percent of affected patients before age 20 underscores the importance of obtaining ECGs as part of the evaluation of patients with congenital deafness in whom the etiology is uncertain. Treatment with propranolol or by ganglionectomy may be helpful in preventing the syncopal episodes.[22]

Pendred syndrome accounts for approximately 1 percent of the congenitally deaf. The sensorineural hearing loss may vary in degree from about 40 to 100 dB. The associated goiter is unusually euthyroid and may not appear until puberty. The goiter results from a specific enzymatic defect in the organification of trapped iodine by the thyroid gland, which may be demonstrated by the prompt release of iodine from the gland following the administration of perchlorate.[23] It is not entirely clear whether the association of thyroid and ear disease results from the chance segregation of two separate genes or whether the two features of the syndrome are pleiotropic effects of the same gene pair. In one report in which the temporal bone history was studied, a Mondini-type aplasia was found.[24]

## X-Linked Transmission

X-linked inheritance displays no male-to-male (father-to-son) transmission. The female with two X chromosomes may be homozygous or heterozygous for a given mutant gene on the X chromosome, but a male with only one X chromosome is hemizygous for all genes on his single X chromosome, with the possible exception of a limited region of sequence homology between the X and Y chromosomes. Thus, a mutant gene on the X chromosome, whether it is dominant or recessive in the female, will always be fully expressed in the male. Among the children of a male affected by an X-linked recessive trait, all sons are unaffected and all daughters are carriers, provided the mother does not also carry the same gene.

The observation that females in general do not express a higher level of gene activity for X-linked loci, in spite of the fact that they carry two doses of these genes, is one important consequence of the phenomenon of the X-inactivation, which was first recognized by the British geneticist, Mary Lyon. Early in embryogenesis, one of a female's two X chromosomes is randomly inactivated in each somatic cell. Heterozygous females generally show an intermediate level of gene expression. However, in rare cases, a heterozygous female might by chance express the X chromosome with the mutant gene in all or most of her cells and could present as symptomatic manifestation of heterozygotes. In several disorders, carrier testing can be done on females who may be shown to have intermediate levels of gene product between those characteristic of unaffected and affected males, respectively. In disorders in which the phenotype is evident at the cellular level, such as in glucose 6-phosphate dehydrogenase (G6PD) deficiency, the underlying mosaicism of heterozygous females may be demonstrated.[25] It is estimated that X-linked disorders associated with deafness account for only about 1 to 2 percent of genetic deafness. One notable example of X-linked inheritance is congenital fixation of the stapes footplate with perilymphatic gusher, a syndrome that has been described in several families.[26] Vestibular disturbances have also been found. In several reported cases, attempted mobilization of the stapes footplate was associated with profuse drainage of perilymph and cerebrospinal fluid (CSF) at the time of operation. These findings suggest an abnormal patency of the cochlear aqueduct.[26] Even in the absence of effective operative intervention, early recognition with sound amplification can do much to promote the habilitation of affected males. In some families, the carrier females have shown a mild, mixed hearing loss.

## Multifactorial Transmission

In multifactorial inheritance, both genetic and environmental factors interact to produce the disease, but the precise nature and relative contributions of these factors may vary from family to family. The term *polygenic* refers to the hereditary component of this multifactorial causation. Many common disorders appear to be multifactorial in etiology. For most such diseases, the empirically derived recurrence risk after the first affected child is within the range of 2 to 5 percent. In striking contrast to mendelian inheritance, however, parents who have had two affected children have an even higher risk. Thus, the risk among couples may vary greatly, depending on the number of disease-predisposing polygenes they carry and transmit to their offspring. Typically, however, there is no way to identify a couple as being at higher than average risk until they have had one or more affected children. Presbycusis may well constitute a phenotype determined by multifactorial inheritance.

Presbycusis is a progressive sensorineural hearing deficit that usually starts at about age 60. Audiometric speech discrimination decreases proportionately with hearing. The audiogram may have a rapidly falling, sloping, or flat contour. Approximately 20 percent of the population over 65 years of age has a hearing impairment.[27] Pathophysiologically, both stiffness of the basilar membrane and degeneration of the cochlea, cochlear nerve, or central nervous system (CNS) may be involved. The relationship between recessive deafness and presbycusis remains controversial. It has been estimated that no fewer than one person in eight is a heterozygous carrier of one or another of the many different forms of recessive deafness. Studies of families with known recessive deafness have shown that in some kindreds, heterozygotes may exhibit minor audiologic abnormalities that can be similar if not indistinguishable from those of presbycusis, except that they can often be detected at an earlier age.[29] It seems reasonable to suppose that some genes for recessive deafness may, in the heterozygous state, either cause or predispose to the development of presbycusis. Conversely, the detection of minor audiologic abnormalities in the parents or collateral relatives of a child with profound deafness can provide support for the possibility of a genetic etiology.

## GENETIC EPIDEMIOLOGY OF DEAFNESS

### Incidence and Demography

The reported incidence of profound hearing loss varies greatly in different parts of the world and exhibits substantial secular trends as well. For example, rubella epidemics have made a major contribution to the incidence of deafness in the past.

The last major epidemic in the United Staes occurred in the spring and summer of 1964, and it is estimated that about 3 per 100 infants born between December 1964 and May 1965, or 20,000 to 30,000 children nationwide, had some evidence of congenital rubella syndrome, including approximately 5,000 to 10,000 with a clinically significant hearing loss.[30] For many years, the Center for Demographic Studies at Gallaudet College has provided a reliable source for data on the demographic characteristics of deafness in childhood and adolescence in this country. Their data have been collected on an annual basis from multiple schools, agencies, and other reporting sources throughout the country and include identifying information permitting the exclusion of duplicate reports on the same individuals. During the 1983 to 1984 reporting year, data were collected for a total of 58,184 hearing-impaired children and youths. The distribution of the reported cases by age is shown in Table 30-2.

It can be seen that the age distribution is relatively stable among the children who were of school age, with the lower proportion among the preschool and postschool ages, probably reflecting incomplete identification and losses from the reporting system, respectively. When related to the age distribution of the general population, the number of affected children aged 6 to 17 can therefore be used to obtain a minimum estimate of $8.9 \times 10^{-4}$ as the incidence in the population of deafness that is either present at birth or that has its onset in childhood.

The distribution of children by the reported severity of the hearing loss (better ear average) is given in Table 30-3. These data quite likely underestimate the prevalence of children with mild or

**Table 30-2. Age Distribution of 53,184 Hearing-Impaired Children, 1983–1984[a]**

| Age of Child (Years) | Percentage of Reported Cases |
| --- | --- |
| <3 | 2.7 |
| 3–5 | 10.4 |
| 6–9 | 20.0 |
| 10–13 | 23.3 |
| 14–17 | 25.4 |
| 18+ | 18.1 |

[a] Age was not reported in 1.4% of the total samples.

Table 30-3. Severity of Reported Loss in 53,184 Hearing-Impaired Children in 1983–1984[a]

| Degree of Hearing Loss | Percentage of Reported Cases |
| --- | --- |
| <27 dB (minimal loss) | 6.4 |
| 27–55 dB (mild-moderate loss) | 16.1 |
| 45–90 dB (moderate-severe loss) | 33.5 |
| >90 dB (profound loss) | 44.0 |

[a] Level of hearing loss was not reported in 2.8% of the total sample.

unilateral losses. Some investigators have estimated that for every child with profound deafness, there are 10 with lesser but clinically significant degrees of hearing loss. The sex ratio among the reported cases was 1.17. If the excess of affected males were entirely attributable to children with X-linked recessive deafness, this etiology would account for 7.7 percent of all cases.

## Analysis of Family Data

Segregation analysis refers to a method by which the genetic components of an etiologically heterogeneous condition can be estimated from the systematic collection and analysis of family history data. First, the sample of family data to be analyzed is divided into two groups, depending on whether the proband, or index case, is an affected child or an affected parent. Families identified through an affected child are said to have been ascertained by truncate selection, because sibships in which the children could have been affected with genetic deafness, but by chance were none not, do not appear among the study families. By contrast, families identified through an affected parent (complete selection) can include data on offspring sibships regardless of whether they contain an affected child. The study families may be further divided by mating type, that is, those arising from hearing × hearing, deaf × hearing, and deaf × deaf matings, respectively. Families consisting of one deaf parent and one or more deaf children may tentatively be identified as showing dominant transmission. When appropriate allowance is made for the fact that each sibship of this type must have had at least one affected child, the segregation ratio or expected proportion of deaf children may readily be estimated among the remaining siblings.

For a fully penetrant dominant trait, the expected value of the segregation ratio would be 0.5, that is, one-half of the children of a person with a rare dominant trait would be expected to inherit the trait. However, dominant forms of deafness are known, such as Waardenburg syndrome, in which bilateral hearing loss occurs in only a small proportion of those who inherit the gene. Therefore, reduced penetrance is the usual explanation invoked to account for the observation of a segregation ratio of less than 0.5 in deaf × hearing matings with at least one deaf child. Once the average penetrance of the dominant genes for deafness has been estimated, the proportion of the hearing × hearing matings that actually represent cases of dominant transmission in which it is one of the parents who is nonpenetrant can also be estimated. The remaining normal × normal matings include genetic cases showing recessive transmission as well as nongenetic forms of deafness. To estimate the relative proportions of each, a basic assumption is made that all sibships containing two or more affected children are necessarily genetic.

Although it would obviously be possible for a couple to have two children with nongenetic deafness, in the overwhelming majority of such multiplex families, an hereditary etiology is likely. From the frequency of multiplex families and the segregation ratio within them, the proportion of genetic and nongenetic cases among the uncertain (or simplex) families in which there is only one affected child can be estimated, along with the overall segregation ratio among the genetic cases by a systematic or iterative trial-and-error process.

Computer programs written to implement these procedures select the combination of parameter values for p (the segregation ratio) and x (the proportion of sporadic or nongenetic cases) that are most consistent with the observed set of family data. Deaf × deaf matings are of particular interest, since they can occur among individuals who have dominant, recessive, or nongenetic deafness in any combination. The risk of having affected offspring from such matings can be as high as 100 percent if, for example, both parents have the same type of recessive deafness. Alternatively, the risk could be virtually nil if the parents have different types of recessive deafness or if both parents have nongenetic deafness. Intermediate risks can arise when one or both parents have a dominant form of deafness. It turns out that the estimated proportion of deaf × deaf matings that can only give rise to deaf offspring is quite low (about 4 percent). This observation tends to confirm other evidence for the heterogeneity of recessive deafness and also suggests that most persons who carry single genes for two different types of recessive deafness have normal hearing.

The separate analysis of the three mating types may be pooled to obtain an overall estimate of the proportion of cases that are genetic and the relative frequency of dominant and recessive deafness among them. When family histories are assembled for a genetic analysis of this type, it is of great importance to collect these data in a systematic manner from a well-defined population and to give careful attention to the identification of the affected persons (or probands) in each family through whom the kinship was identified or ascertained.

Collections of interesting pedigrees or families culled from the literature or of cases referred for treatment to a specialized center are often of limited value for studies of this type because of unknown ascertainment biases that may cause the families to be unrepresentative. For additional details of the analytic methods involved in segregation analysis, original publications should be consulted.[18,31] (Fig. 30-2).

The result of genetic analysis on several large bodies of data on the family histories of deaf probands has previously been reported.[32,33] The most recent large study is that reported by Rose[18] in-

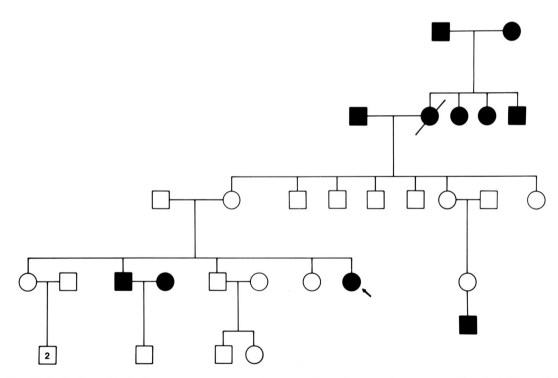

**Fig. 30-2.** Pedigree illustrating complementary and noncomplementary marriages among the deaf. I-1 and I-2 were consanguineous and are presumed to have had the same form of recessive deafness, as indicated by the fact that all their children were deaf (i.e., noncomplementary mating). By contrast, the deafness in II-1 and II-2 must have had different causes, since all their children were hearing (i.e., complementary mating). These children must all be carriers of a recessive gene for deafness of at least one locus, and expectation confirmed by the affected offspring of the marriages between III-1 and III-2.

volving three samples that included data on the hearing status of 65,437 offspring in 15,482 sibships with at least one deaf child.

In one sample, data were collected for 16,471 deaf children in 1968 as part of the Annual Survey of Hearing Impaired Children by the Office of Demographic Studies at Gallaudet College. The second sample involved a reanalysis of the family data collected by Fay[34] at the turn of the century as part of his monumental study of marriage among the deaf in America. The third sample included a series of pedigrees obtained from students at Gallaudet College in 1972.

The final results of the genetic analyses in these three populations are compared in Table 30-4. Although they were collected more than half a century apart, the National Survey and Fay data yielded remarkably similar estimates that about one-half of all deafness is genetic in etiology and that among the genetic cases, recessive transmission is about six times more frequent than dominant inheritance. Marriages among the deaf accounted for 2 to 3 percent of the matings in both samples of fertile couples. However, the total proportion of deaf children arising from such matings increased from 3.8 to 6.0 percent. This reflects an increase in the relative fertility of these marriages during the seven decades between the two studies to more nearly approach that of the hearing population.

In the Gallaudet sample, marriages among the deaf accounted for 12.7 percent of the matings and 18.6 percent of the deaf offspring in all of the families. The estimated proportion of genetic cases was larger in this high-achieving college population, quite likely reflecting the fact that genetic deafness is frequently a discrete or isolated defect, whereas many environmental causes (e.g., congenital rubella syndrome) may be associated with other neurologic defects.

Another important difference is that the National Survey included the 1964 to 1965 rubella cohort, while the age cohort for the Gallaudet students did not include an epidemic year. Bieber[33] showed that when the results of segregation analysis for deaf probands from hearing × hearing matings born in nonepidemic years are compared with those from students born in an epidemic year, the estimated proportion of genetic cases among the former is nearly twice as great: 15 percent versus 29 percent.

## Empirical Risk Figures

The practical importance of these results is that they clearly indicate that the relative frequency of recessive deafness is so high that unless clear evidence for an environmental etiology can be ad-

**Table 30-4.  Summary Estimates from Genetic Analyses in Three Samples of Sibships Ascertained Through Deaf Offspring**

| Mating Types | Total No. and Percentage of Families | Mean No. of Children per Family | Offspring Phenotypes | | | | Distribution of Genetic Cases | |
| --- | --- | --- | --- | --- | --- | --- | --- | --- |
| | | | Hearing (N) | Deaf (N) | Sporadic (%) | Genetic (%) | Dominant (%) | Recessive (%) |
| EA Fay Data (1898) | | | | | | | | |
| Hearing × hearing | 96.2 | 6.01 | 10,243 | 3258 | 48.2 | 51.8 | 4.3 | 95.7 |
| Deaf × hearing | 1.7 | 5.71 | 136 | 91 | 0.0 | 100.0 | 100.0 | 0.0 |
| Deaf × deaf | 2.1 | 3.85 | 55 | 134 | 0.0 | 100.0 | 59.0 | 41.0 |
| Total | 2335 | 5.96 | 10,434 | 3483 | 45.1 | 54.9 | 12.0 | 88.0 |
| National Survey (1968) | | | | | | | | |
| Hearing × hearing | 94.6 | 3.95 | 32,383 | 15,004 | 54.2 | 45.8 | 3.3 | 96.7 |
| Deaf × hearing | 2.1 | 3.84 | 544 | 478 | 0.0 | 100.0 | 100.0 | 0.0 |
| Deaf × deaf | 3.3 | 3.24 | 367 | 989 | 0.0 | 100.0 | 54.4 | 45.6 |
| Total | 12,665 | 3.93 | 33,294 | 16,471 | 49.3 | 50.7 | 14.11 | 85.6 |
| Gallaudet Survey (1972) | | | | | | | | |
| Hearing × hearing | 82.7 | 3.73 | 917 | 571 | 31.2 | 68.8 | 3.3 | 96.7 |
| Deaf × hearing | 4.6 | 3.83 | 35 | 50 | 0.0 | 100.0 | 100.0 | 0.0 |
| Deaf × deaf | 12.7 | 2.97 | 40 | 142 | 0.0 | 100.0 | 47.2 | 57.8 |
| Total | 482 | 3.64 | 992 | 763 | 23.8 | 76.2 | 22.2 | 77.8 |

(Adapted from Rose SP: Genetic Studies of Profound Prelingual Deafness. Doctoral thesis, Indiana University, 1975.)

duced, recessive deafness must be strongly suspected in an affected child, even if there is neither a history of deafness in the family nor clinical findings that permit the diagnosis of a specific recessive syndrome. These results can also be used to quantify the risk in various counseling situations.[35] Two difficult and frequently encountered counseling problems are hearing couples who seek advice after the birth of an affected child and deaf couples who come for counseling either before or after beginning their families. For a hearing couple, whose first child is deaf, the empirical recurrence risk is approximately 9.8 percent. As normal siblings are born into a family, the best estimate of the recurrence risk declines to 4.3 percent after four normal siblings, reflecting the increasing probability that the deafness was not genetic in the first place. If a second affected child is born, recessive inheritance can be assumed and a 25 percent recurrence risk would be appropriate. It is of interest that if there is a remote history of deafness in the family —in a second- or third-degree relative—the initial empiric risk is 20 percent and declines to 13.8 percent when there are four normal siblings. Obviously, if a specific recessive syndrome can be recognized, or if parental consanguinity can be documented, the parents can be counseled appropriately even with only one affected child.

For a deaf × deaf mating, the empirical risk that the first child will be deaf is only about 9.7 percent, but the phenotype of that child has a profound influence on the best estimate of the risks for subsequent children. Thus, if the first child is deaf, the estimated recurrence risk for the next child is about 61 percent and rapidly approaches 100 percent as more deaf children are born into the family. By contrasts, if the first child has normal hearing, the risk for the next child falls to 4.1 percent and rapidly approaches zero as more normal sibs are born. If both hearing and normal children are present in the sibship, the family should be counseled as if the hearing loss were a dominant trait.

These very different alternatives reflect the initial uncertainty about whether a deaf × deaf mating involves parents who have sporadic, dominant, or recessive deafness and, if the latter, whether both parents have the same or a different form of recessive deafness.

Several different forms of X-linked deafness have been clearly delineated; the substantial excess of affected males raises the possibility that as many as 7.7 percent of all cases could result from X-linked recessive traits. When extensive pedigree data are available, the familiar pattern of mother to son transmission of X-linked deafness can readily be recognized. However, in analyses based on isolated sibships, the only difference to be found between autosomal and X-linked deafness is in the sex distribution of the affected offspring. The affected children will all be males in the case of an X-linked recessive trait but may include males as well as females in the case of autosomal inheritance. Even with the latter, however, families can by chance arise in which the affected offspring are either all males or all females. Thus, to the extent that X-linked recessive genes contribute to genetic deafness, there should be an excess of sibships in which all affected offspring are males in comparison with the all-female-affected sibships. Using this approach, Fraser[36] estimated that 1.8 percent of deafness could be attributed to recessive X-linked genes, while Bieber[33] more recently obtained an estimate of 1.9 percent in a series of U.S. families. These data suggest that only about two-thirds of the excess of affected males with deafness can be attributed to X-linked recessive traits.

---

## GENETIC HETEROGENEITY

### Mechanisms of Detection

The heterogeneous nature of hereditary deafness is being defined with increasing precision on the basis of clinical, genetic, and molecular criteria. To date, most of the recognized forms of genetic deafness have been distinguished by their characteristic clinical or audiologic findings. A mutant gene or gene pair can often give rise to several apparently unrelated pleiotropic effects, a phenomenon that has proved of great value in resolving different hereditary deafness syndromes. In some cases, pleiotropism can be explained by a defect in a common cell type or embryologic structure or by a generalized developmental abnormality that occurs at a specific stage of embryologic life. For diseases in which the nature of the biochemical defect is either known with precision or can be inferred with reasonable accuracy, it may be possible to explain a pleiotropism in terms of shared metabolic pathways or by a cascade of primary and sequential abnormalities. Unfortunately, characteristic clinical abnormalities are found in only about one-fourth of patients with genetic deafness, and it seems likely that genetic, biochemical, or molecular criteria will be required for accurate classification of the remaining cases.

## Genetic Linkage Analysis

Characterization of the mode of inheritance and analysis of critical matings are two important approaches to the recognition of heterogeneity that can be of particular relevance for genetic counseling. Linkage analysis is another potentially powerful approach to the recognition of heterogeneity, but to date this method has seldom been applied to the study of hereditary deafness. During the past decade, remarkable progress has been made in determining the chromosomal location of more than 600 human genes.[1] This knowledge has been acquired by a variety of complementary techniques, including analysis of the co-segregation of specific genes and chromosomes in interspecies somatic cell hybrids, the direct in situ hybridization of clones labeled DNA fragments to specific regions on the human karyotype, the study of patients with chromosomal deletions and other rare rearrangements, and classic linkage studies involving analysis of the co-segregation within families of alleles for polymorphic markers with genes at the loci that produce the genetic diseases in question.

The determination of the linear sequences of genes on chromosomes in several species of lower organisms long before anything about the chemical stucture of the gene was known stands as one of the crowning achievements of genetics during the early decades of this century. Were it not for the phenomenon of crossing over—the physical exchange of chromosome parts that regularly occurs between paired homologues at the time of meiosis —all the genes contained on a single chromosome

would invariably be transmitted together to the resulting gametes. However, because of these exchanges, the farther apart two genes are on a single chromosome, the more likely it is that recombination or crossing over will occur between them, leading to a new combination of genes on the resulting daughter chromosomes. Thus, the frequencies of recombination between several genes on the same chromosome may be used to determine their sequence in exactly the same way that the order of three cities along a highway could be mapped from a knowledge of the distances between them.

A linkage study involves a statistical analysis of the tendency of pairs of genes at separate loci to be transmitted together because of their chromosomal propinquity. In general, data on both affected and normal family members in large multigenerational kinships or collections of many small families known to have the same genetic conditions are required for a successful linkage analysis.

Estimates are obtained of the recombination frequency or map distances, which is most consistent with the observed data along with a measure of the strength of or odds favoring the association. This is usually expressed as the logarithm of the odds, or Lod score, favoring linkage at the most likely, or maximum likelihood, value of $\theta$. Thus, a Lod score of 3.0 would imply that the assumption the loci are linked with the given value of $\theta$ is 1,000 times more likely than nonlinkage (i.e., $\theta = 0.5$). Since tests for linkage with multiple markers are often performed in an analysis, a relatively high confidence level (such as the example given) is usually demanded before a linkage can confidently be considered to have been established.

Other than the recognized X-linked syndromes, the only form of deafness for which chromosomal location has been claimed to have been established is the gene for Waardenburg syndrome. On the basis of analysis of normal and affected individuals in three families, Arias et al.[13] concluded that this locus was 20 cM (centimorgans or crossover units, named for the American geneticist Thomas Hunt Morgan) from the ABO locus. However, the Lod score was only implied that the assumption of linkage was 43 times more likely than nonlinkage, and subsequent reports have not supported the original evidence for linkage.[37] Thus, more data will be required to confirm or refute this claim.

It has been suggested on the basis of clinical studies that there are two different types of Waardenburg syndrome, but it is not known whether the clinical variation results from different alleles at the same locus, mutation of different loci, or possibly the influence of genetic modifiers at separate loci. The demonstration that one form of Waardenburg syndrome is closely linked to a genetic marker such as the ABO locus, while the other form that was not so linked would conclusively establish that the two forms were determined by mutations at different loci.

To be useful for a linkage analysis, the marker locus must be highly variable or polymorphic. A major limiation to such studies in the past has been the relatively small number of suitable genetic markers, such as blood groups, HLA type, and serum protein and red cell enzyme polymorphisms, that are available.

However, the recent discovery of DNA restriction fragment length polymorphisms (RFLPs) promises to provde a virtually unlimited supply of markers for such studies. These polymorphisms are detected by digesting a small sample of DNA with a specific endonuclease or DNA restriction enzyme that cleaves each identical DNA strand into identical fragments, depending on the location of specific recognition or restriction sequences of base pairs along the molecule. If the resulting fragments are then separated by electophoresis, the pieces arising from any particular region may be recognized by hybridization with a radioactive probe or clonal copies of that region.

In cases in which one of the specific restriction sites in the region detected by the probe is mutationally altered such that the DNA molecule is no longer cut by the restriction enzyme at that point, a reduced number of hybridizating fragments and/or a longer, more slowly migrating fragment will be observed. These polymorphic difference can then be used like any other genetic marker for linkage analysis. More than 300 potentially useful probes have been described to date,[38] including nearly a dozen polymorphic RFLPs on the X chromosome,[39] which promise to accelerate greatly the detailed mapping of that chromosome. The clinical importance of such studies for otology is that they will ultimately help define additional genetic causes of deafness and, since these tests can be performed on fetal cells, they will provide a generally applicable approach to the antenatal diagnosis of these defects.

Two methods for the antenatal diagnosis of genetic disease by RFLP analysis have been developed that could be applied to hereditary deafness. In families in which a closely linked RFLP has been identified that is segregating with the gene for deafness, detection of the pattern associated with deafness in the fetal cells would identify embryos that had inherited the deafness gene(s) with a degree of certainty that would be related to the frequency of crossing over between the RFLP and deafness locus. Family studies involving tests on affected and normal parents and siblings are generally required and the method is feasible only in those families in which an informative marker is known to be segregating.

The second approach, to antenatal diagnosis of genetic disease by RFLP analysis obviates the need for somewhat cumbersome family studies, since a restriction enzyme is selected which actually recognizes the genetic difference at the site in the gene at which the mutation occurs. This approach has been applied successfully for the antenatal diagnosis of sickle cell disease but requires a detailed knowledge of the structure of the gene and the precise nature and location of the mutation.[40] Furthermore, because of the extreme degree of variation that can occur among mutations, even within a single locus, there is good reason to believe that this method will only be applicable for such conditions as sickle cell anemia, in which natural selection has caused a particular mutation to reach an unusually high frequency in the population.

## The Nature of Mutations

Within a single gene, mutations may involve the addition, deletion, or substitution of one or more base pairs. About 25 percent of all base-pair substitutions will have no effect on the amino acid sequence of the resulting gene product because they merely result in a change between two alternative codons for the same amino acids; 28 percent of all possible point mutations will lead to the substitution of a polar for a nonpolar amino acid, while 45 percent will result in no net change in the electrical charge on the molecule. Whether these substitutions will have a detectable phenotypic effect will depend on the location of the amino acid in the polypeptide and the effect that the substitution has on critical binding sites as the tertiary structure of the molecule. Finally, 2 percent of all possible substitutions will lead to a change in the stop codon or punctuation in the genetic code such that the genetic message will continue to be read through the normal termination site.

Additions or deletions of base pairs have a greater potential for deleterious effects because they can change the reading frame, altering the entire sequence of amino acids distal to the site of the mutation. Mutations involving the intron sequences can affect the activity of the gene without altering the structure of the resulting polypeptide, if they interfere with the normal processing of the nascent message.

## Otologic Examples of Pleiotropism

### Pigmentary Abnormalities

The pigment cells of the body originate along the dorsal lip of the neural groove and migrate throughout the developing embryo to give rise to many structures, including the adrenal medulla, autonomic ganglion cells, Schwann cells, pigment cells, odontoblasts, craniofacial mesenchyme, and elements of the inner ear. The association between pigmentary defects and deafness is widely recognized in nature and presumably results either from a defect in the migration of functioning of these neural crest derivatives.

In most human deafness syndromes with associated pigmentary abnormalities, patches of hypo- and/or hyperpigmentation are observed. Examples include Waardenburg syndrome, the dominant,[41] recessive,[42] and X-linked[43] piebald spotting syndromes that can be associated with deafness, and the multiple lentigenes syndrome in which hearing loss is found in about 25 percent of cases.[44] Generalized oculocutaneous albinism with deafness has been described in an inbred kinship,[45] but it seems likely that the co-occurence of the two traits in the kindred may have represented a chance association of two recessive traits. Dominant pedigrees of

deafness associated with extreme hypopigmentation or albinoidism have also been described.[46] More recently, late-onset hearing loss has been described in males with X-linked ocular albinism.[47] It is not yet clear how frequent this association may be, since systematic audiologic studies have not been performed in previously reported cases.

The precise etiologies of these pleiotropisms are unknown. However, studies of syndromes in which albinism involves the eye have shown that there are striking abnormalities in the decussation of the optic tracts. This finding suggests that pigment cells may play a important role in the ontogeny of the nervous system. During embryonic life, the brain contains an enormous surplus of neural cells enough, for example, to accommodate readily the innervation of the extra digits of polydactylous individuals. It is possible that through surface recognition signals, pigment cells may participate in the normal elimination of neural cells that have either made no peripheral connections with their appropriate end organs or inappropriate synapses.

Pigment cells clearly play a somewhat similar role in normal rod renewal in the adult retina as well as in the progressive depletion of damaged neurosensory cells that occurs in several of the recognized forms of hereditary pigmentary retinopathy. Pigment cell derivatives may well subserve a similar function in the inner ear, as suggested by reports of similar abnormalities in the decussation of the central auditory pathways in individuals with various types of albinism.

### Skeletal Abnormalities

It is perhaps not surprising that a large number of genetic defects involving the osseous system can be associated with hearing loss. Although there are many exceptions, most of these syndromes are associated with conductive or mixed hearing losses, often resulting from abnormalities in the structure or articulation of the auditory ossicles. Most of these syndromes are either generalized, possibly metabolic abnormalities or seemingly localized structural defects involving the cranium, the hands and feet, or both.

Known and possible metabolic abnormalities that can be associated with hearing loss include osteopetrosis, osteogenesis imperfecta, sclerosteosis, and Paget disease of bone.[2] Syndromes in which the bony abnormalities are more or less localized to the skull include the dominant and recessively inherited craniometaphyseal dysplasias, frontometaphyseal dysplasia, and craniofacial dysostosis[2]. Syndromes in which the hands or both the hands and skull are involved include the dominant forms of symphalangism,[48] the X-linked otopalatodigital,[49] and orofaciodigital syndromes,[2] ectroadactyly with deafness,[50] and Apert syndrome.[51]

When present, fixation of the stapes footplate is a potentially remediable form of conductive hearing loss. Stapes fixation has been reported as a finding in at least 14 hereditary syndromes (Table 30-5) and should therefore be considered in patients with these conditions who exhibit hearing loss.

### Renal Disease

Several forms of hereditary deafness have been delineated in which either progressive kidney failure or structural or functional renal abnormalities are found. The syndrome of progressive sensorineural hearing loss with chronis nephritis was first described by Alport[52] in 1927. The syndrome is an autosomal dominant disorder, but males are more severely affected than females, and renal failure is frequently succumbed to in early adult life. Histologic studies have shown degeneration of the stria vasculars and hair cells of the organ of Corti, especially in the basal turn. Early signs of the renal disease include hematuria and later albuminuria.

Renal biopsies typically reveal intestitial fibrosis, epithelial proliferation in the glomeruli, and lipid-laden foam cells in the tubules. In patients with advance disease, the hearing loss has reportedly improved following kidney transplanation.[2]

Alport syndrome bears interesting similarities to Fabry disease, an X-linked deficiency of the enzyme ceramide trihexosidase in which progressive renal failure is associated with lipoid inclusions in the tubules as well as the glomerular cells. A mild sensorineural hearing loss is found in about 50 percent of cases.[2]

In a separate autosomal dominant disease, progressive sensorineural hearing loss has been reported in association with recurrent fever, urticaria, and amyloidosis, ultimately leading to the development of the nephrotic syndrome and chronic uremia during the third or fourth decade of life.[53]

At least two forms of deafness associated with renal tubular acidosis have been reported. Both are inherited as autosomal recessive traits, but in one form the deafness is prelingual in onset,[54] while in the other, progressive sensorineural hearing loss begins in adolescence.[55]

The frequent association of hearing loss with anomalies of the external ears, including prehelical pits, ear tags, and branchial fistulae, has long been recognized[56,57] and had generally been attributed to a localized developmental defect involving the branchial arches. More recently, however, dominant pedigrees have been reported in which a vari-

**Table 30-5.  Genetic Syndromes Associated with Fixation of the Stapes Footplate**

| Syndrome | Mode of Inheritance | Frequency of Association |
|---|---|---|
| Otosclerosis | Autosomal dominant | Incomplete penetrance |
| Congenital fixation of stapes | X-linked | Constant feature |
| Apert syndrome | Autosomal dominant | Occasional finding |
| Craniometaphyseal dysplasia | Autosomal recessive | Frequent finding |
| Symphalangism | Autosomal dominant | Frequent finding |
| Symphalangism-brachydactyly | Autosomal dominant | Frequent finding |
| Crouzon craniofacial dysplasia | Autosomal dominant | Hearing loss in 33% |
| Mitral insufficiency, joint fusions | Autosomal dominant | Frequent finding |
| Mandibulofacial dysostosis | Autosomal dominant | Variable |
| Cleft palate, tarsal, carpal fusions | Autosomal recessive | Constant finding |
| Multiple ossicular malformations | Autosomal recessive | Constant finding |
| Branchio-oto-renal | Autosomal dominant | Occasional |
| Lop ears with micrognathia | Autosomal dominant | Frequent |
| Thickened lobules, incudostapedial anomalies | Autosomal dominant | Occasional finding |

(Adapted from Konigsmark BW, Gorlin RJ: Genetic and Metabolic Deafness. WB Saunders, Philadelphia, 1976.)

**Table 30-6. Incidence of Isolated Ear Anomalies per 10,000 Births in Maternal Collaborative Perinatal Study**

| Anomaly | Race | | Familial Cases (%) |
| --- | --- | --- | --- |
| | White | Black | |
| Preauricular sinus | 17.8 | 148.8 | 6.3 |
| Preauricular tags | 13.6 | 19.1 | 6.7 |
| Microtia | 1.7 | 1.9 | 0.0 |
| Other anomaly of pinna | 8.3 | 7.2 | 16.3 |
| Branchial cleft sinus | 2.1 | 2.4 | 0.0 |

(Adapted from Melnick M: External Ear Malformations: Epidemiology, Genetics and Natural History. Doctoral thesis, Indiana University, 1978.)

ety of structural defects of the kidney have also been found. These defects range from anomalies of the collecting system and cysts to unilateral or bilateral agenesis of the kidneys.[58] Isolated malformations of the external ear are seen in about 1 percent of newborn infants, and a hearing loss can subsequently be documented in 9.3 percent of these infants. Preauricular sinuses are the most commonly observed defects and are familial in about 6.3 percent of cases[59] (Table 30-6).

Fraser et al. found ear pits in 4.5 percent of 421 deaf children, and documented the branchio-oto-renal syndrome in nearly one-half of those in whom detailed clinical and family studies were possible. Their data suggest that about 6 percent of gene carriers have severe renal dysplasia and that the findings of preauricular ear pits at birth is associated with at least a 0.5 percent risk of a severe hearing loss.[60]

The familiar low-set malformed ears characteristic of renal agenesis (Potter syndrome) are thought to result from the associated oligohydramnios, but the causes of other pleiotropisms involving the ear and kidney are obscure. Both the kidney and cochlea contain active cation pumps that maintain active membrane gradients; both can be damaged by a common group of drugs; some investigators have also documented immunologic evidence that the two organs also share common antigens.[2]

## Audiologic Heterogeneity

When multiple affected individuals can be studied, it is often possible to document distinctive audiologic differences among those families in which hearing loss occurs as an isolated abnormality. Fre-

quently, the audiologic pattern of a single subject may not be sufficiently characteristic to permit an unequivocal classification, but when multiple audiograms are available, the similarities can be impressive.

Because of its therapeutic implications, the most important distinction to be made is between conductive and sensorineural hearing loss. Several distinct genetic syndromes can lead to fixation of the stapes footplate, and many others, particularly those involving the head, branchial arch derivatives, or osseous system, can also be associated with conductive losses arising from abnormalities of the other ossicles, the eardrum, or the ear canal. Even among families with sensorineural losses, however, distictive audiologic patterns have been recognized. Thus, families have been described with dominantly inherited low-,[61] mid-,[62] and high-tone losses.[4] Of the three, losses of the latter two types are usually the most significant clinically because they may involve frequencies within the speech range.

Similar studies in families with recessive deafness have shown that in some, residual sound perception throughout most of the hearing range can be documented at 80- to 100-dB thresholds, while in others, no sound perception can be demonstrated beyond that which can reasonably be attributed to tactile responses to vibrations in the low frequency range.

Finally, it is now abundantly clear that genetic deafness need not be congenital in onset. Syndromes that lead to partial hearing loss typically exhibit very slow progression with age, but dominant and recessive, as well as X-linked pedigrees have been documented in which there is a rapid progression in the hearing loss during early childhood or adolescence.[2] These differences can be of enormous clinical significance, since the presence of any residual hearing during infancy can have a profound effect on sound awareness and the development of linguistic skills. In this regard, one cannot help but wonder to what extent genetic heterogeneity might have contributed to the acrimonious controversy over oral versus manual communication during the early decades of the twentieth century. Clearly, children with any residual hearing, even if it is only transient, would have a much greater likelihood of succeeding in a completely oral program.

## CLINICAL MANAGEMENT OF GENETIC DISEASE

For many genetic diseases, therapeutic options are limited to prevention through genetic counseling. Families may elect not to have children, to adopt, or to use artificial insemination, in vitro fertilization, or surrogate mothering. Other couples may choose to have prenatal diagnosis for those disorders with a chromosomal basis, biochemical origin, or known molecular defect diagnosable with new DNA techniques. Specific therapies, from hearing aids to cochlear implants to high-dose vitamins, are available for a number of defects associated with hearing impairment.

### Genetic Counseling

Genetic counseling may be viewed as providing the information and support necessary to help a family understand the diagnosis, prognosis, and recurrence risk associated with a genetic disease. Although cynics may argue that there is no such thing as nondirective counseling, there is a broad consensus that the proper role of the genetic counselor should be to help parents find the solution that is right for them.

Deaf couples often ask "What's wrong with being deaf?" and may sometimes need reassurance about their ability to rear a hearing child. A physician-counselor who is unable to communicate fluently with deaf patients should make use of a certified translator rather than a solicitous relative who may filter the advice that is given. Patients with Usher syndrome, for example, should not be subjected to the dehumanizing experience of being informed for the first time about the nature and prognosis of their visual symptoms in written exchanges on scraps of paper.

Sometimes parents find unexpected solutions that might never occur to a directive counselor. In one case, the hearing parents of a deaf boy desperately wanted another child but could not accept the risk of bringing another deaf child into the world. They solved their dilemma by adopting a deaf child, an act that achieved their goals and was in the best interests of all parties concerned.

In another case, the mother of an antenatally diagnosed pair of twins who were discordant for Kleinfelter syndrome (a chromosome disorder in which males carry two X chromosomes in addition to their Y chromosome) elected not to be informed which twin was affected so as to avoid the possibility that her diminished expectations might adversely effect his psychological development. Such effects have been hypothesized by social scientists, and in the present case, the mother's decision to remain uninformed was sustained by the judge of a domestic relations court.

Hearing parents who have a deaf child may be helped by the knowledge that on the average, all normal individuals carry from two to four deleterious recessive genes. When present in the homozygous state, these genes are responsible for the extensive array of recognized recessive syndromes, including recessive deafness. This insight can do much to reduce the irrational feelings of stigmatization and guilt that all too often accompany the diagnosis of a genetic disease.

### Antenatal Diagnosis

The prenatal diagnosis of genetic disease can be achieved for a variety of disorders by amniocentesis or by chorionic villus sampling. In the former procedure, a small amount of amniotic fluid is withdrawn from the mother's womb at about the sixteenth to eighteenth week of gestation after localization of the placenta by ultrasound. In competent laboratories, the risk of miscarriage is less than one-half of 1 percent (i.e., less than 0.25 percent). In the latter procedure, a small sample of the chorionic villus is removed at about the eighth to tenth week of gestation by one of several different methods. This material is rapidly dividing and may be examined directly within hours, while culture of amniotic cells typically takes 2 to 3 weeks. The risk of complication with the rather new procedure of chorionic villus sampling is approximately 4 percent. Cells grown from either sampling method may be assayed biochemically for a wide range of metabolic disorders or may be tested with labeled probes to detect specific DNA polymorphisms.

## Specific Therapy

Conventional approaches to the treatment of genetic forms of hearing loss include the appropriate management of associated medical conditions, avoidance of complicating medications or environmental risk factors, use of hearing aids, and reconstructive surgery, especially for these conditions showing a mixed or predominantly conductive hearing loss. Early diagnosis of hearing impairment in infancy and childhood can be crucial to facilitating the optimal development of communication skills.

At least one genetic disease is known in which elucidation of the basic metabolic defect has led to the development of an effective and specific therapy to prevent the development of deafness.

Wolf et al.[63] recently showed that the late-onset form of multiple carboxylase deficiency, an unusual autosomal recessive disease in which the activities of all four biotin-dependent carboxylase are diminished, is caused by the absence of biotinidase activity, an enzyme required for the normal recycling of biotin. Affected individuals ultimately develop signs of biotin deficiency, including skin rash, alopecia, seizures, developmental delay, and metabolic acidosis, in addition to sensorineural hearing loss in a high percentage of cases. The results of recently initiated newborn screening programs have suggested that the incidence of biotinidase deficiency may be as high as 1 in 40,000 and that all symptoms of the disease can readily be prevented by the presymptomatic detection of affected children with the subsequent administration of high doses of biotin.[64]

Although deafness is often genetic in origin, much research needs to be done before the actual correction of the relevant gene defects becomes a reality. Those disorders for which these therapeutic approaches have been proposed include Lesch-Nyhan disease, a devastating X-linked neurologic disorder of uric acid metabolism, and adenosine deaminase deficiency, a disease in which severe combined immune deficiency is associated with impaired function of B and T cells. Bone marrow, kidney, and liver transplants have also been used in several genetically determined malignant, enzymatic, and metabolic disorders, with some success. Unfortunately, except in unusual cases, such as Wilson disease, disorders that show extensive or prenatal involvement of the nervous system appear to be least amenable to these forms of treatment. Thus, it is likely that genetic counseling, antenatal diagnosis, prevention, and rehabilitative support services for affected persons will remain important therapeutic approaches for persons with serious hearing impairment, even in the upcoming age of gene therapy.

## ACKNOWLEDGMENTS

This chapter is publication 275 from the Department of Human Genetics of the Medical College of Virginia. The work was supported in part by Human Health Services grant MCJ-111005 to Gallaudet College and by grant AM 25786-06 from the National Institutes of Health to the Medical College of Virginia.

## REFERENCES

1. McKusick VA: Mendelian Inheritance in Man. 6th Ed. Johns Hopkins Press, Baltimore, 1983
2. Konigsmark BW, Gorlin RJ: Genetic and Metabolic Deafness. WB Saunders, Philadelphia, 1976
3. Beighton P, Sellars S: Genetics and Otology. Churchill Livingstone, Edinburgh, 1983
4. Nance WE, McConnell FE: Status and prospects of research in hereditary deafness. Adv Hum Genet 4:173, 1973
5. Watson JD, Crick FHC: Genetical implications of the structure of deoxyribase nucleic acid. Nature (Lond) 171:964, 1953
6. Friedberg C: DNA Repair. WH Freeman, New York, 1985
7. Taylor AI: Autosomal trisomy syndromes: A detailed study of 27 cases of Edward's syndrome and 27 cases of Patan's syndrome. J Med Genet 5:227, 1968
8. deGrouchy J, Turleau C: Clinical Atlas of Human Chromosomes. 2nd Ed. John Wiley & Sons, New York, 1984

9. Waardenburg PJA: A new syndrome combining developmental anomalies of the eyelids, eyebrows and nasal root with pigmentary defects of the iris and head hair with congenital deafness. Am J Hum Genet 3:195, 1951

10. Fisch L: Deafness as part of an hereditary syndrome. J Laryngol 73:335, 1959

11. Marcus RE: Vestibular function and additional findings in Waardenburg's syndrome. Acta Otolaryngol (Stockh) 229[suppl]:5, 1968

12. Arias S: Genetic heterogeneity in the Waardenburg syndrome. Birth Defects 7(4):187, 1971

13. Arias S, Mota M, de Yanez A, et al: Probable loose linkage between the ABO locus and Waardenburg syndrome Type 1. Humangenetik 27:145, 1975

14. Treacher Collins E: Cases with symmetrical congenital notches in the outer part of each lid and defective development of the malar bones. Trans Ophthalmol Soc UK 20:190, 1900

15. Wildervanck LS: Sysostosis mandibulofacialis (Franceschetti-Zwahlen) in four generations. Acta Genet Med 9:447, 1960

16. Larsson A: Otosclerosis, a genetic and clinical study. Acta Otolaryngol (Stockh) 154[suppl]:1, 1960

17. Fowler EP: Otosclerosis in identical twins. A study of 40 pairs. Arch Otolaryngol 83:324, 1966

18. Rose SP: Genetic Studies of Profound Prelingual Deafness. Doctoral thesis, Indiana University, 1975

19. Usher CH: On the inheritance of retinitis pigmentosa with notes of cases. Roy Long Ophthalmol Hosp Rep 19:130, 1914

20. Boughman JA: Population Genetic Studies of Retinitis Pigmentosa. Doctoral Thesis, Indiana University, 1978

21. Fraser GR, Froggatt P, James: Congenital deafness associated with electrocardiographic abnormalities, fainting attacks and sudden death. Q J Med 33:361, 1964

22. Moss AJ, McDonald J: Unilateral cervicothoracic sympathetic ganglionectomy for the treatment of long QT interval syndrome. N Engl J Med 285:903, 1971

23. Fraser GR: Association of congenital deafness with goiter. Ann Hum Genet 28:201, 1965

24. Hvidberg-Hansen J, Jorgensen MB: The inner ear in Pendred's syndrome. Acta Otolaryngol (Stockh) 66:129, 1968

25. DeMars R, Nance WE: Electrophoretic variants of glucose-6-phosphate dehydrogenase and the single-active X in cultivated human cells. Wistar Inst Symp Mong 1:35, 1964

26. Nance WE, Setleff R, McLeod A, et al: X-linked mixed deafness with congenital fixation of the stapes footplate and perilymphatic gusher. Birth Defects 7:64, 1971

27. National Center for Health Statistics: Characteristics of Persons with Hearing Impairment in the United States (Table XVI), July 1962–June 1963, In Public Health Service Publication 1000, Series 10, 35, April 1967

28. Ruben RJ, Kruger B: Hearing loss in the elderly. p. 123. In Katzman R (ed): The Neurology of Aging, FA Davis, Philadelphia, 1983

29. Nance WE, Sweeney A, McLeod AC: Hereditary deafness: A presentation of some recognized types, modes of inheritance, and aids in counseling. South Med Bull 58:41, 1970

30. Shaver KA: Congenital Rubella Syndrome and Diabetes: A Study of Genetic and Epidemiologic Risk Factors. Doctoral thesis, Virginia Commonwealth University, 1983

31. Chung CS, Robinson OW, Morton NE: A note on deaf mutism. Ann Hum Genet 23:357, 1969

32. Fraser GR: The Causes of Profound Deafness in Childhood. Johns Hopkins Press, Baltimore, 1976

33. Bieber FR: Genetic Studies of Questionnaire Data from a Residential School for the Deaf. Doctoral thesis, Virginia Commonwealth University, 1981

34. Fay EA: Marriages of the Deaf in America. Volta Bureau, Washington, DC, 1898

35. Bieber FR, Nance WE: Hereditary hearing loss. p. 443. In Jackson LG, Schimke RN (eds): Clinical Genetics. John Wiley & Sons, New York, 1979

36. Fraser GR: Sex-linked recessive congenital deafness and the excess of males in profound childhood deafness. Ann Hum Genet 29:171, 1965

37. Arias J, Mota M: Current status of the ABO-Waardenburg syndrome type I linkage. Cytogenet Cell Genet 22:291, 1978

38. Beaudet AL: Bibliography of cloned human and other selected DNA's. Am J Hum Genet 37:386, 1985

39. deMartinville B, Kunkel LM, Bruns G, et al: Localization of DNA sequences in region Xp21 of the human X chromosome: Search for molecular markers close to the Duchenne muscular dystrophy locus. Am J Hum Genet 37:325, 1985

40. Chang JC, Kan KW: Prenatal diagnosis of sickle cell anemia by direct analysis of the sickle mutation. Lancet 2:1127, 1981

41. Telfer MA, Sugar M, Jaeger EA, et al: Dominant piebald trait (white forelock and leukoderma) with neurologic impairment. Am J Hum Genet 23:383, 1971

42. Woolf CM, Dolowitz DA, Aldous HE: Congenital

deafness associated with piebaldness. Arch Otolaryngol 82:244, 1965

43. Ziprkowski L, Krakowski A, Adam A, et al: Partial albinism and deaf-mutism due to a recessive sex-linked gene. Arch Dermatol 86:530, 1982

44. Gorlin RJ, Anderson RC, Moller JH: The leopard (multiple lentigines) syndrome revisited. Birth Defects 7(4):110, 1971

45. Ziprkowski L, Adam A: Recessive total albinism and congenital deaf-mutism. Arch Dermatol 89:151, 1964

46. Tietz W: A syndrome of deafmutism associated with albinism showing autosomal dominant inheritance. Am J Hum Genet 15:259, 1963

47. Winship I, Gericke G, Beighton P: X linked inheritance of ocular albinism with late onset sensorineural deafness. Am J Hum Genet 19:797, 1984

48. Strasburger AK, Hawkins MR, Eldridge R et al: Synphalangism: Genetic and clinical aspects. Bull Johns Hopkins Hosp 117:108, 1965

49. Buran DJ, Duvall AJ: The oto-palato-digital syndrome. Arch Otolaryngol 85:394, 1967

50. Robinson GC, Wildervanck LS, Chiang TP: Ectrodactyly, ectodermal dysplasia, and cleft palate: Its association with conductive hearing loss. J Pediatr 82:107, 1973

51. Bergstrom LV, Neblett LM, Hemenway WG: Otologic manifestations of acrocephalosyndactyly. Arch Otolaryngol 96:117, 1972

52. Alport AC: Hereditary familial congenital nephritis. Br Med J 1:504, 1927

53. Muckle TJ, Wells M: Urticaria, deafness and amyloidosis: A new heridofamilial syndrome. J Med 31:235, 1962

54. Nance WE, Sweeney A: Evidence for autosomal recessive inheritance of the syndrome of renal tubular acidosis with deafness. Birth Defects 7(4):70, 1971

55. Walker WG, Ozer FL, Whelton A: Syndrome of perceptive deafness and renal tubular acidosis. Birth Defects 10(4):163, 1974

56. Pritchard E: Case of symmetrical bilateral helical fistulae, unilateral branchial fistula and preauricular tubercle. Proc R Soc Med 2:227, 1908

57. Fourman P, Fourman J: Hereditary deafness in a family with ear pits (fistulas auris congenita) Br Med J 2:1354, 1955

58. Melnick M, Bixler D, Nance WE, et al: Familial branchio-oto-renal dysplasia: A new addition to the branchial arch syndromes. Clin Genet 9:25, 1976

59. Melnick M: External Ear Malformations: Epidemiology, Genetics and Natural History. Doctoral thesis, Indiana University, 1978

60. Fraser FC, Sproule JR, Halal F: Frequency of the branchio-oto-renal (BOR) syndrome in children with profound hearing loss. Am J Med Genet 7:341, 1980

61. Vanderbilt University Hereditary Deafness Study Group: Dominantly inherited low-frequency hearing loss. Arch Otolaryngol 88:242, 1968

62. Martensson B: Dominant hereditary nerve deafness. Acta Otolaryngol (Stockh) 52:270, 1960

63. Wolf B, Grier RE, Secor McVoy JR, et al: Biotinidase deficiency: A novel vitamin recycling defect. J Inher Metab Dis 8[suppl 1]:53, 1985

64. Wolf B, Heard GS, Jefferson LG, et al: Clinical findings in four children with biotinidase deficiency detected through a statewide neonatal screening program. N Engl J Med 313:16, 1985

# Systemic Disease and Otology

**31**

Andrew W. Morrison
John B. Booth

Many systemic diseases can and do involve the different parts of the ear or its central connections. Indeed the subject could merit a textbook to itself. In this chapter many diseases are excluded or touched upon only briefly, since they are covered more appropriately in other chapters. The many causes of severe childhood deafness, be they infective, teratogenic, hereditary, or metabolic, are largely excluded. Secondary involvement of the ear by neoplasms, reticuloses, or leukemia receives little more than a mention. Central nervous system (CNS) and intracranial pathology is touched upon, although most aspects of this important subject are described elsewhere (Chapters 24, 25, 26).

Diseases of the cardiovascular, hemopoietic, and respiratory systems are covered, as are metabolic and endocrine disorders, renal disease, some CNS disorders, and pathology of the musculoskeletal systems. Treponemal disease is given special attention and an attempt is made to describe the role of autoimmunity in sensorineural deafness.

## CARDIOVASCULAR SYSTEM

No significant correlation between sensorineural hearing loss and a variety of risk factors (blood pressure, heart rate, smoking, serum cholesterol, triglyceride and uric acid and glucose tolerance) could be found by Drettner et al.[1] Likewise, studies of the cochlear and vestibular arteries, as well as the labyrinthine arteries, showed that they remain patent at all ages. Similarly, investigators have failed to find any close relationship between the changes in the inner ear and those of the basilar artery, anterior inferior cerebellar artery, and arteries of the internal auditory canal, nor of patients dying from hypertensive disease.

With age, there is a progressive thickening of the tunica adventitia. The small arteries of the internal auditory canal are of a purely muscular type, but they lack an external elastic membrane. Similarly,

855

there is no evidence of atherosclerosis occurring in any of the smaller vessels supplying the ear.

Inflammation of the vessels, as in cranial arteritis,[2] is occasionally seen and probably signifies involvement of the posterior circulation or terminal cochleovestibular vasculature. Nearly 50 percent of patients with the musculoskeletal disorder, polymyalgia rheumatica, have an associated cranial arteritis.

A single case was reported of a patient with von Recklinghausen's disease, who experienced occlusion of the vertebral and basilar arteries, together with a large infarct of the medulla and pons, 17 days before death.[3] An aneurysm of the left vertebral artery showed atherosclerotic walls; the right vertebral artery showed severe atherosclerosis, and the basilar artery very severe atherosclerotic changes.

### Viscosity

Studies in the guinea pig,[4] by perfusion of the ear with high-viscosity blood showed a rise in the action potential (AP) threshold in 56 percent of animals, and in one third of them there was a significant fluctuation of the AP response: the third type of change noted was an increase in the slope of the input/output curve. Injecting normoviscous blood with a reduced (precritical) level of oxygen caused a mild reduction in the $PO_2$ within the scala media of 15.2 percent; hyperviscous blood with the same level of oxygenation reduced the $PO_2$ to 53.5 or normal. However, although the high viscosity of polycythemic blood decreases the rate of blood flow through the cochlear vessels, the high oxygen content of this blood prevented hypoxia of the cochlea. Experimental work with intravenous glycerol in rabbits[5] has shown a significantly increased cochlear and cerebral blood flow after injection.

Investigations into a possible association between the degree of hearing loss and perilymph oxygenation failed to find any significant correlation.[6] However, two different patterns after the inhalation of 5 percent $CO_2$ and 95 percent $O_2$ (carbogen) in cases with sudden deafness yielded low initial values of perilymph oxygenation and a normal response to inhalation; in those with a slowly progressive sensorineural hearing loss, nor-

mal initial values of perilymph oxygenation but a low response to inhalation were obtained.

Experiments in the guinea pig[7] have shown that changes in $PO_2$ within the scala media correlate closely with changes of endocochlear potential and blood pressure. The $PO_2$ in endolymph was directly proportional to the $CO_2$ concentration respired. A direct correlation was found between changes in systemic arterial pressure and the perilymph pressure and this seemed to be mediated by changes in local labyrinthine blood flow.[8] Paradoxically, brief high-intensity noise exposure in the gerbil produced a highly significant elevation in the cochlear blood flow.[9] An increase in the blood flow in the inferior colliculi due to noise exposure has also been described.

### Polycythemia Vera

In polycythemia vera, the viscosity of blood is increased to five to eight times normal; total red blood cell (RBC) count is elevated 20 to 50 percent; the total blood volume is two to three times normal. These alterations in the peripheral blood result in the engorgement of capillaries, venules, and arterioles with high-viscosity, slowly circulating, oxygen-deficient blood.

An earlier report of two patients with sensorineural hearing loss appeared to show that fluctuation in hearing was directly related to the viscosity of peripheral blood and that hearing improved after phlebotomy. A small personal unpublished series of patients with this condition treated by the same procedure, and a separate group with Waldenström's macroglobulinemia, treated by cell separation, showed that while the viscosity changed after treatment, there was no observable change or improvement either in the pure-tone audiogram or in the susceptance or conductance on oto-admittance measurements (220 and 660 Hz).

### Hyperlipoproteinemia

There is no reported association between deafness and primary hyperlipoproteinemia. It is therefore of considerable importance to exclude causes of secondary hyperlipoproteinemia; the most common of which are diabetes mellitus, hypothyroid-

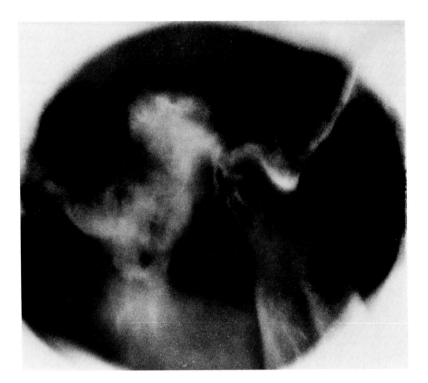

**Fig. 31-1.** Plain radiograph showing lateral view of right temporal bone, with an extensive area of radiodense new bone and areas of osteolysis. (Booth JB: Medical management of sensorineural hearing loss. II. Musculoskeletal system. J Laryngol Otol 96:773, 1982. Print courtesy of Dr. Pauline Emery.)

ism, alcoholism, chronic renal failure, and gout. Likewise, many of the patients who appear to have raised fat levels are obese, some grossly so. When all these separate facts have been taken into account, it appears that the incidence of deafness and hyperlipoproteinemia will prove to be within or near to the incidence of the normal population of that geographic area. Serum lipid levels rise significantly in women over the age of 50.

Xanthomata may very rarely be found in the ear, usually involving the mastoid process.[10] Three cases have been reported in association with hypercholesterolemia (type IIA) one in association with familial hypercholesterolemia, and one with in association with type V hypercholesterolemia[11] (Fig. 31-1). Experimental work on rats[12] using chlorphentermine, an amphophilic agent similar to amphetamine, caused an accumulation of lysosomes containing phospholipids in the inner ear. The inclusions are found mainly in the inner hair cells and nerve fibers, suggesting that the lipid turnover in these structures is especially high. The inclusions lead to changes in the cochlear compound action potential.

## HEMATOPOIETIC SYSTEM

### Erythropoiesis

Anemia of the simple hypochromic microcytic, iron-deficiency type has only rarely been reported as being associated with deafness. Deafness in association with megaloblastic anemia is even more rare. Such cases are usually associated with sudden, bilateral hearing loss that fails to recover. Deafness may be associated with Fanconi's anemia (constitutional anaplastic anaemia).[13]

### Sickle Cell Disease

The sickle cell gene (HbS) is present in approximately 10 percent of the British black population and in a similar proportion of the North American black population.[14] The disease is caused by a genetically inherited hemoglobinopathy, in which valine is substituted for glutamic acid in the sixth position of the β-chain of the hemoglobin molecule. The sickle RBCs are constantly cleared from the circulation, but the RBC life is reduced and patients have a hemolytic anemia with the concomitant sequelae of jaundice and increased bone marrow activity leading to marrow cavity expansion. The latter may affect the skull, and the diploic space between the outer and inner tables becomes obliterated. There is also increased bone marrow activity involving the petrous temporal bones, but this does not give rise to narrowing the internal auditory canal.[15]

A sensorineural hearing loss of apparently gradual onset can occur (22 percent); the extremes of the range, especially the high tones are most frequently involved. It would seem that the frequency of the hemolytic crises may be a factor. The hearing loss may be gradually progressive, fluctuant or sudden in onset; in the last type, partial or almost total recovery may occur.[15] Sensorineural hearing loss in patients with sickle cell disease may also be related to the increased susceptibility to bacterial meningitis. Neurologic involvement is a common complication of sickle cell disease and vestibular dysfunction may occur.

Thalassemia, whether homozygous or trait, has not so far been reported as having an association with deafness but it should be remembered that it can also occur in those with sickle cell disease (sickle β thalassemia).

## Waldenstrom's Macroglobulinemia

This condition, which tends to occur in elderly males, is characterized by retinal hemorrhages, an abnormal bleeding tendency from mucous membranes, generalized weakness and dyspnea. Fundamental to the diagnosis is a raised sedimentation rate and marked increase of serum globulin level in the form of a narrow, dense band in the $B_2$ region. The abnormal macroglobulin coats the platelets and reduces their adhesiveness; it also interferes with fibrin polymerization. A few cases of deafness have been recorded in Waldenström's macroglobulinemia[16,17] although vertigo may be the earliest symptom; immediate diagnosis is essential if the patient is to be prevented from probable permanent bilateral deafness.

Multiple myeloma and leukemia and certain collagen diseases (especially lupus erythematosis and rheumatoid arthritis) may be associated with secondary macroglobulinemia.

## Cryglobulinemia

Cryoglobulins are proteins that precipitate in the cold and redissolve on warming; they are often associated with multiple myeloma and macroglobulinemia but may occur even more commonly in small amounts in systemic lupus erythematosus (SLE) and other connective tissue disorders. Approximately one-fourth are G myeloma proteins, less than 10 percent macroglobulins, and almost two-thirds of mixtures IgG and IgM molecules.

The characteristic clinical signs are purpura, arthralgia, and a Raynaud-like symptom in the lower extremities. Neurologic involvement is low and that affecting the 8th cranial nerve very low, but cases of progressive sensorineural deafness, tinnitus, and vestibular problems have been reported.[18]

## Leukemia

The various forms of leukemia may affect the ear, but it is usually the middle ear that is involved.[19] Otologic complications occur almost invariably in those patients with the acute forms, particularly acute lymphocytic leukemia.

As a general rule, the otologic symptoms appear to be more associated with infiltration and seem to be based on the degree. Leukemic infiltration may occur in the mucoperiosteum of the middle ear following the mucous membrane folds, but this may extend to the ossicles and the sheaths of the tendons of the intratympanic muscles. Infiltration into the bone marrow spaces of the petrous apex frequently occurs and also, to a lesser extent, within the ossicles. Infiltration into the inner ear is uncommon.

Hemorrhagic changes in the temporal bone are more frequently seen in patients with acute lymphocytic leukemia than with the other forms. Sudden deafness and/or vertigo is reported in acute leukemia[20,21] and seems to occur most often in the acute stem cell type. Patients with acute leukemia suffer bone marrow failure with resultant thrombocytopenia, and other coagulation defects, such as hypofibrinogenemia, may occur. Disseminated intravascular coagulation (DIC) and secondary fibrinolysis may also occur.

# RESPIRATORY SYSTEM

## Tuberculosis

While tuberculosis was considered a disease of the past, it has sadly to be acknowledged that this is no longer so and cases, often among immigrant communities, are reappearing in gradually increasing numbers.

As if to illustrate the difficulties, a recent report of 22 cases of tuberculosis otitis media shows that half of the cases occurred under the age of 20.[22] Similarly, in this series, none had a past history of pulmonary tuberculosis (two had tuberculous relatives and four had a past history of the disease at other sites). Subsequent chest radiographs showed pulmonary tuberculosis changes in 8 of 19 patients. Plain radiographs of the mastoid showed a variety of patterns, but in none was bone destruction noted (in 12 there was clouding of the mastoid cellular system).

Clinically, two points should be remembered: the characteristic multiple perforations may coalesce into a single perforation, and secondary infection by other organisms may give little hint as to the real cause unless a biopsy of granulations is obtained; these are often pale and exuberant. The amount of discharge is variable and pain may be present, especially in more active cases. The hearing loss may be disproportionately large; occasionally, there may be no perforation at all. Treatment with streptomycin is well recognized as potentially ototoxic: rifampicin and ethambutol have been reported as being ototoxic, but this is a relatively uncommon occurrence.

## Sarcoidosis

Sarcoidosis may very occasionally affect the ear, but the mechanism by which the deafness is caused is undecided. It is a systemic granulomatous disease of unknown etiology. The disease has a higher incidence among blacks and Puerto Ricans in the United States, and some manifestations of sarcoidosis are known to be associated with certain HLA types. The organs most affected are the lymph nodes, lung, liver, spleen, skin, and eyes, but any tissue may be affected. Neurologic involvement may occur in up to 5 percent of cases. The course of the disease is usually chronic with minimal constitutional upset.

Deafness may be sudden, fluctuating, or progressive. The degree may vary from slight to severe or even total; may affect high or low frequencies; and is usually bilateral, although one side is more severely affected. Caloric testing usually shows reduced or absent responses. From the 35 recorded cases,[23] it would appear that the hearing loss is most probably sensorineural; electrocochleography in two recent cases suggests that the lesion may be retrocochlear with normal hair cell function. No patient has come to postmortem for temporal bone study, but patients with deafness and vertigo have been shown to have adhesive arachnoiditis of the posterior fossa.

Steroids remain the only form of treatment, but their effectiveness is not certain, especially in those with a profound or total hearing loss.

Sarcoidosis involving the ear may be suggested by other signs, such as uveitis, parotid swelling (20 percent), facial nerve palsy (43 percent), (especially if bilateral 17 percent), and lymphadenopathy, including hilar adenopathy (55 percent). However, 40 percent of cases have shown no other neurologic involvement. The trigeminal nerve may be involved in its sensory distribution.

Serum angiotensin-converting enzyme levels are raised in nearly two-thirds of cases of active sarcoidosis, but false-positive elevation of angiotensin-converting enzyme can occur. False-positives are extremely rare in the Kveim test. All patients with the disease should be given liver and renal function tests; abnormalities of calcium metabolism should be excluded in these cases by estimating the serum and urine values. Approximately 10 percent of patients with sarcoidosis have elevation of their serum calcium, thought to be due to hypersensitivity to vitamin D. It is also a characteristic feature of sarcoidosis that infiltration of old scars often occurs; these may provide welcome biopsy material.

## ENDOCRINE SYSTEM

### Diabetes Mellitus

There is a wide variation in the instance of diabetes mellitus; it is evident that this is related to the prevalence of obesity. If diabetes is defined as a blood sugar level of more than 149 mg/dl 2 hours after a glucose load, there is a comparative prevalence of 2 percent in East Pakistan (Bangladesh), 3.3 percent in Malaya, 4.1 percent in Central American, 17 percent in Pennsylvania, and 25 percent in Cherokee Indians.

In spite of efforts to find a causal relationship between diabetes mellitus and deafness, there is almost no evidence supporting it, particularly if it is borne in mind that almost all studies have naturally been done on those sufficiently affected to require insulin treatment. There may be some reduction in the lower frequencies, but this is less in the middle frequencies (1 to 4 kHz) and the same at 8 kHz. Those with a diabetic family history have a significantly better hearing threshold than do those without. So far no correlation has been found between hearing level and insulin requirement.

A recent study in children[24] found no statistically significant differences in auditory function between insulin-dependent diabetics and normal controls, between the diabetics in good or poor control, or between diabetics with or without neurologic or vascular complications. Brain stem responses also showed no difference between the two groups. A small study of patients[25] suffering idiopathic sudden hearing loss and a possible relationship to diabetes also found no correlation in the audiologic pattern; a similar incidence of recovery was noted in the two groups through the middle frequencies; however, the diabetic patients failed to recover as well in the high frequencies. Brain stem evoked responses (BSERs) also showed no abnormality and no evidence of retrocochlear dysfunction or pathology.

Personal experience[26] has shown that while a few middle-aged deaf adults, usually with a premature high tone loss, may show evidence of early diabetes, their fasting blood sugar levels are normal, and there is little evidence of glycosuria during the glucose tolerance test.

In a series of patients with Menière's syndrome,[27] glucose tolerance tests were also carried out, but no increased incidence of primary hypothyroidism or hyperlipoproteinemia.

Glycosuria screening is an insensitive technique for detecting the lesser degrees of glucose intolerance. The renal glucose threshold increases with age, so that false-positive glycosuria is common in the young and produces false-negative results in the old.

### Hypothyroidism

#### Myxedema

A possible association between myxedema and deafness has been argued for many years, but the evidence remains inconclusive. Two recent reports may serve as examples of these conflicting conclusions: Van't Hoff and Stuart[28] in favor, and Parving et al,[29] against.

Delayed mentation on carrying out a subjective test may account for the apparent hearing loss and a subsequent improvement after treatment. However, a recent series[30] appeared to show some relationship. Auditory brain stem responses (ABR) on patients with altered thyroid function have shown two patterns. A good correlation was observed between the brain stem conduction time (BSCT) and the level of sodium tetraiodothyronine (thyroxine, $T_4$). In untreated hyperthyroidism. BSCT was decreased and in some patients ABR was characterized by high amplitude waves, sharp peaks, and jittery contours becoming smoother in pattern and more well defined after treatment.

In untreated hypothyroidism, the ABR was generally characterized by prolonged BSCT, diminished amplitudes, flattened peaks, and poor synchronization; in the older patients, the changes in wave pattern were more pronounced. BSCT appears to be a sensitive index of the $T_4$-dependent cellular status in the neural pathways of the brain stem.

Experimental work on guinea pigs[31] rendered hypothyroid during gestation with either radioactive iodine 131 or propylthiouracil (both methods produced the same auditory results) has shown raised auditory thresholds when the interwave interval for N1 and N2 responses at the round window and vertex response were measured. The interwave intervals for the N1–N2 responses at the round window as well as the interwave intervals for the brain stem response were normal once threshold had been reached.

However, the clinical picture is less well documented in congenital hypothyroidism[32] as human studies have concentrated on two rather isolated topics — endemic cretinism and Pendred's syndrome. These two conditions appear irrelevant for most children with congenital hypothyroidism, because their disease is neither endemic nor hereditary. The hearing in a series of 45 children with thyroid gland agenesis, hypogenesis, or dyshomogenesis, during adequate substitution therapy showed the majority (80 percent) to have normal auditory thresholds, while the remainder exhibited a sensorineural loss of differing degree, in one-half of whom the deafness was important. No relationship between hearing acuity and bone age at diagnosis of hypothyroidism or etiology of thyroid function could be found.

# RENAL SYSTEM

There has been renewed interest in recent years in renal failure, concerning both the use of ototoxic drugs and subsequent treatment by hemodialysis or transplantation.[33] There is now increasing awareness of the potentiation of powerful diuretics and aminoglycoside antibiotics and their ototoxic effect, particularly in patients with renal or liver failure, many of whom require such drugs to survive.

Urea by itself is nontoxic to the cochlear end

organs, but a hearing loss related to the degree of hyponatremia, irrespective of blood urea, has been noted. Such cochlear affections were greatly improved by correcting the renal failure and restoring the serum sodium.

Dialysis patients become more susceptible to cardiovascular disease and premature atherosclerosis, whereas transplant patients are susceptible to complications from immunosuppression and steroid treatment, particularly infections. During hemodialysis, frequent and intense osmotic changes occur. Fluctuations in hearing during a single dialysis period did not appear to have any correlation with corresponding changes in BUN, creatinine, Na, K, Ca, glucose, mean blood pressure level, or weight.

## Alport's Syndrome

Occasionally Alport's syndrome has been mentioned in relation to hearing loss. Alport[34] himself reported a relationship between nephritis and deafness and noted a familial occurrence. The etiology of the hearing loss has never been clearly defined. Characteristically, it varies in severity with the family and is slowly progressive, and the high frequencies are those most severely affected. It has been suggested that there may be as many as five variants: renal disease with the organ of Corti damage, renal disease with spiral ganglion cochlear neuron loss, renal disease and deafness but no histologic ear lesion, renal disease without deafness, and finally deafness without renal disease. Ophthalmologic defects may also be present, although visual acuity is normal or near normal.

Recent assessment of the cochlear abnormalities suggests that strial strophy and vacuolation of the spiral ligament are the most common changes. Varying degrees of degeneration of both population of hair cells and ganglion cells may coexist and may indeed be secondary to strial changes. The most likely explanation of the fundal defect was seen to be an altered metabolism of two glycosides, resulting in the production of faulty basement membrane collagen.

The hearing loss in Alport's syndrome is of a slowly progressive symmetric sensorineural type, which is often not significant until the second decade. Three types of pure-tone audiometric pattern have been described: trough shaped, sloping, and flat. Speech reception thresholds are reported as being in agreement with pure-tone averages and speech discrimination scores consistent with the audiometric configuration. A recent report[35] of 11 patients (from nine families) includes seven with functioning transplants, one on regular hemodialysis, another continuous ambulatory peritoneal dialysis, and two (both female) still with functioning kidneys.

While a family history may indicate the diagnosis, the most common presenting signs are hypertension, proteinuria, and hematuria. Likewise, while patients may have some hearing loss by the time the renal lesion is diagnosed, it has not hitherto been a presenting symptom. The rate of progression of the hearing loss would appear to be slow; the hearing loss was no greater in those receiving hemodialysis or in those showing hypertension. Unequal recruitment was exhibited throughout the auditory range with the trend being greater in the middle frequencies, producing dynamic compression at 2 kHz. Brain stem audiometry showed normal evoked reponses.

## Renal Transplantation

Hearing improvement in sensorineural loss has been reported following renal transplantation. Renal transplantation in those with Alport's syndrome has been shown conflicting results; that is, one report[36] described an improvement, but in another[37] this was less obvious.

# NERVOUS SYSTEM

## Disseminated Sclerosis

Hearing impairment is occasionally an initial, though seldom a prominent, sympton in disseminated sclerosis. When it occurs it is normally unilateral and may be peripheral or central in origin.[38] Rarely, the hearing loss may be sudden in onset.[39]

Deafness seems more likely to occur during the first 4 years of presentation of the condition, but thereafter there is no relationship between the hearing loss and the duration of the disease. Improvement in hearing during remission may occur and occasionally may revert to normal. It appears that in the unilateral case the lesion is likely to lie at the most caudal level of the pathway, involving the intramedullary auditory nerve or cochlear nucleus.

Brain stem evoked responses have been carried out in two groups of patients with disseminated sclerosis: those known to have deafness and those without but exhibiting other signs of the disease.[40] Findings in those with sudden unilateral deafness have shown an absence of waves after wave I. Other abnormalities have included increased latencies or reduced wave amplitudes; such findings may be found in those with normal peripheral hearing levels. The most common abnormality is an absent or low-amplitude wave V (inferior colliculus) or increased III through V separation.[41] No significant correlation has so far been found between the disseminated sclerosis classification and the type of BAER abnormality. A high incidence of BAER abnormalities has been seen in those exhibiting nystagmus or internuclear ophthalmoplegia.

Tests of central auditory dysfunction may be helpful—binaural fusion and dichotic sentences. Some patients have been found to have poor speech discrimination in spite of normal pure-tone testing.[42] Vestibular abnormalities are more common than those in the auditory system, and some 25 percent of patients are troubled by vertigo at some stage during their disease.

## Neurofibromatosis

Neurofibromatosis is a common autosomal-dominant disorder of neural tissue described by von Recklinghausen in 1882. A classic case demonstrates multiple soft elevated cutaneous tumors, cutaneous pigmentation, and neurofibromas of peripheral nerves, which are frequently palpable in the subcutaneous tissue. In addition, elephantoid soft tissue masses on the body and fanlike enlargements of peripheral nerves called plexiform neuromas may occur. Bone lesions occur in about one-half of cases.[43] Skeletal abnormalities include severe scoliosis, defects of the walls of the orbits, erosive defects caused by adjacent neurogenic tumors, bowing and pseudo-arthrosis of the lower leg, and disorders of bone growth. The severe kyphoscoliosis seen in neurofibromatosis is distinguished by the great predominance of the kyphotic element over the scoliotic phase. Acute angulation at the gibbus is typical. The defect of the postero-superior wall of the orbit consists basically of the absence or failure of development of that portion of the membranous bone separating the cranial contents from those of the orbit. The resultant gap in the posterosuperior portion of the orbit, involving the wings of the sphenoid and the orbital plate of the frontal bone, permits direct contact of the temporal lobe of the brain with orbital soft tissue. Bone underlying the soft tissue masses on the head and neck more commonly shows hypoplasia than overgrowth. The facial bones, mandible, and occipital bone may be deformed and hypoplastic. Erosive defects of bone from contiguous neurogenic tumors often involve the ribs, usually on the undersurface. Neurilemmomas and neurofibromas of the cranial and spinal nerves frequently occur in neurofibroma cases.[44] In addition, there is an increased incidence of gliomas and meningiomas, which may be multiple. When the neurofibroma affects the 8th cranial nerve, all the characteristic features of an acoustic neuroma may be found. In von Recklinghausen's disease, they may be bilateral; indeed, if bilateral acoustic neuromas are found, the other stigmata of von Recklinghausen's disease should be sought. Posterior fossa meningiomas may be associated with this disease and may also produce auditory and vestibular symptoms.

## Xeroderma Pigmentosa

Xeroderma pigmentosa is a rare autosomal-recessive condition. Clinically, patients present with an abnormal sensitivity to sunlight, characterized by the appearance of a delayed yet marked erythema of skin exposed to ultraviolet (UV) light. In addition, photophobia is a common symptom, and blepharoconjunctivitis with corneoscleral tumors may also occur. The condition may be associated with mental deficiency, but dwarfism, microcephaly, gonadal hypoplasia, and other neurologic ab-

normalities may occur. Deafness may also be associated with this disease and is usually of the sensorineural type, often associated with other progressive neurologic abnormalities. In a series of three patients[45] with differing forms of the condition, the hearing loss was sensorineural in all, and none had significant tone decay; the speech audiograms were no worse than would be expected from the pure-tone loss at 500 to 2,000 Hz. The stapedius reflex was present and recruited in all patients and BSEPs in two patients showed a normal recording on one and only a mild derangement in the other, suggesting a more peripheral origin to the deafness than the brain stem. Although the deafness was bilateral in all three patients, it was not entirely symmetric. All three patients had normal caloric responses and, from a series of other vestibular tests, it was concluded that (1) the vestibular pathways are involved in xeroderma pigmentosa, but probably to a lesser extent than the auditory pathways, and (2) the vestibulo-ocular reflex suppression is abnormal.

There is no doubt that patients with xeroderma pigmentosa either have an impaired ability to repair damaged DNA (groups A through G) or show slow degeneration of DNA (xeroderma pigmentosa variants). Of the three patients investigated, two were of the former type (complementation groups A and B) and the third was a xeroderma pigmentosa variant.

## Vogt-Koyanagi-Harada Syndrome

The principal feature of Vogt-Koyanagi-Harada syndrome is the prolonged bilateral uveitis, causing blindness.[46] The hearing loss develops at or near the time the blindness occurs;[47] it is also usually bilateral, of varying degree, frequently associated with tinnitus and vertigo. The ear symptoms begin to improve after 1 to 3 weeks as the tinnitus and vertigo subside, greadually returning to normal. Vision often returns to normal in 2 to 6 months, but glaucoma and cataract may continue as complications. Vitiligo, poliosis, and alopecia usually appear when the uveitis begins to improve. Three stages may be recognized in the disease: meningeal, ophthalmic, and convalescent. The meningeal stage is present in at least 50 percent of patients any may last 2 to 4 weeks. The hearing loss may occasionally be unilateral and need not always recover. Most reported cases have been in people of pigmented race. The cause remains unknown.

## Carcinomatous Neuropathy

The highest incidence of carcinomatous neuropathy[48] has been found in patients with carcinoma of the lung, ovary, and stomach and lowest in the rectum, cervix, and uterus. No particular association with either branch of the 8th cranial nerve has been shown thus far, although sudden deafness may occur. Hearing loss has occasionally been reported as the presenting symptom in carcinomatous meningitis.

## MUSCULOSKELETAL SYSTEM

By definition, the temporal bone forms part of the skeletal system but, while it may be affected by many specific conditions, it is relatively infrequently involved in many of the generalized systemic diseases of bone. No single classification is universally acceptable, and the names of many conditions continue to change, and likewise their classification. Table 31-1 lists systemic bone diseases. The biochemical, radiologic, and other characteristics of many of them are summarized in Table 31-2.

## Osteoporosis

An association between primary osteoporosis and sensorineural deafness has been reported, but much larger numbers need to be investigated before the relationship can be established. Of greater interest would be the question of treatment for the osteoporosis and whether this produced any improvement or halted the hearing loss and similarly how the hearing loss related to the stage of the radiologic and clinical picture of the condition.

**Table 31-1.   Systemic Bone Disease**

Otosclerosis
Osteitis deformans (Paget's disease)
Osteogenesis imperfecta (van der Hoeve syndrome)
Fibrous dysplasia
Osteopetrosis
Genetic craniotabular dysplasias
   Craniometaphyseal dysplasia
   Frontometaphyseal dysplasia
Genetic craniotabular hyperostoses
   Hyperostosis corticalis generalisata
   Sclerosteosis
   Congenital hyperphosphatasia
   Progressive diaphyseal dysplasia
Craniofacial dystosis
Osteopathia striata (with sclerotic skull base)
Neurofibromatosis

## Acromegaly

Acromegaly is a chronic disease of middle life that results from excessive secretion of growth hormone by the acidophil cells of the anterior pituitary. A recent study[49] over an 8-year period, found 56 patients (22 male, 34 female) with acromegaly requiring pituitary surgery in a population of 2.5 million. No significant difference between the acromegalics and a matched population control sample could be found, either for air or for bone conduction, at any frequency. Likewise, there was no audiometric change after surgery and no relationship between the hearing and growth hormone levels. (Three ears showed evidence of otosclerosis among the acromegalics and one in the control group.) Radiology in another series[50] of three cases demonstrated massive thickening of the mastoid cortex and posterior bony canal wall with secondary lengthening of the bony external canal; some overgrowth diminishing the lumen may also occur. However, the internal canal, cochlea, and vestibule appeared normal, and the structures of the otic capsule, including the facial nerve, remained in normal relationship.

## Osteomalacia

### Vitamin D Deficiency

Vitamin D deficiency may be seen in a small number of patients and should be considered in those with progressive bilateral sensorineural deaf-

**Table 31-2.   Bony Proteins Associated with Hearing Abnormalities**

| Disorder | Hearing Abnormality | Chemistry | | Radiographic Findings | Other Pathology |
|---|---|---|---|---|---|
| Paget's disease (osteitis deformans) | Conductive and/or sensorineural | Ca<br>PO$_4$<br><br>Alk<br><br>Acid | usually normal<br>hypercalcemia—immobilization<br>phosphatase elevated in active disease<br>phosphatase may be raised<br>Urinary HDP elevated in active disease | Varied—lytic, sclerotic, and mixed phases<br>Skull—great increase in thickness of both tables, particularly outer<br>? patchy sclerosis—wooly appearance<br>Platybasia; basilar impression | X-ray pelvis including femoral heads<br>Osteoporosis circumscripta—patch of reduced density resembling bony defect<br>Pathologic fracture |
| Fibrous dysplasia | Conductive, rarely sensorineural | CA<br>PO$_4$<br>Alk<br><br><br><br>Acid | usually normal<br>always normal<br>phosphatase may be raised in active disease, especially polyostotic form<br>phosphatase normal | Monostotic/polyostotic appearances—same<br>Multiloculated cystic lesion (bone frequently expanded)<br>Occ. lesion more diffuse ground-glass appearance due to multiple fine trabeculae<br>Occ. diffuse sclerotic appearance | Skeletal survey to exclude polyostotic<br>Pathologic fracture<br>Café-au-lait pigmentation may be present (either type) |
| Osteopetrosis<br>Albers-Schönberg | Conductive<br>Occ. mixed | Ca<br>PO$_4$<br>Alk<br>Acid | } normal<br><br>} phosphatase may be markedly elevated<br>Urinary HDP usually normal | Symmetric increase in bone density; bones appear structureless<br>Sclerotic foci—bones within bones<br>Thickening of vertebral end plates (rugger jersey) | Thick dense brittle bones<br>Pathologic fracture<br>Facial palsy<br>Occ. osteomyelitis of mandible after dental extraction<br>Mild anemia |
| Malignant recessive | Sensorineural | As above | | Transverse bands in metaphyseal regions of long bones and longitudinal striations<br>Prox. humerus and distal femur—flask-shaped<br>Vertebrae—rugger jersey | Facial palsy<br>Blindness<br>Pathologic fracture<br>Mental retardation<br>Liver and spleen enlargement<br>Hemolytic anemia and thrombocytopenia |
| Genetic craniotabular hyperosotoses van Buchem's (autosomal-recessive) | Conductive and/or sensorineural | Ca<br>PO$_4$<br>Alk | } normal<br><br>phosphatase frequently raised (50–250%) | Diffuse symmetric increase in bone density<br>Cortical bone—abnormally thick, but bones not increased in size<br>Hyperplasia diaphysis long and short bones<br>Endosteal thickening diaphysis—tubular bones | Normal stature<br>Facial palsy<br>Clavicles—thickened and palpable<br>Overgrowth of brow and mandible |
| Sclerosteosis (autosomal-recessive) | Conductive and/or sensorineural | Ca<br>PO$_4$<br>Alk<br><br><br>Acid | } normal<br><br>phosphatase markedly elevated in nearly all patients<br>phosphatase normal | Bones show increased density but only minor degree of bony modeling, if present<br>Progressive bony thickening | Syndactyly and digital malformation<br>Facial paralysis<br>Tall stature<br>Distortion of face and jaw<br>Chronic headache |

*(Table continues.)*

**Table 31-2.** *(continued)*

| Disorder | Hearing Abnormality | Chemistry | Radiographic Findings | Other Pathology |
|---|---|---|---|---|
| | | | Tubular bones markedly undermodeled with lack of usual diaphyseal constriction | Raised ICP Anosmia Majority Afrikaners |
| Congenital hyperphostasia (autosomal-recessive) | Conductive with decreased bone conduction | Ca PO$_4$ } normal<br>Alk Acid } phosphatases both consistently elevated<br>Urine HDP high | Similar to Paget's Marked irregular thickening of skull ? Narrowing of external auditory canal Tubular bones— width greatly increased, bowing and lack of modeling | Multiple fractures Dwarfing Blue sclerae (? increased serum uric acid and leucine aminopeptidase) |
| Progressive diaphyseal dysplasia (autosomal-dominant) | Combined with large air–bone gap | Ca PO$_4$ Alk phosphatase Acid phosphatase } usually normal | Generalized sclerosis of skull base; vault less commonly/severely affected | Marked thickening of cortices of leg bones medullary canals narrowed; external bony contours irregular |

ICP, intracranial pressure.

ness.[51,52] However, biochemical investigations will be required to unearth such a diagnosis, as there are no characteristic clinical signs. A raised alkaline phosphatase is found in more than 50 percent of those affected and abnormal phosphate levels in perhaps 17 percent, but the serum calcium is seldom raised, although may be at the upper end of the normal range.

Vitamin D refers to a group of steroids that play an essential role with parathyroid hormone in the regulation of calcium and bone metabolism. Vitamin $D_3$ is synthesized in the human skin, and only a small proportion of the body's requirement is obtained from the diet. Vitamin $D_3$ must be metabolized before it becomes physiologically active; the main metabolic pathway is shown in Figure 31-2). The liver and kidney are both important organs involved in the pathology. 25-Hydroxyvitamin $D_3$ (25-OHD) is the main storage form, while 1,25-dihydroxyvitamin $D_3$ produced by the renal tubules mediates most of the actions. The most helpful index of vitamin D status is an assay of serum 25-OHD levels. The hallmark of vitamin D deficiency is a failure of mineralization of bone matrix, which leads to an increased accumulation of osteoid or uncalcified matrix (Fig. 31-3). Low serum levels of vitamin D metabolites frequently leads to secondary hyperparathyroidism and preferential mobilization of calcium from bone.

The biochemical parameters may often be normal due to compensatory metabolic mechanisms; 85 to 100 percent of patients with overt osteomalacia have OHD levels below 5 mg/ml. The 25-OHD lower normal limit varies between different laboratories but is about 8 to 10 ng/ml. The serum 25-OHD is probably the first parameter to be altered in conditions of vitamin D undernutrition.

## Hereditary Primary Hypophosphatemia

When due to an isolated renal tubular leak of phosphate, hereditary primary hypophosphatemia is the most common type of metabolic (vitamin D-resistant) rickets and is nearly always transmitted by an X-linked dominant gene.[53,54] Sporadic cases due to new mutation are not uncommon, and such patients may be expected to transmit the disease to their offspring in the X-linked manner.

## Hypercalcemia

### Primary Hyperparathyroidism

Primary hyperparathyroidism is rarely seen affecting the ear. Involvement of the otic capsule would only seem to occur when the condition has

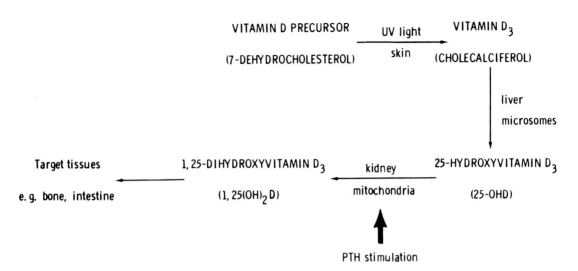

**Fig. 31-2.** The main metabolic pathway of vitamin D. PTH, parathyroid hormone. (Booth JB: Medical management of sensorineural hearing loss. II. Musculoskeletal system. J Laryngol Otol 96:773, 1982. Print courtesy of Mr. G. B. Brookes.)

reached the state of osteitis fibrosa cystica (von Recklinghausen's disease of the bone). Although many patients give evidence of excessive effects of parathyroid hormone on bone, only a few develop clinically evident osteitis fibrosa cystica. For some reason, which is not understood, the incidence of osteitis fibrosa cystica is on the decline.

## Vitamin D Poisoning

One patient with pseudo-hyperparathyroidism who continued to take calciferol, 2.5 mg day, has been reported[55]; he returned 4 years later with a 3-month history of deafness. Examination showed an extensive calcification of the tympanic mem-

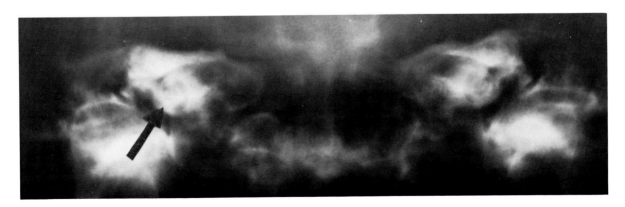

**Fig. 31-3.** Osteomalacia, showing bilateral cochlear demineralization. Arrow indicates obliteration of lumen of basal turn. (Booth JB: Medical management of sensorineural hearing loss. II. Musculoskeletal system. J Laryngol Otol 96:773, 1982. Print courtesy of Mr. G. B. Brookes.)

branes and cornea, with severe conductive deafness. Extensive calcification of the kidneys and blood vessels (renal function tests normal) was seen; radiographs of the mastoids show them to be cellular. Despite treatment, the deafness remained.

## Systemic Bone Disease

### Paget's Disease

There can be few conditions bearing an eponym that are so well known and that have provided such persistent interest as Paget's disease. Sir James Paget described the condition in 1877. It has an unusual racial and geographic distribution, being very common in the United Kingdom, Australia, and New Zealand and in other populations of British origin, such as North America and South Africa. It was therefore considered a disease of Anglo-Saxon origin, but there are now well-documented instances occurring in African and Asian subjects. Surveys have revealed a marked geographic variation in the disease from high to lower levels over very short distances.

Paget himself described the onset of the disease in middle age with slow progression, producing the effect by changing the shape, size, and direction of the diseased bones. He noted the common enlargement of the skull, which nevertheless did not seem to cause brain compression, and drew attention to the very frequent involvement of the femora and tibiae.

Of those with widespread active disease, bone pain is a troublesome symptom and probably occurs in as many as 20 percent of cases, sufficient to warrant treatment. Expansion of bones around foramina at the base of the skull and in the orbit can lead to neurologic defects and optic atrophy. The pelvis is the area most commonly affected by the disease (76 percent), and the skull is involved in 28 percent.

Whereas the precise etiology is unknown, it is now widely accepted that Paget's disease is, pathogenetically, an example of primary osteoclast dysfunction. It is now 10 years since inclusions were noted only in the osteoclast, and they are morpho-logically analogous to those seen in proven paramyxovirus infections — measles or respiratory syncytial virus.[56] Clinicopathologic aspects of Paget's disease have several paramyxovirus-type antigens. There is also an unexplained possibility of a birth-cohort-related cyclic disease incidence. Even more inexplicable is the fact that the incidence of Paget's is apparently declining.

In a series of more than 1,000 patients, Harner et al.[57] found 17 percent of patients to have tinnitus and 21 percent dizziness; the most common type of the latter was postural positional unsteadiness. Sensorineural hearing loss was the most frequent auditory disturbance but was usually not part of the disease process. In those patients whose initial audiogram showed a mixed hearing loss, the mean age was 56 years, and 49 percent showed evidence of the disease before the age of 60. In those with a sensorineural loss, the mean age was 61 years, with 37 percent below the age of 60. In those in whom there was radiologic evidence of skull involvement, the incidence of mixed hearing loss was statistically much greater than expected; the incidence of tinnitus and dizziness was also higher than in the overall group. While increased tortuosity and hypertrophy of the anterior terminal branch of the superfical temporal artery may be seen in many patients with skull involvement in Paget's disease, it is by no means characteristic of the condition.

The radiologic findings are as follows: in the early stages, small areas of lucency and dense patches are seen that fade into one another; there is often a typical mixture of lytic and sclerotic areas, and the skull is thick where it is affected, predominantly over the vertex. Some coarse trabeculae are nearly always visible, except in the most advanced cases.

Tomographic changes in the temporal bone due to Paget's disease vary from minimal demineralization of the petrous apex to demineralization of the entire petrous pyramid, including the otic capsule; they appeared to correlate grossly with the degree of skull involvement. The involvement of the internal auditory canals consisted of demineralization of the walls without evidence of narrowing. In patients with extensive involvement, the internal auditory canal was no longer identifiable as a distinct structure; the margins of the external auditory

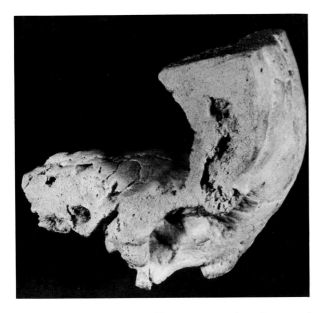

**Fig. 31-4.** Paget's disease. Transverse section of temporal bone showing gross thickening of cortex and petrous areas.

canal and middle ear showed demineralization in those with extensive involvement. Nearly all ears with sensorineural deafness had cochlear radiographic changes.

The medial aspect of the petrous pyramid is the initial site of involvement, followed by progressive involvement of the internal auditory canal, but the otic capsule is spared until advanced changes are present in the remainder of the petrous pyramid (Fig. 31-4). The bone changes in the pyramid begin in areas best supplied with marrow tissue. Involvement of the labyrinthine capsule (Fig. 31-5), when present, begins in the outer periosteal layer; the middle endochondral layer is more resistant, and the greatest resistance is present in the endosteal layer, but with extensive involvement these three layers can no longer be distinguished. Some have attributed the sensorineural loss to platybasia and basilar impression with torsion of the 8th cranial nerve. High-resolution computed tomography (CT) may also be used for more detailed information (Fig. 31-6).

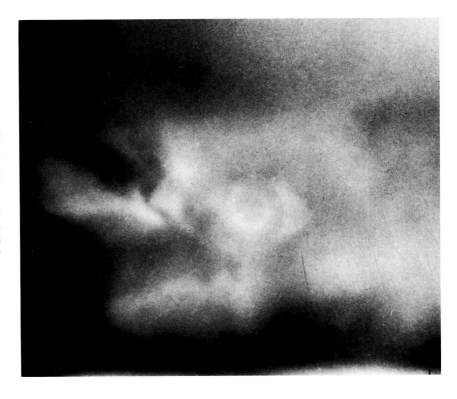

**Fig. 31-5.** Paget's disease. Hypocycloidal tomogram showing pagetoid bone replacing most of the periosteal bone at the petrous pyramid but also involving some of the bone of the labyrinthine capsule. (Booth JB: Medical management of sensorineural hearing loss. II. Musculoskeletal system. J Laryngol Otol 96:773, 1982. Print courtesy of Drs. G. A. S. Lloyd and P. Phelps.)

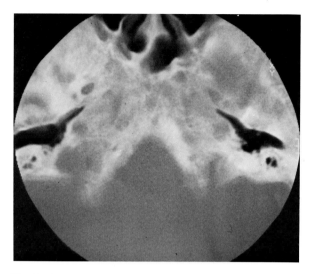

**Fig. 31-6.** Paget's disease. Axial CT scan showing disease affecting the skull base. (Print courtesy of Drs. G. A. S. Lloyd and P. Phelps.)

Serum calcium is usually normal in Paget's disease, but immobilization will lead to greater bone resorption than formation; as a result, hypercalcemia and hypercalciuria can occur. Serum alkaline phosphatase activity is elevated in active disease, particularly if it is widespread. Activity of this enzyme is related to bone formation by osteoblasts and probably by osteocytes as well. Serum acid phosphatase is an index of osteoclastic activity and is often increased in Paget's disease, particularly when the alkaline phosphatase is quite high, but its measurement is of little diagnostic value. Urinary hydroxyproline is an amino acid found exclusively in collagen; in Paget's disease, it may be greatly elevated when the condition is active, reflecting the breakdown of bone collagen.

More recently, treatment was attempted with synthetic human calcitonin, and with porcine calcitonin, and with salmon calcitonin. While such treatment has been associated with a striking reduction in the turnover of diseased bone confirmed by biochemical changes, there has been no significant hearing improvement in any of the patients. A follow-up of 3 years by Walker et al.[58] on 13 patients treated earlier by Solomon and co-workers similarly reported no discernible difference between the treated and untreated groups.

Disodium etidronate diphosphonate (EHDP) seems to possess all the biologic properties of pyrophosphate, including the ability to inhibit bone resorption. The drug appears to inactivate osteoclasts and osteoblasts, properties that have led to its trial in Paget's disease. However, long-term administration may result in histologic osteomalacia associated with pathologic fractures. It has the advantage that it may be taken orally, but so far only one short report by Gennari and Sensini[59] of its use in the deafness of Paget's disease has been published. Five patients were treated whose pure-tone audiograms showed a significant improvement in the air-conduction threshold of greater than 15 dB in three out of five cases.

### Fibrous Dysplasia

Three types of fibrous dysplasia are described[60]:

Type I, monostotic: limited to one bone (usually femur, tibia, ribs or facial bones, particularly mandible and maxilla)

Type II, polyostotic (monomelic): more than one bone involved (most frequently the lower limbs); in the skull, the lesser and greater wings of the sphenoids and the vertical and horizontal processes of the frontal bones mainly affected; frontal and sphenoid sinuses frequently obliterated

Type III: disseminated with extraskeletal manifestations (McCune-Albright syndrome); with bone distribution similar to the polyostotic but commonly unilateral and skin hyperpigmentations and endocrine disturbances

Barrionuevo et al.[61] found the temporal bones affected in 23 recorded cases of the monostotic and in four of the polystotic form. There has been no report of the temporal bone being affected in type III.

The most common symptoms are loss of hearing and increased volume of the temporal region, mostly postauricular. The hearing loss is caused by partial or complete obstruction of the external auditory canal and direct or indirect involvement of the middle ear by fibro-osseous proliferation. When tinnitus is the first symptom, the disease affects the middle ear.

Two cases have shown sensorineural hearing loss, one due to encroachment on the internal auditory canal[62] and the other due to a labyrinthine fistula.[63]

Serum calcium, phosphorus, and alkaline phospatase have been found to be normal in all cases. Both the polyostotic and monostotic lesions are pathologically and radiologically identical. The radiologic appearance of the disease is a function of its histologic structure.[64] A predominance of osseous elements renders the lesion more opaque (Fig. 31-7), while a mixture of fibrous and bony elements produces a ground-glass appearance, and predominance of fibrous elements produces a radiolucent cystlike picture (Fig. 31-8). Malignant change and the possible association between fibrous dysplasia and primary hyperparathyroidism have been reported.[60]

Recently, it has been suggested that primary hyperparathyroidism and fibrous dysplasia may occasionally occur together and that the serum calcium may occasionally be elevated in both the polyostotic form and the disseminated form of fibrous dysplasia, but never in the monostotic unless there is concomitant primary hyperparathyroidism. The serum phosphorus level is always normal. The alkaline phosphatase level is said to be raised in all types of fibrous dysplasia with the presence of an active lesion, and it is always raised in the disseminated type. It would seem that the level of alkaline phosphatase is an indication of the activity of the lesion.

## Osteosclerosis (Osteopetrosis)

Osteosclerosis comprises the two variants of osteopetrosis and pyknodystosis (Toulouse-Lautrec syndrome). Osteopetrosis exists in two forms: the autosomal-dominant (benign), otherwise known as Albers-Schonberg's disease; and the autosomal-recessive (malignant) type. When remodeling of bone involves the cranial foramina, stenosis and compression of emergent nerves and vessels may occur.[65]

In the temporal bone, as elsewhere, it is the endochondral layer that is most severely affected and the entire mastoid air cell system may be absent and filled instead with sclerotic bone. Myers and Stool[66] found no inner ear abnormalities that could be attributed directly to the abnormal bone; likewise, the internal auditory canal may be narrowed, but the otic capsule remains unaffected.[67]

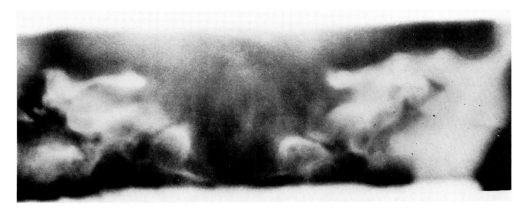

**Fig. 31-7.** Fibrous dysplasia. Dense bone obliterates the external auditory canal on the left side. (Booth JB: Medical management of sensorineural hearing loss. II. Musculoskeletal system. J Laryngol Otol 96:773, 1982. Print courtesy of Drs. G. A. S. Lloyd and P. Phelps.)

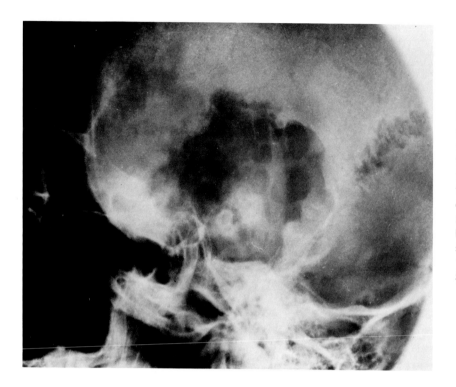

**Fig. 31-8.** Left temporal bone showing extensive area of destruction. Labyrinth remained intact with normal facial nerve function, but a large area of posterior and middle fossa dura was exposed. (Booth JB: Medical management of sensorineural hearing loss. II. Musculoskeletal system. J Laryngol Otol 96:773, 1982. Print courtesy of Mr. M. Sharp.)

In Albers-Schonberg disease, the hearing loss is predominantly conductive but may occasionally be mixed. In the malignant recessive form, the hearing loss is sensorineural. In either form, a facial palsy may occur or be the presenting sign.

Serum calcium, phosphorus, and alkaline phosphatase levels are normal, but the acid phosphatase may be markedly elevated; the urinary hydroxyproline levels are usually within normal limits.

## Hyperostosis Corticalis Generalisata

Hyperostosis corticalis generalisata (van Buchem's disease) was first described by van Buchem et al.[68] in 1955; additional reports have appeared since. This autosomal-recessive condition, associated with normal stature and gross overgrowth of bone in the skull and skeleton, is associated with facial palsy and conductive deafness, but normal digits.

This condition is characterized by osteosclerosis of the skull (Fig. 31-9), mandible, clavicles, and ribs, as well as hyperplasia of the diaphyseal cortex of the long and short bones. The skull and mandible may enlarge from the age of 10 onward, with thickening of the calvaria, the skull base becoming dense, and with thickening of the clavicles, which thereby become palpable. The facial paralysis may be unilateral or bilateral, and a gradually symmetric hearing loss may be noted in patients from the age of about 15. In some cases a sensorineural loss, in others a mixed loss may occur. Optic nerve involvement is a late complication. The serum calcium and phosphorus remain normal, but the alkaline phosphatase is frequently raised by as much as 50 to 250 percent.

## Sclerosteosis

Sclerosteosis is an autosomal-recessive condition in which overgrowth is associated with syndactyly

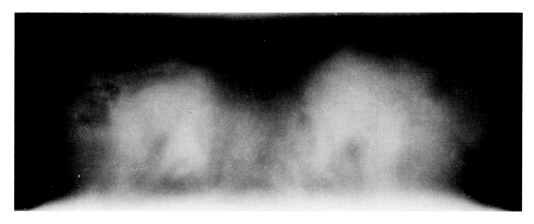

**Fig. 31-9.** van Buchem's disease. Sclerotic bone affecting both petrous pyramids with some tilt due to platybasia and bone softening. (Booth JB: Medical management of sensorineural hearing loss. II. Musculoskeletal system. J Laryngol Otol 96:773, 1982. Print courtesy of Drs. G. A. S. Lloyd and P. Phelps.)

and digital malformation. Facial palsy and deafness are common complications, and raised intracranial pressure may develop.

The hearing loss may be bilateral sensorineural, mixed, or conductive.[69] Facial nerve paralysis is often unilateral in childhood, becoming bilateral in late adolescence. There is also decreased sensory function of the ophthalmic and maxillary divisions of the 5th cranial nerve, anosmia, and chronic headache.

The serum calcium, phosphorus, and acid phosphatase concentrations are within normal limits, but the alkaline phosphatase is markedly elevated in nearly all patients. Parathyroid hormone, calcitonin, growth hormone, thyroid function studies, and prolactin are also normal. Radiologically, the bones show increased density, but abnormalities of bony modeling, if present, are of minor degree. The mastoid air cells are obliterated, but the paranasal sinuses remain intact (Fig. 31-10). The changes involving the temporal bone include a marked increase in overall dimensions, extreme sclerosis, and narrowing and constrictuion of the external ear canal, middle ear cleft, internal auditory canal, and fallopian canal. Early decompression of the internal auditory canal and fallopian canal may help preserve cochlear and facial nerve function.

## Congenital Hyperphosphatasia

Congenital hyperphosphatasia (osteoectasia) is a rare autosomal-recessive condition, with skeletal deformities developing in the second or third year of life. It is associated with dwarfing, fractures, and blue sclerae. There is marked irregular thickening of the skull and enlargement of the calvaria. The external auditory canal may become narrowed, and there is a progressive mixed hearing loss of approximately 60 to 80 dB which becomes evident from the fourth to the fourteenth year. Serum alkaline and acid phosphatase are both consistently elevated.

## Progressive Diaphyseal Dysplasia

Progressive diaphyseal dysplasia (Camurati-Englemann's disease: osteopathia hyperostotica sclerositans multiplex infantilis) is an autosomal-dominant condition principally involving the long bones, but the skull may be mildly affected as well. Generalized sclerosis of the base similar to osteopetrosis may be seen, but the vault bones are less commonly and less severely affected (Fig. 31-11).

Sparks and Graham[70] reported a case of a 26-year-old man with progressive hearing difficulty

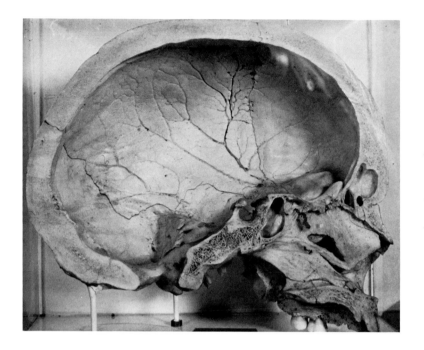

**Fig. 31-10.** Sclerosteosis. The skull of a 30-year-old man, showing sclerosis of an extreme degree. The diploe have been replaced by dense compact tissue, but the sutures remain patent. (Courtesy of the Medical Illustration Department, Royal College of Surgeons of England.)

leading to total deafness on the right side associated with a facial paralysis. Bilateral decompression of the slitlike internal auditory canals was carried out, and some initial improvement was noted.

Recently, two cases of progressive diaphyseal dysplasia were described for which surgery was performed.[71] The first was a 26-year-old man who complained of bilateral hearing loss, right-sided facial paralysis, and chronic unsteadiness. Radiographs showed bilateral massive overgrowth of

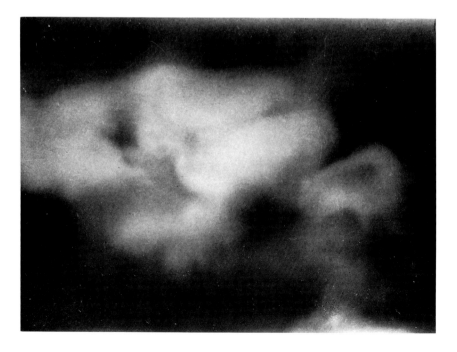

**Fig. 31-11.** Engelmann's disease. Dense bone appears to be narrowing the internal auditory canal. (Booth JB: Medical management of sensorineural hearing loss. II. Musculoskeletal system. J Laryngol Otol 96:773, 1982. Print courtesy of Drs. G. A. S. Lloyd and P. Phelps.)

dense bone involving the petrous apex and mastoid bone. Both internal auditory canals were partially obliterated by this dense bone. The second case was of a 30-year-old woman with bilateral sensorineural hearing loss, occurring suddenly 14 months earlier on the right side, and 9 months later on the left. Both cases were explored surgically by a middle cranial fossa approach, the first to improve the facial nerve function, and the second to decompress the internal auditory canal on the right side. Following surgery, the hearing of the second patient has remained stable and further radiographs showed no evidence of recompression.

## Osteogenesis Imperfecta

Osteogenesis imperfecta or fragilitas osseum is a relatively rare disease having a frequency of two to five per 100,000 of the population.[72-74] It is a dominant hereditary disorder of collagen, usually but not always manifest, therefore carriers exist in some families. Sporadic cases also occur. The severity of the disease varies from family to family. In the most severe surviving cases, multiple fractures date from infancy, leading to considerable deformity of the limbs; in the least severe cases, there may be only a few fractures in response to trivial trauma. In the natural history of the disease, the tendency to fractures disappears in adolescence or early adult life.

The tendency to fractures is encountered in almost all cases, while some 85 percent have blue sclerae and 50 percent develop a hearing loss. Other features are less commonly encountered, such as joint laxity, an increased tendency to bruising, and amelogenesis imperfecta (a yellow staining of the permanent teeth, reminiscent of tetracycline damage).

Important features of this form of deafness are the age of onset and development. Whereas only some 10 percent of affected individuals will be deaf in childhood or adolescence, 50 percent of persons are likely to have hearing loss by middle age.[74] Another interesting feature is the absence of any relationship between the severity of the hearing loss and the severity of the fractures.[73] In some family members, the disease is manifested by blue sclerae and deafness without the tendency to frac-

tures.[75,76] The hearing loss may increase during pregnancy. When multiple fractures, blue sclerae, and deafness occur together, they constitute the syndrome described by van der Hoeve and de Kleyn.[77]

### Otologic Features

The hearing loss in osteogenesis imperfecta normally involves a conductive element, so much so that it resembles otosclerosis. However, there is usually a sensorineural component, and wide air–bone gaps are unusual. In more than 10 percent of those with deafness, the lesion is entirely sensorineural and total deafness may result in a few.[74] Compliance values using a probe tone of 220 Hz tend to be normal or high compared with otosclerosis, in which they tend to fall within the low-normal range. In osteogenesis, fractures of the stapes arch can occur; in affected ears, the compliance values are abnormally high, combined with a stapedius reflex of high amplitude, if there is not too great a conductive loss on the other side (i.e., if the afferent pathway can be stimulated). Carhart notches are not described and, considering the widespread changes in the skull and temporal bones, a Schwartze sign is rarely seen.

Vertiginous symptoms have been reported as rare in fragilitas osseum[73,75,78] and as frequent as 20 percent of affected cases.[74,79-81] One of the temporal bone microdissections reported by Johnsson et al.[82] showed extensive endolymphatic hydrops with severe changes in the pars inferior and superior on both sides. Secondary hydrops appears to be unusual in temporal bones affected by this disease.

Multidirectional tomography demonstrates the widespread changes in the otic capsule with mottled areas of sclerosis and lysis. The decalcification and loss of outline of inner ear structures are not nearly as marked as in Paget's disease of the bone. Histologically, there are similarities to otosclerosis[83] yet these diseases are strikingly different.[84-87]

### Treatment

There is no known curative treatment of osteogenesis imperfecta. Appropriate hearing aids are likely to become necessary in most deafened subjects. Except in the few with total or subtotal deafness, discrimination remains good. If surgery is delayed until several years after the last fracture, stapedectomy results are generally satisfactory[75,76,81,88-90] in those who have an adequate air–bone gap. Care should be taken not to fracture the incus or malleus. Loss of the stapes arch from prior fractures may be encountered during surgery. The stapes footplate tends to be uniformly thick — the type of footplate that can readily float during manipulation.

## Syphilis

Although penicllin and other antitreponemal antibiotics have had a dramatic effect on the prevalence and prognosis of syphilitic disease, otologic manifestations, both early and late, continue to be seen. Awareness of the problem is the first essential. Between 1977 and 1981, approximately 4,500 new cases were reported each year in the United Kingdom.[91] From a population of say 56 million, this indicates an incidence of eight per 100,000 of the population each year. The numbers of new cases of congenital syphilis have fallen dramatically over the past 50 years. In England and Wales,[92-94] for example, the incidence has fallen from 2,439 new cases in 1931, to 1,223 new cases in 1950, and to 137 new cases in 1976. New cases of acquired syphilis are currently about 20 to 25 times as frequent as congenital cases. This has significance for the otologist. Whereas some years ago congenital syphilitic ear disease was encountered three times as often as the acquired variety,[95] the acquired otologic variants of the disease are likely to assume greater importance in the future.

**Early Syphilis.** Neonatal congenital syphilitic otolabyrinthitis and meningoneurolabyrinthitis are not encountered today, at least in Britain, presumably due to screening tests and appropriate therapy during pregnancy. These clincopathologic entities were described in detail by Rodger[96] in 1940.

Secondary syphilis, presenting with otologic features, is encountered today mainly in adult males who are often, although not always, homosexual. There are two similar clinical pictures, both with classic manifestations of secondary disease. The patient is likely to complain of malaise, slight fever,

sore throat with enlarged lymph glands, vague headaches, and classically of skin rashes with some loss of hair. There may be jaundice as well. These symptoms are usually spread over a period of some weeks or even 1 to 2 months. At some stage during this period of malaise, the patient complains of tinnitus and deafness, usually bilateral, although frequently worse on one side, developing rapidly over one or two days. Vestibular symptoms are less usual, but dizziness or transient vertigo may be induced by movement or positional change. It is the acute onset of otologic symptoms that brings the patient to the otologist, the other vague symptoms having been dismissed by the patient due to an upper respiratory infection. The pathologic process is a treponemal labyrinthitis and/or meningitis.

The other variant is very similar in its general manifestations but, in addition, there is an acute meningovascular secondary syphilis. Headache is a more prominent feature and, apart from the sudden otologic features, other cranial nerves may be acutely involved, the 6th being the most common.

In secondary syphilis of the inner ear, the hearing loss is sensorineural, mainly high frequency, and showing either absence, threshold elevation, or decay of the acoustic reflexes for frequencies above 1 kHz. Speech discrimination is relatively poor. The caloric responses are likely to be diminished on both sides. Spontaneous nystagmus may be present after abolishing fixation. Increased latency and/or reduced amplitude on wave V of the auditory brain stem responses has been reported.[97] With appropriate therapy, the cochlear and vestibular changes are partially reversible.

In all cases, serologic tests for syphilis are strongly positive and the VDRL slide test is positive in high dilution, indicating the activity of the disease process. The TPHA and FTA absorbed (ABS) are most commonly used. FTA IgG and IgM analysis will give positive results. In the meningovascular variant, all these tests are positive in the cerebrospinal fluid (CSF), which also shows an elevated protein and white cell count together with a meningitic Lange curve.

Left untreated, the acute infection runs a relatively benign course, although the deafness and tinnitus are likely to persist, and the otologist may see the untreated patient many months later.

Treatment should be energetic and is best carried out by, or in association with, a venereologist. The treatment may involve more than one course and, when there has been syphilitic meningitis and labyrinthitis, it is wise to check the CSF 6 to 12 months later and to repeat therapy if the CSF still shows abnormal findings. Penicillin is best given by an intramuscular high-dose injection over a 3-week period, together with probenecid to block urinary excretion of penicillin. Steroids are probably indicated for the first 10 days of therapy. Should penicillin allergy be present or develop (a more likely problem in late syphilis), alternatives include administration of erythromcyin, cephaloridine, or doxycycline.

**Late Syphilis.** Late syphilis of the temporal bone is a very different disease from early syphilis. Once established, its progress over long periods of time is relentless. Even with present-day antitreponemal and antiinflammatory agents, the prognosis is only somewhat better than it was in 1863 when Hutchinson, a physician at the London Hospital, wrote his treatise on inherited syphilis.[98]

Late syphilis affects the ear 10 to 40 years after the primary infection. Congenital syphilis of the ear is twice as frequent as the acquired variety; the former is somewhat commoner in younger female patients, the latter in older males. The pathologic changes in the temporal bones are similar, beautifully described in 1936 by Mayer and Fraser,[99] including descriptions of the endolymphatic hydrops, antedating the description of hydrops in Menière's disease. Later Goodhill[100] gave histopathologic accounts of the temporal bones in late acquired syphilis. There have since been many good accounts,[101-103] including descriptions of a gummatous osteitis with involvement of all three layers of the otic capsule; obliteration of the endolymphatic duct system, usually in the region of the sinus and sac; hydrops of the pars inferior and superior; and extensive degeneration of the neuroepithelial structures of the inner ear. The later stages are marked by extensive loss of cochlear and vestibular nerve fibers.

In congenital disease, there is likely to be, or to have been, evidence of stigmata of syphilis. Interstitial keratitis with or without choroidoretinitis, sometimes recurrent episodes, occur in about 90

percent of cases. These acute inflammatory attacks date from childhood, adolescence, or early adult life. When the patient presents, usually later, with otologic symptoms there may be no evidence of the previous interstitial keratitis unless the telltale corneal blood vessels are detected on slit-lamp examination. Treponemes can sometimes be recovered from the aqueous humous.

An estimated one in three patients with congenital syphilis develops otologic manifestations,[102] but the figure could well be closer to one in two. At all events, this is the second most frequent manifestation of congenital syphilis. About 20 percent have Hutchinsonian teeth, thickening, and wedge- or screwdriver-shaped permanent incisors. The facies described as typical of congenital syphilis — saddle nose and frontal bossing — are found in only 10 percent.[95,103] Other features, such as Clutton's joints, rhagades at the angles of the mouth, and Dubois sign, are very uncommon.

Neurosyphilis is seen in late congenital and in late acquired disease. Because most patients have had several courses of antitreponemal drugs over the years, there is rarely evidence of florid neurosyphilis, and certainly in the congenital variety the CSF is usually normal. In late acquired syphilis, there may be more evidence of neurologic disease such as one or more of the following symptoms: lightning pains, loss of ankle jerk, and vibration sense, sensory changes, bladder symptoms, Argyll Robertson pupils, or early optic atrophy. In these patients, the CSF protein may be slightly elevated and may show an abnormal Lange curve, together with positive tests for syphilis and even treponemes. However, even in late acquired previously treated syphilis, the CSF is likely to be normal, despite the presence of active otologic disease.

In late disease, the older serologic screening tests for syphilis (e.g., CWR) are often negative. The VDRL test can be positive in more than two-thirds of such patients and is a useful indication of disease activity. The FTA ABS test is likely to be positive in almost 100 percent of cases of late syphilis. In Britain, patients rarely volunteer information about congenital syphilis or about previously treated acquired venereal disease. In addition, they are very unlikely to associate the recent otologic symptoms with a disease that they consider to have been long since cured. One must therefore rely on clinical suspicion and the newer serologic tests to make a diagnosis. Once the blood tests have been doubly confirmed, the patient can usually be told of the findings, and the past history will be volunteered. It is generally wise to involve a venereologist, who is best suited to advise on therapy, follow-up, and examination of relatives and contacts. Patients with congenital syphilis can be reassured that they will not pass on the disease.

The hearing loss in late congenital syphilis is usually symmetric, while in late acquired disease it is often asymmetric and may remain unilateral for many months or years. The associated deafness and tinnitus are of sudden onset in 20 percent of cases, symptoms fluctuate in 30 percent, and in all cases, the hearing loss progresses to a profound degree, usually over many years, but sometimes quite rapidly. The fluctuant deafness is more likely to be seen in the presenting stages of the disorder and may be more obvious by testing speech discrimination.[104-106] Within the first 2 years of onset of hearing loss, the pure-tone audiogram, as expected by the pathologic hydrops, is low tone, peaked, or flat (as in Menière's disease) in 60 percent of cases.[107,108] Once established, there is an increasing percentage of high-tone deafness. For a surprisingly long time, the deafness remains sensory. Transtympanic electrocochleography in ears affected by late syphilis, like many ears affected by hydrops, whatever the cause, shows an enhanced negative summating potential and a cochlear microphonic of diminished amplitude.[109]

Vestibular disturbances can usher in the otologic phase of the disease. Most patients eventually have evidence of peripheral vestibular damage, and in fully 50 percent there is progressive damage leading to varying degress of ataxia. In almost one-half of these patients, there are paroxysms of acute vertigo lasting from 20 minutes to several days. In such cases, especially if there is a low-tone sensory deafness, the clinical differentiation from Meniere's disease can be difficult; bithermal caloric responses are lost at a much earlier stage in late syphilis.

Hennebert's sign,[110] a fistula sign without a perforation or evidence of middle ear disease, is not pathognomonic of syphilitic ear disease. Like the Tullio phenomenon, it is encountered from time to time in idiopathic or secondary endolymphatic hydrops.

There is ample clinical evidence that steroids alone can improve the hearing in late syphilis.[95,101,102,104-106,109,111] Sometimes on withdrawal of steroids the deafness increases, and many patients require long-term steroid therapy to preserve what hearing remains. Some do not respond to steroids at all; in these cases, a clinical decision has to be taken whether or not to continue. Left untreated, the prognosis is dreadful. Penicillin or other antitreponemal antibiotics alone, although indicated and used in these patients because of the systemic disease, does not prevent the relentless destruction of the inner ear. Steroids may be contraindicated for reasons of hypertension, diabetes, peptic ulceration, tuberculosis, glaucoma, depression, or pregnancy. Each case must be treated on its own merits.

In patients treated with antitreponemal drugs and steroids, hearing gains of 20 to 30 dB can be expected in the lower frequencies, although discrimination scores sometimes improve significantly without much pure-tone threshold change. If seen and treated early in the development of the aural disease, about one-half of these patients respond in this way, but the relapse rate is high if or when steroids are withdrawn. Patients with fluctuant deafness are most likely to respond than are those with either sudden or progressive loss. Vestibular symptoms are dramatically controlled in the great majority of patients.

**Autoimmune Disease.** The role of autoimmunity in the etiology of inner ear disease is not fully defined. The subject (which is covered in greater detail in Ch. 29) awaits further study. There may well be several different clinical syndromes. Immunologic responses, whether normal or abnormal, may play a part in the otologic manifestations of several diseases. For example, in late syphilis, the cellular reactions in the temporal bone, the raised levels of circulating immune complexes, and the response to steroids all point to an immunologic factor, even though treponemes may have been responsible for the initial osteitis.

Cogan's disease is now considered autoimmune in origin. Otolaryngologists will find that the clinical picture can be very like that of late syphilis, although the serologic tests are negative. It is characterized by fluctuant and progressive bilateral sensorineural deafness, which in time becomes subtotal or total, by episodic vestibular symptoms and loss of vestibular responses, and by recurrent inflammatory eye changes. Secondary hydrops occurs and transtympanic electrocochleography, if performed before all hearing loss, reveals the abnormal AP/SP waveform characteristic of Meniere's disease or late syphilis. Neo-osteogenesis within the perilymphatic spaces signifies a late stage in the pathologic process. Such new bone formation can also be encountered after inflammatory disease.

The type of autoimmune sensorineural hearing loss described by McCabe[113] seems to be a distinct entity, for there is frequently associated facial paralysis, sometimes inflammatory change in the middle ear and mastoid, and a remarkable response to steroids and cytotoxic drugs. Four of McCabe's 18 patients subsequently developed autoimmune disease, with nonsyphilitic keratitis, Hashimoto's struma, or chronic ulcerative colitis cited.[114] In some of these patients, the lymphocyte inhibition test using inner ear antigen was positive.

Our experience, which dates from 1970,[115-118] suggests that the inner ear may be involved in any of the recognized types of immunologic disease, including the hypersensitivity reactions (type 1), the cytolytic or cytotoxic reactions (type 2), the toxic complex syndrome reactions (type 3), the cell-mediated or delayed hypersensitivity reactions (type 4), and perhaps the antibody-dependent cell-mediated cytotoxic reaction (type 5). The otologic picture is usually one of sudden or rapid bilateral deterioration of hearing, often with tinnitus, with variable vestibular symptoms, and sometimes with fluctuant features. The clinical picture also depends on which type of immunologic reaction is responsible for the inner ear damage. For example, if there has been a hypersensitivity reaction to the administration of a drug or to serum, the patient may be acutely ill. Type 3 reactions of this sort need not be so acute as in the tissue damage from toxic complexes in the collagen diseases.

A remarkable number of diseases are now considered to have an autoimmune basis or to result from the pathologic as opposed to the physiologic effects of immune-complex deposition. Some tissues, such as skin, synovial membranes, blood ves-

sels, kidney glomeruli, and choroid plexus, are recognized sites of the immune-complex injury, presumably because these tissues have the appropriate receptors. Research is required to ascertain whether any of the human inner ear tissues fall within this category. The animal work of Yoo and colleagues[119-121] points in this direction. Some tissues separate from blood and from the reticuloendothelial system provoke no antibody response; when damaged, however, they may release antigenic material that may cause an IgM-mediated response, as in sympathetic ophthalmia, Hashimoto's thyroiditis, some of the acquired hemolytic anaemias, or any of the diseases characterized by cold agglutinins. In the same way, bacterial or vital damage or physical trauma to the inner ear may result in delayed forms of endolymphatic hydrops. The finding of elevated levels of circulating immune complexes in a proportion of patients with idiopathic Menière's disease raises the possibility of this type of pathogenesis.[122,123] Inner ear problems are encountered in patients with many of the diseases that have an immunologic basis, such as hypersensitivity states, temporal arteritis, most of the thyroid diseases, ankylosing spondylitis, recurrent iritis, rheumatoid arthritis, gluten enteropathy, relapsing polychondritis, periarteritis nodosa, midline granuloma, systemic lupus erythematosus, Cogan's disease, psoriasis, pernicious anemia, some acquired hemolytic anemias, disseminated intravascular coagulation disorders, Sjögren's syndrome, patients on renal dialysis who may develop immune complexes from the antigenicity of the membranes in the dialysis machines, and in diabetes mellitus which can be of autoimmune etiology. Whether the association with any or all of these diseases is coincidence or common pathogenesis awaits elucidation.

In the investigation of patients with suspected inner ear autoimmune disease, several lines of inquiry are possible. The levels of circulating immunoglobulins may be estimated, although it is doubtful whether these levels have much relevance in this context. Autoantibodies to the usual tissue components may be sought. Positive findings are not necessarily significant,[118,122] since autoantibodies need not be autoaggressive. The complement system is worthy of investigation. Many of the cascade factors C1 to C9 are ephemeral, but circulating levels of C3c and C1q binding and of the immune complexes of IgG, IgM, and IgA (antigen–antibody complexes) can be measured. Acutely raised levels of these complexes might be a result of inflammatory reaction, but persistently raised levels can be harmful if the complexes are deposited on body tissues when they can precipitate the complement cascade, resulting in cell damage. The ideal would be to examine biopsy material for evidence of deposited complex — presenting problems with inner ear tissue. In some immune-complex diseases, there is a secondary deficiency of circulating complement due to consuming antibody–antigen interactions. In the assessment of cell-mediated immunity, the lymphocyte migration inhibition test, using peripheral blood leukocytes and fresh inner ear tissue as antigen, may be employed.[113,114] Alternatively, a lymphocyte transformation test with specific antigen could be used.[123] Yet another line of inquiry would be HLA tissue typing, since many of the autoimmune diseases, such as systemic lupus erythematosus, psoriasis, Graves' disease, ankylosing spondylitis, or gluten enteropathy, are associated with a preponderance of specific HLA types. This would be useful in specific inner ear syndromes, such as Cogan's disease, the facial palsy syndrome described by McCabe,[113] sudden idiopathic bilateral sensorineural deafness cases, or Meniere's disease, in which preliminary tests indicate such an association.[124]

The place of autoimmunity in the etiology of ear disease awaits further study and quantification. But this is not just an academic exercise. The therapeutic implications are significant and involve immunosuppressants, cytotoxic drugs, and, in selected cases, single therapy or repeat plasma exchange, or plasmapheresis or lymphoplasmapheresis to remove the offending immune complexes from the serum.[118,125]

# REFERENCES

1. Drettner B, Hedstrand H, Klockhoff I, Svedberg A: Cardiovascular risk factors and hearing loss. Acta Otolaryngol (Stockh) 79:366, 1975

2. Sofferman RA: Cranial arteritis in otolaryngology. Ann Otol Rhinol Laryngol 89:215, 1980

3. Kitamura K, Berreby M: Temporal bone histopathology associated with occlusion of vertebrobasilar arteries. Ann Otol Rhinol Laryngol 92:33, 1983

4. Hildesheimer M, Rubinstein M, Nuttal AL, Lawrence M: Influence of blood viscosity on cochlear action potentials and oxygenation. Hearing Res 8:187, 1982

5. Larsen HC, Angelborg C, Hultcrantz E: The effect of glycerol on cochlear blood flow. Otol Rhinol Laryngol 44:101, 1982

6. Nagahara K, Fisch U, Yagi N: Perilymph oxygenation in sudden and progressive sensorineural hearing loss. Acta Otolaryngol (Stockh) 96:57, 1983

7. Prazma J: Perilymph and endolymphatic $PO_2$. Arch Otolaryngol 108:539, 1982

8. Carlborg, B. and Farmer, J.C. Relationships of labyrinthine fluid pressures and blood flow. Laryngoscope 93:998, 1983

9. Prazma J: Cochlear blood flow. Arch Otolaryngol 109:611, 1983

10. Ferlito A, Recher G, Bordin S: Involvement of the temporal bone in hyperlipidemic xanthomatosis. Otolaryngol Head Neck Surg 91:100, 1983

11. Emery PJ, Gore M: An extensive solitary xanthoma of the temporal bone, associated with hyperlipoproteinaemia. J Laryngol Otol 96:451, 1982

12. Bichler E, Wieser M: Experimental lipidosis of the inner ear. Acta Otolaryngol (Stockh) 95:307, 1983

13. Harada T, Sando I, Stool SE, Myers EN: Temporal bone histopatholic features in Fanconi's anemia syndrome. Arch Otolaryngol 106:275, 1980

14. Davies SC, Hewitt, PE: Sickle cell disease. Br J Hos Med 33:440, 1984

15. Donegan JO, Lobel JS, Gluckman JL: Otolaryngologic manifestations of sickle cell disease. Am J Otolaryngol 3:141, 1982

16. Coyle JT, Frank PE, Leonard AL, Weiner A: Macroglobulinemia and its effect upon the eye. Arch Ophthalmol 65:75, 1961

17. Afifi AM, Tawfeek S: Deafness due to Waldenstrom macroglobulinemia. J Laryngol Otol 85:275, 1971

18. Nomura Y, Mori S, Tscuchida M, Sakurai T: Deafness in cryoglobulinemia. Ann Otol Rhinol Laryngol 91:250, 1982

19. Paparella MM, Berlinger NT, Oda M, El Fiky F: Otological manifestations of leukemia. Laryngoscope 83:1510, 1973

20. Schuknecht HF, Igarashi M, Chasin WD: Inner ear haemorrhage in leukemia. A case report. Laryngoscope 75:662, 1965

21. Sklansky BD, Jafek BW, Wiernik PH: Otolaryngol-

ogic manifestations of acute leukemia. Laryngoscope 84:210, 1974

22. Windle-Taylor PC, Bailey CM: Tuberculous otitis media: A series of 22 patients. Laryngoscope 90:1039, 1980

23. Majumdar B, Crowther J: Hearing loss in sarcoidosis. J Laryngol Otol 97:635, 1983

24. Sieger A, Skinner MW, White NH, Spector GJ: Auditory function in children with diabetes mellitus. Ann Otol Rhinol Laryngol 92:237, 1983

25. Wilson WR, Laird N, Soeldner JS, et al: The relationship of idiopathic sudden hearing loss to diabetes mellitus. Laryngoscope 92:155, 1982

26. Booth JB: Hyperlidaemia and deafness. Proc R Soc Med 70:642, 1977

27. Moffat DA, Booth JB, Morrison AW: Metabolic investigations in Meniere's disease. J Laryngol Otol 93:545, 1979

28. Hoff WV, Stuart DW: Deafness in myxoedema. Q J Med 48:361, 1979

29. Parving A, Parving H-H, Lyngsoe J: Hearing sensitivity in patients with myxoedema before and after treatment with L-thyroxine. Acta Otolaryngol (Stockh) 95:315, 1983

30. Himelfarb MZ, Lakretz T, Gold S, Shanon E: Auditory brain stem responses in thyroid dysfunction. J Laryngol Otol 95:679, 1981

31. Meyerhoff WL: Hypothyroidism and the ear: Electrophysiological, morphological and chemical considerations. Laryngoscope 89 [suppl 19], 1979

32. Debruyne F, Vanderschueren-Lodeweyckx M, Bastiens P: Hearing in congenital hypothyroidism. Audiology 22:404, 1983

33. Hutchinson JC, Klodd DA: Electrophysiologic analysis of auditory, vestibular and brain stem function in chronic renal failure. Laryngoscope 92:833, 1982

34. Alport AC: Hereditary familial congenital haemorrhagic hepatitis. Br Med J 1:504, 1927

35. Gleeson MJ: Alport's syndrome: Audiological manifestations and implications. J Laryngol Otol 98:449, 1984

36. Mitschke H, Schmidt P, Kopsa H, Zazgornik J: Reversible uremic deafness after successful renal transplantation. N Engl J Med 292:1062, 1975

37. McDonald TJ, Zincke H, Anderson CF, Ott NT: Reversal of deafness after renal transplantation in Alport's Snydrome. Laryngoscope 88:38, 1978

38. Daugherty WT, Lederman RJ, Nodar RH, Conomy JP: Hearing loss in multiple sclerosis. Arch Neurol 40:33, 1983

39. Jabbari B, Marsh EE, Gunderson CH: The site of the lesion in acute deafness of multiple sclerosis —

Contribution of the brain stem auditory evoked potential test. Clin Electroencephalogr 13:241, 1982

40. Arnold JE, Bender DR: BSER abnormalities in a multiple sclerosis patient with normal peripheral hearing acuity. Am J Otol 4:235, 1983

41. Chiappa KH, Harrison JL, Brooks EB, Young RR: Brainstem auditory evoked responses in 200 patients with multiple sclerosis. Ann Neurol 7:135, 1980

42. Hausler R, Colburn S, Marr E: Sound localization in subjects with impaired hearing. Spatial discrimination and inter aural-discrimination tests. Acta Otolaryngol (Stockh) [suppl]:400, 1983

43. Hunt JC, Pugh DG: Skeletal lesions in neurofibromatosis. Radiology 76:1, 1961

44. Beighton P: Inherited Disorders of the Skeleton. Churchill Livingstone, Edinburgh, 1978

45. Kenyon GS, Booth JB, Prasher DK, Rudge P: Neuro-otological abnormalities in xeroderma pigmentosa with particular reference to deafness. Brain 108:771, 1985

46. Rosen E: Uveitis with poliosis, vitiligo, alopecia and dysacousia (Vogt-Koyanagi Syndrome). Arch Ophthalmol 33:281, 1945

47. Schuknecht HF: Pathology of the ear. Harvard University Press, Cambridge, Ma, 1974

48. Henson RA: Modern Trends in Neurology. Vol. 5. p. 209. Butterworths, London, 1970

49. Doig JA, Gatehouse S: Hearing in acromegaly. J Laryngol Otol 98:1097, 1984

50. Graham MD, Brackmann DE: Acromegaly and the temporal bone. J Laryngol Otol 92:275, 1978

51. Brookes BB: Vitamin D deficiency — A new cause of cochlear deafness. J Laryngol Otol 97:405, 1983

52. Brookes GB: Vitamin D deficiency and deafness — 1984 update. Seventh Shambaugh-Shea International Workshop on Otology, March 4th, 1984

53. Stamp TC, Baker LRI: Recessive hypophosphataemic rickets, and possible aetiology of the vitamin-D-resistant syndrome. Arch Dis Child 51:360, 1976

54. Weir N: Sensorineural deafness associated with recessive hypophosphatemic rickets. J Laryngol Otol 91:717, 1977

55. Cohen HN, Fogelman I, Boyle IT, Doig JA: Deafness due to hypervitaminosis D. Lancet 1:985, 1979

56. Harvey L: Viral aetiology of Paget's disease of bone: A review. J R Soc Med 77:943, 1984

57. Harner SG, Rose DE, Facer GW: Paget's disease and hearing loss. Otol Rhinol Laryngol 86:869, 1978

58. Walker GS, Evanson JM, Canty DP, Gill NW: Effect of calcitonin on deafness due to Paget's Disease of the skull. Br Med J 2:364, 1979

59. Gennari C, Sensini I: Diphosphonate therapy in deafness associated with Paget's Disease. Br Med J 1:331, 1975

60. Williams DML, Thomas RSA: Fibrous dysplasia. J Laryngol Otol 89:359, 1975

61. Barrionuevo CE, Maecallo FA, Coelho A, et al: Fibrous dysplasia and the temporal bone. Arch Otolaryngol 106:298, 1980

62. Chatterji P: Massive fibrous dysplasia of the temporal bone. J Laryngol Otol 88:179, 1974

63. Cohen A, Rosenwasser H: Fibrous dysplasia of the temporal bone. Arch Otolaryngol 89:447, 1969

64. Sharp M: Monostotic fibrous dysplasia of the temporal bone. J Laryngol Otol 84:697, 1970

65. Hamersma H: Osteopetrosis (Marble bone disease) of the temporal bone. Laryngoscope 80:1518, 1970

66. Myers EN, Stool S: The temporal bone in osteopetrosis. Arch Otolaryngol 89:460, 1969

67. Hawke M, Jahn AF, Bailey D: Osteopetrosis of the temporal bone. Arch Otolaryngol 107:278, 1981

68. Van Buchem FSP: Hyperostosis corticalis generalisata. Acta Med Scand 189:257, 1971

69. Nager GT, Stein SA, Dorst JP, et al: Sclerosteosis involving the temporal bone: clinical and radiological aspects. Am J Otolaryngol 4:1, 1983

70. Sparkes RS, Graham CB: Camurati-Engelmann disease: Genetics and clinical manifestations with a review of the literature. J Med Genet 9:73, 1972

71. Miyamoto RT, House WF, Brackmann DE: Neurotologic manifestations of the osteopetroses. Arch Otolaryngology 106:210, 1980

72. Morrison AW: Genetic factors in otosclerosis. Ann R Coll Surg Engl 41:202, 1967

73. Smars G: Osteogenesis Imperfecta in Sweden (Marsden M, trans). Scandinavian University Books, Stockholm, 1961

74. Pedersen U: Hearing loss in patients with osteogenesis imperfecta. A clinical and audiological study of 201 patients. Scand Audiol 13:67, 1984

75. Morrison AW: Diseases of the otic capsule. II, Other disease. p. 465. In (Ballantyne J, Groves J, eds): Scott Brown's Diseases of the Ear, Nose and Throat. 4th Ed. Vol. 2. Butterworths, London, 1979

76. Stoller FM: The ear in osteogenesis imperfecta. Laryngoscope 72:855, 1982

77. van der Hoeve J, de Kleyn A: Blaue sclera knochenkruchig-keit und schwerhorigkeit. Arch Opthalmol 95:81, 1918

78. Quisling RW, Moore GR, Jahrsdoerfer RA: Osteogenesis imperfecta: A study of 160 family members. Arch Otolaryngol 105:207, 1979

79. Riesenman FR, Yates WM: Osteogenesis imperfecta. Arch Intern Med 67:950, 1941

80. McKusick VA: Osteogenesis imperfecta. p. 408. In Heritable Disorders of Connective Tissue. CV Mosby, St. Louis, 1972

81. Shea JJ, Postma DS: Findings and long-term surgical results in the hearing loss of osteogenesis imperfecta. Arch Otolaryngol 108:467, 1982

82. Johnsson LG, Hawkins JE Jr, Rouse RC, Linthicum FH Jr: Cochlear and otoconial abnormalities in capsular otosclerosis with hydrops. Ann Otol Rhinol Laryngol 97 [suppl]:3, 1982

83. Wullstein H, Ogilvie RF, Hall IS: Van der Hoeve's syndrome in mother and daughters. J Laryngol Otol 74:67, 1960

84. Atlmann F, Kornfeld M: Osteogenesis imperfecta and otosclerosis: New investigations. Ann Otol Rhinol Laryngol 76:89, 1967

85. Bretlau P, Jorgensen MB: Otosclerosis and osteogenesis imperfecta. Arch Otolaryngol 90:4, 1969

86. Riley FC, Jowsey J, Brown DM: Osteogenesis imperfecta: Morphologic and biochemical studies of connective tissue. Pediatr Res 7:757, 1973

87. Pedersen U, Nielsen HE, Jensen KJ, et al: Bone mineral content in osteogenesis imperfecta and in otosclerosis. J Laryngol Otol 93:697, 1979

88. Shea JJ, Smyth GDL, Altmann F: Surgical treatment of the hearing loss associated with osteogenesis imperfecta. J Laryngol Otol 77:679, 1963

89. Patterson CN, Stone HB III: Stapedectomy in van der Hoeve's syndrome. Laryngoscope 80:544, 1970

90. Kosoy J, Maddox HE III: Surgical findings in van der Hoeve's syndrome. Arch Otolaryngol 93:115, 1971

91. Editorial: Sexually transmitted disease surveillance 1981. Br Med J 286:1500, 1983

92. Annual Report, Chief Medical Officer for the year 1968: On the state of public health. Appencix C. Her Majesty's Stationery Office, London, 1969

93. Annual Report: Chief Medical Officer for the year 1972: On the state of public health. Her Majesty's Stationery Office, London, 1973

94. Annual Report, Chief Medical Officer for the year 1974: On the state of public health. Her Majesty's Stationery Office, London, 1975

95. Morrison AW: Late syphilis. p. 109. In Management of Sensorineural Deafness. Butterworths, London, 1975

96. Rodger TR: Syphilis as seen by the aural surgeon. J Laryngol Otol 55:168, 1940

97. Rosenhall U, Lowhagen GB, Roupe G: Auditory function in early syphilis. J Laryngol Otol 98:567, 1984

98. Hutchinson J: A Clinical Memoir on Certain Disease of the Eye and Ear Consequent on Inherited Syphilis. J & S Churchill, London, 1963

99. Mayer O, Fraser JS: Pathological changes in late congenital syphilis. J Laryngol Otol 51:755, 1936

100. Goodhill V: Syphilis of the ear: A histopathological study. Ann Otol Rhinol Laryngol 48:676, 1939

101. Perlman HB, Leek JH: Congenital syphilis of the ear. Laryngoscope 62:1175, 1952

102. Karmody CS, Schuknecht HF: Deafness in congenital syphilis. Arch Otolaryngol 83:18, 1966

103. Belal A Jr, Linthicum FH Jr: Pathology of congenital syphilitic labyrinthitis. Am J Otolaryngol 1:109, 1980

104. Hahn RD, Rosin P, Haskins HL: Treatment of neural deafness with prednisone. J Chron Dis 15:395, 1962

105. Dawkins RS, Sharp M, Morrison AW: Steroid therapy in congenital syphilitic deafness. J Laryngol Otol 82:1095, 1968

106. Kerr AG, Smyth GDL, Cinnamond MJ: Congenital syphilitic deafness. J Laryngol Otol 87:1, 1973

107. Morrison AW: Diseases of the otic capsule. p. 478. In Ballantyle J, Groves J eds: Scott-Brown's Diseases of the Ear, Nose and Throat. Butterworths, London, 1979

108. Schuknecht HF: Pathology of the Ear. Harvard University Press, Cambridge MA, 1974

109. Ramsden RT, Moffat DA, Gibson WPR: Transtympanic electrocochleography in patients with syphilis and hearing loss. Ann Otol Rhinol Laryngol 86:827, 1977

110. Hennebert C: Un syndrome nouveau dans la labyrinthite hérédo-syphilitique. Clin Brux 25:545, 1911

111. Morrison AW: Management of severe deafness in adults. Proc R Soc Med 62:959, 1969

112. Adams DA, Kerr AG, Smyth GDL, Cinnamond MJ: Congenital syphilitic deafness — A further review. J Laryngol Otol 97:399, 1983

113. McCabe BF: Autoimmune sensorineural hearing loss. Ann Otol Rhinol Laryngol 88:585, 1979

114. McCabe BF: Treatment of autoimmune inner-ear disease. p. 389. In Proceedings of the Sixth Shambaugh International Workshop on Otomicrosurgery and Third Shea Fluctuant Hearing Loss Symposium. Strode, Huntsville, AL, 1981

115. Morrison AW, Booth JB: Sudden deafness: An otological emergency. Br J Hosp Med 4:287, 1970

116. Morrison AW: Sudden deafness. p. 175. In Management of Sensorineural Deafness. Butterworths, London, 1975

117. Morrison AW: Sudden sensorineural deafness: Outline of management. Proc R Soc Med 69:16, 1976

118. Brookes GB, Immune complex associated deafness; preliminary communication. J R Soc Med 78:47, 1985

119. Yoo TJ, Tomoda K, Stuart JM, et al: Type II collagen-induced autoimmune otospongiosis. A preliminary report. Ann Otol Rhinol Laryngol 92:103, 1983

120. Yoo TJ, Tomoda K, Stuart JM, et al: Type II collagen-induced autoimmune sensorineural hearing loss and vestibular dysfunction in rats. Ann Otol Rhinol Laryngol 92:267, 1983

121. Yoo TJ, Yazawa Y, Tomoda K, Floyd R: Type II collagen-induced autoimmune endolymphatic hydrops in Guinea pig. Science 222:65, 1983

122. Morrison AW: Predictive tests for Meniere's Disease. Paper presented to the Seventh Shambaugh-Shea International Workshop in Otology, Chicago, March 1984

123. Hughes GB, Kinney SE, Barna BP, Calabrese LH: Autoimmune reactivity in Meniere's Disease: A preliminary report. Laryngoscope 93:410, 1983

124. Xenellis J, Morrison AW, McClowsky D, Festenstein H: HLA antigens in the pathogenesis of Menière's disease. J Laryngol Otol 100:21, 1986

125. Hamblin TJ, Mufti GJ, Gracewell A: Severe deafness in systemic lupus erythematosis: Its immediate relief by plasma exchange. Br Med J 284:1374, 1982

# Effects of Hearing Loss in Adults 32

## Jerome D. Schein

The effects of hearing loss in adults has largely been underestimated. That impaired hearing can have grave psychological, sociologic, and economic consequences has been little recognized until recent years. Rather, hearing impairments — except the most severe — often have been looked upon as annoyances rather than as serious health problems. As a result, proportionally less research and service funding has been allocated for the prevention and remediation of hearing impairments than would be warranted by their pernicious effects.

The significance of hearing impairments can be approached in two ways: their frequency and their human costs. How many persons are affected is an important consideration, especially for social-service planners and program administrators. No less important are the consequences of hearing impairments: their psychological, social, and economic effects. Far more difficult to convey is the suffering caused by impaired hearing. No single study can picture the comprehensive effects of decreased and distorted hearing on the lives of those who are affected. The notion that the sole measures of the effects of hearing impairment are in terms of their interference with communication is addressed and, it is hoped, refuted. Estimating the costs of impaired hearing can be done entirely in economic terms, but to do so overlooks its pervasive influences. This chapter considers all three viewpoints, beginning with incidence and prevalence — the numbers of persons afflicted with hearing disabilities — the impact of impaired hearing on communication is then assessed, followed by specific topics that have been studied by psychologists, sociologists, and economists, with both quantitative and qualitative information presented about each.

## AGE AT ONSET AND DEGREE OF IMPAIRMENT

Hearing impairment cannot be understood without specification of the degree of impairment and the age at onset of the affected person. The extent of their disability interacts with the age at which it occurs yielding rather different consequences for the various configurations that arise. Two adults may have identical degrees of hearing impairment, but if age of onset has occurred at different stages in their development, the effects will differ. Similarly, if two persons suffer different degrees of impairment at the same ages, the effects again will not be the same.

While these two points may appear obvious, the literature is unfortunately replete with studies that fail to take into account these two factors, especially age at onset. For example, a recent National Health Survey (NHS) study of hearing impairment failed to gather information about age at onset, rendering the data emerging from the study of limited use to serious students of the disability.[1] The loss of these critical data was due not to the lack of sophistication on the part of the NHS staff, but to budget restrictions limiting the amount of information that could be gathered. As is too often the case, the budgetary constraint in designing that nationwide survey wasted more in informational utility than it saved in dollars. The pertinence of both specifications to any analysis of hearing impairment is supported by additional examples in the sections to follow.

## THE FREQUENCY OF HEARING IMPAIRMENT

Although sometimes not distinguished, *incidence* and *prevalence* are separate concepts in demography and epidemiology — and for good reason. Incidence refers to the number of new cases in a period of time, prevalence to the number of all cases existing at a particular time.[2] A moment's reflection should convince the reader that these are different items, one measuring the rate at which cases are accruing and the other the number that must be treated. Except under special circumstances, the incidence of a chronic condition cannot be determined from successive prevalences. If that point seems unreasonable, recall that affected people die, move from the area being studied, or may recover from the condition; thus, the difference between two prevalences for a given condition may reflect mortality, migration, or remission, masking the addition of new cases, if the rates are the same, or overestimating an increase in the condition, if the increase results from afflicted persons moving into the area. These hints aside, the reader

should appreciate that both types of data are needed for programming and serving disabled persons.

## INCIDENCE

With respect to hearing impairment in the United States, almost no information about incidence is available other than occasional crude estimates. But gathering data about the number of new cases has not captured the attention of investigators of hearing impairments in the United States. For 1935 through 1936, the National Health Survey (ad hoc predecessor to the present organization of the same name) attempted to arrive at the incidence of deafness by taking the differences between successive age groups.[3] That strategy overlooks the fact that incidence is apt to vary with both cause and type of impairment, a fact not taken into consideration in deriving the estimates.

Illustrating the importance of obtaining incidence, changes in incidence rates have been highly dramatic in Switzerland. From 1915 to 1922, the number of deaf neonates ranged from 120 to 170 per 100,000 births. The rate dropped to 40 per 100,000 in 1925 as a result of preventive measures introduced.[4] While the decrease in the incidence rate of from 30 to 60 percent stands out, the corresponding changes in overall prevalences would not immediately reflect the declines, since infants are only a small fraction of the hearing-impaired population.

Spectacular events, such as the rubella epidemics that affect fetuses whose mothers are infected, also call attention to the value of incidence data. In the 1963 through 1965 rubella epidemics in the United States, numbers of deaf and deaf–blind children were added at a far greater rate than would be normally expected. An estimated 35,000 to 40,000 deaf children were added during those years, representing a rate for the period of about 360 per 100,000 live births, as opposed to the rate of 50 to 90 per 100,000 that has often been estimated for deafness at birth in the United States. This marked increase in the incidence of deafness created what has been referred to as the rubella bulge. The term emphasizes the greater-than-usual number of affected children born. The U.S. Congress reacted to the huge increase in the number of deaf children with legislation that has provided more funds with which to deal with the problems created by the bulge as it passes from age group to age group. However, studies of data from 1900 to 1950 make it clear that other epidemics have occurred from time to time in various parts of this country, leading to sharp fluctuations in the numbers of born-deaf children.[5] The search for the single incidence rate for deafness in a given region makes no sense: over any span of years, variation in incidence should be expected.

Why are incidence rates not collected? The answer appears to be a lack of interest, not a lack of methodology. Infant screening programs could provide incidence data for neonates. Such programs would enable intervention to be undertaken early, a strategy urged by most experts on the care of hearing-impaired children. Yet routine neonatal auditory screening has been opposed by many audiologists on the grounds that present procedures lead to too many false-positive results. This peculiar argument implies that practitioners would upset parents by incorrectly advising them about their children's hearing instead of properly alerting them to the possibility of such a problem and urging them to obtain follow-up testing. Expense has also been raised as an objection to routine screening. Again, however, that argument exaggerates the modest amount required, while underplaying the benefits that would be derived from earlier identification.[6]

Critics point to the fact that the low incidence of hearing impairment might mean testing 1,000 children to identify one in need of treatment. However, these critics do not object to putting silver nitrate in every newborn's eyes, even though the rate for maternal syphilis is less than 1 per 3,000. Other potential sources of incidence data are the screening programs in public schools. Reporting the results of such annual efforts would provide useful data, provided they adequately met the standards for such procedures.[7] Even rates of failures to pass audiometric screening levels are seldom found in the literature, indicating a low level of interest in incidence data. Such neglect impedes

research, misleads planners, and ultimately damages the provision of services.

## PREVALENCE

Unlike incidence, prevalence data, the outcomes of special surveys, abound. From 1830 to 1930, the U.S. Bureau of the Census determined the number of deaf persons in each decennial census. Since establishment of the NHS, in 1956, three special studies of the prevalence of hearing impairment have been conducted. The results have shown hearing impairment to be the most frequent chronic physical disability in the United States.

The estimated rates reported by the NHS for hearing impairment have grown from 43.7 per 1,000 noninstitutionalized persons 3 years of age and older, in 1963, to 69.0, in 1971, and 70.2 per 1,000, in 1977.[8] Because similar, though not identical, methods were followed in the three surveys, one may have confidence in positing an increase in the prevalence of hearing impairment over the 14-year period. A careful look at the methods, however, tempers the interpretation of the increases between 1963 and 1971 somewhat. The 1963 screening procedure to reach the hearing supplement, which obtained detailed information about the impairment, asked only, "Does anyone in the family have any of these conditions: Deafness or serious trouble hearing with one or both ears?" That single item was the first of 11 conditions that included serious trouble seeing, cleft palate, and paralysis of any kind. In 1971 and 1977, three screening questions were asked: "Does anyone in the family now have deafness in one or both ears? Any other trouble hearing with one or both ears? Tinnitus or ringing in the ears?" The three questions about hearing were in a list of seven items, the remaining four of which inquired about blindness, cataracts, glaucoma, and colorblindness. The 1963 inquiry clearly emphasizes severity of impairment, while the 1971 and 1977 schedules imply wider ranges of impairments, both in degree and type. Thus, some of the seeming increase in prevalence rates between 1963 and 1971 are likely due to differences in questions and the context in which they were embedded and to procedural changes in administration.

## AGE AND SEX

Two generalizations with respect to age and sex can be made at the outset. First, men experience proportionally more hearing impairment than do women. This finding holds across ages, age at onset, and degree of impairment in almost all studies reviewed for this chapter.[9] The second is that rates for hearing impairment increase with age.

Table 32-1 provides a comparison of rates from the last two NHS reports. For the entire age range, the estimated prevalences rates increased between 1971 and 1977 by a little less than 2 percent, from 690 to 702 per 100,000. Hearing impairment increased for males by about 3 percent, while for females it remained at the same level. Between age

**Table 32-1.   Rates per 1,000 Persons 3 Years of Age and Over Reporting Trouble Hearing, by Age and Sex: United States, 1971 and 1977**

| Sex and Age (years) | Rates per 1,000 Population | |
|---|---|---|
| | 1971 | 1977 |
| Both sexes, all ages 3+ | 69.0 | 70.2 |
| 3–16 | 16.2 | 16.3 |
| 17–24 | 26.5 | 20.5 |
| 25–44 | 44.7 | 41.4 |
| 45–64 | 100.0 | 107.3 |
| 65+ | 274.1 | 261.9 |
| Males, all ages 3+ | 80.9 | 83.2 |
| 3–16 | 17.8 | 18.3 |
| 17–24 | 34.9 | 22.9 |
| 25–44 | 55.7 | 56.4 |
| 45–64 | 128.6 | 141.4 |
| 65+ | 326.2 | 313.4 |
| Females, all ages 3+ | 58.1 | 58.0 |
| 3–16 | 14.5 | 14.1 |
| 17–24 | 18.9 | 18.1 |
| 25–44 | 34.5 | 27.4 |
| 45–64 | 74.1 | 76.4 |
| 65+ | 235.9 | 225.7 |

(Ries PW: Hearing ability of persons by sociodemographic and health characteristics: United States. Vital Health Stat [10], No. 140, 1982.)

groups, the only increases in rates for men, women, and both combined are in the 45-to-64 group. For the other age groups, rates either remained the same or declined somewhat.

For these surveys, the two generalizations about sex and age hold without equivocation: more hearing impairments are reported by men than by women and by older than by younger persons. These points are upheld when comparing each age-by-sex category for either of the 2 years. The contrasts of rates for corresponding categories in the 2 years, however, likely reflect sampling variability, with the exceptions of the overall increase for all ages combined and the sizable increase shown in those 45 to 64 years of age.

What about the future? Do current trends suggest what lies ahead with respect to the prevalence of hearing impairment? The strong relationship between age and hearing impairment presages a continuing increase in the overall prevalence of this disorder. By the year 2000, the overall prevalence rate is projected to be 9,000 per 100,000. For persons 65 years of age and over, the prediction calls for a rate of 46,000 per 100,000. These prognostications should be read with the recognition that they are based largely on the assumption that the current aging trends in the population will continue. At present, 11.60 percent of the population is 65 years of age and over. By 2000, this figure is expected to increase to 12.97. Since a large share of that 10 percent increase will be due to greater longevity, and since the longer people live, the greater the likelihood of hearing impairment, the prediction that the relative prevalence of hearing impairment will grow has strong support. Consider further that for 2050, the forecasted rates are 11.8 percent for hearing impairment in the general population, with a rate of 59 percent for those 65 years of age and over.[10]

## GEOGRAPHIC DISPERSION

Prevalence rates for hearing impairment vary from place to place. Within the United States, there are marked differences between the four regions into which the Bureau of the Census divides the country: Northeast, North Central, South, and West. For the most recent year, 1977, NHS reported the following overall rates of hearing impairment per 1,000 persons for these regions: Northeast, 65.2; North Central, 69.0; South, 72.7; West, 73.6. When degree of impairment is also taken into account, a somewhat more complex picture emerges. Table 32-2 displays data from NHS 1971 and the National Census of the Deaf Population.[11] The relative standings of the four regions were the same for all degrees of hearing impairment: highest in the West, followed by the South, North Central, and Northeast, in that order. When only those who are deaf are considered, the order shifts, with the highest rate in the North Central region, followed by the West, South, and Northeast. Similarly, if age at onset of deafness is considered, the highest prevalence rate is in the North Central region, with the South second, followed by the West, and finally the Northeast. These differences by degree and age at onset highlight further the importance of the two characteristics in any consideration of hearing impairment.

The finding of geographic differences within the United States is reflected in data from other countries. The Peruvian census of 1940 found vast disparities in rates of deafness between its provinces; for example, Amazonas, a rural, mountainous area, had a rate for deafness of 843 per 100,000, and Lima, the coastal area including the cities of Lima and Callao, a rate of 30 per 100,000. Prevalence rates for deafness in Argentina ranged from 64 to 373 per 100,000 for different regions of that country. Even a relatively small nation such as Finland had variations between regions of nearly 50 percent. Neighboring countries often have great disparities in their prevalence rates for deafness: Sweden's 86.9 versus Norway's 53.0 per 100,000; Switzerland's 93.7 versus France's 47. These data demonstrate the fallacy of trying to estimate hearing impairment within one region from rates derived in another region, even when the regions are adjacent areas of the same country.[9]

## RACE OR COLOR

In every decennial census of the United States, from 1830 to 1930, the proportion of white deaf persons has exceeded the proportion of nonwhite deaf persons. The NHS has found similar results for all degrees of hearing impairment in the three special studies it conducted, in 1963, 1971, and 1977. In 1963, the rates per 100,000 for bilateral hearing impairment were 2,300 for whites and 1,510 for nonwhites; in 1977, the corresponding rates were

**Table 32-2.** **Distribution of Prevalence Rates for the Hearing-Impaired Population, by Hearing-Impairment Category and by Region: United States, 1971**

| | Rate per 100,000 | | |
|---|---|---|---|
| United States and Regions[a] | All Types[b] | Deaf[c] | Early Deaf[d] |
| United States | 6,603 | 873 | 203 |
| Northeast | 5,977 | 697 | 173 |
| North Central | 6,563 | 965 | 242 |
| South | 6,807 | 895 | 196 |
| West | 7,170 | 931 | 194 |

[a] Northeast: CN, ME, MA, NH, NJ, NY, PA, RI, VT.
North Central: IL, IN, IA, KS, MC, MN, MO, NB, ND, OH, SD, WI.
South: AB, AR, DE, DC, FL, GA, KY, LA, MD, MI, NC, OK, SC, TN, TX, VA, WV.
West: AL, AA, CA, CO, HA, ID, MT, NE, NM, OR, UT, WA, WY.
[b] All degrees of hearing impairment.
[c] Cannot hear and understand through the ear alone.
[d] Deaf before 19 years of age.
(Schein JD, Delk MT: The Deaf Population of the United States. National Association of the Deaf, Silver Spring, MD, 1974.)

3,865 for whites and 1,770 for nonwhites. These statistically significant differences in rates are very large. While the findings are consistent across studies, attempts to account for them are not. Explanations have varied from genetic,[12] to economic,[13] to methodologic.[11] The evidence so far available would lend support to any of the three hypotheses, suggesting that all contribute in some proportion to the substantial discrepancy in rates of hearing impairment for the two groups.

## DEAFNESS

In the preceding discussion, only oblique references have been made to degree of hearing impairment. While hearing impairment is relatively common in this country, it is relatively rare in its extreme form. The NHS has distinguished between unilateral and bilateral hearing impairments. Roughly one-half of all persons reporting trouble hearing consider themselves to have unilateral impairments. Of those with bilateral involvements, about one-fourth are deaf. Deafness — the inability to hear and understand speech through the ear alone — occurs at a rate of 415 to 873 per 100,000, the latter figure coming from the National Census of the Deaf Population.[11] Research interest has focused on an even rarer group, those deaf persons with a prelingual age at onset, usually considered to be before 3 years of age. The prevalence rate of prelingual deafness is estimated to be about 100 per 100,000. Thus, it would appear that for hearing impairment, there is a "rule" that research occurs in inverse proportion to the size of the population affected: the fewer persons, the more studies. The rule further specifies that as age of onset increases, research interest declines: the earlier the onset of deafness, the more studies. In what follows, then, much of the evidence on the psychological, social, and economic consequences of hearing impairment derive from studies of persons deafened in childhood or at birth. This evidential skew should be borne in mind, since degree of impairment and age at onset are critical factors in determining the effects of hearing impairment.

The frequency of occurrence of deafness is of social–psychological importance, because the relative rarity of early deafness means that those who are so characterized form a minority group in the population. Many aspects of the behavior of early deafened people would be differently construed, if they were not such a small proportion of the population.

## EFFECTS ON SPEECH AND LANGUAGE

A principal consequence of hearing impairment is interference with communication. Much interpersonal behavior revolves about verbal–vocal interchanges. When hearing impairment occurs in early childhood, the effects are much more serious. Speech development will be affected, as will language development. The later hearing impairment occurs in the developmental cycle, the less severe will be its consequences. Similarly, the smaller the degree of impairment, the smaller will be the effects on speech and language.

Maintaining the distinction between speech and language is essential to research on hearing impairment. "That the word *language* derives from *lingua* (tongue) betrays the common confusion about the relation between speech and language."[14] Persons may have speech without language or language without speech — of great concern to those who work with hearing-impaired people.

## SPEECH

Teachers rated the intelligibility of the speech of a national sample of 978 hearing-impaired students, 4 to 23 years of age, whose better-ear-average hearing levels for speech ranged from moderate (less than 70 dB) to severe (71 to 90 dB) to profound (91 dB or greater). The percentages judged to have intelligible or highly intelligible speech were as follows: 86.2 percent of the moderate, 54.8 percent of the severe, and 22.5 percent of the profound.[15] These results, while clearly demonstrating the relationship between degree of impairment and speech intelligibility, should not be construed to mean that prelingually deaf children cannot learn to speak well. Indeed, the results show that about one in five of the profoundly impaired children do develop good speech, as determined by their teachers' ratings. That they have greater difficulty in doing so than those less impaired, however, is patent.

For those whose hearing loss occurs after the development of speech, efforts must be directed at speech maintenance. The habit of speaking, once established, remains strong for most persons. As the age at onset of hearing impairment comes later and later in development, the need for attention to speech lessens, although deafened persons must remain alert for dysfluencies that may emerge insidiously. Speakers of American English must be particularly sensitive about the pronounciation of new words, since orthographic clues are not reliable, as they are in most other written and spoken languages. Unless heard first, such words as *naif* are apt to be pronounced "nafe" instead of "nah-eef," since our written language frequently flaunts its own principles of transcription. These are nonetheless petty points in contrast with the speech problems of prelingually deaf persons who must struggle to acquire even the concept of oral communication.

## LANGUAGE

The imposing barrier to the child's language development erected by early deafness has been recognized and remarked upon since Aristotle wrote *History of Animals* more than 2000 years ago. Present-day authorities believe that his translators, and not the great sage, are guilty of the stigma imposed on deaf people by statements in that book, such as "Those who are born deaf all become senseless and incapable of reason." What Aristotle actually wrote is more correctly read as, "Those who

become deaf from birth also become altogether speechless. Voice is certainly not lacking, but there is no speech."[16] It was the former interpretation, however, that served as the justification for refusing even to try to educate deaf children. The speech impairment was construed as reflecting a language deficit. That the two must be coordinate has been shown to be false; that the two often are coordinate represents pedagogical failure.

What is the magnitude of that failure? The average deaf student graduating from high school obtains reading scores at fourth-grade level, which is to say, these students are illiterate. Using an adaptation of the Stanford Achievement Test, a national sample of 6,873 hearing-impaired students was examined. The grade equivalents for the scores of the 17-year-old sample were all below 7th grade: vocabulary, below 3rd grade; reading comprehension, 4th grade; mathematical concepts, 5th grade; and mathematical computation, 6th grade. These are dismal results for students who should be performing at an 11th-grade level. As shown in Table 32-3, the results are also poor for all other ages and across the four subtests. Beginning below grade level (8-year-old students ought to be performing at 2nd-grade level), the students make very small accretions in scores, in many instances being only one-tenth of a grade per year.

Further analysis of the data in Table 32-3 by the researchers underscores the role of age at onset and the degree of impairment. As hearing impairment increases, scores decline. While this is true, as it has been in similar past studies, the differences are most marked in the tests of English-language skill. The fact that mathematical computation appears least affected deserves attention. It is a finding that has appeared again and again in studies of academic achievement of deaf students. While mathematical computation is also language-dependent, it is not as dependent on English language. To compute, one parses mathematical sentences. The expression $2 + 3 = 5$ is a statement that, in English, translates into "Add the abstract quantity *two* to the abstract quantity *three* and the resulting compound will be *five*." Why do deaf students have less difficulty with such statements than with "Joe hit the ball with his bat"? The answer probably lies in the regularity of mathematical language—it has no exceptions—and with the greater ablility of

**Table 32-3.** Approximate Grade Levels Corresponding to Mean Stanford Achievement Test[a] Scaled Scores Attained by National Sample of Hearing-Impaired Students (N = 6,871), by Subtest and Age: Spring 1974

| Age | Number | Vocabulary | Grade-Equivalent Scores[b] | | |
| --- | --- | --- | --- | --- | --- |
| | | | Reading Comprehension | Math Concepts | Math Computation |
| −8 | 108 | KO[c] | 1.5 | 1.6 | 1.6 |
| 8 | 530 | K2 | 1.6 | 1.5 | 1.6 |
| 9 | 1,395 | K2 | 1.8 | 1.6 | 1.9 |
| 10 | 520 | 0.9 | 2.2 | 2.1 | 2.7 |
| 11 | 436 | 1.1 | 2.4 | 2.4 | 3.1 |
| 12 | 484 | 1.4 | 2.6 | 2.7 | 3.9 |
| 13 | 500 | 1.6 | 2.7 | 3.1 | 4.5 |
| 14 | 580 | 1.8 | 3.0 | 3.2 | 4.9 |
| 15 | 801 | 1.9 | 3.3 | 3.6 | 5.1 |
| 16 | 496 | 2.2 | 3.7 | 4.3 | 5.8 |
| 17 | 394 | 2.4 | 4.0 | 4.8 | 6.1 |
| 18 | 319 | 2.6 | 4.2 | 5.1 | 6.4 |
| 19 | 194 | 2.6 | 4.1 | 5.1 | 6.5 |
| 20+ | 114 | 2.7 | 4.4 | 5.6 | 7.2 |

[a] Special edition for hearing-impaired students.
[b] Estimated from standard scores and rounded to nearest tenth.
[c] Below kindergarten level.
(Jensema C: The relationship between academic achievement and the demographic characteristics of hearing impaired children and youth. Series R, No. 2. Office of Demographic Studies, Gallaudet College, Washington, DC, 1975.)

teachers for whatever reasons, to get across its concepts as opposed to those of English. The language deficits attributed to early deafness appear to be deficits in the native language (here, of English) than some inherent inability to acquire language per se. The same deaf child who can barely communicate in English often communicates at a very high cognitive level in American Sign Language.[17]

The results displayed in Table 32-3 are average, cross-sectional data. Some deaf children do much better than average, and some worse. This simple point, again, serves to illustrate that early deafness need not interfere with (native) language development, as it need not prevent speech development. How, then, does one account for the lags already noted in deaf children's development? Educational practices appear the most likely source of the variance. The odd acceptance of explanations of educational failures that indict only the students has been noted and questioned. That the condition requires special attention and sizable efforts on the part of educators and parents remains intact. What cannot stand the scrutiny of the evidence at hand is a pessimistic attitude toward the speech and language development of children who suffer hearing impairments of whatever degree.

## PSYCHOLOGICAL CONSEQUENCES

The first recorded breakthroughs in public prejudices against educating deaf children came in the Renaissance, first with a challenge from the Italian physician, Girolamo Cardano, to the established wisdom of Aristotle — a step that must have taken courage, although it did not prompt Cardano to act upon his belief — and then by efforts of Spanish clerics to educate deaf children of the nobility. Pedro de Ponce and, later, Juan Pablo Bonet made impressive strides in devising methods for teaching those children previously considered unteachable. Their efforts link directly to France's Abbe de l'Epée and the establishment of the first school generally available to deaf students, not simply those rich or noble, in 1755, in Paris. Once educated, deaf people themselves could counter the linking of deafness and mental retardation to uncover its basis in poor communication.

## INTELLIGENCE TESTS

Despite advances in their status, deaf people found themselves on the defensive again with the growth of the mental testing movement at the turn of the twentieth century. The careless application of the new psychological tests led to erroneous conclusions about the intelligence of deaf people. The conclusions were hardly univocal. A review of 44 studies[18] found most research agreeing that deaf and hearing persons attained the same average scores, but some studies showed deaf persons to have lower and some to have higher averages than comparable groups from the general population. The mixture of results can be easily explained by references to the sampling, the choice of instruments, the procedures followed, and failure to account for inability to meet basic assumptions in the interpretation of the results obtained. From 1960 to the present, opinions held by psychologists have drastically altered. For example, in 1960, the author of a popular text on hearing impairment considered five factors—cognition, memory, convergent thinking, divergent thinking, evaluation—in relationship to early deafness and concluded[19]:

> If we assume that each of these consists of both verbal and nonverbal functions, then all five mental operations would be influenced to some degree by language limitation. But what about generalized involvement; does deafness have an equal effect on each of these mental processes? . . . it appears that deafness does not influence cognition. . . . memory is affected selectively. . . . Convergent thinking also may be affected only selectively. . . . Divergent thinking and evaluation ability both appear to be affected by deafness.

Another prominent psychologist at that time reached a similar and more incisive conclusion: "although the deaf as a group are of average mental endowment, functional lags exist in the areas of conceptual thinking and abstract reasoning."[20]

Today, however, both points of view have been corrected. Less ethnocentric reviews of the research evidence admit of no limitations on cognitive abilities as a sole result of deafness. Rather, the earlier conclusions can be dealt with in terms of their definitions of the concepts studied and their overlooking of unequal conditions that invalidate direct comparisons of deaf and general-population samples. For example, the use of the term *intelligence* varies so widely as to make interpretation of its undefined study hazardous, as note the array of studies yielding conflicting results with respect to deafness. Furthermore, since intelligence tests all implicitly assume equal access to practice with the materials used, the comparisons begin with an unacceptable disadvantage for most deaf children. Once these and similar criticisms are met, the results indicate that the inability to hear, by itself, does not account for the diverse results obtained.[21] Indeed, an even more enlightened view would be to regard the question as meaningless without careful specification of its terms. Neither intelligence nor deafness represents a unitary concept; each covers a sizable congeries of culturally determined behaviors. As holds for all science, the great art lies in asking the questions. Once recognizing why the question is asked, the scientist can safely eschew the study of intelligence in relation to deafness. Since our society now requires an education for all children, regardless of physical or mental condition, the question has no urgency. If a negative answer is sought to justify inadequate instruction, it is unworthy of pursuit. If the scientist hopes an answer will aid in the development of better educational procedures, its pursuit is vain, for more precise information than would result from such studies is needed to aid educators in designing better learning environments and developing improved instructional procedures.

## SHORT-TERM MEMORY

Granting the vagueness of the term *intelligence*, we find such concepts as *cognition* no more precise.

Substituting the less imposing word *thinking* for *cognition* does not help. The problem is that the mental processes are not unitary. Psychologists use *cognition* to cover an easily discriminable set of functions that, while related, are separate. In an effort to answer questions about the relationships between thinking and hearing impairment, psychologists have found it profitable to investigate the individual functions. One of these — a critical one — is memory. In turn, the memory function must be subdivided for purposes of study and ultimate generalization, at least into long term and short term.

Studies of deafness and short-term memory have uncovered a number of important relationships that do point to improved instructional strategies. Deaf people, for instance, typically repeat as many numbers forward as backward on the digit-span test, while persons in general have shorter spans backward than forward. The finding speaks to visual imagery. Stimulus–response compatibility emerges as a major factor affecting deaf children's performance on short-term memory tasks. Various coding strategies have been found to differ among deaf persons and between deaf and other persons. As one psychologist urges, we should "look beyond linguistic and experiential deficits of the deaf as explanatory variables and try to understand the interplay among ability, stimulus–response relationships, and motivational factors. Closer attention to specific factors that obstruct the learning of deaf persons, such as visual imagery suppression, intersensory coordination, and competing associations, may reveal the presence or absence among deaf persons of flexibility and adaptability in using their information-processing strategies to fit the requirement of a particular task."[22]

tion's appeal probably rests on its power to relieve able-bodied people of any guilt they may feel when contemplating those who are disabled. As for the empirical evidence, it is precisely to the contrary.

Not only do deaf people not see better than the general public, but they are more likely to have visual anomalies.[11] As for their visual functions, a synthesis of published research concludes there is no evidence to support this generous idea[23]:

> In some respects, deaf interactants and communicators surely substitute an eye for an ear and perceive and act like their hearing counterparts. But this substitution leads to an overloaded visual system, and deaf–hearing differences appear which increase problems of social misunderstandings. . . . Contrary to popular lore, necessity is not the mother of compensation.

Research on other sensory functions similarly shows that the deaf participants have either the same or lessened abilities. Examinations of the haptic senses of 300 deaf and hearing children found no differences on most of the tests, except that the normally hearing children performed faster on all timed trials and deaf children were somewhat more sensitive to vibrotactile and two-point measures.[24] A study of tactual perception of rhythmic patterns found deaf children to perform poorly compared with normal-hearing and blind children, and the differences persisted after training.[25]

That being unable to hear "sharpens vision" or some such notion does not have research support. Rather than compensation, the loss of hearing tends either to be associated with either no or greater impairment in other sensory modalities. Does this finding hold across degrees and ages at onset of impairment? Systematic data are lacking, yet it would certainly seem to be worth gathering such information.

## PERCEPTION

A cherished belief of many laypeople, and one that persists in the scientific literature as well, is the Doctrine of Compensation. In effect, this dictum alleges that when one bodily function or part is impaired or lost another is strengthened. The no-

## EMOTIONS AND MENTAL ILLNESS

Much has been made of the emotional impact of hearing loss. Ratings by teachers of 516 students in a residential school for deaf children were compared with similar ratings for 532,567 Los Angeles

County public school students. Of the deaf students, 11.6 percent were judged to be severely emotionally disturbed and 19.6 percent to present behavioral problems requiring a disproportionate amount of staff time. The comparable findings for the public school students were 2.4 percent severely emotionally disturbed and 7.3 percent behavioral problems—a startling difference of nearly five times more severe disturbance and nearly three times more difficult behavioral problems among the deaf students. The Annual Survey of Hearing Impaired Children and Youth reported for three consecutive school years, 1969 to 1971, that emotional disturbances and behavioral problems were the most frequently cited additional handicapping condition among more than 25,000 hearing-impaired students in their samples. Almost 1 in 10 students (9.2 percent) were judged by their schools to have emotional/behavioral problems. These startlingly high proportions have suggested that hearing-impaired children are suffering from an epidemic of emotional disturbance.[26]

But, paradoxically, rates for emotional disturbance among early deafened adults do not reflect these extremely high rates in children. The classic study of New York State's early deafened population over 15 years of age concluded, "It would appear from these data that the severe and varied stresses associated with early total deafness do little to increase the chance of developing clinical symptoms of schizophrenia."[27]

A national survey of psychiatric hospitals established a rate of 94 hearing-impaired patients per 1,000 patients. Of these, 79.5 per 1,000 were hard of hearing and 13.5 deaf. These rates contrasted with the hospitals' own reports of 32 hard of hearing per 1,000 and 8 deaf per 1,000 patients. The investigators attribute their higher rates to the more careful procedures and to the hospital staff's confusion between behaviors that are a function of hearing impairment and those due to psychosis. Noting that deafness occurs at a rate of about 8 per 1,000 in the general population, they conclude that the 13.5 deaf patients per 1,000 rate shows a significant correlation between mental illness and deafness. Similarly, they reason, the higher rates for hard of hearing persons in the institutions than in the general population imputes a relationship between hearing impairment and mental illness.[28]

However, this reasoning does not take into account three points: (1) the lengths of stay for hearing-impaired patients, (2) the age distributions of the institutionalized and noninstitutionalized patients, and (3) their ages at onset of hearing impairment. With respect to the first point, the investigators do, indeed, note that hearing-impaired patients stay in hospital longer, on the average, than non-hearing-impaired patients. The New York Psychiatric Institute survey also found this to be true. Thus, the excess prevalence rates may be due solely to the lengths of stay in the hospital, not to differences in the incidence of mental illness, and greater lengths of stay may indicate poorer ability to deal with the hearing-impaired patients rather than greater severity of their conditions. As for the age distributions, the higher proportion of hearing impairment among elderly persons and the higher proportion of elderly persons institutionalized may interact to yield the apparent relationship between mental illness and hearing impairment.

Finally, the ages at onset of the hearing-impaired patients were not provided. This factor is critical in determining the effects of hearing impairment on behavior. Any tendency of hearing impairment to precipitate emotional problems may be limited to the later onsets. Insofar as early deafness is concerned, other mental health workers tend to agree with the summation given four decades ago, "All things considered, cheerfulness may be said to be an attribute of the larger number of the deaf."[29]

If we accept the latter view, how can we reconcile it with the evidence for great emotional/behavioral disturbance among deaf children? For early deafened people, the answer may lie in the deaf community—the associations of and between deaf people. Cut off from their normal-hearing peers by the difficulties in communicating with them and finding concerted action occasionally important, deaf adults have banded together to form a community defined by common interests and methods of communication.[30] In doing so, they have provided a stability for their lives that is often denied in their commerce with the general community. Probably of equal psychological value, the deaf community opens to deaf adults the potential to enjoy high statuses they could not otherwise expect. A born-deaf man may hold a menial job by day, entitling him to little respect from his working associates, and at night he may be an officer in a deaf club. The latter source of self-esteem probably contributes importantly to his psychological good health. The deaf community, then, provides the support group that assists its deaf members to attain and maintain a healthy life adjustment.

What about late-onset hearing impairment? Aside from the national study cited earlier, which only concerns emotional distrubances severe enough to warrant hospitalization, little demographic information is available on this group. Clinical evidence, however, indicates that many people react to the onset of hearing impairment with marked depression. This reaction arises not only from the increased difficulties in communication but also from the loss of background sound — which Ramsdell[31] has named the "primitive" level of hearing.

> It was the constant reiteration, by hard-of-hearing patients at Deshon Army Hospital, of the statement that the world seemed dead that led to the investigation of this third [primitive] level of hearing and of the psychological effect of its loss upon the deaf. . . . It relates us to the world at a very primitive level, somewhere below the level of clear consciousness and preception. The loss of this feeling of relationship with the world is the major cause of the well-recognized feeling of "deadness" and also of the depression that permeates the suddenly deafened and, to a lesser degree, those in whom deafness develops gradually.

Persons who lose hearing in adulthood seldom associate with the deaf community. Is their adjustment poorer as a consequence? How effectively do they find supportive relationships? Self-help groups are a recent addition to the rehabilitation of hearing-impaired persons, so it is untimely to assess their contribution, although experiences in other areas creates optimism about their likely value. Good family relations and supportive counseling from professionals are also important to the persons whose hearing impairment occurs late in life. There is a danger that hearing difficulties may encourage passivity, especially in elderly people; this passivity can increase the difficulties in adjustment to whatever environment — home, workplace, or institution — the hearing-impaired people are in. Why passivity? Because the hearing-impaired person must continually ask that whatever is said be repeated, sometimes several times. Most people react to such requests with patent annoyance, leading hearing-impaired persons to quickly abandon attempts to comprehend what is being said. For them, maintaining tolerable social relations translates into adopting a nonresistant nonparticipatory stance.[32]

Not unexpectedly, the relationship of hearing impairment to emotional adjustment is complex. Age at onset is critical, with the earlier onset being related to better adult adjustment. This appears to be true, despite the opinions of educators that a disproportionately high amount of emotional/behavioral disturbance occurs among hearing-impaired schoolchildren. (One may ponder on the influence on these children of such a dour attitude on the part of those responsible for their education.) The deaf adult appears to gain much support from the deaf community, the network of interpersonal relationships with other deaf people. For hearing impairments of later onset, pertinent demographic data are lacking, but clinicians provide evidence of the condition's severity. As the degree of impairment increases, the amount of stress increases. The loss of hearing interacts with the life stage in which the individual is at its onset. In the years prior to retirement, it often necessitates career changes or substantial modifications; after retirement, it tends to produce a passive attitude that may keep the individual from an optimal adjustment. In all these situations, emotions are aroused that require counseling, whether group or individual, to enable the individual to understand what has happened and to assist in adapting to the alterations in physical status.

## SOCIAL CONSEQUENCES

Impairment of hearing interferes with human interactions. That statement is intended to say more than that hearing impairment disrupts communication between impaired and unimpaired. More is involved: the attenuated communication results in broader social consequences, and these are reflected in several important ways.

## FAMILY LIFE

Three facts dominate any discussion of family life:

1. Ninety percent of deaf children are born to parents who can hear.
2. When they marry, 8 out of 10 early deafened people choose hearing-impaired spouses.
3. Ninety percent of children born of deaf-by-deaf marriages have normal hearing.

Most deaf children grow up without deaf parents, deaf siblings, or deaf near relatives, which means that those closest to deaf children have had no experience with deafness. It is no wonder, then, that parents of deaf children report so much difficulty in adjusting to having a disabled child. Some parents reject them completely; others become overprotective and overcontrolling. Few react by accepting deafness.[33,34] They lack the experience to identify the variations in growth markers that set apart deaf from hearing children. Nor are they apt to have much assistance in accepting their deaf children from the professionals with whom they consult. Most of the professional literature dwells on the horrors of deafness and on maneuvers that will enable the deaf child to become as like normal-hearing children as possible. Seldom do professionals advise parents how to raise a normal deaf child!

For hearing-impaired children, the difficulty arises from the failure to identify their diminished hearing. Moderately impaired children often receive diagnoses of mental retardation, emotional or behavioral disturbance, or learning diability. Of particular concern are those children who suffer from recurrent otitis media, periodically rendering them hearing impaired until the loss becomes chronic. The effects of less severe hearing impairments on language development has appeared in other research. A comparison of two groups of schoolchildren — matched on a variety of factors, such as age and intelligence, and differing in that one group had normal hearing and the other had losses of 15 to 45 dB and histories of otitis media —

showed significant academic retardation, regardless of the degree of impairment.[35] Those with the more severe losses showed the larger deficits, but even those with far less severe losses showed some retardation in their anticipated school performances and, one can assume, some difficulties in their personal life adjustment. Given this study, educators should be especially alert to the possibilities of hearing impairment and should schedule audiologic examinations of all children on an annual basis up to 13 years of age and biennially through high school. If that program cannot be attained, school authorities should at least demand that every child exhibiting an educational handicap or emotional disturbance be carefully examined for sensory disabilities. Parents cannot be depended upon to recognize the effects of hearing impairments, because their own experiences usually leave them unaware of the potential dangers.

Once identified, milder hearing losses in children do not present the disruption of parent–child relations that deafness does. Mildly to moderately hearing-impaired children continue in direct oral–aural contact with their parents, given the modest care their conditions warrant. Deaf children, however, present much greater difficulties, sometimes leading to complete interruption of communication with their parents. This unfortunate circumstance also can be avoided, as will be discussed below.

## MARRIAGE AND DIVORCE

The proportion of single never-married adults is about three times greater in the deaf than in the general population. The discrepancy may be partly accounted for by the fact that early deafened people tend to marry later than persons in general. This may or may not reflect the greater difficulties in gaining satisfactory employment that provides sufficient money to support a family (see the section on income). While the proportion of those who do not marry is greater among deaf people, the fact remains that most early deafened adults do marry.

When deaf children attain marriageable age,

they will typically select a deaf spouse. Propinquity may explain this finding as well as any other; people naturally marry those they know, and they are most likely to know those who are near them. When asked, deaf adolescents say they prefer a spouse with whom they can be comfortable, and they can be most comfortable with other early-deafened people, who share problems and interests and, above all, who communicate easily with them. The decision to marry another deaf person, then, is certainly an expected one. Contrary to the general tendency, the data show that those with later onset and those with more education (the two factors are, as has been shown, correlated) select a normal-hearing spouse more often than other early-deafened persons, although the trend is small. Also, a deaf woman is more likely to have a normal-hearing husband than is a deaf man a normal-hearing wife.

Once married, early-deafened marriages have about the same probability of success as marriages in general. Divorce rates are 3.6 and 3.8 percent, respectively, for the deaf and hearing populations. However, divorce rates are higher in marriages in which one person is normal hearing and the other deaf than in those involving two deaf persons.

Compared with what is known about marriage and divorce in the deaf community, knowledge of civil status in relationship to lesser degrees of impairment and later onsets is sparse. The NHS does not publish data on the civil status of hearing-impaired persons, which may suggest a lack of conviction that a meaningful relationship exists. We are left to speculate as to the contribution of late-onset hearing impairment on courtship, choice of spouse, marital discord, and the breakdown of marriages. While effects can easily be imagined, empirical support for them is lacking. Extrapolation from the rich data available about the early deafened cannot be justified, since their social lives appear to differ so markedly from those of persons with lesser impairments of later onset.

## ORGANIZATIONAL ASPECTS

The preceding discussion of civil status paves the way for a discussion of the deaf community — the tendency of early-deafened people to interact with each other in organized ways. The desire of deaf people to affiliate with each other finds expression in numerous national, state, and local organizations. Indeed, it would appear that deaf people join together at remarkably high rate. If by "join together" we mean to pay dues to a formal organization — one that has established operating procedures, maintains its identity over time, and is recognized by its members as an entity that, in turn, identifies them — then we find, in the one study that gathered such data, that one-half of deaf adults belong to such organizations.[36] That figure, high as it may seem, does not fully describe the extent to which deaf people seek each other's company, but it does indicate the breadth of the deaf community's infrastructure.

With a membership in excess of 15,000, the National Association of the Deaf (NAD) is probably the largest organization in the deaf community. The NAD works *for* deaf people, but it is uniquely an organization *of* deaf people. Founded in 1880, the NAD is also the oldest organization created by a group of disabled people. Those familiar with the history of the education of deaf children will recognize the NAD's founding year as the year in which the Milan Manifesto, the document condemning sign language and prescribing the oral method as the principal means of communication in the classroom, was adopted.[32] A number of deaf adults realized that their jobs in educational institutions would be threatened by that decision: teaching orally was something they could not do very well, if at all. They established the NAD to fight against the trend. Ever since then, the NAD has been a prime advocate for early-deafened people, representing them before Congress and in state legislatures and in efforts to shape administrative decisions affecting its members.

Another example of self-help is the National Fraternal Society of the Deaf (affectionately known in the deaf community as The Frat). The Frat grew out of early-deafened people's frustrations in applying for life insurance. They often faced discriminatory rates or, worse, outright rejection by insurers. In 1901, The Frat began as a fraternal insurance company. Today, it is a highly successful insurer, with a fine assets-to-risk ratio and excellent earnings, leaving no doubt the early deafness does not impair business acumen. The Frat also serves as a social center, through its many local lodges' activities, and as a vehicle for social betterment, offering scholarships to family members' children and organizing charitable events.

The American Athletic Association of the Deaf exemplifies a more purely social organization. It promotes sporting events and, through the International Games for the Deaf, encourages competition between deaf athletes from many nations. There are, incidentally, international analogues of the U.S. organizations (e.g., World Federation of the Deaf, housed in Rome, and Comité Internationale Sports Silenceaux, in Paris). These visible structures, literally, in the case of the NAD and The Frat, both of which own their headquarter's buildings, concretize the tendencies of early deafened people to look inward, toward their deaf peers, for support. That support from others disabled like themselves may in large measure explain why, despite difficult years of child development, deaf adults do not have disproportionately high rates of mental illness (see the section on the emotional impact of early deafness on mental health).

What about persons with milder impairments and later onsets of deafness? Do they share the affiliative drives of those deafened early? Until very recently, the answer appears to be a flat no. Few of the members of the NAD, The Frat, and other such organizations are mildly or moderately impaired, and even fewer are late deafened. Some of the latter regard the deaf community as hostile to them; others are unaware of it or ignore it altogether. The principal basis for these reactions probably will be found in the next section of this chapter, in communication practices.

The largest group of late hearing-impaired people is Self-Help for Hard of Hearing People, which has elected the acronym SHHH. Founded in 1979 by a former CIA agent, Howard "Rocky" Stone, SHHH increased the press run of its bimonthly journal to 15,000 in January 1985. Since the prevalence of deafness of adult onset and hearing impairment less than deafness is, respectively, at ratios of 3:1 and 26:1 early-deafened person, SHHH's membership seems small. Does it reflect its newness (less than 6 years old) or unwillingness on the part of later and less hearing-impaired people to seek each other's company? More than likely the answer to that question is a little bit of both! The growth of SHHH from a cold start has been spectac-

ular, but it has not yet captured a large enough constituency to ensure its long-term future. It will be fascinating to study its course over the next decade or two.

---

## COMMUNICATION

Hearing impairment has been characterized as a communication disorder. The designation is apt but incomplete, as the preceding discussion endeavors to make clear. Granting that point, a discussion of hearing impairment can hardly be complete without exhaustive attention to how it affects communication: proximal, mediated, and distal. The three adjectives, while not completely satisfactory, succinctly delineate the subject, since communication differs when it is between individuals in immediate visual contact, when it is interpreted by a third party, and when it is between one or more individuals at a distance from each other.

---

## PROXIMAL COMMUNICATION

As in most other aspects of life covered in this chapter, the effects of hearing impairment depend on degree and age at onset of the disability. The most dramatic manifestation occurs when the hearing impairment is profound and occurs early. For early-deafened individuals, the communication of choice has tended, and appears to continue to be, manual. Once speech has been securely achieved, it remains for most persons a principal means of expression. Similarly, on the receptive side, speechreading increases as the preferred method as age at onset increases. As hearing ability declines toward deafness, the tendency to use manual methods, expressively and receptively, increases. Numerous other factors might be considered. Prime among these is the amount of education received.

Table 32-4 displays the personal judgments of their communication abilities made by respon-

**Table 32-4. Percentage Distribution of Communication Ability as Judged by Respondent, by Highest School Grade Completed for Respondents 25 to 64 Years of Age: United States, 1972**

| Rating by Communication Mode | Highest School Grade Completed[a] | | | |
|---|---|---|---|---|
| | 1–8 | 9–12 | 13–16 | 17+ |
| Speech | | | | |
| Good | 18 | 31 | 47 | 54 |
| Fair | 42 | 41 | 39 | 27 |
| Poor | 25 | 19 | 12 | 13 |
| None | 16 | 9 | 2 | 6 |
| Lipreading | | | | |
| Good | 24 | 41 | 55 | 54 |
| Fair | 40 | 37 | 37 | 33 |
| Poor | 26 | 15 | 4 | 10 |
| None | 11 | 7 | 4 | 2 |
| Signing | | | | |
| Good | 66 | 70 | 59 | 65 |
| Fair | 22 | 17 | 18 | 10 |
| Poor | 7 | 6 | 4 | 6 |
| None | 7 | 8 | 21 | 21 |

[a] Percentages rounded to nearest whole number.
(Adapted from Schein JD, Delk MT: The deaf population of the United States. National Association of the Deaf, Silver Spring, MD, 1974.)

dents to interviews in the National Census of the Deaf Population. As can be seen, speech and lipreading abilities relate closely to academic achievement: the more education, the better the abilities. Very few persons with only a grade school education consider their speech to be good, while about one-half of those with some college education regard themselves as having good speech. At the other extreme, about one in six of the grade school sample claim no speaking ability, while the ratio for the college group ranges between 1 in 50 and 1 in 17 who are speechless. For the entire group, 1 in 10 state they are functionally mute.

Turning to manual communication, the majority of each educational group claims to be a good signer. The relationship between the ability to sign and education is barely significant: of those with no college experience, about 1 in 12 claims no signing ability; of those with some college through graduate education, about one in five rate their signing ability as nil. However, the grade-school-only and high school samples do not differ from each other, nor do the college and graduate-school samples. Thus, the relationship between education and manual communication is smaller than between education and oral communication. The explanation probably resides in the fact that, to get a college education requires good oral skills, but communi-

cation in the deaf community is largely manual. Furthermore, those with more education tend to have deafness of later onset, which reinforces the relationship. What about other manual methods of communication, such as fingerspelling, and other aspects, such as reading signs and fingerspelling? The data from the National Census of the Deaf Population support those of other studies in showing that judgments of manual communication abilities are highly correlated. Interested readers may wish to consult the original report, which contains the complete results.

Another way to look at communication is to ask deaf people how they communicate in a variety of situations. The data presented in Table 32-5 show some of the responses to that inquiry by the same respondents as in Table 32-4. The most common single method of communicating in a store is by writing, followed closely by speech, with signs and gestures seldom used alone. Speech plus writing is the most common of the combined methods used in commerce. At work, the way the deaf person expresses himself to different persons correlates highly with the way they respond: e.g., if the deaf person speaks to the supervisor and other workers, they tend to respond vocally. A significant exception is the disproportionality in the speech-plus-writing category: deaf people tend to use this com-

Table 32-5. Percentage Distribution[a] of Communication Methods Used by Respondents with Various Categories of Persons: United States, 1972

| Communication Methods | To Sales Clerk | To Supervisor | By Supervisor | To Others at Work | By Others at Work |
|---|---|---|---|---|---|
| Speech | 32 | 26 | 26 | 28 | 27 |
| Manual | 1 | 2 | 2 | 3 | 3 |
| Writing | 37 | 25 | 22 | 18 | 15 |
| Gesture | 4 | 4 | 4 | 3 | 4 |
| Speech + manual | [b] | 2 | 3 | 5 | 5 |
| Speech + writing | 13 | 17 | 13 | 9 | 11 |
| Speech + gesture | 3 | 2 | 4 | 3 | 3 |
| Writing + gesture | 5 | 4 | 6 | 5 | 5 |
| Other combinations | 6 | 12 | 20 | 26 | 26 |

[a] Less than 0.5 percent.

[b] Percentages rounded to nearest whole number.

(Adapted from Schein JD, Delk MT: The deaf population of the United States. National Association of the Deaf, Silver Spring, MD, 1974.)

bination more with supervisors than they use it in return. What this may reflect is the deaf persons' uncertainties about their speaking ability. With colleagues in the workplace, however, this disproportion does not occur, possibly because the deaf person is less concerned about being misunderstood in interchanges with other workers. Notice that, while almost 70 percent of deaf people rated their speech as good or fair, they used that speech only about 30 percent of the time. Many early-deafened adults experience embarassment and confusion when they speak, partly because of their odd voices, sometimes because of their misarticulation (English orthography, from which they learn to pronounce words, is riddled with exceptions), and occasionally because they cannot determine the level of surrounding noise, causing them to speak too softly. Whatever the reason or reasons, deaf people's use of speech does not accord with their expressed confidence in their ability. As for manual communication, its use depends on the ability of both parties to understand it: signing to someone who does not know sign is a futile exercise. Since most people do not understand sign language, deaf people have little occasion to use it in proximal communication with the majority.

## MEDIATED COMMUNICATION

A relatively recent change in communication was brought about during the Civil Rights era: the use of manual interpreters to bridge the gap between those who speak and those who cannot hear. Deaf people's use of a hearing mediator who knows sign language is not new, though history does not accord a precise date when this practice began. What is new is the change of interpreting from a *favor* to a *paid profession*. For interpreters [in what follows, the use of interpreters without qualification means *manual* interpreters], the inception of professionalism dates from 1964, the year in which the federal government sponsored a workshop to establish the Registry of Interpreters for the Deaf (RID). Before 1964, most interpreters performed a friendly gesture: after 1964, interpreters received remuneration for their efforts. The money hardly marked the difference in the service. As a favor, interpreters were undisciplined, following whatever style of behavior suited them. As a profession, they required training, a code of ethics, and a means of monitoring their activities. The change has been dramatic. In 1964, there were only about 300 manual interpreters available to serve nearly half a million deaf people who depended upon sign for communication. By 1980, the number of trained interpreters had increased to more than 3,000. Although still inadequate, that number measures the distance that this country has come in providing for the communication needs of a significant linguistic minority group. Much of the credit for the rapid increase in the numbers of interpreters can be attributed to the Rehabilitation Act of 1973, which contains two landmark provisions. Title V, known as The Bill of Rights for the Handicapped, forbids discrimination against persons on the basis of their disabilities in any activity supported by federal funds. That has been widely interpreted to mean that deaf persons must be provided interpreters at meetings, and many states have followed the federal lead by opening their government-sponsored meetings to deaf people by providing interpreters. In addition, the Act provided that all rehabilitation activities must be conducted in the client's native language or preferred mode of communication. Together, those two provisions have meant a burgeoning demand for interpreters.[32]

For persons dependent on lipreading, another kind of interpreter has arisen, the oral interpreter. Oral interpreters are needed when deaf persons are seated at a distance or in lighting that precludes their being able to clearly discriminate the speaker's facial movements. Second, oral interpreters do not wear mustaches, cover their mouths with their hands, and do other things that make lipreading difficult or impossible. They are usually familiar to the deaf persons whom they serve, which again eases the interpreting process. The oral interpreter also aids the communication through an awareness of words that are difficult to discriminate (e.g., homophenous words such as "time" and "dime"). When ambiguity occurs, the oral interpreter adds gestures and emphases to improve discrimination.

Being so young, interpreting has aroused little research interest. The process seems simple enough: the interpreter signs whatever is said and, in reverse, speaks aloud whatever the deaf person signs (unless the deaf person prefers to speak). At meetings or in classrooms, a single interpreter can sign for as many deaf persons as can see her or him. But what may seem simple and direct has many unstudied aspects that may well complicate the process. Deaf people prefer some interpreters over others. Why? Interpreters encounter many stressful situations, such as two persons speaking at the same time, speakers who speak very rapidly, or speakers who use terms unfamiliar to the interpreter. What techniques do they use to handle these situations? Deaf people vary in their linguistic skills, some having little ability in either English or American Sign Language. How does the interpreter determine and adjust to various linguistic levels? These issues, while having obvious importance to the interpreting process, have had no formal research. As these questions are resolved, others will likely arise, as is characteristic of researched areas. For now, we can only note that interpreting as a professionalized activity is a welcome addition to the deaf community.

## TELECOMMUNICATIONS

When hearing-impaired persons must communicate with persons who are out of sight, the burden of their disability is magnified.[37] Alexander Graham Bell invented the telephone as a device to aid in the rehabilitation of deaf people, as a means of improving their speech. Instead, the telephone created an occupational handicap for deaf people, since its use became critical to many better-paying types of employment. Not being able to use the telephone meant being denied many opportunities. For some hearing-impaired persons, communication is easier over the telephone than it is in many everyday situations; the telephonic conversation is at a volume they prefer, and surrounding noise is usually at a minimun. Amplified handsets further reduce the difficulties they might otherwise have in using the instrument.

For those who are deaf, an adaptation has been invented. Known familiarly as the TTY (because the first equipment consisted of discarded Western Union teletype machines), the devices consist of a modem that converts typed signals into impulses that are transmitted over the telephone lines to a companion modem that decodes the impulses and displays them in print. Two such send–receive devices enable deaf persons to carry on a conversation limited only by the availability of a telephone. While this invention has opened telephonic communication to deaf persons, it is not as poplar as one might expect. For early–deafened people, their poor grasp of the English language inhibits the use of a device that makes patent their inadequacy. They prefer the Picturephone, which transmits images and sound via telephone. Unfortunately, American Telephone & Telegraph Company has withdrawn this product, because its wide bandwidth requirements are too costly in terms of transmission load: 1,000,000-Hz bandwidth for the Picturephone versus 3,000 Hz for ordinary voice transmission. More than 300 voice calls can be carried in the space required by one Picturephone call.

Broadcast television initially held much promise for those who could not hear, but it rapidly proved to be "radio with a few pictures." The comprehension of most programs depends initimately on the spoken portions. Worse, even in roundtable discussions, the camera frequently focusses on the person being spoken to rather than the speaker, thereby eliminating the possibility of lipreading much of the dialogue. Recognizing the importance of television as both entertainment and information source, Public Broadcasting Service began, in 1972, to study the feasibility of captioning programs. The studies culminated in 1980 with the establishment of the National Captioning Institute, a private nonprofit organization formed to provide captions for television. Unfortunately, the government elected to support closed captioning, that is, captions that are invisible except to those who purchase a special decoder. Since decoders cost about as much as the television set, which is also essential, those who wish to receive captions pay for the privilege. The cost is made less palatable by the fact that only a portion of the programs in any broadcast day are captioned and one of the networks has refused to participate until recently.

Again, for the early-deafened population, inserting over the picture on the screen a printed version of the spoken portions of programs does not satisfy many of them, because they have difficulty reading English. However, some experts believe that the presence of captions may, in time, encourage deaf people to improve their reading abilities. Those who depend on sign for basic communication enjoy the occasional presence of interpreters on television and the very rare program that is entirely signed. In the latter case, interpretation of the signs is provided by voice, of which the deaf viewer is unaware. For the moderately hearing-impaired person with average or better English language development, the captions could be a boon. Listening in any situation in which hearing is imperfect creates stress that the supportive captions could relieve. Ironically, all of the emphasis in captioning has been directed toward those who are deaf — the smallest portion of the hearing-impaired population and one that has some reluctance to accept the product.

An exciting innovation that has been tested but has not yet been implemented is radio for deaf people. Radio waves can transmit signals that activate a TTY as well as simulate music or voices. In the former case, a special receiver has been invented that accomplishes the translation of radio signals that can be broadcast over any available frequency. Since the usual radio receivers have no means of receiving the signals, those receiving the voice and music signals would not be bothered by the messages intended for TTY receivers. The system is relatively inexpensive, but it has not captured the interest of those who might bring it to fruition.

The initial introduction of telecommunications devices (telephone, television, radio) have further handicapped many hearing-impaired persons. During the past few decades, steps have been taken to overcome the lack of access to telecommunications. For the most part, the approaches have been sound. However, economic and social factors have, as would be expected, interfered with the full realization of the benefits that could be derived by hearing-impaired persons from the technologic advances.

## ECONOMIC CONSEQUENCES OF HEARING IMPAIRMENT

The financial effects of hearing impairment can be assessed in three domains: labor market participation, occupational conditions, and earnings. Each is discussed in the three sections that follow. The sections begin with definitions that are essential to understanding, in order to compare hearing-impaired persons to the general public.

## LABOR FORCE STATUS

The civilian labor force consists of all persons 16 years of age and older classified as employed or unemployed. Employed persons worked as employees for any pay at all or in their own business, profession, or farm, even if they did not work during the reference period because they were temporarily absent due to illness, bad weather, strike, vacation, or personal reasons. Unemployed persons not only are not employed but are also actively seeking employment during the reference period and are ready to accept it, if found. The criteria "ready, willing, and able" determine labor force status for those who do not hold a job at the time of the interview. For example, a person who has retired at whatever age is not in the labor force. However, an able-bodied person who has become discouraged and is no longer looking for work is not unemployed, hence is not part of the labor force. The data are gathered weekly by the Department of Labor's Bureau of Labor Statistics (BLS) by interviews. To provide data for a part of the population that is comparable to the entire population, the questions asked must be identical.

The National Census of the Deaf Population followed the BLS format in obtaining information about a nationwide sample of people who became deaf before 19 years of age. The results are shown in Table 32-6. Overall, deaf people participated in the labor market at about the same rate as the general population. While deaf men and women had somewhat greater rates of participation in the labor force, this finding reflected the higher rates of participation for white deaf men and women; nonwhite deaf males and females had slightly lower rates than their general population counterparts. The differences, though small, should not be ignored, since they are indicative of persistent trends with respect to the interaction of race and deafness. As will be seen in other economic measures, non-white deaf persons differ more from nonwhite persons in general than white deaf persons differ from white persons in general. The relatively greater economic consequences of deafness among nonwhite than white deaf persons suggests that bearing two handicaps—deafness and minority racial status—compounds, rather than adds to, the individual's problems. Note further that the most extreme differences between deaf and general population peers occurs among nonwhite women. Again, it would appear that factors prejudicial to employment interact in a multiplicative fashion.

This latter statement is exemplified by the unemployment statistics in Table 32-6. White deaf men do better than do men in general, having a low 2.2 percent unemployment rate compared with 4.5 percent for white males. Nonwhite deaf men, however, do more poorly than nonwhite men in general: 10.4 to 8.9 percent, respectively. Deaf women do worse than women in general (10.2 to 6.6 percent), but the differences are greatest for the nonwhite deaf versus general population women, being 16.5 percent for the former and 11.3 percent for the latter.

## OCCUPATIONAL CONDITIONS

With a sizable portion of the deaf population seeking employment and the majority obtaining it, the next questions turn to the positions deaf people hold in industry. On the one hand, deaf people are

**Table 32-6.** Percentage Distribution of Labor-Force Status of Prevocationally Deaf Respondents to the National Census of the Deaf Population, 16 to 64 Years of Age, Compared with the General Population, by Race and Sex: 1972

| Sex and Race | Labor Force Status | | | | | | | | | |
|---|---|---|---|---|---|---|---|---|---|---|
| | Total | | Out | | In | | Unemp. | | Emp. | |
| | Deaf | Gen | Deaf | Gen | Deaf | Gen | Deaf | Gen | Deaf | Gen |
| Males | 100 | 100 | 17.3 | 20.3 | 82.7 | 79.7 | 2.9 | 4.9 | 97.1 | 95.1 |
| White | 100 | 100 | 16.1 | 20.4 | 83.9 | 79.6 | 2.2 | 4.5 | 97.8 | 95.5 |
| Nonwhite | 100 | 100 | 28.2 | 26.3 | 71.8 | 73.7 | 10.4 | 8.9 | 89.6 | 91.1 |
| Females | 100 | 100 | 50.6 | 56.1 | 49.4 | 43.9 | 10.2 | 6.6 | 89.8 | 93.4 |
| White | 100 | 100 | 50.4 | 56.8 | 49.6 | 43.2 | 9.5 | 5.9 | 90.5 | 94.1 |
| Nonwhite | 100 | 100 | 52.3 | 51.3 | 47.7 | 48.7 | 16.5 | 11.3 | 83.5 | 88.7 |

Gen, General population; Unemp, Unemployed; Emp, employed.
(Adapted from Schein JD, Delk MT: The deaf population of the United States. National Association of the Deaf, Silver Spring, MD, 1974.)

found in almost every civilian occupation, from domestics to professionals, and every industry, from agriculture to public administration, except the armed forces. This is true for early- and late-deafened people. It may seem odd that there are prelingually deaf lawyers, physicians, accountants, actors, and actresses and not the least bit odd that professional persons become deaf, which they do. The same may be said of those who are hard of hearing. On the other hand, the distribution of early-deafened persons across occupational categories is not consistent with that for the general public. The proportions in the professional, technical, managerial, sales, and clerical positions are far lower for early-deafened people than for the general public, and conversely, the proportions of early-deafened people in craftsmen, operative, service, and private-household worker, and laborer positions are higher than for the general population.

## UNDEREMPLOYMENT

What this latter finding suggests is considerable underemployment of early-deafened people. Underemployment is a concept that is intuitively simple to grasp, but it has not been defined in a manner that leads readily to quantification. One approach is to compare the level of employment with the amount of education. While education and occupation are highly correlated for early-deafened people, far more are in unexpectedly lower portions of the occupational hierarchy than would be expected from their educational background. For example, almost 43 percent of early-deafened adults who have completed 13 or more years of school hold positions in clerical, transit- and nontransit-operative, farm and nonfarm laboring, and service and private-household occupations. Other evidence supports the notion that early deafened people are more frequently underemployed than persons in general. Promotions, for instance, are often denied deaf employees because management believes that training for the higher position would overly strain communication between trainer and deaf employee. Hence, data have shown deaf peo-

ple remain longer in entry-level positions than the average for those hired at the same time.[11]

## VOCATIONAL REHABILITATION

What about the occupational distribution of persons with lesser degrees of hearing impairment than deafness? The limitations, if any, that mild to moderate degrees of hearing impairment place on employment have not been documented. Nor have large-scale studies been done of the consequences of late-onset hearing impairments, regardless of degree. Such studies are needed to extend information about the likely relations between hearing impairment and vocational adjustment.

Data from the Rehabilitation Services Administration summarizing the experiences of all state agencies provides some suggestions of what might be found by carefully designed studies. As shown in Table 32-7, hearing-impaired clients are more successfully rehabilitated than any other disability, except for those with neoplasms. Hearing-impaired clients are rehabilitated half again as

**Table 32-7. Selected Rehabilitation Ratios[a] for State Agency Clients, by Major Disabling Conditions: United States, Fiscal Year 1970**

| Condition | Rehabilitation Ratio |
|---|---|
| All disabilities | 3.52 |
| Hearing impairments | 8.21 |
|   Deafness | 6.12 |
|     Unable to talk | 4.60 |
|     Able to talk | 7.51 |
|   Other hearing impairments | 10.82 |
| Visual Impairments | 5.81 |
|   Blindness, both eyes | 4.77 |
|   Other visual impairments | 6.50 |
| Orthopedic impairments | 3.23 |
| Absence/amputation of extremities | 5.53 |
| Mental illness | 2.15 |
| Mental retardation | 3.98 |
| Benign/unspecified neoplasms | 11.22 |
| Allergies | 4.25 |
| Endocrine disorders | 4.77 |
| Epilepsy | 2.87 |

[a] Number of clients rehabilitated divided by number not rehabilitated. Cases in process are not included in the calculations.

(Adapted from Schein JD: Model for a state plan for vocational rehabilitation of deaf clients. J Rehabil Deaf Monogr 3:1, 1973.)

often as those with visual impairment (8.21 to 5.81). The least successful group of rehabilitants are those classified as mentally ill. Within the hearing-impaired category, deaf clients have poorer rates than the other degrees of impairment (6.12 to 10.82) and those deaf clients with early onsets ("Unable to talk") less success than those with later onsets: 4.60 to 7.51, respectively.

While these findings support other data relating degree and age at onset of hearing impairment to various social-psychological factors, they must be interpreted cautiously. The sample of clients does not necessarily represent the populations from which they have been drawn. The most severely disabled deaf clients may not know about or apply to their states' vocational rehabilitation agencies or, conversely, those with lesser degrees of impairment may not find it necessary to seek governmental assistance. Employer attitudes contribute heavily to rehabilitation, since clients are not vocationally rehabilitated if they are unemployed; hence, industrial prejudices for or against particular disabilities must be controlled to justify comparisons across categories. Within the agencies, cases rejected as unacceptable for their services (nonfeasible for rehabilitation) are not included in calculating the rehabilitation ratios. Do these potentially biasing factors apply uniformly across disability groups? It is unlikely: the agencies' experiences and their resources may tend to make them select particular client types. Finally, all clients do not conveniently have single disabilities.

The decision to cast a case into one or another rubric has some arbitrary features: In which category should the mentally retarded individual with an amputated limb be placed? What about clients with three disabilities? Obviously, mixing together clients with more than one disability together with those having only that disability reduces the cogency of deductions from relationships between the disability and other factors. Nonetheles, the experience shown in Table 32-7 is in accord with other findings that show that the effects of hearing impairments depend in large measure on their degrees and ages at onset. Compared with other disabilities, hearing-impaired persons as a group tend to be among the best prospects for vocational rehabilitation; however, that finding may not withstand close scrutiny that controls for extraneous factors.

# INCOME

Studies of representative samples of deaf people indicate that their personal earnings from wages and salaries fall below those for relevant groups in the general population. Table 32-8 shows the earnings of early-deafened persons relative to median earnings for the entire population. Figures are shown for two studies involving the same group of deaf adults surveyed in 1971 and 1976. The losses in respondents over the 5 years probably means that the differences are not as great as they would have been had the groups remained intact, since losses tend to be among those whose incomes have severely declined, forcing them to move without great concern for forwarding addresses and so forth.

What the data show is that, in 1971, deaf men and women had earnings that were about three-fourths those of the average for the general population. The difference between the sexes was insignificant. But 5 years later, female earnings had declined sharply (from 75.4 percent of the national average for women to 59.5 percent) while male earnings declined considerably less, from 74.7 percent to 70.3 percent of the national average for men. A possible explanation for the large sex difference is that the worsening economic conditions in 1976 affected women more, because they were forced to enter the labor market by their husband's losses of employment and declines in earnings. Other data bear this point out. For men, unemployment doubled between 1972 and 1977, jumping from a rate of 5.4 to 10.2 percent.[38] For deaf

**Table 32-8.** **Median Person Income from Wages and Salaries of Deaf Adults as a Percentage of Median Income for the General Population, by Sex: United States, 1971 and 1976**

| Sex | Percent | |
| --- | --- | --- |
| | 1971 | 1976 |
| Both sexes | 74.6 | 64.2 |
| Males | 74.7 | 70.3 |
| Females | 75.4 | 59.5 |

(Data from Schein JD: The demography of deafness. In Higgins P, Nash J (eds): The Deaf Community and the Deaf Population. Gallaudet College Press, Washington, DC, 1982.)

women, the rates declined, from 16.5, in 1972, to 12.0 percent, in 1977. Taken together, these findings suggest that women were taking positions in 1977 that they had declined in 1972 — probably at lower pay than they had earlier considered worthwhile. Whatever the explanation, the overall result is that deaf adults' average earnings have fallen to a little less than two-thirds of the national average, a heavy price exacted by early deafness.

What about lesser degrees and later onsets of deafness? Again, systematic studies of these questions have not been done, although they would certainly appear worthwhile. Data within the group labeled deaf indicates that the earlier the onset the lower the earnings. Similarly, the greater the impairment, the lower the earnings. However, there are irregularities in even these data that urge further study. For example, born deaf persons tend to do somewhat better than those deafened between birth and 3 years of age. Neither group does as well as those deafened after 3 years of age, and the correlation between age at onset and earnings, with degree of impairment held constant, continues to rise through age 18 years. One factor that may contribute to this odd curl in the tail of the distribution is that born-deaf children are more likely to have deaf parents. Other studies have shown that deaf parents tend to be more accepting of deaf children and better able to cope with them.[39] This advantage to deaf children may be reflected in their adult performances, as it clearly is in their education. For those whose hearing impairment occurs in adulthood and for those with milder impairments, regardless of age at onset, the relationships may hold further insights that will be exposed by careful inquires.

## CONCLUSIONS

Affecting as it does nearly 7 percent of the U.S. population, hearing impairment is manifestly a major health problem. But its great prevalence alone does not justify the sizable expenditure of scientific resources that ought to, but have not been, expended on it. The psychological, social, and economic conditions associated with hearing impairment should encourage a major effort to reduce its incidence and ameliorate its consequences. Admittedly, funds have been allocated by the federal government for some programs to prevent hearing impairment and to reduce its burdens, but not in proportion to either the numbers affected or the disruption of their lives that hearing impairments cause.

Another reason for greater societal attention to hearing impairment is that its prevalence is increasing. Although the precise amount of the increase is difficult to determine from available data because of methodological inconsistencies, there is no question that the prevalence of hearing impairment has grown. And experts predict continued increases in the near future. The incidence of hearing impairment, however, is unknown, but logic and the little information at hand support an erratic rate of annual occurence. Hearing impairment of epidemic origin would be a major determiner of this lack of smoothness in the data. Particularly conditions like prelingual deafness tend to fluctuate sharply from year to year, which makes all the more important having accurate, up-to-date information about the numbers of deaf children being added each year, if for no other reason than to assist those responsible for educational planning.

Some pertinent generalizations remain firm. Males are more frequently hearing impaired than are females, and the older the individual, the more likely the presence of a hearing impairment. Whites exhibit hearing impairments more frequently than do nonwhites, leading to a variety of explanations, with no one completely accounting for the large differences in proportions affected. Generally, rates for early deafness tend to be lower on the seacoasts than inland. All other considerations aside, the distribution of prevalence rates for hearing impairments differs from place to place, often markedly, even within the same country. Thus, average prevalence rates for any large geographic area cannot be used confidently to estimate rates for smaller regions within the larger area.

In research programming, sufficient attention is not being paid to fundamentals, such as determining the incidence as well as prevalence of hearing impairments, which is essential to understanding them and planning for them. Understanding a hearing impairment also requires specification of the degree of the hearing impairment and the age of the individual at its onset. As has been repeatedly set forth in the preceding exposition, the effects of a hearing impairment are related to its severity and, interacting with that factor, the age at onset; thus, in all that follows results must be qualified with respect to these two considerations. For instance, as degree of hearing impairment increases, disturbances of speech and language development increase. Similarly, the earlier the age at onset of hearing impairment, the more severe the speech and language disturbances (with language referring to English).

Would deaf children's poor academic achievement be tolerated if they were a larger portion of the population? Might their education be more effective if other early-deafened people planned it, rather than the majority group educators who now control the curriculum? The fact that early-deafened children learn American Sign Language so readily, although no school now teaches it to them, must challenge the claim that deafness creates a barrier to language learning. English language learning, yes; vocal language learning, certainly; but language learning per se, no. In short, researchers must consider the politics of deafness along with its demography.

The minority status of early-deafened people arises again in explaining their reactions to rejection by their families, difficulties in adjusting to school, and the buffeting that many encounter as adults. An appealing rationale for the lack of psychosis among them is the support that they gain from the deaf community. That it plays a sizable role in stabilizing the lives of many early-deafened people cannot be doubted by the impartial observer, but the nature of how it functions and of which deaf people are accepted and which rejected by it has not been sufficiently investigated. The demographic paradox remains: the sizable numbers of deaf children labeled emotionally disturbed as not paralleled by their adult status, which is essentially normal.

The economic and vocational findings may also be explained by the prejudices that most develop toward those who differ from them. The physically handicapped people form identifiable minorities who experience discrimination that is not commen-

surate with their abilities to perform useful work. That reasoning led to the passage of the Title V of the Rehabilitation Act Amendments of 1973, which forbids discrimination against persons on the basis of their physical disabilities, the so-called Handicapped Americans' Bill of Rights. Employer prejudice, however, may not be the sole explanation of the reduced earnings of early-deafened people: poorer education, difficulties in communication, and lower self-concepts vis à vis the general population probably contribute as much or more to the observed findings. What must be noted is that, in times of economic stress, the economic status of physically handicapped people worsens.

## TWO NECESSARY CORRECTIVES

In the preceding discussions, such terms as "effect," "consequence," and "impact," have been used in ways that may imply that hearing impairments in and of themselves are causal agents that lead directly to the observed relationships. That position defies logic: the observations may arise from factors other than hearing impairment, but factors are also related to hearing impairment. For instance, persons of low socioeconomic status suffer hearing impairments proportionally more often than those of middle and high status. Since academic achievement is (modestly) correlated with socioeconomic status—the lower the status, the lower the achievement—the poor academic records of hearing-impaired children could be due, in part, to their lower-class background. Thus, to speak of hearing impairments being the cause of the sad academic records associated with deaf children would not be strictly accurate. To establish the extent of the cause–effect relationships between hearing impairment and the various factors considered in this essay requires controlled experiments that have not been done or additional evidence that has not been systematically gathered. That causal relations do exist, then, is a matter of faith held until science catches up with this problem by those who have examined the evidence so far available but who continue to respect the canons of logical inference. In what has been written here, the awkwardness of constantly repeating that "a relationship has been found between" has been avoided, with the admitted risk of misleading some readers. If such has occurred it is unfortunate, mostly because the certainty that comes from establishing causal relations frequently stems the desire for more research, a search for deeper implications. Clearly, given its human costs and its pervasiveness throughout the population, hearing impairment deserves more, not less, study.

Another misunderstanding that sometimes arises from the recitation of demographic information is that the conditions being described are static and/or immutable. Neither position can be acccepted. Insofar as historical data are available, they indicate that many status indicators for hearing impairment have fluctuated, sometimes a little and sometimes a lot. The earnings of early-deafened people just cited provide an instance of a changing condition, especially for women. Along with the changing prevalence of hearing impairment will likely come other changes, both in attitudes toward the problems and in efforts to resolve them. The demography of hearing impairment should be seen as dynamic and, more importantly, negative factors related to hearing impairments should be viewed as subject to remediation. The long view of hearing impairments fosters the belief that, given the effort, the deleterious effects now associated with them can be reduced or avoided altogether.

## REFERENCES

1. Ries PW: Hearing ability of persons by sociodemographic and health characteristics: United States. Vital and Health Statistics, Series 10, No. 140, 1982
2. Hill AB: Principles of Medical Statistics. Oxford University Press, New York, 1961
3. Beasley WC: Characteristics and distribution of impaired hearing in the population of the United States. J Acoust Soc Am 12:114, 1940
4. Trotter WR: The association of deafness with thyroid dysfunction. Br Med Bull 16:92, 1960
5. Fraser GR: The Causes of Profound Deafness in Childhood. Johns Hopkins University Press, Baltimore, 1976
6. Campanelli PA, Schein JD: Inter-observer agreement in judging auditory responses in neonates. Eye Ear Nose Throat Monthly 48:697, 1969
7. Martin FN, Sides DG: Survey of current audiometric practices. ASHA 27(2):29, 1985
8. Gentile A, Schein JD, Haase, K: Characteristics of persons with impaired hearing: United States, July 1962–June 1963. Vital and Health Statistics, Series 10, No. 35, 1967.
9. Schein JD: Hearing disorders. p. 276. In Kurland LT, Kurtzke JF, Goldberg ID (eds): Epidemiology of Neurologic and Sense Organ Disorders. Harvard University Press, Cambridge, MA, 1973
10. Schein JD: Hearing impairment among elderly people. Soundbarrier 1(2):4, 1984
11. Schein JD, Delk MT: The Deaf Population of the United States. National Association of the Deaf, Silver Spring, MD, 1974
12. Post RH: Hearing acuity variation among negroes and whites. Eugen Q 11:65, 1964
13. Georgia's Deaf: Works Project Administration of Georgia, Atlanta, 1942
14. Schein JD: Speaking the Language of Sign: The Art and Science of Sign. Doubleday, New York, 1984
15. Jensema CJ, Karchmer MA, Trybus RJ: The rated speech intelligibility of hearing impaired children: Basic relationships and a detailed analysis. Series R, No. 6. Office of Demographic Studies, Gallaudet College, Washington, DC, 1978
16. Bender RE: The Conquest of Deafness. 3rd Ed. Interstate Printers & Publishers, Danville, IL, 1981
17. Dee A, Rapin I, Ruben RJ: Speech and language development in a parent–infant Total Communication program. Ann Otol Rhinol Laryngol 91[5, suppl 97]:62, 1982
18. Vernon M: Fifty years of research on the intelligence of deaf and hard of hearing children: A review of literature and discussion of implications. J Rehabil Deaf 1:4, 1968
19. Myklebust HR: The Psychology of Deafness. Grune & Stratton, Orlando, FL, 1960
20. Levine ES: The Psychology of Deafness. Columbia University Press, New York, 1960
21. Hoemann HW, Ullman DG: Intellectual development. p. 43. In Bolton B (ed): Psychology of Deafness for Rehabilitation Counselors. University Park Press, Baltimore, 1976
22. Green B: Performance of deaf children on memory tasks. NYU Educ Q 12:20, 1980
23. Schiff W, Thayer S: An eye for an ear? Rehab Psychol 21:50, 1974

24. Schiff W, Dytell RS: Deaf and hearing children's performance on a tactual perception battery. Percept Mot Skills 35:683, 1972

25. Rosenstein J: Tactile perception of rhythmic patterns by normal, blind, deaf, and aphasic children. Am Ann Deaf 102:399, 1957

26. Schein JD: Multiply handicapped hearing-impaired children. p. 357. In Bradford LJ, Hardy WG (eds): Hearing and Hearing Impairment. Grune & Stratton, Orlando, FL, 1979

27. Rainer JD, Altshuler KZ, Kallmann FJ (eds): Family and Mental Health Problems in a Deaf Population. New York State Psychiatric Institute, Columbia University, NY, 1963

28. Hearing impaired patients in public psychiatric hospitals. Gallaudet Res Inst Newsl Spring:1, 1984

29. Best H: Deafness and the Deaf in the United States. Macmillan, New York, 1943

30. Higgins PC: Outsiders in a Hearing World. Sage Publications, Beverly Hills, CA, 1980

31. Schein JD: Society and culture of hearing-impaired people. p. 479. In Bradford LJ, Hardy WG (eds): Hearing and Hearing Impairment. Grune & Stratton, Orlando, FL, 1979

32. Schein JD: Hearing impairment among elderly people. Soundbarrier 1(2):4, 1984

33. Schlesinger HS, Meadow KP: Sound and Sign. University of California Press, Berkeley, 1972

34. Naiman D, Schein JD: For Parents of Deaf Children. National Association of the Deaf, Silver Spring, MD, 1978

35. Ling D: Rehabilitation of cases with deafness secondary to otitis media. In Glorig A, Gerwin KS (eds): Otitis Media. Charles C Thomas, Springfield, IL, 1972

36. Schein JD: The Deaf Community. Gallaudet College Press, Washington, DC, 1968

37. Schein JD, Hamilton RN: Impact 1980. Telecommunications and Deafness. National Association of the Deaf, Silver Spring, MD, 1980

38. Schein JD: The demography of deafness. p. 1. In Higgins P, Nash J (eds): The Deaf Community and the Deaf Population. Gallaudet College Press, Washington, DC, 1982

39. Meadow KP: Deafness and Child Development. University of California Press, Berkeley, 1980

# Otosclerosis (Otospongiosis): General Considerations

# 33

## Ronald E. Gristwood

## DEFINITIONS

Otosclerosis is a term used to describe an idiopathic lesion of bone, first identified and reported by Politzer[1,2] in 1893, that originates in the human labyrinthine capsule and stapes footplate and that may interfere with the function of hearing or balance, depending on the site, size, and histologic activity of the pathologically involved area. Siebenmann[3] in 1912 observed that the newly formed bone is more spongy than the dense ivory-hard bone of the labyrinth capsule that it replaces; he therefore proposed the more accurate name of otospongiosis.

## Histologic Otosclerosis

Histologic otosclerosis refers to the subclinical or asymptomatic variety in which the areas of otosclerotic bone within the otic capsule have not caused stapedial fixation or cochlear degeneration. These patients do not show any hearing loss. This condition is common, the lesions being found in between 5 and 10 percent of the adult white population and can only be diagnosed with certainty by serial sectioning of temporal bones.

## Clinical Otosclerosis

Clinical otosclerosis is found in about 10 percent of those with histologic otosclerosis and denotes patients who have measurable hearing losses from otosclerosis. It may be subclassified into stapedial and cochlear otosclerosis.

### Stapedial Otosclerosis

Stapedial Otosclerosis denotes stapedial fixation from a focus of otosclerosis involving the stapes footplate, annular ligament, or margins of the oval window niche. The patient suffers from a conductive hearing loss but in many cases of stapedial otosclerosis, a sensorineural hearing loss may antedate, develop coincidentally with, or ensue after the conductive hearing loss, resulting in a mixed or combined hearing impairment.

### Cochlear Otosclerosis

Although many patients with stapedial otosclerosis have evidence of varying degrees of cochlear degeneration including subtotal or profound hearing losses, the term cochlear otosclerosis refers to cases of otosclerosis involving the labyrinthine capsule and cochlear endosteum, without associated stapes fixation, but with sensorineural hearing loss occurring in a pure form (without a conductive component). The prevalence of pure cochlear otosclerosis remains a matter of considerable dispute. On the basis of histologic studies, Schuknecht[4] has observed that the incidence of cochlear otosclerosis involving endosteum in 326 ears with progressive sensorineural hearing loss is about 1 percent and that most cases of progressive sensorineural hearing loss are attributable to genetically determined and age-related influences rather than otosclerosis. Others who have studied the problem and have failed to establish an association between otosclerosis and sensorineural hearing impairment include Glorig and Gallo,[5] Schuknecht,[6] and Young et al.[7] Although audiologic evidence to the contrary is also available,[8,9] there is no doubt that sensorineural hearing loss coexists with stapedial otosclerosis and may sometimes be severe.

Gristwood[10] examined 103 patients with unilateral otosclerosis who had normal hearing acuity in the opposite ear. In just over 60 percent of the otosclerotic ears, the average B.C. level (0.5 to 2 kHz) exceeded 25 dB, and in just over 10 percent the bone conduction (BC) level was greater than 40 dB in the speech frequencies.

Analysis of the audiometric data of 1,013 consecutive cases of clinical otosclerosis suitable for surgery in South Australia[10] showed a sensorineural component to the hearing loss, much worse at all ages than the presbyacusis curves for normals measured elsewhere.[11,12] It must be concluded that otosclerosis has an adverse effect on the sensorineural status of the affected ear. Shambaugh[13] and Derlacki and Valvassori[14] have developed several diagnostic criteria for cochlear otosclerosis (although the definition is obviously broadened) including

1. Positive Schwartze sign in one or both ears
2. Family history of stapedial otosclerosis
3. Bilateral symmetrical sensorineural hearing loss and one ear with a conductive loss due to stapes fixation
4. Slowly progressive sensorineural loss which begins insidiously in early or middle adult life with no known etiology

5. Sensorineural loss with an unusual audiometric pattern that is low tone, flat or saucer-shaped with good speech discrimination
6. Development of an additional conductive loss due to stapes fixation in a patient with a progressive sensorineural loss
7. Polytomographic evidence of osteoporotic areas in the cochlear capsule of a patient with progressive sensorineural loss

---

## HISTORICAL

Valsalva[15] in 1704 first described stapes fixation as a cause of hearing loss during the macroscopic dissection of the ear of a deaf person, and Toynbee[16] in 1841 described an ear in which

> "a remarkable pathologic condition is presented in the firm anchylosis of the base of the stapes to the margin of the fenestra ovalis. This appears to be produced by an expansion of the base of the stapes, which projects into the cavity of the vestibule, so as to form within it an oval protuberance, which is smooth, and of an opaque white, and firmly adherent to the vestibular parietes. This anchylosis appears to depend upon a disease of the stapes, the walls of the vestibule being perfectly healthy."

In his textbook of 1868, Toynbee[17] stated that he had found 136 specimens of ankylosis of the base of the stapes to the fenestra ovalis in the dissection of 1,149 diseased ears.

In his writings from 1894, Politzer[1,2] showed that clinical otosclerosis did not present a diseased condition of the mucosa of the tympanic cavity, as had been previously held, but was a primary disease of the labyrinthine capsule with circumscribed new bone growth and tissue changes clearly demonstrable in sections through the stapes and oval window niche and adjacent labyrinthine wall. Various degrees of involvement of the fixed stapes footplate in the new bone formation were recorded: partial ankylosis of the anterior pole: filling in of the angle between anterior crus and footplate, great thickening of the whole of the footplace, and filling in of the entire oval window niche by a bony mass continuous with the pathologic labyrinthine capsule.

Mention must also be made of the pioneering histologic work of Guild, which set the stage for the modern era of histologic and epidemiologic investigation.[18,19]

# ETIOLOGY

The cause of otosclerosis remains obscure despite the renewed interest in its pathogenesis, histopathology, and histochemistry over the past 25 years. Otosclerosis occurs only in humans and lack of a suitable experimental animal has been a great hindrance to research.

Altmann[20] emphasized three elementary rules for experimental otosclerosis:

1. The lesions must be focal and confined to the labyrinthine capsule.
2. The causative factor must be able to produce foci not only in the oval window region but also in other typical locations (e.g., round window, stapes footplate, internal auditory canal, and semicircular canals).
3. Histologic similarity between experimentally produced lesions in the animal labyrinthine capsule and human otosclerosis does not alone permit conclusions about the etiologic factors of human otosclerosis.

Guild[19] pointed out that any attempt to explain the pathogenesis of otosclerosis had to take into account the morphologic facts that otosclerosis is limited to the otic capsule and occurs unilaterally in about 30 percent of cases; that in persons with bilateral otosclerosis, bilateral symmetry is not always present in regard to location, extent and histologic activity; and that in any person both otic capsules have been supplied with blood containing identical nutritional factors for identical periods of time irrespective of temporary or permanent deviations from the normal range.

The following factors have been put forward to explain the pathogenesis of otosclerosis.

## Heredity and Constitution

In many families there is strong evidence of autosomal dominant inheritance with penetrance of the pathologic gene of between 25 and 40 percent.[21-24] The rate of manifestation varies from 10 to 100 percent in different families, and, once manifest, any degree of clinical severity may be encountered. Variable clinical severity is usual among families but there is often a marked similarity in clinical features in affected individuals within the same family, usually within siblings but especially monozygotic twins. In those with no familial history the possibility of an autosomal-recessive inheritance cannot be ruled out. In many cases, the etiology may be multifactorial from the interaction of many genes and exogenous influences.[25] There is no evidence of an association between otosclerosis and the ABO, MN, and rhesus blood groups, the secretor status, the haptoglobin genotypes,[22] or the human leukocyte antigens (HLA) A, B, and C.[26] There is, however, a statistically significant association between otosclerosis and the ability to taste phenylthiocarbamide. The genetic basis of otosclerosis is further described in Chapter 30.

It has been suggested that otosclerosis and osteogenesis imperfecta are related,[27] although this is no longer believed. Both Altmann and Kornfeld[28] and Bretlau and Jorgensen[29] agree that where otosclerosis and osteogenesis imperfecta coexist, the two conditions can be clearly distinguished histologically. The not infrequent coexistence of the two conditions could be explained by osteogenesis imperfecta predisposing to the onset of otosclerosis by way of chemical or ultramicroscopic structural abnormalities.

## Hormonal Factors

The harmful influence of pregnancy on the course of some cases of otosclerosis, presumably by activating or accelerating the development of the process, has long been known and suggests that endocrine factors in the female play a role to account for the preponderance of females over males in clinical otosclerosis.

Juvenile otosclerosis, which becomes manifest during the period of active skeletal growth, is often a fulminating lesion associated with severe and diffuse involvement of the stapedial footplate or with obliteration of the oval window niche. It is likely that hormonal influences are responsible for acceleration of the pathologic process in this age group.

## Autoimmunity to Type 2 Collagen

A possible role for type 2 collagen autoimmunity in the etiology of otosclerosis has been suggested,[30] the type 2 collagen being present in the embryonic cartilage rests of the normal human otic capsule.

## Local Factors

Local factors including inflammatory processes, unstable cartilaginous rests in the fissula ante fenestram, and abnormal mechanical stresses in the base of the skull as a result of the erect human posture have been put forward as possible explanations for the development of otosclerosis. According to Sercer and Krmpotic,[31,32] otosclerosis is caused by intrinsic strains and stresses developing during the growth of the skull and acting on the petrous pyramid as a result of the angulation of the base of the skull at the sphenoidal axis. This angulation gradually increases during childhood and reaches its maximum after puberty. The degree of angulation varies among races and individuals and represents an inherited characteristic which is less marked in blacks than in whites. The forces that produce the rotation of the otic capsule act most strongly on the areas of predilection for the development of the otosclerotic foci, especially if the resistance of the capsule is lowered due to constitutional, endocrine, biochemical, or other factors.

Wright,[33] who examined 401 specimens removed during stapedectomy for otosclerosis, found that 25 percent showed avascular necrosis rather than reactive bone formation. The presence of fat emboli in the stapes mucosal vessels and intravascular rouleaux formation provided additional evidence for the etiologic importance of ischemia. She considered that fixation of the stapes footplate in the oval window was due to expansion of the footplate in reaction to a small ischemic lesion, or to a larger lesion with subsequent subperiosteal deposition of layers of new bone. Wright explained the deterioration of hearing in otosclerosis in many cases of pregnancy with childbirth on the basis of vascular insufficiency and emboli occurring during and after labor.

## Activating Factors

The factors initiating the histologic events in otosclerosis are completely unknown. The finding of intranuclear inclusions in the multinucleated osteoclasts of Paget's[34] disease suggesting a viral etiology requires similar studies to be made in patients, especially juveniles, with an active phase of otosclerosis.

---

# PATHOLOGY OF OTOSCLEROSIS

## Labyrinthine Capsule

During embryonic development, the mesenchyma surrounding the various parts of the membranous epithelial labyrinth is converted into a cartilaginous otic capsule, which finally becomes ossified.[35]

The bony labyrinthine capsule consists of three layers, which differ in thickness, structure, and staining characteristics.[36] The endosteal (innermost) layer is a fairly thin, regular zone of lamellar bone, which is lined on its internal surface by a thin periosteum to which the endosteum, a layer of flattened perilymphatic cells resembling a squamous epithelium, is closely adherent.

The enchondral or endochondral (middle) layer is much thicker than the endosteal layer in most regions and retains a peculiar skein-like structure in which cartilaginous remnants from the embryonic capsule may persist to form "globuli interossei."

The periosteal (outermost) layer is irregular in thickness and consists of distinct Haversian lamellae.

The enchondral layer has usually been considered as metabolically inert in adult life because of the inability of fractured endochondral bone to form a callous. However, perivascular uptake of tetracycline within the enchondral bone of the otic capsule of patients treated with this antibiotic during adult life suggests that osteogenesis is occurring continuously in the adult, that the new bone is lamellar or Haversian in character, and that the process of new bone deposition and simultaneous bone resorption occur normally in a state of dynamic equilibrium within the otic capsule.[37]

## Histogenesis of Otosclerotic Foci

There is general agreement that otosclerosis is a primary, often bilaterally symmetrical, disease of the bony labyrinth capsule.[19,38,39] Circumscribed destruction of the capsule by focal resorption of the hard endochondral bone at certain typical places, usually starting in a cartilaginous area, especially in the area anterior to the oval window between stapes, the upper border of the promontory, and the cochleariform process, is followed by the formation of a highly vascular, excessively cellular, and soft new spongy bone. The new bone has a strong affinity for hematoxylin and carmine dyes and is sharply demarcated from the surrounding normal capsular bone. The otosclerotic focus may retain its abnormally spongy character or may in time be converted by remodeling into dense eosinophilic lamellar bone.[40] The principal histologic features of otosclerosis have been extensively studied and well described since the turn of the nineteenth century by Politzer, Siebenmann, Denker, Manasse, Gray, Meyer, and Wittmaack, among others. Nevertheless, otosclerosis remains an enigma.

The confinement of the otosclerotic lesion to the labyrinthine capsule means that modern histologic and morphometric methods applied with particular success to the investigation of generalized metabolic disorders of bone (such as osteoporosis and Paget's disease) are not applicable. However, the assumption that otosclerosis is confined to the labyrinthine capsule has never been proved beyond doubt because to do so would require serial sections throughout the entire skeleton.

Several developmental stages are described in the otosclerotic lesion (see Ch. 22). They include osteoclastic destruction of old capsular bone with formation of pathologic bone marrow, rich in cells and poor in fibrils within the resorption spaces;

replacement of absorbed old bone by newly formed immature fibrous bone, which is basophil, excessively cellular, and comprising slightly more cement and correspondingly fewer fibers than usual; and a gradual increase in the amount of collagen fibers manufactured by the osteoblasts.

The growth of the otosclerotic focus may occur on a broad front or by means of finger-like projections from the focus into the surrounding capsular bone.

Electron microscopic (EM) studies of the otosclerotic focus in osteoid lamellae or portions of the stapes footplate by Chevance et al.[41,42] indicated that osteoclasts appear to play a subordinate role during the phase of bony resorption. They propose that osteocytic resorption without osteoclasis occurs in otosclerosis. Pericellular lysis of collagen was an invariable finding and lysozymes were often observed in the surrounding osteocytes. The endothelial cells of the capillary network in the focus were normal, however. EM also demonstrated a large number of "microfoci" in the immediate neighborhood of the otosclerotic focus with gaps in the collagen bundles, which become thinner and lose their normal periodic striation before the process of destruction becomes complete.

## Histochemistry of Otosclerosis

Histochemical investigations of the active otosclerotic focus have demonstrated altered polymerization of the mucopolysaccharides[43] and an increased quantity of alkaline phosphatase in the focus, especially in the middle ear mucosa and about the blood vessels, and to a lesser extent in osteocytes in the vicinity of the vessels.[44]

Osteoclasts have a negative reaction for alkaline phosphatase. An intense acid phosphatase reaction has been seen in osteoclasts within the focus, and to a lesser extent in the matrix of otosclerotic bone and in the overlying mucosa.[44] No enzyme defect has been detected to account for the otosclerotic lesion, but within the focus a positive reaction for two intracellular hydrolytic enzyme systems— leucine aminopeptidase and nonspecific esterases —has been noted in the fibrous perivascular tissue and osteocytes and in thickened and vascular mucosa overlying the footplate.[45] Sera from otosclerotic patients show no significant variation from those of control subjects in the distribution of nonspecific esterases, and alkaline and acid phosphatases.[46]

## Histologic Similarities Between Otosclerosis and Other Bone Diseases

The structural features of otosclerosis-osteoclasis, fibrous replacement of bone, and lamellar bone formation are also found in osteogenesis imperfecta, osteitis fibrosa, osteitis deformans, and in the healing of fractures. The more-or-less identical histologic picture in all of these different pathologic conditions at one stage in their development implies similarities in healing processes in the temporal bone damaged by various diseases or trauma.[47] Any statement regarding pathogenetic similarity or dissimilarity of these conditions must depend not on local histologic examination of limited areas of bone alone, but also on a consideration of general features.

## Incidence of Histologic Otosclerosis

Otosclerosis in its asymptomatic histologic form is a common condition in whites and occurs in about 5 to 10 percent of the adult population. The following list shows the findings of several investigators:

1. Weber[48] cited 11 percent of 200 cases.
2. Engstrom[49] cited 12 percent of 100 cases.
3. Schuknecht and Kirchner[50] reported 4.4 percent of 634 temporal bones.
4. Bretlau and Jorgensen[51] and Jorgensen and Kristensen[52] reported 11.4 percent of 237 temporal bones.
5. Guild[18] reported 8.3 percent of 518 temporal bones.

In Guild's series[18] the highest incidence of otosclerosis was 12.6 percent for pooled sexes (18.5 percent for women, 9.6 percent for men) in the age group 30 to 49 years, whereas Jorgensen and Kristensen[52] found the highest incidence of 17.8 percent in the age group 61 to 80 years.

Histologic otosclerosis seems rare in infancy and childhood. Jorgensen and Kristensen[52] found no signs of otosclerosis in 18 temporal bones from nine fetuses or in 138 temporal bones from 71 newborn infants in whom particular care was given to the study of the region of the fissula ante fenestram.

## Guild's Study

Guild's material[18,19] represents a classic study on the prevalence of otosclerosis in a collection of 1,161 serially sectioned temporal bones from unselected cadavers of 585 American whites and 576 American blacks, about one-third of each racial group being female. Guild made the following conclusions:

1. Only 1 of 161 children (0.6 percent) under 5 years of age showed histologic otosclerosis.
2. The histologic, asymptomatic, or nonclinical form of otosclerosis is a common condition in whites, with an incidence of 1 in 12 (8.3 percent) in those over the age of 5 years. After puberty the incidence increases rapidly, reaching its peak between the ages of 30 and 50 years when as many as 18.5 percent of the women and half as many white men have one or more foci of pathologic otosclerotic bone in their labyrinthine capsules.
3. Otosclerosis is rare in American blacks (5/576 = 0.9 percent).
4. A clear distinction must be drawn between clinical otosclerosis with deafness and asymptomatic histologic otosclerosis. Approximately seven out of eight patients with otosclerotic lesions have no symptoms because the stapes footplate is not ankylosed. The presence of the disease is unsuspected until serial sections of the temporal bones are studied microscopically.
5. The effect of the disease on hearing is secondary to its location and extent.

## Size and Number of Otosclerotic Foci

The otosclerotic lesion remains small and asymptomatic in the great majority of cases. Otosclerotic areas differ in size from those less than 1 mm in diameter to those in which the disease process has involved almost the entire otic capsule. Small and moderate-sized areas of otosclerosis occur far more often than extensive ones. Usually only one oto- sclerotic area is present in a temporal bone. Re- porting on 81 temporal bones with evidence of otosclerosis, Guild[18,19] found one lesion in 54 bones (66.7 percent), two anatomically separate lesions in 22 bones (27.2 percent), and three or more independent otosclerotic areas in only five bones (6.2 percent). Nylen[38] reported similar find- ings. Diffuse otosclerosis that involves the greater part of the cochlea and vestibule and areas of the semicircular canals is a relatively rare condition. Other similar studies have been reported by Black et al.,[53] Bretlau and Jorgensen,[51] and Lindsay.[54]

### Site of Otosclerotic Focus

A primary focus of otosclerosis may occur within the stapedial footplate itself independently of any other area in the otic capsule in 5 to 12 percent of cases.

Other areas affected are around the cochlea (25 to 35 percent), the round window niche (33 per- cent), the anterior wall or floor of the internal audi- tory canal (10 to 30 percent), and around the semi- circular canals (15 percent). Rare indeed are otosclerotic foci found outside the otic capsule; but such foci have been reported in the carotid canal, tegmen, cochleariform process, malleus, and incus.[39] Diffuse otosclerosis can develop as such from the beginning or from confluence of multiple, initially independent lesions involving vast areas of the labyrinthine capsule. This is seen in approxi- mately 10 percent of specimens. The diffuse form of otosclerosis can totally obliterate one or both windows. Severe involvement of the basal turn of the cochlea can incite formation of new lamellar bone within the scalae.

### Relationship of Focus to Fissula Ante Fenestram

The fissula ante fenestram, a constant feature of the human otic capsule, is a fibrous tissue-filled perilymphatic fissure or cleft, passing from the me- dial wall of the tympanic cavity to end internally at the junction of vestibule and scala vestibuli, just anterior to the oval window. Anson[55] and Bast[56] consider it an area of histologic instability.

Although any part of the otic capsule may be the site of otosclerosis, about 80 to 90 percent of all otosclerotic foci are in a particular region called the site of predilection for otosclerosis, which lies im- mediately in front of the oval window niche. De- tails of the extension are given by Guild.[18,19]

Because the majority of otosclerotic foci are situ- ated in the antefenestral area, the fissula antefen- estram has been considered as the place where the otosclerotic focus arises. The opinion of Anson[55] and Bast[56] that the cause of otosclerosis is related to changes that occur in the tissues of the fissula ante fenestram is unlikely according to the studies of Guild[18,19] and Bretlau[57] because (1) otosclerosis histologically indistinguishable from that occur- ring in the site of predilection can and does origi- nate in parts of the otic capsule far removed from the fissula antefenestram, and (2) at least some of the otosclerotic areas anterior to the oval window, when still small, are not in any contact with any portion of the fissula.

### Unilateral and Bilateral Otosclerosis

Unilateral otosclerosis has been found in 25 to 30 percent of sectioned temporal bones pairs.[18,19,38] Bilateral symmetry of the otosclerotic foci is usually present in persons with bilateral otoscle- rosis,[18] although the extent and the activity of the lesions may differ.[18,19]

### Activity of the Focus

It is not unusual for an otosclerotic focus to con- tain both histologically active and quiescent re- gions. Opinions differ about the age when foci be- come quiescent.[58] In a histopathologic examination of stapes obtained at surgery, Iyer and Gristwood[59] found (1) that the earlier the age of onset of hearing loss, the greater the probability of diffuse, severe, and active otosclerotic involvement of the foot- plate; (2) that two-thirds of cases with severe and diffuse footplate otosclerosis had signs of active disease; and (3) that healing of the active focus might not always occur, despite a long duration of symptoms.

## Stapedial Ankylosis

Although the majority of otosclerotic lesions develop in the ante fenestral area of the labyrinthine capsule, it is a remarkable and fortunate circumstance that only about one in ten of the lesions in this location causes ankylosis of the stapes. As the otosclerotic focus enlarges, it involves and replaces the cartilage at the margin of the oval window. New bone makes its appearance in the annular ligament and eventually produces bony ankylosis of the stapes. Otosclerotic changes appear in the stapes footplate in varying degrees, mainly at the anterior pole. The otosclerotic lesion can extend posteriorly along the superior and inferior margins of the oval window producing exostoses, which can severely narrow the oval window niche as well as invading the annular ligament and footplate. The focus often grasps the base of the anterior crus when it invades the anterior pole of the stapedial footplate, and the otosclerotic bone may grow into the base of the anterior crus. In some cases, the whole footplate becomes diffusely and greatly thickened by otosclerosis when the focus is primarily in the footplate. Expansion of the footplate then causes it to become wedged into the oval window. In other cases, the whole oval window niche is obliterated by otosclerotic bone. Fixation of the stapes can also result from an otosclerotic focus distorting the contours of the oval window to produce jamming, subluxation, or fibrous immobilization of the footplate.

## Hearing Impairment: Conductive, Sensorineural, and Mixed

Increasing stiffness of the stapediovestibular articulation when it is invaded by the otosclerotic focus leads in most cases to a progressive conductive impairment of hearing. Most cases of stapedial otosclerosis are also accompanied or followed by sensorineural hearing losses, which can be greater than what would be expected from age alone. There is still a striking discrepancy between the supposedly frequent occurrence of sensorineural hearing losses in patients suffering from clinical otosclerosis and the scarcity of histologic evidence on light microscopy to explain such changes.

Schuknecht and Kirchner,[50] from a study of temporal bones with otosclerosis, have concluded that the sensorineural hearing loss that accompanies otosclerosis is almost always caused by pathologic changes unrelated to the otosclerotic lesion. Only in a few rare cases of otosclerosis was the lesion responsible for the sensorineural hearing loss, and in these cases, the pathologic changes were severe and the hearing loss was profound.

Convincing histologic evidence has been presented by many other investigators to show that severe and extensive involvement of the labyrinthine capsule by active otosclerosis not only fixes the stapes footplate but also frequently causes profound sensorineural hearing losses. Pathologic involvement of endosteum or spiral ligament in proximity to the focus has been associated with observed vascular communications between vessels of the focus and those of the inner ear, degenerative changes in the spiral ligament, stria vascularis, organ of Corti or cochlear neurons, rupture of the cochlear duct, obliteration of both windows, and extensive lamellar bone formation in the scala tympani.[60-65]

Causse and colleagues[66-70] have produced evidence for an enzymatic concept to explain the bone destruction and the sensorineural deterioration in otospongiosis. They have established statistical correlations between measurements of trypsin, $\alpha_1$-antitrypsin, and $\alpha_2$-macroglobulin in samples of perilymph removed at stapedectomy in hundreds of patients, and the audiometric progression of the bone conduction audiogram over 1 to 2 years.

In otosclerosis, a breakdown in the normal protease-inhibitor equilibrium occurs, which allows free trypsin and lysosomal proteases to act on the hair cells with consequent depression of cochlear function. The trypsin is inhibited by $\alpha_1$-antitrypsin and $\alpha_2$-macroglobulin. The sensorineural deterioration is said to be directly proportional to the level of trypsin activity and inversely proportional to the levels of $\alpha_1$-antitrypsin and $\alpha_2$-macroglobulin. Sensorineural deterioration was present in 21 percent of 48 patients who had low perilymph concentrations of trypsin (less than $4.5\,\mu g/ml$) and severely in 97 percent of 37 patients who had high perilymph concentrations of trypsin (greater than $7.4\,\mu g/ml$).

## Macroscopic Features of Otosclerotic Focus in Middle Ear

In cases of stapedial ankylosis, the focus of otosclerosis can often be seen with the aid of the operating microscope at the time of stapes surgery. The site of predilection is on the promontory in front of the oval window, and from there the focus passes backward to embrace the anterior crus and anterior pole of the stapes footplate. The otosclerotic lesion appears as a sharply demarcated area of chalky white bone, which contrasts with the normal yellowish bone of the promontory or with the thin bluish bone of the normal stapedial footplate. The mucoperiosteum overlying the lesion may be thin, delicate, and relatively avascular when the disease is inactive, or thickened and highly vascularized when the focus is active.

## Classification of the Footplate Lesion

The macroscopic appearance of the focus around the oval window niche and in the stapes footplate can be classified into several categories of generally increasing severity and surgical difficulty. During stapedectomy, it is not always possible to see the precise localization or morphology of the lesion that fixes the stapes, although in the great majority of cases it is possible to classify them according to the pathologic degree of involvement of the stapes footplate and oval window niche. The classification found most useful by the author is presented here. The figures and percentages relate to 1,013 consecutive surgical cases of stapedial otosclerosis operated on at Adelaide, South Australia.

**Ligamentous Fixation.** A thin blue footplate becomes impacted against the posterior wall of the oval window niche by an expanding focus in front, or the annular ligament at the anterior pole becomes calcified or invaded by new bone. The footplate is easily and often inadvertently mobilized (40 patients; 3.9 percent).

**Anterior Polar Focus (small).** Anterior polar focus involving less than half the footplate area but involving the anterior crus. The remaining portion of the footplate remains thin and blue (504 patients; 49.8 percent).

**Anterior Polar Focus (Large).** The anterior polar focus invades the anterior half, or more, of the footplate area (37 patients; 3.7 percent).

**Posterior Polar Focus.** This relatively rare condition can involve less or more than half of the footplate area (13 patients; 1.3 percent).

**Bipolar Foci.** In this type, foci at both anterior and posterior poles of the footplate leave a thin blue intercrural area (52 patients; 5.1 percent).

**Marginal Obliteration, Annular Focus or Doughnut Footplate.** There is marked annular thickening of the footplate, often with obliteration of the stapediovestibular joint, leading to a doughnut footplate with a small thin central area (46 patients; 4.5 percent).

**Thin Biscuit Footplate.** The footplate is diffusely opaque and thickened to less than 0.5 mm. It is easily punctured by a sharp needle or hook (83 patients; 8.2 percent).

**Solid Delineated, Thick Biscuit, or Rice Grain Footplate.** The focus of otosclerosis in this type begins in the footplate, which becomes diffusely and often greatly thickened to between 1.0 and 1.5 mm. Expansion of the footplate within the oval window niche leads to fixation, but the margins of the oval window are usually well-delineated and normal due to the presence of an intact annular ligament. Surgical extraction of this footplate, when accomplished, leaves a well-defined smooth edge to the oval window frame. When fixation of the footplate is less than expected, inadvertent mobilization can occur during attempts to transect it, unless special care is taken (125 patients; 12.3 percent).

**Solid, Partly Obliterated Footplate.** In this type, the footplate is diffusely and greatly thickened and there is a rim of delineation, which is often spurious over 25 to 50 percent of the circumference, the remainder of the margin being obliterated. A rare variant (5 patients) is the case of a thick solid footplate surrounded by a complete gutter of delineation, the spurious nature of which is only revealed after surgical attempts to bisect and remove either half of the footplate fail because of obliteration deeper in (52 patients; 5.1 percent).

**Truly Obliterated Footplate.** The footplate is greatly thickened and diffusely replaced by a mass of otosclerotic bone, which fills in the oval window niche in varying degree, obliterating the margins of the window niche so that they are not identifiable, and partially burying the crura of the stapes (61 patients; 6.0 percent).

The various categories of footplate pathology are depicted diagrammatically in Figures 33-1 and

## Minor Degrees of Footplate Otosclerosis

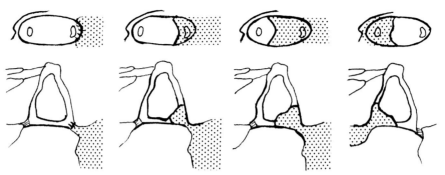

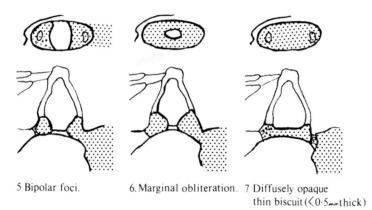

1. Ligamentous fixation.　2. Anterior pole focus (less than ½ footplate)　3. Anterior pole focus (more than ½ footplate)　4. Posterior pole focus.

## Intermediate Degrees of Footplate Otosclerosis

5 Bipolar foci.　6. Marginal obliteration.　7 Diffusely opaque thin biscuit (< 0·5 mm thick)

## Severe Degrees of Footplate Otosclerosis

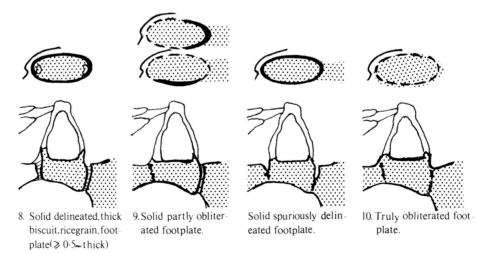

8. Solid delineated, thick biscuit, ricegrain, foot-plate (≥ 0·5 mm thick)　9. Solid partly obliterated footplate.　Solid spuriously delineated footplate.　10. Truly obliterated foot-plate.

**Fig. 33-1.** Diagram of various categories of stapedial footplate involvement in otosclerosis. (Gristwood RE: Deafness from Otosclerosis in South Australia. Ch.M. Thesis, University of Edinburgh, Edinburgh, 1981.)

33-2, and a representative microphotograph of stapedial otosclerosis is shown in Figure 33-3.

## The Narrowed Oval Window Niche

The oval window may be narrowed by peripheral otosclerotic foci forming exostoses which substantially overlap and narrow the niche. This should not be classified as obliterative otosclerosis. The pathologic classification of a case is determined by the degree of involvement of the footplate in the otosclerotic lesion. A narrow niche may occur with a relatively thin footplate or with a severly thickened footplate. In the author's material in South Australia, the oval window niche was narrowed to less than 0.8 mm in 4.1 percent of cases of otosclerosis, and a slitlike niche was rare, occurring in 0.3 percent. The presence of narrowing of the niche or promontory exostoses is more often recorded in the minor forms of footplate pathology than in the severe forms of lesion, possibly due to the relative ease with which narrowing of the niche can be observed in cases with a thin footplate[10] (Fig. 33-4).

## Thickness of the Stapes Footplate

The normal stapes footplate is thin and bluish in appearance and varies from 0.1 to 0.2 mm in thickness in the intercrural region. Of the 1,013 South

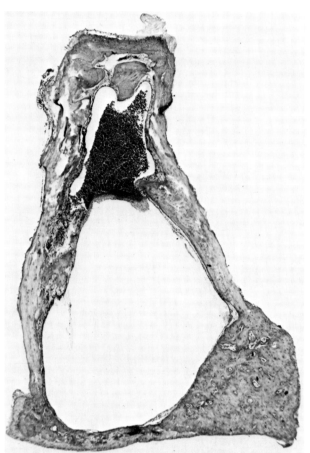

**Fig. 33-3.** Stapedial otosclerosis, anterior pole focus. (×30.) Specimen from a 29-year-old white woman with progressive impairment of hearing for 2 years. Marked expansion of anterior pole of footplate by otosclerotic bone with filling in of angle between base and anterior crus. The otosclerotic focus shows features of quiescence — acidophilic woven bone with increased numbers of osteocytes (but without osteoblasts or osteoclasts) and numerous small vascular spaces. The promontory wall in front of the oval window was also involved by otosclerosis in this patient, but the anterior pole is sharply delineated in this specimen, which mobilized easily and inadvertently. (Gristwood RE: Deafness from Otosclerosis in South Australia. Ch.M. Thesis, University of Edinburgh, Edinburgh, 1981.)

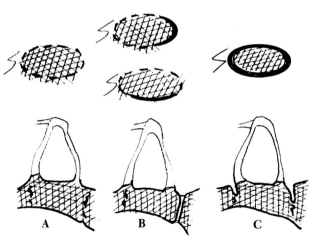

**Fig. 33-2.** Diagram illustrating three variants of the obliterated oval window niche. **(A)** Truly obliterated footplate. **(B)** Partially obliterated footplate in which the limited segment of delineation may be polar or adjacent to the promontory. **(C)** Spuriously delineated footplate. (Gristwood RE, Venables WN: Otosclerotic obliteration of oval window niche: An analysis of the results of surgery. J Laryngol Otol 89:1185, 1975.)

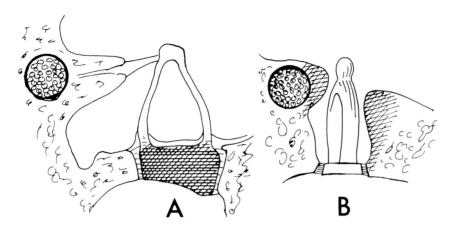

**Fig. 33-4.** Diagram illustrating **(A)** the solid, delineated, "thick-biscuit" or "rice-grain" footplate, and **(B)** oval window niche narrowed by exostoses of promontory and facial canal. Both conditions are excluded by definition from the case of obliterative otosclerosis. (Gristwood RE, Venables WN: Otosclerotic obliteration of oval window niche: An analysis of the results of surgery. J Laryngol Otol 89:1185, 1975.)

Australian otosclerotic footplates analyzed, 692 (68.3 percent) in footplate pathology categories 1 to 6 had some thin area of blueness of the footplate, whereas 319 (31.5 percent) had footplates that presented as diffusely thickened, opaque, and white. Approximately one-half of the thickened footplates were less than 1 mm in depth and half were 1 mm or more in thickness. Seventeen footplates were 2 mm or more in thickness.

### Narrowing and Obliteration of the Round Window Niche

Complete obliteration of the round window niche by otosclerosis is extremely rare (0.2 percent), and severe narrowing of the niche is not common (1.6 percent). In cases with total obliteration of the round window niche, the site of the niche is represented by a mere dimple on the promontory. Only two patients in the author's series were found with this condition. Both patients had greatly thickened footplates (one obliterated and one delineated); both had profound deafness and bone conduction thresholds were not measurable in either patient at the maximum output of the audiometer. Neither patient achieved any hearing improvement after stapes surgery.

### Otosclerotic Obliteration of the Labyrinthine Vestibule

Massive proliferation of the otosclerotic focus with invasion and obliteration of the vestibule is fortunately a most singular phenomenon because it

precludes all possibility of a surgical remedy. Six such bones have been described by Nager and Fraser.[65]

### Mucoperiosteum of Oval Window Niche

The mucoperiosteum overlying the otosclerotic footplate and lining the walls of the oval window niche varies greatly in thickness and vascularity. Mucoperiosteum can be classified at the time of stapes surgery into four groups[10]:

1. Thin, delicate, and transparent and essentially avascular (86 percent)
2. Thin and delicate but considerably congested (2.2 percent)
3. Thickened and avascular (5.4 percent)
4. Thickened and highly vascularized with leashes and loops of abnormally dilated vessels apparent therein over stapes footplate and adjacent promontory (5.9 percent)

There is a highly significant association ($P < .00001$) between stapedial footplate pathology and the characteristics of the mucoperiosteum lining oval window niche and promontory. Thickening of the mucoperiosteum is present in about 40 percent and increased vascularity in about 25 percent of patients with severe footplate otosclerosis. By contrast, patients with minor footplate pathology have thickened mucoperiosteum in 1 percent and excessive vascularity in 2.7 percent.

## Schwartze's Sign

Mucosal congestion on the promontory of the middle ear produces the Schwartze sign of a flamingo pink flush seen through a transparent tympanic membrane. Schwartze's sign has a clear tendency to be associated with abnormal mucoperiosteum, vascular or thickened or both, in the oval window niche or on the adjacent promontory.

## Footplate Pathology and Other Variables

The mean average B.C. thresholds (0.5 to 2 kHz) show slight differences (6.5 dB) among groups, but there is no clear-cut evidence that the more severe grades of footplate pathology have higher average BC thresholds ($P < 0.05$). The mean average AC thresholds (0.5 to 2 kHz) vary significantly with the severity of footplate pathology from 66 dB for ligamentous fixations to 82 dB for obliterated niches ($P < .00001$). The mean average B/A gaps (0.5 to 2 kHz) increase with the severity of the footplate lesion from 31 dB for ligamentous fixations to 42 dB for obliterative cases ($P < .00001$).

In unilateral otosclerosis, the incidence of severe footplate pathology is much less than that of bilateral cases, whereas the incidence of minor footplate pathology is correspondingly increased. Both unilaterality and minor forms of footplate pathology are associated with a later age of onset.

## Comparison of Footplate Pathology in Both Ears

There is a strong tendency to bilateral symmetry of the footplate lesion in patients who have both ears operated on for clinical otosclerosis, although this tendency is not absolute. (Table 33-1)

## Geographic Variations in Stapedial Footplate Pathology

There appear to be wide geographic variations in the pattern of stapedial footplate pathology among continents and among different regions of the same continent. This is illustrated in Table 33-2.

# EPIDEMIOLOGY OF OTOSCLEROSIS

## Definition

Epidemiology is the study of a disease in relation to populations and is an integral part of its basic description.[84] Epidemiology deals with the prevalence, distribution, and control of a disease in a population at risk.

The systematic study of geographic variations in the incidence and prevalence of otosclerosis in population groups living in different environments and separated from one another by race; religion or culture; social, economic, or hygienic standards; and occupation may provide clues to its etiology. There are well-known differences in prevalance of otosclerosis, in age of onset of hearing loss, and in the severity of the pathologic process as it affects the stapedial footplate and sensorineural hearing function. As in most other diseases, genetic, socio-economic, climatic, and geophysical factors must be considered.

**Table 33-1. Comparison of the Footplate Involvement in First and Second Ears of 265 Patients Who Had Both Ears Operated on for Clinical Otosclerosis**

| Footplate Pathology of 1st Ear | Footplate Pathology of Second Ear | | | |
|---|---|---|---|---|
| | Minor | Intermediate | Severe | Totals |
| Minor | 112 | 8 | 7 | 127 |
| Intermediate | 24 | 24 | 11 | 59 |
| Severe | 12 | 12 | 55 | 79 |
| Totals | 148 | 44 | 73 | 265 |

$\chi^2 = 153.3$ on 4 d.f. Significant at .00001 level.
(Gristwood RE· Deafness from Otosclerosis in South Australia. Ch. M. Thesis, University of Edinburgh, Edinburgh, 1981.)

Table 33-2. Geographic Variation in Footplate Pathology

| Study | Country | N | Obliterated (%) | Solid Delineated (%) |
|---|---|---|---|---|
| **United States** | | | | |
| House[a] | California | 800 | 1.2 | 10.3 |
| Farrior[72] | Florida | 700 | 4.5 | 8.0 |
| McGee[73] | Michigan | 555 | 5.7 | N.A. |
| Shea[74] | Tennessee | 1,000 | 4.4 | 10.2 |
| Robinson[75] | Rhode Island | 4,761 | 3.0 | 23.0 |
| Sooy[a] | California | 5,000 | 2.0 | 7.0 |
| **Europe** | | | | |
| Cawthorne[a] | Great Britain | 250 | 6.0 | 22.0 |
| Morrison[76] | Great Britain | 510 | 10.2 | 19.4 |
| Tos[77] | Denmark | 200 | 1.0 | 7.5 |
| Palva[a] | Finland | 250 | 1.6 | 5.6 |
| Plester[a] | Germany | 1,000 | 2.3 | 11.5 |
| Causse[78] | France | 9,570 | 6.7 | 9.2 |
| Feenstra[a] | Netherlands | 100 | 10.0 | 9.0 |
| **South America** | | | | |
| Chiossone[a] | Venezuela | 220 | 4.1 | 10.5 |
| de la Fuente et al[79] | Chile | 119 | 0.9 | 20.1 |
| Velasco[80] | Chile | 135 | 4.5 | 25.1 |
| **Australia** | | | | |
| Halliday[81] | New South Wales | 500 | 6.2 | 25.2 |
| Packer[a] | West Australia | 1,173 | 2.5 | 10.4 |
| Willis[82] | Victoria | 1,450 | 6.3 | 24.3 |
| Gristwood et al[83] | South Australia | 1,013 | 11.2 | 12.3 |

[a] Personal communications, 1965–1984.

## Incidence and Prevalence

It is important to emphasize the distinction between the terms incidence and prevalence. Incidence is the rate at which new cases appear in the population. Prevalance is that fraction of the population affected at a particular time. Since spontaneous recovery from otosclerotic deafness is not possible, and since the condition does not appreciably reduce life expectancy, even a small incidence can accumulate to a relatively large prevalence.

## Prevalence of Otosclerosis in Whites

There is apparently striking evidence that the prevalence of otosclerosis varies enormously in different racial groups and populations. This is apparent even allowing for the scarcity of available data and for the inevitably anecdotal nature of many reports. It appears to be generally established, however, that otosclerosis is frequent only among white populations, uncommon among Mongoloid populations, and extremely rare in black populations (the latter including the black population of the United States, which evidently shares an environment with a large and susceptible white population).

Altmann, et al.[85] combined the data of Engstrom[49] and Guild,[18] which showed that 6 out of 601 white individuals 10 years and older, whose temporal bones had been obtained at autopsy and serially sectioned, had stapedial ankylosis from otosclerosis. This 1 percent prevalence of stapes fixation has generally been accepted among those of European populations. Hinchcliffe,[86,87] on the basis of otologic and audiometric examination of two random samples of the rural population of Great Britain, stratified for ages and sex, found a similar figure.

However, Morrison,[22] reporting on a genetic and clinical study undertaken during the years 1961 to 1964 in the east of London concluded that the prevalence of otosclerosis in adults in east London could not be much higher than 3/1,000.

Hall[88] found that the prevalence of otosclerosis in Norway varied between counties but overall was approximately 3/1,000.

In Lithuania, Gapany-Gapanavicius[24] gives the prevalence of otosclerosis for the age period of risk (16 to 50 years) as 0.44/1,000 (males 0.26 and females 0.58/1,000).

Pearson et al.[89] in their study of the population of Rochester, Minnesota over a 20-year period, reported a total of 126 cases of clinical otosclerosis and estimated the prevalence to be at least 2.4/1,000 (1.51 for males, and 3.13 for females) over all age groups, with a maximum value of 10.2/1,000 for females in the age group 50 to 59 years, and 5.2/1,000 for males in the age group 60 to 69 years.

More recently, Gristwood and Venables[90] estimated a lower limit for the prevalence of clinical otosclerosis within each age group in South Australia, and observed that (1) for women between 45 and 64 years in the 1966 census year, the prevalence for otosclerosis was at least 1 percent; (2) for men between 50 and 64 years, the prevalence was at least 0.5 percent; and (3) for age groups 35 to 70 years the ratio of women to men was very close to 2 : 1.

It is important to emphasize that the figures of Gristwood and Venables are underestimates of the true prevalence of otosclerosis in the South Australian community. (Fig. 33-5)

The foregoing reports indicate marked geographic variations in the prevalence of otosclerosis in those of European origin. However, even conservative estimates of prevalence in different communities can be expected to vary widely for quite different reasons. In a situation where the condition can only be confirmed after elective surgery, some variation must be attributed to different social, cultural, and economic conditions of the community studied. Also, some authors candidly admit that their estimates are based on more-or-less subjective extrapolation from the available data. Comparison of the results of several regional studies where the information is given is presented in Tables 33-3 and 33-4. The apparent decline in the recorded prevalence of otosclerosis with advancing years evident in Table 33-3 must to some extent be due to a reluctance on the part of some elderly patients to undergo surgery on the ear.

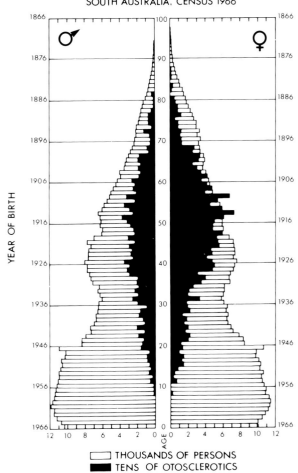

**AGE DISTRIBUTION OF THE POPULATION**
SOUTH AUSTRALIA, CENSUS 1966

☐ THOUSANDS OF PERSONS
■ TENS OF OTOSCLEROTICS

**Fig 33-5.** Surgical cases of otosclerosis in South Australia related to population in 1966 census, by age and sex. (Gristwood RE, Venables WN: Otosclerosis in South Australia. Clin Otolaryngol 9:221, 1984.)

## Prevalence of Otosclerosis in Other Races

Data on the prevalence of otosclerosis in blacks are scarce, even for those living in the United States. In examining serially sectioned temporal bones from cadavers of 576 American blacks, Guild[18] found that histologic otosclerosis was rare (5 cases = 0.9 percent). It has not been observed in the Mabaans of Sudan or among the Bantus of central, southern and eastern Africa.[85]

Table 33-3.   Geographic Variations in Prevalence of Otosclerosis
(Rates per 1,000 Population)

| Age Groups (Years) | Morrison[22] (Lond) | Gristwood & Venables[90] (South Australia) | | | Pearson et al.,[89] (Rochester[89] Minnesota) | | |
|---|---|---|---|---|---|---|---|
| | | Both Sexes | M | F | Both Sexes | M | F |
| 30–34 | 2.15 | 3.48 | 3.2 | 3.8 | 1.48 | 1.45 | 1.50 |
| 35–39 | 1.94 | 4.50 | 3.4 | 5.7 | | | |
| 40–44 | 1.85 | 4.94 | 3.6 | 6.4 | 6.01 | 5.70 | 6.29 |
| 45–49 | 1.85 | 5.83 | 3.6 | 8.2 | | | |
| 50–54 | 1.80 | 7.24 | 5.0 | 9.6 | 7.30 | 3.62 | 10.20 |
| 55–59 | 1.29 | 7.39 | 4.8 | 10.0 | | | |
| 60–64 | 1.38 | 6.57 | 4.8 | 8.3 | 8.22 | 5.17 | 10.33 |
| 65–69 | 0.99 | 5.86 | 4.0 | 7.4 | | | |
| 70–74 | 0.57 | 3.20 | 3.0 | 3.3 | 6.75 | 2.46 | 8.98 |
| 75–79 | 0.77 | 3.05 | 2.4 | 3.5 | | | |
| 80+ | 0.53 | 1.02 | 0.74 | 1.18 | 5.00 | 2.80 | 5.94 |

(Gristwood RE, Venables WN: Otosclerosis in South Australia. Clin Otolaryngol 9:221, 1984.)

Otosclerosis is also extremely rare in the North American Indian.[91-93] According to Tato and Tato[94] the prevalence of otosclerosis in 11,000 South American Indians from Bolivia, Paraguay, and Peru was 0.3/1,000.

Otosclerosis is generally considered to be a common disease in India,[95] but figures for prevalence are not available.

Otosclerosis is considered to be relatively rare in Chinese, but data on prevalence are not available. Choa[85] found 100 cases of otosclerosis (suitable for stapes surgery) in 1,700 southern Chinese who had ear disease and lived in Hong Kong. Joseph and Frazer[96] found 11 Chinese otosclerotics in 220 cases of clinical otosclerosis in their practice in Hawaii.

The prevalence of otosclerosis in Japanese is unknown but Joseph and Frazer[96] found that otosclerosis is not rare among Japanese living in Hawaii. They found 40 Japanese otosclerotics in 220 patients with the disease. They calculated that otosclerosis was 2.1 times as common in whites as in Japanese.

## Environmental Trace Elements and Otosclerosis

Several relationships between environmental trace elements and human disease have been postulated, for example, between zinc and stomach cancer, between iodine deficiency and goiter, and between fluoride concentration in drinking water and mottled enamel and dental caries.[97]

Daniel[98] described an apparently low "incidence" of otosclerosis in a high (1.9 mg/L) fluoride

Table 33-4.   Regional Estimates of Prevalence of Otosclerosis in Whites
(Rates per 1,000 of Population)

| Age Group (Years) | London[22] (United Kingdom) | Rochester[89] (USA) | Adelaide[90] (South Australia) | Lithuania[24] |
|---|---|---|---|---|
| 39–49 | | | | |
| All cases | 2.00[a] | 3.44 | 4.70 | 0.44 |
| Males | 1.69 | 3.22 | 3.43 | 0.26 |
| Females | 2.47 | 3.66 | 6.05 | 0.58 |
| 50–69 | | | | |
| All cases | 1.52[a] | 7.70 | 6.89 | NA |
| Males | NA | 4.26 | 4.74 | NA |
| Females | NA | 10.21 | 9.00 | NA |
| Number of patients | 262 | 126 | 3,138 | 974 |

[a] Approximate figure only.
NA, not available.
(Gristwood RE, Venables WN: Otosclerosis in South Australia. Clin Otolaryngol 9:221, 1984.)

area of Texas and a high "incidence" of clinical otosclerosis in a low (0.6 mg/L) fluoride area of Missouri. He concluded that the "incidence" of footplate otosclerosis was significantly greater (4:1) in the low fluoride area. Daniel's "incidence" rates are not based on whole population studies, so his figures remain ambiguous in establishing whether there is a real difference in the prevalence of otosclerosis in high and low fluoride areas. Nevertheless, the idea that the fluoride ion might affect the distribution of clinical otosclerosis is interesting, in view of the high prevalence of otosclerosis in South Australia and the low fluoride content (0.1 to 0.3 mg/L) of the drinking water in the most populated parts of the country during the period of Gristwood and Venables' study, and deficiencies of other trace elements in the soil.[90]

## CLINICAL FEATURES OF OTOSCLEROSIS

### Introduction

The focus of otosclerosis in the enchondral layer of the otic capsule is asymptomatic until it becomes sufficiently large to involve the annular ligament and stapes footplate. Increasing stiffness and eventual ankylosis of the stapediovestibular joint lead to a progressive conductive hearing impairment, which is often bilateral but not always symmetrical. It is now certain that some cases of otosclerosis involving the cochlea and in which fixation of the stapes has not taken place can present with progressive loss of hearing of pure sensorineural type, but the proportion of such cases is believed (on the basis of the best histologic evidence) to be small.

Typically, the hearing impairment of otosclerosis is noted in early adult life, is insidious and painless in onset, and progresses slowly. There can be marked individual variation, some cases becoming stationary and remaining so for decades, whereas in others, the hearing loss continues to advance relentlessly and sometimes rapidly from the start leading to profound deafness. The onset of symptoms is rare in childhood and after the age of 50 years. Affected individuals are otherwise remark-

ably healthy, and have normal tympanic membranes and patent eustachian tubes. A small proportion of cases (3.8 percent) show a flamingo pink flush through the tympanic membrane, the positive Schwartze sign, due to congestion of promontory mucoperiosteum overlying an active and often rapidly advancing focus of disease.[10] It is more common in young and in male patients. Functional examination in cases with stapes fixation elicits the well-known Bezold's triad: loss of hearing for lower tones, prolongation of hearing by bone conduction, and a negative Rinne test.

In advanced cases, sensorineural deafness is commonly added to the existing middle ear deafness, giving the picture of a mixed middle ear and inner ear deafness. Although most cases presenting for diagnosis are bilateral, otosclerosis may occur unilaterally in from 10 to 20 percent of cases. Tinnitus accompanies the deafness in about two-thirds of the patients, and often patients affected bilaterally can apparently hear better against background noise, the phenomenon of Willis' paracusis. The voice usually remains quiet and well modulated in the deafness from otosclerosis until severe sensorineural deterioration occurs. Recurring transitory sensations of giddiness on stooping are reported by about one-fourth of patients with otosclerosis, but such symptoms may disappear for months on end or even permanently.

Females appear to be affected twice as frequently as males,[21,24,78,89,90,99,100] and a positive familial history of hearing loss in near relatives is obtained in about 50 percent of the cases. Only Larsson[21] and Morrison and Bundey[23] provide evidence for a sex ratio of unity. Between 20 and 65 percent of female otosclerotic patients who bear children experience subjective deterioration of hearing during the later months of one or more of their pregnancies or shortly after parturition.

In rare cases, otosclerosis is associated with fragilitas ossium and blue sclera.

### Sex Distribution in Otosclerosis

In two epidemiologic investigations[89,90] into the prevalence of clinical otosclerosis not only was the rate for women shown to increase with increasing age from about 6/1,000 in the 40- to 49-year-old age group, to about 9 or 10/1,000 in the 50- to

69-year-old age group, but also the rate for men was about half that for women.

## Familial Pattern in Otosclerosis

A familial history of hearing impairment in siblings, parents, or other near relatives is generally reported to be present in about half of the cases of clinical otosclerosis. A full discussion of the genetics of otosclerosis is given in Chapter 30. In summary, there is strong evidence of an autosomal dominant inheritance, with penetrance of the pathologic gene of between 25 and 40 percent.

## Age at Onset of Hearing Impairment

The age at onset of hearing impairment due to otosclerosis is not always easy to determine because the onset is usually gradual and the patient may not become aware of the loss of hearing for some time, especially if only one ear is affected. There is wide variation among individuals, but the general impression is that in the majority of cases the age of onset is between puberty and 45 years.

## Juvenile Otosclerosis

Guild[18] concluded that otosclerosis seldom begins to develop before the age of 5 years. Most authors agree that hearing impairment from clinical otosclerosis under the age of 11 years occurs in less than 2 percent of their cases, while onset under the age of 15 or 16 is found in from 3 to 8.5 percent. Of South Australian cases, 14.6 percent developed onset of symptoms before the age of 16 years.[10]

The importance of an early age of onset of clinical otosclerosis during the period of active skeletal growth lies in the greatly increased chance of contracting a rapidly progressive lesion with severe and diffuse involvement of the stapedial footplate and obliteration of the oval window niche[83] (Table 33-5).

## Age at Surgery

The age at which patients present for advice and surgical treatment is known with accuracy in several series and appears to be between 30 and 60 years. There is no upper age limit for modern stapes surgery providing the patient is fit and willing.

In the younger age groups not only are smaller numbers of suitable patients available, but most surgeons adopt an attitude of caution for those under the age of 20 years (about 2.5 percent of surgical cases), and especially for children under the age of 12 years (0.2 percent in each of three series).

## Tinnitus in Otosclerosis

The subjective sensation of constant ringing, hissing, buzzing, roaring, or pulsing of variable intensity in one or both ears is a common symptom in otosclerosis. Occasionally, tinnitus may precede the onset of hearing impairment by months or years, especially in the younger person. Fortunately, many patients do not appear to be greatly disturbed by this symptom, which may persist for years subject to periods of comparative ameliora-

**Table 33-5. Incidence of Reported Juvenile Otosclerosis**

| Investigators | N | Incidence of Juvenile Otosclerosis |
|---|---|---|
| Cawthorne[99] (United Kingdom) | 2,000 | 1.9% under 11 yr |
| Wullstein[21] (Germany) | 700 | 8.5% under 16 yr |
| Larsson[21] (Sweden) | 262 | 2.3% under 11 yr |
| | | 8.3% under 16 yr |
| Hajek[101] (Israel) | 135 | 3.7% under 16 yr |
| McKenzie[102] (United Kingdom) | 300 | 2.7% under 15 yr |
| Gapany-Gapanavicius[24] (Lithuania) | 634 | 1.3% under 11 yr |
| | | 4.9% under 16 yr |
| Gristwood[10] (South Australia) | 1,013 | 1.9% under 10 yr |
| | | 14.6% under 16 yr |

tion. Infrequently, the intensity of tinnitus is intolerable and causes more concern to the patient than the deafness. Tinnitus may disappear spontaneously, even after many years, but in many cases it continues unabated and may become louder as the hearing loss progresses. The origin of the tinnitus is not clear. It may arise from pathologic vascularization of the otosclerotic lesion within the labyrinthine capsule. Tinnitus can be present in patients with either conductive or mixed deafness. The formal evaluation of tinnitus is complex and time consuming and requires tests of tinnitus matching and masking which rely on the patient's subjective responses. (See Ch. 63.)

## Paracusis Willisii

Patients with stapedial fixation often have an apparent improvement in hearing for conversation against background noise as when traveling by car, bus, or train or when working in noise. The phenomenon is named after Thomas Willis who, in 1672, reported the case of a woman who could only hear her husband speaking when a drum was beaten. The explanation is that, in the presence of background noise, the speaker (with normal hearing) has to raise the intensity of his own voice, which is heard without distortion by the person conductively deaf.

## Vertigo in Otosclerosis

Vertigo is not a particularly prominent feature of otosclerosis, but about 20 to 25 percent of patients will, if questioned, admit to a slight and transitory sensation of giddiness on stooping. The vertigo is not a constant feature but tends to disappear for weeks or months on end, and to some may never reappear. Rarely, a vague history of giddiness without other aural symptoms may be the presenting symptom in otosclerosis and can precede the onset of hearing loss by intervals of up to 5 years.

Otosclerosis is infrequently associated with attacks of severe episodic rotary vertigo, nausea and vomiting, and a sense of fullness and increased tinnitus in one ear indistinguishable from and probably due to classical Meniere's disorder. Since both otosclerosis and Meniere's disease are common

conditions, it is inevitable that both disorders will occur together at some time in the one patient, as has been demonstrated in temporal bone studies.[53]

Vestibular abnormalities recorded by means of electronystagmography (ENG) are more common in clinical otosclerosis than is generally supposed. Fisch[103] reported on the vestibular function of 66 patients with otosclerosis before and after stapedectomy by means of electronystagmography. In 52 preoperative patients vestibular dysfunction was observed in 15 (28.8 percent), spontaneous nystagmus in 8, and a direction fixed positional nystagmus (Nylen II) in 7. Patients with preoperative vestibular disturbances showed audiometric evidence of more impaired cochlear function in comparison with those patients without vestibular signs. Similar findings are reported by Causse et al.,[78] Meurman et al.,[104] and Virolainen.[105]

Sando et al.[106] reported histologic confirmation of vestibular pathology in two patients with otosclerosis. The findings included apposition of the otosclerotic focus to the superior vestibular nerve, invasion of the cribriform area, degeneration of vestibular nerve fibers adjacent and distal to the otosclerotic focus, degeneration of the sensory epithelium of the cristae of the lateral semicircular ducts, and a basophilic deposit in the ampullary end of the posterior semicircular duct. Gussen[107] has also reported histologic changes in the vestibular labyrinth.

## Unilateral Otosclerosis

Clinically, otosclerosis usually involves both ears, but a number of authors have noted unilateral otosclerosis in a number of their patients, varying from about 2 to 30 percent.

A fundamental question concerns the proportion of patients with unilateral stapedial fixation who will ultimately develop bilateral clinical otosclerosis. In longitudinal study of 186 patients with unilateral stapedial fixation, 29 (15.6 percent) eventually developed the condition in both ears at from 6 months to 11 years after the initial assessment.[10] The great majority of those who developed bilateral disease (25 of 29 cases) first demonstrated audiometric or tuning fork evidence of conductive loss in the opposite ear 5 years or more after the initial diagnosis. It was also found that further losses of both conductive and sensorineural types in the opposite ear were more likely when there was preexisting sensorineural impairment in that ear.

## Pregnancy and Otosclerosis

The worsening of hearing during pregnancy in some cases of otosclerosis has long been known. Before modern techniques of stapes surgery had been developed, young women with otosclerosis were often advised to avoid pregnancy.

Many authors have recorded that between 20 and 65 percent of their female otosclerotic patients who have children found that their hearing deteriorated during the later months of one or more of their pregnancies or shortly after parturition (see Table 33-6).[21,24,76,88,99,100,108-115]

Gristwood and Venables[116] reported on a retrospective study of 479 women with deafness from otosclerosis, who were suitable candidates for surgery and for whom a full history of parity was available, classified according to the number of pregnancies they had had and whether there had been a subjective impression of deterioration of hearing during or immediately after at least one pregnancy. The study confirmed previous reports that hearing may worsen during pregnancy in otosclerotics. The chance that a woman with bilateral otosclerosis reports an aggravation of hearing loss in pregnancy rises sharply from about 33 percent after one pregnancy to about 63 percent after six pregnancies. The rising proportion of patients with deterioration of hearing according to numbers of pregnancies could be partially accounted for by the increased proportion of the patients' adult life spent pregnant. However, pregnancies form strong temporal markers for women, and the more pregnancies the higher the chance of an aggravation of deafness either coinciding fortuitously with a pregnancy, or of being remembered as such. The study provided no strong evidence that pregnancies cause any alteration to the actual footplate pathology of female patients. Until a good matched control group is studied the question remains unresolved.

## AUDIOLOGIC FEATURES OF OTOSCLEROSIS

### Introduction

Persons with otosclerosis can present with varied levels of acuity of hearing, ranging from near normal to near total deafness. Asymptomatic cases of

**Table 33-6.   Reports on Subjective Loss of Hearing in Otosclerosis During Pregnancy**

| Study | Loss with Pregnancy | |
| --- | --- | --- |
|  | No. Cases | Percent Worse |
| Hall[88] | 1,266 | 8.5 |
| Nager[100] | 383 | 29.0 |
| Gapany-Gapanvicius[24] | 338 | 21.6 |
| Elbrond and Jensen[110] | 144 | 23.6 |
| Smith[113] | 73 | 37.0 |
| Walsh[115] | 243 | 43.0 |
| House (cited in ref. 115) | 194 | 45.0 |
| Larsson[21] | 104 | 46.0 |
| Allen[108] | 72 | 48.6 |
| Shambaugh[114] | 475 | 50.0 |
| Guggenheim[112] | NA | 50.0 |
| Morrison[76] | NA | 54.0 |
| Barton[109] | 133 | 55.0 |
| Goethals et al.[111] | 375 | 56.2 |
| Cawthorne[99] | 419 | 63.0 |
| Gristwood and Venables[116] | 479 | 16.0–71.0[a] |

[a] According to whether unilateral or bilateral and to number of pregnancies.

histologic otosclerosis show no evidence of hearing impairment and remain undiagnosed in the living. In clinical or symptomatic otosclerosis increasing stiffness and eventual ankylosis of the stapediovestibular joint by pathologic bone formation leads to insidious onset of hearing impairment, which usually is inexorably progressive and bilateral.

During the earliest stages, stiffness of the annular ligament produces a low-frequency conductive loss of hearing with normal bone conduction (BC) thresholds. The air conduction (AC) curve shows a stiffness tilt sloping upward to the higher frequencies, and there is a minor bone-air gap in the lowest frequencies[117-119] (Fig. 33-6).

As stapedial fixation develops the bone-air gap becomes more pronounced, the AC threshold being elevated over all frequencies to produce a flat curve at about 50 to 60 dB International Standards Organization Zero reference level (ISO).[10] The BC curve no longer accurately depicts the level of cochlear reserve but suffers a mechanical distortion known as the Carhart notch, due to oval window obstruction[117] (Fig 33-7).

In many cases of stapedial otosclerosis, a sensori-

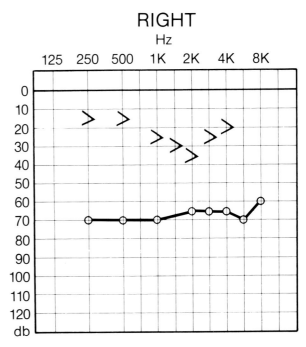

**Fig. 33-7.** Audiogram showing pronounced bone–air gap, flat elevation of air conduction threshold curve to 70-dB level, and distortion of the bone conduction threshold curve (Carhart notch) typical of fully developed stapedial ankylosis from otosclerosis.

neural hearing loss antedates, develops coincidentally with, or develops after the conductive hearing loss. A mixed or combined hearing impairment develops with elevation of both AC and BC thresholds, the AC curve more than the BC, so that the BC curve of the patient lies between the AC curve and the normal threshold level. The AC curve represents the sum of the hearing losses produced independently by the stapedial fixation and by the cochlear lesion[117] (Fig. 33-8).

Sloping high-frequency losses are the most common type of audiometric configuration in sensorineural deterioration associated with classic stapes fixation.[119] The loss of sensorineural function in otosclerosis is markedly age dependent, the older patient showing the greater BC losses.[10] The loss of sensorineural function in many otosclerotics is often much greater than what would be expected from aging processes alone, as has been previously discussed (Fig. 33-9). It has been explained as a consequence of damage to sensorineural elements from substances released into the labyrinthine

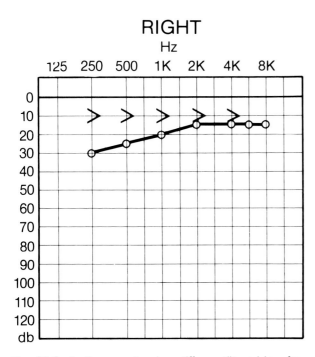

**Fig. 33-6.** Audiogram showing stiffness tilt and low frequency bone–air gap in earliest stages of stapedial otosclerosis.

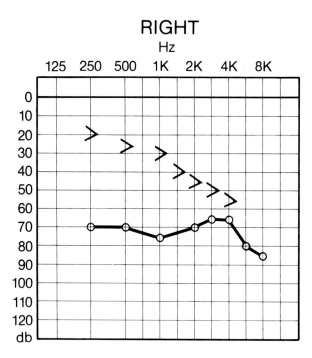

## RIGHT
### Hz

**Fig. 33-8.** Mixed hearing loss in stapedial otosclerosis indicating sensorineural deterioration associated with classic stapes fixation.

fluids from the otosclerotic focus itself. The degree of sensorineural deterioration in otosclerosis may vary in different population groups and geographic localities. Care must be taken not to be misled by an unusually large Carhart notch. Mean air conduction audiograms for a group of otosclerotic patients, classified by age, are shown in Figure 33-10.

## Evaluation of Hearing

Audiologic studies complemented by tuning fork tests and acoustic impedance measurements are an essential part of the investigation of hearing. They are done after aural toilet and otoscopy are completed.

### Tuning Fork Tests

Clinical tuning fork tests — Rinne, Weber, absolute bone conduction, Bing and Gelle — have in no way been outmoded by the advances of audiology but retain their important place in the diagnosis of the type of hearing impairment.

The results of tuning fork tests should always be correlated with the audiometric findings, and any discrepancy between them should cause one to question the accuracy of the audiologic test procedure.

In severe conductive losses a Rinne negative response may be obtained with all tuning forks from 256 to 4096 Hz. In lesser degrees of conductive hearing impairment a Rinne negative response may be demonstrable only with low frequency tuning forks of 128 and 256 Hz. A detailed analysis is given by Gristwood.[10]

### The Audiometric Tests

Basic audiologic tests include the determination of pure tone thresholds for AC and BC, the assessment of the speech reception threshold (SRT) for Spondee word lists, and the maximum discrimination score (PB Max) for a list of phonetically balanced words.

### Acoustic Impedance Measurements

Measurements of acoustic impedance using an electroacoustic impedance meter can provide valuable clinical information including assessment of middle ear pressure, shape and height of the tympanogram, and middle ear muscle reflexes. In otosclerosis middle ear pressures are usually atmospheric and a wide range of compliance values is possible.

Although there are reports of clinical variations in acoustic compliance with otosclerosis,[10,76] they are not sufficiently predictable to be of clinical help. In fixation of the stapes, the stapedius muscle reflex is absent in the affected ear to both ipsilateral and contralateral acoustic stimulation. In the earliest preclinical stages of stapedial otosclerosis in which the AC thresholds show a stiffness tilt and the BC thresholds do not show a Carhart notch,[117] the stapedius reflex is frequently diphasic[120,121] with an on-off effect.

### Bone Conduction Measurements in Prediction

Measurements of BC thresholds in otosclerosis are important to estimate the patient's level of sensorineural reserve, and to predict the postoperative hearing level. The bone-air gap estimates the amount of gain in hearing a patient can expect after

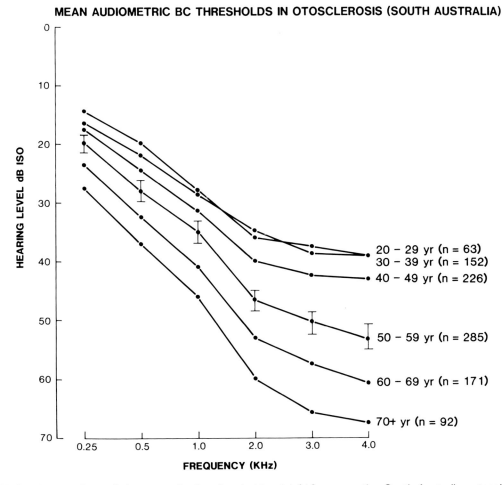

**Fig. 33-9.** Mean audiometric bone conduction thresholds of 1,013 consecutive South Australian otosclerotic patients classified by frequency (kHz) and age group. Note that the 95 percent CI for the means are shown in the 50- to 59-year age group. Differences between groups are significant at the 0.00001 level for all frequencies, above 0.5 kHz (Gristwood RE: Deafness from Otosclerosis in South Australia. Ch.M. Thesis, University of Edinburgh, Edinburgh, 1981.)

successful surgical correction of a lesion in the transmission system of the middle ear, whereas the BC threshold predicts the actual level of hearing that can be anticipated. However, several factors can influence the accuracy of prediction. These include

(a) the many variables that differentiate one otosclerotic lesion from another, as well as one operation from the next and on which the outcome of surgery depends;
(b) an atypical Carhart notch;
(c) the limitations of BC audiometry by which threshold measurements can be in serious

error because of false lateralization of the test tone in the absence of adequate masking, hyperdistractibility in the presence of masking noise, and the fact that masking becomes ineffective when applied to an ear with substantial hearing impairment.[117]

### Carhart Notch Values

The Carhart notch is an artifact of BC testing caused by a stiff ossicular chain, which classically is depressed 5 dB at 500 Hz, 10 dB at 1,000 Hz, 15 dB at 2,000 Hz, and 5 dB at 4,000 Hz.[117,122]

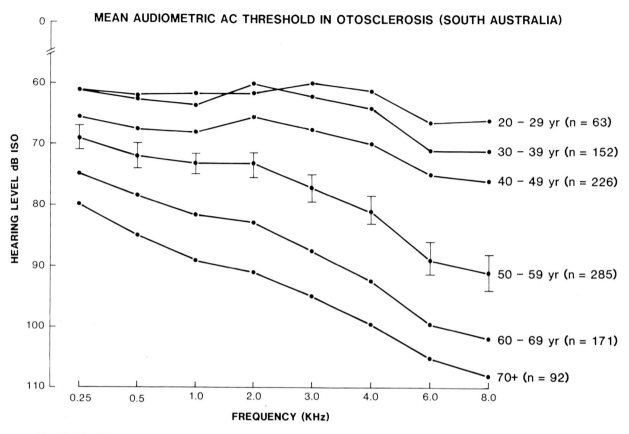

**Fig. 33-10.** Mean audiometric air conduction thresholds at various test frequencies for 1,013 South Australian otosclerotic patients classified by age group. Note that the 95 percent confidence intervals for the means are shown in the 50- to 59-year age group. The differences between means are statistically highly significant (*P* less than 0.00001) for all test frequencies. (Gristwood RE: Deafness from Otosclerosis in South Australia. Ch.M. Thesis, University of Edinburgh, Edinburgh, 1981.)

In a series of 1,013 confirmed otosclerotic patients Gristwood[10] found evidence of a Carhart notch in 54 percent, and no notch in 46 percent of patients. The mean Carhart notch value for all 1,013 patients was 2.4 dB, but if patients without a notch were excluded the mean notch value was 8.7 dB. There was no evidence of an association between the presence of a positive notch value and the average BC level (over 0.5, 1, and 2 kHz.). The mean notch values were not significantly different over various groups of footplate pathology when cases without a notch were excluded from the analysis (F ratio = 1.6 on 9 and 536 df NS).

## Bone-Air Gap in Surgical Cases of Otosclerosis

The mean bone-air gap had its greatest value (49 dB) at the test frequency 0.25 kHz and its smallest value (26-28 dB) at the highest test frequencies 2 to 4 kHz.[102] A bone-air gap of less than 20 dB was exceptional at 0.25 kHz but occurred in one-third of the cases at 2 to 4 kHz. The mean average bone-air gap (0.5 to 2 kHz) increased from 33 dB to about 40 dB, with increasing age of the patient, and from 31 dB in cases with a short history of less than

5 years to about 44 dB in patients with deafness of 50 years duration. There was no sex difference.[10]

### Footplate Pathology, AC Thresholds and Bone-Air Gap

The mean average AC thresholds (0.5 to 2 kHz) varied considerably (by 15.6 dB) over 10 groups of footplate pathology, as did the mean average bone-air gaps (by 11 dB). The less severe forms of footplate pathology have on average somewhat better AC thresholds and smaller bone-air gaps than do the more severe forms of oval window lesions. It seems clear that the severe otosclerotic lesion of longer duration within the oval window increases the rigidity of the stapes footplate, thus raising the AC thresholds and correspondingly increasing the bone-air gap compared with minor footplate lesions.[10]

## RADIOLOGY OF OTOSCLEROSIS

Valvassori,[123] Dulac et al.,[124] and Rovsing[125] have reported on the radiographic interpretation of otosclerosis. Conventional radiography is of little value. Tomography in two projections (AP and lateral) with sections 1 mm in thickness are necessary to demonstrate a focus of otosclerosis at least 2 mm in diameter in the cochlear capsule. The normal cochlear capsule appears as a sharply defined homogeneously dense bony shell outlining the lumen of the cochlea. The views of the capsular regions seen on-end are more informative than those seen on-face because the latter are superimposed on the lumen of the labyrinth. Two types of change are described.

1. *Otospongiotic changes of demineralization.* There is decreased density of the involved portion of the capsule. Changes range from small dehiscences in the normally smooth and homogeneous white line forming the outline of the capsule to larger patchy areas of radiolucency.
2. *Sclerotic changes due to apposition of mature*

*otosclerotic bone increasing the thickness of the capsule.* Roughening and scalloping of the outer and inner margins of the cochlear lumen may be observed. Spongiotic changes are said to correspond to active and vascular foci of otosclerosis, which are commonly observed with a positive Schwartze sign in young patients or in patients with rapidly progressive sensorineural losses.

Applebaum and Shambaugh[126] studied three sets of temporal bones from patients who, during life, had polytomographic examinations suggesting otospongiosis of the cochlea. In one set of temporal bones, no otospongiosis was present. In the other two cases with stapedial otosclerosis, the otospongiosis did not involve the cochlea. These authors concluded that caution must be exercised in the interpretation of subtle polytomographic changes in the cochlear capsule and restraint used in the radiologic diagnosis of pure cochlear otosclerosis until there was evidence of correlation with pathologic material.

Direct multiplanar high-resolution CT of the petrous bone in seven different otoradiologic planes is a recent development. The semilongitudinal plane of Zonneveld[127] is of special interest in visualizing the basal and second turn of the cochlea and the oval and round window niches, and may be of value in diagnosing otospongiotic lesions of these regions.[127,128] Further comments are to be found in Chapter 12.

## DIFFERENTIAL DIAGNOSIS OF STAPEDIAL OTOSCLEROSIS

Several other conditions may resemble otosclerosis in having a normal or near normal tympanic membrane in association with a conductive or mixed hearing impairment. They include congenital stapedial fixation, stapes fixation from tympanosclerosis, osteogenesis imperfecta and Paget's disease, epitympanic fixation of the malleus and incus, and ossicular chain discontinuities or subluxation.

The importance of a detailed history and examination of the structure and mobility of the tympanic membrane with the operating microscope is obvious. Acoustic impedance measurements may provide valuable additional information. In some cases the true diagnosis of the abnormality may only become apparent at exploratory tympanotomy.

## Congenital Stapes Fixation

Congenital stapes fixation is a rare condition. In the adult patient, the differentiation from clinical otosclerosis depends on a history of nonprogressive hearing loss dating from birth or from earliest childhood.[129]

Patients affected bilaterally may have retarded development of speech. The pure-tone audiogram shows a severe flat conductive loss of 60 to 70 dB with good BC thresholds. Successful mobilization of such a congenitally fixed stapes can give long-term hearing gains as refixation is unlikely. If stapedectomy is considered necessary, a preliminary minute needle puncture of the fixed footplate is recommended to rule out the presence of a perilymph gusher. Perilymph flooding is a contraindication to stapedectomy because of the high risk of cochlear deafness.

## Tympanosclerosis

Small plaques of tympanosclerosis are common in the mobile tympanic membrane of patients with a history of previous otitis media. Such changes have been found in about 5 percent of patients with typical stapedial otosclerosis. Infrequently, a patient with an intact and mobile tympanic membrane showing plaques of tympanosclerosis is found to have large middle ear deposits of white amorphous hyaline material on the deep aspect of the drumhead, or involving the oval window region and stapes or the epitympanum. Ossicular fixation with conductive hearing impairment similar to that of otosclerosis is found. Heavy and diffuse tympanosclerotic involvement of the drumhead should alert the surgeon to the possibility of immobilization of any or all of the ossicles in the tympanosclerotic process.

## Fixed Malleus Head Syndrome

Congenital fixation of the malleus head is very rare. More commonly found in 1 to 2 percent of exploratory tympanotomies is acquired fixation of the malleus head by synostosis to one of the epitympanic walls.[131-133] The cause of the condition is unknown. The history of progressive impairment of hearing of conductive or mixed type is similar to that of stapedial otosclerosis. The sensorineural impairment in the higher frequencies has been stressed by several investigators.[134,135] Palpation of the malleus handle through the tympanic membrane or at tympanotomy confirms rigidity of the malleus. Malleus head fixation in association with stapedial otosclerosis has been found in 0.6 percent of 1,281 consecutive cases of stapedectomy.[10] Ensuring that the malleus and incus are not impeded in their normal movement by such coexistent lesions is an essential step before proceeding to stapedectomy.

## Ossicular Discontinuity or Subluxation

Dislocation of the incus after head injury or previous cortical mastoidectomy should be suspected from the history if hearing impairment is unilateral with an audiometric bone-air gap greater than 50 dB and if higher than normal compliance values are obtained on impedance audiometry. Slight scarring of the drumhead is often seen in cases of necrosis of the long process of the incus arising from previous middle ear suppuration.

## Seromucinous Otitis Media

Occasionally, chronic seromucinous otitis media may present with near normal tympanic membranes and be misdiagnosed. The sluggish or absent mobility of the tympanic membrane with Siegle's pneumatic otoscope and tympanometry should make the diagnosis clear.

## Osteogenesis Imperfecta

Osteogenesis imperfecta is a true inherited disorder of collagen characterized by brittle bones. The disorder shows considerable heterogeneity.

The classification of Sillence and colleagues[136] is widely used. Normal-colored sclerae and severe bone disease are often associated. Most patients (80 percent) have mild bone disease inherited as an autosomal-dominant trait (group I) characterized by fragile bones and blue sclerae. The condition is relatively rare, with a prevalence of 3.5/100,000. In these patients, fractures occur mainly in childhood in the preschool-age period, and about 20 percent will show clinical deformity of upper or lower limbs. Eventual stature is near normal. Extraskeletal tissues containing collagen are prominently affected, with blue sclerae, hypermobile joints, thin aortic valves, and rupture of tendons.

A tendency to bruise easily has been observed in 30 to 75 percent of patients. A high proportion (about 40 percent) of adults develop severe hearing impairment of conductive or combined type clinically indistinguishable from that of otosclerosis. Stapes fixation usually occurs from the formation of abnormal new bone, histologically similar to that of otosclerosis. The onset of the deafness is usually in the third decade, but about 20 percent of patients who become deaf have onset of hearing loss before age 20. Stapedectomy can give excellent results in these cases for hearing improvement, but if the long process of the incus is delicate and thin it must be handled with considerable care.

## Paget's Disease of Bone or Osteitis Deformans

This condition can produce progressive hearing loss and vestibular symptoms similar to otosclerosis. The diagnosis is to be suspected in older patients if clinical symptoms develop after the age of 50, especially if there is enlargement of the head and tortuosity of the branches of the superficial temporal artery. Progressive impairment of hearing of sensorineural type is present in up to 50 percent of patients with skull involvement and is often associated with a low-frequency conductive loss. Vestibular dysfunction with dizziness and unsteadiness occurs in about 20 percent of patients.

The pathology of Paget's disease involving the temporal bone has been well described by Davies,[137] Lindsay and Lehman,[138] Schuknecht,[139] Friedmann,[140] and Nager.[141] A number of structural alterations have been described to account for the conductive and sensorineural components of the progressive combined hearing loss that is associated with this condition in 30 to 50 percent of patients. The conductive component mainly involves the low frequencies, is often low grade, and is rarely suitable for stapes surgery even when stapes fixation is found. The results of stapedectomy are disappointing not only because of the predominant high-frequency sensorineural loss but also because other bony abnormalities of epitympanum and other ossicles additional to stapes fixation prejudice the final outcome of surgery.

## REFERENCES

1. Politzer A: Ueber primare Erkrankung der Knochernen Labyrinthkapsel. Ohrenheilkd 25:309, 1894
2. Politzer A: Diseases of the Ear. 5th Ed. Baillíere, London, 1909
3. Siebenmann F: Demonstration mikroskopischer und makroskopischer praparate von otospongiosis progressiva. Int Otol Cong 9:207, 1912
4. Schuknecht HF: Cochlear otosclerosis: An intractable absurdity. J Laryngol Otol 8:[suppl] 81, 1983
5. Glorig A, Gallo R: Comments on sensorineural hearing loss in otosclerosis. p. 63. In Schuknecht HF (ed): Otosclerosis. Henry Ford Hospital International Symposium. Little, Brown, Boston, 1962
6. Schuknecht HF: Panel discussion on sensorineural deafness in otosclerosis: Introductory remarks. Ann Otol Rhinol Laryngol 75:418, 1966
7. Young IM, Mikaelian DO, Trocki IM: Sensorineural hearing level in unilateral otosclerosis. Otolaryngol Head Neck Surg 87:486, 1979
8. Sataloff J, Farb S, Menduke H, Vassallo L: Sensorineural hearing loss in otosclerosis. Trans Am Acad Ophthalmol Otolaryngol 68:243, 1964
9. Linthicum FH, Lalani AS: Sensorineural impairment in unilateral otosclerosis. Ann Otol Rhinol Laryngol 84:11, 1975
10. Gristwood RE: Deafness from Otosclerosis in South Australia. ChM. Thesis, University of Edinburgh, Edinburgh, 1981

11. Hinchcliffe R: The threshold of hearing as a function of age. Acustica 9:303, 1959

12. Glorig A, Nixon J: Hearing loss as a function of age. Laryngoscope 72:1596, 1962

13. Shambaugh GE: Diagnosis and treatment of the otosclerotic lesion. p. 97. In Oto-Rhino-Laryngology: Proceedings of the Ninth International Congress 1969. Excerpta Medica, Amsterdam, 1970

14. Derlacki EL, Valvassori G: Clinical and radiological diagnosis of labyrinthine otosclerosis. Laryngoscope 75:1293, 1965

15. Valsalva AM: De Aure Humana Tractatus. Bononiae: Cap. II, p. 31, 1704 (cited in Nager)

16. Toynbee J: Pathological and surgical observations on the diseases of the ear. Med Chir Trans Med Chir Soc Lond 24:190, 1841

17. Toynbee J: The Diseases of the Ear: Their Nature, Diagnosis and Treatment. HK Lewis, London, 1868

18. Guild SR: Histologic otosclerosis. Ann Otol Rhinol Laryngol 53:246, 1944

19. Guild SR: Incidence, location and extent of otosclerotic lesions. Arch Otolaryngol 52:848, 1950

20. Altmann F: Histopathology and etiology of otosclerosis: A critical review. p. 15. In Schuknecht HF (ed): Otosclerosis. Henry Ford Hospital International Symposium. Little, Brown, Boston, 1962

21. Larsson A: Otosclerosis: A genetic and clinical study. Acta Otolaryngol (Stockh) 154:[suppl] 1, 1960

22. Morrison AW: Genetic factors in otosclerosis. Ann R Coll Surg Engl 41:202, 1967

23. Morrison AW, Bundey SE: The inheritance of otosclerosis. J Laryngol Otol 84:921, 1970

24. Gapany-Gapanavicius B: Otosclerosis: Genetics and Surgical Rehabilitation. Keter, Jerusalem, 1975

25. Fraser GR: Genetical basis for otolaryngological disorders. p. 121. In Hinchcliffe R, Harrison D (ed): Scientific Foundations of Otolaryngology. Heinemann, London, 1976

26. Pedersen U, Madsen M, Lamm LU, Elbrond O: HLA-A, -B, -C antigens in otosclerosis. J Laryngol Otol 97:1095, 1983

27. Ogilvie RF, Hall IS: On the aetiology of otosclerosis. J Laryngol Otol 76:841, 1962

28. Altmann F, Kornfeld M: Osteogenesis imperfecta and otosclerosis: New investigations. Ann Otol Rhinol Laryngol 76:89, 1967

29. Bretlau P, Jorgensen MB: Otosclerosis and osteogenesis imperfecta. Acta Otolaryngol (Stockh) 67:269, 1969

30. Yoo TJ, Stuart JM, Kang AH, et al: Type II collagen autoimmunity in otosclerosis and Meniere's disease. Science 217:1153, 1982

31. Sercer A, Krmpotic J: Further contributions to the development of the labyrinthine capsule. J Laryngol Otol 72:688, 1958

32. Sercer A, Krmpotic J: Thirty years of otosclerosis studies. Arch Otolaryngol 84:598, 1966

33. Wright I: Avascular necrosis of bone and its relation to fixation of a small joint: The pathology and aetiology of "Otosclerosis." J Pathol 123:5, 1977

34. Rebel A, Malkani K, Basle M: Anomalies nucléaires des ostéoclastes de la maladie osseuse de Paget. Nouv Presse Med 3:1299, 1974

35. Anson BJ, Donaldson JA: Surgical Anatomy of the Temporal Bone and Ear. 2nd Ed. WB Saunders, Philadelphia, 1973

36. Engstrom H, Rockert H: Normal histology of the labyrinthine capsule and oval window area. p. 3. In Schuknecht HF (ed): Otosclerosis. Henry Ford Hospital International Symposium. Little, Brown, Boston, 1962

37. Hawke M, Jahn AF: Bone formation in the normal human otic capsule. Arch Otolaryngol 101:462, 1975

38. Nylen B: Histopathological investigations on the localization, number, activity and extent of otosclerotic foci. J Laryngol Otol 63:321, 1949

39. Nager GT: Histopathology of otosclerosis. Arch Otolaryngol 89:341, 1969

40. Ogilvie RF, Hall IS: Observations on the pathology of otosclerosis. J Laryngol Otol 67:497, 1953

41. Chevance LG, Jorgensen MB, Bretlau P, Causse J: Electron microscopic studies of the otosclerotic focus. Acta Otolaryngol (Stockh) 67:563, 1969

42. Chevance LG, Bretlau P, Jorgensen MB, Causse J: Otosclerosis. An electron microscopic and cytochemical study. Acta Otolaryngol (Stockh) 272:[suppl]1, 1970

43. Arslan M, Ricci V: Histochemical investigation of otosclerosis with special regard to collagen disease. J Laryngol Otol 77:365, 1963

44. Albernaz PLM, Covell WP: Otosclerosis of the stapes. A study of the lesion by histochemical procedures and fluorescence microscopy. Laryngoscope 71:1333, 1961

45. Alberti PWRM, Tarkannen JV: Stapedial otosclerosis: Recent histochemical and histopathological observations. Laryngoscope 73:1184, 1963

46. Soifer N, Altmann F, Holdsworth C, Block W: Biochemical studies of otosclerosis. 1. Distribution of serum haptoglobins, esterases, and alkaline and acid phosphatases. Arch Otolaryngol 78:649, 1963

47. Hall IS, Ogilvie RF: The healing process in otosclerosis. Acta Otolaryngol (Stockh) 57:246, 1964

48. Weber M: Otosklerose und Umbau der labyrinthkapsel. Offizin Poeschel und Trepte, Leipzig, 1935

49. Engstrom H: Uber das Vorkommen der Otosklerose nebst experimentellen Studien Uber chirurgische Behandlung der Krankheit. Acta Otolaryngol (Stockh) 43:[suppl]1, 1940

50. Schuknecht HF, Kirchner JC: Cochlear otosclerosis: Fact or fantasy. Laryngoscope 84:766, 1974

51. Bretlau P, Jorgensen MB: Histological investigations of otosclerotic foci. Acta Otolaryngol (Stockh) 65:413, 1968

52. Jorgensen MB, Kristensen HK: Frequency of histological otosclerosis. Ann Otol Rhinol Laryngol 90:83, 1981

53. Black FO, Sando I, Hildyard VH, Hemenway WG: Bilateral multiple otosclerotic foci and endolymphatic hydrops. Ann Otol Rhinol Laryngol 78:1062, 1969

54. Lindsay JR: Histopathology of otosclerosis. Arch Otolaryngol 97:24, 1973

55. Anson BJ: Fissular region of the otic capsule in relation to otosclerosis. Arch Otolaryngol 52:843, 1950

56. Bast TH: Postnatal rebuilding and otosclerotic bone formation in the region of the otic capsule. Arch Otolaryngol 52:882, 1950

57. Bretlau P: Relation of the otosclerotic focus to the fissula ante fenestram. J Laryngol Otol 83:1185, 1969

58. Jorgensen MB, Kristensen HK: Activity of otosclerosis assessed histologically. J Laryngol Otol 81:911, 1967

59. Iyer PV, Gristwood RE: Histopathology of the stapes in otosclerosis. Pathology 16:30, 1984

60. Benitez JT, Schuknecht HF: Otosclerosis: A human temporal bone report. Laryngoscope 72:1, 1962

61. Altmann F: Sensorineural deafness in otosclerosis. Ann Otol Rhinol Laryngol 75:469, 1966

62. Ruedi L: Otosclerotic lesion and cochlear degeneration. Arch Otolaryngol 89:364, 1969

63. Ruedi L, Spoendlin H: Pathogenesis of sensorineural deafness in otosclerosis. Ann Otol Rhinol Laryngol 75:525, 1966

64. Schuknecht HF, Gross CW: Otosclerosis and the inner ear. Ann Otol Rhinol Laryngol 75:423, 1966

65. Nager FR, Fraser JS: On bone formation in the scala tympani of otosclerotics. J Laryngol Otol 53:173, 1938

66. Causse J, Chevance LG, Bel J, Michaux P, et al: L'Otospongiose, maladie enzymatique cellulaire et lysosomale confrontation cyto-clinique. Ann Otolaryngol (Paris) 89:563, 1972

67. Causse J, Chevance LG, Bretlau P, Jorgensen MB, et al: Enzymatic concept of otospongiosis and cochlear otospongiosis. Clin Otolaryngol 2:23, 1977

68. Causse JR, Shambaugh GE, Causse JB, Bretlau P: Enzymology of otospongiosis and NaF therapy. Am J Otol 1:206, 1980

69. Causse J, Shambaugh GE, Chevance LG, Bretlau P: Cochlear otospongiosis etiology, diagnosis and therapeutic implications. Adv Oto-Rhino-Laryngol 22:43, 1977

70. Causse JR, Uriel J, Berges J, Shambaugh GE: The enzymatic mechanism of the otospongiotic disease and NaF action of the enzymatic balance. Am J Otol 3:297, 1982

71. Gristwood RE, Venables WN: Otosclerotic obliteration of oval window niche: An analysis of the results of surgery. J Laryngol Otol 89:1185, 1975

72. Farrior JB: Stapes pathology—drill cases Arch Otolaryngol 78:742, 1963

73. McGee TM: The stainless steel piston. Surgical indications and results. Arch Otolaryngol 81:34, 1965

74. Shea JJ: A technique for stapes surgery in obliterative otosclerosis. p. 199. In Boies LR (ed): Symposium on Hearing Loss—Problems in Diagnosis and Treatment. Otolaryngologic Clinics of North America. WB Saunders, Philadelphia, 1969

75. Robinson M: Total footplate extraction in stapedectomy. Ann Otol Rhinol Laryngol 90:630, 1981

76. Morrison AW: Diseases of the otic capsule. 1. Otosclerosis. p. 405. In Ballantyne J, Groves J (ed): Scott-Brown's Disease of the Ear, Nose and Throat. 4th Ed. Vol. 2. Butterworths, London, 1979

77. Tos M, Barfoed C: Failures and complications in the surgery of otosclerosis. Acta Otorhinolaryngol Ital 2:485, 1982

78. Causse J, Bel J, Michaux P, Cezard R, et al: Apport de L'informatique dans L'Otospongiose. Statistiques sur 15 ans de stapedectomies. Ann Otolaryngol (Paris) 93:149, 393, 543, 1976

79. De La Fuente F, Otte Garcia J: Otoesclerosis. Resultados de su tratamiento quirurgico. Rev Otorrinolaringol (Santiago) 26:79, 1966

80. Velasco R: Consideraciones sobre 135 casos de estapedectomia. Rev Otorrinolaringol (Santiago) 25:1, 1965

81. Halliday GC: The solid footplate in the surgery of otosclerosis. Report: Stapes surgery for otosclerosis. J Laryngol Otol 77:837, 1963

82. Willis RC: Obliterative otosclerosis: An analysis of

the surgical results. J Otolaryngol Soc Aust 1:293, 1964

83. Gristwood RE, Venables WN: A note on progression of the otosclerotic focus. Clini Otolaryngol 7:257, 1982

84. Rose G, Barker DJP: Epidemiology for the uninitiated. Br Med J London, 1979

85. Altmann F, Glasgold A, MacDuff JP: The incidence of otosclerosis as related to race and sex. Ann Otol Rhinol Laryngol 76:377, 1967

86. Hinchcliffe R: Prevalence of the commoner ear, nose and throat conditions in the adult rural population of Great Britain: A study by direct examination of two random samples. Br J Prevent Soc Med 15:128, 1961

87. Hinchcliffe R: Epidemiology and otolaryngology. p. 133. In Hinchcliffe R, Harrison D (ed): Scientific Foundations of Otolaryngology. William Heinemann, London, 1976

88. Hall JG: Otosclerosis in Norway: A geographical and genetical study. Acta Otolaryngol (Stockh) 324:[suppl]1, 1974

89. Pearson RD, Kurland LT, Cody DTR: Incidence of diagnosed clinical otosclerosis. Arch Otolaryngol 99:288, 1974

90. Gristwood RE, Venables WN: Otosclerosis in South Australia. Clin Otolaryngol 9:221, 1984

91. Gregg JB, Holzhueter AM, Steele JP, Clifford S: Some new evidence on the pathogenesis of otosclerosis. Laryngoscope 75:1268, 1965

92. Jaffe BF: The incidence of ear diseases in the Navajo Indians. Laryngoscope 79:2126, 1969

93. Wiet RJ: Patterns of ear disease in South-Western American Indian. Arch Otolaryngol 105:381, 1979

94. Tato JM, Tato JM: Quelques résultats des examens otologiques et audiologiques des Indiens Sud-Americains. Acta Otolaryngol (Stockh) 67:277, 1969

95. Kapur IP, Patt AJ: Otosclerosis in South India. Acta Otolaryngol (Stockh) 61:353, 1966

96. Joseph RB, Frazer JP: Otosclerosis incidence in Caucasians and Japanese. Arch Otolaryngol 80:256, 1964

97. Dean HT, Arnold FA, Elvove E: Domestic water and dental caries. Public Health Rep 57:1155, 1942

98. Daniel HJ III: Stapedial otosclerosis and fluorine in the drinking water. Arch Otolaryngol 90:585, 1969

99. Cawthorne T: Otosclerosis. J Laryngol Otol 69:437, 1955

100. Nager FR: Zur klinik und pathologischen Anato-

mie der Otosklerose. Acta Otolaryngol (Stockh) 27:542, 1939

101. Hajek EF: Juvenile otosclerosis. J Laryngol Otol 75:621, 1961

102. McKenzie W: Otosclerosis in childhood. J Laryngol Otol 62:661, 1948

103. Fisch U: Vestibulare Symptome vor and nach Stapedektomie. Acta Otolaryngol (Stockh) 60:515, 1965

104. Meurman OH, Aantaa E, Virolainen E: Vestibular disturbances in clinical otosclerosis. Arch Otolaryngol 90:756, 1969

105. Virolainen E: Vestibular disturbances in clinical otosclerosis. Acta Otolaryngol (Stockh) 306:[suppl]1, 1972

106. Sando I, Hemenway WG, Miller DR, Black FO: Vestibular pathology in otosclerosis. Temporal bone histopathological report. Laryngoscope 84:593, 1974

107. Gussen R: Otosclerosis and vestibular degeneration. Arch Otolaryngol 97:484, 1973

108. Allen ED: Pregnancy and otosclerosis. Am J Obstet Gynecol 49:32-48, 1945

109. Barton RT: The influence of pregnancy on otosclerosis. N Engl J Med 233:433, 1945

110. Elbrond O, Jensen JJ: Otosclerosis and pregnancy: A study of the influence of pregnancy on the hearing threshold before and after stapedectomy. Clin Otolaryngol 4:259, 1979

111. Goethals PL, Banner EA, Hedgecock LD: Effect of pregnancy on otosclerosis. Am J Obstet Gynecol 86:522, 1963

112. Guggenheim LK: On the diagnosis and treatment of otosclerosis. Am J Surg 42:156, 1938

113. Smith HW: Effect of pregnancy on otosclerosis. Arch Otolaryngol 48:159, 1948

114. Shambaugh GE Jr: Surgery of the Ear. 2nd Ed. WB Saunders, Philadelphia, 1967

115. Walsh TE: The effect of pregnancy on the deafness of otosclerosis. Trans Am Acad Ophthalmol Otolaryngol 58:420, 1954

116. Gristwood RE, Venables WN: Pregnancy and otosclerosis. Clin Otolaryngol 8:205, 1983

117. Carhart R: Effect of stapes fixation on bone conduction response. p. 175. In Schuknecht HF (ed): Otosclerosis. Henry Ford Hospital International Symposium. Little, Brown, Boston, 1962

118. Goodhill V, Moncur JP: The low-frequency air/bone gap. Laryngoscope 73:850, 1963

119. Carhart R: Cochlear otosclerosis: Audiological considerations. Ann Otol Rhinol Laryngol 75:559, 1966

120. Terkildsen K, Osterhammel P, Bretlau P: Acoustic

middle ear muscle reflexes in patients with otosclerosis. Arch Otolaryngol 98:152, 1973

121. Bel J, Causse J, Michaux P, Cezard R, et al: Mechanical explanation of the on – off effect (diphasic impedance change) in otospongiosis. Audiology 15:128, 1976

122. Naunton RF, Valvassori GE: Sensorineural hearing loss in otosclerosis. Arch Otolaryngol 89:372, 1969

123. Valvassori GE: The interpretation of the radiographic findings in cochlear otosclerosis. Ann Otol Rhinol Laryngol 75:572, 1966

124. Dulac GL, Claus E, Barrois J: Otoradiology. Xray Bulletin, Monographia Otoradiologica, Agfa-Gevaert, Belgium, 1973

125. Rovsing H: Otosclerosis: Fenestral and cochlear. Radiol Clin North Am 12:505, 1974

126. Applebaum E, Shambaugh G: Otospongiosis (otosclerosis): Polytomographic and histologic correlation. Laryngoscope 88:1761, 1978

127. Van Waes PFGM, Zonneveld FW, Damsma H, et al: Direct Multi-planar C.T. of the Petrous Bone. Philips, Netherlands, 1982

128. De Groot JAM, Huizing EH, Damsma H, et al: Labyrinthine otosclerosis studied with a new computed tomography technique. Ann Otol Rhinol Laryngol 94:223, 1985

129. House HP, House WF, Hildyard VH: Congenital stapes footplate fixation. Laryngoscope 68:1389, 1958

130. Gristwood RE, Venables WN: Cholesteatoma and tympanosclerosis. p. 133. In Cholesteatoma and Mastoid Surgery. Proceedings of the Second International Conference, Tel Aviv, Israel, March 1981. Kugler, Amsterdam, 1982

131. Goodhill V: External conductive hypacusis and the fixed malleus syndrome. Acta Otolaryngol (Stockh) 217:[suppl]1, 1966

132. Powers WH, Sheehy JL, House HP: The fixed malleus head: A report of 35 cases. Arch Otolaryngol 85:177, 1967

133. Sleeckx JP, Shea JJ, Pitzer FJ: Epitympanic ossicular fixation. Arch Otolaryngol 85:619, 1967

134. Davies DG: Malleus fixation. J Laryngol Otol 82:331, 1968

135. Katzke D, Plester D: Idiopathic malleus head fixation as a cause of a combined conductive and sensorineural hearing loss. Clin Otolaryngol 6:39, 1981

136. Sillence DO, Senn A, Danks DM: Genetic heterogeneity in osteogenesis imperfecta. J Med Genet 16:101, 1979

137. Davies DG: Paget's disease of the temporal bone. Acta Otolaryngol (Stockh) 242:[suppl]1, 1968

138. Lindsay J, Lehman R: Histopathology of the temporal bone in advanced Paget's disease. Laryngoscope 79:213, 1969

139. Schuknecht HF: Pathology of the Ear. Harvard University Press, Cambridge, MA, 1974

140. Friedmann I: Pathology of the Ear. Blackwell Scientific Publications, Oxford, 1974

141. Nager GT: Paget's disease of the temporal bone. Ann Otol Rhinol Laryngol 84[suppl 22]:1, 1975

# Noise and Its Effect on Communication

# 34

Sharon M. Abel
Peter W. Alberti

## INTRODUCTION

Most clinical assessments of hearing routinely include the measurement of pure-tone thresholds, speech reception threshold, and speech discrimination in quiet.[1] The results of these tests, while a good indicator of speech perception under optimal listening conditions, do not reliably predict intelligibility under adverse (i.e., noisy or degraded) or even normal environmental listening situations. Important variables that must be considered, in addition to the individual's audiogram, are age,[2] the level and type of concomitant background noise, the signal-to-noise (S/N) ratio,[3,4] and the speech-testing materials.[5,6]

This chapter provides an overview of investigations of speech discrimination in relation to these variables as well as comments on related practical problems. The foci of special interest are the effects of a noise background and hearing impairment due to a lesion of the peripheral auditory pathway. The relationship of speech perception to more basic measures such as temporal acuity and frequency selectivity is also considered.

## AGING AND SPEECH PERCEPTION

Everyday comments from patients as well as a large number of research studies point to a deterioration in speech perception with aging. According to a recent textbook by Bergman,[7] as well as a report from the National Academy of Sciences in Washington, DC,[2] the ability to understand speech changes gradually with age and in the absence of significant hearing loss. This deficit may not be apparent under optimal listening conditions. However, the effect is observed where there is stimulus degrading, concomitant background noise, or a noisy communication channel. This effect was referred to in the early literature as phonemic regression.[8] One issue is whether phonemic regression is the result of a decrease in intellectual functioning or of changes in the peripheral and central auditory pathway.

### Discrimination in Quiet

One of the earliest reports favoring the possibility that alterations in the CNS affect perception

943

included a histopathologic study of changes in the auditory nervous system with aging.[9]. A comparison of the brains of 11 males and female cadavers aged 68 to 87 years with those of 15 young adults sectioned at various levels of the central auditory pathway (viz., ventral cochlear nucleus, superior olivary nucleus, inferior colliculus, and medial geniculate body) indicated that there were changes at all levels with aging. These data provided morphologic evidence for possible alterations in the central neural encoding of the sound stimulus that might mediate a deterioration in speech perception.

An audiologic investigation described in the same report compared the speech discrimination performance of 10 young adults aged 20 to 30 years with that of older persons aged 50 to 70 years. All had pure-tone thresholds within 10 dB of normal at 250, 500, and 1,000 Hz. The materials used were monosyllables distorted by means of low-pass filtering at 1,200 Hz. For presentation levels of 40, 60, and 80 dB hearing level (HL), the average discrimination scores were 40 percent and 26 percent, respectively, for the two groups. Since the hearing of the two groups was essentially the same for the material presented, the difference was ascribed in part to changes in the auditory nervous system due to aging.

It has been suggested that the essential component of speech perception is good frequency discrimination. In a study of aging, Konig[10] measured difference limens for pure-tone frequencies ranging from 125 to 4,000 Hz presented at a comfortable level to 70 listeners, aged 20 to 89 years, screened for ear disease and difficulty in hearing. The Weber fraction, $\Delta f/f$ (the proportion of change needed for discrimination of a change in frequency), varied from 0.008 in individuals aged 20 to 29 years to 0.060 in those aged 86 to 89 years at 125 Hz, from 0.004 to 0.016 at 1,000 Hz, and from 0.006 to 0.022 (for those 60 to 69 years) at 4,000 Hz. Clearly, frequency discrimination for suprathreshold stimuli deteriorated with aging. A replotting of the data in terms of $\Delta f$ showed that this deterioration was approximately linear from 25 to 55 years of age, with an abrupt increase after 55 years in the frequency region above 3,000 Hz.

## Relation to Temporal Processing

The decreasing ability to understand speech with aging, in spite of relatively normal hearing for pure tones, has also been shown to be related to problems with temporal processing. In a study by Bergman,[11] 282 subjects, ranging in age from 20 to 89 years, and considered normal for understanding conversational speech, listened to speech that had been degraded in various ways or placed in competition with other stimuli. While perception for unaltered speech changed by only 10 percent across the age range studied, discrimination of speech interrupted electronically at the rate of eight interruptions/sec deteriorated linearly from 10 to 65 percent between the ages of 30 to 39 years and 80 to 89 years. The interpretation of this result was that with aging, time sampling provides less effective exposure of the speech stimulus.

The notion that changes in speech intelligibility with aging were related to changes in temporal resolving power was further supported in a study of the effects of time compression of speech signals.[12] The subjects, ranging in age from 54 to 84 years, all had speech discrimination scores of 90 percent or better for normal presentation, that is, 0 percent time compression. Time-compressing lists of words presented at a comfortable listening level by 20, 40, and 60 percent of normal duration resulted in a progressive decrease in performance for all subjects. For a presentation level of 40 dB sensation level (SL) (i.e., 40 dB above threshold), those aged 54 to 60 years showed a decrement of approximately 15 percent as the compression increased from 0 to 60 percent. Those aged 75 to 84 years showed a change of about 27 percent. These decrements increased as sensation level decreased. The effect on the energy spectrum of speeding up the playback of speech produced normally is a shift toward the higher frequencies.[13]

Deterioration in the utilization of dichotic time differences for lateralization have also been shown with aging. Herman and co-workers[14] compared older (60 to 72 years) and younger men (22 to 32 years) on their judgment of the apparent laterality of a train of clicks presented binaurally over headphones. While the two groups were equally sensitive to interaural amplitude differences less than

1.5 dB, the younger group required a shorter interaural onset difference than the older group to identify the ear leading in time, 15 μsec compared with 30 μsec.

### Discrimination in Noise

In contrast to the effects noted above, subjects do not appear to be more susceptible to changes in either the level of competing noise or signal to noise (S/N) ratio, as they age. Smith and Prather[15] compared 10 normal-hearing adults over the age of 60 years with 10 young adults aged 18 to 30 years in their ability to discriminate phonemes, low-pass filtered at 3,120 Hz. The speech stimuli were lists of 16 consonant–vowel monosyllables presented with white background noise of 30 to 55 dB SL in combination with S/N ratios of −5 to +10 dB. Lists were also presented in quiet at levels ranging from 20 to 70 dB SL. The results showed that younger subjects had significantly better discrimination scores by 10 percent on average. Both the variation in level of the background noise and S/N ratio produced significant main effects. However, neither of these variables discriminated the older from the younger listeners. Similar findings were reported in a later study by Townsend and Bess.[16]

### Summary

These studies suggest that decrements in speech discrimination with aging in the face of relatively normal hearing are most likely the result of both poor frequency discrimination and a deterioration in temporal processing in the auditory system. Histopathologic experiments provide evidence for atrophy and degeneration of cells with aging throughout the central auditory pathway.

---

## THE EFFECT OF COMPETING NOISE

### Listeners with Normal Hearing

The simplest measure of the effect of a noise background on speech discrimination is the most comfortable level (MCL) for listening chosen by observers. Beattie and co-workers[17] asked 25 young normal listeners to track their MCL in quiet and in white noise levels of 55, 70, 85, and 100 dB SPL. The observed mean MCL in quiet was 82.5 dB SPL (±11.1 dB). Statistically, there was no difference between the MCL values chosen for listening in quiet and in noise of 55 and 70 dB SPL. Across these three conditions, values ranged from 82.5 to 84.5 dB SPL. For the two higher noise levels, i.e., 85 and 100 dB SPL, the mean MCL across subjects was 90.0 (±6.3) and 100.3 dB (±6.2) SPL, respectively.

The effect of type of noise background was investigated by Danhauser and Leppler.[18] Discrimination scores were obtained using items of the California Consonant Test[19] presented against a four-talker complex, a nine-talker complex, cocktail party noise, and white noise. Across conditions, the mean percentage correct ranged from about 35 percent for a S/N of −3 dB to 90 percent for a S/N of +30 dB. The various backgrounds produced similar effects for S/N ratios ranging from +10 to +30 dB. For lower S/N values of 0 and +5 dB, both the four-talker and nine-talker complex resulted in greater difficulty in discrimination than was found for the cocktail party or white noise backgrounds. Danhauser and Leppler[18] argued that the difference might be due to the fact that these were perceptual rather than peripheral maskers.

Rupp and Phillips[20] contended that individuals with what they termed normal-fragile ears (i.e., with normal scores for pure tone and speech-in-quiet assessments but difficulty with discrimination in noise) could be more easily identified using speech-spectrum noise rather than white noise as a masker. Using both noise backgrounds, Doyle and Rupp[21] tested 20 normal-hearing University students under a variety of listening conditions, using W22-lists presented at 40 dB HL, monaurally over earphones or binaurally using loudspeakers. While speech discrimination in quiet was close to 100 percent, monaural discrimination in noise resulted in a decrement of 19 percent for white noise, and 44 percent for speech-spectrum noise. Tests of binaural speech discrimination in noise, with speech and noise from the same loudspeaker, yielded scores of 79.1 percent and 57.0 percent, respectively, for these two conditions. By contrast, spatial separation of the speech and noise resulted in scores close to those for the quiet condition.

An experiment by Horii and associates[22] attempted to specify the nature of the effect of speech-spectrum noise by studying the discrimination of various articulatory parameters. Speech-spectrum noise was created by multiplying white noise and the amplitude envelope of the speech. The speech materials allowed for both consonant and vowel differentiation. Items were presented at 65 dB SPL under earphones, and the S/N ratio ranged from −20 to +4 dB. The results indicated that for both the white noise and speech-spectrum noise, the slope of the function relating percentage correct and S/N ratio was 2.5 percent/dB for consonants and 4.0 percent/dB for vowels. Vowels were 15 to 25 percent more intelligible than were consonants in continuous white noise. Increasingly, more practice was needed to achieve maximum performance levels with the envelope noise as S/N ratio decreased.

### Listeners with Hearing Impairment

Subjects with relatively normal hearing often show a decrease in speech perception with aging. Dubno and co-workers[23] attempted to discriminate between the effects of aging and hearing loss for speech recognition in noise. Four categories of subjects were defined on the basis of age (under 44 years or more than 65 years) and hearing loss (auditory thresholds $\leq 15$ dB HL for frequencies between 250 and 4,000 Hz or SRT $\geq 35$ dB HL, with word recognition in quiet $\geq 90$ percent). Test materials comprised both high- and low-predictability sentences, and spondee words presented at 56, 72, and 88 dB SPL against a background of multitalker babble or in quiet. Significant differences in quiet were observed between the normal-hearing and hearing-impaired subjects for all three types of test item, with the largest effect for the low-predictability sentences, which lacked redundancy and syntactic cues. For listening in noise, significant main effects included age, level of speech, and hearing loss. There was also a significant difference due to signal-to-babble ratio for the two age groups for each type of material. Pure-tone thresholds did

not accurately predict overall performance either in quiet or in noise, and there was no significant interaction between hearing loss and age.

A recent experiment by Gordon-Salant and Wightman[24] evaluated the comparative masking effects of the phonetic content and spectral content of competing speech on speech perception in noise in young normal and hearing-impaired listeners. Both groups had speech discrimination in quiet scores greater than 90 percent. Competing signals included multitalker babble, continuous speech spectrum noise, a consonant–vowel (CV) masker, and a brief noise masker shaped to resemble the onset spectrum of the CV masker. The speech material comprised two sets of synthesized CV stimuli. The first set consisted of a continuum of 11 three-formant burstless voiced-stop consonants paired with a vowel; the second set comprised voiceless-stop consonants paired with the same vowel. The data indicated that in contradiction to previous studies, continuous speech and noise maskers produced the same amount of interference. With continuous maskers, the performance of normal-hearing and impaired listeners was not significantly different. Hearing-impaired listeners experienced greater interference than did normals with the brief duration maskers, and CV maskers were more disruptive than brief noise maskers despite similar spectra. Finally velar CVs were more effective as maskers than bilabial CVs.

### Occupational Noise Exposure

#### Effect of Listening with Ear Protection

Studies of communication in noise in occupational environments has largely revolved around the issue of possible drawbacks of wearing hearing protectors.[25] Misuse of protectors by workers often reflects concern that the wearing of the device will interfere with the perception of speech, warning signals, and machinery malfunctions in noise, and thus constitute a hazard to safety.

In an effort to explore this possibility Abel and co-workers[26] studied the intelligibility of monosyllabic words presented in quiet or in backgrounds of white or crowd noise of 85 dBA (for definition, see Chapter 8), with and without protectors. There were three groups of subjects: those with normal hearing, those with bilateral noise-induced high-frequency loss, and those with bilateral flat loss. For each of these three categories of hearing, one-half of the subjects were fluent in English and one-half poorly conversant. The results showed that intelligibility decreased with S/N ratio and was poorer in crowd noise than in white noise. While the protector had no effect for the normal listener, those with impairment showed a substantial decrement. In all groups, nonfluency with the language spoken resulted in a further decrement of 10 to 20 percent independent of the degree of hearing loss.

In a subsequent experiment,[27] the effect on detection of a bilateral moderate to severe noise-induced hearing loss in combination with the wearing of ear insert protectors was examined. The signals to be detected were one-third octave bands of noise centered at 1,000 or 3,000 Hz, superimposed on backgrounds of steady-state or intermittent industrial noise of 84 dBA. While listeners with normal hearing showed an advantage of 3 dB with protectors for the 3,000-Hz signals, those with noise-induced loss gave masked detection thresholds well over 100 dBA. In other words, using protectors in noise, these individuals were performing at the limit of the audiometer. Detection of a 1,000-Hz signal by listeners with a mild to moderate loss at 1,000 Hz was similar to normal. Further analysis of these data suggested that as long as the loss was less than some value between 35 and 65 dB HL, the individual would not be seriously handicapped when wearing protectors.

## Auditory Fatigue

The intelligibility of speech in noise may also be significantly affected by auditory fatigue. Sorin and Thouin-Daniel[28] presented normal-hearing subjects with distinctive feature consonant oppositions (e.g., p and t) presented against a background of white masking noise, filtered so that the spectrum was the same as the average speech spectrum. The S/N ratio was|−6 dB. For each consonant opposition, there were four word and four nonword disyllabic items (e.g.,| *talon/palon, pavot/tavot, impôt/intôt,* and po*teau*/po*peau*). Each consonant was positioned in the initial and middle position of each word type. There were two conditions of presentation, one in which presentation of a list of 120

items was preceded by a fatiguing noise giving rise to a temporary threshold shift of 15 dB at 2,000 and 3,000 Hz, and one in which the list was preceded by quiet. Subjects were required to judge whether each item presented was a word or a nonword and to repeat the item. For masked speech presented at a low level, auditory fatigue resulted in a decrease in identification scores, a reduction in correct lexical decisions (word versus nonword), more frequent confusion of fricatives, and a slight increase in reaction time for incorrectly repeated items. Sorin and Thouin-Daniel were unable to conclude whether these effects of auditory fatigue were mediated by peripheral or by central processes.

### Summary

The results of these experiments indicate that when predicting speech understanding in noise, the speech materials, the competing masker, the configuration of the hearing loss, and other conditions of listening must be carefully specified. Their unique interaction will determine the extent of the decrement in intelligibility compared with listening in quiet. For the listener with normal hearing, good performance will likely be maintained to the degree that the listener can separate out phonemic elements of the stimulus from the masker. Familiarity of the test items and practice in focusing on alternate cues available, such as lower frequencies of sound, may be important determinants of perception.

---

## INTELLIGIBILITY OF INTERRUPTED OR TIME-COMPRESSED SPEECH

### Temporal Acuity

It has been suggested that good auditory temporal acuity might underlie the processing of complex time-varying stimuli such as speech.[29,30] One paradigm for assessing the temporal resolving power of the ear is the measurement of the detectability of a brief gap in sound.[29,31,32]

Fitzgibbons and Wightman[29] compared performance in normal-hearing subjects and those with a longstanding moderate bilateral sensorineural hearing loss. A detection paradigm was used. The standard gap was 0 msec, bounded by two temporally adjacent noise markers, each approximately 400 msec in duration. The temporal gap required to distinguish a second pair of markers was measured for each observer. The octave band of the markers was varied across conditions, taking on values of 400 to 800, 800 to 1,600, and 2,000 to 4,000 Hz. With the amplitude of the markers set at 30 dB SL, the gap-detection threshold for normal listeners increased from 6 to 12 msec as the octave-band center frequency of the marker decreased. Average values for hearing-impaired listeners increased from 8 to 17 msec over these same conditions. One hypothesis advanced for better resolution with high-frequency markers was a faster transient response. Since the markers were equally audible for the normal-hearing and hearing-impaired groups, the relatively poorer performance in the hearing-impaired was attributed to changes in processing imposed by damage to the cochlea, perhaps giving rise to the persistence of sensation.

The difference in the detectability of a brief noise burst and temporal gap has also been studied for normal-hearing and hearing-impaired listeners. For example, Irwin and Purdy,[33] compared detection of a brief increment or decrement ($\Delta I$) in the intensity of continuous white noise of 60 dB SPL. For both conditions, the minimum duration detectable for normal listeners decreased as the amount of the increment or decrement ($\Delta I$) increased. At a $\Delta I$ of 10 dB, the minimum detectable burst averaged 1.2 msec; the minimum gap was significantly higher and close to 4 msec. The minimum duration for listeners with sensorineural hearing loss was considerably longer as compared with normal at all levels of increment or decrement. Listeners with conductive loss achieved values observed in normal listeners only for the highest $\Delta I$ values tested (i.e., 15 dB or greater). In both groups, as in normal listeners, bursts were easier to detect than gaps. Irwin and Purdy[33] speculated that such difficulties for simple temporal discriminations in hearing-impaired listeners would degrade the perception of fast-changing signals to a greater degree than an elevation in their thresholds for pure tones might suggest.

## Interrupted Speech

The effect of a temporal gap on intelligibility has been investigated using interrupted speech. Data for normal observers were described by Miller and Licklider.[34] Their speech materials were lists of phonetically balanced monosyllables. Interruption was achieved by periodic 100 percent amplitude modulation using a train of rectangular pulses. Variables included the number of interruptions of the speech per second, the proportion of time the speech was on between successive interruptions, and the degree of regularity of the interruptions. In quiet, conversational speech was easily understood when the rate of interruption was greater than 10 times per second with an on–off ratio of 0.50. In other words, frequently occurring interruptions were hardly noticed. At a very high interruption rate of 10,000 per second the words were as intelligible as if not interrupted. Performance decreased to a minimum of about 40 percent of words correctly repeated when the frequency of interruption was 1 time per second or less. As the speech–time fraction decreased from 0.50, performance deteriorated.

By contrast, under conditions of continuous speech presented against a background of interrupted noise masking with a S/N ratio of 0 dB, the percentage of words correctly repeated was about 80 percent for noise interruption frequencies between 0.10 and 10 per second and decreased to 70 percent for higher rates of interruption. For a S/N ratio of −9 dB, performance increased to a maximum of 80 percent as the interruption rate for the noise increased to 10 times per second and then descended to a plateau of 30 percent at an interruption frequency of 100 times per second.

Many studies have suggested that interrupted speech may be useful for diagnosis of central lesions of the auditory pathway. Bergman,[7,11] for example, showed differences in the ability to understand interrupted speech as a function of aging, as reviewed earlier.

## Time-Compressed Speech

An alternate method for distorting speech is time compression or expansion.[13] With slight speeding up of the playback of speech produced normally, about 110 to 175 words per minute, perception will not be altered. However, as playback is speeded up by a factor of 1.7 or higher, intelligibility of the material deteriorates rapidly. The effect on the energy spectrum of increasing the speech is a shift toward higher frequencies; the effect of slowing the speed is a decrease in frequency.

A recent series of experiments reported by Korsan-Bengtsen[35] compared the perception of distorted speech in normal listeners and patients with peripheral hearing loss and intracranial lesions. Test materials included interrupted speech (7 times per second), frequency-distorted speech, time-compressed speech (290 words per minute), and competing speech. The performance of patients with conductive loss was similar to that for normal-hearing patients as long as the SPL was sufficient to compensate for the hearing loss. The performance of patients with sensorineural loss depended on whether the lesion was congenital or acquired. Those with congenital lesions did not show poorer scores under conditions of distortion. By contrast, those with acquired lesions were affected, possibly because the auditory system had not yet adjusted to processing signals reduced in redundancy.

Experiments with time-compressed monosyllables were performed by Beasley and colleagues.[36,37] Beasley et al.[36] studied the effect on intelligibility of variation in time compression in combination with variation in sensation level. The subjects were young adults with normal hearing. The results showed that for percentages of time compression between 0 and 60 percent, as sensation level increased from 8 to 32 dB, the percentage of words correctly repeated increased from about 60 to 90 percent. For a time compression of 70 percent, the average intelligibility score increased linearly from 10 to 60 percent over the range of levels studied. Beasley and co-workers considered the possibility of improvement in score with adaptation to the task and materials. Such an effect was later documented in the work of Korsan-Bengsten.[35]

## FREQUENCY SELECTIVITY AND SPEECH PERCEPTION

### Definition of Frequency Selectivity

Like temporal processing, frequency selectivity, the ability to distinguish individual pure-tone frequencies within a complex auditory stimulus, has been suggested as a correlate of speech-reception error in hearing-impaired listeners.[38-41] Frequency selectivity in both normal listeners and the hearing-impaired has typically been measured using either a simultaneous or forward masking paradigm. The level of a pure-tone masker required to alter the detectability of a pure-tone probe is measured as a function of the variation in frequency of the former. A plot of the masker level that alters the detection of the probe tone is plotted against the masker frequency; the resulting function is known as a psychophysical tuning curve (see Ch. 8, Fig. 18).

### Effect of a Hearing Loss

Wightman and co-workers[42] compared tuning curves for normal listeners and those with cochlear hearing loss at three pure-tone probe frequencies, 300, 1,000, and 3,000 Hz, which for the hearing-impaired represented regions of normal, transitional, or moderate to severe loss, respectively. The level of the probe was 10 dB SL. Tuning curves for normal listeners had a characteristic V shape, with the minimum masker level required to alter perception located at the frequency of the probe and a steeper slope for the high-frequency leg; that is, detectability was much less affected by higher masker frequencies than those lower than the probe. The tuning curve became broader; that is, selectivity, or the ability to distinguish probe from masker, decreased as the frequency of the probe decreased. Tuning curves for listeners with cochlear lesions were generally broader than normal, even in the region of relatively normal hearing.

In the hearing-impaired listener, the shape of the tuning curve for different probe-tone frequencies will be related to the audiogram. In a study by Carney and Nelson,[38] a subject with moderate to severe hearing loss of 50 dB at 500 Hz produced a tuning curve for 500 Hz that was essentially flat. A subject with a high-tone loss and fairly good hearing at 500 Hz of 35 dB HL produced a characteristically normal V shaped tuning curve that was broader than those observed for normal listeners. For this particular subject, the tuning curve for 1,000 Hz was erratic, showing no clear region of maximum masking. Tuning curves for 2,000 and 4,000 Hz, the regions of greatest loss, were broad and inverted. One explanation given for the inversion was detection on the basis of temporal interaction between the masker and the probe in the region of the probe, giving rise to audible beats for the impaired listener.

### Relationship to Word Discrimination

The relationship between frequency resolution and phonetic errors in speech perception is not always clear.[43,44] A study by Ritsma and colleagues[45] suggests that poor statistical correlations between these two measures may be due to the wide variation in speech scores across subjects with hearing loss. Forty-five patients with cochlear pathology and 13 normal individuals served as subjects. The value of $Q_{10}$ (i.e., the center frequency divided by the width of the tuning curve 10 dB up from the tip) was constant for hearing loss up to 15 dB HL and decreased linearly for loss in the range of 15 to 65 dB HL. The correlation coefficient was $-0.80$. For a mean $Q_{10}$ value above 3 (close to normal), the variation in word discrimination scores based on phonetically balanced word lists was relatively small. By contrast, a mean value for $Q_{10}$ of 2.0, associated with a moderate hearing loss of 50 dB HL, gave rise to speech discrimination scores varying from 25 to 100 percent. Unfortunately, no attempt was made by Tyler and colleagues to relate speech discrimination score to the bandwidth of the tuning curve for a particular pure-tone probe frequency. Rather, the data for 500, 1,000, 2,000, and 4,000 Hz were averaged, which may have resulted in the poor statistical correlations observed.

A more carefully controlled study of the relationship between frequency selectivity and speech discrimination in noise was conducted by Patterson et al.[40] The effect of cochlear pathology was as-

sessed by comparing groups with progressive sensorineural hearing loss due to aging. The question of interest was whether the deterioration in performance generally observed for older listeners was due to a loss in frequency selectivity or to a reduction in the efficiency of processing speech more centrally in the auditory pathway. The speech test used was the four-alternative auditory feature (FAAF) test developed by Foster and Haggard.[46] A list of 100 items were bandpass filtered using an octave-band filter centered 1,800 Hz and presented in noise with a notch centered at 1,800 Hz. The percentage of words correctly identified increased as the width of the notch increased from 0 to 900 Hz. The rate of improvement clearly and consistently decreased with age for subjects ranging from 24 to 76 years. Correlation of the slope of this function with other measures of hearing showed a strong relationship to the audiogram as well as to parameters of frequency selectivity based on pure-tone detection of 500, 2,000, and 4,000 Hz in notched noise. The application of a theoretical model to the data indicated that processing efficiency had little significance for the trends observed.

---

## DISCUSSION

A review of the literature on the effect of noise on communication for normal-hearing and hearing-impaired listeners leads to a number of general conclusions. First, as individuals age, and in the face of relatively normal hearing, decreased speech understanding, likely mediated by decrements in both temporal processing and frequency discrimination, will be evident. The cause of these observed behavioral changes in perception with aging is concomitant with gradual degeneration and atrophy of cells throughout the central auditory pathway. Surprisingly, this degeneration does not appear to give rise to a greater sensitivity to changes in the S/N ratio. Older and young people will be equally affected.

The perception of speech in noise in listeners with normal hearing will depend on the level of the test item, the S/N ratio, and the nature of the background noise. Perceptual maskers appear to be more effective than peripheral maskers. For example, backgrounds similar to the test material in phonetic content are more disruptive than those similar in spectrum. Speech understanding will also be affected by such variables as familiarity of the test items, the context (e.g., a high or low predictability sentence), and auditory fatigue. Persons who have hearing loss, will be particularly adversely affected by test materials comprising low-predictability items, for which redundancy and syntactic cues are lacking. With respect to these effects, studies show that the effects of hearing loss and aging are not additive.

Performance on speech tests by subjects with hearing loss is not well predicted either by detection thresholds for different frequencies or by measures of frequency selectivity. Generally, the bandwidth of the tuning curve does not correlate well with measures of speech discrimination. This may be largely due to the significant variability in the latter across subjects with the same hearing loss. However, positive correlations between the two measures were recently demonstrated by Patterson et al.[40] In contrast to much of the research in this area, this study uses highly similar methods for masking pure tones and speech and compares decrements in performance for the two tasks as a function of aging.

Temporal processing, including detection of a gap and intelligibility of interrupted speech, in individuals with hearing loss is significantly related to speech intelligibility in noise. Both the level of the stimulus presented and the site of lesion are important variables. Patients with conductive loss show improvements in performance with an increase in the level of the stimulus. Those with sensorineural hearing loss are unable to benefit from an increase in perceived loudness.

listening situations, including industrial and nonindustrial occupational environments and educational settings. Noise levels typical of a quiet office equipped with personal computers and air conditioners are in the range of 50 dB SPL. While this level is not considered injurious to hearing and is in fact below the comfortable listening level for speech presented in quiet, it may well provide a deterrant to understanding of speech presented over the telephone, spoken in competition, periodically interrupted, or unpredictable. Listeners over the age of 40 and those with a moderate hearing loss will be at a particular disadvantage.

Amplification devices do not for the most part selectively enhance the message and, for the hearing-impaired, may lead to a greater contribution from the masker. While the presence of noise is a tolerable inconvenience in many situations, it is increasingly providing a potential safety hazard in both occupational and nonoccupational environments. Most of us acknowledge the difficulty of the hearing-impaired miner wearing ear protection in identifying and localizing warning signals, but few realize the potential danger of crossing a busy street with the volume of our personal headsets turned up, missing a garbled message over an air traffic controller's noisy headset, or failing to hear an ambulance siren while driving and listening to a news broadcast. Whereas noise and its effect on communication were once exclusively a problem for occupational safety specialists, increasingly it is rapidly becoming a domain for inquiry of a wide range of health professionals, including such diverse specialties as aviation and geriatric medicine.

## ACKNOWLEDGMENTS

This research was supported in part by contract 97711-4-6897 from the Department of National Defence (DCIEM) and in part by a National Health Research Scholar Award (SMA) from Health and Welfare Canada.

## SUMMARY

The results of the experiments reviewed in this chapter have important implications for everyday

# REFERENCES

1. Katz J (ed): Handbook of Clinical Audiology. Williams & Wilkins, Baltimore, 1972
2. Pickett JN, Bergman M, Berlin C, et al: Speech understanding and aging. Working Group 75. National Academy of Sciences, Washington, DC, 1977
3. Suter AH: The ability of mildly hearing-impaired individuals to discriminate speech in noise. Aerosp Med Res Lab Wright Patterson AFB, Jan. 1978
4. Coleman GJ, Graves RJ, Collier SG, et al: Communication in noisy environments. Report on CEC Contract 7206/00/8/09, Institute of Occupational Medicine, Roxburgh Place, Edinburgh, June 1984
5. Webster JC: Compendium of Speech Testing Material and Typical Noise Spectra for Use in Evaluating Communications Equipment. Naval Electronics Laboratory Center, San Diego, 1972
6. Webster JC, Allen CR: Speech Intelligibility in Naval Aircraft Radios. Naval Electronics Laboratory Center, San Diego, 1972
7. Bergman M: Aging and the Perception of Speech. University Park Press, Baltimore, 1980
8. Gaeth J: A Study of Phonemic Regression Associated with Hearing Loss. Ph.D. Thesis. Northwestern University, Evanston, IL, 1948
9. Kirikae I, Sato T, Shitara T: Study of hearing in advanced age. Laryngoscope 74:205, 1964
10. Konig E: Pitch discrimination and age. Acta Otolaryngol (Stockh) 48:475, 1957
11. Bergman M: Hearing and aging. Audiology 10:164, 1971
12. Konkle D, Beasley D, Bess F: Intelligibility of time-altered speech in relation to chronological aging. J Speech Hearing Res 20:108, 1977
13. Lee FF: Time compression and expansion of speech by the sampling method. J Audiol Eng Soc 20:738, 1972
14. Herman GE, Warren LR, Wagener JW: Auditory lateralization: Age differences in sensitivity to dichotic time and amplitude cues. J Gerontol 32:187, 1977
15. Smith R, Prather W: Phoneme discrimination in older persons under varying signal-to-noise conditions. J Speech Hearing Res 14:630, 1971
16. Townsend TH, Bess FH: Effects of age and sensorineural hearing loss on word recognition. Scand Audiol 9:245, 1980
17. Beattie RC, Zentil A, Svihovec DA: Effects of white noise on the most comfortable level for speech with normal listeners. J Audiol Res 22:71, 1982
18. Danhauer JL, Leppler JG: Effects of four noise competitors on the California Consonant Test. J Speech Hearing Dis 44:354, 1979
19. Owens E, Schubert ED: Development of the California Consonant Test. J Speech Hearing Res 20:463, 1977
20. Rupp RR, Phillips D: The effect of noise background on speech discrimination function in normal-hearing individuals. J Audiol Res 9:60, 1969
21. Doyle KJ, Rupp RR: Validation norms for speech discrimination scores of normal-hearing subjects in wide-band and in speech-spectrum noise at S/N 0 dB. J Audiol Res 17:269, 1977
22. Horii Y, House AS, Hughes GW: A masking noise with speech-envelope characteristics for studying intelligibility. J Acoust Soc Am 49:1849, 1971
23. Dubno JR, Dirks DD, Morgan DE: Effects of age and mild hearing loss on speech recognition in noise. J Acoust Soc Am 76(1):87, 1984
24. Gordon-Salant SM, Wightman FL: Speech competition effects on synthetic stop-vowel perception by normal and hearing impaired listeners. J Acoust Soc Am 73:1756, 1983
25. Abel SM, Haythornthwaite C: The progression of noise-induced hearing loss: A survey of workers in selected industries in Canada. J Otolaryngol 13[suppl 13], 1984
26. Abel SM, Alberti PW, Haythornthwaite C, Riko K: Speech intelligibility in noise: Effects of fluency and hearing protector type. J Acoust Soc Am 71:708, 1982
27. Abel SM, Kunov H, Pichora-Fuller K, Alberti PW: Signal detection in industrial noise: Effects of noise exposure history, hearing loss, and the use of ear protection. Scand Audiol 14:161, 1985
28. Sorin C, Thouin-Daniel C: Effects of auditory fatigue on speech intelligibility and lexical decision in noise. J Acoust Soc Am 74:456, 1983
29. Fitzgibbons PJ, Wightman FL: Gap detection in normal and hearing impaired listeners. J Acoust Soc Am 72:761, 1982
30. Zwicker E, Schorn K: Temporal resolution in hard-of-hearing patients. Audiology 21:474, 1982
31. Abel SM: Discrimination of temporal gaps. J Acoust Soc Am 52:519, 1972
32. Irwin RJ, Hinchcliff LK, Kemp S: Temporal acuity in normal and hearing impaired listeners. Audiology 20:234, 1981
33. Irwin RJ, Purdy SC: The minimum detectable duration of auditory signals for normal and hearing-impaired listeners. J Acoust Soc Am 71:967, 1982
34. Miller GA, Licklider JCR: The intelligibility of interrupted speech. J Acoust Soc Am 22:167, 1950
35. Korsan-Bengtsen M: Distorted speech audiometry. Acta Otolaryngol (Stockh) [suppl] 310, 1973
36. Beasley DS, Schwimmer S, Rintelmann WF: Intelli-

gibility of time-compressed CNC monosyllables. J Speech Hearing Res 15:340, 1972

37. Beasley DS, Forman BS, Rintelmann WF: Perception of time-compressed CNC monosyllables by normal listeners. J Audiol Res 12(1):71, 1972

38. Carney AE, Nelson DA: An analysis of psychophysical tuning curves in normal and pathological ears. J Acoust Soc Am 73:268, 1983

39. Florentine M, Buus S, Scharf B, Zwicker E: Frequency selectivity in normally-hearing and hearing impaired observers. J Speech Hearing Res 23:646, 1980

40. Patterson RD, Nimmo-Smith I, Weber DL, Milroy R: The deterioration of hearing with age: Frequency selectivity, the critical ratio, the audiogram and speech threshold. J Acoust Soc Am 72:1788, 1982

41. Tyler RS, Hall JW, Glasberg BR, et al: Auditory filter asymmetry in the hearing impaired. J Acoust Soc Am 76:1363, 1984

42. Wightman F, McGee T, Kramer M: Factors influencing frequency selectivity in normal and hearing impaired listeners. p. 295. In Evans EF, Wilson JP (eds): Psychophysics and Physiology of Hearing. Academic Press, London, 1977

43. Tyler RS, Wood EJ, Fernandes M: Frequency resolution and hearing loss. Br J Audiol 16:45, 1982

44. Tyler RS, Wood EJ, Fernandes M: Frequency resolution and discrimination of constant and dynamic tones in normal and hearing-impaired listeners. J Acoust Soc Am 74:1190, 1983

45. Ritsma RJ, Wit HP, van der Lans WP: Relations between hearing loss, maximal word discrimination score and width of psychophysical tuning curves. p. 472. In Van den Brink G, Bilsen FA (eds): Psychophysical, Physiological and Behavioral Studies in Hearing. Delft University Press, The Netherlands, 1980

46. Foster JR, Haggard MP: FAAF—An efficient analytical test of speech perception. Proc Inst Acoust 9–12, 1979

# INDEX

Page numbers followed by f designate figures; those followed by t designate tables.